Post-Intensive Care Syndrome

Post-Intensive Care Syndrome

A Practical Approach

Edited by
Brad W. Butcher
University of Pittsburgh School of Medicine

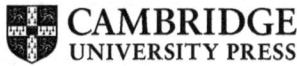

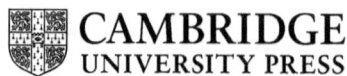

Shaftesbury Road, Cambridge CB2 8EA, United Kingdom

One Liberty Plaza, 20th Floor, New York, NY 10006, USA

477 Williamstown Road, Port Melbourne, VIC 3207, Australia

314–321, 3rd Floor, Plot 3, Splendor Forum, Jasola District Centre,
New Delhi – 110025, India

103 Penang Road, #05–06/07, Visioncrest Commercial, Singapore 238467

Cambridge University Press is part of Cambridge University Press & Assessment,
a department of the University of Cambridge.

We share the University's mission to contribute to society through the pursuit of
education, learning and research at the highest international levels of excellence.

www.cambridge.org
Information on this title: www.cambridge.org/9781009501484

DOI: 10.1017/9781009501477

© Cambridge University Press & Assessment 2026

This publication is in copyright. Subject to statutory exception and to the provisions
of relevant collective licensing agreements, no reproduction of any part may take
place without the written permission of Cambridge University Press & Assessment.

When citing this work, please include a reference to the DOI 10.1017/9781009501477

First published 2026

Cover image: filo / DigitalVision Vectors / Getty Images

A catalogue record for this publication is available from the British Library

A Cataloging-in-Publication data record for this book is available from the Library of Congress

ISBN 978-1-009-50148-4 Paperback

Cambridge University Press & Assessment has no responsibility for the persistence
or accuracy of URLs for external or third-party internet websites referred to in this
publication and does not guarantee that any content on such websites is, or will remain,
accurate or appropriate.

For EU product safety concerns, contact us at Calle de José Abascal, 56, 1°, 28003 Madrid, Spain,
or email eugpsr@cambridge.org

....

Every effort has been made in preparing this book to provide accurate and up-to-date information
that is in accord with accepted standards and practice at the time of publication. Although case
histories are drawn from actual cases, every effort has been made to disguise the identities of the
individuals involved. Nevertheless, the authors, editors, and publishers can make no warranties that
the information contained herein is totally free from error, not least because clinical standards are
constantly changing through research and regulation. The authors, editors, and publishers therefore
disclaim all liability for direct or consequential damages resulting from the use of material contained
in this book. Readers are strongly advised to pay careful attention to information provided by the
manufacturer of any drugs or equipment that they plan to use.

Contents

List of Contributors ix
Foreword xxi
Margaret S. Herridge

Section 1 Introduction

1 **Developing the Concept of PICS: A Historical Narrative** 1
Ramona O. Hopkins and Brad W. Butcher

2 **Fundamentals of PICS** 6
Brad W. Butcher, Lindsey R. Morris, and Michael Baram

3 **The Pathophysiology of PICS** 31
Samantha Bottom-Tanzer, Sarah Kader, and Eric J. Mahoney

Section 2 The Hazards of Hospitalization

4 **Immobility and ICU-Acquired Weakness** 45
Felipe González-Seguel, Sabrina Eggmann, Owen Gustafson, Kirby P. Mayer, and Selina M. Parry

5 **Frailty in the Critically Ill** 61
Joshua I. Gordon and Nathan E. Brummel

6 **Dysphagia in the Critically Ill** 77
Nicole Langton-Frost and Martin B. Brodsky

7 **Nutritional Impairments in the Critically Ill** 88
Kate J. Lambell, Lee-anne S. Chapple, and Emma J. Ridley

8 **Delirium in the Critically Ill** 101
Chukwudi A. Onyemekwu, Kelly M. Toth, Niall T. Prendergast, and Timothy D. Girard

9 **Sleep Impairments in the Critically Ill** 117
Janna R. Raphelson and Robert L. Owens

10 **The Psychological Impacts of Hospitalization** 125
Erin L. Hall-Melnychuk and Dorothy Wade

Section 3 Strategies to Prevent PICS

11 **Bundles and Checklists** 135
Heyi Li, Michael Baram, and Brad W. Butcher

12 **Physical Rehabilitation in the ICU and Hospital** 150
Felipe González-Seguel, Sabrina Eggmann, Owen Gustafson, Kirby P. Mayer, Selina M. Parry, and Dario Villalba

13 **Cognitive Rehabilitation in the ICU and Hospital** 166
Kelly S. Casey

14 **Psychological Care in the ICU and Hospital** 184
Erin L. Hall-Melnychuk, Dorothy Wade, and Teresa Deffner

15 **The Role of Spirituality throughout the Continuum of Critical Care** 197
Maggie Keogh, Arvind V. Murali, Elizabeth B. Hewett, and Neha S. Dangayach

16 **Humanization of the ICU** 208
Gabriel Heras La Calle and José Manuel Velasco Bueno

17 **Family-Centered Care in the ICU and Hospital** 217
Cassiano Teixeira and Regis Goulart Rosa

18 **ICU Diaries** 230
Peter Nydahl, Brigitte Teigeler, and Teresa Deffner

19 **Music as Therapy in the ICU** 246
Sikandar H. Khan, Sophia Wang, and Babar Khan

20 **Animal-Assisted Interventions in the ICU** 255
Kate Tantam, Tania Lovell, and Lyndsey Uglow

21 **The Importance of Fresh Air in Intensive Care** 269
Kate Tantam, Louise Rose, and Natalie Pattison

22 **Transitioning from the ICU to Home** 281
Anna G. Kalema, Ashley A. Montgomery, Brad W. Butcher, and Melissa Soper

Section 4 General Principles of Critical Illness Survivorship and Follow-Up Care

23 **A Holistic Approach to Care** 293
Kehllee L. Popovich and Janet A. Kloos

24 **Health Equity and the Social Model of Disability** 303
Leslie P. Scheunemann, Hiam Naiditch, and Gitouf Elnema

25 **Social Determinants of Health and Their Relationship with Critical Illness** 325
Jessica Nobile, J. Lloyd Allen, and Jared W. Magnani

26 **What Matters Most to Patients and Families** 339
Sarah K. Andersen and Kirsten Fiest

27 **A Brief History of ICU Follow-Up Clinics** 352
John C. Madara and Michael Baram

28 **Fundamentals of ICU Follow-Up Clinics** 359
Brad W. Butcher

29 **Telemedicine-Based ICU Follow-Up Clinics and Digital Health** 373
Neha S. Dangayach and Jenna M. Tosto-Mancuso

30 **Financial Considerations for ICU Follow-Up Clinics** 385
Karen A. Korzick, Ross H. Perfetti, and Janet F. Tomcavage

31 **Best Practices for Interprofessional Teams** 399
Aysar Al-Husseini, Deepali Dixit, and Sugeet Jagpal

Section 5 Diagnosis and Management of PICS

32 **Medication Management across the Continuum of Care** 405
Joanna L. Stollings and Taylor J. Miller

33 **Mortality, Chronic Disease, and Healthcare Utilization in Survivors of Critical Illness** 420
Hiam Naiditch, Florian B. Mayr, and Brad W. Butcher

34 **Quality of Life in Survivors of Critical Illness** 428
Rita Bakhru and Howard Saft

35 **Pulmonary and Diaphragmatic Complications in Survivors of Critical Illness** 437
Megan Trieu, Le T. Ho, and Amy Bellinghausen

36 **Common Somatic Concerns in Survivors of Critical Illness** 446
Hiam Naiditch and Brad W. Butcher

37 **Sleep Impairments in Survivors of Critical Illness** 456
Janna R. Raphelson and Robert L. Owens

38 **Persistent Dysphagia in Survivors of Critical Illness** 463
Lauren Costa, Kirra Mediate, Lauren Tusar Van Fleet, and Veronica Tyszkiewicz

39 **Laryngeal Disorders in Survivors of Critical Illness** 473
Libby J. Smith and Laura Habich

40 **Nutrition Impairments in Survivors of Critical Illness** 485
Kathlene E. Hendon, Melissa A. Jacobs, and Matthew D. Smith

41 **Physical Impairments in Survivors of Critical Illness** 500
Sara U. Dorn, Felipe González-Seguel, Kirby Mayer, Selina Parry, and Hallie Zeleznik

42 **Functional Impairments in Survivors of Critical Illness** 520
Samantha Green, Meg Williamson, Maria Shoemaker, and Avital S. Isenberg

43 **Cognitive Impairments in Survivors of Critical Illness** 535
Patsy Bryant, James C. Jackson, and Ramona O. Hopkins

44 **Resuming Employment and Driving** 547
Dharmanand Ramnarain, Ricarda Pingel, Maria Twichell, and Sjaak Pouwels

45 **The Role of Physiatry Consultation in PICS** 559
Maria Twichell and Jean-Luc Banks

46 **Psychological Outcomes in Survivors of Critical Illness** 569
Jamie L. Tingey, Jessica M. Hampton, and Megan M. Hosey

47 **Palliative Care Needs in Survivors of Critical Illness** 582
Ross H. Perfetti, Jessica Lee, Taylor Lincoln, and Andrew L. Thurston

48 **Post-Intensive Care Syndrome – Family** 600
Ji Won Shin and Judith Tate

49 **Peer Support for Survivors of Critical Illness and Their Loved Ones** 616
Heather Imperato-Shedden, Brad W. Butcher, and Annie B. Johnson

Section 6 PICS in Specific Populations

50 **PICS in Older Survivors of Critical Illness** 625
Chisom A. Ikeji and Leslie P. Scheunemann

51 **PICS in Survivors of Cardiac Arrest** 641
George E. Sayde and Sachin Agarwal

52 **PICS in Survivors of Neurological Insult** 660
Julia M. Carlson and Matthew N. Jaffa

53 **The Long-COVID Syndrome** 670
Samuel K. McGowan, Ann M. Parker, and Lekshmi Santhosh

54 **PICS in Pediatric Survivors of Critical Illness** 682
Ericka L. Fink, Aline B. Maddux, Debbie A. Long, Brenda M. Morrow, Julia A. Heneghan, Trevor A. Hall, Karen Choong, Rubén Eduardo Lasso Palomino, Pei Fen Poh, and Joseph C. Manning

Section 7 Conclusions

55 **PICS Advocacy** 707
Sarah Holler and Michael G. Allison

56 **A Case Study of PICS** 718
Brad W. Butcher

57 **In Their Own Words: Perspectives from Survivors and Their Loved Ones** 729
Franziska Herpich, Scott H. Hommel, Sr., Karen A. Korzick, Constance M. Bovier, and Cori Davis

Afterword 743
Derek C. Angus

Index 745

Contributors

Sachin Agarwal, MD, MPH, FAHA
Associate Professor of Neurology, Division of Neurocritical Care and Hospitalist Neurology
Director, NeuroCardiac Comprehensive Care Clinic
Columbia University College of Physicians and Surgeons, New York, NY, USA

Aysar Al Husseini, MD
Fellow, Division of Pulmonary and Critical Care, Department of Medicine
Rutgers Robert Wood Johnson Medical School, New Brunswick, NJ, USA

Junior Lloyd Allen, PhD, MSW, MPH
Assistant Professor, School of Social Work
Wayne State University, Detroit, MI, USA

Michael G. Allison, MD
Chief, Division of Critical Care Medicine
University of Maryland St. Joseph Medical Center, Towson, MD, USA

Sarah K. Andersen, MD, MS, FRCPC
Assistant Professor, Department of Critical Care Medicine
Faculty of Medicine and Dentistry
University of Alberta, Edmonton, Alberta, Canada

Derek C. Angus, MD, MPH
Distinguished Professor and Chair, Department of Critical Care Medicine
Associate Vice Chancellor for Healthcare Innovation
University of Pittsburgh School of Medicine, Pittsburgh, PA, USA

Rita Bakhru, MD, MS
Associate Professor, Division of Pulmonary, Critical Care, Allergy, and Sleep Medicine
Medical University of South Carolina, Charleston, SC, USA

Jean-Luc Banks, MD
Resident, Department of Physical Medicine and Rehabilitation
University of Pittsburgh Medical Center, UPMC Mercy Hospital, Pittsburgh, PA, USA

Michael Baram, MD
Professor of Medicine, Division of Pulmonary, Allergy, and Critical Care Medicine
Jane and Leonard Korman Respiratory Institute, Thomas Jefferson University Hospital
Sidney Kimmel Medical College, Philadelphia, PA, USA

Amy Bellinghausen, MD
Assistant Professor, Division of Pulmonary and Critical Care Medicine
Co-founder, Post-ICU Recovery Clinic
University of California San Diego School of Medicine, San Diego, CA, USA

Samantha Bottom-Tanzer, BA
MD/PhD Candidate
Tufts University School of Medicine, Boston, MA, USA

Constance M. Bovier
Critical Illness Survivor and PICS Advocate
Society of Critical Care Medicine ICU Hero, 2020
Peer Support Group Facilitator, Critical Illness Recovery Center at UPMC Mercy
Pittsburgh, PA, USA

Martin B. Brodsky, PhD, ScM, CCC-SLP, F-ASHA
Section Head, Speech-Language Pathology, Integrated Surgical Institute, Cleveland Clinic, Cleveland, OH, USA
Adjunct Associate Professor, Department of Physical Medicine and Rehabilitation and Division of Pulmonary and Critical Care Medicine
Johns Hopkins University, Baltimore, MD, USA

Nathan E. Brummel, MD, MSCI, FCCM, ATSF
Associate Professor, Division of Pulmonary, Allergy, Critical Care, and Sleep Medicine
The Ohio State University College of Medicine, Columbus, OH

Patsy Bryant, MS
Research Coordinator, Critical Illness, Brain Dysfunction & Survivorship (CIBS) Center
Vanderbilt University Medical Center, Nashville, TN, USA

Brad W. Butcher, MD, FCCM
Associate Professor, Department of Critical Care Medicine
Founder and Director, Critical Illness Recovery Center, UPMC Mercy
University of Pittsburgh School of Medicine, Pittsburgh, PA, USA

Julia M. Carlson, MD
Assistant Professor of Neurology, Division of Neurocritical Care
Director, Neurorecovery Clinic
University of North Carolina School of Medicine, Chapel Hill, NC, USA

Kelly S. Casey, OTD, OTR/L, BCPR, ATP, CPAM
Occupational Therapist, Rehabilitation Therapy Manager
Director, Johns Hopkins Acute Care Occupational Therapy Fellowship
The Johns Hopkins Hospital, Baltimore, MD, USA

Lee-anne S. Chapple, BMedSci, MNutrDiet, PhD
Associate Professor, Faculty of Health and Medical Sciences, The University of Adelaide
Royal Adelaide Hospital, Adelaide, South Australia, Australia

Karen Choong, MB, BCh, FRCP(C), MSc
Professor, Departments of Pediatrics and Critical Care
Department of Health Research Methods, Evidence and Impact
McMaster University, McMaster Children's Hospital, Hamilton, Ontario, Canada

Lauren Costa, MA, CCC-SLP
Speech Language Pathologist,
Critical Illness Recovery Center at UPMC Mercy
UPMC Rehabilitation Institute, Pittsburgh, PA, USA

Neha S. Dangayach, MD, MSCR, FAAN, FNCS, FCCM, FCCP
Associate Professor, Departments of Neurology, Neurosurgery, and Rehabilitation and Human Performance
Research Director, Neurocritical Care and Recovery
Icahn School of Medicine at Mount Sinai, New York, New York, USA

Cori Davis
Critical Illness Survivor and PICS Advocate
Pittsburgh, PA, USA

Teresa Deffner, Dr. rer.nat. Dipl.-Rehapsych. (FH)
Psychologist, Department of Anaesthesiology and Intensive Care Medicine
Jena University Hospital, Jena, Germany

Deepali Dixit, PharmD, BCCCP, FCCM
Clinical Associate Professor, Ernest Mario School of Pharmacy
Rutgers, The State University of New Jersey, Piscataway, NJ, USA

Sara Uribe Dorn, PT, DPT, CCS
Board-Certified Cardiovascular and Pulmonary Clinical Specialist
Physical Therapist, Duke Critical Care Recovery Center
Department of Rehabilitation Services
Duke University Medical Center, Durham, NC, USA

Sabrina Eggmann, PT, PhD, MSc
Department of Physiotherapy
Inselspital, Bern University Hospital, Bern, Switzerland

Gitouf Elnema, MD
Fellow, Department of Critical Care Medicine
University of Pittsburgh School of Medicine, Pittsburgh, PA, USA

Kirsten Fiest, PhD
Scientific Director, O'Brien Institute for Public Health
Associate Professor, Departments of Critical Care Medicine, Community Health Science, and Psychiatry
Cumming School of Medicine, University of Calgary, Calgary, Alberta, Canada

Ericka L. Fink, MD, MS
Professor, Division of Pediatric Critical Care Medicine, Pediatrics, and Clinical and Translational Science
Associate Director, Safar Center for Resuscitation Research
Director, Critical Illness Recovery for ChiLdrEn (CIRCLE) Program
UPMC Children's Hospital of Pittsburgh, Pittsburgh, PA, USA

Timothy D. Girard, MD, MSCI
Associate Professor, Department of Critical Care Medicine
Director, Clinical Research, Investigation, and Systems Modeling of Acute Illness (CRISMA)
University of Pittsburgh School of Medicine, Pittsburgh, PA, USA

Felipe González-Seguel, PT, MSc
PhD student, Rehabilitation and Health Sciences Program, Department of Physical Therapy, College of Health Sciences, University of Kentucky, Lexington, KY, USA
Adjunct Professor, School of Physical Therapy, Faculty of Medicine
Clínica Alemana Universidad del Desarrollo, Santiago, Chile

Joshua I. Gordon, MD
Clinical Instructor, Division of Pulmonary, Critical Care, and Sleep Medicine
The Ohio State University College of Medicine, Columbus, OH, USA

Samantha Green, MSOT, OTR/L, BCPR, CSRS
Occupational Therapist, Department of Rehabilitation Services
Duke Critical Care Recovery Center
Duke University Medical Center, Durham, NC, USA

Owen Gustafson, MSc, Res, BSc (Hons), FHEA, MCSP
Senior Clinical Academic Physiotherapist, Oxford Allied Health Professions Research & Innovation Unit
Oxford University Hospitals NHS Foundation Trust, Oxford, United Kingdom

Laura Habich, MS, CCC-SLP
Lead Speech Language Pathologist, UPMC Voice Center
University of Pittsburgh Medical Center, Pittsburgh, PA, USA

Trevor A. Hall, PsyD, ABPdN
Professor of Pediatrics, Division of Pediatric Psychology and Pediatric Critical Care
Pediatric Neuropsychologist
Associate Director, Pediatric Critical Care and Neurotrauma Recovery Program
Oregon Health & Science University, Portland, OR, USA

Erin L. Hall-Melnychuk, PsyD, MSCP
Assistant Professor, Department of Psychiatry
Clinical Health Psychologist, Departments of Trauma Surgery and Critical Care Medicine
Geisinger Medical Center and Geisinger Commonwealth School of Medicine, Danville, PA, USA

Jessica M. Hampton, MClinPsych
Senior Clinical Psychologist, Psychology Department, Allied Health
Logan Hospital, Metro South Health
University of Queensland, Brisbane, Australia

Kathlene E. Hendon, RD, LDN, CNSC
Advanced Practice Dietitian
The Johns Hopkins Hospital, Baltimore, MD, USA

Julia A. Heneghan, MD, MS
Assistant Professor, Department of Pediatrics, Division of Pediatric Critical Care
University of Minnesota Medical School, Minneapolis, MN, USA

Gabriel Heras La Calle, MD, PhD
Director, International Research Project for the Humanization of Intensive Care Units (Proyecto HU-CI)
President, Humanizing Healthcare Foundation, Madrid
Intensive Care Unit, Hospital Universitario de Jaén and Hospital HLA Inmaculada, Granada
Francisco de Vitoria University, Madrid, Spain

Franziska Herpich, MD
Clinical Assistant Professor, Department of Neurology
Sidney Kimmel Medical College, Thomas Jefferson University, Philadelphia, PA, USA

Margaret S. Herridge, MSc, MD, FRCPC, MPH
Professor of Medicine, Division of Critical Care and Respiratory Medicine
Senior Scientist, Toronto General Research Institute
Tier 1 Canada Research Chair in Critical Illness Outcomes and the Recovery Continuum
Director, the RECOVER program
University Health Network and University of Toronto, Toronto, ON, Canada

Elizabeth B. Hewett, M.Div, BCC, BCPC
Director of Spiritual Care
Post-ICU Recovery Clinic
University Hospitals Health System, Cleveland Medical Center, Cleveland, OH, USA

Le T. Ho, RRT
Respiratory Therapist, ICU Recovery Clinic
University of California San Diego, San Diego, CA, USA

Sarah Holler, MSN, MS, RN, CCRN
Program Coordinator, Beyond Intensive Care: Surviving & Thriving
University of Maryland, St. Joseph Medical Center, Towson, MD, USA

Scott H. Hommel, Sr.
Critical Illness Survivor
Milton, PA, USA

Ramona O. Hopkins, PhD
Professor of Psychology and Neuroscience

Brigham Young University, Provo, UT, USA

Megan M. Hosey, PhD
Assistant Professor, Department of Physical Medicine and Rehabilitation, Division of Rehabilitation Psychology and Neuropsychology and Department of Medicine, Division of Pulmonary and Critical Care Medicine
Johns Hopkins University School of Medicine, Baltimore, MD, USA

Chisom A. Ikeji, MD
Assistant Professor, Department of Critical Care Medicine
University of Pittsburgh School of Medicine, Pittsburgh, PA, USA

Heather Imperato-Shedden, MSW, LCSW
Program Manager, ICU and Post-ICU Support Social Work Team
Morristown Medical Center, Morristown, NJ, USA

Avital S. Isenberg, CScD, MS, OTR/L
Assistant Professor, Department of Occupational Therapy
School of Health and Rehabilitation Sciences, University of Pittsburgh, Pittsburgh, PA, USA

James C. Jackson, MA, PsyD
Research Professor of Medicine and Psychiatry
Director of Behavioral Health, ICU Recovery Center
Vanderbilt University Medical Center, Nashville, TN, USA

Melissa A. Jacobs, MS, RD, CSO, LDN, CNSC
Advanced Practice Dietitian
The Johns Hopkins Hospital, Baltimore, MD, USA

Matthew N. Jaffa, DO
Assistant Professor, Department of Neurology

University of Connecticut School of Medicine, Farmington, CT, USA
Director, Neuro Recovery Clinic
Ayer Neuroscience Institute, Hartford Hospital, Hartford, CT, USA

Sugeet Jagpal, MD
Associate Professor, Division of Pulmonary and Critical Care
Rutgers Robert Wood Johnson Medical School, New Brunswick, NJ, USA

Annie B. Johnson, APRN, CNP, FCCM
Critical Care Nurse Practitioner
Director, Mayo Clinic ICU Recovery Program
Mayo Clinic, Rochester, MN, USA

Sarah Kader, MD, MBA
Resident, Department of General Surgery
Lahey Hospital and Medical Center
Beth Israel Lahey Health, Burlington, MA, USA

Anna G. Kalema, MD
Associate Professor, Division of Pulmonary, Critical Care, and Sleep Medicine
University of Kentucky College of Medicine, Lexington, KY, USA

Maggie Keogh, M.Ed, BCC
ICU Spiritual Care Provider, Center for Spirituality and Health
Mount Sinai Hospital System, New York, NY, USA

Babar Khan, MD, MS
Professor of Medicine
Indiana University School of Medicine, Indianapolis, IN, USA
Indiana University Center for Aging Research
Regenstrief Institute, Inc., Indianapolis, IN

Sikandar H. Khan, DO, MS
Assistant Professor of Medicine

Indiana University School of Medicine,
Indianapolis, IN, USA
Indiana University Center for Aging
Research
Regenstrief Institute, Inc.,
Indianapolis, IN

Janet A. Kloos, RN, PhD, APRN-CCNS, CCRN
Senior Clinical Nurse Specialist, Post-ICU
Recovery Clinic
University Hospitals Health System,
Cleveland Medical Center,
Cleveland, OH

Karen A. Korzick, MD, MA, FCCP, FACP, FCCM
Professor of Critical Care Medicine
Geisinger Medical Center, Danville, PA, USA
Geisinger College of Health Sciences,
Scranton, PA, USA

Kate J. Lambell, BHSc, MNutrDiet, PhD
Senior ICU Dietitian and ICU Allied
Health Lead, Alfred Health
Affiliate Research Fellow, Australian and
New Zealand Intensive Care Research Centre
Monash University, Melbourne, Victoria,
Australia

Nicole Langton-Frost, MA, CCC-SLP, BCS-S
Rehabilitation Therapy Manager, Acute
Care Therapy Services, The Johns Hopkins
Hospital
Assistant Professor, Department of
Physical Medicine and
Rehabilitation
The Johns Hopkins University School of
Medicine, Baltimore, MD, USA

Rubén Eduardo Lasso Palomino, MD
Professor, Division of Pediatric Critical
Care Medicine
Director, CRECEP PICU Program,
Fundación Valle del Lili
Universidad ICESI, Cali, Colombia

Jessica Lee, DO
Fellow, Department of Critical Care
Medicine
University of Pittsburgh School of
Medicine, Pittsburgh, PA, USA

Heyi Li, MD
Assistant Professor of Medicine,
Division of Pulmonary and Critical Care
Montefiore Medical Center
Albert Einstein College of Medicine,
New York, NY, USA

Taylor Lincoln, MD, MS
Assistant Professor, Department of Critical
Care Medicine and Section of Palliative
Care and Medical Ethics
University of Pittsburgh School of
Medicine, Pittsburgh, PA, USA

Debbie A. Long, BN, MNurs (Critical Care), PhD
Professor, Churchill Fellow
Queensland University of Technology,
Brisbane, Queensland, Australia
Children's Health Queensland, Hospital
and Health Services

Tania Lovell, BN, MPH, MHM
Clinical Nurse, Intensive Care Unit,
Division of Surgery
Princess Alexandra Hospital, Metro
South Health, Brisbane, Queensland,
Australia

John C. Madara, MD
Assistant Professor of Medicine
Penn State Health Milton S. Hershey
Medical Center
Penn State College of Medicine, Hershey,
PA, USA

Aline B. Maddux, MD, MSCS
Associate Professor of Pediatrics, Section of
Critical Care
Children's Hospital of Colorado,
Aurora, CO
University of Colorado School of Medicine,
Aurora, CO, USA

Jared W. Magnani, MD, MSc, FAHA
Associate Professor of Medicine,
Division of Cardiology, Department of Medicine
Heart, Lung, Blood, and Vascular Medicine Institute
University of Pittsburgh School of Medicine, Pittsburgh, PA, USA

Eric J. Mahoney, MD, FACS
Director, Critical Care Outpatient Center
Surgeon/Intensivist, Lahey Hospital and Medical Center
Beth Israel Lahey Health, Burlington, MA, USA
Assistant Professor of Surgery
Tufts University School of Medicine, Boston, MA, USA

Joseph C. Manning, PhD, MNursSci (Hons), PGCert Paeds Crit Care, RN
Professor of Nursing and Child Health
Nottingham Children's Hospital,
Nottingham University Hospitals NHS Trust
School of Healthcare, College of Life Sciences, University of Leicester, Leicester, United Kingdom

Kirby P. Mayer, PT, DPT, PhD
Assistant Professor of Physical Therapy
Director of Research, University of Kentucky ICU Recovery Clinic
College of Health Sciences, University of Kentucky, Lexington, KY, USA

Florian B. Mayr, MD, MPH
Associate Professor, Department of Critical Care Medicine
Center for Research, Investigation, and Systems Modeling of Acute Illness (CRISMA)
VA Pittsburgh Healthcare System
University of Pittsburgh School of Medicine, Pittsburgh, PA, USA

Samuel K. McGowan, MD
Assistant Professor, Division of Pulmonary and Critical Care Medicine
Director, UCSF OPTIMAL clinic
University of California San Francisco
School of Medicine, San Francisco, CA, USA

Kirra Mediate, MA, CCC-SLP
Program Director for Speech Outpatient Services
UPMC Rehabilitation Institute, Pittsburgh, PA, USA

Taylor J. Miller, PharmD
Clinical Pharmacist, Critical Illness Recovery Center
UPMC Mercy Hospital, Pittsburgh, PA, USA

Ashley A. Montgomery, MD, FCCM
Associate Professor, Division of Pulmonary, Critical Care, and Sleep Medicine
Director, ICU Recovery Clinic
University of Kentucky College of Medicine, Lexington, KY, USA

Lindsey R. Morris, MD
Assistant Professor, Division of Pulmonary and Critical Care Medicine
University of Texas Southwestern Medical Center, Dallas, TX, USA

Brenda M. Morrow, PhD, BSc (PT)
Professor, Department of Pediatrics and Child Health
Physiotherapist
University of Cape Town, Cape Town, South Africa

Arvind V. Murali, MSCR
ORISE Research Fellow, Centers for Disease Control and Prevention, Roybal Campus

Research Assistant, Neuroemergencies Management and Transfers (NEMAT) Group
Icahn School of Medicine at Mount Sinai, New York, NY, USA

Hiam Naiditch, MD, MHS
Clinical Instructor and Post-Doctoral Scholar, Division of Pulmonary, Allergy, Critical Care, and Sleep Medicine
University of Pittsburgh School of Medicine, Pittsburgh, PA, USA

Jessica Nobile, PhD, MSW, LCSW
Senior Social Worker, Critical Illness Recovery Center
UPMC Mercy Hospital, Pittsburgh, PA, USA

Peter Nydahl, RN, PhD
Nursing Research, University Hospital of Schleswig-Holstein, Kiel, Germany
Institute of Nursing Science and Practice, Paracelsus Medical University, Salzburg, Austria

Chukwudi A. Onyemekwu, DO
Post-Doctoral Scholar, Division of Pulmonary, Allergy, Critical Care, and Sleep Medicine
University of Pittsburgh School of Medicine, Pittsburgh, PA, USA

Robert L. Owens, MD, ATSF
Professor of Medicine, Division of Pulmonary, Critical Care, and Sleep Medicine
Co-founder, Post-ICU Recovery Clinic
University of California San Diego School of Medicine, San Diego, CA, USA

Ann M. Parker, MD, PhD
Assistant Professor, Departments of Medicine and Physical Medicine and Rehabilitation
Director, Johns Hopkins Post-Acute Critical Care Team (JH PACT)
The Johns Hopkins University School of Medicine, Baltimore, MD, USA

Selina M. Parry, B. Physio (Hons), PhD, Grad Cert in University Teaching, FACP
Associate Professor, Department of Physiotherapy
The University of Melbourne, Melbourne, Victoria, Australia

Natalie Pattison, RN, BSc(Hons), MSc, DNSc, AFHEA
Professor of Clinical Nursing
Clinical Lead for Critical Care Recovery Clinic
University of Hertfordshire, Hertfordshire, United Kingdom

Ross H. Perfetti, MSc
PhD candidate, University of Pennsylvania, Department of Anthropology, Philadelphia, PA, USA
MD candidate, Harvard Medical School, Boston, MA, USA

Ricarda Pingel, BScN, RN
Department of Intensive Care Medicine
University Hospital Goettingen, Goettingen, Lower Saxony, Germany

Pei Fen Poh, RN, MSN
Nurse Clinician, ECMO Nurse Specialist, Children's Intensive Care Unit
KK Women's and Children's Hospital, Singapore

Kehllee L. Popovich, MSN, ACNP-BC
Clinical APP, Post ICU Recovery Clinic
Senior Nurse Practitioner, System Lead Advanced Practice Education
University Hospitals Health System, Cleveland Medical Center, Cleveland, OH, USA

Sjaak Pouwels, MD, PhD (mult)
Department of Surgery, Marien Hospital
Herne, University Hospital of Ruhr
University Bochum, Herne, NRW,
Germany
Department of Intensive Care Medicine,
Elisabeth-Tweesteden Hospital, Tilburg,
The Netherlands

Niall T. Prendergast, MD
Assistant Professor of Medicine, Division
of Pulmonary, Allergy, Critical Care, and
Sleep Medicine
University of Pittsburgh School of
Medicine, Pittsburgh, PA, USA

Dharmanand Ramnarain, MD, MSc
Department of Intensive Care Medicine,
Elisabeth-Tweesteden Hospital, Tilburg,
The Netherlands
Department of Intensive Care Medicine,
Saxenburgh Medical Center, Hardenberg,
The Netherlands

Janna R. Raphelson, MD, CM
Fellow, Division of Pulmonary, Critical
Care, and Sleep Medicine
University of California San Diego School
of Medicine, San Diego, CA, USA

**Emma J. Ridley, BNutriDietet, APD,
MPH, PhD**
Associate Professor (Research), Acute and
Critical Care
Dietetics and Nutrition, Alfred Health,
Melbourne, Victoria, Australia
School of Public Health and Preventive
Medicine, Monash University, Melbourne,
Victoria, Australia

Regis Goulart Rosa, MD, MSc, PhD
Internal Medicine Department, Hospital
Moinhos de Vento
Porto Alegre (RS), Brazil

Louise Rose, MBE, RN, PhD
Professor of Critical Care Nursing, Faculty
of Nursing, Midwifery, and Palliative Care
King's College London, London, United
Kingdom

Howard Saft, MD, MSHS
Associate Professor, Division of Pulmonary
and Critical Care Medicine
National Jewish Health
University of Colorado School of Medicine,
Aurora, CO, USA

Lekshmi Santhosh, MD, MAEd
Associate Professor of Clinical
Medicine
Medical Director, UCSF Post-COVID
OPTIMAL Clinic
University of California San Francisco
School of Medicine, San Francisco,
CA, USA

George E. Sayde, MD, MPH
Clinical and Research Fellow,
Department of Psychiatry, Division
of Consultation-Liaison
Psychiatry
Columbia University College of Physicians
and Surgeons, New York, NY, USA

Leslie P. Scheunemann, MD, MPH
Assistant Professor, Divisions of
Geriatrics and Pulmonary, Allergy,
Critical Care, and Sleep
Medicine
University of Pittsburgh School of
Medicine, Pittsburgh, PA, USA

Ji Won Shin, PhD, RN
Assistant Professor
The Ohio State University College of
Nursing, Columbus, OH, USA

Maria Shoemaker, MS, OTR/L
Senior Occupational Therapist, Critical
Illness Recovery Center at UPMC Mercy
UPMC Rehabilitation Institute, Pittsburgh,
PA, USA

Libby J. Smith, DO
Professor, Department of Otolaryngology

Division Chief, Laryngology and Director,
UPMC Voice Center
University of Pittsburgh School of
Medicine, Pittsburgh, PA, USA

Matthew D. Smith, MS, RD, LDN, CNSC
Advanced Practice Dietitian
The Johns Hopkins Hospital, Baltimore,
MD, USA

Melissa Soper, MSN, APRN, ACNP-BC
Medical ICU and ICU Recovery Clinic
Nurse Practitioner
University of Kentucky Medical Center,
Lexington, KY, USA

Joanna Stollings, PharmD, FCCM, FCCP
MICU Clinical Pharmacy Specialist
ICU Recovery Center at Vanderbilt
Pharmacist
Vanderbilt University Medical Center,
Nashville, TN, USA

**Kate Tantam, RN, BSc(Hons), MRes
PGCE BEM**
Specialist Sister ICU, Rehabilitation Team
University Hospitals Plymouth NHS Trust,
Plymouth, United Kingdom

Judith Tate, PhD, RN, ATS-F, FAAN
Associate Professor
The Ohio State University College of
Nursing, Columbus, OH, USA

Brigitte Teigeler, RN
Diploma in Nursing Science
Journalist and Author, Redaktionsbüro
Teigeler, Wiesbaden, Germany

Cassiano Teixeira, MD, PhD
Internal Medicine Department,
Rehabilitation Department
Univeridade Federal de Ciências da Saúde
de Porto Alegre (UFCSPA) Medical
School
Nora Teixeira Hospital, Santa Casa de
Porto Alegre, Brazil

Andrew L. Thurston, MD, FAAHPM
Medical Director of Palliative Care,
UPMC Mercy
Clinical Associate Professor of Medicine,
Division of General Internal Medicine
UPMC Section of Palliative Care and
Medical Ethics
University of Pittsburgh School of
Medicine, Pittsburgh, PA, USA

Jamie L. Tingey, PhD
Clinical Assistant Professor, Department of
Psychiatry and Behavioral Sciences,
Division of Sleep Medicine
Stanford University School of Medicine,
Palo Alto, CA, USA

Janet F. Tomcavage, MSN, RN
Executive Vice President, Chief Nurse
Executive
Geisinger Health, Danville, PA, USA

Jenna M. Tosto-Mancuso, PT, DPT, NCS
Clinical Director, Division of
Rehabilitation Innovation, Department of
Rehabilitation and Human Performance
Icahn School of Medicine at Mount Sinai,
New York, NY, USA

Kelly M. Toth, PhD, RN
Research Assistant Professor, Department
of Critical Care Medicine
Center for Research, Investigation, and
Systems Modeling of Acute Illness (CRISMA)
University of Pittsburgh School of
Medicine, Pittsburgh, PA, USA

Megan Trieu, MD
Fellow, Division of Pulmonary and Critical
Care Medicine
University of California San Diego School
of Medicine, San Diego, CA, USA

Lauren Tusar Van Fleet, MA, CCC-SLP, CBIS
Speech Language Pathologist, Certified
Brain Injury Specialist
Critical Illness Recovery Center at UPMC
Mercy

UPMC Rehabilitation Institute,
Pittsburgh, PA

Maria Twichell, MD
Assistant Professor, Department
of Physical Medicine and
Rehabilitation
University of Pittsburgh School of
Medicine, Pittsburgh, PA, USA

Veronica Tyszkiewicz, MS, CCC-SLP
Speech Language Pathologist
UPMC Rehabilitation Institute, Pittsburgh,
PA, USA

Lyndsey Uglow
Certificate in Animal Assisted
Therapy Activities and Learning
Founder, Southampton Children's
Hospital Animal Assisted Intervention
Team
Abu Dhabi, United Arab Emirates

José Manuel Velasco Bueno
International Research Project for the
Humanization of Intensive Care Units
(Proyecto HU-CI)
Patron of Humanizing Healthcare
Foundation, Madrid
Hospital Virgen de la Victoria, Málaga,
Spain

Dario Villalba, PT, RT
Director, Post-ICU Follow-up and
Rehabilitation Committee, Argentine
Society of Intensive Care
Respiratory Therapist, Santa Catalina
Neuro Rehabilitación Clínica, CABA,
Argentina
Chivilcoy Hospital, Buenos Aires,
Argentina

Dorothy Wade, PhD
Honorary Associated Professor
Consultant Health Psychologist, Critical
Care, Royal Free Hospital Trust
University College London, London,
United Kingdom

Sophia Wang, MD, MS
Associate Professor of Clinical
Psychiatry
Indiana Alzheimer's Disease Research
Center
Indiana University School of Medicine,
Indianapolis, IN, USA

Louise (Meg) Williamson, MOT, OTR/L, BCPR
Senior Occupational Therapist,
Department of Rehabilitation Services
Duke University Medical Center,
Durham, NC

Hallie Zeleznik, PT, DPT
Board-Certified Neurologic Clinical
Specialist
Critical Illness Recovery Center at UPMC
Mercy
Vice Chair, Department of Physical
Therapy
University of Pittsburgh, Pittsburgh,
PA, USA

Foreword

Margaret S. Herridge

After I finished my critical care clinical training, I wanted to quit. I was physically exhausted, emotionally burned out, and felt that I had made a terrible mistake in choosing a subspecialty in which so many patients died. And those who didn't die left us abruptly and were never seen by us again. We simply assumed that these folks enjoyed a full recovery and resumed the lives that they were leading prior to critical illness, but this was not entirely clear.

I returned to a faculty position in Toronto following my research training in Boston, where I had the privilege of working with Frank Speizer at the Channing Laboratory. Frank was the founder of the Nurses' Health study, and he taught me about the potent impact of carefully conducted, granular, longitudinal research. Conducting longitudinal research after critical illness seemed to me to be the best way to understand what happened to patients and their families following hospital discharge. I had a particular interest in patients with the acute respiratory distress syndrome (ARDS), and I believed that their long-term outcomes would surely be instructive and indicative of what happened to other survivors with similar or lesser degrees of illness.

I first met Gord in December 1998. He had severe gallstone pancreatitis complicated by ARDS, requiring four weeks in the intensive care unit (ICU). He was the first patient recruited to our five-year ARDS long-term outcomes cohort in Toronto. When he completed his five-year follow-up appointment, he asked me if he could keep in touch through email because the clinic had provided him with a sense of continuity, security, and comfort – a safety net going forward. Once or twice each year, an email would appear in my inbox entitled "Gord's big adventure." This made me smile but also brought concern, since these updates were typically bittersweet, with some wonderful family events coupled with new health challenges. We remained in touch for the next 23 years until his death in 2022. I had the privilege to learn how his episode of severe critical illness had altered the course of his life and the life of his family. His story highlights so many aspects of the relatively new construct of post-intensive care syndrome (PICS) and the vital importance of both engagement throughout the critical illness care continuum and standardized post-ICU longitudinal care.

Through our study, and the work of others in the international community similarly caring for survivors of critical illness, I learned that Gord's recovery over the subsequent years was quite typical for a survivor of severe ARDS. I was surprised, however, by how durable the sequelae of his critical illness were over the following decades and by how truly transformative they were for both him and his family.

There were many pivotal events in Gord's journey that would now be viewed as commonplace and expected. His muscle wasting and weakness were profound, necessitating extensive inpatient and outpatient rehabilitation, and severe neuropathic pain in his legs and feet made regaining mobility excruciating. After transitioning back to the community, he was challenged with a new diagnosis of diabetes, complicated and infected foot ulcers, a Charcot joint necessitating protracted casting of his left leg, complex pressure injuries, new-onset depression, and difficulty returning to work because of these functional limitations. His family physician often reached out to me to discuss how best to manage these critical illness-related health consequences. This reinforced to me how fundamental it is for intensivists and primary care physicians to talk – communication that virtually never occurs.

Gord's post-ICU course was also illustrative of some less common, but nevertheless devastating, health consequences. At 18 months, he underwent surgery for tracheal stenosis, which also required a protracted recovery. He was diagnosed with bladder cancer and, in 2015, with colon cancer. Although a common diagnosis in the general population, I often reflected on how Gord had vastly exceeded his lifetime radiation dose from abdominal CT scans and wondered if these malignancies were late consequences of his critical illness. Gord ultimately succumbed to metastatic colon cancer in 2022. A few days before he died, we spoke on the phone while he was in palliative care, and he again reflected on how much the longitudinal relationship with the post-ICU clinic had meant to him and his family. He told me that we were their lifeline.

In 2003, during our five-year ARDS follow-up program, Toronto experienced an outbreak of a novel coronavirus that caused the severe acute respiratory syndrome (SARS). We used our ARDS outcomes study platform to quickly establish a one-year follow-up program for this new population of patients and then extended the study to involve family caregivers. The one-year SARS follow-up findings reinforced the robust multidimensional and durable nature of post-ICU sequelae for patients and their families, which were similar to those described in our five-year ARDS cohort. The outbreak also highlighted an urgency to establish formal follow-up for survivors of pandemics, both for the delivery of needed clinical care and for the generation of new knowledge. Long-term symptoms in survivors of SARS were often debilitating and met with helplessness and skepticism from both the lay public and many in the healthcare system. Severe acute respiratory syndrome also provided early insight into the mental health sequelae for families resulting from isolation from their loved ones during hospitalization, disrupted communication with the medical team, and the stigma experienced by virtue of being related to a patient with SARS. Indeed, this outbreak from decades ago was a potent harbinger of COVID-19-related critical illness and its attendant constellation of persistent symptoms and disabilities. The COVID-19 pandemic recapitulated the mental health consequences of isolation (for both the patient and their loved ones), poor access to healthcare for many, and the exhausted resilience of healthcare professionals. And, as with the SARS outbreak, for many survivors of the illness, ICU follow-up programs often served as the only outpatient medical resource for those unable to access primary or other specialty care.

The COVID-19 pandemic produced the most survivors of critical illness in history and focused attention on outcomes resulting from the intersection of ARDS, sepsis, and chronic critical illness. It underscored the health consequences of heightened technological support, such as extracorporeal membrane oxygenation (ECMO) and its companion complications from cannulation, anticoagulation, and the immobility that accompanies paralytic infusions and prolonged deep sedation. The systematic "de-adoption" of ICU "best practices" during the COVID-19 pandemic compromised long-term functional and neuropsychological outcomes and highlighted the harm created by such divergence from practice standards.

The final members of the baby boom generation turned 60 in 2024. Future ICU outcomes clinical and research work will be dominated by older survivors of critical illness who carry a greater burden of chronic disease and by their older family members. These patients will have longer ICU lengths of stay, heightened case complexity, and consequently compromised outcomes. Post-intensive care syndrome will increasingly be influenced by the challenges of ageing and its attendant loss of organ resilience; post-ICU care and research will further elucidate the impact of critical illness on older survivors with multiple comorbid conditions, providing invaluable data as outcome expectations are managed and ongoing consent to treatment is deliberated during a complex ICU stay.

Patients and families have informed the breadth of multidimensional healthcare needs after critical illness for over 30 years. Their volunteerism, investment, and commitment to enroll in ICU follow-up programs have transformed our understanding of long-term outcomes and rehabilitation trajectories after severe illness. Patients and loved ones have called attention to several robust themes about PICS and follow-up after critical illness that are instructive for our ICU community.

They have consistently endorsed longitudinal care as an essential practice standard within the ICU care continuum. Patients and families want to be followed. Their health is fragile, and they seek advocacy for ongoing and future healthcare needs. They want continuity of care from ICU healthcare providers. They need opportunities to frequently debrief with critical illness experts to process their trauma. They want to know exactly what happened to them, to share the impact of their illness, and to give feedback on the care they received. They want and need advocacy for ongoing mental health and subspecialty care, return to work, and navigation of the myriad barriers to resume their life before critical illness. Many wish to teach medical trainees and members of the interprofessional team by sharing their experiences; indeed, several of our post-ICU patients and families participate in educational seminars for critical care trainees. Some wish to fundraise and to educate our broader medical community, government agencies, and the lay public about their transformative life event.

Surviving critical illness is a dynamic journey that may last years to decades, and the legacy may be permanent. The multidimensional physical, neuropsychological, and economic sequelae for patients and families will continue to evolve, to expand and reflect temporal changes in ICU case-mix and increased use of advanced technological support. Post-intensive care syndrome is a dynamic construct. Critical illness survivorship has and will continue to have important public health ramifications, but these are still largely unknown to funding agencies, our medical colleagues, and the lay community. This important and timely textbook led and edited by Dr. Butcher will provide a crucial, comprehensive, state-of-the-art review on what we know about PICS for patients and their families and how to move this burgeoning aspect of critical care forward and fully integrate it into mainstream, contemporary critical care management.

Section 1 Introduction

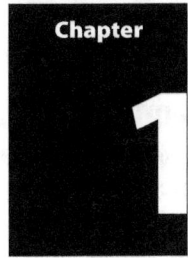

Developing the Concept of PICS: A Historical Narrative

Ramona O. Hopkins and Brad W. Butcher

Introduction

Since the development of intensive care units (ICUs) in the 1950s as a response to the polio epidemic and its need for the provision of specialized ventilation [1], the principal focus of critical care has been to rescue patients from impending death. Perhaps unsurprisingly, as research in the nascent field of critical care medicine began to develop, survival was the primary outcome assessed in the earliest studies of interventions administered in the ICU. This focus on survival stimulated the remarkable development of novel treatments, sophisticated technologies, and improvements in processes of care, which have collectively led to a significant increase in the number of patients surviving previously fatal illnesses and injuries [2]. For decades, the belief in the critical care community was that survival alone was a good outcome, and although that remains somewhat true today, it is also clear that survivors of critical illness face numerous debilitating symptoms, physical and neuropsychological morbidities, and functional impairments that require long-term management. As both the number of survivors and recognition of the burden of survivorship have increased significantly over the last 25 years, clinicians and researchers have paid considerably more attention to outcomes beyond mortality [3]. Between the 1970s and the 1990s, there were few studies of outcomes in the critically ill after hospital discharge, but, coincident with a paradigm shift in the thought leaders of critical care research, this number began to increase dramatically in the 2000s [4].

The Beginnings of Long-Term Outcomes Research

In the early 1990s, Dr. Hopkins's research was focused on neuropsychological outcomes following hypoxia, primarily in the setting of carbon monoxide poisoning [5]. Colleagues in the ICU caring for hypoxemic patients with acute respiratory failure engaged her in several conversations regarding the available data and the merit of exploring cognitive outcomes in this patient population. These conversations ultimately led to the authors' first cognitive outcomes study in survivors of the acute respiratory distress syndrome (ARDS), in which they found new cognitive impairments, depression, anxiety, chronic pain, and fatigue that persisted one year after hospital discharge [6]. Around the same time, a small number of other research groups were focusing on additional long-term outcomes following critical illness. For example, McHugh and colleagues found that survivors of ARDS had durable impairments in pulmonary function and self-perceived health scores [7], while Herridge and colleagues identified numerous physical impairments in a similar patient population, including muscle wasting, weakness, shorter distances achieved during the six-minute walk test, reduced ability to resume employment, and impaired health-related quality of life, particularly in the physical domain [8].

Increasing International Attention to Long-Term Outcomes

In 2001, the American Thoracic Society annual scientific meeting held a session entitled "What Happens to Survivors of ARDS." While data had been presented at previous scientific meetings, to Dr. Hopkins's knowledge, this was the first session that gathered critical care outcomes researchers together to discuss the morbidities of critical illness survivorship. Held in a small room, the session had only about 10 attendees alongside a handful of presenters. Her presentation was entitled "Neuropsychological sequelae in ARDS survivors," highlighting her work in the field [6,9,10]. Fortunately, influential leaders in critical care research were present, which bolstered the importance of this work and laid the foundation for additional exploration of critical care survivorship through advocacy for long-term outcomes sessions at future international critical care conferences and support of young investigators.

As interest in long-term outcomes following critical illness continued to increase, it became clear that certain key questions needed to be addressed. In 2002, the Brussels Roundtable was one of the first international meetings that assembled content experts to focus solely on outcomes in survivors of critical illness [11]. Importantly, this meeting suggested the novel idea that an episode of critical illness ends only when a patient's risk of late complications has returned to that of a similar person who had not fallen ill. A call was made to encourage future observational, interventional, and methodological studies to broaden their scope and include patient-centered outcomes in addition to mortality. Furthermore, specific research objectives were suggested, including elucidation of the etiologies and risk factors for impairments in physical, cognitive, and psychological health; strategies for their prevention; interventions to improve them; and their financial implications to both individuals and society at large. Specific, patient-centered outcomes of interest, including functional status, quality of life, and the ability to return to work, and the need to determine the tools best-suited to evaluate long-term outcomes, were identified as research priorities [11].

Over the next eight years, interest in long-term outcomes research expanded geometrically. In addition to published research, poster presentations and invited speaker sessions addressing long-term outcomes at national and international critical care conferences became increasingly popular. Certain conferences, such as the International Sepsis Forum 6th Annual Summer Colloquium, held in 2007 and entitled "The Sepsis Aftermath: Repair, Recurrence, Recovery, and Rehabilitation," were largely devoted to the topic. Interest in the impact of critical illness on particularly vulnerable patient populations, such as the elderly, also began to grow, highlighted by a meeting held by the National Institute on Aging to identify knowledge gaps in long-term outcomes in elderly survivors of critical illness and to develop a cohesive research plan to address them [12]. Such knowledge gaps included identification of impairments in physical, cognitive, and psychological health and the effective provision of patient-centered care and rehabilitation therapies. In addition to traditional research methods, innovative approaches studying molecular, pathological, and pathophysiological interactions were recommended to better understand the effects of critical illness in the elderly [12].

Developing the Term Post-Intensive Care Syndrome

This period of increased recognition and research, as remarkable as it was, was impeded by lack of a unifying terminology to describe the clinical phenotype being studied. In 2010, a conference was convened by the Society of Critical Care Medicine (SCCM) "to inform stakeholders from the rehabilitation, outpatient, and community care settings of the long-term consequences of critical illness and to initiate improvements across the continuum of care for survivors and their families" [13]. The goals of the SCCM meeting were to increase awareness of long-term outcomes among clinicians, patients and their families, and the general public; to increase screening for specific impairments occurring after critical illness; and to facilitate further research [14]. The 31 invited international experts and stakeholders agreed that, given the prevalence of multiple and significant impairments following critical illness, awareness of such adverse long-term outcomes would be improved by developing terminology to signify the presence of one or more of these impairments. Post-intensive care syndrome (PICS) was the term chosen, defined as "new or worsening impairments in physical, cognitive, or mental health status arising after critical illness and persisting beyond acute care hospitalization"; the term could be applied to either a survivor or their family members [13]. The term PICS covers diverse outcomes resulting from critical illness, including an unspecified number of impairments across its three primary domains, but importantly, it was *not* intended to be used as a medical diagnosis [13].

A PubMed search confirms that the development and use of the term PICS has increased both the number of studies investigating its associated impairments and the consistency of terminology used in those studies. In the first 12 years since the term PICS was coined, over 350 studies using the term were published, including 81 studies in 2024 alone.

Limitations of the Term PICS

Although coining the term PICS was critical for coalescing clinical and research endeavors under a unifying term, its definition does not encompass every aspect of the long-term impairments with which patients and their families contend. The definition of PICS does not include criteria for duration or severity of impairments, and given the multidimensional nature of the syndrome, efforts to ascribe degrees of severity, although attempted [15], are difficult. Similarly, the fairly inclusive definition of the syndrome makes screening for PICS challenging, and little expert consensus exists regarding the most appropriate screening tools for its assessment [16,17,18]. It seems unlikely that a single screening question or test will be able to predict PICS in all survivors of critical illness, but use of a limited number of brief screens may indicate the need for more detailed assessment [19]. Lastly, despite the benefits of such an inclusive definition, there are also potential drawbacks; for example, should every new symptom or outcome identified in survivors of critical illness be considered a manifestation of PICS? A variety of somatic concerns (e.g., alopecia, sensory impairments, fatigue, and pain) and vulnerabilities to adverse health outcomes (e.g., hospital readmission and development of new chronic diseases) are common in survivors of critical illness, but should patients with these concerns or susceptibilities be classified as having PICS in the absence of impairments in the three defined domains? Moreover, although the difficulties reintegrating into previous social roles, the inability to resume employment, and worsened social determinants of health are common themes in PICS-related research, should the original definition of PICS be amended to include impairments in social and functional domains of health that extend beyond discrete physical, cognitive, or psychological impairments, while acknowledging that such impairments may directly or indirectly impact social and functional roles?

Conclusions

The last quarter of a century has greatly expanded our knowledge of adverse long-term outcomes in survivors of critical illness. A growing body of research has not only characterized these outcomes, collectively labeled as PICS, but has also sought to address their pathophysiological basis, risk factors for their development, and prediction tools to identify those most vulnerable. While significant progress has been made, important knowledge gaps remain, particularly with respect to determining severity, identifying the best tools for screening and assessment, and exploring the relationship between PICS and other important health outcomes. Given the significant need to improve the lives of an ever-increasing population of survivors of critical illness, hope burns bright that the next quarter century will substantially increase our understanding of PICS and our ability to both prevent and treat it as effectively as possible.

Key Points

1. It took nearly 50 years for the field of critical care medicine to complement studies solely focused on decreasing mortality of the critically ill with studies comprehensively examining patient-centered, long-term outcomes in survivors.
2. Key meetings in 2001 and 2002, including the American Thoracic Society annual scientific meeting and the Brussels Roundtable, respectively, shined a light on the nascent field of long-term outcomes research, leading to a paradigm shift in the research agenda of critical care medicine.
3. In 2010, during a stakeholders conference held by SCCM, the term post-intensive care syndrome was coined and defined as "new or worsening impairments in physical, cognitive, or mental health status arising after critical illness and persisting beyond acute care hospitalization."
4. Despite the utility of the term PICS to enhance awareness and education and to organize research endeavors, vagueness in the definition highlights challenges in determining the severity of PICS, the most appropriate methods of screening for it, and deciding whether new impairments fall within its scope.

References

1. P.G. Berthelsen, M. Cronqvist. The first intensive care unit in the world: Copenhagen 1953. *Acta Anaesthesiol Scand* 2003; **47**(10): 1190–5.
2. Z. Zhang, P.M. Spieth, D. Chiumello, et al. Declining mortality in patients with acute respiratory distress syndrome: an analysis of the acute respiratory distress syndrome network trials. *Crit Care Med* 2019; **47**(3): 315–23.
3. N.E. Brummel. Measuring outcomes after critical illness. *Crit Care Clin* 2018; **34**(4): 515–26.
4. A.E. Turnbull, A. Rabiee, W.E. Davis, et al. Outcome measurement in ICU survivorship research from 1970 to 2013: a scoping review of 425 publications. *Crit Care Med* 2016; **44**(7): 1267–77.

5. L.K. Weaver, R.O. Hopkins, K.J. Chan, et al. Hyperbaric oxygen for acute carbon monoxide poisoning. *N Engl J Med* 2002; **347**: 1057–67.
6. R.O. Hopkins, L.K. Weaver, D. Pope, et al. Neuropsychological sequelae and impaired health status in survivors of severe acute respiratory distress syndrome. *Am J Respir Crit Care Med* 1999; **160**(1): 50–6.
7. L.G. McHugh, J.A. Millbert, M. E. Whitcomb, et al. Recovery of function in survivors of the acute respiratory distress syndrome. *Am J Respir Crit Care Med* 1994; **150**(1): 90–4.
8. M.S. Herridge, A.M. Cheung, C.M. Tansey, et al. One-year outcomes in survivors of the acute respiratory distress syndrome. *N Engl J Med* 2003; **348**(8): 683–93.
9. R.O. Hopkins. Neuropsychological sequelae in ARDS survivors. Oral presentation at the American Thoracic Society 97th International Conference. San Francisco, CA, USA. May 20, 2001.
10. R.O. Hopkins, V. Larson-Lohr, L. K. Weaver, E.D. Bigler. Neuropsychological impairments following hantavirus pulmonary syndrome. *J Int Neuropsychol Soc* 1998; **4**(2): 190–6.
11. D.C. Angus, J. Carlet. Surviving intensive care: a report from the 2002 Brussels roundtable. *Intensive Care Med* 2003; **29**(3): 386–77.
12. E.B. Milbrandt, B. Eldadah, S. Nayfield, et al. Toward an integrated research agenda for critical illness in aging. *Am J. Respir Crit Care Med* 2010; **182**(8): 995–1003.
13. D.M. Needham, J. Davidson, H. Cohen, et al. Improving long-term outcomes after discharge from intensive care unit: Report from a stakeholders' conference. *Crit Care Med* 2012; **40**(2): 502–9.
14. S.L. Hiser, A. Fatima, M. Ali, D. M. Needham. Post-intensive care syndrome (PICS): recent updates. *J Intensive Care* 2023; **11**(1): 23.
15. M.A. Narváez-Martínez, Á.M. Henao-Castaño. Severity classification and influencing variables of the post-intensive care syndrome. *Enferm Intensiva (Engl Ed)* 2024; **35**(2): 89–96.
16. D.M. Needham, K.A. Sepulveda, V. D. Dinglas, et al. Core outcome measures for clinical research in acute respiratory failure survivors: an international modified Delphi consensus study. *Am J Respir Crit Care Med* 2017; **196**(6): 1122–1130.
17. M.E. Mikkelsen, M. Still, B.J. Anderson, et al. Society of Critical Care Medicine's international consensus conference on prediction and identification of long-term impairments after critical illness. *Crit Care Med* 2020; **48**(11): 1670–9.
18. L. Sutton, E. Bell, S. Every-Palmer, et al. Survivorship outcomes for critically ill patients in Australia and New Zealand: a scoping review. *Aus Crit Care* 2024; **37**(2): 354–68.
19. C.D. Spies, H. Krampe, N. Paul, et al. Instruments to measures outcomes of post-intensive care syndrome in outpatient care settings: results of an expert consensus and feasibility field test. *J Intensive Care Soc* 2021; **22**(2): 159–74.

Chapter 2
Fundamentals of PICS

Brad W. Butcher, Lindsey R. Morris, and Michael Baram

Introduction and Definition

Because of advances in technology and the provision of critical care, an increasing number of patients are surviving critical illness, exemplified by a 35% relative mortality decrease from 1988 to 2012 [1]. More than 5.7 million adults in the United States require intensive care annually, accounting for approximately 20% of all acute care admissions [2]; roughly 85% of these patients will survive, and an increasing number of them will live for years following their index critical illness. This growing population of survivors is characterized by heightened vulnerability to a host of adverse health outcomes and by the development of multidimensional impairments that significantly impact their quality of life and societal participation.

This protracted vulnerability challenges the idea that critical illness ends with discharge from the intensive care unit (ICU). For many, the need for critical care is not a transient phenomenon but instead the beginning of a significant burden of chronic illness and debility that far exceeds the time spent in the hospital. The report generated by the 2002 Brussels Roundtable suggested that an episode of critical illness ends only when a patient's risk of late complications has returned to that of a similar person who had not fallen ill [3]. Recognition of this premise not only inspired a focus on long-term outcomes in research but also fostered increased interest in optimizing clinical care for survivors of critical illness. Indeed, improving survivorship has been considered the defining challenge of critical care medicine in the twenty-first century [4].

In 2010, a conference was convened by the Society of Critical Care Medicine (SCCM) to "inform stakeholders from the rehabilitation, outpatient, and community care settings of the long-term consequences of critical illness and to initiate improvements across the continuum of care for intensive care survivors and their families" [5]. Participants agreed that given the burden of impairments following critical illness, awareness would be improved by use of one term to identify the presence of one or more of these impairments. The term chosen was "post-intensive care syndrome," or PICS, which is defined as "new or worsening impairments in physical, cognitive, or mental health status arising after a critical illness and persisting beyond acute care hospitalization." PICS can also impact family members and loved ones, who may develop physical, psychological, and social impairments in the face of caregiver burden, changing family dynamics, and socioeconomic pressures [5]. Importantly, PICS was not intended to be used as a medical diagnosis but instead as a construct for raising awareness among clinicians and the lay public, increasing screening for impairments following critical illness, and facilitating further research [6].

Clinical Manifestations

Survivors of critical illness are a heterogeneous patient population, and considerable variation exists with respect to the breadth, depth, duration, and mutability of their symptoms and impairments. Indeed, the burden of survivorship is both complex and unique to each individual, preventing a "one-size-fits-all" approach to caring for these patients [7]. Physical impairments consistent with PICS, which are often driven by the development of ICU-acquired weakness (ICU-AW; see Chapter 4 for additional information), are considerable and include: persistent dyspnea (see Chapter 35 for additional information); impaired exercise tolerance, endurance, strength, and balance (see Chapter 41 for additional information); chronic dysphagia (see Chapter 38 for additional information); laryngeal disorders (see Chapter 39 for additional information); malnutrition (see Chapter 40 for additional information); and neuropathy, pressure injuries, joint contractures, heterotopic calcification, procedure-related trauma (e.g., incontinence), and cosmetic concerns (see Chapter 36 for additional information). Cognitive impairments include difficulties with memory, executive function, visuospatial skills, language, attention, processing speed, and concentration (see Chapter 43 for additional information). Mental health concerns include anxiety, depression, post-traumatic stress disorder (PTSD), suicidality, and substance use disorders (see Chapter 46 for additional information). Family members, loved ones, and caretakers of survivors of critical illness may develop PICS-Family (PICS-F), which includes anxiety, depression, PTSD, complicated grief, caregiver burden, reduced attention to their own physical health, compromised employment, and financial stress (see Chapter 48 for additional information) [7,8]. Selected clinical manifestations, along with selected risk factors, preventative strategies, screening tools, and treatment modalities for PICS and PICS-F are summarized in Table 2.1.

Some have argued that the definition of PICS should be broadened to include additional conditions that are frequently described in survivors of critical illness (see Figure 2.1) [9]. Patients with PICS have increased vulnerability to adverse health outcomes, including heightened risks of hospital readmission, healthcare resource utilization, development or worsening of chronic diseases, and long-term mortality (see Chapter 33 for additional information). They also commonly develop functional impairments, including dependence in activities of daily living (ADLs) and instrumental activities of daily living (IADLs; see Chapter 42 for additional information), which may compromise the ability to live independently; social health impairments, including worsened quality of life (see Chapter 34 for additional information), difficulties resuming driving and employment (see Chapter 44 for additional information), and failure to reintegrate into previous familial, vocational, and community roles [10]; and chronic pain, chronic fatigue, and sleep disorders, among others, which defy classification into one of the three discrete domains in the original definition of PICS (see Chapters 36 and 37 for additional information) [9]. The validity of such an expanded definition requires rigorous assessment before its widespread adoption [9].

Lack of Communication About Post-ICU Problems

Despite the growing appreciation of the significant challenges that survivors of critical illness face, this topic is insufficiently addressed by intensivists with patients and their surrogate decision-makers. In a survey of intensivists in 73 hospitals in Michigan, only 34% reported having discussions with "almost every" or "many but not all" of their patients about post-ICU challenges; 27% reported "almost never" communicating these issues to

Table 2.1 An overview of selected clinical manifestations, risk factors, preventative strategies, screening tools, and treatment modalities for PICS

PICS domain	Selected clinical manifestations	Selected risk factors	Selected preventative strategies	Selected screening tools	Selected treatment modalities
Physical	Impaired strength Impaired exercise tolerance Impaired endurance Impaired balance Persistent dyspnea Chronic dysphagia Laryngeal disorders Malnutrition Neuropathy Pressure injuries Heterotopic calcifications Procedure-related trauma Cosmetic concerns	**Patient-related** Pre-existing frailty Pre-existing functional impairment Pre-existing cognitive impairment Older age **Hospital-related** ICU-AW Prolonged bed rest Severity of illness	ABCDEF bundle Inpatient physical therapy Inpatient occupational therapy	**Exercise capacity** 6MWT 2MWT **Strength** Handgrip strength dynamometry MRC sum score **Composite** SPPB Timed up and go **Other** Gait speed Balance assessment	Outpatient physical therapy Pulmonary rehabilitation Swallowing therapy Nutritional therapy Referral to ENT and other specialists as appropriate
Functional	Inability to perform ADLs Inability to perform IADLs	Similar to physical and cognitive impairments	ABCDEF bundle Inpatient physical therapy Inpatient occupational therapy Inpatient cognitive therapy	**ADLs** Katz ADLs Barthel Index FIM **IADLs** Lawton IADLs	Outpatient occupational therapy

	Symptoms	Risk factors	Assessment	Treatment/Prevention
Cognitive	Impaired memory Impaired executive function Impaired visuospatial skills Impaired attention Impaired processing speed Impaired concentration Language difficulties	**Patient-related** Pre-existing cognitive dysfunction Older age **Hospital-related** Delirium Receipt of sedation Benzodiazepine exposure Sepsis Shock Hypoxemic respiratory failure Receipt of life support Length of stay	ABCDEF bundle Inpatient occupational therapy Inpatient cognitive therapy	**Cognition** MoCA RBANS MMSE SMQ Trail Making Test Mini Cog	Outpatient cognitive therapy Neuropsychology follow-up
Psychiatric	Depression Anxiety PTSD Suicidality Substance use disorders	**Patient-related** Pre-existing mental health concerns Female sex **Hospital-related** Memories of frightening experiences	ABCDEF bundle Inpatient psychological therapy ICU diaries	**Depression** HADS PHQ–9 PHQ–4 BECK DEPRESSION INVENTORY **Anxiety** HADS GAD–7 PHQ–4 **PTSD** IES-R IES–6	Psychotherapy Review of ICU diary Participation in peer support group

Table 2.1 (cont.)

PICS domain	Selected clinical manifestations	Selected risk factors	Selected preventative strategies	Selected screening tools	Selected treatment modalities
Social	Reduced quality of life Impaired ability to drive Impaired ability to return to work Difficulty resuming familial, avocational, and community roles	Not well defined	ABCDEF bundle	**Quality of life** EQ–5D–5L EQ–5D–3L EQ-VAS SF–36 SF–12 WHODAS 2.0	Vocational rehabilitation Driving rehabilitation programs Participation in peer support group
PICS-F	Depression Anxiety PTSD Sleep disturbances Prolonged grief Impaired physical health Caregiver burden Compromised employment Financial stress	**Person-related** Female sex Younger age Being the patient's spouse **Hospital-related** Psychological distress during hospitalization Fear of loss of a loved one Poor communication with medical team Sleep deprivation Personal and family conflict Restricted visiting hours	ABCDEF bundle ICU diaries Flexible visitation policies Promotion of family presence Educational programs Enhanced communication strategies Social work, palliative care, spiritual care, and psychology consultations	**Depression** HADS PHQ–9 PHQ–4 Beck DEPRESSION INVENTORY **Anxiety** HADS GAD–7 PHQ–4 **PTSD** IES-R IES–6 **Caregiver burden** Zarit CAREGIVER burden scale **Sleep disorders** PSQI	Psychotherapy Review of ICU diary Grief counseling Participation in peer support group

Other	Persistent fatigue Sleep disorders Chronic pain Metabolic disorders Endocrine disorders	Not well defined	ABCDEF bundle
Sleep disorders	PSQI		
Pain	BPI		Outpatient physical and occupational therapy Referral to sleep specialist Referral to chronic pain specialist Referral to other specialists as appropriate Pharmacotherapy for insomnia and pain management Energy conservation strategies Complementary medicine approaches

Note that this is not meant to be comprehensive and not all components of the table are evidence-based.

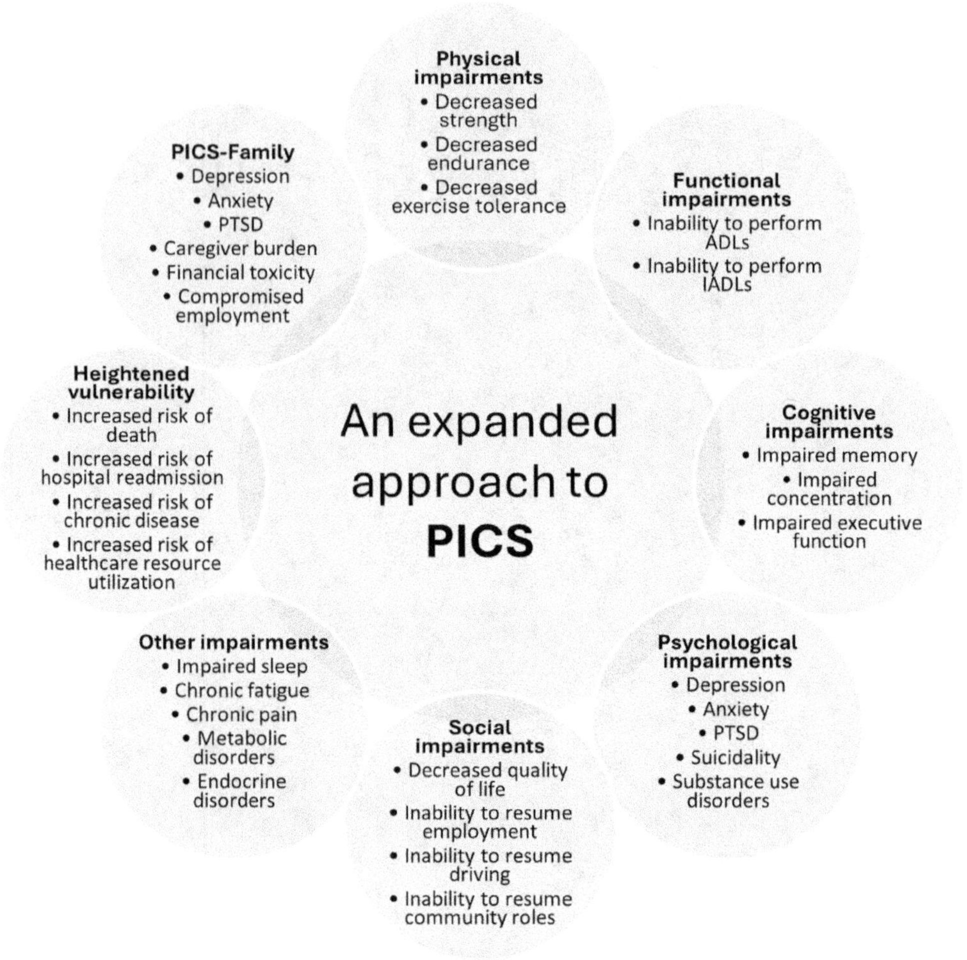

An expanded approach to PICS

- **Physical impairments**
  - Decreased strength
  - Decreased endurance
  - Decreased exercise tolerance

- **Functional impairments**
  - Inability to perform ADLs
  - Inability to perform IADLs

- **Cognitive impairments**
  - Impaired memory
  - Impaired concentration
  - Impaired executive function

- **Psychological impairments**
  - Depression
  - Anxiety
  - PTSD
  - Suicidality
  - Substance use disorders

- **Social impairments**
  - Decreased quality of life
  - Inability to resume employment
  - Inability to resume driving
  - Inability to resume community roles

- **Other impairments**
  - Impaired sleep
  - Chronic fatigue
  - Chronic pain
  - Metabolic disorders
  - Endocrine disorders

- **Heightened vulnerability**
  - Increased risk of death
  - Increased risk of hospital readmission
  - Increased risk of chronic disease
  - Increased risk of healthcare resource utilization

- **PICS-Family**
  - Depression
  - Anxiety
  - PTSD
  - Caregiver burden
  - Financial toxicity
  - Compromised employment

Figure 2.1 An expanded conceptualization of post-intensive care syndrome. This depiction includes additional categories of impairments or vulnerabilities that survivors of critical illness and their loved ones may face along with selected examples of each.

patients [11]. Moreover, irrespective of the presence of communication, surrogate decision-makers and physicians often have misaligned expectations for patients' long-term outcomes. In a study of 126 patients requiring tracheotomy for prolonged mechanical ventilation, surrogate decision-makers and physicians were interviewed at the time of tracheotomy about their expectations for one-year patient survival, functional status, and quality of life, which were then compared with observed one-year outcomes. Agreement regarding expectations between physicians and surrogates was low, and accuracy in outcome prediction was poor, with surrogates being overly optimistic and physicians slightly pessimistic [12]. In a study involving surrogate decision-makers and physicians caring for patients at high risk of death, discordance in prognosis between physicians and surrogates, defined as a difference in prognostic estimates of at least 20%, occurred 53% of the time [13]. Given that intensivists rarely see patients in the outpatient setting, that knowledge of PICS among intensivists is inconsistent, and that prediction tools for long-term impairments are lacking, it must be asked how adequately clinicians are prepared to accurately predict patient recovery trajectories and long-term outcomes.

On the Nature of Disability

Functional Status

Functional status is a broad term that describes one's ability to perform the physical, cognitive, and social tasks necessary to meet basic needs, fulfill usual roles, and maintain health and well-being. It is characterized by four components: functional capacity, functional performance, functional reserve, and functional capacity utilization [14]. While functional capacity describes what one *can do* when maximally performing an activity in a *standardized* environment (e.g., lifting the heaviest weight possible during one repetition), functional performance represents what one *actually does* during daily living in their *usual* environment (e.g., ADLs and IADLs, including bathing and shopping). Functional performance below the level necessary for independent living is one means of conceptualizing disability (see Figure 2.2) [14,15].

Functional reserve and functional capacity utilization are related terms whose sum is equivalent to the patient's functional capacity. Functional reserve describes the *potential* ability that can be harnessed to perform a task, while functional capacity utilization describes the fraction of maximal performance required to accomplish a task. Patients

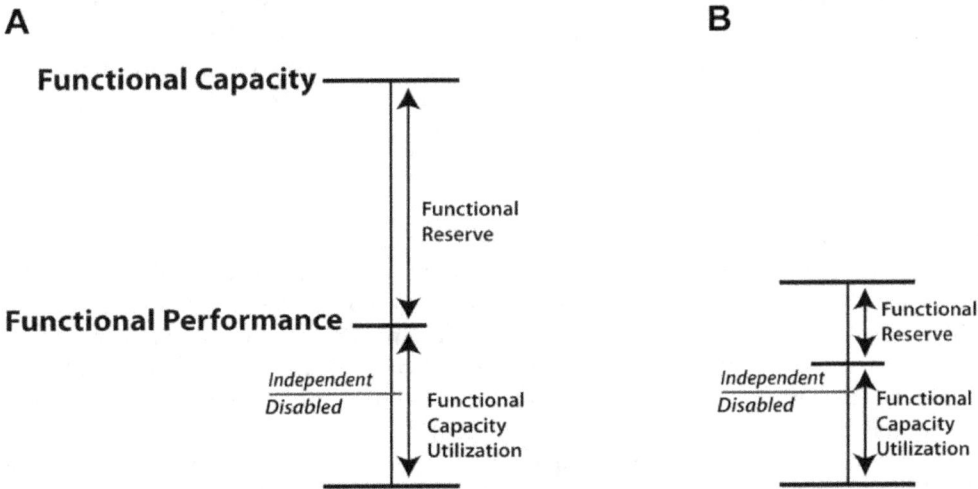

Figure 2.2 A comparison of functional status between two patients. (A) depicts the functional status of a 35-year-old healthy person while (B) depicts the functional status of a 65-year-old survivor of critical illness. Note that the functional capacity for patient (A) is considerably higher than the functional capacity for patient (B). Although functional performance differs slightly between the two, patient (B) is much closer to the threshold for dependence. Patient (A) has greater functional reserve, indicating that they are capable of performing more strenuous tasks, while patient (B) has very little reserve. Moreover, patient (B) is using much more of their functional capacity (i.e., high functional capacity utilization) and is exerting themselves more to perform daily activities. Reproduced from: N.E. Brummel. Measuring outcomes after critical illness. *Crit Care Clin* 2018; **34**: 515–26 with permission from Elsevier.

with high functional capacity utilization (i.e., significant effort is required to perform an activity), have limited functional reserve (i.e., the ability to perform additional activities), while patients with low functional capacity utilization (i.e., little effort is required to perform an activity) have greater functional reserve [14]. Patients with high functional capacity utilization (and therefore limited functional reserve) may need to decrease the frequency or intensity with which daily activities are performed or may need to stop some activities altogether, which may result in a transition from independent to disabled [14]. Interventions designed for survivors of critical illness with impaired functional capacity could either augment functional capacity (e.g., physical and cognitive therapy) or minimize functional capacity utilization (e.g., using assistive devices for mobilization), both of which could improve functional performance and mitigate the risk of disability [14].

The Biomedical Model

Disability is considered "a state of decreased functioning associated with disease, disorder, injury, or other health conditions, which, in the context of one's environment, is experienced as an impairment, activity limitation, or participation restriction" [16]. Disability is therefore not a personal characteristic but instead the difference between personal capabilities and environmental demands [15]. An instructive biological model describing how an acute illness can lead to disability was proposed by Nagi [17] and subsequently modified by Verbrugge and Jette to include risk factors, intra-individual factors (e.g., coping skills, lifestyle changes, and activity accommodations), and extra-individual factors (e.g., rehabilitative therapies, external supports, and environmental modifications) [15]. In this framework, illness and injuries that disrupt normal physiological processes (pathologies) lead to dysfunction in physical, cognitive, or emotional processes (impairments), which can in turn reduce the ability to perform physical and cognitive tasks (limitations) and ultimately preclude participation in socially defined roles (disability). Figure 2.3 demonstrates how this scheme can be applied to a survivor of critical illness. An alternative to the biomedical model of disability, the social model of disability, which emphasizes barriers in the physical and social environment, is explored in Chapter 24.

Incidence and Prevalence

Quantifying the incidence of PICS is challenging for many reasons, including the frequent absence of baseline status prior to critical illness, the numerous screening tools used, and the inconsistent criteria by which PICS is diagnosed [7]. For a given PICS domain, several different outcomes can be measured, and, for any given outcome, there are multiple ways of measuring it, considerably influencing the reported incidence [9]. This variability also impacts clinical research, affecting the reproducibility and interpretation of results as well as the ability to make comparisons across studies [9].

In a study that relied on proxy completion of the 36-Item Short Form Survey (SF-36) at the time of ICU admission and patient or proxy completion of the SF-36 and the Short Memory Questionnaire (SMQ) six months following ICU admission, the incidence of PICS, in this case defined as a decline in physical or mental status by virtue of at least a 10-point decrease in scores on these questionnaires, was 63.5% [18]. In a more comprehensive study by Geense and colleagues, data was collected via patient- or proxy-completed questionnaires before or at the time of ICU admission and repeated one year following ICU discharge, assessing frailty (using the Clinical Frailty Scale), fatigue (using the Checklist

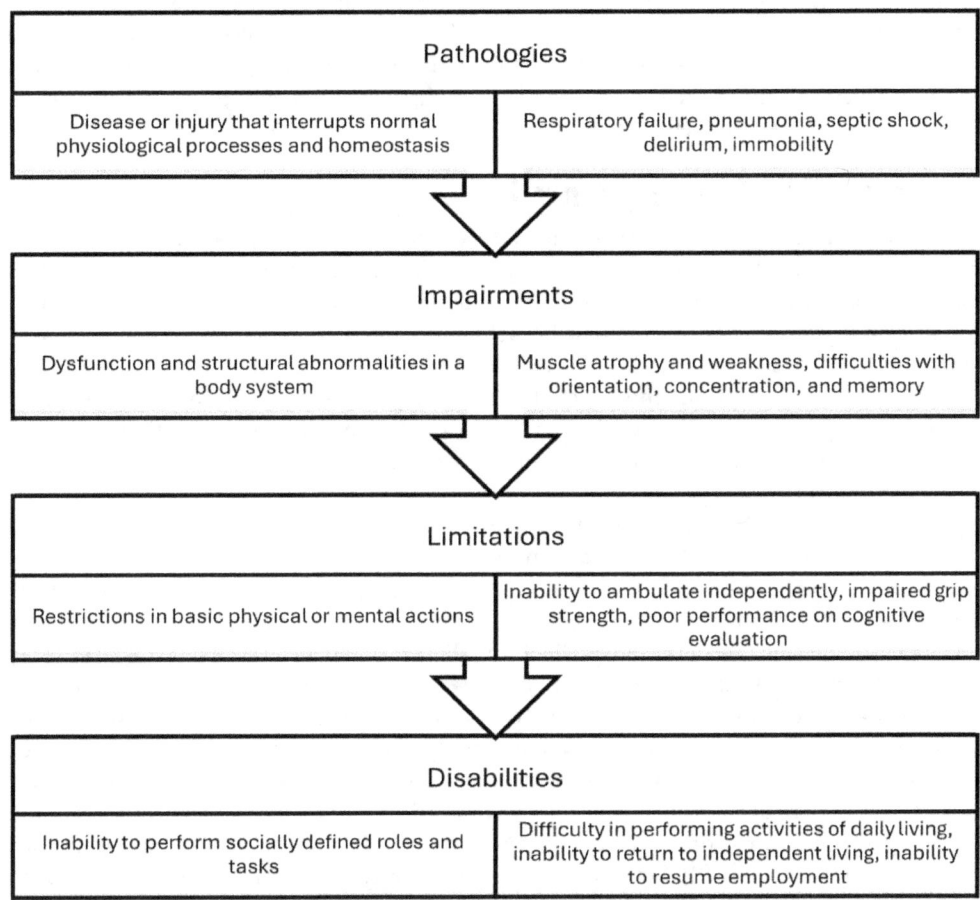

Figure 2.3 A model of disability as applied to a survivor of critical illness. The left side of the diagram displays the conceptual definitions of pathologies, impairments, limitations, and disabilities, while the right side of the diagram applies these concepts to a survivor of critical illness. Adapted and reproduced from: N.E. Brummel. Measuring outcomes after critical illness. *Crit Care Clin* 2018; **34**: 515–26 with permission from Elsevier.

for Individual Strength), new or worsened physical problems (using a non-validated questionnaire), anxiety and depression (using the Hospital Anxiety and Depression Scale [HADS]), cognitive health (using the Cognitive Failure Questionnaire), and quality of life (using the SF-36). One year after admission, 58% of patients admitted to the medical ICU, 64% admitted to the surgical ICU for emergency surgery, and 43% admitted to the surgical ICU for elective surgery were suffering from new physical, cognitive, and/or mental health problems [19].

More commonly, given the lack of baseline status prior to critical illness, most studies measure the prevalence of PICS, which varies considerably based on the study consulted. Analysis of data collected over 24 months in 289 sepsis survivors requiring admission to the ICU showed a remarkably high prevalence of PICS, with 98.6% of patients experiencing difficulties in at least one of six PICS components: depression and/or PTSD (mental health domain); cognitive impairment (cognitive domain); and chronic pain, neuropathic symptoms, and/or dysphagia (physical domain). When more conservative definitions of PICS were considered, such as requiring deficits in both the physical domain and a combined neuropsychiatric domain or deficits in all three distinct domains, the prevalence fell to 81.7% and 32.9%, respectively [20].

Co-occurrence of Impairments

The presence and severity of deficits in the three classic domains of PICS may vary over time, and the importance of specific deficits to individual patients may also shift as they learn to cope with their limitations and their life circumstances change. Manifestations of PICS are infrequently restricted to an isolated impairment in a single domain and commonly involve challenges across all three domains. Moreover, the *interactions* between physical function, cognition, and psychological health define the survivorship experience, and viewing symptoms through a holistic, biopsychosocial lens to ensure that all factors contributing to the patient's experience are addressed is paramount (see Chapter 23 for additional information) [7].

In a widely cited study on the prevalence of PICS, Marra and colleagues assessed survivors of critical illness at 3 and 12 months after discharge for combinations of cognitive impairment, depression, and limitations in performing ADLs. One or more PICS problems were present in 64% and 56% of the cohort at 3 and 12 months, respectively, and problems in 2 or more domains were present in 25% and 21% at 3 and 12 months, respectively [21]. Importantly, however, this study is limited by a relatively modest approach to screening for PICS; had a more comprehensive evaluation been performed, including a 6-minute walk test (6MWT), screening for impairments in performing IADLs, and assessments of anxiety and PTSD, the percentage of patients with impairments in multiple domains would have likely been higher [21]. These limitations were partially addressed in the aforementioned study of 289 sepsis survivors requiring admission to the ICU, where a more comprehensive screening approach for PICS-related challenges revealed a much higher prevalence of impairments across multiple domains through 24 months of follow-up [20].

A secondary analysis of the ALTOS study, in which 430 survivors of the acute respiratory distress syndrome (ARDS) were assessed with a battery of physical, emotional, and cognitive health screening tools, reinforced the idea that physical and mental health challenges commonly occur together. In this study, four distinct subtypes of disability were identified: mildly impaired physical and mental health in 22%, moderately impaired physical and mental health in 39%, severely impaired physical health and moderately impaired mental health in 15%, and severely impaired physical and mental health in 24% [22].

Duration of Impairments

The duration of PICS-related impairments is difficult to quantify, as comparatively few studies have investigated outcomes beyond two years after hospital discharge. A landmark study by Herridge and colleagues found that, five years after discharge, survivors of ARDS had persistent physical impairments, evidenced by a decreased median distance achieved during a 6MWT (76% of the predicted distance) and physical component scores on the SF-36 quality of life questionnaire below those of age- and sex-matched controls [23]. This finding was corroborated by a meta-analysis of 1700 survivors of critical illness, which demonstrated that the mean 6MWT distance achieved at 3 months, 12 months, and 60 months post-hospitalization was considerably below population norms, emphasizing persistent deficits in exercise capacity in this patient population [24]. Handgrip strength dynamometry, along with the distance achieved on the 6MWT and physical component scores on the SF-36, is similarly impaired up to five years following critical illness, particularly in those patients who had an ICU length of stay of eight or more days [25]. Furthermore, patients with ICU-AW, as diagnosed by the Medical Research Council (MRC) sum score, were also prone to durable impairments in handgrip strength dynamometry, 6MWT distance, and physical component scores on the SF-36 at five years of follow-up [26].

A systematic review of 46 studies assessing cognitive impairment in survivors of critical illness found that the prevalence of cognitive impairment was dependent on the type of cognitive instrument used. Objective rather than subjective assessments and comprehensive cognitive batteries rather than the Mini-Mental State Examination (MMSE) both revealed a higher prevalence of cognitive impairment. The presence of cognitive impairment measured by comprehensive cognitive batteries was 43% at 12 months and 46% at 24 months following discharge. Six of the included studies evaluated cognitive function at two or more years following hospital discharge, and although limited by small sample sizes, they demonstrated similar rates of cognitive dysfunction [27]. Survivors of sepsis had decrements in cognitive function and functional capacity (i.e., the ability to perform ADLs and IADLs) that persisted in up to eight years of follow-up [28].

In a five-year longitudinal study of psychiatric symptoms in 186 survivors of ARDS, Bienvenue and colleagues found that prolonged symptoms of anxiety, depression, and PTSD were common, affecting 38%, 32%, and 23% of survivors, respectively. Fifty-two percent of survivors had prolonged psychiatric morbidity in at least one of the three mental health outcomes, and perhaps surprisingly, the most common pattern of prolonged psychiatric morbidity involved symptoms of all three [29]. Large meta-analyses of studies investigating symptoms of depression [30], anxiety [31], and PTSD [32] in survivors of critical illness over 12 months of follow-up found a prevalence of approximately 30%, 33%, and 20%, respectively [30].

Severity

The protean nature of PICS has made attempts to delineate it into degrees of severity challenging. Results from certain screening tools assessing individual domains of PICS can be divided into degrees of severity; for example, the Montreal Cognitive Assessment (MoCA) tool and the HADS can be categorized into degrees of mild, moderate, and severe cognitive impairment and depression/anxiety, respectively. To characterize the severity of PICS as a whole, Narváez-Martinez and colleagues analyzed data from 135 patients who completed the Healthy Aging Brain Care (HABC) tool, developed by the Indianapolis Discovery Network for Dementia, which assesses PICS in four domains: cognitive status, functional status, behavior and mood, and caregiver stress. Clustering determined by Gaussian mixture models allowed for classification of PICS presentations as mild, moderate, or severe, with cutoffs on the HABC tool of 9 or fewer points, 10 to 42 points, and 43 or more points, respectively. Patients were more likely to have moderate or severe PICS if they were male, older, had longer ICU lengths of stay, had higher APACHE II scores, and were exposed to sedation, analgesia, and/or neuromuscular blockers [33]. Given that the

HABC tool is not broadly utilized, additional studies are needed to clarify degrees of PICS severity using more commonly applied screening tools.

Prediction Tools and Risk Factors

An improved ability to predict impairments following critical illness could guide clinical decision-making during hospitalization and care coordination following discharge, inform enrollment in clinical trials, and ultimately facilitate patient rehabilitation [34]. Given the often-fragmented care that survivors of critical illness face following discharge, provided by clinicians with variable abilities to recognize the sequelae of critical illness, there is considerable need to be able to predict those at greatest risk for developing PICS [34]. Only three studies have focused on the development of tools to predict either physical or mental health outcomes following critical illness [35,36,37]; no studies have developed a prediction tool for cognitive function after discharge. Collectively, these tools and clinical judgment are insufficient to reliably predict PICS-related problems in all survivors of critical illness, but certain patient- and illness-related risk factors can reasonably identify those at highest risk [34]. Given the limited evidence base regarding risk prediction, however, clinicians should acknowledge during goals of care conversations the uncertainty with which PICS can be currently predicted. Clearly, there is a need to develop rigorous prediction models to predict post-ICU impairments that can be used to inform clinical decision-making [34].

Although comprehensive prediction tools for the development of PICS have remained elusive, more considerable work has been done in attempting to elucidate risk factors for the specific domains of PICS. Such risk factors are commonly divided into patient-related factors and illness- or hospitalization-related factors. Patients at risk for physical impairment following critical illness include those with pre-existing frailty, functional disability, and cognitive impairment and those whose critical illness was complicated by significant bed rest and the development of ICU-AW [38]. Patients at risk for cognitive impairments following critical illness include those with pre-existing cognitive dysfunction and those whose critical illness was characterized by delirium, receipt of sedation (particularly with benzodiazepines), sepsis, shock, hypoxemic respiratory failure, and receipt of life support, including mechanical ventilation. Patients at risk for psychological impairments following critical illness include those with pre-existing mental health concerns, including depression, anxiety, and PTSD, and those whose hospitalization was complicated by memories of frightening experiences [38].

Additionally, a systematic review and meta-analysis of 89 studies of risk factors for the development of PICS impairments identified 60 unique risk factors, including 33 patient-related and 27 ICU-related factors. Of these, significant risk factors for physical impairment included older age, higher severity of illness, and female sex, and significant risk factors for mental health impairment included a history of mental health concerns, negative ICU experiences, and female sex [39]. Although the only significant risk factor for cognitive impairment identified in this analysis was delirium [39], a German study of sepsis survivors requiring ICU admission also found higher age and longer durations of ICU treatment and mechanical ventilation were significant risk factors for cognitive impairment [20]. Section 2 of this text, entitled the Hazards of Hospitalization, thoroughly reviews key known and potential risk factors for PICS, including immobility and ICU-AW (see Chapter 4 for additional information), frailty (see Chapter 5 for additional information), nutritional impairments (see Chapter 7 for additional information), delirium (see Chapter 8 for additional information), sleep impairments (see Chapter 9 for additional information), and negative psychological experiences during hospitalization (see Chapter 10 for additional information).

Prevention

Although studies examining interventions to prevent the development of PICS are lacking, the ABCDEF bundle (Assess, prevent, and manage pain; Both spontaneous awakening trials (SAT) and spontaneous breathing trials (SBT); Choice of analgesia and sedation; Delirium: assess, prevent, and manage; Early mobility and exercise; and Family engagement and empowerment), as recommended by the SCCM, has demonstrated the ability to improve short-term outcomes in critically ill patients, with the potential for ultimately reducing the incidence of PICS (see Chapter 11 for additional information). In a study of more than 15,000 patients across 68 ICUs, complete ABCDEF bundle performance was associated with lower likelihood of: hospital death within 7 days, need for next-day mechanical ventilation, coma, delirium, use of physical restraints, readmission to the ICU, and discharge to a facility other than home. Moreover, there was a consistent dose-dependent relationship between the number of individual bundle elements performed and improvements in each of these clinical outcomes [40].

The provision of physical and occupational therapy during hospitalization is commonly recommended to prevent or minimize the physical and functional impairments associated with ICU-AW and PICS (see Chapters 12 and 13 for additional information) [41]. While findings from two meta-analyses examining physical rehabilitation during hospitalization suggest that, when compared with the standard of care, patients receiving physical rehabilitation have improved muscle strength and mobility status at the time of hospital discharge, consistent improvements in long-term physical functioning are lacking, and more research is needed to better understand the efficacy of rehabilitation strategies in the ICU and hospital [42,43]. The SCCM ABCDEF bundle includes early mobility and exercise as one of its core provisions based in part on the study of Schweikert and colleagues, in which 104 previously functionally independent patients requiring mechanical ventilation were randomly assigned to early exercise and mobilization performed by physical and occupational therapists during SATs or to usual care. Return to independent functional status at hospital discharge, as defined by the ability to perform six ADLs and walk independently, occurred in 59% of patients in the intervention group compared with 35% of patients in the control group; those in the intervention group also had less delirium and were extubated more quickly [44].

Few studies regarding the role of psychological intervention in the ICU have been performed, but the SCCM [38] and the National Institute for Health and Clinical Excellence (NICE) in the United Kingdom (UK) [45] have recommended that all critically ill patients be assessed for a history of psychological problems and be screened for psychological symptoms prior to discharge to help determine risk for future psychological morbidity (see Chapter 14 for additional information). ICU diaries, typically composed by staff caring for the patient and the patient's loved ones, are compilations of notes, thoughts, and feelings that can be used by the patient following discharge to fill in memory gaps, process difficult emotions, and reconstruct their illness narrative, particularly when reviewed with healthcare professionals in ICU follow-up programs. In multiple meta-analyses, ICU diaries have had variable impact on the development of depression, anxiety, and PTSD in both patients and their loved ones, but they are generally seen as a constructive tool for patients who are struggling to make meaning of their illness experience and for families struggling to cope with a loved one's critical illness (see Chapter 18 for additional information) [46,47].

In addition to providing ICU diaries, other strategies can be used to minimize the development of PICS-F, including the provision of psychological care to families (see Chapter 14 for additional information), spiritual care (see Chapter 15 for additional information), humanizing the ICU experience (see Chapter 16 for additional information), and practicing family-centered care. Components of family-centered care include flexible visitation policies and the promotion of family presence and engagement; educational programs and enhanced communication strategies between healthcare providers and loved ones; and family support through social work, palliative care, spiritual care, and psychology consultations (see Chapter 17 for additional information).

Section 3 of this book, entitled Strategies to Prevent PICS, further explores other potential modalities for preventing the development of or mitigating the severity of PICS, including the roles of spiritual therapy (see Chapter 15 for additional information), music therapy (see Chapter 19 for additional information), animal assisted therapy (see Chapter 20 for additional information), and fresh air therapy (see Chapter 21 for additional information).

Screening and Diagnosis

Guidelines

The UK NICE guidelines recommend that adults who required critical care for more than four days have a clinical evaluation within three months of hospital discharge [45]. Following publication of these guidelines, outpatient services for survivors of critical illness were present at 74% of sites in the UK, typically co-delivered by two or more healthcare professionals, including intensivists, nurses, and physiotherapists. Although post-discharge physical rehabilitation programs were present in only 17.6% of institutions, peer support services were available in nearly half [48]. Similarly, the French central health authority recommends that survivors of critical illness at high risk for PICS receive an evaluation conducted by an intensivist that includes a battery of screening instruments [49]. Despite the presence of these guidelines, however, only 28.6% of French ICUs offer the recommended follow-up visit, most commonly conducted three to six months following discharge. Of those ICUs not offering follow-up services, nearly half indicated an intention to start in the next year but cited a lack of available staff and equipment and not viewing PICS as a priority as barriers [50]. In Australia, only two ICU follow-up clinics have been implemented [51], while follow-up in Scandinavian countries ranged from 17% to 30%, with visits largely focused on the human experience of critical illness and understanding the past rather than looking toward the future [52].

Similarly, the SCCM International Consensus Conference on prediction and identification of long-term impairments after critical illness recommends serial and dynamic assessments of patients at heightened risk for PICS beginning within two and four weeks of hospital discharge and following important health and life changes, both anticipated and unanticipated [38]. Serial assessments establish a longitudinal framework to more effectively prepare survivors to reengage with employment and society, mitigate the sense of isolation and abandonment that often accompany survivorship, address patient needs in a timely manner, and prevent complications through a deliberate, coordinated, longitudinal approach to care [38]. In some ICU follow-up programs, serial assessments occur at specified time points (e.g., at 3 months, 6 months, and 12 months after discharge), and in others, assessments are variable and based on patients' rehabilitation needs or following setbacks, such as hospital readmission. In a scoping review of 754 studies of PICS evaluations, appointments were most commonly conducted at 3 months (25% of follow-ups), 12 months (21%), and 6 months (21%) [53].

ICU Follow-Up Clinics

Building a collaborative, multidisciplinary team to longitudinally follow and treat patients with PICS is often essential to support this medically fragile population. A holistic, coordinated, and personalized approach is important to manage the complex, interconnected impairments in physical, cognitive, and psychological health that survivors of critical illness face and may enhance recovery, quality of life, and patient satisfaction with their care (see Chapter 23 for additional information).

Such multidisciplinary teams are the therapeutic core of ICU follow-up clinics, which are the most comprehensive vehicle to support survivors of critical illness and their loved ones, screen them for PICS-related impairments, and provide treatment (see Chapter 28 for additional information). Despite the paucity of evidence demonstrating consistent clinical and financial benefit, ICU follow-up clinics are becoming increasingly popular, as multiple guidelines now suggest that survivors of critical illness receive a comprehensive assessment of PICS-related impairments soon after discharge [38,45,49]. ICU follow-up clinics vary widely with respect to the composition of the multidisciplinary team, patient recruitment strategies, timing and duration of follow-up, and approaches to screening for PICS. Although the vast majority of ICU follow-up clinics are led by intensivists, given that many primary care physicians and specialists lack sufficient knowledge and time to manage the complexities of this syndrome, close collaboration between intensivists, primary care physicians, and other providers is essential [9].

Telemedicine-based interventions, including ICU follow-up clinics, tele-rehabilitation, and tele-therapy, have promise in providing care to patients who are otherwise unable to overcome physical, logistical, and socioeconomic barriers to care (see Chapter 29 for additional information). Section 4 of this text, entitled General Principles of ICU Aftercare, further explores the history of, fundamentals of, and financial considerations for ICU follow-up clinics (see Chapters 27, 28, and 30, respectively) as well as other important aspects of caring for these patients, such as exploring social determinants of health (see Chapter 25 for additional information) and eliciting what matters most to patients and their families (see Chapter 26 for additional information).

Screening Tools and Approaches

The rapid growth in research publications regarding long-term outcomes in survivors of critical illness has made comparison and synthesis of the results particularly difficult, with one scoping review documenting the use of 250 unique instruments across 425 publications from 1970 to 2013 [54] and a second documenting the use of 107 instruments across 754 publications from 2014 to 2022 [55]. Having a core outcome measures set, defined as "a group of patient outcomes, health-related conditions, or aspects of healthcare that are essential to evaluate in all studies within a specific clinical field," could facilitate comparisons and meta-analyses, allowing clinicians and researchers to more easily and accurately answer questions of clinical importance [56]. Although a core outcome measures set does not yet exist for patients with PICS and may be premature given the dynamic state of evolving PICS research, a three-round modified Delphi consensus process generated one for survivors of acute respiratory failure. Among 75 measurement instruments that were evaluated, the following met criteria for inclusion in the core outcome measures set: EuroQol-5D-5L (EQ-5D) and SF-36 for the "satisfaction with life and personal enjoyment" and pain outcomes and both the HADS and the Impact of Events Scale-Revised (IES-R) for the mental health outcome. No measures reached consensus for the cognition, muscle and/ or nerve function, physical function, and pulmonary function outcomes [56].

Screening tools, or outcome measurement instruments, can be broadly divided into two categories: patient-reported outcome measures and performance-based outcome measures. Patient-reported outcome measures usually involve the completion of a questionnaire, during which patients *rate* their performance on a set of functional tasks, whereas performance-based outcome measures require the patient to *perform* a set of functional tasks, during which data is objectively collected and compared against control populations. Patient-reported measures identify the patient's *perceived* level of function, while performance-based measures determine an *objective* level of function. Patient-reported outcomes are generally convenient and easy to measure, and for that reason, are frequently preferred, but agreement between patient-reported outcome measures and performance-based outcome measures is often modest, highlighting the need for performance-based measures to complement patient-reported measures [57].

Of the numerous screening tools that can be administered in a clinic setting (see Chapter 29, Table 29.1 and Chapter 48, Table 48.2), the aforementioned SCCM International Consensus Conference recommends the following based on degree of consensus from the expert participants: the MoCA for assessment of cognitive impairment (strong consensus), the HADS for assessment of both anxiety and depression (strong consensus), the IES-R or the abbreviated IES-6 for assessment of PTSD (weak consensus), and the 6MWT and/or the EQ-5D-5L for assessment of physical impairment (weak consensus) [38]. A subsequent modified Delphi approach of 23 members of the Japanese Society of Intensive Care Medicine PICS committee reached consensus on a broader battery of 20 PICS assessment instruments, including: the 6MWT, MRC score, and grip strength dynamometry for assessment of the physical domain; the MoCA, MMSE, and SMQ for assessment of the cognitive domain; the HADS, IES-R, and the Patient Health Questionnaire-9 (PHQ-9) for assessment of the mental health domain; the Barthel Index, IADL screening tool, and Functional Independence Measure (FIM) for assessment of independence in ADLs; the SF-36, EQ-5D-5L, EQ-5D-3L, EQ-Visual Analog Scale (VAS), and SF-12 for assessment of quality of life; the Pittsburgh Sleep Quality Index (PSQI) for assessment of sleep; the Brief Pain Inventory for assessment of pain; and the SF-36, HADS, and IES-R for assessment of PICS-Family [58]. The authors included a broad range of instruments to circumvent concerns regarding the need for specific training, equipment, and cost, as well as the ability to administer screening tools over the telephone [58].

Using a combination of expert consensus and feasibility field testing, a German group proposed a two-step PICS screening process that involves a combination of patient-reported and performance-based outcome measures [59]. The first step of the screening process is brief (requiring approximately 20 minutes per patient), free, and easily administered by healthcare professionals without specialized training. It includes the Patient Health

Questionnaire-4 (PHQ-4), Mini Cog and animal naming, Timed Up-and-Go (TUG) and handgrip strength, and the EQ-5D-5L to assess mental health, cognition, physical health, and quality of life, respectively. Patients reporting new or worsening health problems or those with impairments identified during the initial screen then undergo a second, more comprehensive assessment administered by a specialized healthcare provider familiar with PICS, which requires between 85 and 110 minutes. This assessment includes: the Patient Health Questionnaire-8 (PHQ-8), Generalized Anxiety Disorder Scale-7 (GAD-7), and IES-R to assess mental health; the Repeatable Battery for the Assessment of Neuropsychological Status (RBANS) and the Trail Making Test (TMT) A and B to assess cognitive function; the 2-minute walk test (2MWT), handgrip strength, and Short Physical Performance Battery (SPPB) to assess physical function; and the EQ-5D-5L and the WHO Disability Assessment Schedule (WHODAS 2.0) to assess quality of life [59].

More detailed information regarding these and other screening tools can be found in Chapters 15 (spiritual concerns), 34 (quality of life), 35 (pulmonary disorders), 37 (sleep disorders), 38 (swallowing disorders), 40 (nutritional disorders), 41 (physical impairments), 42 (functional impairments), 43 (cognitive impairments), 46 (psychiatric impairments), and 48 (PICS-Family).

Functional Trajectories

The way in which patients recover from PICS is not uniform. Understanding how recovery unfolds over time and the factors that influence this recovery could inform the timing and intensity of therapeutic interventions and provide prognostic information about the likelihood, rate, and anticipated course of functional recovery [60]. Based on thoughtful analysis of existing clinical data, Iwashyna conceptually divided functional trajectories following critical illness into three pathways, one consistent with recovery and two that are more commonly associated with chronic illness (see Chapter 33, Figure 33.1). Understanding which pathway a patient is on may better inform how to care for them in the outpatient setting [61]. In the "Big Hit" trajectory, patients have an acute loss of function as a consequence of their critical illness but gradually recover over the course of months to years, occasionally to their pre-morbid level of function. When caring for these patients, efforts are made to limit the degree of disability, enhance the rapidity of the functional recovery, and minimize any residual deficit they might sustain. In the "Slow Burn" trajectory, patients fail to completely recover from critical illness and instead follow a path of persistent, more rapid decline. When caring for these patients, the goal is to minimize the pace and depth of this decline. In the "Relapsing Recurring" trajectory, patients have multiple acute exacerbations with varying degrees of partial recovery in between (e.g., repeated hospital admissions). When caring for these patients, the goal is to maximize the interval between exacerbations, shorten their duration, or prevent them altogether [61].

More formal analyses generally align with this conceptual framework with some modest variations. Gandotra and colleagues studied physical function in 260 survivors of acute respiratory failure at hospital discharge and two, four, and six months thereafter using the SPPB, a composite assessment of balance, gait speed, and lower extremity strength that is predictive of disability, hospitalization, institutionalization, and mortality in older patients [62]. Four distinct recovery trajectories emerged, distinguished by both the degree and rate of physical function recovery. Group 1 included patients discharged with physical function disability who showed no improvement over six months, while Group 2 showed minimal improvement and remained functionally disabled at six months. Group 3 had low physical function at discharge and improved to intermediate physical function, while Group 4 had intermediate physical function at discharge with rapid improvement to normal function at two months, which was sustained at six months. Group 4 consisted primarily of younger women with shorter ICU lengths of stay, while Group 1 consisted primarily of older patients with more exposure to sedating medications and longer ICU lengths of stay. The greatest change in physical function occurred during the first two months following discharge, highlighting the importance of expedited outpatient evaluation and initiation of rehabilitative therapies [62].

A multicenter Canadian cohort study showed that functional status seven days after ICU discharge, as measured by the FIM, determined four disability outcome trajectories based on patient age and ICU length of stay in a diverse sample of critically ill patients who were mechanically ventilated for more than two weeks [63]. Trajectories, which were independent of the presenting diagnosis and illness severity, predicted discharge disposition, need for hospital and ICU readmission, and mortality at one year of follow-up. Patients less than 42 years of age with ICU lengths of stay less than two weeks had the best functional status and lowest mortality at one year compared with patients older than 66 years of age with ICU lengths of stay greater than two weeks, who experienced the worst disability and highest mortality. Each additional decade of age and each additional week in the ICU beyond two weeks were independently associated with increased multidimensional disability and mortality at one year [8,63].

Importantly, the potential for recovery following critical illness is not only impacted by age, sex, ICU length of stay, and severity of illness but also by the patient's degree of disability prior to critical illness. In a prospective cohort study of 754 community-dwelling persons older than 70, one quarter of patients with minimal pre-ICU disability became severely disabled or died within 30 days after critical illness. Of those with mild to moderate pre-ICU disability, 39.5% became severely disabled, and more than one-quarter died. Of those with severe pre-ICU disability, one third experienced early death, and the rest remained severely disabled. Overall, 53.4% of the sample experienced functional decline or early death after critical illness, and patients with mild to moderate or severe disability prior to critical illness had more than double and triple the risk of death within one year of ICU admission, respectively [64].

Treatment

To date, there is contradictory literature on the efficacy of ICU follow-up and rehabilitation programs. Patient heterogeneity and differences with respect to pre-ICU health status and post-ICU recovery trajectories are significant challenges to the development and testing of these programs, in that results may be more profoundly influenced by patients' baseline health and nutritional status than the nature of the follow-up or rehabilitative interventions [8]. Furthermore, existing studies have risk of bias from incomplete reporting, loss to follow-up, and lack of standardization in the instruments used to measure outcomes [6]. A systematic review of 36 studies evaluated the effectiveness of six categories of nonpharmacological interventions for improving long-term outcomes following critical illness, including early mobilization and physical rehabilitation, post-ICU follow-up, psychosocial programs, ICU diaries, informational and educational activities, and "other" interventions; only 31% of these studies included interventions following hospital discharge. Although many outcomes favored the interventions, significant differences were only found for ICU diaries in reducing depression and anxiety and exercise programs in improving the mental health component score on the SF-36 [65].

A second systematic review of nonrandomized studies of ICU follow-up interventions similarly found variable and inconsistent benefits in survival; functional status; symptoms of anxiety, depression, and PTSD; and patient and family satisfaction [66]. In a companion meta-analysis of randomized controlled trials of ICU follow-up models focusing on psychological interventions, no significant differences were appreciated in symptoms of anxiety and depression, but symptoms of PTSD were improved in the three-to-six-month period of follow-up [66].

Specific interventions to improve impaired physical function have had variable efficacy, and randomized controlled trials of both intensive inpatient and outpatient physical therapy interventions and multidisciplinary approaches seeking to increase physical function have failed to consistently improve long-term physical function [60], although some have resulted in improvements in symptoms of depression and mental health-related quality of life [66]. Because patients respond differently to physical therapy, a single prescriptive approach for all patients may be ineffective and a principal reason that trials to date have failed to consistently demonstrate benefit in improving functional recovery. A targeted rehabilitation approach directed at specific subgroups based on patient-specific predictors may be a superior approach [60].

In an effort to develop a multidisciplinary and professional guideline for rehabilitative therapy in survivors of critical illness, 15 healthcare professionals applied a structured, evidence-based approach to address questions related to the management of PICS. Recommendations with the strongest evidence were in the domain of rehabilitation of psychological health and included the following: (1) critically ill patients with depression and anxiety benefit from psychological interventions, which should begin in the ICU and continue through early rehabilitation, (2) access to professional support and aftercare should be offered in the first twelve months after discharge, (3) post-traumatic stress reactions should be treated by interventions such as psychoeducation and psychotherapy, and (4) ICU diaries, if available, should be read and processed with healthcare professionals [10]. Additionally, although not addressed in this study, peer support has long been utilized by patients with various chronic diseases to help meet their complex recovery needs, and despite a lack of definitive evidence, there is little reason to doubt that the same is true for survivors of critical illness who participate in peer support groups. There is no "one-size-fits-all" approach to developing peer support groups for survivors of critical illness; variety and flexibility promote adaptation across a wide range of settings and help meet individual participant needs. Peer support can improve psychological empowerment, self-advocacy, social support, and shared coping while reducing feelings of loneliness and depression (see Chapter 49 for additional information) [67].

The design and evaluation of non-pharmacological interventions to treat manifestations of PICS is at an early stage and requires further investigation to improve our understanding of potential efficacy [6]. High-quality randomized controlled trials designed to evaluate complex interventions and powered to detect clinically meaningful differences in relevant outcomes are essential to elucidate the efficacy of these types of intervention and ultimately guide clinical practice. It is important to develop follow-up models and interventions based on individual risk factors for long-term disabilities rather than models directed to a general cohort of subjects, given that the heterogeneity of the general ICU population may mitigate the potential benefits of ICU follow-up interventions [66].

Section 5 of this text, entitled Diagnosis and Management of PICS, further explores specific treatment modalities for patients with PICS, including physical therapy (see Chapter 41 for additional information), occupational therapy (see Chapter 42 for additional information), cognitive therapy (see Chapter 43 for additional information), and psychotherapy (see Chapter 46 for additional information). Additional chapters in this section address management of pulmonary disorders (see Chapter 35 for additional information), common somatic complaints (see Chapter 36 for additional information), sleep disorders (see Chapter 37 for additional information), dysphagia (see Chapter 38 for additional information), laryngeal disorders (see Chapter 39 for additional information), and malnutrition (see Chapter 40 for additional information), as well as rehabilitation specifically addressed at resuming employment and driving (see Chapter 44 for additional information).

Conclusion

Observations of the durable and diverse complications following critical illness are robust, yet dissemination of this knowledge has been limited, even within the field of critical care medicine [8]. Moreover, despite the flurry of research that began in the late 1990s and accelerated with the publication of the definition of PICS in 2012, tools to prevent, predict risk for, screen for, diagnose, and treat PICS remain in their infancy. The continuum of critical illness lends itself to a complementary continuum of tailored care that is focused on longitudinal follow-up and individualized rehabilitation plans based on patient values, preferences, and goals. Intensivists cannot handle this responsibility alone, necessitating a focus on educational engagement with colleagues, including trainees, interprofessional team members, outpatient therapy providers, and primary care physicians, as well as the lay public. As eloquently stated by Herridge and Azoulay, divorcing ourselves from the historic compartmentalization of critical illness into pre- and post-ICU care and adopting a multi-year timeline as the standard for assessing the consequences of critical care provide opportunities for continuity of care, education, advocacy, and accountability for critically ill patients, their caregivers, and our healthcare system [8].

Key Points

1. Because of advances in technology and the provision of critical care, an increasing number of patients are surviving critical illness; this growing population of survivors of critical illness is characterized by heightened vulnerability to a host of adverse health outcomes and by the development of multidimensional impairments that significantly impact their quality of life and societal participation.
2. PICS is defined as new or worsening impairments in physical, cognitive, or mental health status arising after a critical illness and persisting beyond acute care hospitalization. PICS-F describes the psychological and social impairments that family members, loved ones, and caregivers can develop as a consequence of their loved one's critical illness.

3. Survivors of critical illness are a heterogeneous patient population, and considerable variation exists with respect to the breadth, depth, duration, and mutability of their symptoms and impairments. The burden of survivorship is both complex and unique to each individual, preventing a "one-size-fits-all" approach to caring for these patients.
4. Given the marked heterogeneity in screening tests for PICS and criteria for its diagnosis, it is difficult to synthesize the growing literature on incidence and prevalence, co-occurrence of impairments, severity, duration, and prediction tools. Various guidelines exist regarding approaches to screening patients for PICS impairments, but a core outcome measures set for clinical research does not yet exist.
5. Many risk factors for the development of PICS impairments have been described, and studies describing interventions to either prevent or treat PICS have failed to show consistent benefit, although the literature is limited by significant variability regarding patient population and timing, duration, and success of employing the interventions being tested. Referrals to physical, occupational, cognitive, and psychological therapies and participation in support groups are the current mainstays of treatment, often delivered through participation in an ICU follow-up clinic.

References

1. The Society of Critical Care Medicine. https://sccm.org/communications/critical-care-statistics. Accessed February 1, 2025.
2. E.M. Viglianti, T.J. Iwashyna. Toward the ideal ratio of patients to intensivists: finding a reasonable balance. *JAMA Intern Med* 2017; **177**(3): 396–8.
3. D.C. Angus, J. Carlet. Surviving intensive care: a report from the 2002 Brussels Roundtable. *Intensive Care Med* 2003; **29**(3): 368–77.
4. T.J. Iwashyna. Survivorship will be the defining challenge of critical care in the 21st century. *Ann Intern Med* 2010; **153**: 204–5.
5. D.M. Needham, J. Davidson, H. Cohen, et al. Improving long-term outcomes after discharge from intensive care unit: report from a stakeholders' conference. *Crit Care Med* 2012; **40**(2): 502–9.
6. S.L. Hiser, A. Fatima, M. Ali, D. Needham. Post-intensive care syndrome (PICS): recent updates. *J Intensive Care* 2023; **11**: 23.
7. L.M. Cagino, K.S. Seagly, J.I. McSparron. Survivorship after critical illness and post-intensive care syndrome. *Clin Chest Med* 2022; **43**: 551–61.
8. M.S. Herridge, E. Azoulay. Outcomes after critical illness. *N Engl J Med* 2023; **388**(10): 913–24.
9. A.-F. Rousseau, H.C. Prescott, S.J. Brett, et al. Long-term outcomes after critical illness: recent insights. *Crit Care* 2021; **25**: 108.
10. C. Renner, M-M Jeitziner, M. Albert, et al. Guideline on multimodal rehabilitation for patients with post-intensive care syndrome. *Crit Care* 2023; **27**: 301.
11. S. Govindan, T.J. Iwashyna, S.R. Watson, et al. Issues of survivorship are rarely addressed during intensive care unit stays: baseline result from a statewide quality improvement collaborative. *Ann Am Thorac Soc* 2014; **11**(4); 587–91.
12. C.E. Cox, T. Martinu, S.J. Sathy, et al. Expectations and outcomes of prolonged mechanical ventilation. *Crit Care Med* 2009; **37**(11): 2888–94.
13. D.B. White, N. Ernecoff, P. Buddadhumaruk, et al. Prevalence of and factors related to discordance about prognosis between physicians and surrogate decision makers of critically ill patients. *JAMA* 2016; **315**(19): 2086–94.

14. N.E. Brummel. Measuring outcomes after critical illness. *Crit Care Clin* 2018; **34**: 515–26.
15. L.M. Verbrugge, A.M. Jette. The disablement process. *Soc Sci Med* 1994; **38**: 1–14.
16. M. Leonardi, J. Bickenbach, T.B. Ustun, et al. The definition of disability: what is in a name? *Lancet* 2006; **368**(9543): 1219–21.
17. S.Z. Nagi. A study in the evaluation of disability and rehabilitation potential: concepts, methods, and procedures. *Am J Public Health Nations* Health 1964; **54**: 1568–79.
18. D. Kawakami, S. Fujitani, T. Morimoto, et al. Prevalence of post-intensive care syndrome among Japanese intensive care unit patients: a prospective, multicenter, observational, J-PICS study. *Crit Care* 2021; **25**: 69.
19. W.W. Geense, M. Zegers, M.A.A. Peters, et al. New physical, mental, and cognitive problems 1 year after ICU admission: a prospective multicenter study. *Am J Resp Crit Care Med* 2021; **203**(12): 1512–21.
20. R.P. Kosilek, K. Schmidt, S.E. Baumeister, et al. Frequency and risk factors of post-intensive care syndrome components in a multicenter randomized controlled trial of German sepsis survivors. *J Crit Care* 2021; **65**: 268–73.
21. A. Marra, P.P. Pandharipande, T.D. Girard, et al. Co-occurrence of post-intensive care syndrome problems among 406 survivors of critical illness. *Crit Care Med* 2018; **46**: 1393–401.
22. S.M. Brown, E.L. Wilson, A.P. Presson, et al. Understanding patient outcomes after acute respiratory distress syndrome: identifying subtypes of physical, cognitive, and mental health outcomes. *Thorax* 2017; **72**(12): 1094–103.
23. M.S. Herridge, C.M. Tansey, A. Matte, et al. Functional disability 5 years after acute respiratory distress syndrome. *N Engl J Med* 2011; **364**: 1293–304.
24. S.M. Parry, S.R. Nalamalapu, K. Nunna, et al. Six-minute walk discharge after critical illness: a systematic review and meta-analysis. *J Intensive Care Med* 2021: **36**(3): 343–51.
25. G. Hermans, N. Van Aerde, P. Meersseman, et al. Five-year mortality and morbidity impact of prolonged versus brief ICU stay: a propensity score matched cohort study. *Thorax* 2019; **74**(11): 1037–45.
26. N. Van Aerde, P. Meersseman, Y. Debaveye, et al. Five-year impact of ICU-acquired neuromuscular complications: a prospective, observational study. *Intensive Care Med* 2020; **46**: 1184–93.
27. K. Honarmand, R.S. Lalli, F. Priestap, et al. Natural history of cognitive impairment in critical illness survivors: a systematic review. *Am J Respir Crit Care Med* 2020; **202**(2): 193–201.
28. T.J. Iwashyna, E.W. Ely, D.M. Smith, et al. Long-term cognitive impairment and functional disability among survivors of severe sepsis. *JAMA* 2010; **304**: 1787–94.
29. O.J. Bienvenue, L.A. Friedman, E. Colantuoni, et al. Psychiatric symptoms after acute respiratory distress syndrome: a 5-year longitudinal study. *Intensive Care Med* 2017; **44**(1): 38–47.
30. A. Rabiee, S. Nikayin, M.D. Hashem, et al. Depressive symptoms after critical illness: a systematic review and meta-analysis. *Crit Care Med* 2016; **44**(9): 1744–53.
31. S. Nikayin, A. Rabiee, M.D. Hashem, et al. Anxiety symptoms in survivors of critical illness: a systematic review and meta-analysis. *Gen Hosp Psychiatry* 2016; **43**: 23–9.
32. A.M. Parker, T. Sricharoenchai, S. Raparla, et al. Posttraumatic stress disorder in critical illness survivors: a meta-analysis. *Crit Care Med* 2015; **43**(5): 1121–9.
33. M.A. Narváez-Martinez, A.M. Henao-Castaño. Severity classification and influencing variables of the postintensive care syndrome. *Enferm Intensiva* 2024; **35**(2): 89–96.
34. K.J. Haines, E. Hibbert, J. McPeake, et al. Prediction models for physical, cognitive, and mental health impairments after

critical illness: a systematic review and critical appraisal. *Crit Care Med* 2020; **48** (12): 1871–80.

35. A. Milton, A. Schandl, I.W. Soliman, et al. Development of an ICU discharge instrument predicting psychological morbidity: a multinational study. *Intensive Care Med* 2018; **44**: 2038–47.

36. M.E. Detsky, M.O. Harhay, D.F. Bayard, et al. Six-month morbidity and mortality among intensive care unit patients receiving life-sustaining therapy: a prospective cohort study. *Ann Am Thorac Soc* 2017; **14**: 1562–70.

37. A. Schandl, M. Bottai, U. Holdar, et al. Early prediction of new-onset physical disability after intensive care unit stay: a preliminary instrument. *Crit Care* 2014; **18**: 455.

38. M.E. Mikkelsen, M. Still, B.J. Anderson, et al. Society of Critical Care Medicine's International Consensus Conference on prediction and identification of long-term impairments after critical illness. *Crit Care Med* 2020; **48**(11): 1670–9.

39. M. Lee, J. Kang, Y.J. Jeong. Risk factors for post–intensive care syndrome: a systematic review and meta-analysis. *Aust Crit Care* 2020; **33**: 287–94.

40. B.T. Pun, M.C. Balas, M.A. Barnes-Daly, et al. Caring for critically ill patients with the ABCDEF bundle: results of the ICU Liberation Collaborative in over 15,000 adults. *Crit Care Med* 2019; **47**(1): 3–14.

41. J.W. Devlin, Y. Skrobik, C. Gelinas, et al. Clinical practice guidelines for the prevention and management of pain, agitation/sedation, delirium, immobility, and sleep disruption in adult patients in the ICU. *Crit Care Med* 2018; **46**: e825–e73.

42. C.J. Tipping, M. Harrold, A. Holland, et al. The effects of active mobilisation and rehabilitation in ICU on mortality and function: a systematic review. *Intensive Care Med* 2017; **43**: 171–83.

43. R. Fuke, T. Hifumi, Y. Kondo, et al. Early rehabilitation to prevent postintensive care syndrome in patients with critical illness: a systematic review and meta-analysis. *BMJ Open* 2018; **8**: e019998.

44. W.D. Schweickert, M.C. Pohlman, A.S. Pohlman, et al. Early physical and occupational therapy in mechanically ventilated, critically ill patients: a randomised controlled trial. *Lancet* 2009; **373**(9678): 1874–82.

45. National Institute for Health and Care Excellence (NICE). 2018 surveillance of rehabilitation after critical illness in adults (NICE guideline CG83). www.nice.org.uk/guidance/cg83. Accessed: December 6, 2024.

46. P.A. McIlroy, R.S. King, M. Garrouste-Orgeas, et al. The effect of ICU diaries on psychological outcomes and quality of life of survivors of critical illness and their relatives: a systematic review and meta-analysis. *Crit Care Med* 2019; **47**(2): 273–9.

47. X. Sun, D. Huang, F. Zeng, et al. Effect of intensive care unit diary on incidence of posttraumatic stress disorder, anxiety, and depression of adult intensive care unit survivors: a systematic review and meta-analysis. *J. Adv Nurs* 2021; **77**(7): 2929–41.

48. B. Connolly, R. Milton-Cole, C. Adams, et al. Recovery, rehabilitation, and follow-up services following critical illness: an updated UK national cross-sectional survey and progress report. *BMJ Open* 2021; **11**(10): e052214.

49. Diagnostic et prise en charge des patients adultes avec un syndrome post-réanimation (PICS) et de leur entourage – Haute Autorité de Santé – Juin 2023. www.has-sante.fr/jcms/p_3312530. Accessed: February 6, 2025.

50. M. Agbakou, M. Combet, M. Martin, et al. Post-intensive care syndrome screening: a French multicentre study. *Ann Intensive Care* 2024; **14**: 109.

51. K. Cook, R. Bartholdy, M. Raven, et al. A national survey of intensive care follow-up clinics in Australia. *Aust Crit Care* 2020; **33**(6): 533–7.

52. I. Egerod, S.S. Risom, T. Thomsen, et al. ICU-recovery in Scandinavia: A comparative study if intensive care follow-up in Denmark, Norway, and Sweden. *Intensive Crit Care Nurs* 2013; **29**(2): 103–11.

53. N. Nakanishi, K. Liu, A. Kawauchi, et al. Instruments to assess post-intensive care syndrome assessment: a scoping review and modified Delphi method study. *Crit Care* 2023; **27**: 430.

54. A.E. Turnbull, A. Rabiee, W.E. Davis, et al. Outcome measurement in ICU survivorship research from 1970 to 2013: a scoping review of 425 publications. *Crit Care Med* 2016; **44**: 1267–77.

55. N. Nakanishi, K. Liu, A. Kawauchi, et al. Instruments to assess post-intensive care syndrome assessment: a scoping review and modified Delphi method study. *Crit Care* 2023; **27**: 430.

56. D.M. Needham, K.A. Sepulveda, V.D. Dinglas, et al. Core outcome measures for clinical research in acute respiratory failure survivors. *Am J Resp Crit Care Med* 2017; **196**(6): 1122–30.

57. L.M. Shulman, I. Pretzer-Aboff, K.E. Anderson, et al. Subjective report versus objective measurement of activities of daily living in Parkinson's disease. *Mov Disord* 2006; **21**(6): 794–9.

58. N. Nakanishi, K. Liu, A. Kawauchi, et al. Instruments to assess post-intensive care syndrome assessment: a scoping review and modified Delphi method study. *Crit Care* 2023; **27**: 430.

59. C.D. Spies, H. Krampe, N. Paul, et al. Instruments to measure outcomes of post-intensive care syndrome in outpatient care settings: results of an expert consensus and feasibility field test. *J Intensive Care Soc* 2021; **22**(2): 159–74.

60. A. Neumeier, A. Nordon-Craft, D. Malone, et al. Prolonged acute care and post-acute care admission and recovery of physical function in survivors of acute respiratory failure: a secondary analysis of a randomized controlled trial. *Crit Care* 2017; **21**: 190.

61. T.J. Iwashyna. Trajectories of recovery and dysfunction after acute illness, with implications for clinical trial design. *Am J Respir Crit Care Med* 2012; **186**(4): 302–4.

62. S. Gandotra, J. Lovato, D. Case, et al. Physical function trajectories in survivors of acute respiratory failure. *Ann Am Thorac Soc* 2019; **16**(4): 471–7.

63. M.S. Herridge, L.M. Chu, A. Matte, et al. The RECOVER program: disability risk groups and 1-year outcomes after 7 or more days of mechanical ventilation. *Am J Resp Crit Care Med* 2016; **194**(7): 831–44.

64. L.E. Ferrante, M. Pisani, T.E. Murphy, et al. Functional trajectories among older persons before and after critical illness. *JAMA Int Med* 2015; **175**(4): 523–9.

65. W.W. Geense, M. van den Boogaard, J. can der Hoeven, et al. Nonpharmacologic interventions to prevent or mitigate adverse long-term outcomes among ICU survivors: a systematic review and meta-analysis. *Crit Care Med* 2019; **47**(11): 1607–18.

66. R.G. Rosa, G.E. Ferreira, T.W. Viola, et al. Effects of post-ICU follow-up on subject outcomes: a systematic review and meta-analysis. *J Crit Care* 2019; **52**: 115–25.

67. J. McPeake, T.J. Iwashyna, L.M. Boehm, et al. Benefits of peer support for intensive care unit survivors: sharing experiences, care debriefing, and altruism. *Am J Crit Care* 2021; **30**(2): 145–9.

Chapter 3
The Pathophysiology of PICS

Samantha Bottom-Tanzer, Sarah Kader, and Eric J. Mahoney

Introduction

To provide a comprehensive overview of the pathophysiologic underpinnings of post-intensive care syndrome (PICS), we present a pathophysiological pathway that includes a disordered inflammatory response and an exaggerated genomic response. We explore how these perturbations interact deleteriously with organ systems by addressing inflammation and immunosuppression, genomic storm, transcriptomic perturbations, and disruptions in the gut microbiome. Key terms related to the pathophysiology of PICS are defined in Table 3.1.

Immunologic Perturbation: Simultaneous Inflammation and Immunosuppression

A pathophysiological model that provides a mechanistic rationale for PICS and chronic critical illness (CCI) is the persistent inflammation, immunosuppression, and catabolism syndrome (PIICS). This paradigm incorporates two concepts, the systemic inflammatory response syndrome (SIRS) and the compensatory anti-inflammatory response syndrome (CARS), which describe the simultaneous occurrence of inflammation and immunosuppression in critically ill patients [1]. This leads to a maladaptive cycle of organ injury mediated via the release of immune-activating proteins, which perpetuate inflammation and muscle wasting, culminating in CCI [2] Moreover, PIICS describes the critical illness-induced immune system deficiencies that predispose patients to additional infectious complications (see Figure 3.1) [3].

Inflammation

Acutely following illness or injury, inflammatory mediators, such as cytokines, chemokines, damage-associated molecular patterns (DAMPs), and alarmins, are released, which act to either induce or inhibit inflammation. Studies have found that increased levels of pro-inflammatory cytokines and chemokines are associated with increased mortality and functional impairments following a prolonged intensive care unit (ICU) stay. In their study of inflammatory biomarkers in critically ill patients during the first 14 days of sepsis, Darden and colleagues found that survivors fell into two broad cohorts: those who recovered rapidly and those who experienced CCI [4]. Patients who developed CCI had more elevated biomarkers of both inflammation and immunosuppression than those who recovered, which was associated with a clinical phenotype of worsened functional outcomes at both 3 and 12 months.

Table 3.1 Definitions of key syndromes related to PICS

Syndrome	Description
Sepsis	Life-threatening organ dysfunction caused by a dysregulated host response to infection [68]. Delano and Ward described how "sepsis ... alters the innate and adaptive immune response for sustained periods of time after [apparent] clinical recovery" through impaired immunity and inflammation [69].
Chronic critical illness (CCI)	A subacute disease state requiring high intensity of care for a protracted period of time, characterized by lengthy hospital stays, intense suffering, persistent organ dysfunction, high mortality rates, and substantial resource consumption [70].
Persistent inflammation, immunosuppression, and catabolism syndrome (PIICS)	The sequelae of immune perturbation that frequently occur after critical illness leading to a vicious cycle of organ failure and nosocomial infections and eventually manifesting as the PICS phenotype [3]. The underlying pathobiology that drives PIICS and CCI occurs in a maladaptive self-perpetuating cycle in which organ injury results in the release of alarmins, which promote ongoing inflammation, muscle wasting, and further progression of CCI [2]. It is associated with a prolonged stay in the ICU and is characterized by malnutrition, protein catabolism, impaired wound healing, immunosuppression (with defective innate and adaptive immunity), and recurrent infections [1].
Post-intensive care syndrome (PICS)	New or worsening impairments in physical, cognitive, or psychological domains originating after critical illness and persisting beyond acute care hospitalization [71]. These impairments negatively affect quality of life and function in long-term survivors of critical illness [72].
ICU-acquired weakness (ICU-AW)	The loss of both muscle mass and function due to combined myopathy and polyneuropathy.

In a study of patients with abdominal sepsis, Cox and colleagues found more secondary infections and organ failures in patients who later developed CCI [5]. These patients had persistently elevated biomarkers of dysregulated immunity and metabolism 14 days after sepsis; poorer functional status at 3, 6, and 12 months; and increased 30-day and 1-year mortality compared to those who had rapid improvement, consistent with the subsequent development of PICS. Cox and colleagues proposed a "genomic or cytokine storm" at the time of illness onset as a driving factor in the subsequent development of CCI [2]. Persistent inflammation, demonstrated by elevated plasma cytokine levels, and increased immunosuppression proteins, including soluble programmed death ligand 1 (sPD-L1) and interleukin-10 (IL-10), have been found in survivors of sepsis who developed CCI [6]. Among inflammatory mediators, C-reactive protein (CRP) and matrix metalloproteinase-9 (MMP-9) are the most strongly associated with impaired mobility and inability to perform activities of daily living [7,8]. Of note, there are currently no direct causal links between individual cytokines and the development of PICS.

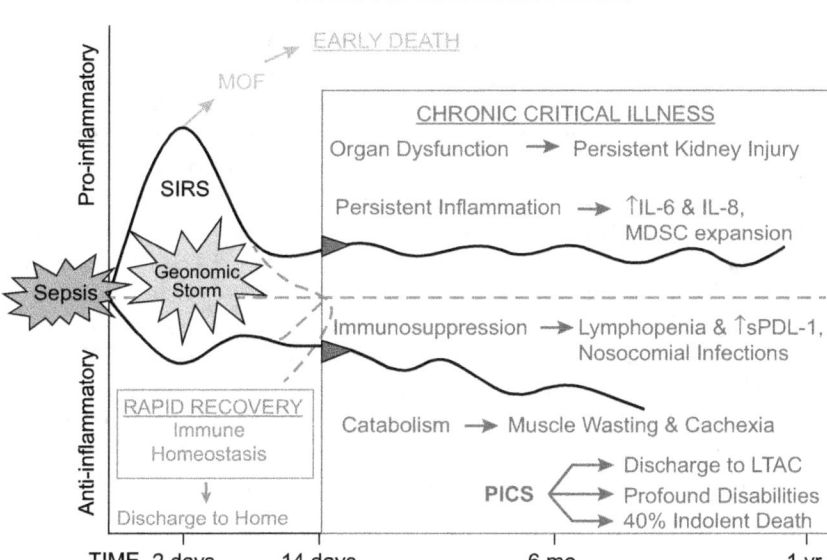

Figure 3.1 The inflammatory response is an underlying mechanism for PICS. From: R.B. Hawkins, S.L. Raymond, J.A. Stortz, et al. Chronic critical illness and the persistent inflammation, immunosuppression, and catabolism syndrome. *Front Immunol* 2018; **9**: 1511. Reproduced with permission from Frontiers under the CC-BY Creative Commons attribution license.

Inflammation and Cognition

The relationship between inflammation and the cognitive and psychological domains of PICS requires specific consideration [9]. First, many patients with PICS initially present with the acute respiratory distress syndrome (ARDS), and approximately 30% of patients with ARDS have cognitive impairment one year after discharge. Preclinical, observational, and case series suggest that ARDS induces, or is highly associated with, neuroinflammation. Lung injury and alveolar stretching elicit the release of inflammatory mediators that can severely damage neurons and disrupt the blood–brain barrier (BBB). ARDS also increases S100 calcium-binding protein B, a marker of both focal and global brain injury [10,11,12]. Second, sepsis induces both pro- and anti-inflammatory mediators that impair neurotransmission by altering neurotransmitter concentration and receptor expression in neurons and resident immune cells. Reduced recycling of the excitatory neurotransmitter glutamate combined with additional glutamate release from resident neuroinflammatory cells leads to excitotoxicity, which is associated with epilepsy [13]. These findings suggest that sepsis and its associated systemic inflammation can induce central nervous system (CNS) injury [9].

Approximately 40% of sepsis patients develop delirium, which is associated with impaired long-term cognitive function and psychiatric symptoms (see Chapters 8 and 43 for additional information) [14,15,16]; importantly, the duration of delirium directly correlates with worsened global cognitive and executive function at 3 and 12 months following hospital discharge [17]. This temporal relationship between delirium and cognitive impairment has a neuroanatomical basis, with longer durations of delirium associated with reduced brain volume and increased white matter abnormalities three months after discharge [18,19], implicating delirium-associated brain atrophy as a putative mechanism in the development of long-term cognitive impairment. White matter disruption in the internal capsule and the corpus callosum in survivors of critical illness is associated with poor cognitive outcomes and working memory impairment [19,20]. Another study demonstrated that 64% of critically ill patients with neurological changes had abnormalities on neuroimaging, nearly half of whom developed long-term cognitive impairment [21].

Cognitive impairment may be associated with BBB dysfunction and direct neuronal damage, indicated by elevated neuro-specific biomarkers, including S100B, neuron-specific enolase, and phosphorylated neurofilament heavy subunit [9,22,23]. Pro-inflammatory cytokines enter the brain through receptor-mediated endocytosis independent of direct CNS damage [24]. Microglia are activated and produce additional inflammatory cytokines and reactive oxygen species, leading to direct brain injury and increased BBB permeability, which, in turn, causes vasogenic edema and white matter abnormalities. Moreover, circulating cytokines directly affect endothelial function, which is directly correlated with delirium duration [9,25]. Sepsis-induced vascular endothelial dysfunction and impaired cerebral blood flow are common in septic shock and lead to cerebral hypoxia, ischemia, and white matter changes.

Immunosuppression

As previously noted, patients with CCI have sustained increases in anti-inflammatory mediators [4]. Prolonged decreases in monocyte human leukocyte antigen-DR (mHLA-DR), an innate immune marker of immunosuppression, is associated with more ICU-acquired infections, while faster recovery of mHLA-DR after ICU admission predicts survival in patients with septic shock [26]. In a separate study, markers of immunosuppression were measured in patients with rapid recovery from sepsis and in patients who developed sepsis-induced CCI; although the concentrations of biomarkers were similar between the two groups initially, patients who developed CCI had prolonged immunosuppression compared to those who had rapid recovery [27]. These studies suggest that an initial phenotype of immunosuppression is common among ICU patients, but it is the trajectory of these biomarkers in the following weeks that is predictive of both short- and long-term outcomes.

Several caveats are important. While a subacute inflammatory profile appears to be strongly associated with mortality and worsened long-term outcomes, this finding is not universal [28]. Moreover, other conditions present in critically ill patients may have impacts beyond inflammation and immunosuppression alone; for example, while mechanical ventilation increases circulating cytokines, it also independently increases the risk of developing hypoxic brain injury and its attendant long-term cognitive and psychological impairments [10]. Finally, measurement of inflammatory markers at a single time point is not predictive of outcomes; rather, multiple measurements are necessary to delineate a patient's risk for CCI [4].

Genomic Storm and Transcriptomic Alterations Contribute to Disease Severity

Transcriptomic analysis allows for assessment of aberrant gene expression in a variety of tissues at numerous time points, providing insight into the molecular underpinnings of acute and chronic deficits consistent with PICS. One of the first transcriptomic studies performed found that severe trauma caused a massive shift in the leukocyte transcriptome, with altered expression of nearly 80% of genes. The genes most upregulated were involved in the inflammatory response and innate immune system, while the genes most suppressed dealt with T-cell activation, reinforcing theories suggesting immunologic perturbation after traumatic injury [29].

Analysis of transcriptomic changes suggests common mechanisms across many types of traumas. Genomic changes early after admission were remarkably similar between severe blunt trauma and burn injury patients; however, when blunt trauma and burn injury patients were grouped by complicated versus uncomplicated hospital courses, the degree of gene expression was remarkably different despite the fact that similar genes had been altered. The magnitude of change in gene expression and the time required for gene expression to return to baseline were most closely associated with illness severity, irrespective of the original mechanism of trauma [29].

Transcriptomic perturbation may also contribute to several risk factors for the development of PICS. For example, ICU-acquired weakness (ICU-AW), which often complicates critical illness and increases the risk for developing physical impairments associated with PICS (see Chapter 4 for additional information), is characterized by a distinct expression signature, particularly notable for the upregulation of extracellular matrix genes. This dysregulation was correlated with collagen deposition in muscle, leading to reduced muscle strength clinically [30].

Transcriptomic analyses from multiple studies show common patterns of perturbation in gene expression, particularly related to the inflammatory response, which accurately predict which patients develop ICU-related complications, including infection and severe sepsis. High-risk patients had markers of immunosuppression, again linking genomic data to the inflammatory domain [31,32]. Not only do these gene expression data suggest clear etiologies of ICU-related complications, but they may also allow for early prediction of heightened risk of PICS and ultimately lead to improvements in the ICU course and long-term outcomes.

Disruption to Microvasculature

The association between severe sepsis, microvascular dysfunction, and increased mortality was first described in 2005 [33]. Since then, sepsis and its associated inflammatory cytokine milieu have been demonstrated to disrupt the barrier function of endothelial cells [34] by directly affecting endothelial expression of adhesion molecules, signaling pathways, and nitric oxide production [25,35]. Endothelium is activated by multiple mediators, including lipopolysaccharide (LPS), pro-inflammatory cytokines, pathogen-associated molecular patterns (PAMPs), and DAMPs [39], leading to impaired release of nitric oxide, which, in turn, increases vasoconstriction, further secretion of Pro-inflammatory mediators, and thrombotic risk. This endothelial dysfunction persists even beyond the successful resuscitation phase [36]. Persistence of these microcirculatory alterations is associated with incident organ failure and worsened mortality in patients with septic shock [37].

Additionally, there has been considerable research describing endothelial dysfunction in the context of vascular aging. While developed in parallel, it appears that many of the features of both PIICS and PICS are similar to the concept of "inflamm-ageing," referring to the "low-grade and chronic inflammation that progressively increases with age" [38]. Key characteristics include chronic activation of the innate immune system; persistently elevated pro-inflammatory mediators; progressive loss of immunologic function; and predisposition to infection, cellular senescence, and mitochondrial dysfunction.

Microvascular disruption can also contribute to ICU-AW. Critical illness-induced pathological interactions between the endothelium and myocytes lead to impaired muscle regeneration, satellite cell dysfunction, and ineffective nutrient, metabolite, and oxygen transfer. Subsequent mismatches in oxygen supply and demand cause further dysfunction, including damaged lung parenchyma; cardiac dysfunction; impaired homeostasis; distorted skeletal muscle, endothelial, and blood flow dynamics; and impaired mitochondrial function, all of which precipitate and perpetuate ICU-AW. Approximately 79% and 37% of survivors of critical illness have impaired exercise capacity at six months and five years following discharge, respectively [39,40].

Myopathy, Catabolism, Sarcopenia, and Cachexia

Sepsis alters the membrane properties of skeletal muscle, with decreased action potential amplitudes and prolonged muscle kinetics [41]. The myopathy precipitated by critical illness and sepsis occurs rapidly, suggesting an active process that is not caused by disuse atrophy alone [42]. Etiologies include cytokine-mediated activation of ubiquitin-proteasomes, reduced insulin-like growth factor (IGF) effects, impaired myosin synthesis, increased protein turnover, muscle atrophy and apoptosis, impaired muscle repair mechanisms, mitochondrial dysfunction, peroxidative stress, and acquired channelopathies. Since muscle contraction and force generation require a complex cascade of events, disruption at any point along the pathway can cause clinical weakness (see Figure 3.2).

Skeletal muscle dysfunction, rather than changes in neural pathways, is thought to be the main mechanism driving persistent ICU-AW [43], and muscle weakness may persist despite restoration of muscle mass following the period of critical illness [44]. Prospective studies have demonstrated that myopathies and muscle mass loss continue even after ICU discharge, suggesting that this catabolic state remains for a prolonged period of time. Furthermore, the cytokine-driven cellular injury stress response is associated with cachexia and lean tissue wasting in CCI [45]. Inflammatory genes within muscle tissue are upregulated up to six months after resolution of the inciting illness, which is associated with a decrease in muscle performance on clinical examination [46]. This pro-inflammatory environment following acute injury also activates the ubiquitin-proteasome system, which further contributes to muscle wasting and weakness. The ubiquitin-proteasome system is essential for muscle homeostasis, as it provides substrates to maintain host energy levels. The activity of this pathway is upregulated by pro-inflammatory factors, accelerating skeletal muscle catabolism, and overload of this system leads to accumulation of toxins, nonfunctional proteins, and ultimately muscle necrosis (see Figure 3.3) [47].

Myeloid-derived suppressor cells (MDSCs), a heterogeneous group of immature myeloid cells that accumulate during sepsis or other pathological conditions, are associated with adverse clinical outcomes in septic patients [48,49]. Despite being functionally immunosuppressive, MDSCs infiltrate skeletal muscle and are associated with tissue injury and sepsis-associated muscle injury [47,50,51]. In addition, satellite cells in skeletal muscle tissue, which are essential for muscle fiber maintenance, repair, and remodeling, may play an important role in skeletal muscle dysfunction. They are responsible for growth and development of skeletal muscle, with the capacity to expand and differentiate to provide an ongoing source of nuclei to growing myofibers, and their cell content is decreased in

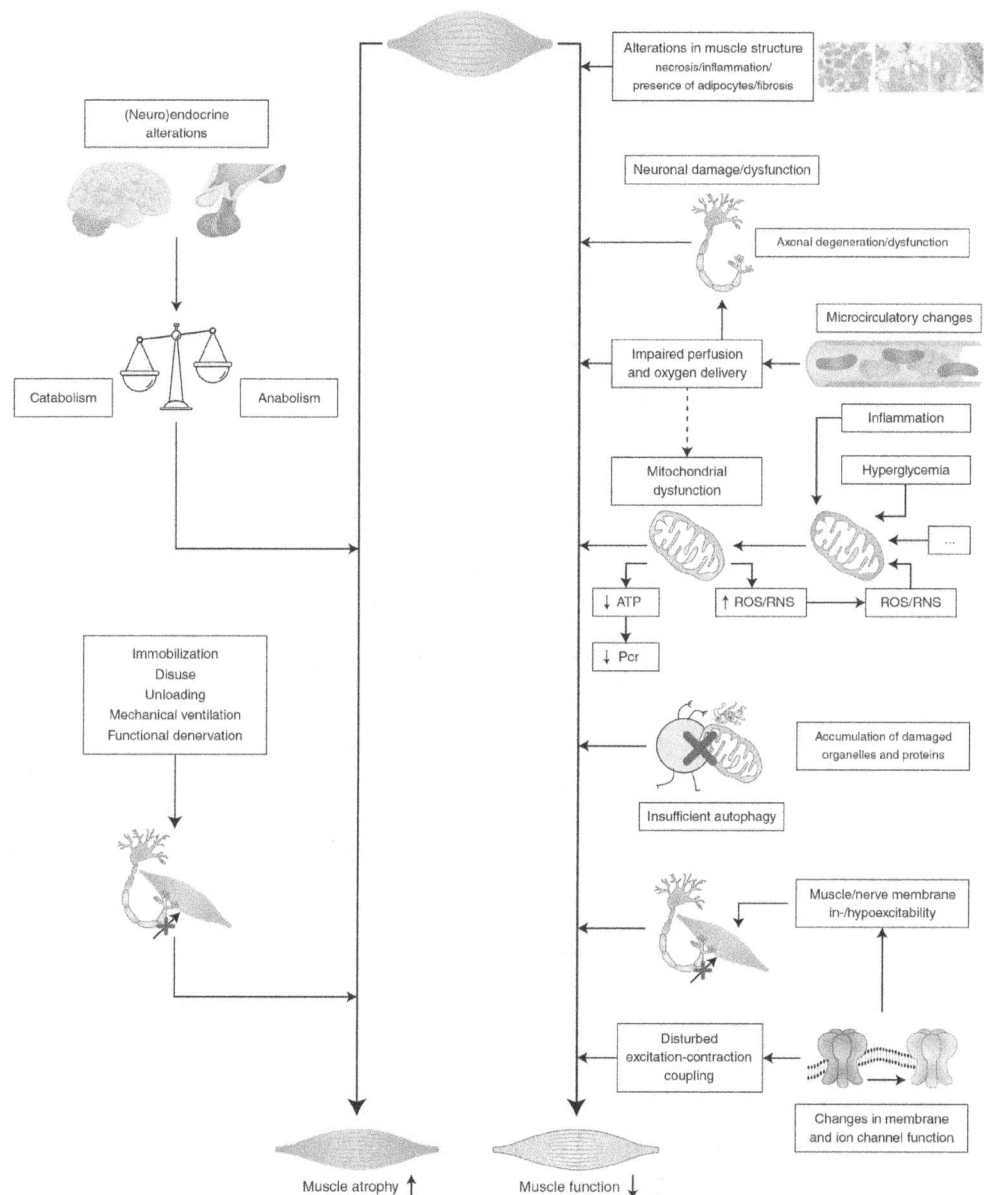

Figure 3.2 Mechanisms implicated in the development of ICU-acquired weakness. From: I. Vanhorebeek, N. Latronico, G. van den Berghe. ICU-acquired weakness. *Intensive Care Med* 2020; **46(4)**: 637–53. Reproduced with permission from Springer Nature.

survivors of critical illness [52]. Other key cellular functions are disrupted, with pathological upregulation of muscle development genes and mitochondrial dysfunction [30,53]. Mitochondrial dysfunction is multifactorial and related to the accumulation of oxidized proteins, calcium overload secondary to calcium channel dysfunction and dysregulated

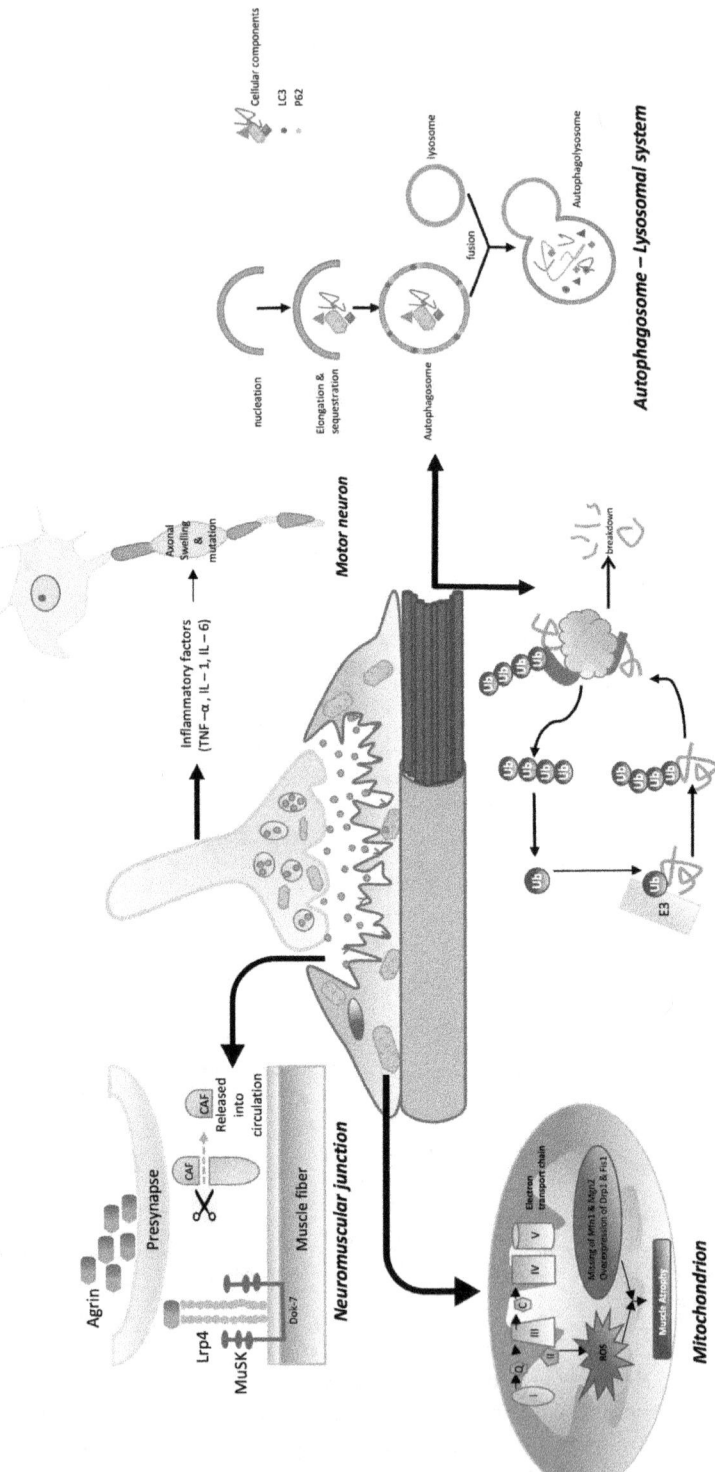

Figure 3.3 Inflammation, the ubiquitin-proteasome pathway, and autophagy contribute to muscle dysfunction.

homeostasis, and the release and accumulation of mitochondrial DAMPs [54], which are thought to further propagate inflammation [55,56].

This injury-induced proteolysis is accompanied by disrupted autophagy, a catabolic process essential for skeletal muscle homeostasis [57]. Autophagy is important for the elimination of damaged cellular products (e.g., mitochondria and toxic protein products) that accumulate during critical illness and is upregulated with fasting, oxidative stress, inflammation, and sepsis, leading to muscle protein degradation. Clinically, several myopathies and muscle wasting conditions have been associated with impaired autophagy, including Pompe and Danon diseases [58,59]. Patients with prolonged critical illness have disrupted muscle autophagy and accumulate cellular damage [46].

Disruptions to the Gut Microbiome in Critical Illness

The human gut microbiome is composed of a vast assortment of microorganisms, both commensal and pathogenic, including bacteria, viruses, fungi, and parasites. Collectively, these microorganisms perform many roles, including regulation of metabolism and immune function, supporting the gut barrier, modulating enteric and CNS activity, synthesizing vitamins and amino acids, and fermenting non-digestible fibers into short chain fatty acids. As a result, the human gut microbiome is now recognized as an important contributing factor along the continuum of critical illness, from predisposition to long-term recovery. Current research is exploring the adverse effects that critical care interventions have on the microbiome and how this, in turn, impacts long-term patient outcomes.

The release of pro-inflammatory cytokines into systemic circulation disrupts tight junction proteins of the intestinal barrier, resulting in increased bacterial translocation and a shift in the microbiome population toward more pathogenic bacteria. Gut microbiome changes can be exacerbated by the catabolic state, glucose and electrolyte imbalances, and hypoperfusion commonly found in critically ill patients. Moreover, many ICU interventions, such as antibiotics, gastric acid suppression, antipsychotic medications, parenteral nutrition, laxatives, and corticosteroids, further reduce gut microbial diversity [60].

Skeletal muscle atrophy and the development of ICU-AW may also be influenced by the gut microbiome. Recent studies have shown that dysbiosis and loss of microbiome-delivered metabolites result in changes to skeletal muscle metabolism; for example, mice lacking gut microbiota exhibited significant muscle atrophy, reduced expression of insulin-like growth factor, and decreased transcription of genes associated with skeletal muscle growth and mitochondrial function [61]. Another study in humans demonstrated that a short period of severe physical inactivity had a significant effect on leg mass as well as significant decreases in the volume of bacteria associated with bile acid breakdown [62]. This connection, named the "gut-muscle axis," is another example of how changes in the gut microbiome contribute to pathological outcomes.

Translational research has shown that the gut microbiome plays an important role in sepsis and the maintenance of basal body temperature. Decreased microbiome diversity impairs temperature regulation and increases the risk of hypothermia in patients with sepsis. Additional research in human and animal models has shown a link between gut microbiome dysbiosis and increased susceptibility to nosocomial infections through multiple mechanisms, including decreased neutrophil activity [63,64].

Changes in the intestinal microbiome are also implicated in the development of delirium. Such alterations can disturb the "gut-brain axis," a physiological connection between the gut microbiota and the nervous system composed of immune modulating, endocrine signaling, and neural signaling pathways. In animal models, changes in bacterial ratios within the gut microbiome were associated with cognitive impairment [65].

The role of the microbiome in mental illness has also been examined, with several animal studies linking changes in the gut microbiome to increases in anxious and depressive behaviors [66]. It has been hypothesized that the microbiome produces neurochemicals which affect the brain (e.g., gamma-aminobutyric acid [GABA] produced by Lactobacillus species) and that microbiome disruption may precipitate neuroinflammation, which subsequently impacts mental health [67].

Conclusion

PICS is the downstream manifestation of innumerable impaired biochemical processes that develop after septic insult, critical illness, or traumatic injury. This syndrome develops as a complex pathological cascade. The initial insult causes excess production of pro-inflammatory cytokines and alarmins, which in turn activate a destructive inflammatory cascade. Additional clinical injuries, such as nosocomial infections, mechanical ventilation, gut dysbiosis, and neurohormonal changes, trigger further elevations in pro- and anti-inflammatory markers, leading to the propagation of a dysregulated immunologic response in an already increasingly susceptible host. This process leads to worsening organ failures, including endothelial, muscular, and neurologic dysfunction. Although the patient may seem to recover from the initial insult, they are left with underlying metabolic and physiologic impairments that serve as the pathophysiological basis for the development of PICS.

Key Points

1. PICS describes the late phenotypic sequelae that develop in a large percentage of survivors of critical illness or injury.
2. The development of PICS is a consequence of perturbations in multiple systems, including innate and adaptive immunity, the endothelium, the brain, skeletal muscle, and the gut microbiome, which lead to a self-perpetuating cycle of ongoing impaired immunity, organ failure, inflammation, cell loss, and functional decline.
3. The road to PICS begins early during critical illness, with certain factors predisposing specific patient populations to its development.

References

1. L.F. Gentile, A.G. Cuenca, P.A. Efron, et al. Persistent inflammation and immunosuppression: a common syndrome and new horizon for surgical intensive care. *J Trauma Acute Care Surg* 2012; **72**: 1491–501.
2. R.B. Hawkins, S.L. Raymond, J.A. Stortz, et al. Chronic critical illness and the persistent inflammation, immunosuppression, and catabolism syndrome. *Front Immunol* 2018; **9**: 1511.
3. S. Inoue, J. Hatakeyama, Y. Kondo, et al. Post-intensive care syndrome: its pathophysiology, prevention, and future directions. *Acute Med Surg* 2019; **6**: 233–46.
4. D.B. Darden, S.C. Brakenridge, P.A. Efron, et al. Biomarker evidence of the persistent inflammation, immunosuppression and catabolism syndrome (PICS) in chronic

critical illness (CCI) after surgical sepsis. *Ann Surg* 2021; **274**: 664–73.

5. M.C. Cox, S.C. Brakenridge, J.A. Stortz, et al. Abdominal sepsis patients have a high incidence of chronic critical illness with dismal long-term outcomes. *Am J Surg* 2020; **220**: 1467–74.

6. J.A. Stortz, J.C. Mira, S.L. Raymond, et al. Benchmarking clinical outcomes and the immunocatabolic phenotype of chronic critical illness after sepsis in surgical intensive care unit patients. *J Trauma Acute Care Surg* 2018; **84**: 342–9.

7. D.M. Griffith, S. Lewis, A.G. Rossi, et al. Systemic inflammation after critical illness: relationship with physical recovery and exploration of potential mechanisms. *Thorax* 2016; **71**: 820–9.

8. N.E. Brummel, C.G. Hughes, J. L. Thompson, et al. Inflammation and coagulation during critical illness and long-term cognitive impairment and disability. *Am J Respir Crit Care Med* 2021; **203**: 699–706.

9. C.G. Hughes, A. Morandi, T.D. Girard, et al. Association between endothelial dysfunction and acute brain dysfunction during critical illness. *Anesthesiology* 2013; **118**: 631–9.

10. M. Huang, A. Gedansky, C.E. Hassett, et al. Pathophysiology of brain injury and neurological outcome in acute respiratory distress syndrome: a scoping review of preclinical to clinical studies. *Neurocrit Care* 2021; **35**: 518–27.

11. M. Fries, J. Bickenbach, D. Henzler, et al. S-100 protein and neurohistopathologic changes in a porcine model of acute lung injury. *Anesthesiology* 2005; **102**: 761–7.

12. I. Galea. The blood-brain barrier in systemic infection and inflammation. *Cell Mol Immunol* 2021; **18**: 2489–501.

13. M.F. Beal. Role of excitotoxicity in human neurological disease. *Curr Opin Neurobiol* 1992; **2**: 657–62.

14. D. Bulic, M. Bennett, E. N. Georgousopoulou, et al. Cognitive and psychosocial outcomes of mechanically ventilated intensive care patients with and without delirium. *Ann Intensive Care* 2020; **10**: 104.

15. M.F. Newman, J.L. Kirchner, B. Phillips-Bute, et al. Longitudinal assessment of neurocognitive function after coronary-artery bypass surgery. *N Engl J Med* 2001; **344**: 395–402.

16. J.T. Moller, P. Cluitmans, L.S. Rasmussen, et al. Long-term postoperative cognitive dysfunction in the elderly ISPOCD1 study. ISPOCD investigators. International study of post-operative cognitive dysfunction. *Lancet* 1998; **351**: 857–61.

17. N.E. Brummel, J.C. Jackson, P. P. Pandharipande, et al. Delirium in the ICU and subsequent long-term disability among survivors of mechanical ventilation. *Crit Care Med* 2014; **42**: 369–77.

18. M.L. Gunther, A. Morandi, E. Krauskopf, et al. The association between brain volumes, delirium duration, and cognitive outcomes in intensive care unit survivors: the VISIONS cohort magnetic resonance imaging study. *Crit Care Med* 2012; **40**: 2022–32.

19. A. Morandi, B.P. Rogers, M.L. Gunther, et al. The relationship between delirium duration, white matter integrity, and cognitive impairment in intensive care unit survivors as determined by diffusion tensor imaging: the VISIONS prospective cohort magnetic resonance imaging study. *Crit Care Med* 2012; **40**: 2182–9.

20. E.M. Palacios, D. Fernandez-Espejo, C. Junque, et al. Diffusion tensor imaging differences relate to memory deficits in diffuse traumatic brain injury. *BMC Neurol* 2011; **11**: 24.

21. M.R. Suchyta, A. Jephson, R.O. Hopkins. Neurologic changes during critical illness: brain imaging findings and neurobehavioral outcomes. *Brain Imaging Behav* 2010; **4**: 22–34.

22. D.A.S. Taskforce, R. Baron, A. Binder, et al. Evidence and consensus based guideline for the management of delirium, analgesia, and sedation in intensive care medicine. Revision 2015 (DAS-Guideline 2015): short version. *Ger Med Sci* 2015; **13**: Doc19.

23. K. Mietani, M. Sumitani, T. Ogata, et al. Dysfunction of the blood-brain barrier in postoperative delirium patients, referring to the axonal damage biomarker phosphorylated neurofilament heavy subunit. *PLoS One* 2019; **14**: e0222721.

24. N. Sekino, M. Selim, A. Shehadah. Sepsis-associated brain injury: underlying mechanisms and potential therapeutic strategies for acute and long-term cognitive impairments. *J Neuroinflammation* 2022; **19**: 101.

25. N.I. Shapiro, P. Schuetz, K. Yano, et al. The association of endothelial cell signaling, severity of illness, and organ dysfunction in sepsis. *Crit Care* 2010; **14**: R182.

26. G. Monneret, A. Lepape, N. Voirin, et al. Persisting low monocyte human leukocyte antigen-DR expression predicts mortality in septic shock. *Intensive Care Med* 2006; **32**: 1175-83.

27. J.A. Stortz, T.J. Murphy, S.L. Raymond, et al. Evidence for persistent immune suppression in patients who develop chronic critical illness after sepsis. *Shock* 2018; **49**: 249-58.

28. M.D. Hashem, R.O. Hopkins, E. Colantuoni, et al. Six-month and 12-month patient outcomes based on inflammatory subphenotypes in sepsis-associated ARDS: secondary analysis of SAILS-ALTOS trial. *Thorax* 2022; **77**: 22-30.

29. W. Xiao, M.N. Mindrinos, J. Seok, et al. A genomic storm in critically injured humans. *J Exp Med* 2011; **208**: 2581-90.

30. C.J. Walsh, J. Batt, M.S. Herridge, et al. Transcriptomic analysis reveals abnormal muscle repair and remodeling in survivors of critical illness with sustained weakness. *Sci Rep* 2016; **6**: 29334.

31. S.C. Brakenridge, P. Starostik, G. Ghita, et al. A transcriptomic severity metric that predicts clinical outcomes in critically ill surgical sepsis patients. *Crit Care Explor* 2021; **3**: e0554.

32. M. Bodinier, G. Monneret, M. Casimir, et al. Identification of a sub-group of critically ill patients with high risk of intensive care unit-acquired infections and poor clinical course using a transcriptomic score. *Crit Care* 2023; **27**: 158.

33. J.L. Vincent, D. De Backer. Microvascular dysfunction as a cause of organ dysfunction in severe sepsis. *Crit Care* 2005; **9 Suppl 4**: S9-12.

34. L. Gupta, M.N. Subair, J. Munjal, et al. Beyond survival: understanding post-intensive care syndrome. *Acute Crit Care* 2024; **39**: 226-33.

35. W.C. Aird. The role of the endothelium in severe sepsis and multiple organ dysfunction syndrome. *Blood* 2003; **101**: 3765-77.

36. A. Zeineddin, F. Wu, W. Chao, et al. Biomarkers of endothelial cell dysfunction persist beyond resuscitation in patients with hemorrhagic shock. *J Trauma Acute Care Surg* 2022; **93**: 572-8.

37. Y. Sakr, M.J. Dubois, D. De Backer, et al. Persistent microcirculatory alterations are associated with organ failure and death in patients with septic shock. *Crit Care Med* 2004; **32**: 1825-31.

38. G. Pacinella, A.M. Ciaccio, A. Tuttolomondo. Endothelial dysfunction and chronic inflammation: The cornerstones of vascular alterations in age-related diseases. *Int J Mol Sci* 2022; **23**: 15722.

39. K.C. Ong, A.W. Ng, L.S. Lee, et al. Pulmonary function and exercise capacity in survivors of severe acute respiratory syndrome. *Eur Respir J* 2004; **24**: 436-42.

40. N. Van Aerde, P. Meersseman, Y. Debaveye, et al. Aerobic exercise capacity in long-term survivors of critical illness: secondary analysis of the post-EPaNIC follow-up study. *Intensive Care Med* 2021; **47**: 1462-71.

41. D.D. Trunkey, H. Illner, I.Y. Wagner, G.T. Shires. The effect of septic shock on skeletal muscle action potentials in the primate. *Surgery* 1979; **85**: 638-43.

42. O. Friedrich, M.B. Reid, G. Van den Berghe, et al. The sick and the weak: neuropathies/myopathies in the critically ill. *Physiol Rev* 2015; **95**: 1025-109.

43. C. Goossens, R. Weckx, S. Derde, et al. Impact of prolonged sepsis on neural and muscular components of muscle contractions in a mouse model. *J Cachexia Sarcopenia Muscle* 2021; **12**: 443–55.

44. J. Segers, I. Vanhorebeek, D. Langer, et al. Early neuromuscular electrical stimulation reduces the loss of muscle mass in critically ill patients: a within subject randomized controlled trial. *J Crit Care* 2021; **62**: 65–71.

45. M.G. Jeschke, D.L. Chinkes, C.C. Finnerty, et al. Pathophysiologic response to severe burn injury. *Ann Surg* 2008; **248**: 387–401.

46. I. Vanhorebeek, J. Gunst, S. Derde, et al. Insufficient activation of autophagy allows cellular damage to accumulate in critically ill patients. *J Clin Endocrinol Metab* 2011; **96**: E633–45.

47. Z.A. Puthucheary, J. Rawal, M. McPhail, et al. Acute skeletal muscle wasting in critical illness. *JAMA* 2013; **310**: 1591–600.

48. J.A. Chesney, R.A. Mitchell, K. Yaddanapudi. Myeloid-derived suppressor cells-a new therapeutic target to overcome resistance to cancer immunotherapy. *J Leukoc Biol* 2017; **102**: 727–40.

49. B. Mathias, A.L. Delmas, T. Ozrzagat-Baslanti, et al. Human myeloid-derived suppressor cells are associated with chronic immune suppression after severe sepsis/septic shock. *Ann Surg* 2017; **265**: 827–34.

50. D. Burzyn, W. Kuswanto, D. Kolodin, et al. A special population of regulatory T cells potentiates muscle repair. *Cell* 2013; **155**: 1282–95.

51. R.R. Flores, C.L. Clauson, J. Cho, et al. Expansion of myeloid-derived suppressor cells with aging in the bone marrow of mice through a NF-kappaB-dependent mechanism. *Aging Cell* 2017; **16**: 480–7.

52. C. Dos Santos, S.N. Hussain, S. Mathur, et al. Mechanisms of chronic muscle wasting and dysfunction after an intensive care unit stay: a pilot study. *Am J Respir Crit Care Med* 2016; **194**: 821–30.

53. D. Brealey, M. Brand, I. Hargreaves, et al. Association between mitochondrial dysfunction and severity and outcome of septic shock. *Lancet* 2002; **360**: 219–23.

54. E. Balboa, F. Saavedra-Leiva, L.A. Cea, et al. Sepsis-induced channelopathy in skeletal muscles is associated with expression of non-selective channels. *Shock* 2018; **49**: 221–8.

55. X. Yao, D. Carlson, Y. Sun, et al. Mitochondrial ROS induces cardiac inflammation via a pathway through mtDNA damage in a pneumonia-related sepsis model. *PLoS One* 2015; **10**: e0139416.

56. W. Zhang, K.J. Lavine, S. Epelman, et al. Necrotic myocardial cells release damage-associated molecular patterns that provoke fibroblast activation in vitro and trigger myocardial inflammation and fibrosis in vivo. *J Am Heart Assoc* 2015; **4**: e001993.

57. P. Grumati, L. Coletto, A. Schiavinato, et al. Physical exercise stimulates autophagy in normal skeletal muscles but is detrimental for collagen VI-deficient muscles. *Autophagy* 2011; **7**: 1415–23.

58. E. Masiero, L. Agatea, C. Mammucari, et al. Autophagy is required to maintain muscle mass. *Cell Metab* 2009; **10**: 507–15.

59. E. Masiero, M. Sandri. Autophagy inhibition induces atrophy and myopathy in adult skeletal muscles. *Autophagy* 2010; **6**: 307–9.

60. J. Sung, S.S. Rajendraprasad, K. L. Philbrick, et al. The human gut microbiome in critical illness: disruptions, consequences, and therapeutic frontiers. *J Crit Care* 2023; **79**: 154436.

61. C. Liu, W.H. Cheung, J. Li, et al. Understanding the gut microbiota and sarcopenia: a systematic review. *J Cachexia Sarcopenia Muscle* 2021; **12**: 1393–407.

62. C. Lefevre, L.B. Bindels. Role of the gut microbiome in skeletal muscle physiology and pathophysiology. *Curr Osteoporos Rep* 2022; **20**: 422–32.

63. K.S. Bongers, R. Chanderraj, R.J. Woods, et al. The gut microbiome modulates body temperature both in sepsis and health. *Am J Respir Crit Care Med* 2023; **207**: 1030–41.

64. J. Schlechte, A.Z. Zucoloto, I.L. Yu, et al. Dysbiosis of a microbiota-immune metasystem in critical illness is associated with nosocomial infections. *Nat Med* 2023; **29**: 1017–27.
65. J.F. Cryan, K.J. O'Riordan, C.S.M. Cowan, et al. The microbiota-gut-brain axis. *Physiol Rev* 2019; **99**: 1877–2013.
66. J.R. Kelly, Y. Borre, E. Patterson, et al. Transferring the blues: depression-associated gut microbiota induces neurobehavioural changes in the rat. *J Psychiatr Res* 2016; **82**: 109–18.
67. P. Strandwitz, K.H. Kim, D. Terekhova, et al. GABA-modulating bacteria of the human gut microbiota. *Nat Microbiol* 2019; **4**: 396–403.
68. M. Singer, C.S. Deutschman, C.W. Seymour, et al. The third international consensus definitions for sepsis and septic shock (sepsis-3). *JAMA* 2016; **315**: 801–10.
69. M.J. Delano, P.A. Ward. The immune system's role in sepsis progression, resolution, and long-term outcome. *Immunol Rev* 2016; **274**: 330–53.
70. J.E. Nelson, C.E. Cox, A.A. Hope, S.S. Carson. Chronic critical illness. *Am J Respir Crit Care Med* 2010; **182**: 446–54.
71. D.M. Needham, J. Davidson, H. Cohen, et al. Improving long-term outcomes after discharge from intensive care unit: report from a stakeholders' conference. *Crit Care Med* 2012; **40**: 502–9.
72. G. Voiriot, M. Oualha, A. Pierre, et al. Chronic critical illness and post-intensive care syndrome: from pathophysiology to clinical challenges. *Ann Intensive Care* 2022; **12**: 58.

Section 2 **The Hazards of Hospitalization**

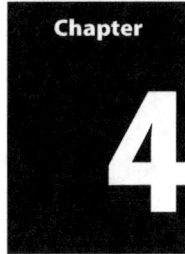

Chapter 4
Immobility and ICU-Acquired Weakness

Felipe González-Seguel, Sabrina Eggmann, Owen Gustafson, Kirby P. Mayer, and Selina M. Parry

Introduction

Regular use of bed rest can be traced back to the time of Hippocrates and was routinely used as a treatment in the nineteenth century [1]. The first intensive care units (ICUs) were established in the 1950s, largely in Denmark, because of the polio epidemic and its demand for respiratory support using mechanical ventilation [2]. Since that time, the sophistication of intensive care practice has grown significantly, with most patients now surviving critical illness. In the 1980s, Bolton and colleagues first described a "severe motor and sensory polyneuropathy at the peak of critical illness." In 2009, the term intensive care unit-acquired weakness (ICUAW) [3] was developed to describe "clinically identifiable weakness acquired in a critical care patient that is directly attributable to their critical care stay where other causes of weakness have been excluded" [4]. It is estimated that almost 50% of critically ill patients will develop muscle weakness because of their intensive care admission [5]. Part I of this chapter provides an overview of the deleterious impact of bed rest on body systems, and Part II contextualizes the hazards of critical illness and associated risk factors for the development of ICUAW.

Part I Impact of Bed Rest and Immobility

Impact of Bed Rest and Immobility on Body Systems

Prolonged periods of bed rest and immobility have significant multisystem consequences, with a particularly detrimental impact on the cardiovascular, respiratory, metabolic, neurological, and musculoskeletal systems (see Figure 4.1) [6].

Patients with critical illness remain inactive for approximately 97% of the total time spent in the ICU, and the duration of inactivity strongly correlates with the ICU length of stay [7]. Inactivity and prolonged bed rest have been shown to result in deconditioning that affects both the central and peripheral cardiovascular systems [8]. In healthy adults, stroke volume can be reduced by 30% within the first month of bed rest, with a clinically relevant compensatory increase in resting heart rate evident after seven days [9]. Orthostatic intolerance can also develop within 72 hours of inactivity, which is attributed to multiple physiological changes, including hypovolemia, hormonal and metabolic changes, and modifications in cardiovascular regulation by the autonomic nervous system [10]. Other cardiovascular and hematologic consequences include an increased risk of venous thromboembolic events and a reduction in red blood cell mass and oxygen carrying capacity [11,12].

The musculoskeletal system is especially vulnerable during periods of immobilization, as gravitational loading is necessary for it to maintain its integrity. Skeletal tissue is

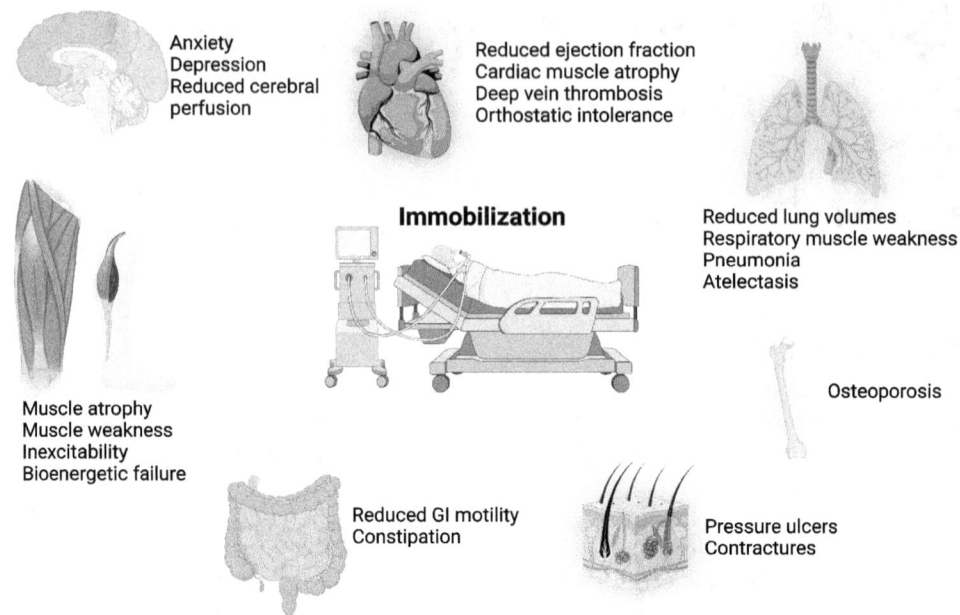

Figure 4.1 Potential complications of immobility.

affected as bone resorption exceeds formation, resulting in reduced bone integrity and demineralization, which subsequently increase the risk of fractures [8,13]. The rate of change in skeletal integrity is relatively slow, with reductions of 1% in bone density of the vertebral column reported after one week of immobilization [14]; despite these slow rates of change, however, studies have demonstrated an increased fracture risk of approximately 20% following immobilization during critical illness [15,16]. Loss of muscle mass occurs within days of microgravity-simulated bed rest, with anti-gravity muscles, such as leg extensors and the trunk musculature, preferentially affected compared to muscles of the upper limb and hand [17,18]. Immobility also increases the production of pro-inflammatory cytokines, with subsequent muscle proteolysis and promotion of overall muscle mass loss [19]. In addition to a generalized decrease in muscle mass, there is also a reduction in muscle fiber size and an accelerated reduction in the strength of fast-twitch (type II) fibers compared to slow-twitch (type I) fibers, resulting in lower fatigue resistance capacity [8]. Reductions in muscle force generation capacity also result from changes in neuron and muscle membrane excitability [20]. The combination of these physiological changes results in reported decrements in muscle strength of up to 40% within the first four weeks of bed rest [21].

The respiratory, metabolic, and neurological systems are also negatively affected. Given altered respiratory mechanics, aerobic capacity is reduced and atelectasis develops, increasing the risk of developing complications such as pneumonia [8,12,22]. Insulin resistance can be present after five days of bed rest and is associated with dyslipidemia and a reduction in protein synthesis and utilization [23,24]. Immobility can also alter sleep patterns and impair cognitive function, particularly executive function and short-term memory [25].

Impact of Critical Illness on the Musculoskeletal System

In addition to the detrimental effects of immobilization alone, critical illness provides a further negative impact on the musculoskeletal system. The etiology by which critical illness leads to muscle dysfunction is complicated, involving multiple processes that vary over time; these processes can be categorized into early and late phases [26]. Meta-analysis data from muscle ultrasound studies demonstrate that critically ill patients experience approximately 2% of peripheral skeletal muscle loss per day in the ICU [27]. A significant contributor to early-phase muscle dysfunction in critical illness is muscle atrophy, which is more pronounced in older rather than younger adults [28]. Muscle atrophy results from an imbalance between muscle protein synthesis (MPS) and muscle protein breakdown (MPB), with MPB drastically overwhelming the muscle's synthetic capacity [29]. Muscle atrophy occurs rapidly during this early phase, with critically ill patients losing approximately 10–14% of skeletal muscle mass during the first week of an ICU admission [27]. The quality of muscle also deteriorates significantly within the first 10 days, with infiltration of non-contractile tissues, such as fat, collagen, and edema [27]. These early changes in muscle mass and muscle quality have been correlated with measures of reduced strength and impaired function [27]. Additionally, as with immobility alone, there is a reduction in muscle fiber size, with selective myosin loss specifically impacting muscle contraction filaments [30].

The catabolic state of critical illness, with reduced anabolic effector hormones, increased catabolic hormones, and mechanical unloading due to immobilization, contribute to this profound and rapid muscle atrophy [31]. The predominant system that mediates MPB in critically ill individuals is the ubiquitin proteasome system (UPS; see Chapter 3 for additional information) [32]. Immobilization and multiple stimuli characteristic of critical illness, including systemic inflammation and oxidative stress, activate the UPS [33]. Additionally, dysregulation of autophagy and upregulation of protein degradation molecules (e.g., calpains and caspases) have also been associated with early phase MPB due to the accumulation of damaged and toxic proteins and modification of myofilament protein structure, respectively [32].

Exercise and nutrition are important regulators in MPS, with nutrient delivery, muscle loading, and activity allowing a balance between MPS and MPB; however, in critical illness, rates of MPS are decreased beyond those seen in immobilization alone and are resistant to an increase in protein delivery [8]. MPS in critical illness is compromised by multiple processes. Muscle mitochondrial function is altered due to direct damage aggravated by inflammation, hyperglycemia, and free radicals [33]. Mitochondrial dysfunction leads to both adenosine triphosphate depletion, which compromises energy provision, and amplification of free radical production, eliciting a vicious cycle of macromolecular damage [31]. Additionally, altered microcirculation leads to ischemic hypoxia of the muscle, with a heterogeneous reduction of perfused capillaries in striated muscle, which is further worsened in patients with severe sepsis [34]. The loss of muscle contractile function is disproportionate to the muscle loss seen during critical illness alone, as there are mechanisms in addition to atrophy that contribute to muscle dysfunction [35]. Nerve microcirculation is also impaired due to increased permeability and activation of leukocytes within the endoneural space [33]. Sodium channel inactivation is also thought to contribute to the inexcitability of nerve and muscle membranes [36].

The late phase of muscle dysfunction refers to the ongoing impairment that begins following resolution of the systemic inflammation that characterizes the early phase [26], and the long-term weakness characterizing this phase has a different etiology compared to the early phase. Although significant MPB contributes to weakness early in critical illness, this is not the case for individuals with long-term weakness following critical illness, in whom neither the UPS or autophagy are activated beyond normal levels [37]. Following the overwhelming MPB in the early phase, muscle atrophy in the long term is due to impaired regrowth and is associated with decreased satellite cell content [37]. Additionally, long-term muscle dysfunction can result following peripheral nerve injury, either through direct trauma or as a result of prolonged neuropathy due to endoneural edema, bioenergy failure, and ion channel dysfunction [38].

Part II Intensive Care Unit-Acquired Weakness: Prevalence, Diagnosis, and Associated Risk Factors

Defining ICUAW and Its Prevalence

Neuromuscular disorders in critical illness have been studied since the late 1970s, but it was not until 2009 that the umbrella term ICUAW was proposed to describe the clinically detectable weakness in critically ill patients in whom there is no plausible etiology other than critical illness. This weakness may persist for months to years after hospital discharge. Three subclassifications of ICUAW, including critical illness polyneuropathy (CIP), critical illness myopathy (CIM), and critical illness neuromyopathy (CINM), have been described [39]. Accurate nosological diagnosis of polyneuropathy and myopathy is challenging in the ICU, as electromyography, nerve conduction studies, and muscle biopsies are required but rarely performed in critical care settings. Moreover, several studies [40,41,42,43] including one landmark study by Latronico and colleagues [44], have demonstrated that CIP and CIM rarely occur in isolation and more commonly present as CINM. Given the complex modalities needed to diagnose CIM, CIP, and CINM, in 2002, De Jonghe and colleagues suggested relying on clinical determination of muscle weakness alone to diagnose what they referred to as ICU-acquired paresis [41].

The prevalence of ICUAW in patients with critical illness ranges from 10% to 86% [45,46], depending on several factors, including study design, the assessment tool used, the timing of evaluation, the underlying etiology, and illness severity. The pooled prevalence of ICUAW reported in two systematic reviews including more than 30 studies has been 33% and 40% when detected clinically by manual muscle testing [47,48]. With respect to the timing of evaluation, a systematic review showed a prevalence of ICUAW of 45% during the first week of critical illness, in which patients lost 1.75% (95% CI -2.05, -1.45) of their rectus femoris thickness or 2.10% (95% CI -3.17, -1.02) of rectus femoris cross-sectional area daily [27]. Importantly, the prevalence of ICUAW may be underreported due to failed completion of clinical and diagnostic testing in several studies and in distinct subpopulations, such as patients requiring renal replacement therapy or extracorporeal membrane oxygenation. Patients with prolonged mechanical ventilation (defined as greater than seven days) and patients with severe sepsis or septic shock have a higher prevalence of ICUAW. Mortality in patients with ICUAW is 30% higher compared to patients without ICUAW at both 6 and 12 months following hospital discharge [49,50].

Diagnosis of ICUAW and Assessment of Physical Functioning in the Clinical Setting

Early identification of patients at risk for ICUAW is relevant for both research and clinical practice to recognize who may require rehabilitation interventions and to subsequently monitor responsiveness to such interventions [51,52]. While clinical diagnosis of ICUAW by manual muscle testing has been established, adjunct physical functioning tools can also help to identify patients at risk for or with ICUAW by complementing the physical evaluation (see Table 4.1) [51,52].

Clinical Examination and Diagnosis of ICUAW

The current gold standard approach for the clinical diagnosis of ICUAW is manual muscle testing using the Medical Research Council Sum-Score (MRC-SS; see Chapter 45 for additional information). Given that the test is dependent on patient effort, screening for alertness and comprehension is essential; additionally, delirium, fatigue, and the patient's mood may impact performance. The assessment of the MRC-SS should occur once the patient is able to follow simple questions and commands; the Standardized Five Questions (S5Q) may be used to assess a patient's ability to cooperate [41]. The MRC-SS uses a 6-point ordinal scale to score muscle strength, from no visible or palpable muscle contraction (0 points) to normal strength (5 points). This scale is used to score 12 peripheral muscle groups (6 in the lower limbs and 6 in the upper limbs), with total scores ranging between 0 and 60 points. The most common categorical interpretation of this scale is using the total score, where fewer than 48 points and fewer than 36 points are interpreted as significant and severe ICUAW, respectively; notably, these cut-offs were chosen empirically rather than based on evidence [41,53]. The primary limitation of the MRC-SS is its subjectivity, with scores depending on the evaluator's judgment. While the inter-rater reliability of MRC-SS is strong, the reliability of the diagnosis of ICUAW (MRC-SS <48 points) is moderate in the early stages of critical illness, suggesting that diagnosing ICUAW is largely examiner-dependent [53].

This limitation of the MRC-SS highlights the need for other, more objective measurements to diagnose ICUAW. One such measurement is handgrip strength assessed using a handheld dynamometer, where the generation of <7 and <11 kilograms of force define ICUAW for females and males, respectively [54]. Assessing handgrip strength may be a reasonable initial approach to screen for ICUAW, particularly in resource-limited settings; those with ICUAW can then be referred to a physiotherapist for a more thorough clinical evaluation using the MRC-SS and other physical functioning measures to ascertain the patient's rehabilitation needs [53].

Electrophysiological Assessment of ICUAW

Electrophysiological studies that evaluate the peripheral nervous system, including nerve conduction studies (NCS), needle electromyography (EMG), neuromuscular junction testing, isometric force assessment, compound muscle action potential, and sensory nerve action potential, are also used in the diagnosis of ICUAW [34]. EMG and NCS identify whether weakness is predominantly myopathic, neuropathic, or a combination of both. Although useful to diagnose ICUAW, these modalities are comparatively costly and invasive, and as such, are rarely employed in the ICU and typically reserved for the diagnosis of complex neuromuscular disorders or research [52,55].

Table 4.1 Diagnostic and surrogate tools of intensive care unit acquired weakness

Domain	Instrument	Brief description	Time required	Main advantages	Main limitations	Interpretation	Language availability*
Muscle strength	MRC-SS	Standardized manual muscle strength testing of 12 pre-defined bilateral muscle groups: shoulder abductors, elbow flexors, wrist extensors, hip flexors, knee extensors, foot dorsiflexors. 6-point ordinal scale, ranging from 0 = no muscle contraction to 5 = normal strength against full resistance, with total score of 0–60. Clinical standard for diagnosing ICUAW.	5–10 minutes	Quick and simple peripheral muscle strength testing. Involves proximal and distal muscle groups.	Ordinal scale may increase bias. Concerns about inter-rater reliability.	Higher scores indicate better muscle strength: <48/60 points = significant ICUAW, <36/60 points = severe ICUAW.	English
	Handgrip dynamometry (HGD)	Evaluates handgrip strength (force generated). Standardized position recommended.	<1 minute per muscle group	Quick and simple. Continuous units in kilograms or pounds of force improves objectivity.	Limited to flexor muscles of the hand/forearm. Specific device required.	Likely ICUAW with <11 kg (males) and <7 kg (females). Cut-off values according to age and gender.	N/A
	Handheld dynamometry (HHD)	Evaluates strength (force generated) of a selected muscle group (e.g., knee extensors, elbow flexors). Standardized position recommended.	<1 minute per muscle group	Quick and simple. Continuous units in kilograms or pounds of force improves objectivity.	Difficult to standardize resistance. Specific device required.	Cut-offs not established for ICUAW diagnosis.	N/A
	MIP/MEP	Global inspiratory/expiratory muscle strength. Patients are asked to perform a forceful inspiration after an	<1 minute	Quick and simple. Continuous units in cmH$_2$O improves objectivity.	Diaphragmatic force cannot be isolated from other respiratory muscles.	Likely ICUAW with MIP <−36 cmH$_2$O. Based on reference values in healthy adults	N/A

Category	Scale	Description	Time	Advantages	Disadvantages	Interpretation	Languages
		expiration to residual volume level (MIP) or expiration after a full inspiration to total lung capacity (MEP) with an open glottis against an occluded mouthpiece.			Specific device required.	and cut-offs for respiratory muscle weakness (Lista-Paz et al 2023).	
Mobility-based scales	IMS	A simple, one-question scale to quantify mobility status on an 11-point scale ranging from 0 (nothing – lying in bed) to 10 (walking independently without a gait aid).	<1 minute	Quick and simple mobility scoring.	Lack of details on physical assistance.	Higher scores indicate better physical functioning.	English, Portuguese, Spanish, Japanese, German [ongoing]
	CPAx	Comprised of 10 components: respiratory function, cough, bed mobility, supine to sitting on the edge of the bed, sitting balance, sit to stand, transfers from bed to chair, standing balance, stepping, and grip strength. 6-point Guttman scale from complete dependence (0) to independence (5). Total score ranges from 0 to 50.	2–10 minutes	Comprehensive peripheral and respiratory muscle function assessment.	Requires additional device (HGD). Thorough in-person evaluation. Walking not evaluated.	Higher scores indicate better physical functioning.	English, Portuguese, Spanish, Danish, German, Chinese, Norwegian, Swedish
	FSS-ICU	Examines the patient's ability to perform 5 functional activities: rolling, transfer from supine to sit, sitting at the edge of bed, transfer from sit to stand, and walking. Each activity is evaluated using an 8-point ordinal scale ranging from 0 (unable to perform) to 7 (complete independence). Total score ranges from 0 to 35.	10–30 minutes	Comprehensive mobility assessment. Detailed physical assistance scoring for all activities.	Limited to mobility activities. Thorough in-person evaluation.	Higher scores indicate better physical functioning.	English, Portuguese, Spanish, Japanese, Korean, Chinese, Turkish, Italian

Table 4.1 (cont.)

Domain	Instrument	Brief description	Time required	Main advantages	Main limitations	Interpretation	Language availability*
	PFIT-s	Comprised of 4 tasks: sit to stand level of assistance, marching on the spot cadence, shoulder flexion strength, and knee extensor strength (strength evaluated via physical examination using the Oxford grading scale). Each item is scored from 0 to 3, with a total maximum score of 12. This ordinal score is then converted to a score out of 10 (interval scale) based on Rasch analytical principles.	10–15 minutes	Balance between exhaustive and quick assessment. Marching in place assessment.	Walking not evaluated.	Higher scores indicate better physical functioning.	English, Portuguese
Imaging tools	CT scan MRI	Imaging technique with accurate measures of muscle mass and composition. Cross-sectional area of psoas by CT at L3 and pectoral muscles most commonly used in ICU.	~1 hour for patients in the ICU	Three-dimensional muscle volume quantification. Image contrast is sharp, and muscle boundaries are relatively clear.	Specific equipment and training required. Expensive and with radiation exposure. Requires significant planning in ICU for scheduling and for patient safety.	Psoas major muscle mass appears representative of whole-body muscle and predictive of patient outcomes	N/A
	Ultrasonography	Image acquisition and analysis of respiratory and peripheral skeletal muscles, including muscle thickness, cross-sectional area, pennation angle, fascicle length, elastography, and echointensity.	<2 minutes per muscle	Objective evaluation of muscle size and quality. Can be used regardless of the patient's level of consciousness.	Specific equipment and training required. Heterogeneity in reported techniques, positioning, and landmarking.	Likely ICUAW during the first week of ICU with <20% in muscle thickness, <10% in cross-sectional area, <5% in pennation angle, and >8% in echointensity.	N/A

Others	EMG, NCS	Diagnostic procedure to assess the health of muscles, neurons, and neuromuscular junction. Non-volitional measurements of motor axon depolarization (evoked force) by either electrical or magnetic stimuli. Objective measure of evoked force using an ergometer.	30–90 minutes	Although not often performed, it is the gold standard for the diagnosis of critical illness neuropathy.	Expensive. Stimuli may cause discomfort (commonly invasive). Specific equipment and training required.	Comparison with healthy controls or followed longitudinally. No standardized values.	N/A
	Muscle biopsy	Procedure used to diagnose diseases involving muscle tissue. Most commonly obtained from vastus lateralis and performed with local anesthesia. Immunohistochemical, histochemical, and biochemical examinations performed on muscle samples.	~1 hour	Determine the source of the disease process.	Expensive, invasive, and with risk of complications. Specific equipment and training required.	Comparisons with healthy controls or followed longitudinally. No standardized values.	N/A

Muscle Mass and Morphological Investigation of ICUAW

Most instruments measuring muscle strength require patient cooperation, both physically and cognitively, which can limit early detection of ICUAW and delay the start of physical rehabilitation. Imaging studies, however, permit muscle assessment in patients that are unable to follow commands. Computed tomography (CT) and magnetic resonance imaging (MRI) can quantify muscle size and quality but are rarely used clinically for this purpose. Muscle ultrasound, a noninvasive, low-cost, and radiation-free modality, has similarly been proposed as a diagnostic tool to assess muscle quantity and quality [56]. Although limited by the training required to reproducibly acquire quality images, muscle ultrasonography shows excellent clinimetric properties and could lead to earlier detection of ICUAW in patients where physical examination is unreliable [56]. Compared to other tests, muscle biopsy plays an integral role in determining the source of muscle dysfunction in critical illness and identifying cellular and molecular mechanisms involved in ICUAW [32,57]. Since muscle biopsy is an invasive and expensive technique, it has limited use in patients with critical illness and is also primarily reserved for research purposes.

Respiratory Muscle Weakness

The muscles of respiration are skeletal muscles that are similarly susceptible to the development of ICUAW. Weakness of respiratory muscles (e.g., the diaphragm and intercostal muscles) is common in the ICU, particularly in mechanically ventilated patients, and is measured by determining maximal inspiratory pressure (MIP) and maximal expiratory pressure (MEP) using a unidirectional pressure valve method. Although a MIP less than -36 cmH_2O has been reported as consistent with the diagnosis of ICUAW (i.e., comparable with an MRC-SS score of <48 points) [58], the relationship between peripheral and respiratory muscle strength is not strong, suggesting that diaphragmatic dysfunction and ICUAW have different risk factors and different impacts on both failure to wean from mechanical ventilation and mortality [59,60]. In a nonselected population of patients deemed ready to perform a spontaneous breathing trial, the prevalence of diaphragm dysfunction was twofold higher than the prevalence of ICUAW; diaphragm dysfunction, but not ICUAW, influenced the success of weaning [61]. In a prospective cohort of 40 patients with ICUAW, 80% had concurrent diaphragmatic dysfunction as evaluated by phrenic nerve magnetic stimulation, ultrasound, and pulmonary function testing. Half of the patients were weaned from the ventilator without requiring reintubation within 72 hours, and the mortality rate in those patients who failed the weaning process was 50% [62].

Physical Functioning and Activity Limitations Related to ICUAW

In addition to the evaluation of peripheral and respiratory muscles as described above, other physical consequences of ICUAW may be detected with tests that examine specific domains of physical functioning developed for the ICU setting. Activity occurs when a coordinated combination of multiple muscle groups works to perform a task with a certain purpose. Physical activities are usually captured by functional scales, and the ones with the most robust clinimetric properties for use in the ICU include the Intensive Care Unit Mobility Scale (IMS), Chelsea Critical Care Physical Assessment Tool (CPAx), Functional Status Score for the Intensive Care Unit (FSS-ICU), and the Physical Function in Intensive Care Test-Scored (PFIT-s) [51]. Although all of these scales evaluate mobility, they differ in their underlying constructs and clinimetric properties, timing of the assessment, and the time and equipment required. These scales are more thoroughly described in Chapter 12.

Physical Functioning Instrument Use in Clinical Practice

Measurement instruments for detecting ICUAW were developed for clinical practice, but their use has largely been restricted to research. A nationwide survey on the clinical use of physical functioning instruments in 93 Chilean ICUs reported that the MRC-SS, FSS-ICU, and muscle ultrasound were used in 89%, 70%, and 44% of the surveyed ICUs, respectively [63], consistent with an Argentinian survey, where the use of MRC-SS was reported in 72% of ICUs surveyed [64]. Additionally, a Japanese survey identified that 21% of clinicians reported the performance of ultrasound-based muscle mass assessment [65]. As these findings are limited to few countries, the actual use of ICUAW measurement instruments in clinical practice is still unknown, challenging clinicians and researchers to identify the most suitable instrument for muscle strength assessment [63].

Risk Factors Associated with ICUAW

Risk factors for ICUAW include patient- and critical illness-related factors (see Figure 4.2), and they are classified as modifiable and nonmodifiable [31,66]. Modifiable risk factors provide clinicians opportunities to directly intervene or to adapt treatments to reduce the risk of ICUAW. The examination of non-modifiable risk factors is also imperative in clinical practice, as early awareness of higher risk can lead to individualized care to prevent or mitigate the severity of ICUAW [66].

Patient-related risk factors (e.g., demographics and social determinants of health) are known to contribute to, influence, and predict health outcomes in a diverse population of patients. Additionally, there are certain critical-illness related risk factors with stronger (e.g., sepsis, multi-system organ failure, and prolonged ICU stay) and weaker (e.g., hypoalbuminemia, need for parenteral nutrition, and need for renal replacement therapy) associations with ICUAW [67,68].

Older age, duration of mechanical ventilation and bed rest, duration of the systemic inflammatory response syndrome, presence and duration of multi-system organ failure, and hyperglycemia are considered probable risk factors for the development of ICUAW. Additionally, female gender, severity of illness on admission, hypoalbuminemia, hyperosmolality, parenteral nutrition, renal replacement therapy, vasopressors, corticosteroids, neuromuscular blocking agents, and aminoglycosides are considered possible risk factors for the development of ICUAW [68]. Clinical interpretation of ICUAW risk factors should cautiously consider interacting confounders, mediators, and collider bias variables to avoid overestimation of causality. The design of direct acyclic graphs could guide clinicians and researchers in understanding the relationship between risk factors and ICUAW [69].

Conclusions

The combined impact of prolonged bed rest and critical illness can significantly impact patients' long-term recovery. ICUAW is common, affecting approximately 50% of patients with critical illness, and is associated with worse short-term and long-term physical functioning and higher rates of mortality. Identifying patients early in their ICU admission using both nonvolitional and volitional-based tests is essential to mitigating risk and initiating early physical rehabilitation.

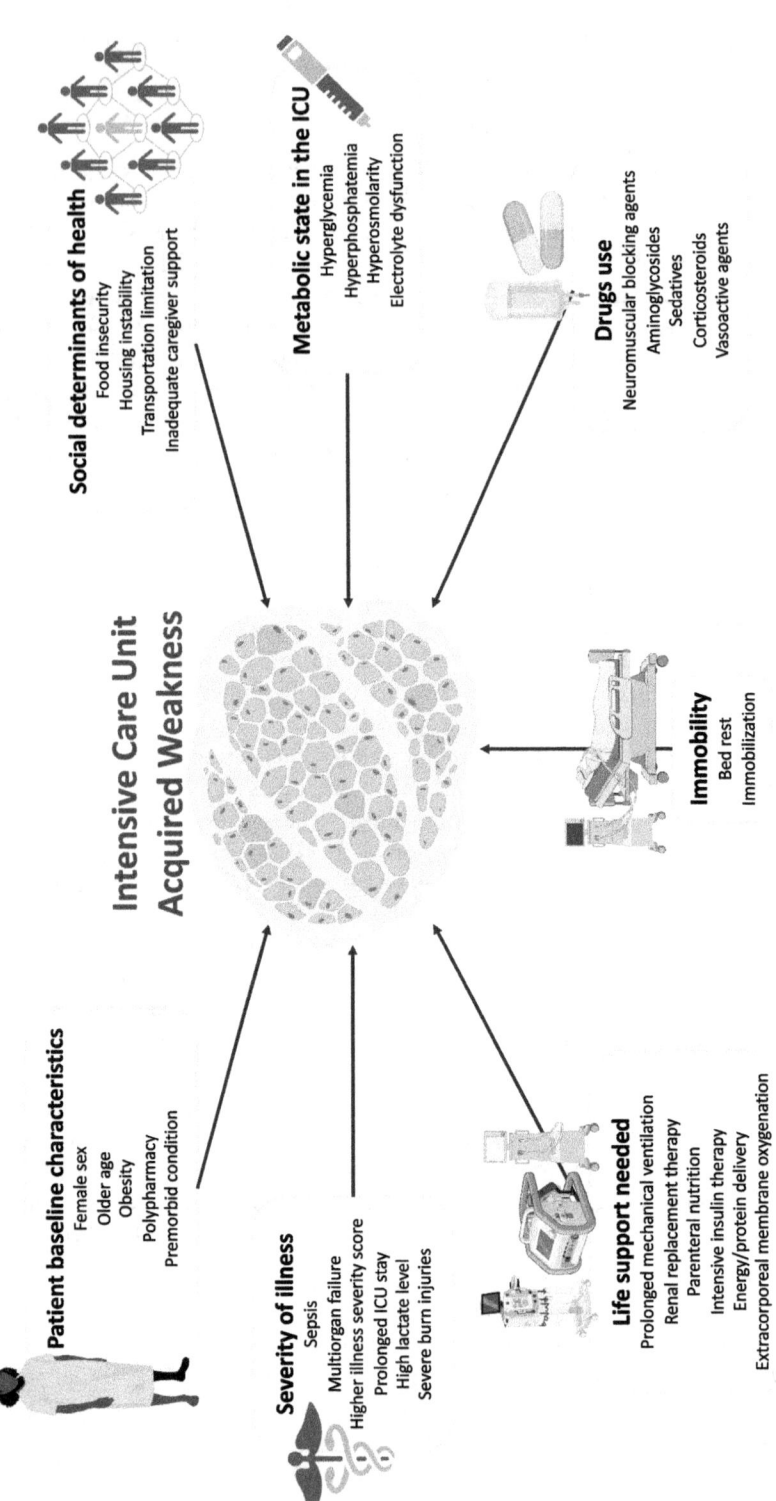

Figure 4.2 Risk factors for the development of intensive care unit-acquired weakness. Abbreviations: ICU=intensive care unit

Key Points

1. Survivors of a critical illness commonly experience severe weakness negatively affecting their recovery and functioning.
2. Prolonged bed rest is associated with cardiovascular, respiratory, metabolic, neurological, and musculoskeletal impairments.
3. Intensive care unit-acquired weakness (ICUAW) is generally diagnosed once patients are able to follow commands using clinical muscle strength tests for 6 major bilateral muscles and is defined as a score of 48 or fewer points out of 60 points on the Medical Research Council Sum-Score.
4. Limitations in physical function and activity can further be assessed with the Chelsea Critical Care Physical Assessment Tool (CPAx), Functional Status Score for the Intensive Care Unit (FSS-ICU), and the Physical Function in Intensive Care Test-Scored (PFIT-s).

References

1. A.E. Sprague. The evolution of bed rest as a clinical intervention. *J Obstet Gynecol Neonatal Nurs* 2004; 33: 542–9.
2. F.E. Kelly, K. Fong, N. Hirsch, J.P. Nolan. Intensive care medicine is 60 years old: the history and future of the intensive care unit. *Clin Med (Lond)* 2014; 14: 376–9.
3. C.F. Bolton, J.J. Gilbert, A.F. Hahn, W.J. Sibbald. Polyneuropathy in critically ill patients. *J Neurol Neurosurg Psychiatry* 1984; 47: 1223–31.
4. C. Taylor. Intensive care unit acquired weakness. *Anaesth Intensive Care Med* 2021; 22: 81–4.
5. N. Latronico, M. Herridge, R.O. Hopkins, et al. The ICM research agenda on intensive care unit-acquired weakness. *Intensive Care Med* 2017; 43: 1270–81.
6. S.A. Thomovsky. The physiology associated with "bed rest" and inactivity and how it may relate to the veterinary patient with spinal cord injury and physical rehabilitation. *Front Vet Sci* 2021; 8: 601914.
7. F. González-Seguel, A. Camus-Molina, M. Leiva-Corvalán, et al. Uninterrupted actigraphy recording to quantify physical activity and sedentary behaviors in mechanically ventilated adults: a feasibility prospective observational study. *J Acute Care Phys Ther* 2022; 13: 190–7.
8. S.M. Parry, Z.A. Puthucheary. The impact of extended bed rest on the musculoskeletal system in the critical care environment. *Extrem Physiol Med* 2015; 4: 16.
9. J. Spaak, S. Montmerle, P. Sundblad, D. Linnarsson. Long-term bed rest-induced reductions in stroke volume during rest and exercise: cardiac dysfunction vs. volume depletion. *J Appl Physiol (1985)* 2005; 98: 648–54.
10. V. Convertino, J. Hung, D. Goldwater, R.F. DeBusk. Cardiovascular responses to exercise in middle-aged men after 10 days of bedrest. *Circulation* 1982; 65: 134–40.
11. C. Capelli, G. Antonutto, M. Cautero, et al. Metabolic and cardiovascular responses during sub-maximal exercise in humans after 14 days of head-down tilt bed rest and inactivity. *Eur J Appl Physiol* 2008; 104: 909–18.
12. C. Winkelman. Bed rest in health and critical illness: a body systems approach. *J Anim Sci* 2009; 20: 254–66.
13. D.M. Griffith, T.S. Walsh. Bone loss during critical illness: a skeleton in the closet for the intensive care unit survivor? *Crit Care Med* 2011; 39: 1554–6.

14. A.D. LeBlanc, H.J. Evans, V.S. Schneider, et al. Changes in intervertebral disc cross-sectional area with bed rest and space flight. *Spine* 1994; **19**: 812–17.

15. N.R. Orford, K. Saunders, E. Merriman, et al. Skeletal morbidity among survivors of critical illness. *Crit Care Med* 2011; **39**: 1295–300.

16. J. Rawal, M.J. McPhail, G. Ratnayake, et al. A pilot study of change in fracture risk in patients with acute respiratory distress syndrome. *Crit Care* 2015; **19**: 165.

17. A.A. Ferrando, C.A. Stuart, D.G. Brunder, G.R. Hillman. Magnetic resonance imaging quantitation of changes in muscle volume during 7 days of strict bed rest. *Aviat Space Environ Med* 1995; **66**: 976–81.

18. A. Pavy-Le Traon, M. Heer, M.V. Narici, et al. From space to Earth: advances in human physiology from 20 years of bed rest studies (1986–2006). *Eur J Appl Physiol* 2007; **101**: 143–94.

19. Z. Puthucheary, H. Montgomery, J. Moxham, et al. Structure to function: muscle failure in critically ill patients. *J Physiol* 2010; **588**: 4641–8.

20. H.E. Berg, L. Larsson, P.A. Tesch. Lower limb skeletal muscle function after 6 wk of bed rest. *J Appl Physiol (1985)* 1997; **82**: 182–8.

21. S.A. Bloomfield. Changes in musculoskeletal structure and function with prolonged bed rest. *Med Sci Sports Exerc* 1997; **29**: 197–206.

22. V.A. Convertino. Cardiovascular consequences of bed rest: effect on maximal oxygen uptake. *Med Sci Sports Exerc* 1997; **29**: 191–6.

23. G. Biolo, B. Ciocchi, M. Lebenstedt, et al. Short-term bed rest impairs amino acid-induced protein anabolism in humans. *J Physiol* 2004; **558**: 381–8.

24. N.M. Hamburg, C.J. McMackin, A.L. Huang, et al. Physical inactivity rapidly induces insulin resistance and microvascular dysfunction in healthy volunteers. *Arterioscler Thromb Vasc Biol* 2007; **27**: 2650–6.

25. D.M. Lipnicki, H.C. Gunga. Physical inactivity and cognitive functioning: results from bed rest studies. *Eur J Appl Physiol* 2009; **105**: 27–35.

26. D.C. Files, M.A. Sanchez, P.E. Morris. A conceptual framework: the early and late phases of skeletal muscle dysfunction in the acute respiratory distress syndrome. *Crit Care* 2015; **19**: 266.

27. B. Fazzini, T. Märkl, C. Costas, et al. The rate and assessment of muscle wasting during critical illness: a systematic review and meta-analysis. *Crit Care* 2023; **27**: 2.

28. R.E. Tanner, L.B. Brunker, J. Agergaard, et al. Age-related differences in lean mass, protein synthesis and skeletal muscle markers of proteolysis after bed rest and exercise rehabilitation. *J Physiol* 2015; **593**: 4259–73.

29. Z.A. Puthucheary, J. Rawal, M. McPhail, et al. Acute skeletal muscle wasting in critical illness. *JAMA* 2013; **310**: 1591–600.

30. S. Derde, G. Hermans, I. Derese, et al. Muscle atrophy and preferential loss of myosin in prolonged critically ill patients. *Crit Care Med* 2012; **40**: 79–89.

31. I. Vanhorebeek, N. Latronico, G. Van den Berghe. ICU-acquired weakness. *Intensive Care Med* 2020; **46**: 637–53.

32. J. Batt, M.S. Herridge, C.C. dos Santos. From skeletal muscle weakness to functional outcomes following critical illness: a translational biology perspective. *Thorax* 2019; **74**: 1091–8.

33. O. Friedrich, M.B. Reid, G. Van Den Berghe, et al. The sick and the weak: neuropathies/ myopathies in the critically ill. *Physiol Rev* 2015; **95**: 1025–109.

34. N. Latronico, C.F. Bolton. Critical illness polyneuropathy and myopathy: a major cause of muscle weakness and paralysis. *Lancet Neurol* 2011; **10**: 931–41.

35. M. Llano-Diez, G. Renaud, M. Andersson, et al. Mechanisms underlying ICU muscle wasting and effects of passive mechanical loading. *Crit Care* 2012; **16**: R209.

36. W.J. Z'Graggen, C.S. Lin, R.S. Howard, et al. Nerve excitability changes in critical illness polyneuropathy. *Brain* 2006; **129**: 2461–70.

37. C. dos Santos, S.N.A. Hussain, S. Mathur, et al. Mechanisms of chronic muscle

wasting and dysfunction after an intensive care unit stay. *Am J Respir Crit Care Med* 2016; **194**: 821–30.

38. J. Batt, C.C. dos Santos, J.I. Cameron, M.S. Herridge. Intensive care unit-acquired weakness: clinical phenotypes and molecular mechanisms. *Am J Respir Crit Care Med* 2013; **187**: 238–46.

39. R.D. Stevens, S.A. Marshall, D.R. Cornblath, et al. A framework for diagnosing and classifying intensive care unit-acquired weakness. *Crit Care Med* 2009; **37**: S299–308.

40. D. Lacomis, J.T. Petrella, M.J. Giuliani. Causes of neuromuscular weakness in the intensive care unit: a study of ninety-two patients. *Muscle Nerve* 1998; **21**: 610–17.

41. B. De Jonghe, T. Sharshar, J.P. Lefaucheur, et al. Paresis acquired in the intensive care unit: A prospective multicenter study. *JAMA* 2002; **288**: 2859–67.

42. J. Bednarik, Z. Lukas, P. Vondracek. Critical illness polyneuromyopathy: the electrophysiological components of a complex entity. *Intensive Care Med* 2003; **29**: 1505–14.

43. W. Trojaborg, L.H. Weimer, A.P. Hays. Electrophysiologic studies in critical illness associated weakness: myopathy or neuropathy – a reappraisal. *Clin Neurophysiol* 2001; **112**: 1586–93.

44. N. Latronico, F. Fenzi, D. Recupero, et al. Critical illness myopathy and neuropathy. *Lancet* 1996; **347**: 1579–82.

45. J.V. Campellone, D. Lacomis, D.J. Kramer, et al. Acute myopathy after liver transplantation. *Neurology* 1998; **50**: 46–53.

46. M. Tepper, S. Rakic, J.A. Haas, A.J. Woittiez. Incidence and onset of critical illness polyneuropathy in patients with septic shock. *Neth J Med* 2000; **56**: 211–14.

47. E. Fan, F. Cheek, L. Chlan, et al. An official American Thoracic Society Clinical Practice guideline: the diagnosis of intensive care unit-acquired weakness in adults. *Am J Respir Crit Care Med* 2014; **190**: 1437–46.

48. R.T. Appleton, J. Kinsella, T. Quasim. The incidence of intensive care unit-acquired weakness syndromes: A systematic review. *J Intensive Care Soc* 2015; **16**: 126–36.

49. L. Wieske, D.S. Dettling-Ihnenfeldt, C. Verhamme, et al. Impact of ICU-acquired weakness on post-ICU physical functioning: a follow-up study. *Crit Care* 2015; **19**: 196.

50. G. Hermans, H. Van Mechelen, B. Clerckx, et al. Acute outcomes and 1-year mortality of intensive care unit-acquired weakness: a cohort study and propensity-matched analysis. *Am J Respir Crit Care Med* 2014; **190**: 410–20.

51. S.M. Parry, M. Huang, D.M. Needham. Evaluating physical functioning in critical care: considerations for clinical practice and research. *Crit Care* 2017; **21**: 249.

52. F. González-Seguel, E.J. Corner, C. Merino-Osorio. International classification of functioning, disability, and health domains of 60 physical functioning measurement instruments used during the adult intensive care unit stay: a scoping review. *Phys Ther* 2019; **99**: 627–40.

53. S.M. Parry, S. Berney, C.L. Granger, et al. A new two-tier strength assessment approach to the diagnosis of weakness in intensive care: an observational study. *Crit Care* 2015; **19**: 52.

54. N.A. Ali, J.M. O'Brien, Jr., S.P. Hoffmann, et al. Acquired weakness, handgrip strength, and mortality in critically ill patients. *Am J Respir Crit Care Med* 2008; **178**: 261–8.

55. S.M. Parry, C.L. Granger, S. Berney, et al. Assessment of impairment and activity limitations in the critically ill: a systematic review of measurement instruments and their clinimetric properties. *Intensive Care Med* 2015; **41**: 744–62.

56. M. Mourtzakis, S. Parry, B. Connolly, Z. Puthucheary. Skeletal muscle ultrasound in critical care: a tool in need of translation. *Ann Am Thorac Soc* 2017; **14**: 1495–503.

57. N.C. Joyce, B. Oskarsson, L.W. Jin. Muscle biopsy evaluation in neuromuscular disorders. *Phys Med Rehabil Clin N Am* 2012; **23**: 609–31.

58. G. Tzanis, I. Vasileiadis, D. Zervakis, et al. Maximum inspiratory pressure, a surrogate parameter for the assessment of ICU-acquired weakness. *BMC Anesthesiol* 2011; **11**: 14.

59. M. Dres, B. Jung, N. Molinari, et al. Respective contribution of intensive care unit-acquired limb muscle and severe diaphragm weakness on weaning outcome and mortality: a post hoc analysis of two cohorts. *Crit Care* 2019; **23**: 370.

60. C. Saccheri, E. Morawiec, J. Delemazure, et al. ICU-acquired weakness, diaphragm dysfunction and long-term outcomes of critically ill patients. *Ann Intensive Care* 2020; **10**: 1.

61. M. Dres, B.P. Dubé, J. Mayaux, et al. Coexistence and impact of limb muscle and diaphragm weakness at time of liberation from mechanical ventilation in medical intensive care unit patients. *Am J Respir Crit Care Med* 2017; **195**: 57–66.

62. B. Jung, P.H. Moury, M. Mahul, et al. Diaphragmatic dysfunction in patients with ICU-acquired weakness and its impact on extubation failure. *Intensive Care Med* 2016; **42**: 853–61.

63. F. González-Seguel, C. Cáceres-Parra. Physical functioning assessment tools in critical care: a wide national survey in Chile during the COVID-19 pandemic. *Rev Med Chil* 2022; **150**: 1565–74.

64. M.N. Bertozzi, S. Cagide, E. Navarro, M. Accoce. Description of physical rehabilitation in intensive care units in Argentina: usual practice and during the COVID-19 pandemic. Online survey. *Rev Bras Ter Intensiva* 2021; **33**: 188–95.

65. K. Nawata, N. Nakanishi, S. Inoue, et al. Current practice and barriers in the implementation of ultrasound-based assessment of muscle mass in Japan: a nationwide, web-based cross-sectional study. *PLoS One* 2022; **17**: e0276855.

66. T. Yang, Z. Li, L. Jiang, et al. Risk factors for intensive care unit-acquired weakness: a systematic review and meta-analysis. *Acta Neurol Scand* 2018; **138**: 104–14.

67. B. De Jonghe, J.-C. Lacherade, M.-C. Durand, T. Sharshar. Critical illness neuromuscular syndromes. *Neurologic Clinics* 2008; **26**: 507–20.

68. R. Fuentes-Aspe, R. Gutierrez-Arias, F. González-Seguel, et al. Which factors are associated with acquired weakness in the ICU? An overview of systematic reviews and meta-analyses. *J Intensive Care* 2024; **12**: 33.

69. D.J. Lederer, S.C. Bell, R.D. Branson, et al. Control of confounding and reporting of results in causal inference studies. Guidance for authors from editors of respiratory, sleep, and critical care journals. *Ann Am Thorac Soc* 2019; **16**: 22–8.

Chapter 5

Frailty in the Critically Ill

Joshua I. Gordon and Nathan E. Brummel

Introduction

Millions of Americans survive critical illness each year, only to be faced with new life-altering impairments in physical, cognitive, and mental health function that alter their ability to live independently and lead to poor health-related quality of life and financial toxicity [1,2,3,4,5,6,7]. The mechanisms underlying these sequelae of critical illness are incompletely understood but are believed to be multifactorial and develop as a function of the severity of the critical illness, the care delivered in the intensive care unit (ICU), and the patient's underlying vulnerability [4].

While severity of illness scores and the iatrogenic harms of factors such as sedation, delirium, and immobility are known to most ICU clinicians, many providers are less well-versed in appreciating patients' pre-existing vulnerability. Clinically, this underlying vulnerability can be understood as the syndrome of frailty [8,9]. Over the past decade, emerging data have demonstrated how common frailty is among those admitted to the ICU, the independent association between frailty and worse outcomes in those with critical illness, and the role of critical illness in the development of newly acquired frailty, highlighting the importance of this under-recognized syndrome.

This chapter defines frailty and describes its impact on outcomes in critically ill patients. We explore two different conceptual models of this syndrome, review validated tools used to assess frailty, and discuss their application to those with critical illness and survivors of critical illness. Finally, because there are limited data on interventions to reduce frailty in those with critical illness and survivors, we will discuss interventions shown to reduce frailty in community-dwelling older adults and their potential use in those affected by critical illness.

Defining Frailty

Frailty is a multidimensional syndrome that is characterized by the loss of physiologic reserve, leading to the inability to maintain or restore homeostasis in the setting of an acute stressor [10]; consequently, frailty often leads to a more consequential worsening of health status following an illness or injury. As demonstrated in Figure 5.1, a fit patient (dashed line) who develops a minor illness, such as a urinary tract infection, may suffer a slight decline in their functional abilities but soon returns to their baseline functional status. In contrast, a patient with frailty (solid line) who suffers the same minor illness not only begins with a lower baseline functional status but also suffers a much larger decline, which is slower to recover and may never return to the previous baseline [11,12].

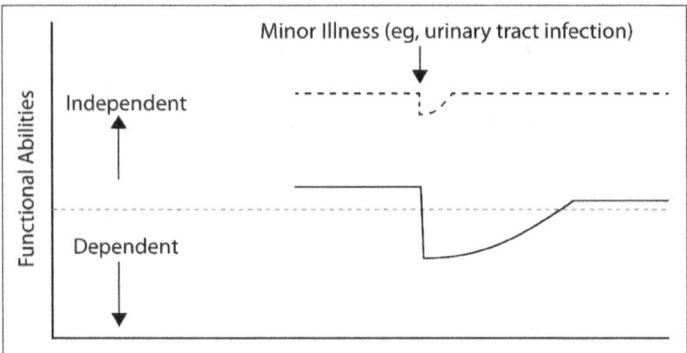

Figure 5.1 Change in function according to frailty status in response to a minor insult.
The dashed line represents a fit person, who, in response to a minor illness (e.g., a urinary tract infection), suffers a small decrement in their functional status but recovers quickly to their baseline functional status. In contrast, the solid line represents a person with frailty, who experiences a much larger impairment in their physical function from the same minor illness, is much slower to recover, and does not return to their pre-illness baseline.[11] From: A. Clegg, J. Young, S. Iliffe, et al. Frailty in elderly people. *Lancet* 2013; **381**: 752–62. Reproduced with permission from Elsevier.

Epidemiology

In community-dwelling older adults aged 65 years and older, the prevalence of frailty ranges between 4% and 16% and increases with age [13,14,15,16,17]. Although historically viewed as an age-related syndrome, emerging data suggest that even younger people can develop frailty; a study of participants enrolled in the UK Biobank study showed the prevalence of frailty in middle-aged adults (i.e., 37 to 65 years old) to be 3% [18].

Over the past decade, studies have shown frailty to be common among those admitted to the ICU. Data from a systematic review and meta-analysis of 10 observational cohort studies including over 3000 patients admitted to the ICU showed that frailty was present in 30% [19]. Additionally, one cohort study reported that half of the patients with frailty at the time of ICU admission were younger than 65 years old [20]. The high prevalence of frailty in those admitted to the ICU suggests that those with frailty are less likely to tolerate insults and injuries before developing organ failures that are pathognomonic of critical illness. While frailty is common among those admitted to an ICU, emerging data also show that critical illness leads to a rapid acceleration in the development of frailty. Recent cohort studies that measured frailty at ICU admission and during follow-up show that frailty is present in 20% to 40% of survivors of critical illness, including up to 60% of those who were not frail before their ICU admission [21,22,23]. Thus, the relationship between frailty and critical illness is bi-directional: frailty increases susceptibility to critical illness, and critical illness, in turn, can drive the development of frailty.

Outcomes Associated with Frailty Present at ICU Admission

Those with frailty who develop critical illness suffer worse outcomes, both during and after their critical illness. For example, those with frailty have longer hospital lengths of stay and are also more likely to be institutionalized following hospital discharge [20,23,24,25,26,27,28]. Furthermore, the presence of frailty at ICU admission is associated with greater mortality, even after accounting for traditional mortality risk factors, such as age, comorbidities, and severity of illness. A Canadian cohort study found that frailty was associated with a near doubling of the odds of dying in the hospital (32% versus 16%; adjusted odds ratio [OR] 1.81, 95% CI 1.09–3.01). A second French cohort study showed that in-hospital mortality increased with the severity of frailty (p=0.003) [29,30], and a third from southeast Asia found that those with frailty had a greater 30-day mortality compared to those who were not frail (49% versus 28.5%, p=0.02) [30]. Frailty is also associated with longer-term mortality; multiple cohorts demonstrate that those with frailty who become critically ill have 1.5 to 1.8 times greater odds of death in the year following hospital discharge [20,29,31,32,33,34,35].

Those with frailty who become critically ill are also more likely to suffer new or worsened dependencies in activities of daily living (ADLs) and instrumental activities of daily living (IADLs) [20,26,35]. In a study of over 300 patients who had been admitted to the ICU during the Precipitating Events Project, Ferrante and colleagues found that frailty and pre-frailty (i.e., frailty symptoms that do not meet the full syndromal definition of frailty) were associated with a 1.4 times greater risk and a 1.3 times greater risk of developing worsened dependencies in ADLs, respectively, when compared to those who were not frail [26]. Similarly, combined data from the BRAIN-ICU and MIND-ICU studies reported that more severe frailty was associated with a 1.2 times greater risk of new or worsened disabilities in IADLs [20]. Finally, Heyland and colleagues found that frailty was an independent predictor of poor recovery (e.g., reduced physical function or death) in a cohort of Canadian older adults admitted to the ICU, such that those with more severe frailty were 68% less likely to achieve functional recovery [34].

Critical Illness-Associated Frailty

Though most frailty research in those with critical illness is focused on the presence of frailty at the time of ICU admission, emerging data suggest that frailty is worsened or newly acquired in a large number of survivors. A Dutch study of 1,300 survivors of critical illness demonstrated higher frailty scores after ICU admission, which peaked at hospital discharge and modestly improved over the ensuing months [21]. Among those whose frailty scores improved, the majority had a planned ICU admission (e.g., following elective surgery), while those with an unplanned ICU admission (e.g., unexpected critical illness) were more likely to have higher frailty scores (i.e., more severe frailty) in the year after their ICU stay [21]. A second multicenter cohort of 567 survivors of critical illness enrolled from ICUs at academic, community, and Veterans Administration (VA) hospitals in the United States found that 40% had frailty at one year, 60% of whom were not frail before ICU admission [23]. In a multicenter Canadian study, frailty was present in 45%, 68%, and 43% at ICU admission, hospital discharge, and six months after discharge, respectively [22]. While the similar percentages of patients with frailty at ICU admission and at six-month follow-up seem to suggest no effect of critical illness on the development of frailty, 50% of those with frailty at ICU admission died. Therefore, because half of those who were frail at ICU admission died (and therefore did not participate in follow-up), the similar proportion of frailty at six months represents an increase in the number who developed frailty as a result of their critical illness [33].

Conceptual Models of Frailty

There are two conceptual models to describe frailty: the physical frailty phenotype model and the deficit accumulation model (see Figure 5.2) [36]. The physical frailty

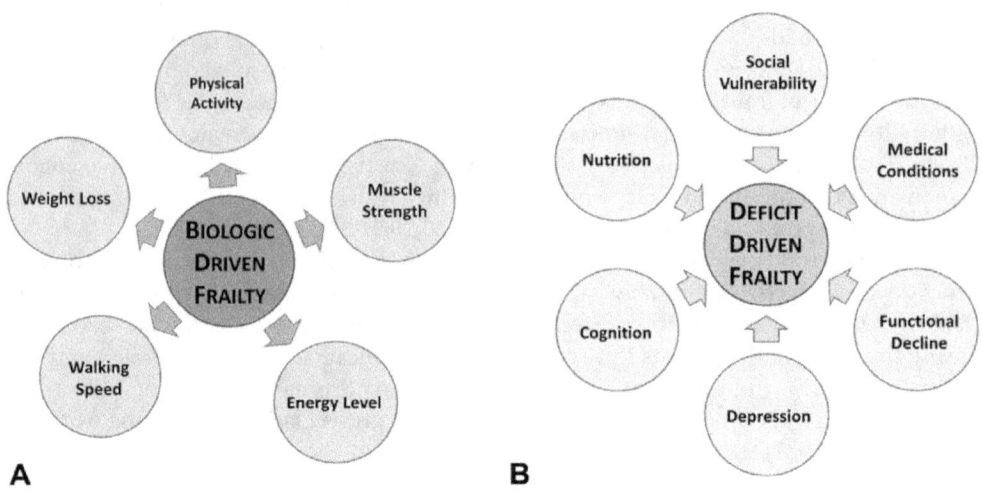

Figure 5.2 Conceptual models of frailty.
Panel A illustrates the frailty phenotype model. In this model, an underlying syndrome leads to the characteristics of frailty: low muscle strength, low energy levels, slow walking speed, weight loss, and low physical activity. Panel B illustrates the deficit accumulation model. This model suggests that frailty is driven by an accumulation of deficits, such that the more deficits one has, the less likely one is able to tolerate additional deficits. Note the different directions of the arrows between the two panels. The arrows in panel A point outward, suggesting that frailty arises from a biological process leading to specific physical manifestations. In contrast, the arrows in panel B point inwards, suggesting that frailty arises from outside factors [36]. From: T.N. Robinson, J.D. Walston, N.E. Brummel, et al. Frailty for surgeons: Review of a national institute on aging conference on frailty for specialists. *J Am Coll Surg* 2015; **221**: 1083–92. Reproduced with permission from Wolters Kluwer Health, Inc.

phenotype model hypothesizes that frailty arises as the result of an underlying biological syndrome that manifests as a combination of unintentional weight loss, exhaustion, muscle weakness, slow walking speed, and low physical activity [8]. In contrast, the deficit accumulation model hypothesizes that frailty is the result of the accumulation of health deficits, including chronic diseases, cognitive and physical impairments, poor nutritional status, abnormal laboratory values, and disabilities, such that the more deficits one has, the less likely one is able to tolerate additional deficits, and the more likely one is to be frail [37].

While both of these definitions represent the multiple dimensions of frailty, they identify different populations. Xue and colleagues analyzed data collected from over 5,000 participants enrolled in the Longitudinal Cardiovascular Health Study, which assessed both the physical frailty phenotype and deficit accumulation models and found that 7% of participants were identified as frail using the phenotype model and 8% were identified as frail using the deficit accumulation model [38]. Of those identified as having frailty by either model, only 12% were classified as having frailty by both, and agreement between which participants were frail according to both models was poor (Kappa = 0.16 [95% CI 0.12 to 0.20]). Participants with discrepant frailty (i.e., frail by one model but not the other) differed in important ways with respect to age, sex, health status, and cognitive function. While both models were associated with greater mortality and disability, associations were stronger among those considered frail by the physical phenotype model [38]. Thus, although both models of frailty are valid means with which to identify this syndrome, they cannot be used interchangeably.

Assessing Frailty

There are numerous tools that have been validated to measure frailty in community-dwelling older adults. As interest in capturing frailty in those admitted to the ICU has grown, however, several tools have been studied to assess frailty in those affected by critical illness, reflecting both the frailty phenotype and deficit accumulation approaches. A systematic review of 57 studies conducted by Bertschi and colleagues found that 19 different methods were used to assess frailty in critically ill patients. The most commonly used tool was the Clinical Frailty Scale (CFS; n=35, 60.3%), followed by the Frailty Phenotype (n=6, 10.3%) and the Frailty Index (n=5, 8.6%) [39]. We describe here these methods and highlight important nuances for their use in assessing frailty in the critically ill and survivors of critical illness.

Assessing Frailty Using the Phenotypic Approach

The frailty phenotype assesses five different symptoms of frailty emanating from the underlying biological syndrome: unintentional weight loss, muscle weakness, slow walking speed, self-reported exhaustion, and low physical activity (see Table 5.1). As originally derived by Fried and colleagues using data from the Cardiovascular Health Study, each criterion is scored as being present or absent according to specific cut-points (e.g., weight loss of more than 5% in the past year, fatigue present on four or more days per week, and handgrip strength, walking speed, and/or physical activity in the bottom quintile). The presence of three or more of these criteria is suggestive of frailty.

Classically, the first three symptoms are assessed using performance-based measures (i.e., measuring body weight using a scale, handgrip strength using handgrip dynamometry, and walking speed using the time it takes to walk four meters), while the latter two symptoms are measured using questionnaires. Though the frailty phenotype has been applied to the critically ill [26], few patients will have undergone the necessary performance-based measures shortly before developing critical illness. Moreover, because performance-based measures are confounded by critical illness and its treatment, it is difficult, if not impossible, to assess the frailty phenotype as it was originally conceived in the critically ill [8].

To overcome this obstacle, several questionnaire-based approaches have been used [29,31]. Le Maguet and colleagues adapted the frailty phenotype by substituting measurements of handgrip strength and walking speed with questions about difficulty rising from a chair and a subjective slowing in walking speed over the prior six months, respectively (see Table 5.1) [29]. Hope and colleagues also assessed for muscle weakness by asking about difficulty rising from a chair without using the arms, and in lieu of measuring walking speed, they assessed for impaired mobility by asking whether the patient had fallen in the past year [31]. These questionnaire-based approaches to measuring the frailty phenotype in those with critical illness show predictive validity for both mortality and disability in survivors of critical illness, suggesting that they are a reasonable approach to identifying preexisting frailty in the critically ill. Nevertheless, further studies are needed to validate this approach, including questionnaires that can be answered by well-chosen surrogates for patients incapable of participating in the assessment [40].

Assessing Frailty Using the Deficit Accumulation Approach

There are two major tools that assess frailty using the deficit accumulation approach: the Clinical Frailty Scale and its parent tool, the frailty index.

Table 5.1 The frailty phenotype

Frailty Characteristic	Frailty Phenotype (using performance-based measures)	Questionnaire-based Frailty (for use in those with critical illness)	Score
Weight Loss	Unintentional (not due to dieting or exercise) weight loss of ≥10 lbs (4.5 kg) or more than 5% of body weight in the prior year	Unintentional (not due to dieting or exercise) weight loss of ≥10lbs (4.5 kg) or more than 5% of body weight in the prior year	Yes = 1 No = 0
Muscle Weakness	Handgrip strength measured by dynamometer (adjusted for gender and body mass index) in the lowest 20% of cohort	Difficulty rising from a chair	Yes = 1 No = 0
Slow Walking Speed	Time to walk 4 meters (adjusted for gender and standard height) in the slowest 20% of cohort	Subjective slowing of walking speed (during the last 6 months, with difficulties walking and with an aid/assistive device) and/or the occurrence of fall(s)	Yes = 1 No = 0
Low Physical Activity	Kilocalories expended per week in the lowest 20% of cohort	Discontinued daily leisure activities, such as walking or gardening, and/or a weekly athletic activity.	Yes = 1 No = 0
Exhaustion	How often in the past 3 months did one feel that everything one does is an effort and/or that one cannot get going: Rarely or not at all = 0; Occasionally = 1; Often = 2; Usually = 3	How often in the past 3 months did one feel that everything one does is an effort and/or that one cannot get going: Rarely or not at all = 0; Occasionally = 1; Often = 2; Usually = 3	Score of 2 or 3 to either question = 1

The first column presents the phenotypic symptom of frailty. The second column presents the original criteria developed and validated by Fried and colleagues (from: L.P. Fried, C.M. Tangen, J. Walston, et al., Frailty in older adults: evidence of a phenotype. *J Geron Med Sci* 2001; **56A**: M146–156). The third column presents a questionnaire-based frailty phenotype assessment used in patients with critical illness where performance-based assessments of body weight, handgrip strength, and walking speed are difficult. For either assessment, a point is assigned for each positive criteria. A score of 3 or more indicates frailty, scores of 1 or 2 indicates pre-frailty, and scores of 0 indicate robustness [29]. From: P. Le Maguet, A. Roquilly, S. Lasocki, et al. Prevalence and impact of frailty on mortality in elderly ICU patients: a prospective, multicenter, observational study. *Intensive Care Med* 2014; **40**: 674–82. Reproduced with permission from Springer Nature.

Clinical Frailty Scale

Developed in 2005 using data from the Canadian Study of Health and Aging, the CFS is a widely used and validated judgment-based frailty assessment tool that can be completed using routinely collected clinical data [37,41,42]. The CFS considers multiple domains leading to frailty, including chronic illnesses, physical function and disability, and cognition. Each of these are synthesized to generate a score ranging from 1 (very fit) to 9 (severely frail) [37]. Descriptions of each level of frailty are provided in Figure 5.3.

The CFS is the most widely used frailty assessment tool in the ICU setting given its ability to be measured using data from the patient, their surrogate, and/or clinical data, thereby overcoming the obstacle of obtaining reliable information for patients who are incapable of participating in the assessment. Nevertheless, several important nuances to assessing frailty with the CFS warrant further discussion. First, though the CFS is judgment-based, it must be described using clinical data and not supposition. Second, the CFS should be used to reflect a patient's baseline health status (i.e., how the patient was doing *before* they became ill), as even the most fit persons can appear frail when acutely ill. Third, the CFS is not designed to be used with persons whose disabilities reflect a single-system problem (e.g., spinal cord injury) or developmental delay rather than an age-related accumulation of health deficits. Finally, although most patients are easily categorized by a single score, some may meet two categories equally well; if this is the case, then it is best to assign the patient a higher (i.e., greater) frailty score.

Frailty Index

The frailty index is the parent tool of the CFS and consists of an assessment of anywhere from 30 to 70 potential deficits. The index is calculated as the ratio of deficits that are present in the patient to the total number of deficits assessed [43]. The higher the frailty index, the more likely the patient is to be frail. In most studies, an index at or above 0.2 is consistent with frailty. As with all frailty tools, the frailty index was originally derived and validated in community-dwelling older adults, although the frailty index has been adapted for use in those with critical illness (see Table 5.2) [34]. Lower scores on the frailty index are associated with improved physical recovery following critical illness [34]; in contrast, higher scores are associated with higher ICU and long-term mortality and a lower likelihood of being discharged home [28,44].

A recent multicenter Canadian study found that, compared to the CFS, the frailty index identified a higher proportion of patients as frail both during critical illness and afterwards (30% versus 45%, 55% versus 68%, and 34% versus 43% at ICU admission, hospital discharge, and six-month follow-up, respectively), suggesting that the more detailed approach of the frailty index may detect more subtle cases of frailty and may be more suitable for research studies. In contrast, the CFS may be more rapidly assessed and is thus more suitable for a busy ICU environment. Nevertheless, a second important point when deciding between these two approaches is that even though the frailty index is more cumbersome, the CFS does not provide insight into the mechanisms by which frailty develops, making it difficult to derive interventions. In contrast, by measuring individual deficits, the frailty index can identify specific potential targets for intervention.

Frailty Management and Interventions

To date, the study of frailty in the setting of critical illness is largely confined to observational cohort studies describing the prevalence and outcomes of this syndrome. Thus,

CLINICAL FRAILTY SCALE

	1	**VERY FIT**	People who are robust, active, energetic and motivated. They tend to exercise regularly and are among the fittest for their age.
	2	**FIT**	People who have **no active disease symptoms** but are less fit than category 1. Often, they exercise or are very **active occasionally**, e.g., seasonally.
	3	**MANAGING WELL**	People whose **medical problems are well controlled**, even if occasionally symptomatic, but often **not regularly active** beyond routine walking.
	4	**LIVING WITH VERY MILD FRAILTY**	Previously "vulnerable," this category marks early transition from complete independence. While **not dependent** on others for daily help, often **symptoms limit activities**. A common complaint is being "slowed up" and/or being tired during the day.
	5	**LIVING WITH MILD FRAILTY**	People who often have **more evident slowing**, and need help with **high order instrumental activities of daily living** (finances, transportation, heavy housework). Typically, mild frailty progressively impairs shopping and walking outside alone, meal preparation, medications and begins to restrict light housework.
	6	**LIVING WITH MODERATE FRAILTY**	People who need help with **all outside activities** and with **keeping house**. Inside, they often have problems with stairs and need **help with bathing** and might need minimal assistance (cuing, standby) with dressing.
	7	**LIVING WITH SEVERE FRAILTY**	**Completely dependent for personal care**, from whatever cause (physical or cognitive). Even so, they seem stable and not at high risk of dying (within ~ 6 months).
	8	**LIVING WITH VERY SEVERE FRAILTY**	Completely dependent for personal care and approaching end of life. Typically, they could not recover even from a minor illness.
	9	**TERMINALLY ILL**	Approaching the end of life. This category applies to people with a **life expectancy <6 months**, who are **not otherwise living with severe frailty**. Many terminally ill people can still exercise until very close to death.

SCORING FRAILTY IN PEOPLE WITH DEMENTIA

The degree of frailty generally corresponds to the degree of dementia. Common **symptoms in mild dementia** include forgetting the details of a recent event, though still remembering the event itself, repeating the same question/story and social withdrawal.

In **moderate dementia**, recent memory is very impaired, even though they seemingly can remember their past life events well. They can do personal care with prompting.

In **severe dementia**, they cannot do personal care without help.

In **very severe dementia** they are often bedfast. Many are virtually mute.

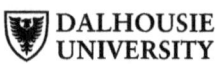 DALHOUSIE UNIVERSITY

Clinical Frailty Scale ©2005–2020 Rockwood, Version 2.0 (EN). All rights reserved. For permission: www.geriatricmedicineresearch.ca Rockwood K et al. A global clinical measure of fitness and frailty in elderly people. CMAJ 2005;173:489–495.

Figure 5.3 Clinical frailty scale.
The Clinical Frailty Scale is a 9-point judgment-based frailty assessment tool that uses clinical data collected from a patient, their surrogate, clinical assessments, and the medical record to assign a score based on the descriptions provided. For those with critical illness, it is important to remember to assess a patient in relation to how they were doing in the weeks before they became critically ill [37]. From: K. Rockwood, X. Song, C. MacKnight, et al. A global clinical measure of fitness and frailty in elderly people. *CMAJ* 2005; **173**: 489–95. Reproduced with permission.

interventions to improve outcomes in those with frailty who are admitted to the ICU and in those with newly acquired frailty as the result of critical illness have not been tested. In community-dwelling older adults, interventions are largely tailored around three key areas: physical activity, nutrition, and palliative care, which have been, alone or in combination, shown to reduce the burden of frailty. This section discusses how these different interventions can be used to meaningfully help patients with pre-existing or newly acquired frailty.

Physical Activity Interventions

Given the strong link between frailty and poor physical function, it stands to reason that those with frailty who become critically ill would be the least likely to withstand further loss of muscle mass and strength and therefore would be the most likely to benefit from interventions such as early mobility. Nevertheless, most studies of early mobility have not evaluated the effects of this intervention specifically in those with frailty [45,46,47,48,49] A single observational cohort study, however, evaluated the effect of early mobility according to frailty status in 264 patients admitted to a cardiovascular ICU [50]. Those with frailty not only safely tolerated early mobility interventions, but they also experienced similar improvements in level of function as their non-frail counterparts. While further study is needed, these data suggest that frailty should not serve as a barrier to early mobility and that the potential benefits to early mobility extend to those with frailty.

Though not directly studied in survivors of critical illness who develop frailty, two lines of evidence suggest that physical activity interventions could improve or reverse frailty, thereby reducing the burden of ICU survivorship. For example, a meta-analysis of ten randomized controlled trials by Kidd and colleagues found that physical activity interventions, either alone or in combination with other therapies (e.g., nutrition), were effective at helping community-dwelling older adults with frailty maintain independence [51]. A randomized controlled trial by Fiatarone and colleagues demonstrated an improvement in muscle strength and stair-climbing power in community-dwelling older adults with frailty who received resistance training compared with those who did not [52].

In patients with both chronic lung disease and frailty, pulmonary rehabilitation offers a means by which to reduce frailty [53]. In six studies reviewed as part of an American Thoracic Society workshop on pulmonary rehabilitation in those with chronic lung disease, all six demonstrated benefits of pulmonary rehabilitation on gait speed and sit-to-stand performance in those with frailty, and those with frailty showed greater improvements than those without frailty [53]. While these data suggest that interventions directed at increasing physical activity in those with frailty related to age and chronic lung disease may improve outcomes, no study to date has specifically evaluated the effects of this intervention on recovery from critical illness-related frailty, an area in need of future study. Nevertheless, given the safety of these interventions in other populations with frailty, a personalized approach to physical rehabilitation focused on improving the physical symptoms of frailty (i.e., muscle weakness, fatigue, and slow walking speed) should be considered in survivors of critical illness with frailty.

Nutrition Interventions

In community-dwelling older adults, most of those with frailty have a poor nutritional status, and most of those with malnutrition are frail. Thus, those with preexisting frailty who become critically ill are at greater risk of becoming malnourished, and because critical

Table 5.2 A frailty index for patients with critical illness

#	Item
1	Overall health of the patient?
2	Do you think the patient was depressed?
3	Do you think the patient worried a lot or got anxious?
4	Do you think the patient felt exhausted or tired all the time?
5	Did the patient have sleep problems?
6	Did the patient have problems with memory or thinking?
7	Did the patient have any problems speaking to make him/herself understood?
8	Did the patient have difficulty hearing?
9	Did the patient have problems with eyesight (even when wearing glasses)?
10	Did the patient having problems with balance?
11	Did the patient complain of feeling dizzy or lightheaded?
12	Did the patient need assistance of a person or aid to prevent falling?
13	Did the patient hold onto furniture to keep from failing?
14	Was the patient able to walk alone?
15	Was the patient able to get out of a bed or chair alone?
16	Did the patient have problems with bowel control?
17	Did the patient have problems with bladder control?
18	Did the patient experience any unplanned weight loss in the last 6 months?
19	What was the patient's food intake in the week prior to ICU admission?
20	Was the patient able to carry out some day-to-day tasks?
21	Was the patient able to feed himself/herself?
22	Was the patient able to take a bath or shower?
23	Was the patient able to dress himself/herself?
24	Was the patient able to drive?
25	Was the patient able to look after his/her own medications?
26	Was the patient able to do day-to-day shopping?
27	Was the patient able to do day-to-day household cleaning?
28	Was the patient able to cook well enough to maintain his/her nutrition?
29	Was the patient able to look after his/her own banking and financial affairs?
30	Overall health of the patient?
31	Did the patient have a myocardial infarction?
32	Does the patient have congestive heart failure?
33	Does the patient have peripheral vascular disease?
34	Does the patient have cerebrovascular disease +/- hemiplegia?

Table 5.2 (cont.)

#	Item
35	Does the patient have dementia?
36	Does the patient have chronic pulmonary disease?
37	Does the patient have connective tissue disease?
38	Does the patient have ulcer disease?
39	Does the patient have any liver disease?
40	Does the patient have diabetes?
41	Does the patient have moderate or several renal disease?
42	Does the patient have diabetes with end organ damage?
43	Does the patient have any tumor?

For the Frailty Index, Heyland and colleagues created a list of 43 potential health deficits. Each item is scored as present/absent. The total number of deficits that are present is then divided by 43 to generate the index. Scores of 0 to 0.19 indicate mild frailty, 0.2 to 0.39 indicate moderate frailty, and scores of 0.4 or more indicate severe frailty. For example, if a patient had nine deficits present, the index would be 9/43= 0.2. [34] From: D.K. Heyland, A. Garland, S.M. Bagshaw, et al. Recovery after critical illness in patients aged 80 years or older: a multi-center prospective observational cohort study. *Intensive Care Med* 2015; **41**: 1911–20. Reproduced with permission from Springer Nature.

illness leads to an inherently catabolic state, poor nutritional status may be an important driver of the development of critical illness-associated frailty. Therefore, nutrition is a potentially important area of intervention to combat physical decline and frailty (see Chapters 7 and 40 for additional information).

Rahman and colleagues explored the effects of nutritional intake among those at high nutritional risk using the Nutritional Risk in Critically Ill (NUTRIC) score and found that six-month survival was greater among those at high nutritional risk who received a larger proportion of prescribed nutrition (as defined according to expert guidelines) [54]. Although the NUTRIC score does not specifically identify those with frailty, persons with higher NUTRIC scores in this study were older, and three-fourths had more than two comorbidities, suggesting a population at high risk for frailty. This research group then built on this work by exploring the effects of nutrition in those with high nutritional risk, sarcopenia, and frailty in an observational cohort study [55]. Among those with all three syndromes, mortality was greater than those with any one syndrome alone. In those with more severe nutritional risk, sarcopenia, and frailty, greater caloric and protein intake were associated with 30–40% greater odds of being discharged alive from the hospital by day 60 (hazard ratio [HR] 1.3 [95% CI 1.04 to 1.6], p=0.02 and 1.4 [95%CI 1.04 to 1.8], p=0.03, for calories and protein, respectively). These data suggest that identifying those with frailty at ICU admission and providing adequate nutritional intake (i.e., meeting caloric and protein needs as defined by expert guidelines) may improve mortality, although further study is needed.

Nutritional supplementation has been used to prevent the development of frailty in community-dwelling older adults, suggesting that similar strategies could be used during critical illness to prevent the development of critical illness-associated frailty. For example, several studies show the benefits of augmented protein intake, omega-3 fatty acid supplementation, and vitamin D supplementation in the prevention of sarcopenia (i.e., loss of muscle mass and strength) and functional decline [56]. Nevertheless, data from interventional nutritional studies investigating increased protein provision or supplementation with omega-3 fatty acids or vitamin D in the critically ill have shown either no benefit or worse long-term outcomes in survivors [57,58,59]. To date, interventional nutrition studies have not specifically explored the effects of these supplemental nutritional interventions on those with frailty, highlighting an important research gap.

Finally, among survivors of critical illness with frailty, nutritional interventions could serve as a means by which to aid in recovery. For example, a scoping review of interventions in community-dwelling older adults found that nutritional education, the Mediterranean diet, and protein supplementation, deployed as part of multicomponent interventions (e.g., along with physical activity, psychological interventions, social skills, and reducing polypharmacy), were effective at improving frailty symptoms [60]. Though the multicomponent interventions mirror many of those already in place across ICU follow-up and long-COVID clinics, few of these programs report use of nutritional interventions [61]. Further study is needed to evaluate whether interventions shown to reduce age-related frailty may also be effective in mitigating critical illness-associated frailty.

Palliative Care Interventions

Given the strong association between frailty and mortality in those with critical illness, frailty may serve as a useful trigger to screen patients for palliative care needs. Hope and colleagues used the CFS to explore the additive benefit of frailty status compared to other common triggers for palliative care consultation in those with critical illness (e.g., two or more comorbidities, advanced malignancy, cardiac arrest, intracranial hemorrhage treated with mechanical ventilation, and anoxic brain injury) [62]. In this cohort, those with frailty were nearly twice as likely to have a specialty palliative care consultation than those without frailty. Despite the higher rate of specialty palliative care in those with frailty, consultation rates were still lower than those with traditional palliative care triggers, despite having similar rates of six-month mortality. These data indicate that frailty is potentially an underutilized trigger for palliative care consultation in those with critical illness.

Perhaps surprisingly, even those with the most severe forms of frailty are more likely to survive than die in the year following a critical illness [20]; therefore, while end-of-life discussions are an important component of palliative care, symptom management and tailoring ICU treatments to a patient's values and preferences are equally important palliative care interventions. For example, in an observational cohort study of those admitted to ICUs in the Canadian province of Alberta, Montgomery and colleagues observed that frail patients were less likely to receive vasoactive medications and invasive mechanical ventilation than their non-frail counterparts, suggesting that frailty status is an important data point that influences specific treatments received in the ICU [63]. Moreover, use of frailty status to guide discussions about long-term functional decline and disability after hospital discharge may aid patients and their families in their decisions to receive or forgo specific ICU treatments, particularly in those who are wary of a high burden of treatments or interventions [64].

After ICU discharge, those with frailty continue to have palliative care needs. Pollack and colleagues assessed symptom burden prior to hospital discharge among older survivors of critical illness with frailty as measured by the frailty phenotype [65]. On average, those with frailty had significantly higher physical and emotional symptoms than those without frailty, including greater fatigue, drowsiness, and anxiety, and worse overall well-being; in the majority, these symptoms persisted or worsened after hospital discharge. These data suggest a large burden of palliative care needs present in survivors of critical illness with frailty, supporting the idea that survivors of critical illness should undergo routine symptom screening, and if warranted, referral to palliative care specialists (see Chapter 47 for additional information).

Conclusions

Frailty is increasingly recognized as a syndrome that affects large numbers of both the critically ill and survivors of critical illness. Validated tools exist to identify frailty in those affected by critical illness based on both the frailty phenotype and the deficit accumulation models of frailty. While effective interventions such as physical activity, nutritional support, and palliative care can reduce age-related frailty among community-dwelling older adults, the efficacy of these interventions in those along the continuum of critical illness is an area of ongoing study.

Key Points

1. Frailty is present in one out of three patients admitted to an ICU.
2. The presence of frailty at ICU admission is associated with greater mortality, and among survivors of critical illness, greater disability in activities of daily living and instrumental activities of daily living.
3. Frailty is present in 40% of survivors of critical illness, the majority of whom were not frail before they became critically ill, suggesting a rapidly accelerated, critical illness-associated form of frailty.
4. Interventions adopted from those used in community-dwelling older adults may be a means by which to reduce the burdens of frailty in survivors of critical illness, but further study is needed.

References

1. D.C. Angus, A.F. Shorr, A. White, et al. Critical care delivery in the United States: distribution of services and compliance with Leapfrog recommendations. *Crit Care Med* 2006; **34**: 1016–24.
2. T.J. Iwashyna, E.W. Ely, D.M. Smith, K.M. Langa. Long-term cognitive impairment and functional disability among survivors of severe sepsis. *JAMA* 2010; **304**: 1787–94.
3. H. Wunsch, C. Guerra, A.E. Barnato, et al. Three-year outcomes for medicare beneficiaries who survive intensive care. *JAMA* 2010; **303**: 849–56.
4. N.E. Brummel, M.C. Balas, A. Morandi, et al. Understanding and reducing disability in older adults following critical illness. *Crit Care Med* 2015; **43**: 1265–75.
5. T.J. Iwashyna, C.R. Cooke, H. Wunsch, J.M. Kahn. Population burden of long-term survivorship after severe sepsis in older

Americans. *J Am Geriatr Soc* 2012; **60**: 1070–7.

6. O.J. Bienvenu, E. Colantuoni, P. A. Mendez-Tellez, et al. Depressive symptoms and impaired physical function after acute lung injury: a 2-year longitudinal study. *Am J Respir Crit Care Med* 2012; **185**: 517–24.

7. K.E. Covinsky, L. Goldman, E.F. Cook, et al. The impact of serious illness on patients' families. SUPPORT Investigators. Study to understand prognoses and preferences for outcomes and risks of treatment. *JAMA* 1994; **272**: 1839–44.

8. L.P. Fried, C.M. Tangen, J. Walston, et al. Frailty in older adults: evidence for a phenotype. *J Gerontol A Biol Sci Med Sci* 2001; **56**: M146–56.

9. J. Walston, E.C. Hadley, L. Ferrucci, et al. Research agenda for frailty in older adults: toward a better understanding of physiology and etiology: summary from the American Geriatrics Society/National Institute on Aging Research Conference on Frailty in Older Adults. *J Am Geriatr Soc* 2006; **54**: 991–1001.

10. J.E. Morley, B. Vellas, G.A. van Kan, et al. Frailty consensus: a call to action. *J Am Med Dir Assoc* 2013; **14**: 392–7.

11. A. Clegg, J. Young, S. Iliffe, et al. Frailty in elderly people. *Lancet* 2013; **381**: 752–62.

12. C.K. Liu, A. Lyass, M.G. Larson, et al. Biomarkers of oxidative stress are associated with frailty: the Framingham Offspring Study. *Age (Dordr)* 2016; **38**: 1.

13. R.M. Collard, H. Boter, R.A. Schoevers, R. C. Oude Voshaar. Prevalence of frailty in community-dwelling older persons: a systematic review. *J Am Geriatr Soc* 2012; **60**: 1487–92.

14. S.A. Sternberg, A. Wershof Schwartz, S. Karunananthan, et al. The identification of frailty: a systematic literature review. *J Am Geriatr Soc* 2011; **59**: 2129–38.

15. N.F. Woods, A.Z. LaCroix, S.L. Gray, et al. Frailty: emergence and consequences in women aged 65 and older in the Women's Health Initiative Observational Study. *J Am Geriatr Soc* 2005; **53**: 1321–30.

16. K. Bandeen-Roche, Q.L. Xue, L. Ferrucci, et al. Phenotype of frailty: characterization in the women's health and aging studies. *J Gerontol A Biol Sci Med Sci* 2006; **61**: 262–6.

17. D.K. Kiely, L.A. Cupples, L.A. Lipsitz. Validation and comparison of two frailty indexes: the MOBILIZE Boston Study. *J Am Geriatr Soc* 2009; **57**: 1532–9.

18. P. Hanlon, B.I. Nicholl, B.D. Jani, et al. Frailty and pre-frailty in middle-aged and older adults and its association with multimorbidity and mortality: a prospective analysis of 493 737 UK Biobank participants. *Lancet Public Health* 2018; **3**: e323–e32.

19. J. Muscedere, B. Waters, A. Varamballly, et al. The impact of frailty on intensive care unit outcomes: a systematic review and meta-analysis. *Intensive Care Med* 2017; **43**: 1105–22.

20. N.E. Brummel, S.P. Bell, T.D. Girard, et al. Frailty and subsequent disability and mortality among patients with critical illness. *Am J Respir Crit Care Med* 2017; **196**: 64–72.

21. W. Geense, M. Zegers, P. Dieperink, et al. Changes in frailty among ICU survivors and associated factors: results of a one-year prospective cohort study using the Dutch Clinical Frailty Scale. *J Crit Care* 2020; **55**: 184–93.

22. J. Muscedere, S.M. Bagshaw, M. Kho, et al. Frailty, outcomes, recovery and care steps of critically ill patients (FORECAST): a prospective, multi-centre, cohort study. *Intensive Care Med* 2024; **50**: 1064–74.

23. N.E. Brummel, T.D. Girard, P. P. Pandharipande, et al. Prevalence and course of frailty in survivors of critical illness. *Crit Care Med* 2020; **48**: 1419–26.

24. M. Hamidi, M. Zeeshan, V. Leon-Risemberg, et al. Frailty as a prognostic factor for the critically ill older adult trauma patients. *Am J Surg* 2019; **218**: 484–9.

25. S.M. Fernando, D.I. McIsaac, J.J. Perry, et al. Frailty and associated outcomes and resource utilization among older ICU

patients with suspected infection. *Crit Care Med* 2019; **47**: e669–e76.

26. L.E. Ferrante, M.A. Pisani, T.E. Murphy, et al. The association of frailty with post-ICU disability, nursing home admission, and mortality: a longitudinal study. *Chest* 2018; **153**: 1378–86.

27. L.E. Ferrante, T.E. Murphy, L.S. Leo-Summers, et al. The combined effects of frailty and cognitive impairment on post-ICU disability among older ICU survivors. *Am J Respir Crit Care Med* 2019; **200**: 107–10.

28. F.G. Zampieri, T.J. Iwashyna, E. M. Viglianti, et al. Association of frailty with short-term outcomes, organ support and resource use in critically ill patients. *Intensive Care Med* 2018; **44**: 1512–20.

29. P. Le Maguet, A. Roquilly, S. Lasocki, et al. Prevalence and impact of frailty on mortality in elderly ICU patients: a prospective, multicenter, observational study. *Intensive Care Med* 2014; **40**: 674–82.

30. M.S. Kalaiselvan, A. Yadav, R. Kaur, et al. Prevalence of frailty in ICU and its impact on patients' outcomes. *Indian J Crit Care Med* 2023; **27**: 335–41.

31. A.A. Hope, S.J. Hsieh, A. Petti, et al. Assessing the usefulness and validity of frailty markers in critically ill adults. *Ann Am Thorac Soc* 2017; **14**: 952–9.

32. S.M. Bagshaw, J. Muscedere. Is this intensive care unit patient frail? Unraveling the complex interplay between frailty and critical illness. *Am J Respir Crit Care Med* 2017; **196**: 4–5.

33. J. Muscedere, S.M. Bagshaw, M. Kho, et al. Frailty, outcomes, recovery and care steps of critically ill patients (FORECAST): a prospective, multi-centre, cohort study. *Intensive Care Med* 2024; **50**: 1064–74.

34. D.K. Heyland, A. Garland, S.M. Bagshaw, et al. Recovery after critical illness in patients aged 80 years or older: a multi-center prospective observational cohort study. *Intensive Care Med* 2015; **41**: 1911–20.

35. S.M. Bagshaw, H.T. Stelfox, R. C. McDermid, et al. Association between frailty and short- and long-term outcomes among critically ill patients: a multicentre prospective cohort study. *CMAJ* 2014; **186**: E95–102.

36. T.N. Robinson, J.D. Walston, N. E. Brummel, et al. Frailty for surgeons: review of a national institute on aging conference on frailty for specialists. *J Am Coll Surg* 2015; **221**: 1083–92.

37. K. Rockwood, X. Song, C. MacKnight, et al. A global clinical measure of fitness and frailty in elderly people. *CMAJ* 2005; **173**: 489–95.

38. Q.L. Xue, J. Tian, J.D. Walston, et al. Discrepancy in frailty identification: move beyond predictive validity. *J Gerontol A Biol Sci Med Sci* 2020; **75**: 387–93.

39. D. Bertschi, J. Waskowski, M. Schilling, et al. Methods of assessing frailty in the critically ill: a systematic review of the current literature. *Gerontology* 2022; **68**: 1321–49.

40. N.E. Brummel. R03AG083556 "Surrogate Assessment of Frailty using Electronic Tools (SAFE-T)," 2024 Available from: https://reporter.nih.gov/search/91IV13mnAkqqCBuA0FicQA/project-details/10725607.

41. S. Church, E. Rogers, K. Rockwood, O. Theou. A scoping review of the Clinical Frailty Scale. *BMC Geriatr* 2020; **20**: 393.

42. R.J. Pugh, A. Ellison, K. Pye, et al. Feasibility and reliability of frailty assessment in the critically ill: a systematic review. *Crit Care* 2018; **22**: 49.

43. A.B. Mitnitski, A.J. Mogilner, K. Rockwood. Accumulation of deficits as a proxy measure of aging. *ScientificWorldJournal* 2001; **1**: 323–36.

44. M.C. Kizilarslanoglu, R. Civelek, M. K. Kilic, et al. Is frailty a prognostic factor for critically ill elderly patients? *Aging Clin Exp Res* 2017; **29**: 247–55.

45. W.D. Schweickert, M.C. Pohlman, A. S. Pohlman, et al. Early physical and occupational therapy in mechanically ventilated, critically ill patients: a randomised controlled trial. *Lancet* 2009; **373**: 1874–82.

46. M. Moss, A. Nordon-Craft, D. Malone, et al. A randomized trial of an intensive physical therapy program for patients with acute respiratory failure. *Am J Respir Crit Care Med* 2016; **193**: 1101–10.

47. P.E. Morris, M.J. Berry, D.C. Files, et al. Standardized rehabilitation and hospital length of stay among patients with acute respiratory failure: a randomized clinical trial. *JAMA* 2016; **315**: 2694–702.

48. S.J. Schaller, M. Anstey, M. Blobner, et al. Early, goal-directed mobilisation in the surgical intensive care unit: a randomised controlled trial. *Lancet* 2016; **388**: 1377–88.

49. C.L. Hodgson, M. Bailey, R. Bellomo, et al. Early active mobilization during mechanical ventilation in the ICU. *N Engl J Med* 2022; **387**: 1747–58.

50. M. Goldfarb, J. Afilalo, A. Chan, et al. Early mobility in frail and non-frail older adults admitted to the cardiovascular intensive care unit. *J Crit Care* 2018; **47**: 9–14.

51. T. Kidd, F. Mold, C. Jones, et al. What are the most effective interventions to improve physical performance in pre-frail and frail adults? A systematic review of randomised control trials. *BMC Geriatr* 2019; **19**: 184.

52. M.A. Fiatarone, E.F. O'Neill, N.D. Ryan, et al. Exercise training and nutritional supplementation for physical frailty in very elderly people. *N Engl J Med* 1994; **330**: 1769–75.

53. M. Maddocks, L.J. Brighton, J.A. Alison, et al. Rehabilitation for people with respiratory disease and frailty: an official American thoracic society workshop report. *Ann Am Thorac Soc* 2023; **20**: 767–80.

54. A. Rahman, R.M. Hasan, R. Agarwala, et al. Identifying critically-ill patients who will benefit most from nutritional therapy: further validation of the "modified NUTRIC" nutritional risk assessment tool. *Clin Nutr* 2016; **35**: 158–62.

55. Z.Y. Lee, M.S. Hasan, A.G. Day, et al. Initial development and validation of a novel nutrition risk, sarcopenia, and frailty assessment tool in mechanically ventilated critically ill patients: the NUTRIC-SF score. *JPEN J Parenter Enteral Nutr* 2022; **46**: 499–507.

56. A.J. Tessier, S. Chevalier. An update on protein, leucine, omega-3 fatty acids, and vitamin D in the prevention and treatment of sarcopenia and functional decline. *Nutrients* 2018; **10**.

57. J.L.M. Bels, S. Thiessen, R.J.J. van Gassel, et al. Effect of high versus standard protein provision on functional recovery in people with critical illness (PRECISe): an investigator-initiated, double-blinded, multicentre, parallel-group, randomised controlled trial in Belgium and the Netherlands. *Lancet* 2024; **404**: 659–69.

58. D.M. Needham, V.D. Dinglas, P.E. Morris, et al. Physical and cognitive performance of patients with acute lung injury 1 year after initial trophic versus full enteral feeding. EDEN trial follow-up. *Am J Respir Crit Care Med* 2013; **188**: 567–76.

59. A.A. Ginde, R.G. Brower, J.M. Caterino, et al. Early high-dose vitamin D. *N Engl J Med* 2019; **381**: 2529–40.

60. P.Y. Khor, R.M. Vearing, K.E. Charlton. The effectiveness of nutrition interventions in improving frailty and its associated constructs related to malnutrition and functional decline among community-dwelling older adults: a systematic review. *J Hum Nutr Diet* 2022; **35**: 566–82.

61. V. Danesh, L.M. Boehm, T. L. Eaton, et al. Characteristics of post-ICU and post-COVID recovery clinics in 29 U.S. health systems. *Crit Care Explor* 2022; **4**: e0658.

62. A.A. Hope, O.M. Enilari, E. Chuang, et al. Prehospital frailty and screening criteria for palliative care services in critically ill older adults: an observational cohort study. *J Palliat Med* 2021; **24**: 252–6.

63. C.L. Montgomery, D.J. Zuege, D.B. Rolfson, et al. Implementation of population-level screening for frailty among patients admitted to adult intensive care in Alberta, Canada. *Can J Anaesth* 2019; **66**: 1310–19.

64. T.R. Fried, E.H. Bradley, V.R. Towle, H. Allore. Understanding the treatment preferences of seriously ill patients. *N Engl J Med* 2002; **346**: 1061–6.

65. L.R. Pollack, N.E. Goldstein, W. C. Gonzalez, et al. The frailty phenotype and palliative care needs of older survivors of critical illness. *J Am Geriatr Soc* 2017; **65**: 1168–75.

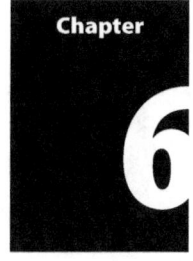

Chapter 6

Dysphagia in the Critically Ill

Nicole Langton-Frost and Martin B. Brodsky

Epidemiology

Endotracheal intubation is an indispensable treatment for airway protection and respiratory compromise in the intensive care unit (ICU). As many as 20 million people across the globe are intubated in ICUs each year. Of patients who survive more than 24 hours of intubation with mechanical ventilation, 50% will develop swallowing disorders (dysphagia), 75% will develop voice disorders (dysphonia), and nearly all patients will have some form of laryngeal injury upon extubation [1]. The ability to breathe, phonate, and swallow share common anatomical and physiological pathways, each requiring specialized attention following extubation. This chapter focuses on screening and assessing hospitalized patients for dysphagia after extubation, with an emphasis on the complexities and considerations in the immediate post-extubation period and during the remainder of the patient's hospitalization.

Admitting Diagnosis and Hospital Course

Pneumonitis and pneumonia resulting from aspiration events are common causes of acute respiratory failure, especially in patients with dysphagia. Pneumonia is named among the five condition-specific mortality measures by the Centers for Medicare & Medicaid Services used to calculate hospital-level 30-day risk-standardized mortality rates. This is a particularly common reason that speech-language pathologists (SLP) are asked to evaluate patients in the ICU.

Before evaluating a patient, the SLP should complete a focused chart review to identify possible causes of and contributors to dysphagia. The patient's admitting diagnosis can help identify pertinent information in the medical record to establish risk factors for dysphagia and to offer a basis for prognosis. The patient's medical history should be reviewed to identify additional risk factors for physiologic swallowing impairments, including a history of dysphagia; surgeries of the head, neck, and thorax; altered nutritional intake/maintenance; gastroesophageal reflux disease; aspiration pneumonia; and chronic respiratory disease.

Chart review should also include a review of nursing, physical therapy, and occupational therapy notes to understand the patient's current level of function and precautions that may influence the SLP session. Helpful data include safety precautions, vital signs fluctuations with positioning changes (e.g., significant changes in blood pressure with head of bed elevation), evidence of autonomic dysreflexia, the current level of mobility, results of delirium screening tools and other measures of cognitive status, and the amount of assistance required for completion of activities of daily living, such as feeding and performing oral care.

Respiratory Disease

Risk factors for the development of dysphagia in patients who require mechanical ventilation due to acute respiratory distress syndrome (ARDS) include older age, severity of illness (as defined by APACHE score), an endotracheal tube (ETT) size ≥8.0, duration of intubation, and number of intubations [1]. For patients in the ICU, surgical interventions, manipulation of the anatomy, and reduced functional reserve due to the dysfunction of multiple organ systems may also be present, increasing the risk for the development of dysphagia.

Endotracheal Intubation

While intubation is a necessary and lifesaving intervention for many, there are risks associated with it, including laryngeal injury (see Chapter 39 for additional information), dysphagia, and aspiration. Patients with ETTs larger than 8.0 are especially at risk. Intubation duration also plays a role in the likelihood of developing dysphagia, with an 80% increased odds of experiencing dysphagia symptoms at hospital discharge for each day of intubation up to six days [1]. Patients requiring intubation for 48 hours or longer often develop neuromuscular weakness, as evidenced by a 35% reduction in tongue strength at 48 hours of mechanical ventilation [2], a decline in diaphragmatic strength after 18 hours of mechanical ventilation, and a delay in laryngeal vestibular closure (LVC) in patients with ARDS as compared to healthy controls [3].

High-Flow Nasal Cannula

Currently, there are limited data on the impact of high-flow nasal cannula on swallow function [4]. For healthy adults, the flow rate appears to be correlated with the duration of LVC, with higher flow rates resulting in a longer duration of LVC [5]. Use of high-flow nasal cannula has also been shown to improve respiratory-swallow coordination when compared to low-flow nasal cannula in patients recently extubated in the ICU [6]. Swallow evaluation and treatment of patients that require high-flow nasal cannula should be individualized, with close attention paid to the patient's respiratory status over time and the incorporation of instrumental swallow assessments, such as flexible endoscopic evaluation of swallowing, when appropriate.

Tracheostomy Tubes

Patients who require creation of a tracheostomy are at increased risk of dysphagia and aspiration, and the presence of dysphagia in patients with tracheostomy is often multifactorial. Most tracheostomies are performed following a prolonged period of intubation and mechanical ventilation, with its attendant risks of laryngeal injury, swallowing dysfunction, generalized deconditioning, and ICU-acquired weakness, which results from both critical illness and prolonged immobility. Risks attributable to the placement of a tracheostomy tube include changes in laryngeal (i.e., subglottic) and pharyngeal pressures due to the creation of an opening by the tracheostomy tube in the pathway from the mouth to the lungs. A one-way speaking valve (OWSV) can be helpful to improve pressure equilibrium and sensation, including smell and taste, by temporarily closing the opening during swallowing and expiration, approaching normal physiology. An instrumental swallow assessment can be completed despite the presence of a tracheostomy tube, regardless of the need for ventilatory support or whether an OWSV is in place. Due to the high rates of silent aspiration identified for patients with a tracheostomy tube in place, instrumental assessments are considered best practice before starting an oral diet.

Chest Imaging

Chest imaging can provide important details regarding lung pathology and any precautions or restrictions for the swallow evaluation or intervention. Patients with an untreated pneumothorax, for example, may not be candidates for respiratory muscle strength training (RMST).

Specific Patient Populations

Neurology and Neurosurgery Patients

Reviewing neuroimaging studies is an important component of the SLP evaluation in patients admitted with neurological insults or following neurosurgery. Such studies may identify neural pathways that may have been affected by the neurological injury or its related surgery and may help determine the likelihood of dysphagia and the types of functional impairments associated with it. For example, a patient with a stroke involving the internal capsule may have a higher likelihood of dysphagia due to disruptions associated with the corticobulbar tract, which directly impacts swallowing. Sequelae from neurological insults, such as edema, herniation, hydrocephalus, or midline shift, may influence treatment recommendations and prognosis. Medical interventions, such as administration of tissue-type plasminogen activator (tPA) or tenecteplase (TNK), thrombectomy, placement of an external ventricular drainage (EVD) device, or hemicraniectomy may also impact prognosis related to dysphagia. For example, a patient's condition may decline before improving if they are deemed to not be a candidate for thrombectomy but present with a perfusion deficit.

Neurosurgeries will have direct bearing on the patient's prognosis and recovery of dysphagia. Operative notes should be reviewed with a specific focus on the manipulation of cranial nerves, particularly the trigeminal (V), facial (VII), glossopharyngeal (IX), vagus (X), and/or hypoglossal (XII) nerves, which may increase the risk of dysphagia. The presence of tumor adherent to nerves and the treatment thereof are of vital importance. Whereas a patient with a retracted nerve may suffer temporary changes, sacrificed nerves are permanent. Dysphagia outcomes from spinal surgery depend on the location of the surgery and the number of levels of the spine involved. In general, higher and multilevel spinal surgery yields a greater risk for the development of dysphagia [7].

Cardiovascular Surgery Patients

Medical interventions that may influence swallow function in patients admitted to the Cardiovascular Surgery ICU include extracorporeal membrane oxygenation (ECMO), Impella devices, and intra-aortic balloon pumps (IABP) because these devices may necessitate activity restrictions that may limit safe positioning for swallowing.

Other factors relevant to this patient population should be considered, such as recurrent laryngeal nerve manipulation, New York Heart Association classification of heart failure severity, intubation duration, and transesophageal echocardiography [8]. Patients with a lower body mass index, chronic lung disease, and history of stroke, and patients who require more complex procedures (e.g., ventricular assist device implantation and heart transplantation), use of hypothermic circulatory arrest, and longer operative times, are more likely to develop dysphagia after cardiac surgery [8,9].

Lung and Liver Transplant Recipients

After organ transplantation, patients receive immunosuppression to reduce the likelihood of rejection, which places them at increased risk of developing infection. Although even healthy patients aspirate while sleeping, recipients of lung transplantation are at heightened risk for the development of aspiration pneumonia given their immunocompromised state. Further, an aspiration event may increase the patient's risk of lung rejection or other complications, requiring a more conservative approach for diet recommendations and advancement.

Patients before and after liver transplantation have comorbidities such as ascites, hepatic encephalopathy, malnutrition, and limited mobility. These comorbidities may result in complications if dysphagia is also present, as multiple medical diagnoses, reduced functional status, and impaired level of alertness have been found to be predictors of aspiration pneumonia [10,11]. Further complicating their clinical picture, patients often present with cognitive impairments due to hepatic encephalopathy, which may impact swallow function.

General Considerations Prior to the SLP Evaluation

Medications

Numerous medications that may be administered during critical illness can influence swallowing function, including neuromuscular blockers, opioid analgesics, and benzodiazepines, among others. Neuromuscular blockers can lead to severe deconditioning and weakness that can impact the muscles of respiration and swallowing. Morphine, a commonly used opioid analgesic, can result in impaired oral coordination, impaired laryngeal protection, and reduced spontaneous swallow frequency in healthy adults. Midazolam, a commonly used benzodiazepine, results in similar deficits as morphine, reduces pharyngeal contraction forces, and increases pharyngeal retention in healthy adults [12]. To date, there are no clinical studies describing the impact of opioid analgesics or benzodiazepines on swallow function in patients specifically admitted to the ICU; however, it is plausible that critically ill patients receiving central nervous system depressants may experience reduced pharyngeal sensation and/or muscle weakness and thus have an increased risk of dysphagia and aspiration.

Moreover, benzodiazepines increase the risk of developing both hypoactive and hyperactive delirium (see Chapter 8 for additional information). Impaired attention and memory, a decreased level of arousal, or intermittent hyperactivity may all increase the risk of developing dysphagia [13]. To date, the specific pathophysiology of swallow impairments typically observed in patients with delirium are unknown; however, it is plausible that impaired arousal and attention may impact bolus control and the cortical control of swallow function.

Swallow Screen

A bedside swallow screen, generally performed by nursing staff, can be completed as soon as the patient is appropriate (i.e., awake, alert, and able to accept oral intake) after extubation. Exclusions for completion of the swallow screen vary between facilities and may include new lung transplantation, new esophagectomy, presence of a tracheostomy tube, presence and/or history of head and neck cancer, or history of dysphagia. It is important to utilize a validated swallow screen, such as the Yale Swallow Protocol (YSP) [14], the post-extubation dysphagia (PED) swallow screen [15], or the Gugging Swallow Screen-Intensive Care Unit (GUSS-ICU) [16], each of which has clearly defined pass and fail criteria. For example, if the patient has any of the exclusion criteria noted in the YSP, the patient should remain nil per os (NPO) until their condition improves or an SLP consult is performed. If the patient does not meet any of the exclusion criteria, the patient should drink three ounces of water consecutively. If the patient demonstrates interrupted drinking, coughing, or choking during or immediately after completion of drinking, this is considered failure, and an SLP consult is recommended.

Discussion with Medical Team

Prior to completing an initial swallow evaluation, a brief discussion between the SLP and the patient's multidisciplinary care team is beneficial. This discussion allows for clarification of any questions developed from the chart review and provides opportunities to gain insights into the nurse's perspective on the patient's current function and medical status.

Bedside Swallow Evaluation

Current Mentation

Level of alertness can influence swallowing function and should be assessed during the bedside swallow evaluation. This may include the ability to maintain adequate arousal, answer biographical and orientation questions, follow simple commands, and communicate basic wants and needs. A comparison with the medical team's recent observations is often helpful.

Vital Signs and Current Respiratory Status

For patients in the ICU, current vital signs and goal vital signs set by the primary team, including heart rate, blood pressure, oxygen saturation, and respiratory rate, should be closely monitored, as they may fluctuate due to the patient's medical acuity. For example, the medical team may be utilizing permissive hypertension to increase the likelihood of improved perfusion to at-risk brain tissue following an acute ischemic stroke. If the patient's blood pressure drops below the goal, discontinuation of the swallow evaluation may be necessary.

Social History and History of Dysphagia

Obtaining the patient's social history is necessary to understand the patient's baseline functional status, including cognitive impairments (e.g., attention, memory, and problem solving) and independence (or dependence) in activities of daily living and instrumental activities of daily living. This may include mobility status and need for assistive devices, support at home, access to follow-up services at home, and access to resources for diet modifications if needed. Focusing on the patient's history of dysphagia provides information on the patient's baseline swallow function. Important factors include: a history of gastroesophageal reflux and laryngopharyngeal reflux, a history of modified oral diet or alternate nutrition, the current oral diet, signs of aspiration (e.g., coughing during meals), and regurgitation during or after meals. Similarly, understanding a patient's priorities for their care is imperative to develop appropriate recommendations.

Cranial Nerve Examination

A cranial nerve examination focusing on cranial nerves V–XII should be completed during the bedside swallow evaluation. This will assess the integrity of these areas within the central and peripheral nervous systems and their potential involvement in swallowing difficulties (see Table 6.1). Impairments to swallowing-related musculature may not be observed during the cranial nerve exam.

Table 6.1 Cranial nerves and their functions related to swallowing

Cranial Nerve	Normal Function
Trigeminal Nerve (CN V)	<ul><li>Facial sensation</li><li>Sensation of anterior 2/3 of tongue</li><li>Muscles of mastication</li><li>Velar elevation</li><li>Hyoid elevation</li></ul>
Facial Nerve (CN VII)	<ul><li>Sensation of anterior 2/3 of tongue</li><li>Hyoid elevation</li></ul>
Glossopharyngeal Nerve (CN IX)	<ul><li>Sensation and taste of posterior 1/3 of tongue</li><li>Sensation of pharyngeal plexus</li><li>Elevation of pharynx and larynx</li></ul>
Vagus Nerve (CN X): Pharyngeal Branch	<ul><li>Elevation of posterior tongue</li><li>Elevation of pharynx</li><li>Elevation of soft palate</li><li>Shortens pharynx</li></ul>
Vagus Nerve (CN X): Internal Branch of the Superior Laryngeal Nerve	<ul><li>Sensation to the<ul><li>Vocal cords and above the level of the vocal cords</li><li>Valleculae</li><li>Epiglottis</li><li>Aryepiglottic folds</li><li>Pyriform sinuses</li><li>Upper and middle pharyngeal constrictors</li></ul></li></ul>
Vagus Nerve (CN X): External Branch of the Superior Laryngeal Nerve	<ul><li>Lengthens vocal cords</li><li>Shortens pharynx</li><li>Relaxes upper esophageal sphincter during swallow</li></ul>
Vagus Nerve (CN X): Recurrent Laryngeal Nerve	<ul><li>Sensation to the<ul><li>Vocal cords and below the level of the vocal cords</li><li>Inferior pharyngeal constrictor</li><li>Upper esophagus</li></ul></li><li>Shortens vocal cords</li><li>Vocal cord opening and closing</li></ul>
Accessory Nerve (CN XI)	<ul><li>Head and neck motion/stability that may be necessary for compensatory strategies</li></ul>
Hypoglossal Nerve (CN XII)	<ul><li>Lingual Movement</li></ul>

Oral Health

Aspiration of oral contents includes aspiration of resident bacteria, and proper oral care reduces bacterial load in the oral cavity. An inspection of the oral cavity, including the patient's gingiva, teeth, and hard palate, provides information regarding the patient's overall oral health. The presence of multiple decayed teeth, swollen gums, and dried secretions may indicate an increased risk of bacterial burden in the oral cavity. Frequent and detailed oral care during each assessment and treatment session is important, and collaboration with nursing and occupational therapy can assist the patient in completing oral care and improving oral hygiene in between treatment sessions.

Instrumental Swallow Evaluation

Although the identification of aspiration may be an observation that is made during instrumental swallow evaluations, it is never the goal. Instead, the goals of instrumental swallow evaluations are to: assess the patient's swallowing safety and efficiency, assess the effectiveness of compensatory strategies, identify and describe physiologic swallowing impairments, and guide the development of a physiologic-based treatment plan that includes diet recommendations (see Table 6.2).

Videofluoroscopic Swallow Study

Videofluoroscopic swallow study (VFSS), also known as the modified barium swallow study (MBSS) or dynamic swallow study, allows for visualization of the oral, pharyngeal, and esophageal phases of swallowing during a real-time video X-ray. A VFSS may be the assessment to visualize and evaluate concerns for esophageal impairment. This evaluation is completed with various barium consistencies that mimic food and drink to improve visualization in the radiographic technique.

Table 6.2 Benefits of VFSS and FEES for patients in the ICU

VFSS	FEES
Visualization of the oral, pharyngeal, and esophageal phases of the swallow	Direct visualization of the vocal cords
Completion of kinematic analysis of swallow	Direct visualization of pharyngeal and laryngeal mucosa
	Assessment of secretion management
	Can be completed when patients are unable to sit fully upright
Assessment of swallow physiology	
Assessment of swallow safety (penetration and aspiration)	
Assessment of swallow efficiency (pharyngeal residue)	

Flexible Endoscopic Evaluation of Swallowing

Flexible endoscopic evaluation of swallowing (FEES) provides direct visualization of the pharyngeal and laryngeal mucosa and is portable, allowing it to be completed at the patient's bedside. This assessment may be beneficial for patients after extubation and for patients who are unable to sit fully upright due to medical acuity. Although standardized in its presentation of foods, this evaluation may be completed with any food and drink. Food coloring is encouraged to improve visualization with water and other transparent/light-colored consistencies (e.g., applesauce).

Best Practice in the ICU

Patients admitted to the ICU are medically fragile, requiring continuous monitoring and care from specialized healthcare providers. Although both VFSS and FEES are considered gold standards for swallowing assessment and are complementary in their findings, FEES has been identified as the preferred swallowing assessment for patients in the ICU because it can be completed at the bedside with continuous monitoring and readily available medical personnel throughout the assessment. It is also able to provide a superior assessment of laryngeal function compared with VFSS. VFSS is, however, an alternative option provided that resources are available to monitor and transport the patient to and from radiology.

Decision Making/Synthesis for Recommendations

Following completion of the chart review, discussion with the multidisciplinary team, discussion with the patient and family, and the bedside swallow evaluation, the SLP must synthesize all of the pertinent information, develop overall recommendations, and establish a plan of care. Considerations should include: the patient's current cognitive status; the patient's and family's goals of care; the patient's nutritional status and access for essential medications; and concerns for laryngeal trauma, altered oral and/or laryngeal sensation, and neuromuscular weakness. Current coordination of breathing and swallowing, signs of aspiration at the bedside, and overall risk factors for the development of pneumonia, including medical frailty, immune status, and oral health, should also be considered. If pharyngeal dysphagia is suspected, recommendations should include an instrumental assessment to confirm or exclude dysphagia, guide diet recommendations, and allow for identification of physiologic impairments to guide the treatment plan.

Treatment

Following confirmation of dysphagia on an instrumental swallow assessment, the SLP should develop a treatment plan in collaboration with the patient, family, and medical team. Interventions should consider both the underlying medical cause(s) of the dysphagia as well as the specific physiological deficits identified on the instrumental assessment. Swallow treatment should begin in the ICU and continue when the patient transitions to the ward. If dysphagia persists upon hospital discharge, swallow treatment should continue at the next level of care (see Chapter 38 for additional information).

Treatment interventions may focus on compensation or restoration. Historically, treatment in the ICU has focused primarily on compensation [17]; however, there is now emerging evidence to support initiating restorative treatment in the acute care setting [18]. Compensation includes strategies to support continued oral intake while compensating for the current physiologic swallow deficits. Some examples include use of a chin tuck to compensate for incomplete LVC or use of a head turn to compensate for unilaterally reduced pharyngeal contraction. Restorative treatment may focus on strength, sensation, coordination, or a combination thereof. Example exercises include an effortful swallow or the Shaker exercise to target strength, pharyngeal electrical stimulation to target sensation, and use of biofeedback to target coordination (see Chapter 38 for additional information).

Case Example

Mr. S. was admitted to the medical ICU for ARDS, where he required intubation and mechanical ventilation for seven days, with a continuous infusion of fentanyl provided for analgesia. Following extubation, the patient did not pass the nurse swallow screen administered by the bedside nurse, and SLP was consulted for a bedside swallow evaluation. During the evaluation, the patient demonstrated a dysphonic vocal quality, poor oral health, an inability to independently complete oral care and feed himself due to upper extremity weakness, and consistent coughing with drinking thin liquids. Nursing, physical therapy, and occupational therapy reported limited functional mobility. A subsequent FEES revealed reduced vocal cord adduction, concern for laryngeal injury, impaired swallow safety with inconsistent cough response to aspiration, and impaired swallow efficiency with thicker viscosities.

It is likely that the underlying cause of the patient's dysphagia was multifactorial, including ICU-acquired weakness suggested by the prolonged bedrest, prolonged intubation, upper extremity weakness, and reduced functional mobility. These factors, along with the pharyngeal residue observed with thicker consistencies on the instrumental assessment, suggested reduced strength in the muscles associated with swallowing. Further, the prolonged intubation, concern for laryngeal injury, and inconsistent cough response to aspiration suggested a potential sensory impairment.

Physiologically, the patient presented with deficits in both swallow safety and swallow efficiency due to reduced anterior hyoid excursion, incomplete LVC, prolonged time to LVC, reduced tongue base retraction, and reduced pharyngeal contraction.

When developing a treatment plan, the SLP considers both the underlying causes of the dysphagia and the physiologic deficits, all in the context of the patient's and family's goals and preferences. An example treatment plan for this patient is provided in Table 6.3.

Table 6.3 Example of a treatment plan for a patient with dysphagia following extubation

	Underlying Deficit	Physiologic Impairments	Frequency/Intensity
Effortful swallow in conjunction with surface electromyography (sEMG) Biofeedback	• Strength	• Reduced hyoid excursion • Incomplete laryngeal vestibular closure • Reduced pharyngeal contraction • Reduced tongue base retraction	• Sets of 10 • sEMG effortful swallow goal set at 110% off 3 baseline typical swallows
Pharyngeal electrical stimulation	• Sensation	• Reduced sensation	• 10 minutes per day for 3 consecutive days
Shaker exercise	• Strength	• Reduced hyoid excursion	• 3 isometric head lifts; sustain for 60 seconds • 30 isokinetic head lifts; sustain for 1 second

Key Points

1. Dysphagia is common in critically ill patients, requiring thorough assessment and treatment to reduce the risks of aspiration and related complications.
2. A multidisciplinary approach to assessment and treatment of dysphagia is necessary, requiring collaboration between patients, their caregivers, and the healthcare team.
3. Instrumental assessments such as the video fluoroscopic swallow study (VFSS) and flexible endoscopic evaluation of swallowing (FEES) are recommended to identify the physiologic disorder(s) related to swallowing and to guide the development of a comprehensive treatment plan that includes diet recommendations.
4. Dysphagia treatment focusing on compensation or restoration can begin in the intensive care unit (ICU).

References

1. M.B. Brodsky, M.J. Levy, E. Jedlanek, et al. Laryngeal injury and upper airway symptoms after oral endotracheal intubation with mechanical ventilation during critical care: a systematic review. *Crit Care Med* 2018; **46**(12): 2010–17.
2. H. Su, T. Hsiao, S. Ku, et al. Tongue weakness and somatosensory disturbance following oral endotracheal extubation. *Dysphagia* 2015; **30**(2): 188–95.
3. M.B. Brodsky, I. De, K. Chilukuri, et al. Coordination of pharyngeal and laryngeal swallowing events during single liquid swallows after oral endotracheal

intubation for patients with acute respiratory distress syndrome. *Dysphagia* 2018; **33**(6): 768–77.

4. M.J. Flores, E. Kortney, G. Elisabeth, et al. Initiation of oral intake in patients using high-flow nasal cannula: a retrospective analysis. *Perspectives of the ASHA Special Interest Groups* 2019; **4**(3): 522–31.

5. K. Allen and K. Galek. The influence of airflow via high-flow nasal cannula on duration of laryngeal vestibule closure. *Dysphagia* 2021; **36**(4): 729–35.

6. P. Rattanajiajaroen and N. Kongpolprom. Effects of high flow nasal cannula on the coordination between swallowing and breathing in postextubation patients, a randomized crossover study. *Crit Care* 2021; **25**(1): 365.

7. G. Tsalimas, D.S. Evangelopoulos, I. S. Benetos, et al. Dysphagia as a postoperative complication of anterior cervical discectomy and fusion. *Cureus* 2022; **14**(7): e26888.

8. E.K. Plowman, A. Anderson, J.D. York, et al. Dysphagia after cardiac surgery: prevalence, risk factors, and associated outcomes. *J Thorac Cardiovasc Surg* 2023; **165**(2): 737–746.e3.

9. J.C. Grimm, J.T. Magruder, R. Ohkuma, et al. A novel risk score to predict dysphagia after cardiac surgery procedures. *Ann Thorac Surg* 2015; **100**(2): 568–74.

10. S.E. Langmore, M.S. Terpenning, A. Schork, et al. Predictors of aspiration pneumonia: how important is dysphagia? *Dysphagia* 1998; **13**(2): 69–81.

11. J. Almirall, R. Boixeda, M.C. de la Torre, et al. Aspiration pneumonia: a renewed perspective and practical approach. *Respir Med* 2021; **185**: 106485.

12. C. A. Hårdemark, E. Sundman, K. Bodén, et al. Effects of morphine and midazolam on pharyngeal function, airway protection, and coordination of breathing and swallowing in healthy adults. *Anesthesiology* 2015; **122**(6): 1253–67.

13. E. Grossi, C. Rocco, L. Stilo, et al. Dysphagia in older patients admitted to a rehabilitation setting after an acute hospitalization: the role of delirium. *Eur Geriatr Med* 2023; **14**(3): 485–92.

14. D.M. Suiter, J. Sloggy, S.B. Leder. Validation of the yale swallow protocol: a prospective double-blinded videofluoroscopic study. *Dysphagia* 2014; **29**(2): 199–203.

15. K.L. Johnson, L. Speirs, A. Mitchell, et al. Validation of a postextubation dysphagia screening tool for patients after prolonged endotracheal intubation. *Am J Crit Care* 2018; **27**(2): 89–96.

16. C. Troll, M. Trapl-Grundschober, Y. Teuschl, et al. A bedside swallowing screen for the identification of post-extubation dysphagia on the intensive care unit: validation of the gugging swallowing screen (GUSS)-ICU. *BMC Anesthesiol* 2023; **23**(1): 122–6.

17. M. Macht, T. Wimbish, B.J. Clark et al. Diagnosis and treatment of post-extubation dysphagia: results from a national survey. *J Crit Care* 2012; **27**(6): 578–86.

18. G.S. Turra, I.V.D. Schwartz, S. Almeida, et al. Efficacy of speech therapy in post-intubation patients with oropharyngeal dysphagia: a randomized controlled trial. *Codas* 2021; **33**(2): e20190246–1782/20202019246.

Chapter 7

Nutritional Impairments in the Critically Ill

Kate J. Lambell, Lee-anne S. Chapple, and Emma J. Ridley

Introduction

Significant muscle wasting of approximately 2% per day occurs in the first week of an intensive care unit (ICU) stay [1], continues over the first two to three weeks (although at a slower rate) [2,3], and plateaus after discharge from the ICU [4]. This muscular atrophy contributes to persistent weakness and functional deficits that represent substantial burden for patients, caregivers, and the healthcare system [5,6]. Reasons for muscle wasting are multifactorial, and while immobility plays an important role, muscle loss in the ICU is five times greater than in studies of healthy volunteers undergoing bed rest [7], highlighting the impact of physiological drivers in critical illness.

Nutrition is considered an important element for recovery from critical illness, particularly for patients who have a protracted hospital stay. In general clinical populations, optimizing nutrition enhances muscle anabolism, reduces catabolism, and improves outcomes in patients with muscle depletion and malnutrition [8]. Maintaining or building muscle requires both adequate provision of energy to spare muscle protein from breakdown and amino acids to provide a substrate for muscle protein synthesis [8]; however, given the severe inflammation, anabolic resistance, and immobility characteristic of critical illness, enhanced nutrition interventions have not been able to consistently improve muscle outcomes [9]. This may be due to the inability of the body to effectively utilize delivered nutrition during critical illness or to trial factors, such as the timing and dose of nutrition provided in previously tested interventions.

Despite the lack of definitive evidence, prolonged under-provision of nutrition likely contributes to weight and muscle loss and the development of malnutrition, which is associated with increased risk of infection and prolonged hospitalization in the critically ill [10]. In clinical practice, nutrition delivery is frequently inadequate in both the ICU and post-ICU periods [11,12]. This is attributed to many factors, including increased metabolic requirements, delayed initiation of nutrition, interruptions to nutrition with fasting, and gastrointestinal intolerance [12]. Furthermore, critically ill patients who can consume food orally often experience nutrition-related symptoms, such as poor appetite, post-extubation dysphagia (see Chapter 6 for additional information), abdominal discomfort, and nausea, all of which can significantly impair nutritional intake [13]. Accordingly, clinical guidelines recommend early identification of critically ill patients at high nutrition risk and referral to a trained nutrition professional for an individualized nutrition plan and ongoing monitoring of nutrition outcomes [10].

The aims of this chapter are to summarize the current evidence of nutrition care for critically ill patients during hospitalization, with a focus on the complex metabolic

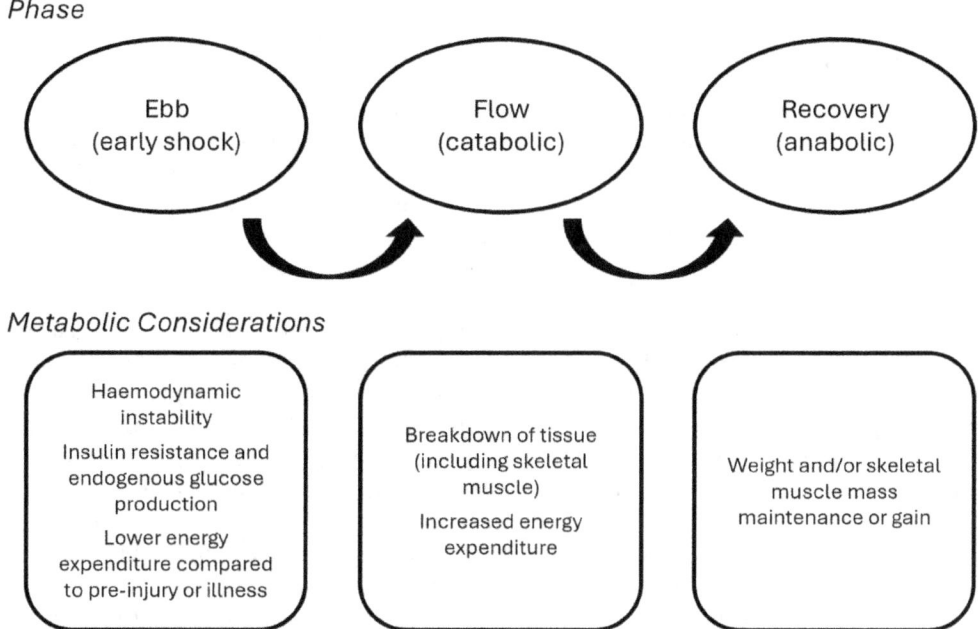

Figure 7.1 Phases of critical illness and key metabolic consequences.

response to injury and utilization of delivered nutrition, and to make practical recommendations for clinicians to attenuate muscle wasting and prevent the progression or development of malnutrition, which may contribute to or exacerbate post-intensive care syndrome (PICS) symptoms and recovery (see Chapter 40 for additional information).

Metabolic Response to Critical Illness

Appreciating the metabolic response to illness, as first described by Sir David Cuthbertson in 1942, is essential to understand the shifting nutrition needs for patients with critical illness. Two distinct sequential metabolic phases of critical illness occur: the "ebb" phase and "flow" phase [14]; more recently, a later "anabolic" recovery phase has been described [15]. Key metabolic characteristics of each phase are displayed in Figure 7.1. The duration of each phase depends on the type and severity of illness, effectiveness of therapies, and clinical complications. There are no validated biomarkers or bedside measures to reliably determine what phase a patient is in; however, the European Society of Clinical Nutrition and Metabolism (ESPEN) clinical guidelines suggest the "ebb" phase typically occurs at ICU days one to two, the "flow" phase between ICU days three to seven, and the "anabolic" recovery phase after day seven [16].

Energy, Protein, and Micronutrients

This section discusses energy, protein, and micronutrient requirements for critically ill patients throughout hospitalization and outlines current clinical recommendations.

Energy

Expenditure

Energy expenditure (EE) changes dynamically across the different phases of critical illness, in parallel with changing clinical condition and therapies, and is influenced by pre-morbid physical condition, with lean body mass being the biggest driver of metabolism [16]. For example, EE can be decreased by hypothermia, analgesia, sedation, muscle relaxants, and fasting, and increased by fever, shivering, increased work of breathing, physical activity, and illness severity (with the degree of hypermetabolism proportional to the degree of injury/illness) [17].

Due to inaccuracies estimating energy requirements using weight-based equations, clinical guidelines recommend measuring EE using indirect calorimetry (IC) [10,18]. IC can be used in both mechanically ventilated and self-ventilating patients and involves measuring gas exchange (VO_2 and VCO_2) when ideal test conditions are present [19]. Given variations in EE, IC results are only accurate at the time of measurement, requiring regular reassessment and consideration of factors that might alter metabolism. When possible, IC should be performed weekly or with changes in clinical condition.

Despite IC being widely recommended, the cost of the device and consumables, need for trained personnel, time necessary for measurement, and requirement for ideal test conditions limit routine use in clinical practice [20]. There is also a lack of definitive evidence supporting targeting energy needs via IC compared with estimations [21]. As such, predictive equations (e.g., 20–25 kcal/kg/day) remain the most common method for estimating energy needs at the bedside [20]. Clinical judgment is paramount when using predictive equations; the limitations of the equation, underlying body composition, clinical parameters, and physical activity must be considered [22].

Delivery

Despite measuring EE, the optimal percentage of energy requirements to provide at each phase of illness is unknown. Due to elevated metabolic requirements and severe muscle loss induced by critical illness, traditional care was to provide early, aggressive nutrition, assuming it may attenuate loss and improve outcomes; however, this strategy has not been shown to influence clinical and functional outcomes in several definitive randomized controlled trials (RCTs) conducted over the past decade [23,24,25,26]. The largest of these, The Augmented versus Routine approach to Giving Energy Trial (TARGET), enrolled 3957 patients and compared 50% higher energy delivery in the intervention group (~30 kcal/kg ideal body weight/day) with standard care over the median 6-day intervention period and found no difference in mortality or secondary clinical and self-reported functional outcomes between groups [24,27]. These results, along with new understanding of the early response to critical illness (e.g., hypometabolism and endogenous glucose production), have led to recommendations for the gradual increase of energy delivery over the first week of critical illness, independent of EE [16,18]. Specifically, ESPEN recommends targeting 70% of the measured or estimated EE for the first week [16], and the American Society for Parenteral and Enteral Nutrition (ASPEN) recommends providing between 12 and 25 kcal/kg/day in the first 7 to 10 days [18].

The later period of critical illness may be the optimal time for nutrient delivery to support recovery; however, data to support this is sparse. With known energy deficits leading to significant weight and muscle loss in healthy people and other clinical populations, it seems appropriate to target 100% of the measured EE in the later phases of critical illness, as recommended by ESPEN guidelines (based on expert opinion) [16], with close monitoring of clinical and nutrition-related parameters as detailed below.

Both under- and overprovision of energy have clinical consequences. Overfeeding may result in hyperglycemia requiring insulin administration, hypertriglyceridemia, hypercapnia, and delayed weaning from mechanical ventilation [17], while prolonged and significant underfeeding may contribute to muscle wasting and malnutrition, as the maintenance or building of skeletal muscle requires adequate provision of energy [8]. Energy underfeeding is common: a post-hoc analysis of prospectively collected data from 17,154 critically ill patients reported that energy delivered was 15±8 kcal/kg (mean±SD), half of what was prescribed [12]. This inadequacy persists on the ward, with reports of patients receiving between 64% and 83% of their energy requirements [11,28–30]. As such, routine monitoring of energy adequacy, inclusive of non-nutritional sources (e.g., intravenous glucose and propofol administration), is imperative throughout hospitalization for high-risk patients.

Protein

Requirements

In health, muscle maintenance relies on the balance between protein degradation and synthesis via the availability of amino acids from dietary protein [31]. In critical illness, skeletal muscle is catabolized to provide precursor amino acids for gluconeogenesis [32,33]; such elevated muscle breakdown results in a negative protein balance that subsequently leads to muscle loss [34]. Dietary protein supplementation delivered intravenously or enterally has been shown to improve whole body protein balance [35,36]; therefore, augmenting dietary protein provision during critical illness may attenuate skeletal muscle wasting.

Clinical guidelines recommend a progressive increase in protein dose to a target of ~1.2–2 g/kg/day, with higher doses provided to patients with burns, multi-trauma, obesity, and those receiving continuous renal replacement therapy (CRRT) [16,18]. Despite these recommendations, conflicting data exist regarding the role of augmented protein delivery on attenuation of muscle mass, with some suggesting benefit [37,38] and others suggesting no effect [3,39]. Two definitive randomized trials of protein dose have now been published. EFFORT Protein, a single-blinded RCT, randomized 1301 mechanically ventilated adult patients at nutritional risk to receive either usual-dose ($\leq$1.2 g/kg/day) or high-dose ($\geq$2.2 g/kg/day) protein. No difference in the primary outcome (time to discharge alive) was observed; however, high-dose protein was associated with worse outcomes in patients with acute kidney injury or a higher baseline SOFA score ($\geq$9) [40]. The second RCT, NUTRIREA-3, randomized 3036 mechanically ventilated adult patients who were receiving vasoactive therapy to either a low-calorie, low-protein intervention (6 kcal/kg/day and 0.2–0.4 g protein/kg/day) or to control (25 kcal/kg/day and 1.0–1.3 g protein/kg/day). The authors reported no difference in all-cause 90-day mortality but a longer "time to readiness for ICU discharge" with greater nutrition delivery [41]. To date, there are no published interventional studies of protein dose that extend after, or are conducted solely, following ICU discharge.

Delivery

Similar to energy delivery, protein delivery in practice is well below prescription and international recommendations, both in the ICU (<50% adequacy, mean±SD 0.6±0.4 g/kg/day) [12] and on conventional wards, where patients meet only 72–83% of estimated protein requirements [11,28,29,30].

In addition to dose, the method of protein delivery may also be important. In a study of 121 patients receiving either intermittent (bolus) or continuous delivery of enteral nutrition (EN), the intermittent delivery group achieved greater protein adequacy than the continuous delivery group; despite this, both groups had similar rates of muscle loss [42].

Interpretation of RCTs of augmented protein delivery in critical illness should consider the timing of delivery, given the significantly blunted amino acid utilization observed early in critical illness [43] and the improved muscle protein balance that occurs over time [34]. Future studies should assess the impact of protein delivered for longer periods, including after ICU discharge, where protein metabolism is likely to be optimized.

Micronutrients

Micronutrients, including trace elements and vitamins, play a key role in the immune response, tissue repair, and energy metabolism. Pre-morbid malnutrition, the illness itself, therapies provided during critical illness (including prolonged CRRT), lack of natural sunlight, and inadequate nutrition provision may all contribute to micronutrient depletion [44]. High-risk micronutrients for critically ill patients include copper, selenium, zinc, and vitamins B1, C, and D [44]. There are a limited number of intervention trials for specific micronutrients in critically ill patients, yielding low-level evidence for high-dose supplementation [44]; however, clinicians should consider patients at high risk of depletion and monitor and supplement as necessary. For a comprehensive discussion on micronutrients, readers should refer to the ESPEN micronutrient guideline [44].

Current Clinical Recommendations

- Commence trophic EN within 24–48 hours of ICU admission.
- *Energy:* Gradual increase during the acute phase to avoid overfeeding. Use IC to measure EE, ideally weekly or with changes in clinical condition. If unavailable, use a predictive equation (e.g., 20–25 kcal/kg/day). Aim for 70% of estimated or measured EE for the first week and 80–100% thereafter.
- *Protein:* Progressively increase protein dose over days 3–7, with the aim to provide 1.3 g/kg/day. Be cautious with protein dose in patients with acute kidney injury.
- Routinely review clinical parameters and therapies that may impact nutrition requirements.
- Monitor energy and protein adequacy (delivery compared to requirements), inclusive of non-nutritional sources.
- Consider micronutrient testing and supplementation for patients who are pre-morbidly malnourished, receive prolonged CRRT (> two weeks), have a prolonged hospital stay, and/or have poor nutrition provision during hospitalization.

Patients at High Risk for Impaired Nutrition Provision

The ability of nutrition to influence patient outcomes is likely dependent on pre-existing nutritional status, medical comorbidities, and length of hospitalization. It is important to be able to identify high-risk patients in whom nutrition is likely to be of the greatest benefit. There are a range of nutrition screening tools available to clinicians, although none have been validated for use in the ICU [10]. A pragmatic approach is to consider patients at high nutrition risk if they spend more than 48 hours in the ICU, require mechanical ventilation, are underfed for five days, or have a chronic disease (e.g., diabetes, pre-existing malnutrition, chronic kidney disease, chronic obstructive pulmonary disease, and/or cirrhosis) [10]. These patients should be referred to a trained nutrition professional, ideally a dietitian, to complete a comprehensive nutrition assessment. This should include a detailed review of their medical, weight, and diet histories; anthropomorphic measurements, such as height, weight, and body mass index; and a general assessment of body composition and physical ability [10]. This data can then be used to formulate and document an individualized nutrition plan. Although there is a paucity of data investigating nutrition interventions in patients with malnutrition on admission, clinical guidelines recommend that these patients receive early nutrition support, and electrolytes should be monitored closely for refeeding syndrome until nutrition is at target [10].

Two emerging populations at high nutrition risk are patients who eat orally and patients with obesity.

Patients Who Eat Orally

A growing number of ICU patients consume nutrients orally, whether exclusively from ICU admission, following extubation, and/or in addition to EN or parenteral nutrition (PN). Nutrition provision in patients receiving an oral diet alone has been shown to be substantially less than prescribed targets in both the ICU (<50% of prescribed targets) and on the ward, with deficits up to twofold greater than when EN and/or PN is provided [45,46,47]. Use of oral nutritional supplements is effective in improving nutrient intake in survivors of critical illness [11] and reducing hospital length of stay (LOS) in general hospitalized patients [48].

Multiple barriers to adequate oral intake exist throughout hospitalization, and these have been classified into patient-, system-, and clinician-related barriers [13]. Patient factors include physical symptoms, such as reduced appetite, post-extubation dysphagia, nausea, and abdominal pain, and psychological factors, including delirium, anxiety, poor sleep, reduced motivation, and fatigue, all of which commonly occur across the recovery trajectory [13]. System issues stem from hospital food systems failing to meet the needs of patients (e.g., timing of delivery and lack of culturally appropriate options). Clinician issues result from poor nutrition education in the health workforce, which can result in premature removal of feeding tubes before establishment of usual dietary intake [49].

Clinical recommendations:
- Following extubation, avoid early removal of feeding tubes until oral adequacy is established.
- Identify and address individual barriers to oral intake.
- Escalate to oral nutrition support (e.g., specialized nutrition drinks/supplements), and/or EN or PN in a timely manner when there is ongoing poor nutrition provision (i.e., <70% estimated requirements for >3–7 days) [10].

Patients with Obesity

The prevalence of obesity is increasing in ICUs worldwide (~20%) and contributes to increased resource utilization [50]. Patients with obesity are more likely to present with pre-existing medical comorbidities and to experience metabolic derangements that have nutritional implications, such as impaired glucose and fat metabolism, insulin resistance, and a pro-inflammatory state [50]. They may also experience management bias, with a tendency for delayed nutrition initiation [51].

The ESPEN and 2016 ASPEN guidelines provide specific recommendations for the nutrition management of patients with obesity, promoting isocaloric and hypocaloric feeding, respectively [10,52]. These discrepant recommendations likely result from the sparsity of data; indeed, the optimal calorie target for obese critically ill patients remains uncertain. Predictive equations have poor agreement with measured EE by IC in obesity, commonly underestimating energy needs [53], and accordingly, IC is preferred to define energy targets for obese patients. Regardless of the method used, it is important that routine monitoring occurs throughout hospitalization to optimize nutrition therapy for recovery.

Clinical recommendations:
- Use IC to measure EE, and if not available, use a predictive equation with an adjusted body weight.
- Monitor biochemistry, particularly glucose and triglyceride levels (especially for patients receiving prolonged periods of propofol and/or PN).
- Monitor nutrition adequacy, weight, muscle mass, and nutritional status.
- Consider targeted weight loss once medically stable.

Optimizing Nutrition Therapy During Hospitalization: The Clinician's Role

All clinicians play an important role in optimizing nutrition therapy. As depicted in Figure 7.2, this involves early identification of patients at high risk of malnutrition and referral to a trained nutrition professional. Clinicians can optimize nutrition delivery by avoiding unnecessary fasting, identifying and addressing barriers to nutrition intake, and, for patients receiving oral diet and fluids, ensuring that they receive the food they like at meal times [13]. Monitoring of nutrition therapy should occur at least weekly in stable patients and more frequently in unstable patients, those at high nutrition risk, and those who are already malnourished. If nutrition provision remains inadequate (e.g., <70% requirements for >3-7 days), then escalation of therapy to either oral nutrition support, EN, and/or total or supplemental PN should occur [10]. The use of PN early in critical illness, when delivered at the same energy dose as EN (~18-20 kcal/kg/day and 0.6-0.8 g/kg/day protein), is safe, with two large RCTs reporting no differences in mortality, length of stay, and infectious complications compared with EN [54,55].

The continuation of nutrition care at transition points during hospitalization (i.e., ICU to ward, ward to rehabilitation) has been identified as a point of failure [49]. A clearly documented nutrition plan, including nutrition status and adequacy, should be provided to relevant staff on transition from ICU to the ward. On discharge from the ward to home or another healthcare service, there should be well-coordinated discharge planning according to individual needs. Please refer to Chapter 40 for nutritional considerations after hospital discharge.

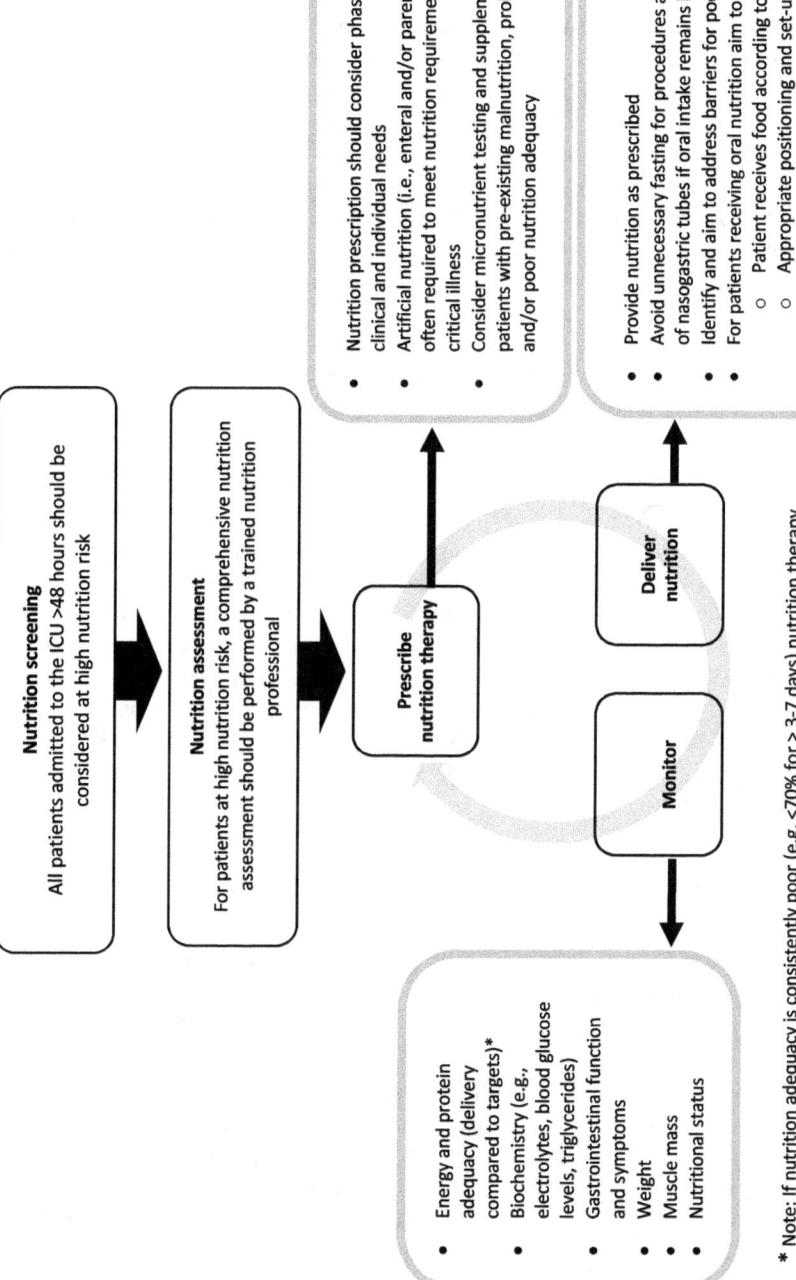

Figure 7.2 Process for optimizing nutrition care for critically ill patients.

Future Directions

Future nutrition trials should appreciate the complexity of nutrition as a therapy, moving beyond early energy or protein dose attainment, to consideration of mode, timing of nutrition delivery, and type of nutrients provided. For example, protein intervention studies may consider the impact of formulation (hydrolyzed versus whole proteins) or protein source (plant- versus animal-derived protein) on outcomes. Another aspect to this complexity is that nutrition interventions are unlikely to work in isolation, and the role of synergistic therapies (e.g., physical activity) must be considered [56].

Furthermore, examination of nutrient utilization across metabolic phases of care is required. In particular, studies may include an adaptable intervention that changes in response to the patient's clinical and metabolic course. The use of biomarkers that could be measured at the bedside to guide the nutrition intervention would be revolutionary.

The conduct of larger definitive RCTs over the last decade has provided data sets that can be used to explore the impact of interventions in a variety of subgroups. This has made us consider that not all ICU patients will respond to a nutrition intervention in the same manner. Future trials may need to consider the study of more homogenous populations, with clinical practice following suit.

Finally, we need to understand the lived experience of nutrition care during hospitalization and include consumers in all aspects of future nutrition research to ensure that research focuses on what matters most to patients and that resources are appropriately utilized.

Conclusion

Nutrition therapy of critically ill patients during hospitalization does not follow a one-size-fits-all model of care. Metabolic needs change during the course of illness and recovery, and the importance of nutrition is likely to be influenced by severity of illness, pre-morbid conditions, and length of hospitalization. International data has consistently demonstrated that nutrition delivery in the ICU and post-ICU is significantly less than prescribed. All clinicians can play an important role in optimizing nutrition therapy across the recovery continuum by identifying patients at nutritional risk, referring to a trained nutrition professional, identifying and addressing barriers to nutrition delivery, and monitoring nutrition adequacy and status.

Key Points

1. Nutrition requirements change dynamically across the different phases of critical illness, along with changing clinical condition and therapies, and they are influenced by pre-morbid physical condition, with lean body mass being the biggest driver of metabolism.
2. Critically ill patients who can consume food orally often experience nutrition-related symptoms, such as poor appetite, post-extubation dysphagia, abdominal discomfort, and nausea, all of which can significantly impair nutritional intake.
3. In clinical practice, nutrition delivery is frequently less than prescription and international guideline recommendations in both the ICU and on the post-ICU ward.

4. Despite the lack of definitive evidence, prolonged under-provision of nutrition likely contributes to weight and muscle loss and the development of malnutrition and impaired recovery following critical illness.
5. All clinicians can play an important role in optimizing nutrition therapy across the recovery continuum by identifying patients at nutritional risk, referring to a trained nutrition professional, identifying and addressing barriers to nutrition delivery, and closely monitoring nutrition adequacy and status.

References

1. B. Fazzini, T. Markl, C. Costas, et al. The rate and assessment of muscle wasting during critical illness: a systematic review and meta-analysis. *Crit Care* 2023; **27**: 2.
2. W. Gruther, T. Benesch, C. Zorn, et al. Muscle wasting in intensive care patients: ultrasound observation of the M. quadriceps femoris muscle layer. *J Rehabil Med* 2008; **40**: 185–9.
3. K.J. Lambell, G.S. Goh, A.C. Tierney, et al. Marked losses of computed tomography-derived skeletal muscle area and density over the first month of a critical illness are not associated with energy and protein delivery. *Nutrition* 2021; **82**: 111061.
4. L.A.S. Chapple, A.M. Deane, L.T. Williams, et al. Longitudinal changes in anthropometrics and impact on self-reported physical function after traumatic brain injury. *Crit Care Resus* 2017; **19**: 29–36.
5. M.S. Herridge, A.M. Cheung, C.M. Tansey, et al. One-year outcomes in survivors of the acute respiratory distress syndrome. *N Engl J Med* 2003; **348**: 683–93.
6. M.S. Herridge, C.M. Tansey, A. Matte, et al. Functional disability 5 years after acute respiratory distress syndrome. *N Engl J Med* 2011; **364**: 1293–304.
7. M.L. Dirks, D. Hansen, A. Van Assche, et al. Neuromuscular electrical stimulation prevents muscle wasting in critically ill comatose patients. *Clin Sci* 2015; **128**: 357–65.
8. C.M. Prado, S.D. Anker, A.J.S. Coats, et al. Nutrition in the spotlight in cachexia, sarcopenia and muscle: avoiding the wildfire. *J Cachexia Sarcopenia Muscle* 2021; **12**: 3–8.
9. Z.Y. Lee, C.S.L. Yap, M.S. Hasan, et al. The effect of higher versus lower protein delivery in critically ill patients: a systematic review and meta-analysis of randomized controlled trials. *Crit Care* 2021; **25**: 260.
10. P. Singer, A.R. Blaser, M.M. Berger, et al. ESPEN practical and partially revised guideline: Clinical nutrition in the intensive care unit. *Clin Nutr* 2023; **42**: 1671–89.
11. E.J. Ridley, R.L. Parke, A.R. Davies, et al. What happens to nutrition intake in the post-intensive care unit hospitalization period? An observational cohort study in critically ill adults. *J Parenter Enteral Nutr* 2019; **43**: 88–95.
12. E.J. Ridley, S.L. Peake, M. Jarvis, et al. Nutrition therapy in Australia and New Zealand intensive care units: an international comparison study. *J Parenter Enteral Nutr* 2018; **42**: 1349–57.
13. E.J. Ridley, L.S. Chapple, M.J. Chapman. Nutrition intake in the post-ICU hospitalization period. *Curr Opin Clin Nutr Metab Care* 2020; **23**: 111–15.
14. D. Cuthbertson. Post-shock metabolic response. *Lancet* 1942; **239**: 433–7.
15. P.E. Wischmeyer. Tailoring nutrition therapy to illness and recovery. *Crit Care* 2017; **21**: 316.
16. P. Singer, A.R. Blaser, M.M. Berger, et al. ESPEN guideline on clinical nutrition in the intensive care unit. *Clin Nutr* 2019; **38**: 48–79.
17. L. Sobotka. *Basics in Clinical Nutrition.* 2019. Prague; Publishing House Galen.
18. C. Compher, A.L. Bingham, M. McCall, et al. Guidelines for the provision of

nutrition support therapy in the adult critically ill patient: The American Society for Parenteral and Enteral Nutrition. *J Parenter Enteral Nutr* 2022; **46:** 12–41.
19. S.A. McClave, D.A. Spain, J.L. Skolnick, et al. Achievement of steady state optimizes results when performing indirect calorimetry. *J Parenter Enteral Nutr* 2003; **27:** 16–20.
20. K.J. Lambell, E.G. Miller, O.A. Tatucu-Babet, et al. Nutrition management of obese critically ill adults: a survey of critical care dietitians in Australia and New Zealand. *Aust Crit Care* 2021; **34:** 3–8.
21. O.A. Tatucu-Babet, K. Fetterplace, K. Lambell, et al. Is energy delivery guided by indirect calorimetry associated with improved clinical outcomes in critically ill patients? A systematic review and meta-analysis. *Nutr Metab Insights* 2020; **13:** 1178638820903295.
22. R.N. Walker, R.A. Heuberger. Predictive equations for energy needs for the critically ill. *Respir Care* 2009; **54:** 509–21.
23. National Heart, Lung, and Blood Institute Acute Respiratory Distress Syndrome Clinical Trials, T. W. Rice, et al. Initial trophic vs full enteral feeding in patients with acute lung injury: the EDEN randomized trial. *JAMA* 2012; **307:** 795–803.
24. TARGET Investigators, for the ANZICS Clinical Trials Group; M. Chapman, S. L. Peake, et al. Energy-dense versus routine enteral nutrition in the critically ill. *N Engl J Med* 2018; **379:** 1823–34.
25. M.P. Casaer, D. Mesotten, G. Hermans, et al. Early versus late parenteral nutrition in critically ill adults. *N Engl J Med* 2011; **365:** 506–17.
26. M.J. Allingstrup, J. Kondrup, J. Wiis, et al. Early goal-directed nutrition versus standard of care in adult intensive care patients: the single-centre, randomised, outcome assessor-blinded EAT-ICU trial. *Intensive Care Med* 2017; **43:** 1637–47.
27. A.M. Deane, L. Little, R. Bellomo, et al. Outcomes six months after delivering 100% or 70% of enteral calorie requirements during critical illness (TARGET): a randomized controlled trial. *Am J Respir Crit Care Med* 2020; **201:** 814–22.
28. L.S. Chapple, A.M. Deane, D.K. Heyland, et al. Energy and protein deficits throughout hospitalization in patients admitted with a traumatic brain injury. *Clin Nutr* 2016; **35:** 1315–22.
29. K. Wittholz, K. Fetterplace, M. Clode, et al. Measuring nutrition-related outcomes in a cohort of multi-trauma patients following intensive care unit discharge. *J Hum Nutr Diet* 2020; **33(3):** 414–22.
30. R. Slingerland-Boot, I. van der Heijden, N. Schouten, et al. Prospective observational cohort study of reached protein and energy targets in general wards during the post-intensive care period: The PROSPECT-I study. *Clin Nutr* 2022; **41:** 2124–34.
31. A.M. Horstman, S.W. Olde Damink, A.M. Schols, L.J. van Loon. Is cancer cachexia attributed to impairments in basal or postprandial muscle protein metabolism? *Nutrients* 2016; **8.**
32. H. Barle, F. Hammarqvist, B. Westman, et al. Synthesis rates of total liver protein and albumin are both increased in patients with an acute inflammatory response. *Clin Sci* 2006; **110:** 93–9.
33. A. Januszkiewicz, M. Klaude, K. Lore, et al. Enhanced in vivo protein synthesis in circulating immune cells of ICU patients. *J Clin Immunol* 2007; **27:** 589–97.
34. L. Gamrin-Gripenberg, M. Sundstrom-Rehal, D. Olsson, et al. An attenuated rate of leg muscle protein depletion and leg free amino acid efflux over time is seen in ICU long-stayers. *Crit Care* 2018; **22:** 13.
35. M. Sundstrom Rehal, F. Liebau, I. Tjader, et al. A supplemental intravenous amino acid infusion sustains a positive protein balance for 24 hours in critically ill patients. *Crit Care* 2017; **21:** 298.
36. M. Sundstrom Rehal, F. Liebau, J. Wernerman, O. Rooyackers. Whole-body protein kinetics in critically ill patients during 50 or 100% energy provision by enteral nutrition:

a randomized cross-over study. *PLoS One* 2020; **15**:e0240045.

37. K. Fetterplace, A.M. Deane, A. Tierney, et al. Targeted full energy and protein delivery in critically ill patients: a pilot randomized controlled trial (FEED trial). *J Parenter Enteral Nutr* 2018; **42**: 1252–62.

38. S. Ferrie, M. Allman-Farinelli, M. Daley, K. Smith. Protein requirements in the critically ill: a randomized controlled trial using parenteral nutrition. *J Parenter Enteral Nutr* 2016; **40**: 795–805.

39. E. Dresen, C. Weisbrich, R. Fimmers, et al. Medical high-protein nutrition therapy and loss of muscle mass in adult ICU patients: A randomized controlled trial. *Clin Nutr* 2021; **40**: 1562–70.

40. D.K. Heyland, J. Patel, C. Compher, et al. The effect of higher protein dosing in critically ill patients with high nutritional risk (EFFORT Protein): an international, multicentre, pragmatic, registry-based randomised trial. *Lancet* 2023; **401**: 568–76.

41. J. Reignier, G. Plantefeve, J.P. Mira, et al. Low versus standard calorie and protein feeding in ventilated adults with shock: a randomised, controlled, multicentre, open-label, parallel-group trial (NUTRIREA-3). *Lancet Respir Med* 2023; **11**: 602–12.

42. A.S. McNelly, D.E. Bear, B.A. Connolly, et al. Effect of intermittent or continuous feed on muscle wasting in critical illness: a phase 2 clinical trial. *Chest* 2020; **158**: 183–94.

43. L.S. Chapple, I.W.K. Kouw, M. J. Summers, et al. Muscle protein synthesis after protein administration in critical illness. *Am J Respir Crit Care Med* 2022; **206**: 740–9.

44. M.M. Berger, A. Shenkin, A. Schweinlin, et al. ESPEN micronutrient guideline. *Clin Nutr* 2022; **41**: 1357–424.

45. S.J. Peterson, A.A. Tsai, C.M. Scala, et al. Adequacy of oral intake in critically ill patients 1 week after extubation. *J Am Diet Assoc* 2010; **110**: 427–33.

46. L.L. Moisey, J. Pikul, H. Keller, et al. Adequacy of protein and energy intake in critically ill adults following liberation from mechanical ventilation is dependent on route of nutrition delivery. *Nutr Clin Pract* 2021; **36**: 201–12.

47. E. Viner Smith, E.J. Ridley, C.K. Rayner, L. S. Chapple. Nutrition management for critically ill adult patients requiring non-invasive ventilation: a scoping review. *Nutrients* 2022; **14**.

48. T.J. Philipson, J.T. Snider, D. N. Lakdawalla, et al. Impact of oral nutritional supplementation on hospital outcomes. *Am J Manag Care* 2013; **19**: 121–8.

49. J. Merriweather, P. Smith, T. Walsh. Nutritional rehabilitation after ICU – does it happen: a qualitative interview and observational study. *J Clin Nurs* 2014; **23**: 654–62.

50. M. Schetz, A. De Jong, A.M. Deane, et al. Obesity in the critically ill: a narrative review. *Intensive Care Med* 2019; **45**: 757–69.

51. A.L. Borel, C. Schwebel, B. Planquette, et al. Initiation of nutritional support is delayed in critically ill obese patients: a multicenter cohort study. *Am J Clin Nutr* 2014; **100**: 859–66.

52. B.E. Taylor, S.A. McClave, R. G. Martindale, et al. Guidelines for the provision and assessment of nutrition support therapy in the adult critically ill patient: Society of Critical Care Medicine (SCCM) and American Society for Parenteral and Enteral Nutrition (A. S.P.E.N.). *Crit Care Med* 2016; **44**: 390–438.

53. K.J. Lambell, O.A. Tatucu-Babet, E.G. Miller, E.J. Ridley. How do guideline recommended energy targets compare with measured energy expenditure in critically ill adults with obesity: a systematic literature review. *Clin Nutr* 2023; **42**: 568–78.

54. S.E. Harvey, F. Parrott, D.A. Harrison, et al. Trial of the route of early nutritional support in critically ill adults. *N Engl J Med* 2014; **371**: 1673–84.

55. J. Reignier, J. Boisrame-Helms, L. Brisard, et al. Enteral versus parenteral early nutrition in ventilated adults with shock: a randomised, controlled, multicentre, open-label, parallel-group study (NUTRIREA-2). *Lancet* 2018; **391**: 133–43.

56. D.K. Heyland, A. Day, G.J. Clarke, et al. Nutrition and Exercise in Critical Illness Trial (NEXIS Trial): a protocol of a multicentred, randomised controlled trial of combined cycle ergometry and amino acid supplementation commenced early during critical illness. *BMJ Open* 2019; **9**:e027893.

Chapter 8

Delirium in the Critically Ill

Chukwudi A. Onyemekwu, Kelly M. Toth, Niall T. Prendergast, and Timothy D. Girard

Introduction

Delirium, which affects a large percentage of critically ill patients, is a key risk factor for the development of the post-intensive care syndrome (PICS), particularly with respect to long-term cognitive impairment, which can be debilitating for many survivors of critical illness [1,2]. This chapter will describe delirium during critical illness, including its risk factors, mechanisms, detection, prevention, and management.

Definition

Delirium, derived from the Latin word *deliriare*, translates literally to *de* (go off) and *liriare* (the furrow), a plowing metaphor suggesting a shift from a normal to an abnormal state. In modern health care, delirium is an acute neuropsychiatric disorder that occurs in the setting of acute illness, intoxication, or withdrawal. In 1980, the American Psychological Association (APA) added delirium to the third edition of the Diagnostic and Statistical Manual of Mental Disorders [3,4], defining it as a "clouding of consciousness – reduced clarity of awareness of the environment – with reduced capacity to shift, focus, and sustain attention to environmental stimuli." The full list of diagnostic criteria is shown in Table 8.1. Over the past 50 years, the APA has revised these criteria several times but has consistently defined delirium as acute disturbances in both attention and cognition.

Though the key features of delirium have remained unchanged since its introduction into medical parlance, the terminology used by critical care clinicians has varied widely. "Intensive care unit (ICU) psychosis" and "ICU syndrome" were often used in the past, but these phrases imply that delirium is an expected and insignificant outcome of intensive care. The large and growing body of research investigating delirium during critical illness and the attention delirium has received in prominent evidence-based clinical practice guidelines, such as those published by the Society of Critical Care Medicine (SCCM) [5], has led many clinicians to abandon older terms (e.g., ICU psychosis) in favor of delirium. Nevertheless, "encephalopathy" is still often used to describe hypoactive delirium (which is characterized by reduced arousal and psychomotor activity) and delirium in the setting of specific medical conditions (e.g., "hepatic encephalopathy" and "septic encephalopathy"), but we recommend the use of "delirium" in all cases where the APA diagnostic criteria are met.

Prevalence

Delirium occurs frequently in the critically ill, with the overall prevalence ranging from 20% to 80% [6,7,8], depending on the patient population studied; typically, the most severely ill patient populations have the highest prevalence of delirium. Among hospitalized adults,

Table 8.1 Changes in the American Psychiatric Association diagnostic criteria for delirium

DSM-III (1980)	DSM–5-TR (2022)
A. Clouding of consciousness (reduced clarity of awareness of the environment), with reduced capacity to shift, focus, and sustain attention to environmental stimuli	A. A disturbance in attention (i.e., reduced ability to direct, focus, sustain, and shift attention) and awareness (reduced orientation to the environment)
B. At least two of the following features: perceptual disturbance (misinterpretations, illusions, or hallucinations); speech that is at times incoherent; disturbance of sleep-wakefulness cycle, with insomnia or daytime drowsiness; and increased or decreased psychomotor activity	B. The disturbance develops over a short period of time (usually hours to a few days), represents a change from baseline attention and awareness, and tends to fluctuate in severity during the course of a day
C. Disorientation and memory impairment (if testable)	C. An additional disturbance in cognition (e.g., memory deficit, disorientation, language, visuospatial ability, or perception)
D. Clinical features that develop over a short period (usually hours to days) that tend to fluctuate over a day	D. The disturbances in Criteria A and C are not better explained by another preexisting, established, or evolving neurocognitive disorder and do not occur in the context of a severely reduced level of arousal, such as coma
E. Evidence from the history, physical examination, or laboratory tests of a specific factor judged to be etiologically related to the disturbance	E. There is evidence from the history, physical examination, or laboratory findings that the disturbance is a direct physiological consequence of another medical condition, substance intoxication or withdrawal (i.e., due to a drug of abuse or to a medication), or exposure to a toxin, or is due to multiple etiologies

delirium occurs more often in the critically ill than in the non-critically ill [9]. In the ICU, those with acute respiratory failure who require mechanical ventilation are more likely to experience delirium than non-mechanically ventilated patients; many studies indicate that up to 80% of mechanically ventilated patients are delirious at some point during their critical illness [10,11,12].

Outcomes

Delirium is associated with numerous adverse outcomes, both in the hospital and after discharge. Patients with delirium are more likely to remove indwelling medical devices (including endotracheal tubes and catheters), and delirium – whether hyperactive or hypoactive – often interferes with medical treatments, including physical therapy. Delirium is also associated with increased risk of falls and infections during hospitalization [13]. Consequently, is it unsurprising that delirium is associated with delayed liberation from mechanical ventilation, longer lengths of stay in the ICU and hospital, and increased healthcare costs. Finally, the most serious and immediate consequence of delirium is its association with increased in-hospital mortality [14,15,16]. Not only are mortality rates higher among those who ever experienced delirium compared with those who were never delirious, but each additional day that a patient is delirious is associated with an increase in mortality, even after adjusting for numerous potential confounders [11,15,17].

Even among patients who recover from critical illness, are no longer delirious, and are discharged from the hospital, delirium is associated with multiple components of PICS, including persistent cognitive impairment and disability (see Chapter 43 for additional information). In multiple studies, the duration of delirium during critical illness predicted the severity of cognitive impairment a full year after hospital discharge [2,18]. This cognitive impairment is, for many patients, as severe as that seen in patients with traumatic brain injury or Alzheimer's disease [18]. Notably, the cognitive impairment associated with delirium can be mild but clinically important. Critical illness survivors, their caregivers, and even their primary care providers may not immediately recognize post-critical illness cognitive deficits, but they often sense something is different. Mild cognitive impairment post-critical illness can result in missed appointments, non-adherence to medications, and hospital readmission, with a consequent increase in morbidity in these patients. Multiple studies and meta-analyses have shown that delirium is associated with new or worsening dementia [19], which is especially true among patients who had known cognitive impairment prior to their critical illness [20,21].

Patients with post-delirium cognitive impairment are also at risk for related problems, including functional disability, depression and anxiety, and social isolation, because of an inability to return to their prior level of function or from shame resulting from new physical or cognitive limitations [22], ultimately leading to further isolation [23].

Detection of Delirium

Because of its high prevalence in the ICU, the acute distress it causes patients and their loved ones, and its association with adverse short- and long-term outcomes, evidence-based clinical practice guidelines recommend that all critically ill patients be routinely monitored for delirium [5]. Traditionally, delirium was detected with examination by an expert clinician (e.g., a psychiatrist or neuropsychologist), who assessed level of consciousness, orientation, cognition, attention, memory, and psychomotor agitation to determine whether the diagnostic criteria described in the DSM were met. Over time, a number of structured tools were developed and validated that streamlined the detection of delirium and facilitated reliable application in both clinical and research settings.

The earliest of these delirium assessment tools was the Delirium Rating Scale (DRS), which was first published by Trzepacz and colleagues in 1988 and later updated to the Revised Delirium Rating Scale (DRS-R-98) [24,25]. The DRS is a 13-item tool that can be used to assess for the presence of delirium and to generate a severity score. The Confusion Assessment Method (CAM), which was published in 1990 [26], is probably the most widely known and accepted delirium assessment tool. The CAM relies on four features to quickly and accurately diagnose delirium: (1) acute onset and fluctuating course, (2) inattention, (3) disorganized thinking, and (4) altered level of consciousness; a diagnosis of delirium requires the presence of features 1 and 2 along with either feature 3 or 4.

A major limitation of these and many other delirium assessment tools [27] is that they require verbal responses from the patient, which are often not possible during critical illness due to the presence of an endotracheal tube or aphasia. Additionally, these tools were not validated in the ICU, where patients are often managed with sedating medications. Consequently, several new delirium assessment tools were developed and validated in cohorts of critically ill patients, including those who were sedated and mechanically ventilated. Based on these validation studies, two tools, the Intensive Care Delirium Screening Checklist (ICDSC) [28] and the Confusion Assessment Method for the ICU (CAM-ICU) [6,29], are currently recommended by clinical practice guidelines.

The ICDSC is an eight-item checklist that relies on bedside observations by the clinical team (typically the bedside nurse) during a typical working shift to determine whether delirium is present [28]. The eight items evaluated with the ICDSC are: altered level of consciousness, inattention, disorientation, hallucination (delusion or psychosis), psychomotor agitation (or retardation), inappropriate speech or mood, sleep-wake cycle disturbances, and symptom fluctuation; a score of ≥ 4 indicates the presence of delirium (see Table 8.2). The CAM-ICU, alternatively, is a structured assessment that a clinician (or researcher) can employ during a two-minute examination (see Figure 8.1) [6,29]. Similar to the original CAM, the CAM-ICU includes four features of delirium and requires that features 1 and 2 be present along with either feature 3 or 4 to detect the presence of delirium [6,29].

Both the ICDSC and CAM-ICU have been validated in numerous studies involving heterogeneous populations of critically ill patients, including those patients who are mechanically ventilated, sedated, and/or severely ill. Although coma (whether due to the underlying disease process or heavy sedation) precludes the detection of delirium, these tools are sensitive, specific, and reliable when used by trained clinicians or researchers in the ICU.

Pathophysiology

The underlying cause of delirium is often multifactorial, arising from a combination of predisposing and precipitating risk factors, and its pathophysiology, though still poorly understood, is likely mediated through multiple mechanisms, which include neuroinflammation, metabolic insufficiency, vascular permeability, and neuronal dysfunction with associated neurotransmitter disturbance (see Figure 8.2). Depending on the patient's risk factors and clinical condition, there are likely other cellular mechanisms underlying the onset of delirium [30,31], and certain risk factors may predispose persons to one or more of these specific mechanisms. Sepsis, for example, causes profound systemic inflammation, characterized by increased secretion of inflammatory mediators, including tumor necrosis factor, interleukin (IL)-1, IL-6, and other cytokines. These inflammatory mediators cross the blood–brain barrier and interact with microglia; activated microglia increase reactive oxygen species and signal astrocytes to produce chemokines, leading to the recruitment of inflammatory cells into the brain. The presence of an increased number of inflammatory cells in turn results in a decrease in metabolic substrates, ultimately impairing neuronal crosstalk [31].

In addition to inflammation, other mechanisms known to occur during critical illness have been linked to delirium (see Figure 8.2), but a detailed description of these pathways is beyond the scope of this chapter (see Chapter 19 for additional information). Delirium likely occurs with only some of these mechanisms being present. For instance, studies have shown that hypotension is associated with delirium, a mechanism that may induce metabolic insufficiency and neuronal dysfunction more than inflammation and vascular permeability. Hypotension leads to a decrease in regional cerebral blood flow, which results in

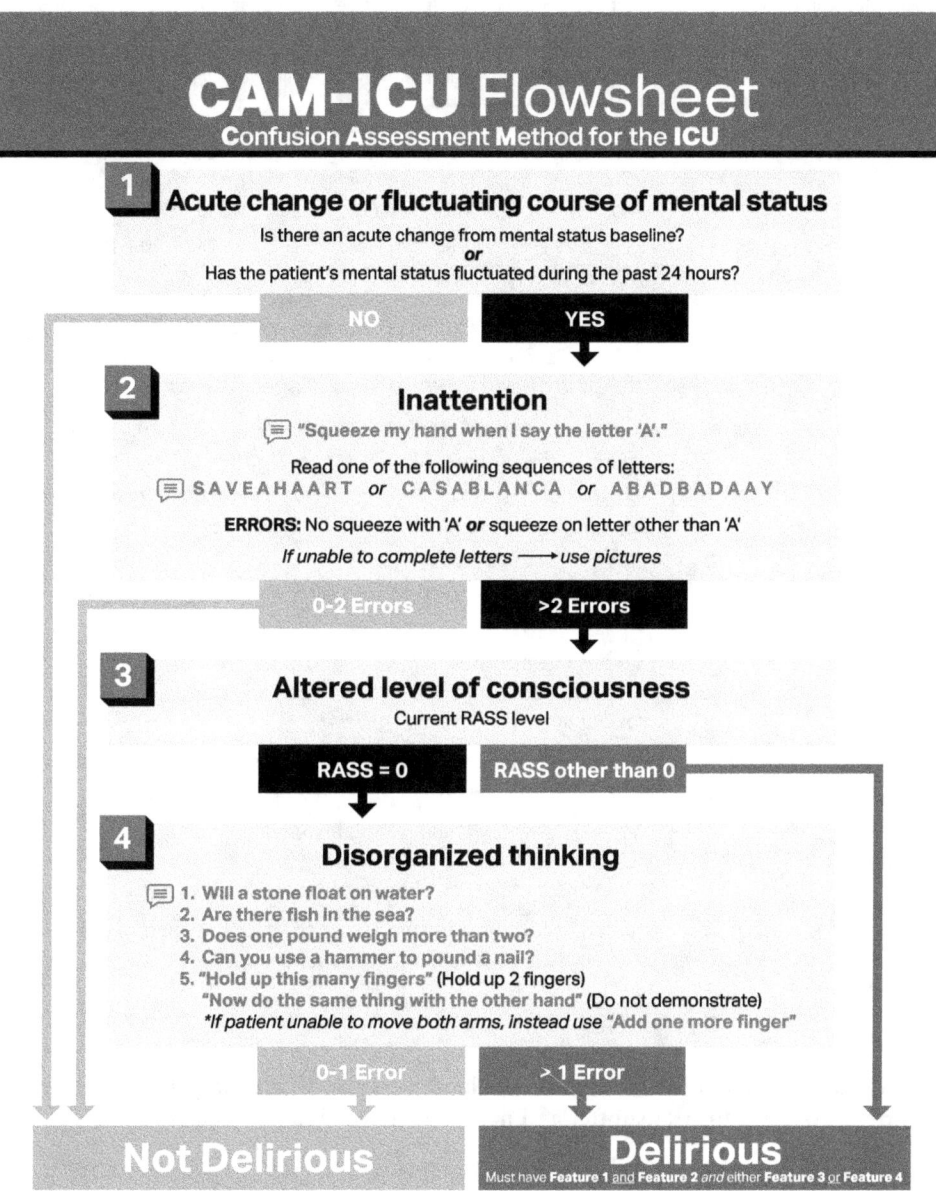

Figure 8.1 Confusion Assessment Method for the ICU (CAM-ICU) flowsheet. A patient screens positive for delirium if features 1 and 2 and either feature 3 or feature 4 are present. Copyright © 2002, E. Wesley Ely, MD, MPH and Vanderbilt University, all rights reserved. Reproduced with permission from www.ICUDelirium.org.

reduced cerebral perfusion and brain hypoxia. Reduction in regional blood flow is associated with delirium and may underlie a possible etiology of delirium [32,33]. Importantly, several medications, including benzodiazepine-induced gamma-aminobutyric acid

Table 8.2 The Intensive Care Delirium Screening Checklist. The scale is completed based on information obtained from an 8-hour shift or the previous 24 hours. Obvious manifestations of an item score 1 point; no manifestations of an item or no assessment possible score 0 points. From: N. Bergeron, M.J. Dubois, M. Dumont, et al. Intensive Care Delirium Screening Checklist: evaluation of a new screening tool. *Intensive Care Med* 2001; 27: 859–64. Reproduced with permission from Springer Nature.

Altered level of consciousness	A) No response or B) the need for vigorous stimulation in order to obtain any response signifies a severe alteration in the level of consciousness precluding evaluation. If there is coma (A) or stupor (B) most of the time period then a dash (-) is entered and there is no further evaluation during that period. C) Drowsiness or requirement of a mild to moderate stimulation for a response implies an altered level of consciousness and scores 1 point. D) Wakefulness or sleeping state that could easily be aroused is considered normal and scores no point. E) Hypervigilance is rated as an abnormal level of consciousness and scores 1 point.
Inattention	Difficulty in following a conversation or instructions. Easily distracted by external stimuli. Difficulty in shifting focus. Any of these scores 1 point.
Disorientation	Any obvious mistake in time, place, or person scores 1 point.
Hallucination, delusion, or psychosis	The unequivocal clinical manifestation of hallucination or of behavior probably due to hallucination (e.g., trying to catch a non-existent object) or delusion. Gross impairment in reality testing. Any of these scores 1 point.
Psychomotor agitation or retardation	Hyperactivity requiring the use of additional sedative drugs or restraints in order to control potential danger to oneself or others (e.g., pulling out IV lines, hitting staff). Hypoactivity or clinically noticeable psychomotor slowing. Any of these scores 1 point.
Inappropriate speech or mood	Inappropriate, disorganized, or incoherent speech. Inappropriate display of emotion related to events or situation. Any of these scores 1 point.
Sleep/wake cycle disturbance	Sleeping less than 4 h or waking frequently at night (do not consider wakefulness initiated by medical staff or loud environment). Sleeping during most of the day. Any of these scores 1 point.
Symptom fluctuation	Fluctuation of the manifestation of any item or symptom over 24 h (e.g., from one shift to another) scores 1 point.

(GABA) agonism, have been associated with increased risk of delirium and exert their effect primarily through neurotransmitter and neuronal crosstalk disturbances [31].

Risk Factors for Delirium

Delirium is an acute organ dysfunction syndrome that results from stress placed on a brain of variable resilience. Factors that make a patient less able to withstand such stress and therefore predisposed to delirium include advanced age, dementia or other forms of preexisting cognitive impairment, comorbid disease (especially cardiovascular and respiratory diseases), and sensory impairments (including vision or hearing impairment [see Table 8.3]) [34]. Elements that stress the brain and may precipitate delirium can be divided into two groups: those related to the patient's presenting illness and those occurring after hospital or ICU admission. The former includes illness severity, major and/or emergent

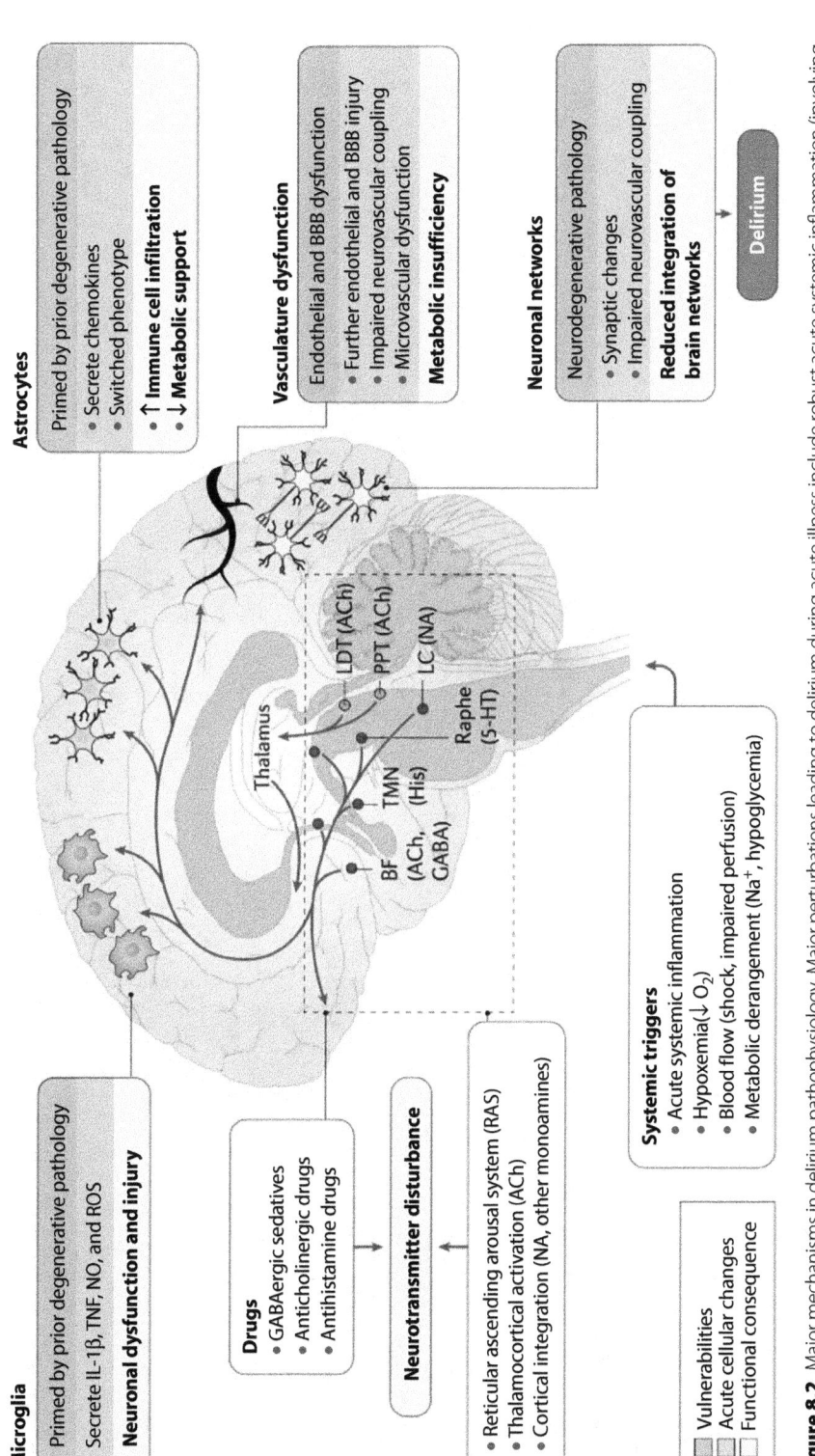

Figure 8.2 Major mechanisms in delirium pathophysiology. Major perturbations leading to delirium during acute illness include robust acute systemic inflammation (involving increased circulating pro-inflammatory cytokines, such as IL-1, IL-1β, and tumor necrosis factor (TNF), pathogen-associated molecular patterns and damage-associated molecular patterns), hypoxemia, impaired blood flow and tissue perfusion, and impaired metabolism (hyponatremia, hypernatremia, and hypoglycemia). Given the altered arousal states present in different subtypes of delirium, it is widely assumed that alteration of function in the ascending arousal system may be involved. These distributed mid-brain and brainstem nuclei include strong cholinergic drive from the tegmentum to the thalamus to activate cortical arousal and multiple monoaminergic nuclei that activate the cortex to modulate and integrate cortical activation. Medications, including but not limited to GABAergic sedatives, anesthetics, anticholinergic, and antihistamine drugs, can therefore

Caption for Figure 8.2 (cont.)

substantially alter arousal and are known to contribute to delirium. Microglia can be primed by existing pathology in the brain and further activated by acute inflammatory stimuli, secreting pro-inflammatory cytokines, reactive oxygen species (ROS), and reactive nitrogen species into the surrounding brain tissue. These mediators can directly affect neuronal function but also act directly on astrocytes. Astrocytes can also be primed during chronic brain pathology, becoming hypersensitive to acute inflammatory stimulation and secreting increased levels of chemokines, which can drive the recruitment of additional peripheral inflammatory cells to the brain. Activated astrocytes may also lose aspects of the energy metabolism support that they provide to neuronal function. The vasculature may become impaired, both by existing degenerative pathology and by superimposed stressors such as systemic inflammation, leading to endothelial injury and blood–brain barrier (BBB) damage, but vascular supply of oxygen and glucose may also become impaired owing to microvascular dysfunction and/or impaired neurovascular coupling, contributing to a metabolic (bioenergetic) insufficiency. All of these mechanisms contribute to the most obvious proximate cause of delirium: acute neuronal dysfunction and network disintegration. 5-HT, 5-hydroxytryptamine; ACh, acetylcholine; BF, basal forebrain; His, histamine; LC, locus coeruleus; LDT, laterodorsal tegmental nucleus; NA, noradrenaline; NO, nitric oxide; PPT, pedunculopontine tegmentum; RAS, reticular activating system; TMN, tuberomammillary nucleus. From: J.E. Wilson, M.F. Mart, C. Cunningham, et al. Delirium. *Nat Rev Dis Primers* 2020; **6**: 90.

Reproduced with permissions from Nature Publishing Group.

Table 8.3 Risk factors for delirium

Premorbid	Presenting Illness	Post-admission
Advanced age	Acute kidney injury	Anticholinergic medications
Alcohol use disorder	Alcohol or drug withdrawal	Benzodiazepines
Comorbid illness	Dehydration	Immobility
Dementia	Electrolyte imbalance	Infection
Depression	Heart failure	Lack of communication
Frailty	Liver dysfunction	Noise
Low educational level	Major surgery	Pain
Malnutrition	Multiple organ dysfunction	Physical restraints
Substance use disorder	Respiratory failure	Psychoactive medications
Visual and hearing impairment	Sepsis	Sleep disruption

surgery, sepsis, inflammation, SARS-CoV-2 infection, organ (especially hepatic and renal) dysfunction, alcohol or drug withdrawal, and mechanical ventilation; the latter includes pain, immobility, blood transfusion, use of sedative medications (particularly benzodiazepines), deep sedation (regardless of the chosen sedative), sleep deprivation, and polypharmacy, among others [31,35,36].

Heterogeneity of Delirium

A key challenge in understanding, managing, and preventing the negative sequelae of delirium is its heterogeneity. Delirium does not present uniformly; instead, it manifests in various forms that can differ in underlying etiology, presentation, and clinical trajectory. Researchers and clinicians must recognize and understand these differences to tailor appropriate treatment strategies and improve long-term outcomes.

Multiple approaches can be used to identify and understand delirium subtypes. Traditionally, including in the APA DSM, subtypes of delirium are defined based on psychomotor symptoms, with patients classified into hyperactive delirium, hypoactive delirium, and mixed delirium (i.e., fluctuating between hyperactive and hypoactive states) [37]. During critical illness, the most common psychomotor subtype is the hypoactive subtype, which affects over half of all ICU patients with delirium [38] and is associated with worse global cognition at 3 months and worse executive functioning at 3 and 12 months [39].

Delirium during critical illness has also been subtyped by both clinicians and researchers according to clinical risk factors or organ dysfunctions; these include delirium induced by hypoxia, sepsis, sedatives, uremia, hepatic dysfunction, alcohol withdrawal, and other clinical subtypes. Studies have shown that longer duration of sedative-induced delirium, the most common clinical risk factor-based subtype, is associated with worse long-term cognitive impairment up to 12 months after hospital discharge [40]. Notably, though most sedatives are considered to have transient effects limited to the ICU, the duration of sedative-associated delirium (a directly modifiable clinical delirium subtype) predicted long-term cognitive impairment in a large heterogeneous cohort of ICU patients [40], suggesting there is still much to learn about what causes long-term harm in survivors of critical illness and that PICS risk may be directly influenced by treatment decisions made by critical care clinicians.

Recent research in delirium heterogeneity used machine learning to identify data-derived delirium subtypes, which may further elucidate delirium's diverse mechanisms and thereby lead to personalized treatments [41,42,43,44]. These advanced analytics overcome some of the challenges of prior subtyping methods, including the reliance on clinician diagnosis for symptom subtype and the frequent co-occurrence of multiple delirium risk factors, which are exceedingly difficult for the clinician to disentangle. Data-driven methods can also leverage additional data, such as serum biomarkers, electroencephalography tracings, and imaging findings, which may help identify treatable traits that are amenable to personalized interventions for delirium and PICS.

Management

Management strategies, which can be used to prevent and/or treat delirium, are often divided into nonpharmacologic and pharmacologic approaches.

Nonpharmacologic

Nonpharmacologic management of delirium is centered around the identification and treatment of modifiable risk factors and triggers for delirium. The management of medical comorbidities (e.g., infection, fluid and electrolyte imbalances, and hypoxemia) is vital and usually self-evident. Beyond this, many evidence-based nonpharmacologic practices are grouped into the ABCDEF bundle promoted by the Society for Critical Care Medicine (see Chapter 11 for additional information). ABCDEF stands for the combination of Assessing, preventing, and managing pain; Both spontaneous awakening and spontaneous breathing trials for those receiving pharmacologic sedation and mechanical ventilation; careful Choice of analgesics and sedatives; Delirium prevention, assessment, and management; Early mobility and exercise; and Family engagement and empowerment. Each element of the bundle has been studied in isolation, and the bundle has also been assessed as a whole.

Spontaneous awakening trials (SATs), spontaneous breathing trials (SBTs), and paired SAT and SBT protocols have been shown to reduce exposure to benzodiazepines, thereby reducing the risk of deep sedation, coma, and prolonged mechanical ventilation. There is extensive literature linking heavy sedation and benzodiazepine use to delirium. Indeed, lighter sedation protocols using propofol or dexmedetomidine are associated with lower delirium risk than sedation strategies using benzodiazepines [45,46,47].

Delirium is frequently missed if not specifically screened for, and early detection of delirium facilitates management [48,49]. Recommended practices to prevent delirium include regulation of sensory input, limitation of inappropriate sensory stimulation with earplugs, providing patients with their usual sensory accessories (e.g., glasses and hearing aids), and day/night-concordant light/dark cycles. Early mobilization of ICU patients, even during mechanical ventilation, reduces ICU delirium [50].

Family engagement has not been studied in randomized trials (and it may be unethical to randomize patients to limited family engagement), but a relationship between family presence and delirium has been suggested in observational studies. A study of patients with SARS-CoV-2 infection, for example, found that restricted family engagement was associated with increased rates of delirium [7]. Another observational study showed that complete

ABCDEF bundle performance was associated with a lower likelihood of next-day delirium, next-day mechanical ventilation, death within seven days, and discharge to a nursing facility rather than to home, and each outcome exhibited a consistent dose-response relationship with performance of the full bundle [51]. More recent studies in the post-COVID-19 era have shown similar results [52].

Pharmacologic

The most common class of medications used to treat delirium is antipsychotics, with the most commonly used medication being haloperidol [53,54,55]. Whereas more than half of delirious ICU patients may receive haloperidol [56], there is now sufficient evidence against its efficacy, with three high-quality, placebo-controlled randomized trials finding no difference in delirium duration between patients who received haloperidol and those who received placebo [57,58,59,60]. Multiple systematic reviews and meta-analyses have similarly found no significant differences in various delirium outcomes between recipients of haloperidol and placebo [60,61,62]. As haloperidol is not without its risks, current guidelines recommend against the routine use of haloperidol for either the prevention or treatment of delirium in the ICU [5]. Similarly, ziprasidone, an atypical antipsychotic, had no significant benefit when used to treat delirium during critical illness [58]. A meta-analysis of atypical antipsychotics, such as ziprasidone and quetiapine, also failed to find a difference in delirium/coma-free days in adults with delirium in the ICU, and as such, guidelines also recommend against their use for prevention or treatment of delirium in the ICU [5].

Certain sedatives used in the ICU are more deliriogenic than others. Whereas benzodiazepines have the strongest association with delirium, other sedatives, especially dexmedetomidine, are less deliriogenic and may have some benefit for treatment of those with hyperactive delirium [45,46,63,64]. In one randomized trial, dexmedetomidine reduced delirium when used at night to promote sleep during mechanical ventilation for acute respiratory failure [65]. In another trial, dexmedetomidine was used to treat agitated delirium that presented a barrier to extubation and was found to increase ventilator-free hours and to hasten the resolution of delirium in the seven-day study period [66]. Ketamine is an analgesic and sedative that has seen increasing use in the ICU over the last decade, but it has not been shown to reduce the incidence of delirium [67,68]. Current guidelines recommend avoiding benzodiazepines as general sedatives, using either dexmedetomidine or propofol as a first-line sedative, and using dexmedetomidine specifically to treat delirium in patients for whom agitation precludes ventilator weaning and extubation. Nevertheless, the current guidelines stop short of recommending the general use of dexmedetomidine to prevent delirium. Ketamine is not currently recommended as a delirium therapy [5].

Other agents, including 3-hydroxy-3-methylglutaryl-coenzyme A reductase inhibitors (statins), melatonin and melatonin receptor agonists, and rivastigmine, have been studied in the prevention and/or treatment of delirium; none has shown a consistent positive signal, and therefore none are currently recommended [69,70,71,72,73].

Conclusions

Delirium is common in the critically ill and contributes to multiple negative outcomes, including longer durations in the ICU and hospital and long-term cognitive impairment. These adverse outcomes contribute to physical deconditioning and impaired cognition, which are hallmarks of PICS. Addressing delirium in the critically ill may help to decrease the sequelae seen in survivors; existing evidence, however, supports only nonpharmacological prevention of delirium. More research and a deeper understanding of the mechanisms underlying delirium are needed before effective pharmacological therapies for delirium can be identified.

Key Points

1. Delirium during critical illness is common and is associated with multiple adverse outcomes that contribute to PICS, including longer ICU and hospital stays and long-term cognitive impairment.
2. Two well-validated tools can be used to detect delirium in the ICU: the Confusion Assessment Method for the ICU and the Intensive Care Delirium Screening Checklist.
3. The underlying mechanism of delirium is unclear, but studies have posited multiple potential mechanisms, including neuroinflammation, vascular permeability, metabolic insufficiency, neuronal dysfunction, and neurotransmitter disturbance.
4. There are multiple risk factors for delirium, including advanced age, preexisting cognitive impairment, severe illness, mechanical ventilation, deep sedation, and sleep deprivation.
5. Management of delirium include pharmacological methods, which are largely ineffective, and nonpharmacological methods, which focus on prevention.

References

1. T.J. Iwashyna, E.W. Ely, D.M. Smith, K.M. Langa. Long-term cognitive impairment and functional disability among survivors of severe sepsis. *JAMA* 2010; **304**: 1787–94.
2. T.D. Girard, J.C. Jackson, P.P. Pandharipande, et al. Delirium as a predictor of long-term cognitive impairment in survivors of critical illness. *Crit Care Med* 2010; **38**: 1513–20.
3. D.J. Cameron, R.I. Thomas, M. Mulvihill, H. Bronheim. Delirium: a test of the Diagnostic and Statistical Manual III criteria on medical inpatients. *J Am Geriatr Soc* 1987; **35**: 1007–10.
4. J.M. Ellison. DSM-III and the diagnosis of organic mental disorders. *Ann Emerg Med* 1984; **13**: 521–8.
5. J.W. Devlin, Y. Skrobik, C. Gélinas, et al. Clinical practice guidelines for the prevention and management of pain, agitation/sedation, delirium, immobility, and sleep disruption in adult patients in the ICU. *Crit Care Med* 2018; **46**: e825–e73.
6. E.W. Ely, S.K. Inouye, G.R. Bernard, et al. Delirium in mechanically ventilated patients: validity and reliability of the confusion assessment method for the intensive care unit (CAM-ICU). *JAMA* 2001; **286**: 2703–10.
7. B.T. Pun, R. Badenes, G. Heras La Calle, et al. Prevalence and risk factors for delirium in critically ill patients with COVID-19 (COVID-D): a multicentre cohort study. *Lancet Respir Med* 2021; **9**: 239–50.
8. F. Sadaf, M. Saqib, M. Iftikhar, A. Ahmad. Prevalence and risk factors of delirium in patients admitted to intensive care units: a multicentric cross-sectional study. *Cureus* 2023; **15**: e44827.
9. R.S. Al Farsi, A.M. Al Alawi, A.R. Al Huraizi, et al. Delirium in medically hospitalized patients: prevalence, recognition and risk factors: a prospective cohort study. *J Clin Med* 2023; **12;** 3897.

10. P. Mesa, I.J. Previgliano, S. Altez, et al. Delirium in a Latin American intensive care unit: a prospective cohort study of mechanically ventilated patients. *Rev Bras Tera Intensiva* 2017; **29**: 337-45.

11. E.W. Ely. Delirium as a predictor of mortality in mechanically ventilated patients in the intensive care init. *JAMA* 2004; **291**: 1753-62.

12. P. Pandharipande, B.A. Cotton, A. Shintani, et al. Motoric subtypes of delirium in mechanically ventilated surgical and trauma intensive care unit patients. *Intensive Care Med* 2007; **33**: 1726-31.

13. C. Dziegielewski, C. Skead, T. Canturk, et al. Delirium and associated length of stay and costs in critically ill patients. *Crit Care Res Pract* 2021; **2021**: 6612187.

14. J. McCusker, M. Cole, M. Abrahamowicz, et al. Delirium predicts 12-month mortality. *Arch Intern Med* 2002; **162**: 457-63.

15. D.K. Kiely, E.R. Marcantonio, S.K. Inouye, et al. Persistent delirium predicts greater mortality. *J Am Geriatr Soc* 2009; **57**: 55-61.

16. K.M. Fiest, A. Soo, C. Hee Lee, et al. Long-term outcomes in ICU patients with delirium: a population-based cohort study. *Am J Respir Crit Care Med* 2021; **204**: 412-20.

17. M.A. Pisani, S.Y.J. Kong, S.V. Kasl, et al. Days of delirium are associated with 1-year mortality in an older intensive care unit population. *Am J Respir Crit Care Med* 2009; **180**: 1092-7.

18. P.P. Pandharipande, T.D. Girard, J.C. Jackson, et al. Long-term cognitive impairment after critical illness. *N Engl J Med* 2013; **369**: 1306-16.

19. S.P. Leighton, J.W. Herron, E. Jackson, et al. Delirium and the risk of developing dementia: a cohort study of 12 949 patients. *J Neurol Neurosurg Psychiatr* 2022; **93**: 822-7.

20. T.G. Fong, R.N. Jones, P. Shi, et al. Delirium accelerates cognitive decline in Alzheimer disease. *Neurology* 2009; **72**: 1570-5.

21. A. Müller, J. von Hofen-Hohloch, M. Mende, et al. Long-term cognitive impairment after ICU treatment: a prospective longitudinal cohort study (Cog-I-CU). *Sci Rep* 2020; **10**: 15518.

22. C.S. Vrettou, V. Mantziou, A.G. Vassiliou, et al. Post-intensive care syndrome in survivors from critical illness including COVID-19 patients: a narrative review. *Life* 2022; **12**: 107.

23. D. Nagarajan, D.-C.A. Lee, L.M. Robins, T.P. Haines. Risk factors for social isolation in post-hospitalized older adults. *Arch Gerontol Geriatr* 2020; **88**: 104036.

24. P.T. Trzepacz, R.W. Baker, J. Greenhouse. A symptom rating scale for delirium. *Psychiatry Res* 1988; **23**: 89-97.

25. P.T. Trzepacz, D. Mittal, R. Torres, et al. Validation of the Delirium Rating Scale-revised-98: comparison with the delirium rating scale and the cognitive test for delirium. *J Neuropsychiatry Clin Neurosci* 2001; **13**: 229-42.

26. S.K. Inouye, C.H. van Dyck, C.A. Alessi, et al. Clarifying confusion: the confusion assessment method: a new method for detection of delirium. *Ann Intern Med* 1990; **113**: 941-8.

27. M.J. Schuurmans, L.M. Shortridge-Baggett, S.A. Duursma. The Delirium Observation Screening Scale: a screening instrument for delirium. *Res Theory Nurs Pract* 2003; **17**: 31-50.

28. N. Bergeron, M.J. Dubois, M. Dumont, et al. Intensive Care Delirium Screening Checklist: evaluation of a new screening tool. *Intensive Care Med* 2001; **27**: 859-64.

29. E.W. Ely, R. Margolin, J. Francis, et al. Evaluation of delirium in critically ill patients: validation of the Confusion Assessment Method for the Intensive Care Unit (CAM-ICU). *Crit Care Med* 2001; **29**: 1370-9.

30. M.L. Gunther, A. Morandi, E.W. Ely. Pathophysiology of delirium in the intensive care unit. *Crit Care Clin* 2008; **24**: 45-65.

31. J.E. Wilson, M.F. Mart, C. Cunningham, et al. Delirium. *Nat Rev Dis Primers* 2020; **6**: 90.

32. H. Yokota, S. Ogawa, A. Kurokawa, Y. Yamamoto. Regional cerebral blood flow in delirium patients. *Psychiatry Clin Neurosci* 2003; **57**: 337–9.

33. J. Kealy, C. Murray, E.W. Griffin, et al. Acute inflammation alters brain energy metabolism in mice and humans: role in suppressed spontaneous activity, impaired cognition, and delirium. *J Neurosci* 2020; **40**: 5681–96.

34. S.K. Inouye, P.A. Charpentier. Precipitating factors for delirium in hospitalized elderly persons. Predictive model and interrelationship with baseline vulnerability. *JAMA* 1996; **275**: 852–7.

35. R. Kaushik, G.J. McAvay, T.E. Murphy, et al. In-hospital delirium and disability and cognitive impairment after COVID-19 hospitalization. *JAMA Netw Open* 2024; **7**: e2419640.

36. N.T. Prendergast, C.A. Franz, C. Schaefer, et al. Inflammatory subphenotype is associated with acute brain dysfunction in mechanically ventilated patients. *Ann Am Thorac Soc* 2024; **21**: 1329–33.

37. J.F. Peterson, B.T. Pun, R.S. Dittus, et al. Delirium and its motoric subtypes: a study of 614 critically ill patients. *J Am Geriatr Soc* 2006; **54**: 479–84.

38. K.N. la Cour, N.C. Andersen-Ranberg, S. Weihe, et al. Distribution of delirium motor subtypes in the intensive care unit: a systematic scoping review. *Crit Care* 2022; **26**: 53.

39. C.J. Hayhurst, P.P. Pandharipande, C.G. Hughes. Intensive care unit delirium: a review of diagnosis, prevention, and treatment. *Anesthesiology* 2016; **125**: 1229–41.

40. T.D. Girard, J.L. Thompson, P.P. Pandharipande, et al. Clinical phenotypes of delirium during critical illness and severity of subsequent long-term cognitive impairment: a prospective cohort study. *Lancet Respir Med* 2018; **6**: 213–22.

41. K.M. Potter, J.N. Kennedy, C. Onyemekwu, et al. Data-derived subtypes of delirium during critical illness. *EBioMedicine* 2024; **100**: 104942.

42. K.M. Potter, N.T. Prendergast, J. G. Boyd. From traditional typing to intelligent insights: a narrative review of directions toward targeted therapies in delirium. *Crit Care Med* 2024; **52**: 1285–94.

43. E.M.L. Bowman, E.L. Cunningham, V. J. Page, D.F. McAuley. Phenotypes and subphenotypes of delirium: a review of current categorisations and suggestions for progression. *Crit Care* 2021; **25**: 334.

44. E.M.L. Bowman, N.E. Brummel, G. A. Caplan, et al. Advancing specificity in delirium: The delirium subtyping initiative. *Alzheimers Dement* 2024; **20**: 183–94.

45. P.P. Pandharipande, R.D. Sanders, T. D. Girard, et al. Effect of dexmedetomidine versus lorazepam on outcome in patients with sepsis: an a priori-designed analysis of the MENDS randomized controlled trial. *Crit Care* 2010; **14**: R38.

46. R.R. Riker, Y. Shehabi, P.M. Bokesch, et al. Dexmedetomidine vs midazolam for sedation of critically ill patients: a randomized trial. *JAMA* 2009; **301**: 489–99.

47. S.S. Carson, J.P. Kress, J.E. Rodgers, et al. A randomized trial of intermittent lorazepam versus propofol with daily interruption in mechanically ventilated patients. *Crit Care Med* 2006; **34**: 1326–32.

48. J.W. Devlin, F. Marquis, R.R. Riker, et al. Combined didactic and scenario-based education improves the ability of intensive care unit staff to recognize delirium at the bedside. *Crit Care* 2008; **12**: R19.

49. P.E. Spronk, B. Riekerk, J. Hofhuis, J.H. Rommes. Occurrence of delirium is severely underestimated in the ICU during daily care. *Intensive Care Med* 2009; **35**: 1276–80.

50. W.D. Schweickert, M.C. Pohlman, A. S. Pohlman, et al. Early physical and occupational therapy in mechanically ventilated, critically ill patients: a randomised controlled trial. *Lancet* 2009; **373**: 1874–82.

51. B.T. Pun, M.C. Balas, M.A. Barnes-Daly, et al. Caring for critically ill patients with the ABCDEF bundle: results of the ICU

liberation collaborative in over 15,000 adults. *Crit Care Med* 2019; **47**: 3–14.

52. J. Barr, B. Downs, K. Ferrell, et al. Improving outcomes in mechanically ventilated adult ICU patients following implementation of the ICU liberation (ABCDEF) bundle across a large healthcare system. *Crit Care Explor* 2024; **6**: e1001.

53. E.W. Ely, R.K. Stephens, J.C. Jackson, et al. Current opinions regarding the importance, diagnosis, and management of delirium in the intensive care unit: a survey of 912 healthcare professionals. *Crit Care Med* 2004; **32**: 106–12.

54. R.P. Patel, M. Gambrell, T. Speroff, et al. Delirium and sedation in the intensive care unit: survey of behaviors and attitudes of 1384 healthcare professionals. *Crit Care Med* 2009; **37**: 825–32.

55. A. Morandi, S. Piva, E.W. Ely, et al. Worldwide survey of the "assessing pain, both spontaneous awakening and breathing trials, choice of drugs, delirium monitoring/management, early exercise/mobility, and family empowerment" (ABCDEF) bundle. *Crit Care Med* 2017; **45**: e1111–e22.

56. M.O. Collet, J. Caballero, R. Sonneville, et al. Prevalence and risk factors related to haloperidol use for delirium in adult intensive care patients: the multinational AID-ICU inception cohort study. *Intensive Care Med* 2018; **44**: 1081–9.

57. M. van den Boogaard, A.J.C. Slooter, R.J.M. Brüggemann, et al. Effect of haloperidol on survival among critically ill adults with a high risk of delirium: the REDUCE randomized clinical trial. *JAMA* 2018; **319**: 680–90.

58. T.D. Girard, M.C. Exline, S.S. Carson, et al. Haloperidol and ziprasidone for treatment of delirium in critical illness. *N Engl J Med* 2018; **379**: 2506–16.

59. N.C. Andersen-Ranberg, L.M. Poulsen, A. Perner, et al. Haloperidol for the treatment of delirium in ICU patients. *N Engl J Med* 2022; **387**: 2425–35.

60. N.C. Andersen-Ranberg, M. Barbateskovic, A. Perner, et al. Haloperidol for the treatment of delirium in critically ill patients: an updated systematic review with meta-analysis and trial sequential analysis. *Crit Care* 2023; **27**: 329.

61. L.D. Burry, W. Cheng, D.R. Williamson, et al. Pharmacological and non-pharmacological interventions to prevent delirium in critically ill patients: a systematic review and network meta-analysis. *Intensive Care Med* 2021; **47**: 943–60.

62. S.F. Herling, I.E. Greve, E.E. Vasilevskis, et al. Interventions for preventing intensive care unit delirium in adults. *Cochrane Database Syst Rev* 2018; **11**: CD009783.

63. C.G. Hughes, P.T. Mailloux, J.W. Devlin, et al. Dexmedetomidine or propofol for sedation in mechanically ventilated adults with sepsis. *N Engl J Med* 2021; **384**: 1424–36.

64. Y. Shehabi, B.D. Howe, R. Bellomo, et al. Early sedation with dexmedetomidine in critically ill patients. *N Engl J Med* 2019; **380**: 2506–17.

65. Y. Skrobik, M.S. Duprey, N.S. Hill, J.W. Devlin. Low-dose nocturnal dexmedetomidine prevents ICU delirium: a randomized, placebo-controlled trial. *Am J Respir Crit Care Med* 2018; **197**: 1147–56.

66. M.C. Reade, G.M. Eastwood, R. Bellomo, et al. Effect of dexmedetomidine added to standard care on ventilator-free time in patients with agitated delirium: a randomized clinical trial. *JAMA* 2016; **315**: 1460–8.

67. J.A. Hudetz, K.M. Patterson, Z. Iqbal, et al. Ketamine attenuates delirium after cardiac surgery with cardiopulmonary bypass. *J Cardiothorac Vasc Anesth* 2009; **23**: 651–7.

68. M.S. Avidan, H.R. Maybrier, A.B. Abdallah, et al. Intraoperative ketamine for prevention of postoperative delirium or pain after major surgery in older adults: an international, multicentre, double-blind, randomised clinical trial. *Lancet* 2017; **390**: 267–75.

69. D.M. Needham, E. Colantuoni, V.D. Dinglas, et al. Rosuvastatin versus placebo for delirium in intensive care and subsequent cognitive impairment in

patients with sepsis-associated acute respiratory distress syndrome: an ancillary study to a randomised controlled trial. *Lancet Respir Med* 2016; **4**: 203–12.

70. V.J. Page, A. Casarin, E.W. Ely, et al. Evaluation of early administration of simvastatin in the prevention and treatment of delirium in critically ill patients undergoing mechanical ventilation (MoDUS): a randomised, double-blind, placebo-controlled trial. *Lancet Respir Med* 2017; **5**: 727–37.

71. H.N. Vijayakumar, K. Ramya, D.R. Duggappa, et al. Effect of melatonin on duration of delirium in organophosphorus compound poisoning patients: a double-blind randomised placebo controlled trial. *Indian J Anaesth* 2016; **60**: 814–20.

72. J.V. Gandolfi, A.P.A. Di Bernardo, D.A.V. Chanes, et al. The effects of melatonin supplementation on sleep quality and assessment of the serum melatonin in ICU patients: a randomized controlled trial. *Crit Care Med* 2020; **48**: e1286–e93.

73. M. Nishikimi, A. Numaguchi, K. Takahashi, et al. Effect of administration of ramelteon, a melatonin receptor agonist, on the duration of stay in the ICU: a single-center randomized placebo-controlled trial. *Crit Care Med* 2018; **46**: 1099–105.

Chapter 9: Sleep Impairments in the Critically Ill

Janna R. Raphelson and Robert L. Owens

Introduction

Sleep impairment in the intensive care unit (ICU) and its role in the development of post-intensive care syndrome (PICS) is not well understood. For those practicing in the critical care setting, it is not difficult to imagine that this exciting and adrenaline-fueled space is not conducive to quality sleep. After a hospitalization requiring critical care, patients commonly report sleeping difficulties that persist well into their recovery, and they often remember their ICU stay as marked by exhaustion and frequent sleep interruptions [1]. Sleep directly and indirectly intersects with all domains of PICS (physical, cognitive, and psychological), and understanding how sleep patterns are influenced by critical illness can help inform care in both the ICU and ICU follow-up clinics. This chapter will address what we know about sleep in critical illness, how this compares to "normal" sleep, links between sleep and delirium, and common ICU interventions intended to promote sleep.

Sleep in the ICU

Sleep problems are prevalent and distressing in the ICU, and sleep quality in the critically ill is subjectively poor. In a study of 203 patients interviewed at discharge after a hospitalization that included time in the ICU, patients unanimously felt that their sleep in the ICU was poorer in quality than sleep at home [2]. Sleep in the ICU has been repeatedly shown to be fragmented, characterized by altered sleep architecture, and marked by profound sleep deprivation, with noise as a commonly perceived driver of these disturbances [2,3]. Patients with preexisting sleep difficulties are at particularly high risk for sleep problems in the ICU and during recovery [4]. Based on estimates from subjective data, healthy sleep patterns take up to 6 to 12 months after discharge to be restored [4].

Sleep in the ICU Compared to Normal Sleep

To better understand sleep disruption in the ICU, knowledge of the normal sleep cycle is essential [5]. Normal sleep is a stepwise progression through three stages of non-rapid eye movement (NREM) sleep (N1 → N2 → N3), often with a brief return to N1/N2 sleep before entering a period of rapid eye movement (REM) sleep. This cycle repeats throughout the course of a night with slight variations in the length and sequence of various stages. At the beginning of a typical eight-hour sleep period, a healthy person will transition from wakefulness to light sleep, or N1 sleep, and remain in this state for one to seven minutes. They next enter N2 sleep for approximately 10–25 minutes, and from here, if allowed to continue sleeping, progress to deep sleep, N3, for 20–40 minutes. After this period of deep sleep, they will briefly return to N1 or N2 sleep before passing into their first period of REM sleep. This first period of REM sleep is generally the shortest, lasting only one to five minutes, but subsequent REM sleep periods become steadily longer throughout the course of the night. One full sleep cycle generally takes 70–100 minutes and may last up to 120 minutes later in the night. Periods of N3 sleep become progressively shorter over the course of the night as the periods of REM sleep lengthen. Given the length of one sleep cycle, it is easy to appreciate that it may be difficult for an ICU patient to complete even one sleep cycle, let alone sleep throughout the night. The ICU's deleterious effects on sleep are thought to arise from disturbance of the normal sleep architecture (see Figure 9.1), sleep fragmentation, and overall decreased sleep duration, but which of these abnormalities predominantly drives poor outcomes is unknown [6].

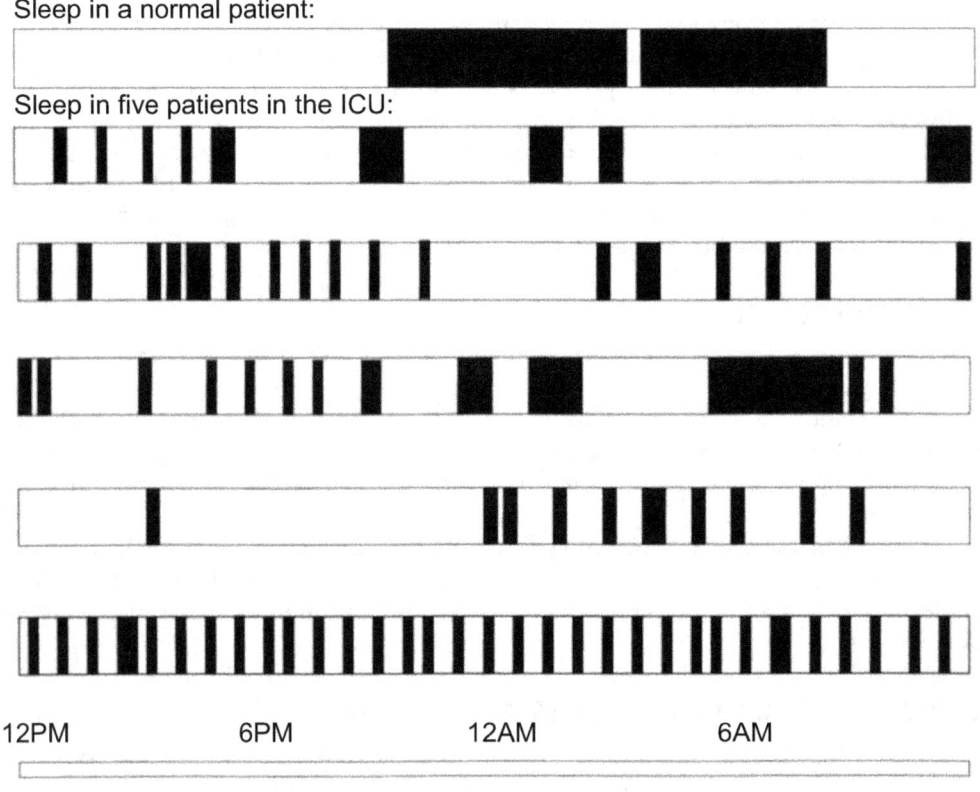

Figure 9.1 Sleep fragmentation in five ICU patients. Black areas represent episodes of sleep and white areas represent wakefulness. Reprinted with permission of the American Thoracic Society. Copyright © 2024 American Thoracic Society. All rights reserved. From: N.S. Freedman, et al. 2001. Abnormal sleep/wake cycles and the effect of environmental noise on sleep disruption in the intensive care unit. *Am J Respir Crit Care Med.* 163; 451–7. The American Journal of Respiratory and Critical Care Medicine is an official journal of the American Thoracic Society.

Reasons for Poor Sleep in the ICU

Knowing that normal sleep is a series of cycles through light, deep, and REM sleep over the course of a night, it is easy to understand how this is frequently interrupted by the interventions, clinical events, and ambient disruptors that occur at nighttime in the ICU.

Environmental factors, particularly noise, are frequently cited as causes of poor sleep. A prospective study [7] found that daily peak noise levels in a surgical ICU averaged 75.6 dB(A) over a six-week period, equivalent to the sound intensity of a coffee grinder or garbage disposal [8]. Similar corroborating studies [9] have determined that sound intensity in ICUs nearly always exceeds 45 dB(A), averages 50–60 dB(A), and often peaks as high as 85 dB(A). For context, the World Health Organization's *Community Guidelines for Noise* [10] recommends that sound levels not exceed 35 dB(A) at night for good quality sleep. A small questionnaire-based study [2] of ICU patients at the time of discharge found that talking and telemetry alarms were significantly more disturbing than other noises, such as televisions, pagers, and IV pump and ventilator alarms (p = 0.003). Even in a relatively calm ICU environment, ambient noise alone has enough potential to arouse patients from sleep.

Noise is not the only factor responsible for sleep disturbances in the ICU. Light patterns are often highly erratic, causing further disruption of circadian sleep–wake cycling [10,13]. Bright lights are frequently on at nighttime, particularly in the rooms of the most critically ill patients, while lights are often turned off during daytime, and rooms may lack windows that allow for natural light. Clinical interventions and interactions for diagnostic purposes can also cause sleep interruptions [1,11,12]. "Morning labs" and other care tasks of unclear clinical value are often performed at night for the convenience of clinicians over patients, and a desire not to pass on procedures to daytime physicians may also cause painful and nonurgent disruptions of sleep. In lower acuity settings, the utility of overnight vital sign checks has been debated [11]. Although it is not realistic to abandon continuous monitoring in the critically ill, a culture of sleep prioritization may justify deferral of nonurgent interventions overnight. In some patients, pain, anxiety, and dyspnea further contribute to sleep disruption; this phenotype that "won't sleep" due to illness-related factors is perhaps more difficult to treat clinically than the "can't sleep" phenotype driven by environment-related factors.

Sleep and Delirium

Delirium is associated with increased mortality, ICU length of stay, and long-term cognitive impairment (see Chapter 8 for additional information) [12,13]. Sleep deprivation and delirium have a similar constellation of symptoms, including sleep–wake cycle disruptions, inattention, and fluctuating mental status, leading many to posit poor sleep as a risk factor for delirium. Although the direct pathologic connection is unclear, lack of sleep may increase risk for delirium; moreover, poor sleep is often treated with deliriogenic medications (e.g., benzodiazepines). A study of ICU patients aged 65 and older found that nighttime sleep duration and total sleep time was equivalent between delirious and non-delirious patients; however, sleep fragmentation was more commonly severe in delirious patients [14]. A study in postoperative ICU patients by the same group found decreased inter-daily stability in actigraphy measurements in delirious patients compared with non-delirious patients, suggesting a trend toward decreased day–night differentiation, even before delirium is clinically recognized [15]. Benzodiazepines and sedatives such as propofol, which are commonly prescribed in the ICU setting, alter sleep structure, which may further drive delirium in some patients. Pharmacologic treatment of sleep to prevent delirium is an active area of study; however, several major trials investigating melatonin, ramelteon, and overnight dexmedetomidine infusions have largely shown no benefit [14,15,16].

Regardless of the exact mechanism, multiple studies have shown that improving sleep can reduce ICU delirium. Kamdar and colleagues [17,18] showed that a multicomponent intervention (including eye masks, soft music, room temperature optimization, daytime wakefulness promotion, and reduction of nighttime alarms and lighting) to improve sleep was associated with a 20% reduction in ICU delirium, a finding since repeated in other ICUs. Given that pharmacological trials to date have shown little benefit in augmenting sleep in the ICU, non-pharmacological interventions seem more useful to promote sleep and thereby reduce delirium. In a study of 171 critically ill patients by Patel and colleagues, for example, implementation of bundled interventions to reduce noise and light in the ICU led to increased sleep efficiency, reduced awakenings, and lower incidence of delirium [19]. The most beneficial interventions remain unknown.

Things That We Do to Improve Sleep: Some Harmful, Some Useless

There is often pressure to provide sedation to critically ill patients on mechanical life support [20], and while such sedation is often equated to sleep, mounting evidence shows that it is not comparable to normal sleep architecture. Sedation is often maintained throughout the day as well, robbing patients of important wakefulness during the day, which in turn, typically promotes natural sleep at night.

Medications

Again, sedation is not equivalent to sleep, and those wishing to help their patients rest must seek alternative strategies. Natural sleep at night requires a buildup of sleep debt during the day, and providing daytime sedation delays the restoration of natural circadian drivers by minimizing daytime activity, preventing development of physiological tiredness at bedtime, and disturbing day/night recognition. It is important when safe and feasible to allow wakefulness during the day to help promote sleep at night; high-quality ICU care with spontaneous awakening trials and physical therapy can help achieve this goal.

Propofol is a common anesthetic agent administered in the ICU. Data are mixed on whether it truly promotes sleep, with a Cochrane review [21] finding insufficient evidence to answer this question. Polysomnography studies of patients appearing to sleep while receiving a propofol infusion found decreased REM sleep and disrupted sleep architecture [22], questioning whether this sleep is truly restorative.

Exogenous melatonin supplementation to promote sleep and prevent delirium has been evaluated, but current data on efficacy are mixed [14]. Melatonin administration also suffers from lack of FDA regulation given its status as a supplement rather than a medication in the United States. A 2018 Cochrane review [23] found insufficient evidence to determine the usefulness of melatonin in the ICU setting but noted several ongoing studies at the time of publication. Similarly, the 2018 Clinical Practice Guidelines from the Society of Critical Care Medicine for the Prevention and Management of Pain, Agitation/Sedation, Delirium, Immobility, and Sleep Disruption in Adult Patients in the ICU [5] made no recommendation for or against the use of melatonin in the ICU for sleep promotion or delirium prevention.

A subsequent trial of 203 critically ill patients randomized to receive 10 mg of melatonin or placebo found significantly improved sleep quality based on self-reported answers to the Richards-Campbell Sleep Questionnaire (RCSQ) in patients receiving melatonin (p = 0.029), but no change in nursing-observed sleep hours [24]. Furthermore, a 2022 randomized control trial of melatonin versus placebo to prevent delirium in ICU patients did not find a significant difference in delirium rates with melatonin administration; sleep outcomes were not assessed [25]. Although mixed, these newer data suggest possible efficacy for melatonin or ramelteon as a subjective sleep-promoting intervention in the ICU but lack of effectiveness for delirium prevention.

Conversely, the alpha-2 agonist dexmedetomidine has been shown to reduce ICU delirium when administered in a low-dose continuous infusion (maximum rate of 0.7 μg/kg/h) at nighttime [26]. Unlike propofol, dexmedetomidine may preserve sleep architecture during nocturnal usage and does not suppress REM sleep, yet in a placebo-controlled trial, dexmedetomidine was not associated with improved sleep quality per patient report [26]. Larger studies using dexmedetomidine for sedation (not sleep) have not consistently shown a reduction in delirium [27,28,29].

Non-pharmacological Factors

Non-pharmacological interventions, including ear plugs, eye masks [30], and cycled lighting [31] to promote circadian cycling, have been investigated. These interventions have been received positively by both patients and staff in study hospitals; however, many studies are limited by difficulty with assessing sleep objectively, recall bias from participants surveyed, and survivor bias when patients are asked about their experience after an ICU stay. Patient acceptance of some of these interventions may be low, but the low cost and lack of adverse effects make such interventions low-risk and potentially high-yield in some patients.

Mechanical Ventilation Considerations

A common strategy in critical care is to "rest" mechanically ventilated patients on assist-control ventilation (ACV) overnight rather than to allow continued pressure support ventilation (PSV). There is a sense from ICU providers that "rest" settings are preferable in patients who are approaching readiness for extubation. Three studies [32,33,34] addressing this issue, including a total 61 patients, found that "resting" on ACV at nighttime, compared with continued PSV, is associated with longer time spent in REM sleep but not with increased total sleep time. This finding, along with the low risk associated with this strategy and its congruence with common clinical practice, led the 2018 Clinical Practice Guidelines for the Prevention and Management of Pain, Agitation/Sedation, Delirium, Immobility, and Sleep Disruption in Adult Patients in the ICU [5] to suggest nocturnal ACV over PSV to promote sleep in the ICU (conditional recommendation, low quality of evidence). We suggest a more individualized approach that considers patient comfort as well: if a patient is comfortable on PSV, we may not necessarily switch to ACV, especially if they report good sleep.

Conclusions

There are many challenges in attempting to promote sleep in the ICU, including high noise levels, competing clinical priorities, and necessary alarms and diagnostic interventions. While interactions between sleep and the development of PICS are not clearly understood, sleeping difficulties are common in patients after an ICU stay. Patients often recall major distress around difficulty sleeping during their hospitalization. Sleep architecture alterations, fragmentation, and deprivation appear to contribute to delirium and are important risk factors for PICS. Despite these challenges, sleep is an actionable target to improve the patient experience in the ICU and long-term outcomes.

Key Points

1. Sleep in the ICU is subjectively poor and objectively characterized by fragmentation and deprivation.
2. Common ICU interventions may drive sleep disruption.
3. An emphasis on promoting sleep has been shown to reduce ICU delirium.
4. Sleep is a potentially modifiable risk factor for the development of PICS.
5. Pharmacological sleep aids are often used to promote sleep but may produce more harm than benefit.
6. Efforts to promote wakefulness during the day (e.g., daily interruptions of sedation and physical therapy) benefit patients and may improve natural sleep.

References

1. M. Zhou, J. Zhang, Z. Xu, et al. Incidence of and risk factors for post-intensive care syndrome among Chinese respiratory intensive care unit patients: A cross-sectional, prospective study. *Aust Crit Care* 2023; **36**: 464–9.
2. N. S. Freedman, N. Kotzer, R. J. Schwab. Patient perception of sleep quality and etiology of sleep disruption in the intensive care unit. *Am J Respir Crit Care Med* 1999; **159**: 1155–62.
3. D. Georgopoulos, E. Kondili, B. Gerardy, et al. Sleep architecture patterns in critically ill patients and survivors of critical illness: A retrospective study. *Ann Am Thorac Soc* 2023; **20**: 1624–32.
4. M. T. Altman, M. P. Knauert, M. A. Pisani. Sleep disturbance after hospitalization and critical illness: A systematic review. *Ann Am Thorac Soc* 2017; **14**: 1457–68.
5. J. W. Devlin, Y. Skrobik, C. Gélinas, et al. Clinical practice guidelines for the prevention and management of pain, agitation/sedation, delirium, immobility, and sleep disruption in adult patients in the ICU. *Crit Care Med* 2018; **46**: e825–73.
6. M. P. Knauert, N. T. Ayas, K. J. Bosma. Causes, consequences, and treatments of sleep and circadian disruption in the ICU: An official American Thoracic Society research statement. *Am J Respir Crit Care Med* 2023; **207**: e49–68.
7. M. Guisasola-Rabes, B. Solà-Enriquez, A. M. Vélez-Pereira, M. de Nadal. Noise levels and sleep in a surgical ICU. *J Clin Med Res* 2022; **11**. http://dx.doi.org/10.3390/jcm11092328.
8. J. Cochary. Noise Awareness Day. Center for Hearing and Communication; 2021 (accessed February 2, 2024). Common Noise Levels. https://noiseawareness.org/info-center/common-noise-levels/.
9. J. L. Darbyshire, J. D. Young. An investigation of sound levels on intensive care units with reference to the WHO guidelines. *Crit Care* 2013; **17**: R187.
10. A. M. Pfister. WHO Guidelines for Community Noise – Executive summary [Internet] (accessed February 2, 2024). www.ruidos.org/Noise/WHO_Noise_guidelines_summary.html.
11. N. M. Orlov, V. M. Arora. Things We Do For No ReasonTM: Routine overnight vital sign checks. *J Hosp Med* 2020; **15**: 272–4.

12. J. J. Dorsch, J. L. Martin, A. Malhotra, et al. Sleep in the intensive care unit: Strategies for improvement. *Semin Respir Crit Care Med* 2019; **40**: 614–28.
13. G. Mistraletti, E. Carloni, M. Cigada, et al. Sleep and delirium in the intensive care unit. *Minerva Anestesiol* 2008; **74**: 329–33.
14. S. J. Jaiswal, T. J. McCarthy, N. E. Wineinger, et al. Melatonin and sleep in preventing hospitalized delirium: A randomized clinical trial. *Am J Med* 2018; **131**: 1110–17.
15. S. J. Jaiswal, S. R. S. Bagsic, E. Takata, et al. Actigraphy-based sleep and activity measurements in intensive care unit patients randomized to ramelteon or placebo for delirium prevention. *Sci Rep* 2023; **13**: 1450.
16. O. Huet, T. Gargadennec, J. F. Oilleau, et al. Prevention of post-operative delirium using an overnight infusion of dexmedetomidine in patients undergoing cardiac surgery: a pragmatic, randomized, double-blind, placebo-controlled trial. *Crit Care* 2024; **28**: 64.
17. B. B. Kamdar, J. Yang, L. M. King, et al. Developing, implementing, and evaluating a multifaceted quality improvement intervention to promote sleep in an ICU. *Am J Med Qual* 2014; **29**: 546–54.
18. J. E. Tonna, A. Dalton, A. P. Presson, et al. The effect of a quality improvement intervention on sleep and delirium in critically ill patients in a surgical ICU. *Chest* 2021; **160**: 899–908.
19. J. Patel, J. Baldwin, P. Bunting, S. Laha. The effect of a multicomponent multidisciplinary bundle of interventions on sleep and delirium in medical and surgical intensive care patients. *Anaesthesia* 2014; **69**: 540–9.
20. G. L. Weinhouse, P. L. Watson. Sedation and sleep disturbances in the ICU. *Crit Care Clin* 2009; **25**: 539–49.
21. S. R. Lewis, O. J. Schofield-Robinson, P. Alderson, A. F. Smith. Propofol for the promotion of sleep in adults in the intensive care unit. *Cochrane Database Syst Rev* 2018; **1**: CD012454.
22. E. Kondili, C. Alexopoulou, N. Xirouchaki, D. Georgopoulos. Effects of propofol on sleep quality in mechanically ventilated critically ill patients: A physiological study. *Intensive Care Med* 2012; **38**: 1640–6.
23. S. R. Lewis, M. W. Pritchard, O. J. Schofield-Robinson, et al. Melatonin for the promotion of sleep in adults in the intensive care unit. *Cochrane Database Syst Rev* 2018; **5**: CD012455.
24. J. V. Gandolfi, A. P. A. Di Bernardo, D. A. V. Chanes, et al. The effects of melatonin supplementation on sleep quality and assessment of the serum melatonin in ICU patients: A randomized controlled trial. *Crit Care Med* 2020; **48**: e1286–93.
25. B. Wibrow, F. E. Martinez, E. Myers, et al. Prophylactic melatonin for delirium in intensive care (Pro-MEDIC): A randomized controlled trial. *Intensive Care Med* 2022; **48**: 414–25.
26. Y. Skrobik, M. S. Duprey, N. S. Hill, J. W. Devlin. Low-dose nocturnal dexmedetomidine prevents ICU delirium. A randomized, placebo-controlled trial. *Am J Respir Crit Care Med* 2018; **197**: 1147–56.
27. P. P. Pandharipande, B. T. Pun, D. L. Herr, et al. Effect of sedation with dexmedetomidine vs lorazepam on acute brain dysfunction in mechanically ventilated patients: The MENDS randomized controlled trial. *JAMA* 2007; **298**: 2644–53.
28. J. Z. Qu, A. Mueller, T. B. McKay, et al. Nighttime dexmedetomidine for delirium prevention in non-mechanically ventilated patients after cardiac surgery (MINDDS): A single-centre, parallel-arm, randomised, placebo-controlled superiority trial. *EClinicalMedicine* 2023; **56**: 101796.
29. Y. Shehabi, D. Howe, R. Bellomo, et al. Early Sedation with Dexmedetomidine in Critically Ill Patients. *N Engl J Med* 2019; **380**: 2506–17.
30. H. Locihová, K. Axmann, H. Padyšáková, J. Fejfar. Effect of the use of earplugs and

eye mask on the quality of sleep in intensive care patients: A systematic review. *J Sleep Res* 2018; **27**: e12607.

31. M. Engwall, I. Fridha, L. Johansson, et al. Lighting, sleep and circadian rhythm: An intervention study in the intensive care unit. *Intensive Crit Care Nurs* 2015; **31**: 325–35.

32. C. Andréjak, J. Monconduit, D. Rose, et al. Does using pressure-controlled ventilation to rest respiratory muscles improve sleep in ICU patients? *Respir Med* 2013; **107**: 534–41.

33. B. Cabello, A. W. Thille, X. Drouot, et al. Sleep quality in mechanically ventilated patients: Comparison of three ventilatory modes. *Crit Care Med* 2008; **36**: 1749–55.

34. B. Toublanc, D. Rose, J. C. Glérant, et al. Assist-control ventilation vs. low levels of pressure support ventilation on sleep quality in intubated ICU patients. *Intensive Care Med* 2007; **33**: 1148–54.

Chapter 10
The Psychological Impacts of Hospitalization

Erin L. Hall-Melnychuk and Dorothy Wade

Introduction

Admission to an intensive care unit (ICU) because of severe illness, complications of surgery, or a serious accident can be an upsetting and frightening life event with a profound psychological impact on patients and their relatives, loved ones, and friends. Studies indicate that at least 40% of patients experience distress [1] and 30–80% develop delirium during an ICU admission [2]. Furthermore, up to 50% of patients experience long-term psychological difficulties, including depression, anxiety, and post-traumatic stress disorder (PTSD), after hospital discharge (see Chapter 46 for additional information).

For several decades, it was common practice for patients to be kept heavily sedated, with comparatively little consideration given to the impact of such an intervention on their psychological state. Clinicians erroneously believed that, because patients were sedated, they would not recall upsetting memories of their time in intensive care; however, pioneering studies suggested that many patients suffered from significant symptoms of depression, anxiety, and PTSD, including disturbing memories of delusions and hallucinations, both during and after discharge from the ICU [3]. This led clinical researchers, including nurses, psychiatrists, and psychologists, to investigate the causes of patients' distress in the ICU. In qualitative studies, patients described a wide range of negative experiences while critically ill, including confusion, fear, worry, nightmares, hallucinations, and an altered sense of reality; some, however, also reported positive experiences, such as gratitude for the kindness and support of staff, post-traumatic growth, and having a second lease on life [4,5].

It is important for ICU staff to understand that experiencing distress, hallucinations, or delusions in the ICU is a risk factor for adverse psychological outcomes following hospital discharge [1,3,6]. Aiming to alleviate patients' distress should be a normal part of the humane, person-centered care that ICUs strive to deliver and a strategy to prevent long-term psychological difficulties. Embedding clinical health psychologists in the ICU team to provide psychological assessments, support, and interventions for patients and families is becoming increasingly common, particularly in the United Kingdom (see Chapter 14 for additional information).

Although it is intuitive that an ICU experience may be associated with negative emotions, it is important to remember that many patients survive their ICU admission without showing signs of severe distress or being traumatized. There is much to learn from these patients about the coping strategies that help them and the factors that support their resilience. Little research has been conducted in this area; however, learning more about positive psychological outcomes following ICU admission and the coping mechanisms associated with them could inform future strategies to help people who are distressed or traumatized by their time in intensive care.

Understanding the psychological impact of ICU admission is incomplete without considering the effects on the families and friends of patients. ICU admissions are often stressful for loved ones, particularly when their relative is deteriorating, delirious, or admitted for a prolonged period [7]. Much like the patient who requires critical care, family members and loved ones may also experience psychological difficulties, including anxiety, depression, and PTSD, for months following a loved one's discharge from the ICU. All ICU staff should aim to reduce psychological distress for families by providing them with education about common intensive care procedures and conditions, including delirium, to improve their understanding of what they are seeing and experiencing and to help them provide optimal support for their relative (see Chapter 17 for additional information).

Psychological Experiences in the ICU

In the ICU, patients commonly experience new or worsened psychological difficulties, including symptoms of depression, anxiety, acute stress, and delirium. These problems may present alone, concurrently, or disguised as physical problems, and they may be difficult to distinguish from one other. Though most studies of critically ill patients have reported symptoms following ICU discharge or later, some qualitative and quantitative studies have evaluated patient psychological symptoms during ICU admission.

Critically ill patients frequently experience symptoms of anxiety, acute stress, and depression, and these are especially prevalent in those who require mechanical ventilation. More than 60% of patients report clinically significant anxiety during ICU admission, which may be associated with distressing physical experiences, the need for procedures, mechanical ventilation and ventilator weaning, invasive lines and tubes, being connected to drips and machines, or experiences associated with delirium [8]. Symptoms of acute stress may manifest as fear, panic, sleep disturbances, and nightmares. Feelings of sadness, isolation, alienation, and loneliness are also among the most common emotional experiences during an ICU admission. Patients may struggle with the lack of control and autonomy associated with treatment in an ICU, profound physical debility or pain, and the inability to perform self-care activities [9]. Being restrained and unable to sit up, eat and drink, or move for long periods of time increases overall distress.

Additionally, many patients experience symptoms of delirium, a syndrome characterized by intermittent confusion, disorientation, and disturbances in attention, concentration, cognition, and psychomotor behavior (either hypoactive or hyperactive; see Chapter 8 for additional information). During ICU admission, up to half of patients who are not mechanically ventilated and up to 80% of those who are experience delirium [5]. Patients who have been delirious often report memories of frightening delusional experiences or hallucinations during hospitalization, a sense of blurred reality, or paranoia. The inability to understand what is happening around them and failure to recall details or periods of time during or prior to ICU admission often increase patient distress.

Early psychological symptoms, both during and following ICU admission, have been linked to long-term psychological morbidity in survivors of critical illness. Given the frequency of psychological challenges in the ICU and their potential long-term repercussions (see Chapter 46 for additional information), it is crucial that clinicians recognize symptoms and their potential causes and initiate efforts to mitigate their impact.

Table 10.1 Risk factors for post-ICU psychological distress

Clinical Factors	Psychological Factors	Sociodemographic Factors
• Prolonged mechanical ventilation [4,11] • Prolonged duration of sedation [1,4,11] • Use of benzodiazepines during ICU admission [4,10,11]	• Acute stress symptoms during ICU admission [4,6,11] • Symptoms of delirium [4,11] • Recall of intrusive [4], frightening, or delusional memories [1,10] • Psychiatric history [1,4,6,10] • Premorbid psychological distress [10] • History of trauma [6]	• Younger age [10] • Female sex [10] • Lower level of education [10] • Unemployment • Lower socioeconomic position [4]

Table includes risk factors identified in the literature associated with post-ICU depression, anxiety, and PTSD

A more sophisticated understanding of the psychological distress experienced by critically ill patients will help ICU clinicians detect distress earlier and provide necessary support.

Risk Factors for Long-Term Psychological Distress

Myriad risk factors for long-term psychological distress following critical illness have been identified. Although risk factors are often considered in relation to long-term psychiatric symptoms of post-intensive care syndrome (PICS), recognition of these factors during ICU admission is important. Risk factors for long-term psychological morbidity in survivors of critical illness can be divided into three categories: clinical factors, psychological factors, and sociodemographic factors (see Table 10.1). Clinical factors include prolonged mechanical ventilation, prolonged duration of sedation, and administration of benzodiazepines [1,4,10,11]. Psychological factors include experience of acute stress symptoms and fear during ICU admission, delirium, and recall of frightening or delusional memories [1,4,6,11]. Psychiatric history and premorbid psychological distress are nonmodifiable risk factors for adverse psychological outcomes [1,10,11]. Sociodemographic risk factors for psychological morbidity include unemployment, lower educational attainment, lower socioeconomic status[4], and being younger and female [10,11].

Stressors Experienced in the ICU

Stressors experienced in the ICU are numerous and impactful; they may be the result of life-threatening illness or injury, treatments provided, and both real or delusional experiences associated with delirium. Earlier recognition of common stressors encountered during ICU admission combined with an understanding of risk factors for later psychological distress may help to mitigate the potential impact of these stressors on patients' recovery.

Illness-Related Stressors

Critically injured or ill patients may experience pain, acute or repeated surgeries or procedures, severe infections, metabolic disturbances, blood loss, and dysfunction of one or more organ systems. Patients frequently undergo uncomfortable, invasive medical procedures and tests, require indwelling lines and tubes, and are often connected to machines, including mechanical ventilators and dialysis machines, all of which can induce pain and anxiety. Many patients experience severe weakness associated with their illness or the immobility that often accompanies it, and they may go for days without eating or drinking, reliant instead on enteral or parenteral nutrition. Patients may be administered medications that are deliriogenic and may be subjected to multiple interventions, including hourly vital sign checks, blood draws, and nighttime light and noise, that cause significant sleep and circadian rhythm disruption. Collectively, the insults to patients' physical integrity and bodily functioning caused by critical illness and hospitalization are a profound source of physiological and psychological stress.

Patients who are receiving noninvasive and invasive mechanical ventilation often experience distress associated with both physical discomfort and communication difficulties. Many patients report discomfort due to pain, xerostomia, thirst, or a sensation of dyspnea while intubated or wearing a noninvasive ventilation mask. Some also experience claustrophobia, increased anxiety associated with the pressure of oxygen delivery, or symptoms of panic, suffocation, or impending death [12]. Tolerating changes to ventilator settings, including spontaneous breathing trials, and adjusting to a new tracheostomy are causes of increased subjective distress for many patients [13]. The inability to communicate is also a significant source of distress and is associated with feelings of fear and isolation [8]. Anxiety associated with mechanical ventilation increases the likelihood of dyssynchrony with the ventilator, compromises a patient's overall stability, and may prevent earlier extubation. In addition, patients with anxiety may receive more sedating and analgesic medications to keep them calm, which can then increase the risk of prolonged mechanical ventilation, immobility, delirium, and other complications.

As mentioned previously, delirium is a common and significant stressor experienced by critically ill patients and is associated with numerous adverse sequelae. For some, delirium is experienced as frightening symptoms of confusion, disorientation, visual hallucinations, and delusional memories. Some of these delusional experiences are persecutory in nature and may include themes of being kidnapped, held hostage, or sexually assaulted. These experiences are commonly associated with significant fear, mistrust of staff or family, and concerns about safety [12]. Patients with delirium also frequently experience disturbances in memory and attention that make it difficult to interpret events around them and to process the passage of time. Many patients do not have insight into their delirium or confusion, but for those who do, recognition of this often induces anxiety about its cause and the possibility of its permanence. Delirium also relates to the emotional distress patients experience, sometimes increasing emotional lability, and, at other times, resulting in patients appearing apathetic or with a flattened affect.

The inability to sleep is a related, widespread problem in the ICU, and its disruption is a source of both physiologic and psychological distress (see Chapter 9 for additional information). Environmental-, illness-, and medication-related factors result in disruptions of patients' sleep and circadian rhythms. Many ICU patients recall frightening nightmares, which can exacerbate the fear associated with falling asleep and increase confusion about experiences that are occurring in reality versus those that are occurring in disturbing dreams. Along with nightmares, discomfort, and noise, worry that falling asleep may result in worsening clinical status commonly contributes to sleep disturbances during critical illness.

In many parts of the world, physical restraint devices such as wrist restraints or mitts may be used with agitated patients (i.e., patients experiencing hyperactive delirium or those who exhibit otherwise challenging behavior) or to prevent self-extubation. Agitation in the ICU is often multifactorial and may be contributed to by physiologic instability, the sensation of breathlessness, pain or other physical discomfort, and anxiety, and it typically occurs in the context of delirium. Agitation can also be precipitated by certain medications, substance intoxication or withdrawal, or frustration. When physical restraints are used, patients may fail to understand the rationale for their use and may feel as if they are in danger, being punished, being tortured, or have been kidnapped. For many, this increases fear, paranoia, or distrust of medical staff [12]. Chemical restraints may also be used for sedation if a patient is demonstrating agitated behavior that increases the risk of medical decompensation or the chance of harm to self or others.

Environment-Related Stressors

The unpredictable environment of the ICU itself contributes to distress for many critically ill patients and families [9]. Patients commonly have little control over their daily routine, limited personal autonomy, and are subjected to frequent unscheduled visits from various medical providers throughout the day and night. Though the layout and organization of ICUs vary across the world – from small rooms to large, shared wards – commonalities exist. Many ICU environments are noisy, with a variety of sounds from machines, staff, and other patients contributing to the overall volume [9]. Patients may be exposed to bright lights throughout the day and night and often have little control over the ambient temperature, increasing general discomfort and impairing sleep at nighttime.

Furthermore, the lack of privacy characteristic of many ICUs can be problematic for several reasons. Due to the proximity of rooms and shared spaces, it is common for patients or visiting family members to witness other patients receiving emergent medical care, suffering, or dying. They may also observe other families in distress. These events can be anxiety provoking, confusing, and traumatic to witness, particularly for patients with delirium and disorientation [9]. Inadequate privacy can also increase stress for patients and families of patients who are actively dying. Though ICU staff often do their best to prioritize privacy under these circumstances, this can be challenging in shared spaces. Similarly, witnessing another family grieving can inspire increased fear and distress in others, given their common experiences and relationships developed in waiting rooms and shared spaces. Feelings of guilt and existential distress can also be experienced by the loved ones of patients who survive after witnessing another family coping with a patient's death.

Interpersonal Stressors

An ICU admission is associated with many experiences that are potentially dehumanizing for patients and often presents a threat to their sense of identity, safety, and self-respect. Patients experience repeated invasive medical procedures, are subjected to invasive lines and tubes, and often must be bathed and have personal hygiene attended to by others. The lessened ability to move and perform basic activities of daily living and personal care increases the sense of demoralization and helplessness [9]. Additionally, having one's naked body exposed and examined by strangers is often stressful and humiliating for patients.

During an ICU stay, many patients experience significant feelings of isolation and loneliness. Feelings of isolation occur due to limited opportunities to engage with others and challenges with communication resulting from medical conditions (e.g., aphasia due to a stroke) or treatment (e.g., the presence of an endotracheal tube) [9]. Difficulty with movement and strength may also prevent nonverbal forms of communication, such as writing or gesturing. Loneliness, the emotional distress that often accompanies feelings of isolation, results from patients missing family and friends or from a lack of visitors while they are hospitalized. Some patients have no or few visitors for multiple reasons: homelessness, advanced age, or distance between the hospital and their community. Many patients have trouble coping with being alone, especially during overnight hours, and these feelings may be intensified by concerns about their health or fears of dying. The presence of loved ones helps to orient patients with delirium and often fuels a sense of hope, determination, and motivation to get better. Patients may have a drastically different experience when visitors are not regularly present.

Sometimes conflict between patients or families and ICU staff is a source of interpersonal stress in intensive care. This may be associated with the quality of communication from ICU clinicians or nurses, cultural differences, or medical treatment. Conflict may also occur related to perceived biases in care, which may be associated with the race, cultural background, gender identity, or sexual orientation of patients and providers. Circumstances surrounding end-of-life decision-making, transitioning to comfort-focused care, and religious beliefs or rites associated with death are common sources of stress and dissension. In the high-stakes environment of the ICU, where the understanding of patients and families is often low and stress is high, conflict may more readily occur.

Other Stressors

One of the most significant psychological challenges that patients face in the ICU is coping with new or worsened medical problems. This may include dealing with a new diagnosis or disability, adjusting to a serious medical illness, or facing an advancing illness at the end of life. Patients often worry about the future, wondering whether they will ever leave the hospital, if they will have a meaningful recovery, and what life will look like after hospital discharge. Those who have experienced delirium may be fearful that their mind may not recover or that they have developed dementia. Some patients may also experience transfer anxiety, the development of concerns about leaving the comparatively protective environment of the ICU, where they have grown comfortable with the care team and routine. Transfer anxiety tends to increase as patients stabilize and are eligible for transfer out of the ICU [14]. A patient's preexisting mental health history, their current psychological state, and the presence of delirium may all impact how they cope with such stressors. This coping will also be affected by the patient's support system, health literacy level, and the ability to understand information provided about their medical condition.

ICU admission may also introduce distress associated with changes in patients' roles and identities. Patients often worry about loved ones seeing them sick or taking time out of their lives to visit them. Many patients fear becoming a burden to their family if family members must assume the role of caregiver once the patient returns home. Financial stress associated with the inability to work or pay bills and the potential need for loved ones to reduce or end their employment to act as caregiver can cause additional worry.

Positive Reactions and Coping

It is remarkable that in the face of the multiple stressors discussed above, around 50% of patients do not show signs of serious distress in the ICU or develop psychological difficulties after hospital discharge. Most clinicians working in an ICU setting have encountered patients with an impressive ability to remain positive and to cope well with their admission.

Research in this area is inadequate, but a cohort study of 416 patients in a Dutch hospital sought to evaluate the impact of positive coping styles on mental health-related quality of life (HRQL) using the Sickness Insight in Coping Questionnaire (SICQ) [15], a tool previously validated for use in the ICU [14]. The SICQ measures five dimensions of coping – positivism (having a positive attitude), redefinition (seeing advantages of the medical situation, such as personal growth), toughness, fighting spirit, and nonacceptance (of the current medical condition and its possible outcome). The study found that positivism, redefinition, and fighting spirit were associated with better mental HRQL after hospital discharge. Correlations with mental HRQL were largest for positivism, and positivism was also associated with better physical HRQL after hospital discharge.

In a study of the psychological impact of ICU admission on patients [1], although negative emotions were more prominent, positive feelings were also present for many, with 49% experiencing a mild/moderate to high/very high level of positive mood. Among other positive factors measured in the study, "emotional support received from others" was rated highly, but scores were low for "sense of personal control." It is worth noting that coping with serious illness relies on a balance between receiving support from other people and having a sense of personal control, and crucially, this balance changes at different points in the illness trajectory. There is a wider debate suggesting that being able to relinquish personal control and receive increased support from other people can be adaptive in coping with the acute phase of serious illness [17].

Certainly, receiving emotional and social support from staff is also highly valued by patients during an ICU admission, a time when most people feel extremely vulnerable [12]. Patients often report that talking to staff, being open about their feelings, asking questions, and getting information about their condition help them cope with their ICU stay. Being able to voice their fears and receive reassurance from a caring staff member enhances coping [4,5,12]. Family support is equally important. Patients benefit from having loved ones at their side to calm and distract them by engaging in casual conversation, performing massage, holding hands, or providing a safe space for self-expression. Loved ones also help by bringing in family photos, cards, familiar items from home, and a patient's own clothes to help them feel more connected to people and life outside the hospital.

As patients improve, regaining a sense of personal control becomes a priority. Health psychology research suggests that people who regain more personal control tend to recover better from sickness [18]. Critically ill patients may recapture a sense of control through performing self-care activities (e.g., brushing their teeth or combing their hair), mobilizing as much as feasible, and keeping in touch with family and friends via electronic devices. They may communicate with the staff caring for them in the ICU and seek information about their condition and treatments from doctors. If they are religious, they may pray and maintain other spiritual practices. They may enjoy receiving visits from family or friends in the hospital but regulate the number of visitors to ensure adequate rest and to avoid being overwhelmed.

In addition to regaining personal control, some people cope with the ICU experience by using familiar strategies that have helped in their daily lives or with prior difficult experiences, including progressive relaxation, mindfulness or breathing exercises, listening to calming music, visualizing pleasant scenes, or focusing on positive thoughts or affirmations [19]. Psychologists and other staff can gently remind people to use their familiar coping strategies or coach them in new ones.

Psychological Impact on Families

The family members and loved ones of a critically ill relative often develop adverse psychological outcomes, with studies suggesting that 25–50% of family members experience psychological symptoms, including anxiety, depression, PTSD, acute stress disorder, sleep disturbances, and complicated grief, both during and after the critical illness of a loved one; these conditions can persist for over four years following discharge [7]. These adverse psychological outcomes have been classified under the umbrella term of post-intensive care syndrome – family (PICS-F; see Chapter 48 for additional information).

A scoping review [20] identified risk factors for PICS-F, including female sex, younger age, being the patient's spouse, unsympathetic interactions with and a lack of communication from ICU staff, and restricted visiting hours. Consistent and informative updates from staff, flexible visiting hours, and family involvement in decision-making were factors associated with reduced anxiety, sleep disturbances, and fatigue in family members.

Conclusions

Admission to an ICU for treatment of a critical illness or injury is associated with significant acute and long-term physical, cognitive, and psychological morbidity. Ample evidence suggests that survivors of critical illness have a heightened risk of experiencing depression, anxiety, and PTSD following ICU admission. Consideration of the psychological impact of an ICU stay and the role of risk factors associated with long-standing distress has become an important focus of research. A better understanding of stressors experienced by patients in intensive care, including illness-related, environment-related, and interpersonal stressors, and earlier recognition of patients at risk for the psychological impairments associated with PICS are crucial to the development of strategies and interventions to mitigate distress. The role of positive coping and the impact of the critical illness on the family's mental health are also important considerations in the overall experience and recovery of the patient.

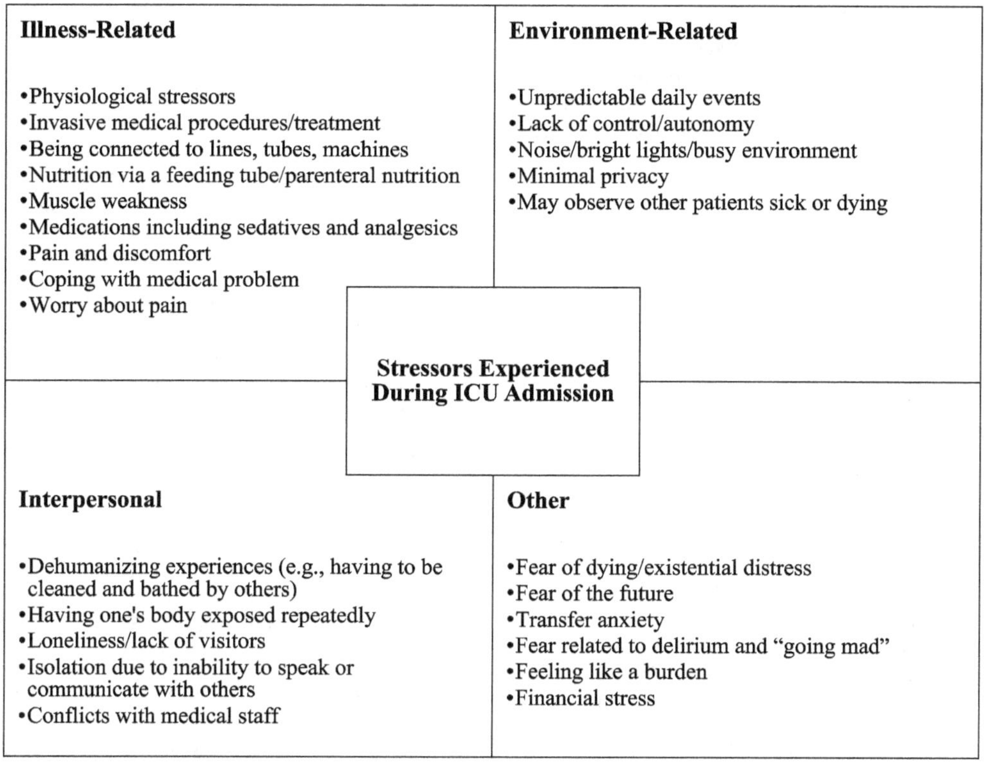

Stressors Experienced During ICU Admission

Illness-Related
- Physiological stressors
- Invasive medical procedures/treatment
- Being connected to lines, tubes, machines
- Nutrition via a feeding tube/parenteral nutrition
- Muscle weakness
- Medications including sedatives and analgesics
- Pain and discomfort
- Coping with medical problem
- Worry about pain

Environment-Related
- Unpredictable daily events
- Lack of control/autonomy
- Noise/bright lights/busy environment
- Minimal privacy
- May observe other patients sick or dying

Interpersonal
- Dehumanizing experiences (e.g., having to be cleaned and bathed by others)
- Having one's body exposed repeatedly
- Loneliness/lack of visitors
- Isolation due to inability to speak or communicate with others
- Conflicts with medical staff

Other
- Fear of dying/existential distress
- Fear of the future
- Transfer anxiety
- Fear related to delirium and "going mad"
- Feeling like a burden
- Financial stress

Figure 10.1 Common stressors experienced by patients and families during ICU admission.

Key Points

1. Psychological distress, including depression, anxiety, acute stress, and delirium, frequently affects critically ill patients and is associated with the development of long-term psychological impairments.
2. Patients face a multitude of stressors during ICU admission including illness- and environment-related stressors, interpersonal stressors, and others.
3. Earlier recognition of stressors experienced by patients and consideration of risk factors associated with psychological distress may help to mitigate long-term psychological impairments.
4. Patients who recover from critical illnesses or injuries without significant psychological distress are important sources of information that may help to better inform understanding of resiliency in ICU survivors.

References

1. D.M. Wade, D.C. Howell, J.A. Weinman, et al. Investigating risk factors for psychological morbidity three months after intensive care: a prospective cohort *study*. *Crit Care* 2012; **16**(5): R192.

2. R. Cavallazzi, M. Saad, P.E. Marik. Delirium in the ICU: an overview. *Ann Intensive Care* 2012; **2**(1): 49.

3. C. Jones, C. Backman, M. Capuzzo, et al. Precipitants of post-traumatic stress disorder following intensive care: a hypothesis generating study of diversity in care. *Intensive Care Med* 2007; **33**(6): 978–85.

4. D.M. Wade, C.R. Brewin, D.C. Howell, et al. Intrusive memories of hallucinations and delusions in traumatised intensive care patients: an interview study. *Br J Health Psychol* 2015; **20**(3): 613–31.

5. M.D. Hashem, A. Nallagangula, S. Nalamalapu, et al. Patient outcomes after critical illness: a systematic review of qualitative studies following hospital discharge. *Crit Care* 2016; **20**(1): 345.

6. D.S. Davydow, D. Zatzick, C.L. Hough, W.J. Katon. A longitudinal investigation of posttraumatic stress and depressive symptoms over the course of the year following medical-surgical intensive care unit admission. *Gen Hosp Psychiatry* 2013; **35**: 226–32.

7. J.E. Davidson, C. Jones, O.J. Bienvenu. Family response to critical illness: postintensive care syndrome – family. *Crit Care Med* 2012; **40**(2): 618–24.

8. J.E. Nelson, D.E. Meier, A. Litke, et al. The symptom burden of chronic critical illness. *Crit Care Med* 2004; **32**(7): 1527–34.

9. J.L. Darbyshire, P.R. Greig, S. Vollam, et al. "I can remember sort of vivid people ... but to me they were plasticine." Delusions on the intensive care unit: what do patients think is going on? *Plos One* 2016; **11**(7): e0160296.

10. D. Davydow, J.M. Gifford, S.V. Desai, et al. Posttraumatic stress disorder in general intensive care unit survivors: a systematic review. *Gen Hosp Psychiatry* 2008; **30**: 421–34.

11. D. Wade, R. Hardy, D. Howell, M. Mythen. Identifying clinical and acute psychological risk factors for PTSD after intensive care: a systematic review. *Minerva Anesesiologica* 2013; **79**: 1–20.

12. L.M. Boehm, A. Jones, A.A. Selim, et al. Delirium-related distress in the ICU: a qualitative meta-synthesis of patient and family perspectives and experiences. *Int J Nurs Studies* 2021; **122**: 104030.

13. H. Carruthers, T. Gomershall, F. Astin. The work undertaken by mechanically ventilated patients in intensive care: a qualitative meta-ethnography of survivors' experiences. *Int J Nurs Stud* 2018; **86**: 60–73.

14. M.A. Coyle. Transfer anxiety: preparing to leave intensive care. *Intensive Crit Care Nurs* 2001; **17**(3): 138–43.

15. E.J. Boezeman, J.G. Hofhuis, C.E. Cox, et al. SICQ Coping and the health-related quality of life and recovery of critically ill ICU patients: a prospective cohort study. *Chest* 2022; **161**(1): 130–9.

16. E.J. Boezeman, J.G. Hofhuis, A. Hovingh, et al. Measuring adaptive coping of hospitalized patients with a severe medical condition: The Sickness Insight in Coping Questionnaire. *Crit Care Med* 2016; **44**(9): e818–e826.

17. I. Aujoulat, B. Young, P. Salmon. The psychological processes involved in patient empowerment. *Orphanet J Rare Dis* 2012; 7 (Suppl 2): A31.

18. B.T. Mausbach, T.L. Patterson, R.V. Känel, et al. The attenuating effect of personal mastery on the relations between stress and Alzheimer caregiver health: a five-year longitudinal analysis. *Aging Ment Health* 2007; **11**(6): 637–44.

19. K.M. Shaffer, E. Riklin, J.M. Jacobs, et al. Mindfulness and coping are inversely related to psychiatric symptoms in patients and informal caregivers in the neuroscience ICU: implications for clinical care. *Crit Care Med* 2016; **44**(11): 2028–36.

20. A.A. Halain, L.Y. Tang, M.C. Chong, et al. Psychological distress among the family members of intensive care unit (ICU) patients: a scoping review. *J Clin Nurs* 2022; **31**(5–6): 497–507.

Section 3 **Strategies to Prevent PICS**

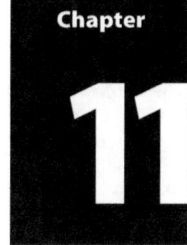

Chapter 11

Bundles and Checklists

Heyi Li, Michael Baram, and Brad W. Butcher

Introduction

A care bundle is a set of evidence-informed practices collectively and consistently performed to improve the quality of care, and they are used widely across healthcare settings to either prevent or manage different conditions. Although based on low-quality evidence, a meta-analysis of 37 randomized trials and controlled before-after studies suggested that care bundles may reduce the risk of negative outcomes when compared with usual care [1]. The Society of Critical Care Medicine (SCCM) launched the Intensive Care Unit (ICU) Liberation Campaign in 2014 as a project to improve patient- and family-centered care that packaged key concepts from the 2013 clinical practice guidelines for the management of pain, agitation, and delirium [2] and their 2018 update [3] into a six-element bundle delivered by an interprofessional team at the bedside.

The goals of the bundle are several and include: optimizing pain management, shortening the duration of mechanical ventilation, minimizing the use of sedating medications, and reducing the incidence and duration of delirium and ICU-acquired weakness by keeping the patient as physically and cognitively engaged as possible through early mobilization and family engagement. In addition to these short-term goals, incorporation of the ABCDEF bundle is one major strategy to decrease the risk of long-term physical, cognitive, and psychiatric impairments, collectively known as the post-intensive care syndrome (PICS), that frequently develop in survivors of critical illness [4]. The **ABCDEF** bundle includes: Assess, prevent, and manage pain; Both spontaneous awakening trials (SAT) and spontaneous breathing trials (SBT); Choice of analgesia and sedation; Delirium: assess, prevent, and manage; Early mobility and exercise; and Family engagement and empowerment (see Figure 11.1). The ABCDEF bundle is one component of well-rounded patient care and optimal resource utilization that results in more interactive ICU patients, who can safely engage with their healthcare providers and families in higher-order physical and cognitive activities as soon as possible in their critical illness [5].

The SCCM A–F Bundle

A Assess, Prevent, and Manage Pain

Many patients in the ICU experience pain, whether it is a part of their disease process, a consequence of procedures performed or required interventions (e.g., arterial line insertion or mechanical ventilation, respectively) [6], or a chronic condition with which they live. Uncontrolled pain is associated with a higher incidence of chronic pain, post-traumatic stress disorder symptoms, and a lower health-related quality of life following hospital

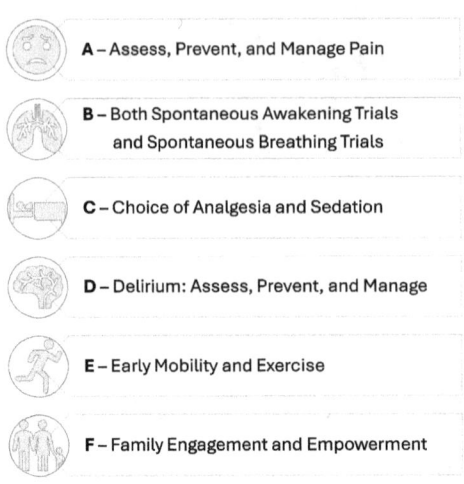

Figure 11.1 The SCCM ABCDEF bundle.

discharge [7]. Often considered the fifth vital sign, pain should be assessed at least every two hours in critically ill patients, and additional assessments should occur both before and after the administration of analgesia. Routine pain assessments should be performed with validated tools, including visual or verbal administration of the numeric rating scale (NRS) [8] in patients capable of self-reporting pain and administration of the Critical Care Pain Observation Tool (CPOT) [9] or the Behavioral Pain Scale (BPS) [10] (see Table 11.1) in patients who are incapable of reporting pain. When appropriate, if the patient is unable to report pain, the patient's family may be involved in their loved one's pain assessment [11]. Importantly, vital sign aberrations, such as tachycardia, tachypnea, and hypertension, are not valid indicators for pain in critically ill adults, but they may prompt administration of a validated pain assessment tool [2].

Opioid analgesics are considered the first-line drug class for treatment of pain, and all intravenous opioids are equally effective when titrated to similar pain scores. To minimize exposure to opioids and their attendant negative effects, including nausea, constipation, respiratory depression, and dependency, utilization of an assessment-driven, protocol-based, stepwise approach for pain management that includes provision of non-opioid analgesics is advised [3]. Non-opioid analgesics include acetaminophen, non-steroidal anti-inflammatory drugs, nefopam, neuropathic pain medication (e.g., gabapentin, carbamazepine, and pregabalin), ketamine, and lidocaine; of these, the quality of evidence is greatest for neuropathic pain medications as an adjunct to opioid analgesics [3,12]. In addition to pharmacotherapy, nonpharmacological interventions can be used to manage pain in the ICU, including relaxation and distraction techniques, massage, playing music that the patient enjoys, and family presence for support and distraction, although the quality of evidence is low [3].

In mechanically ventilated patients, the SCCM 2018 Clinical Practice Guidelines for the Prevention and Management of Pain, Agitation/Sedation, Delirium, Immobility, and Sleep Disruption in Adult Patients in the ICU (PADIS) recommend that analgesic medications should be administered prior to or instead of sedating medications (analgesia-first sedation or analgesia-based sedation, respectively), and for both analgesic and sedating medications, bolus administration should precede initiation of continuous infusions [3].

Table 11.1 The behavioral pain scale

Item	Description	Score
Facial expression	Relaxed	1
	Partially tightened (e.g., brow lowering)	2
	Fully tightened (e.g., eyelid closing)	3
	Grimacing	4
Upper limbs	No movement	1
	Partially bent	2
	Fully bent with finger flexion	3
	Permanently retracted	4
Compliance with ventilation	Tolerating movement	1
	Coughing but tolerating ventilation for most of the time	2
	Fighting ventilator	3
	Unable to control ventilation	4

From: J.F. Payen, O. Bru, J.L. Bosson, et al. Assessing pain in critically ill sedated patients by using a behavioral pain scale. *Crit Care Med* 2001; **29**: 2258–63. [10] Reproduced and adapted with permissions from Wolters Kluwer Health, Inc.

B Both Spontaneous Awakening Trials and Spontaneous Breathing Trials

In a randomized controlled trial of 128 patients receiving mechanical ventilation and continuous infusions of sedative medications, Kress and colleagues demonstrated that daily interruption of sedative infusions decreased the duration of mechanical ventilation and length of stay in the ICU when compared with usual care [13]. In a subsequent trial of 336 mechanically ventilated patients, patients receiving protocolized daily SATs and SBTs were extubated 3.1 days earlier, were discharged from the ICU and hospital earlier, and required fewer tracheotomies than those who received a daily SBT alone. Furthermore, patients who received paired SATs and SBTs were less likely to die in the year following hospitalization than the control group, with a number needed to treat of seven [14].

Based on these studies, most mechanically ventilated patients should have a coordinated SAT and SBT performed at least once daily [3]. Criteria to withhold SATs and SBTs are institution-dependent: criteria that preclude an SAT may include continuous infusion of a paralytic or elevated intracranial pressure, and criteria that preclude an SBT may include high amounts of positive end-expiratory pressure or fraction of inspired oxygen necessary to maintain an acceptable oxygen saturation.

C Choice of Analgesia and Sedation

Sedatives are commonly administered to critically ill patients to reduce the stress associated with mechanical ventilation, to relieve anxiety, and to prevent harm associated with agitation [2]. While it is important that patients receive safe and effective medications for the management of agitation, given the impact that sedative medications have on both short- and long-term outcomes in critically ill patients, the least amount of medication required to ensure patients' comfort is preferred. As above, the SCCM 2018 PADIS guidelines suggest an analgesia-first or analgesia-based approach, in which the primary goal is to adequately treat pain and only add sedating medications if the patient remains agitated based on a protocolized assessment. If additional sedating medication is required, light sedation is preferred to deep sedation based on studies demonstrating an increased duration of mechanical ventilation, increased tracheotomy rate, higher incidence of delirium, and increased hospital and six-month mortality when deep sedation strategies are employed [5,15,16]. Of note, deeper sedation may be required in certain clinical contexts, such as in patients receiving a continuous infusion of a paralytic, patients with elevated intracranial pressure, or patients being managed for status epilepticus.

In addition to the provision of daily SATs, in which sedating medications are completely discontinued for a period of time and restarted at half the previous rate if necessary, a nurse-driven, protocolized sedation strategy can be implemented to titrate medications to achieve prescription-targeted sedation scores [3]. Using such a strategy, the degree of sedation should be assessed every one to two hours using a validated tool, including the Richmond Agitation Sedation Scale (RASS) [17] and the Riker Sedation Agitation Scale (SAS) [18]. The RASS is a 10-point scale, with positive numbers (+1 to +4) representing escalating agitation, 0 representing an alert and calm state, and negative numbers (-1 to -5) representing deepening sedation and coma. The SAS has seven levels, ranging from 1, denoting a patient that is completely unarousable, to 7, a dangerously agitated patient; a level of 4 represents a calm and comfortable patient and is the target for most clinical situations (see Table 11.2).

Table 11.2 The Riker Sedation Agitation Scale (SAS)

Score	Description	Explanation
7	Dangerous agitation	Pulling at endotracheal tube (ET) tube, trying to remove catheters, climbing over bed rail, striking at staff, thrashing side-to-side
6	Very agitated	Does not calm despite frequent verbal reminders of limits, requires physical restraints, biting ET tube
5	Agitated	Anxious or mildly agitated, attempting to sit up, calms down to verbal instructions
4	Calm and cooperative	Calm, awakens easily, follows commands
3	Sedated	Difficult to arouse, awakens to verbal stimuli or gentle shaking but drifts off again, follows simple commands
2	Very sedated	Arouses to physical stimuli but does not communicate or follow commands, may move spontaneously
1	Unarousable	Minimal or no response to noxious stimuli, does not communicate or follow commands

From: R.R. Riker, J.T. Picard, G.L. Fraser. Prospective evaluation of the sedation-agitation scale for adult critically ill patients. *Crit Care Med* 1999; **27**(7): 1327. [18] Reproduced and adapted with permissions from Wolters Kluwer Health, Inc.

Sedation using propofol or dexmedetomidine is preferred over sedation using benzodiazepines in mechanically ventilated adults. When compared with benzodiazepine-based sedation, sedation using propofol demonstrated a shorter time to light sedation and decreased duration of mechanical ventilation, and sedation using dexmedetomidine demonstrated a shorter duration of mechanical ventilation, shorter ICU length of stay, and less delirium [3].

D Delirium: Assess, Prevent, and Manage

Delirium is an acute state of confusion, disorientation, and impaired attention, and it is common in patients in the ICU, arising in 50–80% of mechanically ventilated patients and 20–50% of those who are not (see Chapter 8 for additional information) [19,20]. Delirium is a waxing and waning process, and patients may be phenotypically described as either hyperactive or hypoactive. Delirium is associated with increased risk of several adverse outcomes, including longer length of mechanical ventilation, longer ICU and hospital lengths of stay, increased use of restraints, and death. In a study of 275 mechanically ventilated patients, patients with delirium required a longer period of mechanical ventilation, spent 10 more days in the hospital, and had higher 6-month mortality rates (34% versus 15%) than patients without delirium [21]. Additionally, incident delirium during the ICU stay and its duration are associated with long-term cognitive impairment. In a study of a diverse population of critically ill patients, Pandharipande and colleagues found that at both 3 and 12 months following hospital discharge, across all age groups, approximately one-third of patients with delirium had global cognition scores similar to patients with moderate traumatic brain injury and one-quarter of patients with delirium had scores similar to patients with mild Alzheimer's disease [22].

Given the profound short- and long-term adverse effects associated with delirium, critically ill adults should be regularly assessed for delirium using a validated tool, most commonly the Intensive Care Unit Delirium Screening Checklist (ICDSC; see Chapter 8, Table 8.1) [23] and the Confusion Assessment Method – Intensive Care Unit (CAM-ICU; see Chapter 8, Figure 8.1) [24]. Importantly, the patients level of arousal may influence whether a delirium assessment is able to be performed [3]. In light of the many potential etiologies of delirium, there is no specific treatment other than to address its underlying cause(s). Accordingly, the 2018 PADIS guidelines suggest not using haloperidol, atypical antipsychotics, statins, ketamine, or dexmedetomidine to prevent delirium and suggest not using haloperidol or atypical antipsychotics to treat subsyndromal delirium in critically ill adults [3]. Dexmedetomidine may, however, be used for management of delirium in mechanically ventilated patients in whom agitation is thought to preclude ventilator weaning or extubation [25]. The best approach to manage delirium is to use a multicomponent bundle of non-pharmacologic strategies that is focused on reducing modifiable risk factors [3], including removing catheters and lines as soon as possible; bundling care, particularly at nighttime to minimize interruptions and promote a normal sleep/wake cycle; cognitive stimulation during the daytime with familiar music and television programs or puzzles and games if appropriate; frequent re-orientation; early mobilization; use of sensory aids, including hearing aids and glasses; and visitation by loved ones.

E Early Mobility and Exercise

Early mobilization includes a spectrum of activity that may be as simple as passive range of motion exercises for patients who are unable to engage to more complex functional and resistance exercises (see Chapter 12 for additional information). Early mobilization is a safe and feasible strategy in the ICU and may impact a number of important outcomes, including improved muscle strength at the time of ICU discharge, decreased length of mechanical ventilation, decreased incidence of delirium, decreased ICU and hospital lengths of stay, accelerated functional recovery, increased chance of returning to independent functional status, and improved quality of life [3,26].

Mobility is important to help prevent ICU-acquired weakness, which is present in 25–50% of critically ill patients and is associated with increased duration of mechanical ventilation, prolonged hospital and ICU lengths of stay, impaired physical functioning, a decreased ability to be discharged home, and increased mortality (see Chapter 4 for additional information) [27]. Muscle wasting is most significant in the initial week of critical illness and is influenced by age, the presence of sepsis, systemic inflammation, and immobilization, highlighting the need for exercise to begin as soon as feasible.

In a study by Fan and colleagues, the duration of bed rest during critical illness was the single most important factor associated with persistent muscle weakness throughout two years of follow-up. After adjusting for all other risk factors, muscle strength was 3–11% lower for every additional day of bed rest, highlighting the importance of identifying ICU-acquired weakness and initiating early mobilization [28].

Early mobilization has been shown to be feasible and safe in critically ill patients [29], even those who are mechanically ventilated or receiving vasopressors, continuous renal replacement therapy, and/or extracorporeal membrane oxygenation therapy. In a randomized controlled trial, 104 previously functionally independent patients requiring mechanical ventilation were randomly assigned to early exercise and mobilization performed by physical and occupational therapy during SATs or to usual care by the primary team. Return to independent functional status at hospital discharge occurred in 59% of patients in the intervention group compared with 35% of patients in the control group, and patients in the intervention group also had fewer days of delirium and required less mechanical ventilation than patients in the control group [30].

F Family Engagement and Empowerment

Efforts should be made to promote family presence in the ICU and identify strategies to engage and empower families (see Chapter 17 for additional information). Families play a vital role in the emotional support of the patient and often help the care team ensure that the patient's values and preferences are being heard and honored. Most family dissatisfaction with care is related to either poor communication with the care team or restricted access to the patient. Enhanced family engagement can help limit the negative effects that families may experience because of their loved one's ICU stay, including anxiety, anger, sadness, and frustration [31].

Interventions to enhance family presence may include remaining present during procedures, assisting with patient care activities, participating in daily work rounds with the critical care team, and establishing unrestricted visitation policies. Including families during rounds gives them an opportunity to hear data and the plan of care as it is being formulated, ask any questions that they may have, correct information regarding the patient's history that may be inaccurate, and engage in conversations about the patient's healthcare values and preferences. Frequent meetings with the family can also help manage expectations about what the patient's recovery following hospital discharge might look like. Through actively engaging family members via unrestricted visitation policies and inclusion in patient care activities, including bathing or massage, family members perceive heightened respect and support, which can in turn decrease the incidence of psychological stress, anxiety, depression, and post-traumatic stress disorder after patient discharge or death [32] and increase patient and family satisfaction with care [33].

The Power of the ABCDEF Bundle

Over the past decade, the ABCDEF bundle has demonstrated its ability to improve short-term outcomes in critically ill patients, with the potential for reducing the incidence of PICS, although studies specifically addressing this potential have not yet been performed. In a study of more than 15,000 patients across 68 ICUs, complete ABCDEF bundle performance was associated with lower likelihood of: hospital death within seven days, need for next-day mechanical ventilation, coma, delirium, use of physical restraints, readmission to the ICU, and discharge to a facility other than home; moreover, there was a consistent dose-dependent relationship between the number of individual bundle elements performed and improvements in each of these clinical outcomes [34]. Indeed, the elements of the bundle are highly interdependent and synergistic, and the impact of the complete bundle is greater than the impacts of its individual parts performed separately. For instance, as previously described, deep sedation is associated with delayed extubation [15]; as such, when the "C" element is missing, implementing the "B" element would be difficult. Similarly, patients who had access to early physical and occupational therapy (the "E" element) had a shorter duration of delirium (the "D" element) and more ventilator-free days (the "B" element) [30].

Difficulty in Implementing a Complex Care Bundle

With respect to implementation of the ABCDEF bundle, there has been a long-standing gap between the evidence and real-world practice. Despite widespread awareness and strong international promotion, implementation of the bundle has been poor, particularly during the COVID-19 global pandemic. In a one-day point-prevalence study including 135 ICUs from 54 countries, Liu and colleagues found that, regardless of COVID-19 status, implementation rates for both the complete ABCDEF bundle and for each individual bundle component were remarkably low. Compliance with the complete bundle was performed in 2 out of 1229 patients; coordinated spontaneous awakening and breathing trials occurred in only 12% of patients, mobilization in only 14% of patients (and only 6% of those who were mechanically ventilated), and family engagement in only 23% of patients [35].

According to the Institute for Healthcare Improvement (IHI), the fidelity of care bundle completion should be at least 95%, and all eligible patients should receive all of the elements of the bundle [36]. The most formidable barriers to achieving perfect compliance with best practices are likely the workload in the ICU and the lack of an ICU culture that prioritizes minimization of sedation, mobility, and family engagement. Human cognitive function is often compromised with increasing levels of stress and fatigue, and care providers in the ICU are particularly prone to prospective memory loss when they are handling highly complex information or performing complicated tasks while being frequently interrupted [37]. In a survey across 268 care providers from 10 intensive care units, Boehm and colleagues discovered that for every unit increase in workload burden, bundle adherence decreased by 53%, while factors that are commonly considered barriers to implementation, such as "perceived safety," "confidence," and "perceived strength of evidence," were not associated with bundle adherence [38]. More consistent implementation of the ABCDEF bundle requires carefully designed strategies that suit local resources and cultures. Indeed, critical care teams must develop a culture that prioritizes application of the ABCDEF bundle (often referred to as an "Awake and Walking Intensive Care Unit") to address sedative use, delirium, sleep, and early mobility holistically, which not only leads to better outcomes but also humanizes the ICU experience [39].

Effective Rounding: An Opportunity to Achieve Best Care Delivery

High-quality interprofessional teamwork is important to prioritize and implement consistent bundle use (see Chapter 31 for additional information). Daily structured interdisciplinary rounds are an effective means to improve bundle compliance, hospital costs, and patient outcomes [40], while inadequate interprofessional care team coordination is considered a significant barrier to bundle implementation [41]. An effective interprofessional team collaborating during ICU rounds may involve intensivists, trainees, nurses, respiratory therapists, physical therapists, pharmacists, and, as much as possible, patients and their family members. A structured approach is used to discuss current conditions, facilitate shared decision-making, and formulate a patient-centered care plan. Key factors for effective ICU rounds that facilitate compliance with the ABCDEF bundle include: tools, such as a rounding script, to aid the team in visualizing, performing, and documenting the elements of the bundle; information technology, if available, to track bundle compliance and provide feedback; and a patient-centered and collaborative discussion among the team members [42].

Checklists: From Aviation to Medicine

In 1999, the Institute of Medicine reported that medical errors were responsible for 98,000 preventable deaths per year [43], and in light of the urgent need for a safer healthcare system, the medical industry turned to the aviation industry as a role model. High Reliability Organizations (HROs), such as the nuclear power and aviation industries, are characterized by high complexity and time sensitivity as well as high reliability and impeccable safety. The aviation industry has a long history of using "cockpit checklists" as a cognitive aid and compliance tool. A well-developed, operationally suited checklist serves as a memory aid and frees the operator's mental capacity to perform essential operations. In an effort to remediate the unacceptable and growing number of medical errors, medical experts rapidly adopted the concept of "checklists" to improve the safety of medicine.

A successful example of implementing a checklist in medicine is the WHO Safe Surgery Checklist, which identifies the high-risk steps of a surgery and classifies them into three stages: "check-in," "time-out," and "sign-out." The checklist tool mandates that the operating room staff pause and ensure compliance to these high-standard practices. The WHO Safe Surgery Checklist was rapidly disseminated worldwide and has demonstrated both efficacy in improving safety and team communication and adaptability to different cultures and levels of resources [44].

Types of ICU Checklists

A checklist can serve different functions depending on the scenario in which it is being used; in the field of critical care medicine, checklists are commonly used as safety tools, goal-setting tools, performance and quality improvement tools, and communication tools. In the aviation industry, checklists are classified as either "boldface" or "non-boldface" [45]. The "non-boldface" checklists are designed for conventional procedures, such as take-off and landing, and are used to standardize daily performance and limit bias among different operators. "Non-boldface" checklists are especially useful when the series of tasks is too long to be committed to memory or when interruptions that interfere with memory retrieval are likely. In critical care, checklists are widely used for routine procedures, such as daily patient rounds and transportation of patients to other departments. Many other operational bundles, such as central line insertion or mechanical ventilation care bundles, have served as effective quality improvement solutions and have been adopted widely [46]. "Boldface" checklists, in contrast, are designed to help the operator react to nonroutine and occasionally emergent procedures. The most well-known "boldface" checklist in medicine is the A(airway)-B(breathing)-C(circulation) life support checklist. When a "boldface" situation occurs, time is often critical, and the environment does not usually accommodate the use of a physical list; accordingly, the operator must complete the checklist from memory.

In a guide for medical checklist development, Burian and colleagues [47] recommended that before the actual development process, designers should determine (1) *when* the checklist will be used and (2) *how* the checklist will be used. Checklists can be used in real time during a procedure to standardize the actions taken and the information gathering and sharing process or they can be used after a series of actions are completed as a compliance or evaluation tool. Checklists can be used as either a memory aid (e.g., using A-B-C mnemonics during a cardiac arrest) or to facilitate decision making (e.g., reviewing the ABCDEF bundle during rounds). Accordingly, checklists can be divided into four categories:

1) Real-time memory aid: handover checklist, drug lists
2) After-fact memory aid: operating room "sign out" checklist
3) Real-time decision-making aid: checklist for critical event
4) After-fact decision-making aid: questionnaires, treatment planning guide

Life Cycle of a Checklist

Checklist development methods are often based on the opinions of local experts and may lack a robust methodological foundation, thereby limiting dissemination and penetration of these tools. Reasons for failed checklist initiatives include: poor design, inadequate introduction and training, redundancy with other lists, poor integration with existing workflow, and cultural barriers [47]. In contrast, factors associated with a high-performing checklist include: use of closed loop communication, clearly defined language and text, and a clearly defined context for use of the checklist. Checklist development teams should include "sharp-end" users, departmental leaders, some indirectly affected parties, and a well-recognized chairperson [48]. The "life cycle" of a checklist is presented in Table 11.3 [47].

Table 11.3 Life cycle of a checklist

Stage	Description
Conception	Recognize a problem, analyze its causes
Determination of content and design	Gather experts to decide on tasks, levels of details, and the layout. Multimodal methods (focus groups, Delphi consensus, etc.) are favored over a single method
Testing and validation	Conduct pilot tests or simulation studies
Induction, training, implementation	Inform and educate the pertinent staff to use the checklist
Ongoing evaluation, revision, and possible retirement	Identify roadblocks and capture opportunities for improvement

Stories of Success

Having a patient-centered rounding checklist frees healthcare providers from responding to acute events passively; instead, it creates a space for the team to have a structured, goal-directed conversation focusing on the patient's progress and recovery [49,50]. In 2015, Vukoja and colleagues described an international initiative to disseminate the use of a checklist-based decision support tool for critical care healthcare workers worldwide, including those in low-income countries and resource-limited hospitals, to deliver high-quality, low-cost care and minimize preventable deaths and expensive complications. This tool, the CERTAIN (Checklist for Early Recognition and Treatment of Acute Illness) checklist, consists of a structured, standardized approach to managing acute illness, including use of the ABCDEF bundle, accompanied by a series of faculty training and performance evaluation tools [51]. Six years later, this group reported that the CERTAIN decision support approach has been disseminated to 34 ICUs across 15 countries. The implementation effort was associated with improvement in adherence to best practices, including, but not limited to, better compliance with daily sedation assessments, spontaneous breathing trials, and family conferences as well as decreased ICU and hospital lengths of stay and hospital mortality [52].

The E-Checklist

A common reality of checklist development in healthcare is the ongoing addition of elements that results in a checklist that is inefficient and unappealing. To relieve the time and burden required to employ multiple or lengthy checklists, medical informatics experts have automated and integrated checklists and care bundles into electronic health records (EHR) systems. Moreover, the content of a checklist can be programmed to be dynamic, and traceable clinical processes in EHRs can be used to derive intelligent checklists. Instead of using a "one-size-fits-all" checklist for all patients, De Bie and colleagues reported a novel method for developing individualized rounding checklists for each patient, using an intelligent decision tree based on general clinical and pharmacological rules. The authors reported that in a simulation setting, the access to the intelligent checklist improved human providers' clinical adherence to best practices [53].

The success of using E-checklists embedded in the EHR has been variable. Thongprayoon and colleagues reported that in a simulated setting, providers who were randomized to use E-checklists made fewer errors and had a reduced workload compared with their colleagues who used only paper checklists; however, the E-checklist was not able to be completed more quickly [54]. In another randomized controlled study on an E-checklist, Weiss and colleagues reported that automated E-checklist "pop-ups" on computer screens were less effective than face-to-face prompting during patient rounds, suggested that E-checklists may fail to serve their decision-facilitating purpose if not implemented properly [55]. A common explanation is "checklist fatigue," in which providers simply "tick the boxes" rather than engage in thoughtful deliberation.

Critics and Caveats

A common concern regarding the use of care bundles and checklists is that they may reduce care providers' autonomy and deprive them of an opportunity to apply their individual expertise. Providers may also become less vigilant when they turn on their "autopilot" mode and rely exclusively on checklists rather than critical and deliberate thinking. Improvements in the quality of care associated with checklists is likely not related to the checklist itself but to the attitude and culture change realized during the implementation process. When implementing a checklist, its designers should engage frequently with its users and make considerable effort to understand the details of the work environment (e.g., who is responsible for completing the checklist? Does it require one person or the whole team to pause other tasks to complete it?). Feedback should be monitored, and a "psychological safe space" for the users should be maintained to allow prompt feedback and modifications. Lastly, the length of a checklist is crucial to its feasibility; serial additions for the goal of creating a "comprehensive list" could ultimately lead to its failure.

Conclusions

The ABCDEF bundle, whose elements are interdependent and synergistic, has demonstrated significant efficacy in improving several outcomes in critically ill patients and may be the best tool available to prevent or mitigate the development of PICS. Despite such compelling evidence, compliance with the bundle is still suboptimal worldwide. Accordingly, many institutions utilize "checklists" as cognitive aides to enhance bundle adherence with modest success. The content, format, and implementation processes of ICU checklists are variable, and integration of checklists into the EHR is a current focus of study. When developing an ICU checklist, designers should adapt the checklist to local surroundings; successful implementation is dependent on vigorous teamwork and may require a cultural change.

Key Points

1. A care bundle is a set of evidence-informed practices collectively and consistently performed with the goal of improving quality of care, and they are used widely across healthcare settings to either prevent or manage different conditions.
2. The ABCDEF bundle is a six-element bundle that seeks to keep patients as cognitively and physically engaged as possible by adequately managing pain; minimizing deep sedation and length of mechanical ventilation; preventing, identifying, and managing delirium; encouraging early physical activity; and engaging with and empowering family members.

3. Although compliance with the bundle is poor, when used properly, it results in dose-dependent improvements in numerous clinical outcomes, including hospital mortality, length of mechanical ventilation, incidence of coma and delirium, use of physical restraints, readmission to the ICU, and discharge to a facility other than home. As such, the ABCDEF bundle may be the best tool available to prevent or mitigate the development of PICS.
4. Many institutions utilize "checklists" as cognitive aides to enhance bundle adherence with modest success.

References

1. J.F. Lavallée, T.A. Gray, J. Dumville, et al. The effects of care bundles on patient outcome: a systematic review and meta-analysis. *Implement Sci* 2017; **12**(1): 142.
2. J. Barr, G.L. Fraser, K. Puntillo, et al. Clinical practice guidelines for the management of pain, agitation, and delirium in adult patients in the intensive care unit. *Crit Care Med* 2013; **41**(1): 263–306.
3. J.W. Devlin, Y. Skrobik, C. Gelinas, et al. Clinical practice guidelines for the prevention and management of pain, agitation/sedation, delirium, immobility, and sleep disruption in adult patients in the ICU. *Crit Care Med* 2018; **46**: e825–873.
4. M.E. Mikkelsen, J.W. Devlin. The A2F bundle: quantity and quality matter. *Crit Care Med* 2021; **49**(2): 380–2.
5. A. Marra, E.W. Ely, P.P. Pandharipande, M.B. Patel. The ABCDEF bundle in critical care. *Crit Care Clin* 2017; **33**(2): 225–43.
6. K.A. Puntillo, A. Max, J.F. Timsit, et al. Determinants of procedural pain intensity in the intensive care unit. The Europain® study. *Am J Respir Crit Care Med* 2014; **189**: 39–47.
7. T.J. Gan. Poorly controlled post-operative pain: prevalence, consequences, and prevention. *J Pain Res* 2017; **10**: 2287–98.
8. M. McCaffrey, A. Beebe. *Pain: Clinical Manual for Nursing Practice.* St Louis, MO: Mosby: 1989.
9. C. Gelinas, L. Fillion, K.A. Puntillo, et al. Validation of the critical-care pain observation tool in adult patients. *Am J Crit Care* 2006; **15**: 420–7.
10. J.F. Payen, O. Bru, J.L. Bosson, et al. Assessing pain in critically ill sedated patients by using a behavioral pain scale. *Crit Care Med* 2001; **29**: 2258–63.
11. N.A. Desbiens, N. Mueller-Rizner. How well do surrogates assess the pain of seriously ill patients? *Crit Care Med* 2000; **28**: 1347–52.
12. A. Pesonen, R. Suojaranta-Ylinen, E. Hammarén, et al. Pregabalin has an opioid-sparing effect in elderly patients after cardiac surgery: a randomized placebo-controlled trial. *Br J Anaesth* 2011; **106**: 873–81.
13. J.P. Kress, A.S. Pohlman, M.F. O'Connor, J.B. Hall. Daily interruption of sedative infusions in critically ill patients undergoing mechanical ventilation. *N Engl J Med* 2000; **342**: 1471–7.
14. T.D. Girard, J.P. Kress, B.D. Fuchs, et al. Efficacy and safety of a paired sedation and ventilator weaning protocol for mechanically ventilated patients in intensive care (Awakening and Breathing Controlled trial): a randomised controlled trial. *Lancet* 2008; **371**(9607): 126–34.
15. Y. Shehabi, L. Chan, S. Kadiman, et al. Sedation depth and long-term mortality in mechanically ventilated critically ill adults: a prospective longitudinal multicentre cohort study. *Intensive Care Med* 2013; **39**(5): 910–18.
16. Y. Shehabi, R. Bellomo, S. Kadiman, et al. Sedation intensity in the first 48 hours of mechanical ventilation and 180-day mortality: a multinational prospective longitudinal cohort study. *Crit Care Med* 2018; **46**(6): 850–9.

17. C.N. Sessler, M.S. Gosnell, M.J. Grap, et al. The Richmond Agitation-Sedation scale: validity and reliability in adult intensive care unit patients. *Am J Resp Crit Care Med* 2002; **166**(10): 1338–44.
18. R.R. Riker, J.T. Picard, G.L. Fraser. Prospective evaluation of the sedation-agitation scale for adult critically ill patients. *Crit Care Med* 1999; **27**(7): 1325-9.
19. F. Sadaf, M. Saqib, M. Iftikhar, A. Ahmad. Prevalence and risk factors of delirium, in patients admitted to intensive care units: a multicentric cross-sectional study. *Cureus* 2023; **15**(9): e44827.
20. E.W. Ely, S.K. Inouye, G.R. Bernard, et al. Delirium in mechanically ventilated patients: validity and reliability of the confusion assessment method for the intensive care unit (CAM-ICU). *JAMA* 2001; **286**(21): 2703–10.
21. E.W. Ely, A. Shintani, B. Truman, et al. Delirium as a predictor of mortality in mechanically ventilated patients in the intensive care unit. *JAMA* 2004; **291**(14): 1753–62.
22. P.P. Pandharipande, T.D. Girard, J.C. Jackson, et al. Long-term cognitive impairment after critical illness. *N Engl J Med* 2013; **369**(14): 1306–16.
23. N. Bergeron, M.J. Dubois, M. Dumot, et al. Intensive care delirium screening checklist: evaluation of a new screening tool. *Intensive Care Med* 2001; **27**(5): 859–64.
24. E.W. Ely, R. Margolin, J. Francis, et al. Evaluation of delirium in critically ill patients: validation of the Confusion Assessment Method for the Intensive Care Unit (CAM-ICU). *Crit Care Med* 2001; **29**(7): 1370–9.
25. M.C. Reade, G.M. Eastwood, R. Bellomo, et al. Effect of dexmedetomidine added to standard care on ventilator-free time in patients with agitated delirium: a randomized clinical trial. *JAMA* 2016; **315**: 1460–8.
26. J.P. Kress, J.B. Hall. ICU-acquired weakness and recovery from critical illness. *N Engl J Med* 2014; **371**(3): 287–8.
27. D.A. Kelmenson, N. Held, R.R. Allen, et al. Outcomes of ICU patients with a discharge diagnosis of critical illness polyneuromyopathy: a propensity-matched analysis. *Crit Care Med* 2017; **45**(12): 2055–60.
28. E. Fan, D.W. Dowdy, E. Colantuoni, et al. Physical complications in acute lung injury survivors: a two-year longitudinal prospective study. *Crit Care Med* 2014; **42**(4): 849–59.
29. P. Nydahl, T. Sricharoenchai, S. Chandra, et al. Safety of patient mobilization and rehabilitation in the intensive care unit: systematic review with meta-analysis. *Ann Am Thorac Soc* 2017; **14**(5): 766–77.
30. W.D. Schweickert, M.C. Pohlman, A.S. Pohlman, et al. Early physical and occupational therapy in mechanically ventilated, critically ill patients: a randomised controlled trial. *Lancet* 2009; **373**(9678): 1874–82.
31. G. Wang, R. Antel, M. Goldfarb. The impact of randomized family-centered interventions on family-centered outcomes in the adult intensive care unit: a systematic review. *J Intensive Care Med* 2023; **38**: 690–701.
32. Y. Ito, M. Tsubaki, M. Kobayashi, et al. Effect size estimates of risk factors for post-intensive care syndrome-family: a systematic review and meta-analysis. *Hear Lung.* 2023; **59**: 1–7.
33. R.G. Rosa, M. Falavigna, D.B. da Silva, et al. Effect of flexible family visitation on delirium among patients in the intensive care unit: the ICU visits randomized clinical trial. *JAMA* 2019; **322**: 215–28.
34. B.T. Pun, M.C. Balas, M.A. Barnes-Daly, et al. Caring for critically ill patients with the ABCDEF bundle: results of the ICU Liberation Collaborative in over 15,000 adults. *Crit Care Med* 2019; **47**(1): 3–14.
35. K. Liu, K. Nakamura, H. Katsukawa, et al. Implementation of the ABCDEF bundle for critically ill ICU patients during the COVID-19 pandemic: a multi-national 1-day point prevalance study. *Front Med (Lausanne)* 2021; **8**: 735860.

36. R. Resar, F. Griffin, C. Haraden, T. Nolan. Using care bundles to improve health care quality. IHI innovation series white paper. Cambridge, MA: Institute for Healthcare Improvement: 2012.

37. P. Dieckmann, S. Reddersen, T. Wehner, M. Rall. Prospective memory failures as an unexplored threat to patient safety: results from a pilot study using patient simulators to investigate the missed execution of intentions. *Ergonomics* 2006; **49**(5–6): 526–43.

38. L.M. Boehm, M.S. Dietrich, E. E. Vasilevskis, et al. Perceptions of workload burden and adherence to the ABCDE bundle among intensive care providers. *Am J Crit Care* 2017; **26**(4): e38–e47.

39. K. Dayton, H. Lindroth, H.J. Engel, et al. Creating a culture of an awake and walking intensive care unit: in-hospital strategies to mitigate post-intensive care syndrome. *Crit Care Clin* 2025; **41**(1): 121–40.

40. S.J. Hsieh, O. Otusanya, H.B. Gershengorn, et al. Staged implementation of awakening and breathing coordination, delirium monitoring and management, and early mobilization bundle improves patient outcomes and reduces hospital costs. *Crit Care Med* 2019; **47**(7): 885–93.

41. D.K. Costa, M.R. White, E. Ginier, et al. Identifying barriers to delivering the awakening and breathing coordination, delirium, and early exercise/mobility bundle to minimize adverse outcomes for mechanically ventilated patients: a systematic review. *Chest* 2017; **152**(2): 304–11.

42. J.L. Stollings, J.W. Devlin, J.C. Lin, et al. Best practices for conducting interprofessional team rounds to facilitate performance of the ICU Liberation (ABCDEF) Bundle. *Crit Care Med* 2020; **48**(4): 562–70.

43. L.T. Kohn, J.M. Corrigan, M.S. Donaldson. *To Err Is Human: Building a Safer Health System*. Washington, DC: Committee on Quality Health Care in America, Institute of Medicine: National Academy Press: 1999.

44. T.E.F. Abbott, T. Ahmad, M.K. Phull, et al. The surgical safety checklist and patient outcomes after surgery: a prospective observational cohort study, systematic review, and meta-analysis. *Br J Anaesth* 2018; **120**(1): 146–55.

45. R. Clay-Williams, L. Colligan. Back to basics: checklists in aviation and healthcare. *BMJ Qual Saf* 2015; **24**(7): 428–31.

46. E. Ista, B. van der Hoven, R.F. Kornelisse, et al. Effectiveness of insertion and maintenance bundles to prevent central line-associated bloodstream infections in critically ill patients of all ages: a systematic review and meta-analysis. *Lancet Infect Dis* 2016; **16**(6): 724–34.

47. B.K. Burian, A. Clebonne, K. Dismukes, K.J. Riskin. More than a tick box: medical checklist development, design, and use. *Anesth Analg* 2018; **126**(1): 223–32.

48. O. Thomassen, A. Espeland, E. Softeland, et al. Implementation of checklists in health care; learning from high-reliability organisations. *Scand J Trauma Resusc Emerg Med* 2011; **19**: 53.

49. J.E. Centofani, E.H. Duan, N.C. Hoad, et al. Use of a daily goals checklist for morning ICU rounds: a mixed-methods study. *Crit Care Med* 2014; **42**(8): 1797–803.

50. M.C. Byrnes, D.J. Schuerer, M.E. Schallom, et al. Implementation of a mandatory checklist of protocols and objectives improves compliance with a wide range of evidence-based intensive care unit practices. *Crit Care Med* 2009; **37**(10): 2775–81.

51. M. Vukoja, R. Kashyap, S. Gavriloc, et al. Checklist for early recognition and treatment of acute illness: international collaboration to improve critical care practice. *World J Crit Care Med* 2015; **4**(1): 55–61.

52. M. Vukoja, Y. Dong, N.K.J Adhikari, et al. Checklist for early recognition and treatment of acute illness and injury: an exploratory multicenter international quality-improvement study in the ICUs with variable resources. *Crit Care Med* 2021; **49**(6): e598–e612.

53. A.J.R. De Bie, S. Nan, L.R.E. Vermeulen, et al. Intelligent dynamic clinical checklists improved checklist compliance in the intensive care unit. *Br J Anaesth* 2017; **119** (2): 231–8.
54. C. Thongprayoon, A.M. Harrison, J. C. O'Horo, et al. The effect of an electronic checklist on critical care provider workload, errors, and performance. *J Intensive Care Med* 2016; **31**(3): 205–12.
55. C.H. Weiss, D. Dibardino, J. Rho, et al. A clinical trial comparing physician prompting with an unprompted automated electronic checklist to reduce empirical antibiotic utilization. *Crit Care Med* 2013; **41**(11): 2563–9.

Chapter 12: Physical Rehabilitation in the ICU and Hospital

Felipe González-Seguel, Sabrina Eggmann, Owen Gustafson, Kirby P. Mayer, Selina M. Parry, and Dario Villalba

Introduction

The deleterious impacts of immobility, sedation, and associated critical care interventions and their contributions to the development of post-intensive care syndrome (PICS) have been extensively documented. In the previous chapter, readers were introduced to the multicomponent ABCDEF care bundle developed by the Society of Critical Care Medicine to enhance the quality of care provided to critically ill patients. This chapter will provide a more in-depth discussion regarding **E: Early Mobility and Exercise** in the context of physical rehabilitation in the intensive care unit (ICU) and hospital.

This chapter defines physical rehabilitation and early mobilization, reviews the latest evidence regarding its efficacy, discusses how to operationalize and implement physical rehabilitation in the ICU and hospital, and addresses current areas of controversy in the field.

Defining Physical Rehabilitation and Early Mobility within the ICU Setting

The World Health Organization defines rehabilitation as "a set of interventions designed to optimize functioning and reduce disability in individuals with health conditions in interactions with their environment" [1]. Physical rehabilitation focuses on interventions that are designed to improve any International Classification of Functioning, Disability, and Health (ICF) domain of physical functioning, including those targeting muscle strength, power, exercise capacity, endurance, mobility, and the ability to perform daily activities [2]. Early mobilization is a component of physical rehabilitation that includes in-bed and out-of-bed mobility activities in the ICU. Critical care literature often considers early mobilization as a mobility intervention that occurs within the first 72 to 96 hours of an ICU admission, but there is significant variability in both its timing and definition.

The terms mobilization and physical rehabilitation are often used interchangeably in the literature. Significant heterogeneity in the terminology used and in the characteristics of the intervention, particularly with respect to frequency, intensity, type, and timing, reduces the ability to synthesize the literature and determine the effectiveness of interventions to improve patient outcomes [3,4]. For example, some guidelines define early mobilization as only *active* interventions (i.e., the patient is volitionally able to participate), while others include *passive* interventions (i.e., the patient is unable to volitionally participate) to be a component of early mobilization strategies [5]. The distinction between passive and active engagement is important clinically, as energy expenditure, perceived benefit, and the practice of delivering the intervention are different. More importantly, most ICU early mobilization and physical rehabilitation randomized controlled trials (RCTs) have used a progressive mobility approach, gradually progressing from passive range of motion exercises to functional activities, such as sitting or standing [4,6,7].

The purpose of this chapter is to understand how physical rehabilitation delivered in the ICU may improve outcomes for survivors of critical illness. As detailed throughout this textbook, patients surviving an ICU admission commonly suffer long-term physical, cognitive, psychological, and social health impairments and disabilities [8,9,10,11,12]. For this chapter, we will refer to physical rehabilitation as any passive or active exercise or mobilization that is *planned* and *structured* with the goal of mitigating deficits and improving short- and long-term physical functioning.

Delivery of physical rehabilitation for patients in the ICU should be personalized to each patient and, if physiologically possible, initiated within the first few days of ICU admission. Individualized physical rehabilitation emphasizes patient-centered care by taking into consideration the patient's values and preferences [13]. A personalized approach considers the dose of the intervention and promotes communication with the patient, their family, and the interdisciplinary care team to foster trust, enhance participation, and optimize outcomes [13]. Therefore, the implementation of physical rehabilitation in the ICU setting requires a coordinated effort among members of the multi-professional team, including physicians, nurses, respiratory therapists, dietitians, and physical and occupational therapists. A "sequential steps" protocol has been proposed for clinicians to adapt ICU physical rehabilitation interventions to specific institutional characteristics, clinical practices, and patient populations (see Figure 12.1).

Evidence for Physical Rehabilitation

Early Physical Rehabilitation in the ICU

Physical rehabilitation is one of the most recommended strategies to prevent and minimize the physical impairments associated with intensive care unit-acquired weakness (ICUAW) and PICS [14]. Data from multiple meta-analyses and RCTs, however, suggest that more research is required to understand the efficacy of physical rehabilitation in the ICU [15,16,17,18,19,20,21,22,23]. Findings from a meta-analysis of 14 studies examining 1753 patients support physical rehabilitation when compared to the standard of care for improving muscle strength at ICU discharge, mobility status at hospital discharge, and the number of days alive and out of hospital at day 180 [24]. Data from another meta-analysis of five studies demonstrate that physical rehabilitation initiated within three days of ICU admission improves muscle strength during hospitalization compared to the standard of care [25]. Findings in both of these systematic reviews, however, fail to show consistent effects on the patient-centered outcomes of mortality and long-term physical functioning [24,25]. Cautious interpretation of the findings is imperative, as heterogeneity in the study designs, protocol delivery, and patient populations may explain the lack of definitive benefits on outcomes.

Schweickert and colleagues performed an RCT to examine if early (within 72 hours) physical rehabilitation paired with sedation interruption improved physical functioning at hospital discharge compared to the standard of care [6]. The rehabilitation protocol emphasized daily sedation interruptions, providing an opportunity for patients to be

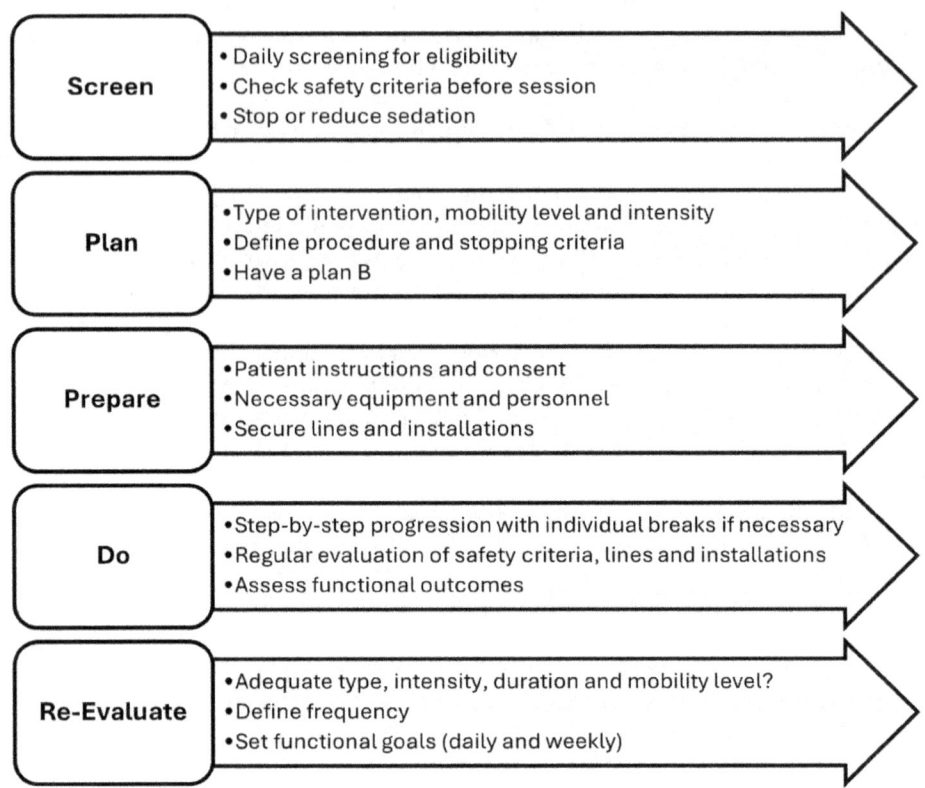

Figure 12.1 Sequential steps for physical rehabilitation strategies.

maximally alert and capable of participating in physical and occupational therapy interventions. The findings strongly support early physical rehabilitation by demonstrating a significant increase in the percentage of patients returning to independent functional status, as defined by the ability to perform six activities of daily living and ambulate independently, at the time of hospital discharge (59% vs 35%, p=0.02, Odds Ratio [OR] 2.7 [95% CI 1.2–6.1]); furthermore, patients who received the rehabilitation intervention had less delirium and more ventilator-free days [6]. This landmark study was one of the first trials of ICU rehabilitation and one of the only studies that specifically paired rehabilitation with sedation interruptions in mechanically ventilated patients. Data from several RCTs that have been conducted since this study are conflicting, and many are perceived as "negative," as demonstrated by recent systematic reviews (see Table 12.1).

The TEAM study, the largest RCT to date with 750 participants, compared early, active, high-dose physical rehabilitation with conventional, low-dose physical rehabilitation in the ICU, with a primary endpoint of days alive and out of the hospital [17]. Importantly, both groups received early physical rehabilitation in this trial, but the time to highest physical rehabilitation level and active physical rehabilitation duration (dose) differed significantly between the two groups. Perhaps surprisingly, the trial found an increase of (serious) adverse events with early, active, high-dose physical rehabilitation; while most of these

Table 12.1 Main findings of recent systematic reviews on physical rehabilitation interventions in the intensive care unit

Year of publication	First author	No. studies included	Design of studies included	Meta-analysis	Population	Intervention	Main findings
2024	O'Grady	33	RCTs	Yes (Updated from Takaoka 2020)	Adults admitted to the ICU	Leg cycle ergometry	Cycling may improve physical function at ICU discharge and after hospital discharge, may reduce ICU/hospital length of stay, with no effect on other outcomes, including mortality and adverse events.
2024	Jiroutková	58	RCTs	Yes (Updated from Waldauf 2020)	Adults admitted to the ICU	Any physical rehabilitation modality, including cycling, NMES, protocolized physical rehabilitation, or functional electrical stimulation-assisted cycle ergometry	None of the rehabilitation intervention strategies influenced mortality. Both duration of mechanical ventilation and ICU length of stay were shortened by physical rehabilitation; however, no early rehabilitation interventions in passive patients seem to have clinical benefits. Regarding long-term functional outcomes, the results remain inconclusive.
2024	Vanderlelie	8	RCTs, non RCTs, and observational studies	No	Adults admitted to the ICU	Arm cycle ergometry	Arm cycle ergometry initiated in the ICU is likely a safe intervention. Its utility is promising, and more rigorous studies could examine its impact on short- and long-term physical function and other patient-important outcomes.
2024	Xu	23	RCTs	Yes	Adults who required invasive mechanical	NMES or NMES + physical therapy	NMES appears to be a straightforward and safe modality. When combined with physical

Table 12.1 (cont.)

Year of publication	First author	No. studies included	Design of studies included	Meta-analysis	Population	Intervention	Main findings
					ventilation in the ICU		therapy, it significantly improved the extubation success rate.
2023	Nakanishi	18	RCTs	Yes	Adults admitted to the ICU	NMES	NMES may result in a lower occurrence of ICUAW in patients with critical illness, but its use may have little to no effect on pricking sensation in patients.
2022	Vollenweide	5	RCTs	No	Sedated and ventilated adults in the ICU	Passive motion of lower extremities	Passive movement shows a slight tendency for beneficial changes on a cellular level in sedated and ventilated patients in the ICU within the first days of admission. This may indicate a reduction of muscle wasting and could prevent the development of ICUAW.
2022	Paton	11	RCTs	Yes	Adults who required invasive mechanical ventilation in the ICU	Early active mobilization	Early active mobilization did not significantly affect days alive and out of hospital at day 180 but was associated with improved physical function in survivors at 6 months. The possibility that it might increase adverse events needs to be considered when interpreting this finding.
2021	Wang	60	RCTs and controlled clinical trials	Yes	Adults admitted to the ICU	Any physical rehabilitation modality	Physical rehabilitation in the ICU improves physical function at hospital discharge and reduces ICU and hospital lengths of stay.

adverse events were transient, the authors suggest the need for a cautious approach to early physical rehabilitation in this patient population. Nevertheless, the TEAM trial should not discourage clinicians from mobilizing patients with critical illness early because the study did not test the *effectiveness* of early physical rehabilitation but rather investigated the required *dose* of physical rehabilitation [26].

The lack of "positive" results in meta-analyses may be explained by the heterogeneity of interventional strategies and by improvements in the control groups over time. Control groups (comparator groups) of RCTs have been changed from "no mobilization" to either lower dose, unstructured mobilization or to other rehabilitation interventions as part of "usual care" [27]. It is important to recognize that RCTs of physical rehabilitation strategies that deliver only passive intervention have very limited or no benefits on patient-centered outcomes [19]. Additionally, physical rehabilitation interventions may incorporate exercise equipment or assistive technology to deliver the intervention, such as neuromuscular electrical stimulation, cycling, and upright tilting. Variation in the type of rehabilitation intervention increases the likelihood of inconsistent results. Heterogeneous patient populations, with RCTs frequently enrolling "all-comers," may also contribute to the lack of definitive benefits; this is highlighted in a post-hoc analysis of the aforementioned TEAM trial, in which the effects of high-dose mobilization were apparent in the subset of patients with diabetes [28]. Finally, intra-individual response variability leading to "responders" and "non-responders" may also explain lack of benefits seen in RCTs [29]. Future physical rehabilitation RCTs must address these issues by performing personalized instead of protocolized interventions and by minimizing heterogeneity in both the patient population and in the intra-individual response to intervention.

Progressive Stepwise Physical Rehabilitation and Physical Activity in the ICU

Although the timing of physical rehabilitation is an important consideration in an early rehabilitation strategy, other studies have highlighted the relevance of progressive physical rehabilitation in the ICU. One of the first studies addressing this concept was by Morris and colleagues, who emphasized the stepwise physical rehabilitation approach from passive to active to resistance training based on improvements in level of arousal and muscle strength [30]. This stepwise physical rehabilitation approach was feasible, safe, cost-effective, and was associated with decreased ICU (5.5 vs. 6.9 days; $p = 0.025$) and hospital (11.2 vs. 14.5 days; $p = 0.006$) lengths of stay when compared with those who received usual care.

This stepwise approach guided by muscle strength was followed by the concept of goal-directed physical rehabilitation using functional activity levels as milestones to progress physical rehabilitation [7]. In a population of surgical ICU patients, early, goal-directed physical rehabilitation shortened ICU length of stay and improved patients' functional mobility at hospital discharge. Similarly, a Brazilian study of goal-directed physical rehabilitation reported better functional status at ICU discharge (as measured by the Barthel index), enhanced mobility (as measured by the ICU Mobility Scale), improved pulmonary function (as measured by forced vital capacity), and shorter ICU length of stay in patients who received a progressive mobility program in which the level and intensity of the physical rehabilitation was adjusted daily based on patient performance [31]. This trial also measured physical activity level with accelerometers, showing that the patients receiving a progressive mobility program had significantly less inactive time while in the ICU.

Use of Assistive Technology within Physical Rehabilitation

Use of assistive technology can assist early physical rehabilitation, but it does not necessarily translate into a clinical benefit. The earliest studies using assistive technology included in-bed cycling devices [20,21,23,32,33,34], which were followed by studies combining in-bed cycling with synchronous neuromuscular electrical stimulation (NMES), a combination termed functional electrical simulation (FES) or FES-cycling [35,36,37]. Other studies have performed in-bed cycling and electrical muscle stimulation separately [38], yet none have found any clear physical or clinical benefits from in-bed leg cycling when compared to standard care as shown by a recent systematic review and meta-analysis of 12 RCTs and 2 non-randomized studies [39]. This was also confirmed by an RCT published in 2024, in which adding early in-bed cycling to usual physiotherapy did not improve physical function, as measured by the Physical Function in Intensive Care Test, three days after ICU discharge when compared with usual physiotherapy alone [23]. The same is also true for arm cycling in patients with critical illness [20]. An updated meta-analysis published in 2024 of 33 RCTs including 3274 patients, however, showed that cycling may improve physical function at both ICU discharge and after hospital discharge and may reduce ICU and hospital lengths of stay but had no impact on other outcomes, including mortality [21]. In-bed cycling, the safety of which has been established [39], can be performed early due to its feasibility in non-responsive, unconscious patients, but its use should be re-evaluated regularly, and it should not prevent progression to active physical rehabilitation [34]. This paradigm also applies to NMES, which has been suggested to improve muscle mass and decrease the occurrence of ICUAW in patients with critical illness, although its effect on functional outcomes and mortality has not been clearly established [40,41]. Based on the available evidence, early progressive physical rehabilitation seems superior to the use of automated devices such as NMES, in-bed cycling, and the combination thereof, and routine use of these therapies instead of early physical rehabilitation is not recommended [37].

Robotic devices are receiving increased attention given their abilities to assist lifting patients out of bed, start interventions earlier, and increase exercise duration, all of which may reduce the number of healthcare professionals required for rehabilitation. Despite their attractiveness, however, a recent feasibility study found that using robotics instead of conventional physical rehabilitation did not save time or reduce the number of healthcare professionals needed [42]. In other studies, robotic devices neither shortened time to first physical rehabilitation nor improved mobility levels [43], although patients were mobilized for longer periods of time [44]. Current evidence does therefore not support robotic devices over progressive physical rehabilitation, yet more studies are needed.

Safety of Physical Rehabilitation in the ICU

Active rehabilitation of patients with critical illness comes with inherent risk. The nature of critical illness, the dependency of the patient, and indwelling lines and tubes increase the risk of adverse events during rehabilitation. A recent systematic review and meta-analysis of 67 trials, of which 52 reported on adverse events during physical rehabilitation sessions in the ICU, demonstrated that less than 3% of physical rehabilitation sessions in the ICU resulted in an adverse event (693 events in 23,395 interventions sessions), with no significant difference between the incidence of adverse events in physical rehabilitation and control groups [16].

Table 12.2 Summary of safety criteria to initiate active mobilization in the ICU

System	Parameter
Cardiovascular	Heart rate > 40 and < 130bpm Systolic arterial pressure > 90 and < 200mmHg Mean arterial pressure > 65 and < 110mmHg Adrenaline/epinephrine < 0.5mcg/kg/min No sub-massive/massive pulmonary embolus, untreated acute aortic dissection, active cooling
Respiratory	Respiratory rate < 40 Peripheral oxygen saturation ≥ 90% $FiO_2 < 0.6$ $PEEP \geq 10 cmH_2O$ No Nitric Oxide, prostacyclin, neuromuscular blocking agents
Neurological	RASS −2 to +2 No elevated intracranial pressure, uncontrolled seizures, open lumbar drain
Orthopedic	No unstable major fracture, orthopedic contraindications
Other	Temperature < 38.5°C No active bleeding, large open abdominal/sternal wound, femoral artery sheath

PEEP: Positive end expiratory pressure; RASS: Richmond agitation and sedation scale
Adapted from references [45,46,47,48].

Although the occurrence of adverse events during physical rehabilitation in patients with critical illness is low, healthcare staff participating in rehabilitation activities should aim to mitigate this risk through appropriate patient selection, properly trained staff, and an adequately prepared environment. For this purpose, expert recommendations on safety criteria for active physical rehabilitation of mechanically ventilated, critically ill adults can guide clinicians to minimize the occurrence of adverse events [45,46]. Table 12.2 provides a summary of published recommendations on initiating active mobilization in the ICU; however, this table does not represent an exhaustive list, and the heterogeneity of the ICU patient population requires that safety parameters should be individualized [45,46,47,48].

Rehabilitation Across the Hospital

Following ICU discharge, patient activity levels in the hospital remain low [49,50]. Rehabilitation, including physiotherapy, occupational therapy, and speech therapy, should continue after ICU discharge, particularly in patients with persistent and profound disabilities. In a feasibility study by Berney and colleagues, exercise training commenced in the ICU and continued through to an outpatient program was safe and feasible for survivors of critical illness, and the intervention group received substantially greater physical rehabilitation than the standard of care, highlighting the benefits of a quantitative approach to exercise training in hospital wards after an ICU stay. While physical rehabilitation interventions following hospital discharge have been associated with improvements in aerobic capacity, depression, and the physical component score of health-related quality of life questionnaires in survivors of critical illness [49], there are multiple challenges in delivering physical rehabilitation in conventional hospital wards. A human factors analysis of mobilization of formerly critically ill patients on hospital wards identified multiple barriers [51]. Patients transferred out of the ICU must compete for priority with patients requiring assessment for hospital discharge and those on enhanced recovery pathways following surgery. Additionally, those patients who are unable to stand and transfer to a chair or who need additional equipment to mobilize are particularly susceptible to missing interventions. Sufficient multidisciplinary staffing levels and skill mix (including experience working with ICU patients) of health staff on hospital ward units are regarded as facilitators to mobilization of formerly critically ill patients who remain hospitalized.

Few studies have evaluated post-ICU rehabilitation in the general hospital wards. The largest study to do so was the RECOVER trial [52], which aimed to deliver higher levels of mobilization, dietetic therapy, occupational therapy, and speech therapy through the use of additional rehabilitation assistants compared with usual ward-based care. The intervention failed to improve physical function at three months, in part because the mobilization component was predominantly delivered to patients who were already more mobile, but patients were generally satisfied with the intervention delivered [53]. Availability of data regarding the efficacy of hospital-based rehabilitation programs after an ICU stay is limited [52,54], and more research is required before definitive recommendations can be made [55].

Assessing Physical Functioning in the ICU

Early and longitudinal assessment of physical functioning in the ICU is important to identify patients at risk of poor physical outcomes, to monitor rehabilitation efficacy, and to predict recovery trajectories. The evaluation of physical functioning is complex and is influenced by multiple interrelated factors, including muscle strength, range of motion, mobility, proprioception, balance, cognition, psychological issues, and environmental factors. Determining the specific purpose for assessing physical functioning is important when selecting an appropriate instrument [56]. Although more than 60 physical functioning instruments have been reported for use in the ICU, not all have been designed or validated for the ICU setting [2]. Several of these instruments have demonstrated robust clinimetric properties in patients with critical illness. Figure 12.2 highlights several physical functioning instruments currently used in the ICU and across the continuum of care stratified by domain and purpose of the assessment. For further details on the evaluation of physical functioning of patients in the ICU, please see Chapter 4.

Additional Effects of Physical Rehabilitation Beyond Physical Functioning

The impact of physical rehabilitation in the ICU is not limited to improvement in measures of physical function alone. Early physical rehabilitation has been shown to decrease delirium [14,57], positively impact cognitive functioning three months after ICU discharge [58], and improve post-ICU neuropsychiatric outcomes [59]. In a study of 200 mechanically ventilated patients, early physical rehabilitation in the ICU demonstrated positive results on cognitive functioning as assessed by the Montreal Cognitive Assessment tool, emphasizing the importance of avoiding delays in initiating physical rehabilitation [60]. Notably, while

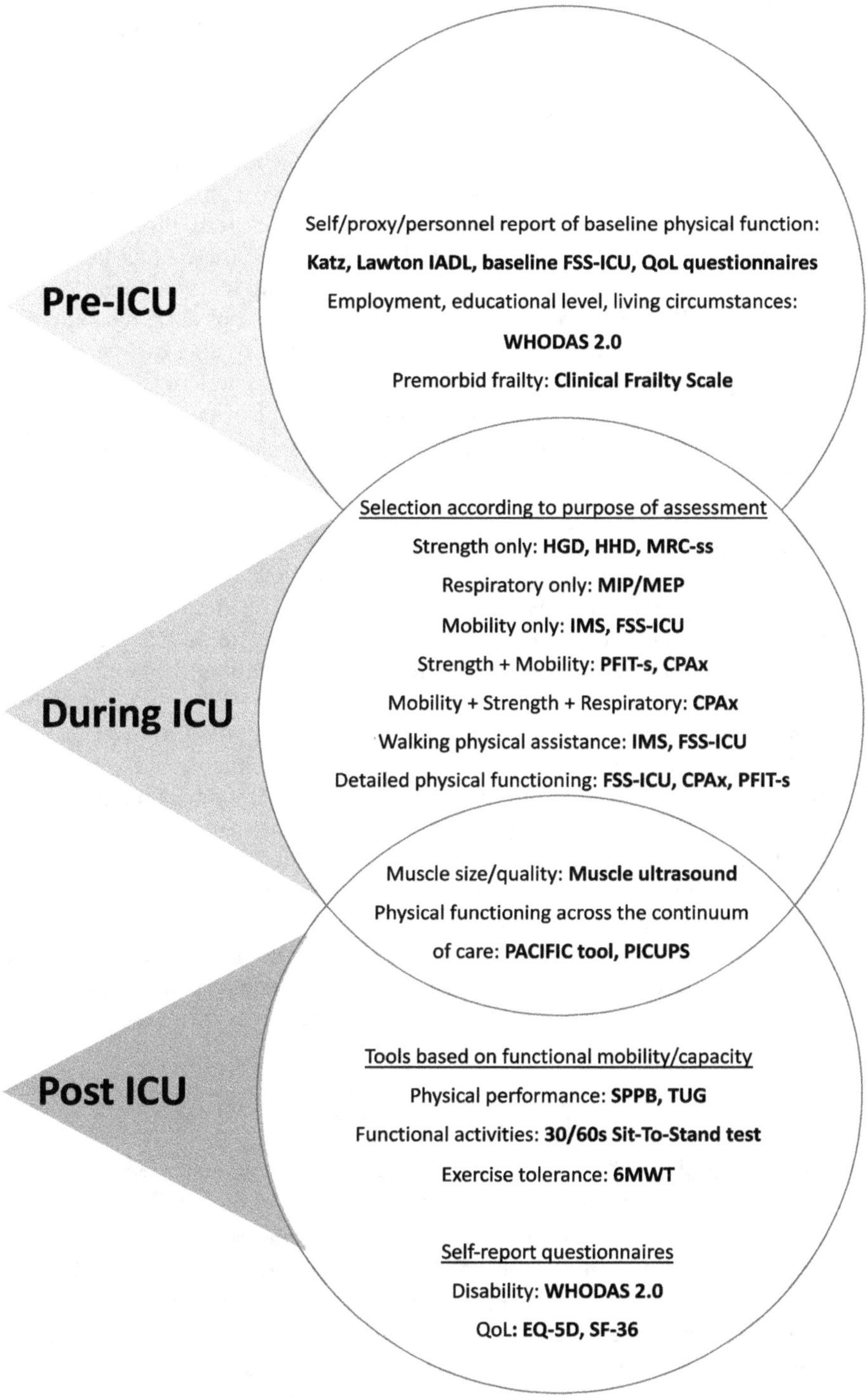

Pre-ICU

Self/proxy/personnel report of baseline physical function:

Katz, Lawton IADL, baseline FSS-ICU, QoL questionnaires

Employment, educational level, living circumstances:

WHODAS 2.0

Premorbid frailty: **Clinical Frailty Scale**

During ICU

Selection according to purpose of assessment

Strength only: **HGD, HHD, MRC-ss**

Respiratory only: **MIP/MEP**

Mobility only: **IMS, FSS-ICU**

Strength + Mobility: **PFIT-s, CPAx**

Mobility + Strength + Respiratory: **CPAx**

Walking physical assistance: **IMS, FSS-ICU**

Detailed physical functioning: **FSS-ICU, CPAx, PFIT-s**

Muscle size/quality: **Muscle ultrasound**

Physical functioning across the continuum of care: **PACIFIC tool, PICUPS**

Post ICU

Tools based on functional mobility/capacity

Physical performance: **SPPB, TUG**

Functional activities: **30/60s Sit-To-Stand test**

Exercise tolerance: **6MWT**

Self-report questionnaires

Disability: **WHODAS 2.0**

QoL: **EQ-5D, SF-36**

Figure 12.2 Physical functioning instruments and common domains assessed before, during, and after the ICU.

the intervention group received early physical and occupational therapy, the comparator group received the local standard of ICU care, which very rarely included physical or occupational therapy in the ICU.

Implications for Clinical Practice

Physical rehabilitation in the ICU seems more effective when using *functional exercises* instead of non-functional exercises alone, such as NMES or cycling [15]. Functional exercises progressively range from in-bed exercises (e.g., rolling and head lifting) to sitting up, standing, transferring, and ultimately walking. When possible, these tasks should be combined with daily activities that matter to the patient, including hair combing, foot bathing, and tooth brushing. Alternative strategies, such as NMES, passive physical rehabilitation with cycle ergometers, and use of other assistive technologies can be used in early stages of critical illness, when the patient is still sedated and functional exercises are not feasible; however, as soon as possible, active physical rehabilitation should be the priority in the ICU. Despite the potential benefits of physical rehabilitation, implementation can be challenging considering certain institutional, clinician, and patient issues in the ICU (see Figure 12.3) [61].

Future Directions and Areas of Controversy

The conflicting results on the effectiveness of early physical rehabilitation highlight evidence gaps related to timing, dose, fidelity, and individualization of the intervention [29,62,63]. First, timing and dosing of exercise interventions have been proposed as a research and clinical challenge. To address the dosage of physical rehabilitation, the seven principles of exercise from the Consensus on Exercise Reporting Template (CERT) must be considered, including individuality, specificity, progression, overload, adaptation, recovery, and reversibility [27,64]. Individuality and specificity are principles that remain challenging for physical rehabilitation in the ICU setting, as interventions in early physical rehabilitation trials usually treat all patients as a homogeneous group and are rarely patient-specific. Second, lack of intervention fidelity in current RCTs is problematic, as the delivered dose of the intervention does not always reach the prescribed dose. Finally, the conflicting results on the effectiveness of early physical rehabilitation have promoted individualization of mobility interventions, which has shown promising results in RCTs based on progressive mobility protocols. To optimize long-term outcomes, a continuum of rehabilitation needs to be established from ICU to hospital discharge and beyond to support patients across their recovery trajectory.

Key Points

1. Physical rehabilitation is one of the most recommended strategies to prevent and minimize physical impairments associated with ICUAW and PICS.
2. Progressive mobilization and the use of assistive technology devices provide opportunities for physical rehabilitation in the ICU and across the hospitalization.
3. Conflicting results on the effectiveness of physical rehabilitation have revealed evidence gaps related to timing, dose, fidelity, and individualization of the intervention.
4. A continuum of rehabilitation strategies needs to be established from ICU to hospital discharge to optimize long-term outcomes of patients across their recovery trajectory.

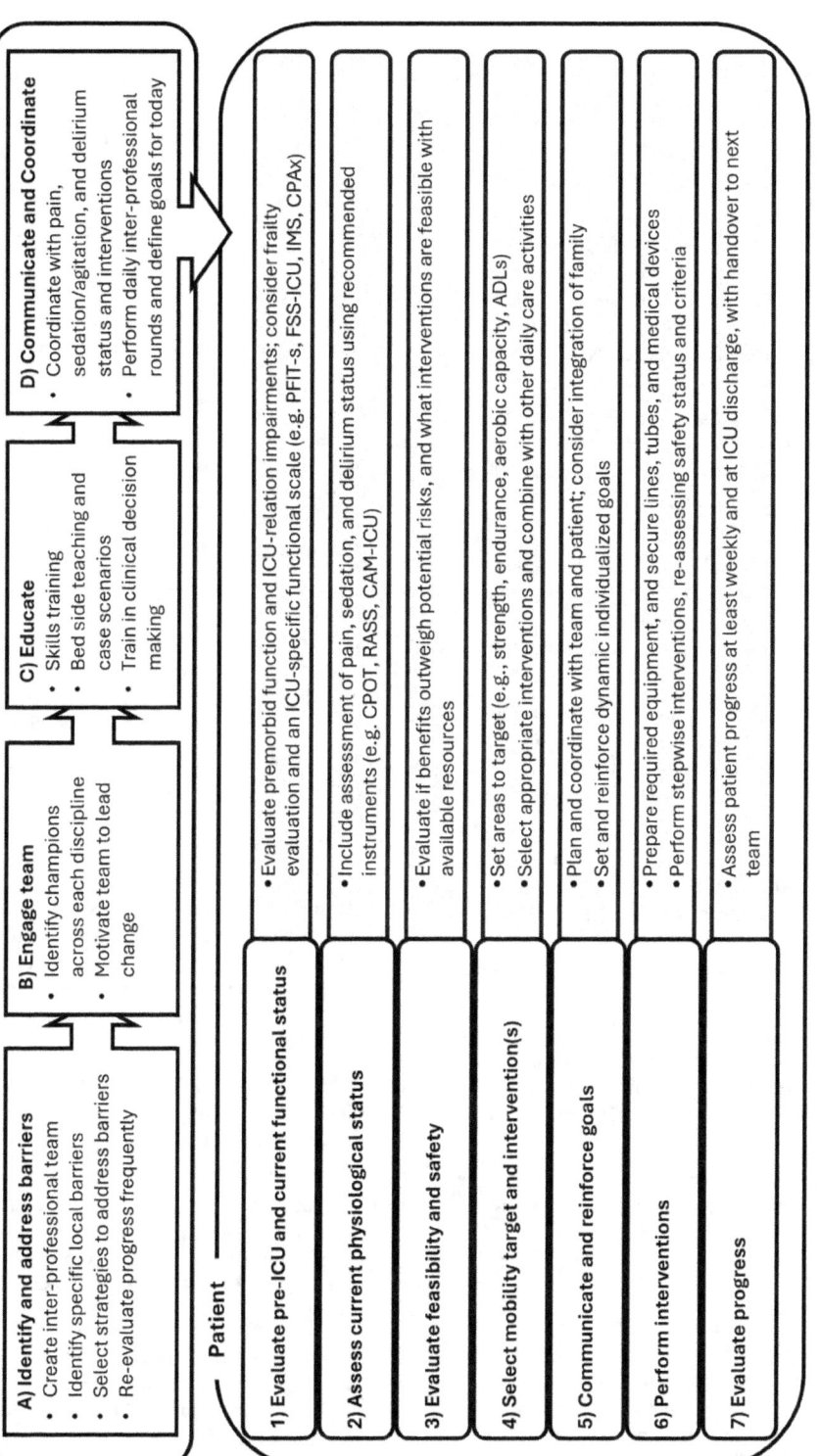

Figure 12.3 Implementation of physical rehabilitation in the ICU. From: S.M. Parry, P. Nydahl, D.M. Needham. Implementing early physical rehabilitation and mobilisation in the ICU: institutional, clinician, and patient considerations. *Intensive Care Med* 2018; **44**: 470–3. Reproduced with permissions from Springer Nature.

References

1. B.H. Sjölund. Rehabilitation. In: Gellman MD, Turner JR, (eds.), *Encyclopedia of Behavioral Medicine*. New York, NY: Springer New York: 2013. pp. 1634–8.

2. F. González-Seguel, E.J. Corner, C. Merino-Osorio. International classification of functioning, disability, and health domains of 60 physical functioning measurement instruments used during the adult intensive care unit stay: a scoping review. *Phys Ther* 2019; **99**: 627–40.

3. C. Clarissa, L. Salisbury, S. Rodgers, S. Kean. Early mobilisation in mechanically ventilated patients: a systematic integrative review of definitions and activities. *J Intensive Care* 2019; **7**: 3.

4. C. Farley, A.N.L. Newman, J. Hoogenes, et al. Treatment fidelity in 94 randomized controlled trials of physical rehabilitation in the ICU: a scoping review. *Crit Care Med* 2024; **52**: 717–28.

5. J.K. Lang, M.S. Paykel, K.J. Haines, C.L. Hodgson. Clinical practice guidelines for early mobilization in the ICU: a systematic review. *Crit Care Med* 2020; **48**: e1121–e8.

6. W.D. Schweickert, M.C. Pohlman, A.S. Pohlman, et al. Early physical and occupational therapy in mechanically ventilated, critically ill patients: a randomised controlled trial. *Lancet* 2009; **373**: 1874–82.

7. S.J. Schaller, M. Anstey, M. Blobner, et al. Early, goal-directed mobilisation in the surgical intensive care unit: a randomised controlled trial. *Lancet* 2016; **388**: 1377–88.

8. B. Fazzini, T. Märkl, C. Costas, et al. The rate and assessment of muscle wasting during critical illness: a systematic review and meta-analysis. *Crit Care* 2023; **27**: 2.

9. K.C. Higa, K. Mayer, C. Quinn, et al. Sounding the alarm: what clinicians need to know about physical, emotional, and cognitive recovery after venoarterial extracorporeal membrane oxygenation. *Crit Care Med* 2023; **51**: 1234–45.

10. O.D. Gustafson, M.A. Williams, S. McKechnie, et al. Musculoskeletal complications following critical illness: a scoping review. *J Crit Care* 2021; **66**: 60–6.

11. B.B. Kamdar, R. Suri, M.R. Suchyta, et al. Return to work after critical illness: a systematic review and meta-analysis. *Thorax* 2020; **75**: 17–27.

12. O.J. Bienvenu, L.A. Friedman, E. Colantuoni, et al. Psychiatric symptoms after acute respiratory distress syndrome: a 5-year longitudinal study. *Intensive Care Med* 2018; **44**: 38–47.

13. Z. van Willigen, C. Ostler, D. Thackray, R. Cusack. Patient and family experience of physical rehabilitation on the intensive care unit: a qualitative exploration. *Physiotherapy* 2020; **109**: 102–10.

14. J.W. Devlin, Y. Skrobik, C. Gelinas, et al. Clinical practice guidelines for the prevention and management of pain, agitation/sedation, delirium, immobility, and sleep disruption in adult patients in the ICU. *Crit Care Med* 2018; **46**: e825–e73.

15. Y.T. Wang, J.K. Lang, K.J. Haines, et al. Physical rehabilitation in the ICU: a systematic review and meta-analysis. *Crit Care Med* 2022; **50**: 375–88.

16. M. Paton, S. Chan, A. Serpa Neto, et al. Association of active mobilisation variables with adverse events and mortality in patients requiring mechanical ventilation in the intensive care unit: a systematic review and meta-analysis. *Lancet Respir Med* 2024; **12**: 386–98.

17. C.L. Hodgson, M. Bailey, R. Bellomo, et al. Early active mobilization during mechanical ventilation in the ICU. *N Engl J Med* 2022; **387**: 1747–58.

18. M. Paton, S. Chan, C.J. Tipping, et al. The effect of mobilization at 6 months after critical illness: meta-analysis. *NEJM Evidence* 2023; **2**: EVIDoa2200234.

19. K. Jiroutkova, F. Duska, P. Waldauf. Should new data on rehabilitation interventions in critically ill patients change clinical practice? Updated meta-analysis of randomized controlled trials. *Crit Care Med* 2024; online ahead of print.

20. L. Vanderlelie, S. Bosich, H. O'Grady, et al. Arm cycle ergometry in critically ill patients: a systematic review. *Aust Crit Care* 2024; **37**: 985–93.

21. H.K. O'Grady, H. Hasan, B. Rochwerg, et al. Leg cycle ergometry in critically ill patients: an updated systematic review and meta-analysis. *NEJM Evid* 2024: EVIDoa2400194.

22. N. Daum, N. Drewniok, A. Bald, et al. Early mobilisation within 72 hours after admission of critically ill patients in the intensive care unit: a systematic review with network meta-analysis. *Intensive Crit Care Nurs* 2024; **80**: 103573.

23. M.E. Kho, S. Berney, A.M. Pastva, et al. Early in-bed cycle ergometry in mechanically ventilated patients. *NEJM Evid* 2024; **3**: EVIDoa2400137.

24. C.J. Tipping, M. Harrold, A. Holland, et al. The effects of active mobilisation and rehabilitation in ICU on mortality and function: a systematic review. *Intensive Care Med* 2017; **43**: 171–83.

25. R. Fuke, T. Hifumi, Y. Kondo, et al. Early rehabilitation to prevent postintensive care syndrome in patients with critical illness: a systematic review and meta-analysis. *BMJ Open* 2018; **8**: e019998.

26. S. Eggmann, P. Nydahl, R. Gosselink, B. Bissett. We need to talk about adverse events during physical rehabilitation in critical care trials. *eClinicalMedicine* 2024; **68**.

27. H.K. O'Grady, J.C. Reid, C. Farley, et al. Comparator groups in ICU-based studies of physical rehabilitation: a scoping review of 125 studies. *Crit Care Explor* 2023; **5**: e0917.

28. A. Serpa Neto, M. Bailey, D. Seller, et al. Impact of high-dose early mobilization on outcomes for patients with diabetes: a secondary analysis of the TEAM trial. *Am J Respir Crit Care Med* 2024; **210**: 779–87.

29. B.H. Cuthbertson. The faltering evidence base for early rehabilitation. *Am J Respir Crit Care Med* 2023; **208**: 7–8.

30. P.E. Morris, A. Goad, C. Thompson, et al. Early intensive care unit mobility therapy in the treatment of acute respiratory failure. *Crit Care Med* 2008; **36**: 2238–43.

31. D.S. Schujmann, T. Teixeira Gomes, A.C. Lunardi, et al. Impact of a progressive mobility program on the functional status, respiratory, and muscular systems of ICU patients: a randomized and controlled trial. *Crit Care Med* 2020; **48**: 491–7.

32. C. Burtin, B. Clerck, C. Robbeets, et al. Early exercise in critically ill patients enhances short-term functional recovery. *Crit Care Med* 2009; **37**: 2499–505.

33. C.E. Hickmann, D. Castanares-Zapatero, L. Deldicque, et al. Impact of very early physical therapy during septic shock on skeletal muscle: a randomized controlled trial. *Crit Care Med* 2018; **46**: 1436–43.

34. S. Eggmann, M.L. Verra, G. Luder, et al. Effects of early, combined endurance and resistance training in mechanically ventilated, critically ill patients: a randomised controlled trial. *PLoS One* 2018; **13**: e0207428.

35. S. Berney, R.O. Hopkins, J.W. Rose, et al. Functional electrical stimulation in-bed cycle ergometry in mechanically ventilated patients: a multicentre randomised controlled trial. *Thorax* 2021; **76**: 656–63.

36. T. de Gomes Figueiredo, M. Frazão, L.A. Werlang, et al. Functional electrical stimulation cycling-based muscular evaluation method in mechanically ventilated patients. *Artif Organs* 2024; **48**: 254–62.

37. P. Waldauf, N. Hrušková, B. Blahutova, et al. Functional electrical stimulation-assisted cycle ergometry-based progressive mobility programme for mechanically ventilated patients: randomised controlled trial with 6 months follow-up. *Thorax* 2021; **76**: 664–71.

38. G. Fossat, F. Baudin, L. Courtes, et al. Effect of in-bed leg cycling and electrical stimulation of the quadriceps on global muscle strength in critically ill adults: a randomized clinical trial. *JAMA* 2018; **320**: 368–78.

39. A. Takaoka, R. Utgikar, B. Rochwerg, et al. The efficacy and safety of in-intensive care unit leg-cycle ergometry in critically ill

adults: a systematic review and meta-analysis. *Ann Am Thorac Soc* 2020; **17**: 1289–307.

40. N.A. Maffiuletti, M. Roig, E. Karatzanos, S. Nanas. Neuromuscular electrical stimulation for preventing skeletal-muscle weakness and wasting in critically ill patients: a systematic review. *BMC Med* 2013; **11**: 137.

41. N. Nakanishi, S. Yoshihiro, Y. Kawamura, et al. Effect of neuromuscular electrical stimulation in patients with critical illness: an updated systematic review and meta-analysis of randomized controlled trials. *Crit Care Med* 2023; **51**: 1386–96.

42. A. Warmbein, L. Hübner, I. Rathgeber, et al. Robot-assisted early mobilization for intensive care unit patients: feasibility and first-time clinical use. *Int J Nurs Stud* 2024; **152**: 104702.

43. L. Huebner, A. Warmbein, C. Scharf, et al. Effects of robotic-assisted early mobilization versus conventional mobilization in intensive care unit patients: prospective interventional cohort study with retrospective control group analysis. *Crit Care* 2024; **28**: 112.

44. M. Lorenz, F. Baum, P. Kloss, et al. Robotic-assisted in-bed mobilization in ventilated ICU patients with COVID-19: an interventional, randomized, controlled pilot study (ROBEM II study). *Crit Care Med* 2024; **52**: 683–93.

45. C.L. Hodgson, K. Stiller, D.M. Needham, et al. Expert consensus and recommendations on safety criteria for active mobilization of mechanically ventilated critically ill adults. *Crit Care* 2014; **18**: 658.

46. H.R. Woodbridge, C.J. McCarthy, M. Jones, et al. Assessing the safety of physical rehabilitation in critically ill patients: a Delphi study. *Crit Care* 2024; **28**: 144.

47. T. Conceição, A.I. Gonzáles, F. Figueiredo, et al. Safety criteria to start early mobilization in intensive care units: systematic review. *Rev Bras Ter Intensiva* 2017; **29**: 509–19.

48. R. Yang, Q. Zheng, D. Zuo, et al. Safety assessment criteria for early active mobilization in mechanically ventilated ICU subjects. *Respir Care* 2021; **66**: 307–15.

49. T.C. Rollinson, B. Connolly, D.J. Berlowitz, S. Berney. Physical activity of patients with critical illness undergoing rehabilitation in intensive care and on the acute ward: an observational cohort study. *Aust Crit Care* 2022; **35**: 362–8.

50. C.E. Baldwin, A.V. Rowlands, F. Fraysse, K.N. Johnston. The sedentary behaviour and physical activity patterns of survivors of a critical illness over their acute hospitalisation: an observational study. *Aust Crit Care* 2020; **33**: 272–80.

51. O.D. Gustafson, S. Vollam, L. Morgan, P. Watkinson. A human factors analysis of missed mobilisation after discharge from intensive care: a competition for care? *Physiotherapy* 2021; **113**: 131–7.

52. T.S. Walsh, L.G. Salisbury, J.L. Merriweather, et al. Increased hospital-based physical rehabilitation and information provision after intensive care unit discharge: the RECOVER randomized clinical trial. *JAMA Intern Med* 2015; **175**: 901–10.

53. P. Ramsay, G. Huby, J. Merriweather, et al. Patient and carer experience of hospital-based rehabilitation from intensive care to hospital discharge: mixed methods process evaluation of the RECOVER randomised clinical trial. *BMJ Open* 2016; **6**: e012041.

54. R. Porta, M. Vitacca, L.S. Gilè, et al. Supported arm training in patients recently weaned from mechanical ventilation. *Chest* 2005; **128**: 2511–20.

55. S. Taito, K. Yamauchi, Y. Tsujimoto, et al. Does enhanced physical rehabilitation following intensive care unit discharge improve outcomes in patients who received mechanical ventilation? A systematic review and meta-analysis. *BMJ Open* 2019; **9**: e026075.

56. S.M. Parry, M. Huang, D.M. Needham. Evaluating physical functioning in critical care: considerations for clinical practice and research. *Crit Care* 2017; **21**: 249.

57. S. Liang, J.P.C. Chau, S.H.S. Lo, et al. Effects of nonpharmacological delirium-prevention interventions on critically ill

patients' clinical, psychological, and family outcomes: a systematic review and meta-analysis. *Aust Crit Care* 2021; **34**: 378–87.

58. J.C. Jackson, E.W. Ely, M.C. Morey, et al. Cognitive and physical rehabilitation of intensive care unit survivors: results of the RETURN randomized controlled pilot investigation. *Crit Care Med* 2012; **40**: 1088–97.

59. R.O. Hopkins, M.R. Suchyta, T.J. Farrer, D. Needham. Improving post-intensive care unit neuropsychiatric outcomes: understanding cognitive effects of physical activity. *Am J Respir Crit Care Med* 2012; **186**: 1220–8.

60. B.K. Patel, K.S. Wolfe, S.B. Patel, et al. Effect of early mobilisation on long-term cognitive impairment in critical illness in the USA: a randomised controlled trial. *Lancet Respir Med* 2023; **11**: 563–72.

61. S.M. Parry, P. Nydahl, D.M. Needham. Implementing early physical rehabilitation and mobilisation in the ICU: institutional, clinician, and patient considerations. *Intensive Care Med* 2018; **44**: 470–3.

62. S. Eggmann, K.T. Timenetsky, C. Hodgson. Promoting optimal physical rehabilitation in ICU. *Intensive Care Med* 2024; **50**: 755–7.

63. H.J. Engel, N.E. Brummel. What exactly is recommended for patient physical activity during an ICU stay? *Crit Care Med* 2024; **52**: 842–7.

64. F. González-Seguel, R. Letelier-Bernal. Early mobilization dose reporting in randomized clinical trials with patients who were mechanically ventilated: a scoping review. *Phys Ther* 2024; **104**: pzae048.

Chapter 13
Cognitive Rehabilitation in the ICU and Hospital

Kelly S. Casey

Introduction

Cognitive impairment is often unidentified or under-diagnosed in acute care hospital settings [1]. Cognitive impairment and hospitalization have a bi-directional relationship with one another: patients with chronic cognitive impairment are more likely to be hospitalized, and hospitalization increases the risk of acute and chronic cognitive impairment [1]. According to a four-year observational analysis examining patients in both inpatient and outpatient settings, 92% of mild cognitive impairment is undiagnosed [2]. A second study found that 27% of hospitalized patients had cognitive impairment, but only 61.5% of them carried the diagnosis prior to admission [3], and a complementary study found that 38% of older hospitalized patients with delirium had previously undiagnosed cognitive impairment [4]. A systematic approach to addressing cognition in the intensive care unit (ICU) and hospital empowers providers to address the often-concerning cognitive impairment that can be diagnosed at the bedside. Identifying cognitive dysfunction with frequent and consistent assessments is essential to promptly address deficits early, decrease their duration, and ideally prevent long-term functional impairment. Using objective measures allows providers to capture cognitive dysfunction, including delirium, more frequently and consistently [5].

Evaluating Cognition

Common screening tools for delirium in the ICU include the Confusion Assessment Method-ICU (CAM-ICU) [6] and the Intensive Care Delirium Screening Checklist (ICDSC) [7] (see Chapter 8 for additional information) [8]. Beyond identifying the presence and severity of delirium, other common screening tools, including the Mini Mental Status Exam (MMSE) [9] and the Montreal Cognitive Assessment (MoCA) tool, are used to assess cognitive function and impairment in the hospital [10]. Another reliable and validated tool, the Activity Measure for Post-Acute Care (AM-PAC) Applied Cognitive Inpatient Short Form (ACISF) [11,12] has demonstrated an excellent combination of performance and feasibility characteristics for the acute care setting [11]. Although discrete guidelines for the frequency of cognitive screening in the hospital do not exist, some facilities have incorporated using a cognitive screening tool, such as the AM-PAC ACISF, with every occupational therapy and speech-language pathology session.

Cognitive screens are an important first step in addressing cognition in the ICU, but they only measure patient performance at a discrete time point and do not provide a comprehensive assessment of the identified impairment(s) impacting functional cognitive performance (see Table 13.1 and Table 13.2). Once cognitive impairment has been

Table 13.1 Standardized cognitive evaluation tools

Tool	Area of Measurement	Type	Time Required	Administration and Scoring	Score Interpretation	Score Range	Cognitive Domain Assessed
Confusion Assessment Method-ICU (CAM-ICU)	Delirium	Screen	1 min	Series of questions and commands that can be completed even if a patient cannot speak	CAM-ICU positive for delirium if features 1 and 2 and either feature 3 or 4 are present	Positive or negative	Acute onset of mental status change or a fluctuating course, inattention, cognitive disturbances, altered level of consciousness
Intensive Care Delirium Screening Checklist (ICDSC)	Delirium	Screen-behavioral observation	Completed in minutes after observing a patient over a period of 8–24 hours	Each item is rated based on the patient's behavior over the previous 12 hours	0 = Normal 1–3 = Subsyndromal Delirium 4–8 = Delirium	0–8	Altered level of consciousness, inattention, delusion or hallucination, disorientation, inappropriate mood or speech, psychomotor agitation or retardation, sleep/wake cycle disturbance, symptom fluctuation
Activity Measure for Post-Acute Care (AM-PAC) Applied Cognitive Inpatient Short Form (ACISF)	IADL, Social Participation	Self-report or by proxy, screen	1 minute	Assesses how much difficulty a person has completing six cognitive tasks: following a speech or presentation, understanding ordinary conversation, taking medications, remembering where things were placed	6: Total functional impairment 24: Total absence of impairment	6–24	Communication, memory, complex task management

Table 13.1 (cont.)

Tool	Area of Measurement	Type	Time Required	Administration and Scoring	Score Interpretation	Score Range	Cognitive Domain Assessed
				or put away, remembering a list of four to five errands, and taking care of complicated tasks			
Coma Recovery Scale – Revised (CRS-R)	Consciousness and functional status	Neurobehavioral assessment	15–30 min	Providing systematic, hierarchical stimulation for each area of function while observing for reflexive to purposeful responses	Lower scores indicate reflexive behaviors and higher scores indicate more cognitively mediated behaviors	0–23	Auditory, visual, motor, oromotor, communication, arousal function
Montreal Cognitive Assessment tool (MoCA)	Multiple domains of cognitive function	Paper and pencil screen	10 min	Alternating trail making, cube and clock drawing, naming, word recall, digit span, sentence repetition, verbal fluency, abstraction, delayed recall, orientation	26–30 = Normal 19–25 = Mild cognitive impairment (MCI) 10–18 = Moderate cognitive impairment <10 = Severe cognitive impairment	30	Attention, concentration, visuospatial and executive function, memory, conceptual thinking/abstraction, orientation
Kettle Test	ADL, IADL	Occupation-based Performance-based	10–30 min	Preparation of 2 hot drinks 13 discrete steps scored on a 4-point scale	Higher scores indicate greater need for assistance	0–52	IADL, Functional Cognition

| | | | | Intact performance
Slow or trial and error
Received general cueing
Received specific cueing
Incomplete or deficient performance
Received physical demonstration or assistance | | | |
|---|---|---|---|---|---|---|---|
| Menu Task | IADL | Performance-based | 5 min | Meal selections using a menu for breakfast, lunch, and dinner with set rules. | Each item scored
1 = performance
0 = error
12 item scores are summed | 0–12 | IADL, Functional cognition |

Table 13.2 Standardized cognitive evaluation tools

Tool	Area of Measurement	Type	Time Required	Administration and Scoring	Score Interpretation	Score Range	Cognitive Domain Assessed
Assessment of Language Related Functional Activities (ALFA)	Assesses language related functional tasks	Performance-based	30–90 min	Telling time, counting money, addressing an envelope, solving math problems, writing a check/balancing a checkbook, understanding medicine labels, using a calendar, reading instructions, using the telephone, and writing a phone message	Independent Function Rating 1. Independent in completing task 2. Needs some assistance with task 3. Unable to complete task independently		Functional Cognition
Hopkins Medication Schedule	IADL	Performance-based	6–10 minutes	Part 1 – Plan a schedule for taking medications, meals, and water during the course of a day. Part 2 – Filling a common pill dispenser labelled morning, lunch, dinner, and bed following the same instructions as the schedule	Part 1: Accurate timing of doses, method, and daily dosage of antibiotics (3 points) and aspirin (3 points) and proper intake of snacks and water (3 points). If completed < 4min = 1 extra point. Part 2: Placement of the proper numbers of antibiotics (1 point) and aspirin (1 point). If completed in <2min = 1 point extra	0 to 10 on the schedule; 0 to 3 on the pillbox	IADL, Functional Cognition

Cognitive Assessment of Minnesota (CAM)	Multiple domains of cognitive function	Pencil/paper and performance-based	40 min	29 item battery	Scores are recorded as either: 3 = mild to no impairment, 2 = moderate impairment, 1 = severe impairment or 2 = intact, 1 = impaired	Each subtest provides specific criteria for a given score	Attention span, memory, orientation, visual neglect, temporal awareness, recall/recognition, auditory memory and sequencing, simple math skills, safety, problem solving and judgment
Repeatable Battery for the Assessment of Neuropsychological Status (RBANS)	Multiple domains of cognitive function	Cognitive/linguistic assessment	20–30 min	Battery	Raw scores correspond with index scores for each domain; global cognition scores correspond with the following classifications: Extremely Low: 69 and below Borderline: 70 to 79 Low Average: 80 to 89 Average: 90 to 109 High Average: 110 to 119 Superior: 120 to 129 Very Superior: 130 and above	40–160	Immediate memory, visuospatial/constructional, language, attention, delayed memory

Table 13.2 (cont.)

Tool	Area of Measurement	Type	Time Required	Administration and Scoring	Score Interpretation	Score Range	Cognitive Domain Assessed
Cognitive Linguistic Quick Test Plus (CLQT+)	Multiple domains of cognitive function	Cognitive/linguistic assessment	15–30 min	Personal facts/orientation, symbol cancellation, confrontation naming, clock drawing, story retelling, symbol trails, generative naming, design memory, mazes, design generation	Raw scores for each item correspond with age-based scaled scores. Each item has a cut score determining impairment. There is a composite severity rating for each domain. Higher scores correspond to better cognitive performance.	Looking at the individual's scaled score can indicate whether the scores are within the normal range or are mild, moderately, or severely impaired	Attention, memory, executive function, language, visuospatial skills

identified via a screening tool, further standardized assessments are needed to more sharply define the type and degree of impairment. Information gleaned from these more targeted standardized assessments allows practitioners to employ interventions that address specific areas of need. Standardized functional cognition assessments, such as the Menu Task [13], the Kettle Test [14], the Executive Function Performance Test (EPFT) [15], the Assessment of Language Related Functional Activities (ALFA) [16], and the Hopkins Medication Schedule [17], help demonstrate the patient's performance with real-life daily tasks. As patients progress, more demanding tools, such as the Weekly Calendar Planning Activity (WCPA) [18], can assess performance in complex instrumental activities of daily living (IADLs), such as planning and managing daily scheduling demands. Other standardized assessments addressing cognition include the Cognitive Linguistic Quick Test Plus (CLQT +) [19], the Repeatable Battery for the Assessment of Neuropsychological Status (RBANS) [20], and the Cognitive Assessment of Minnesota (CAM) [21]. Selection of the standardized assessment used, as well as subsequent interventions, should consider social determinants of health, such as selection of tasks familiar to the patient, health literacy level, and economic implications of follow-up recommendations. These assessments can be used by a variety of professionals during the patient's hospitalization, including occupational therapists, speech-language pathologists, psychologists, and neuropsychologists. A multidisciplinary approach to addressing cognition within the ICU and acute hospital setting smooths transitions along the continuum of care and better prepares the patient for hospital discharge and further outpatient management if needed.

Disorders of Consciousness

Patients may remain unconscious until they recover from their acute neurological insult or critical illness [22]. Interacting with patients experiencing disorders of consciousness can seem daunting. Studies have shown that care for unconscious patients is often performed by healthcare professionals in silence, minimizing interaction with and stimulation of patients who are comatose [22,23]. Performing skilled, intentional interventions in a systematic manner while eliciting and measuring responses can be difficult. Following consistent procedures for administering standardized assessments, such as the Coma Recovery Scale – Revised (CRS-R), is key to detecting even minute changes or responses. The CRS-R is a standardized neurobehavioral assessment measure designed for use in patients with disorders of consciousness that is used to establish diagnosis, monitor behavioral recovery, assess treatment effectiveness, and predict outcomes [24]. The CRS-R consists of 23 hierarchically arranged items assessing auditory, visual, motor, oromotor/verbal function, communication, and arousal. Assessment of patients with disorders of consciousness should occur at regular intervals and with changes in a patient's responsiveness (see Figure 13.1).

Orientation assessment, an essential component to screening for delirium and other cognitive impairment, should occur frequently throughout a patient's hospital stay [25]. Several times a day, clinicians should inquire about the patient's awareness of self, location, date, and situation. If the patient answers incorrectly, active reorientation is helpful to prevent the patient from recalling, repeating, or perseverating on incorrect information. Active reorientation involves stating the patient's name, location, date, and situation several times, for example: "Your name is___," "You are at ___," "Today is___," and "You are in the hospital because ___." This is often followed by a statement of reassurance, such as: "We are taking good care of you" or "Your wife is coming in this evening." Such repeated verbal

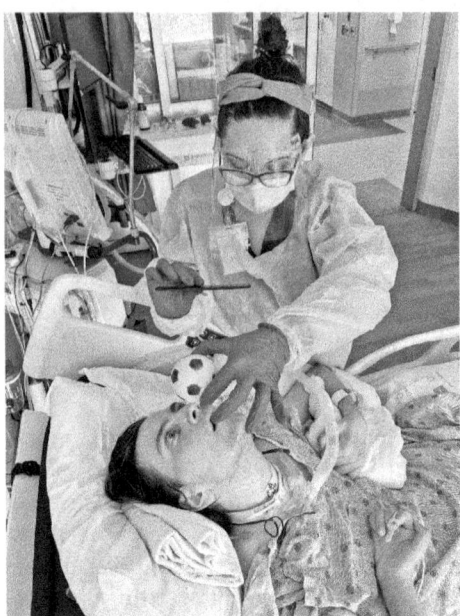

Figure 13.1 An occupational therapist asking the patient to look at the identified item on command while administering the CRS-R.

reorientation is a simple strategy to decrease delirium and cognitive impairment, increase arousal, and decrease agitation, even if the patient's level of consciousness is impaired [25,26]. Indeed, patients report hearing and recalling more than they are able to acknowledge [22,27,28,29].

Along with consistent assessment, ongoing interventions should be guided by the patient's response. Interventions provided can be more or less stimulating or challenging based on the patient's response. For example, patients who are not initially responding may need more stimulation or a longer time after stimulation to respond. If a patient has their eyes opened and is tracking, then the stimulation may be more purposeful, such as visually scanning for an object or visually attending to items for a grooming task. Interventions can include commands that require interacting with objects (object related), such as grasping a ball, or making movements (non-object related), such as with the eyelids or the tongue. Other treatment interventions include cuing a patient for looking at or purposeful reaching toward an identified object. Physical assistance may be provided to the patient's arm or hand to help initiate the movement. Multiple trials and locations or directions of stimuli may be required to obtain a response. Use of salient or meaningful stimuli, such as a picture of a family member or a child's stuffed animal, can further enhance a response; familiar voices also tend to elicit a more powerful and sustained response [25]. If family members or loved ones cannot be present, calling them on the telephone or using applications for video chatting are often helpful.

Modulating Stimulation

The level of stimulation a patient experiences in the ICU can vary significantly on an hourly basis. Modulating the intensity, amount, and duration of various stimuli helps to prevent both overstimulation and understimulation. Overstimulation can result in habituation to the stimulus, ultimately leading to diminished or absent responses when subsequent stimuli are provided by a therapist, nurse, provider, or family member. One strategy to decrease overstimulation is to limit the patient's exposure to excessive ambient noise, examples of which include conversations between providers that do not engage the patient, visitors' telephone conversations in the patient's room, a television being left on when it is no longer being attended to, or the sounds of machines and monitor alarms. Strategies to minimize overstimulation include responding to alarms quickly, stepping outside of the room to have a conversation or take a phone call, and turning off televisions and radios that are not being attended to. In contrast, television and radio stimulation can be helpful if the programs are familiar, meaningful, or favorites of the patient, particularly when the patient is actively engaged with the television or radio program.

Conversely, a hospital room devoid of stimulation can rob the patient of opportunities to respond to or engage with their environment [30,31]. Recommendations to increase stimulation include:

- opening the blinds if natural light is available
- increasing the head of the bed when medically appropriate
- removing covering blankets completely at times throughout the day
- removing splints or boots (if appropriate) combined with stimulation of the limb, passive range of motion, and attempts at active movement
- targeting timing of familiar voices to when the patient is the most alert, either in person or via telephone, video chat, or recording
- providing tactile stimulation, such as hair brushing, bathing, and oral care
- providing hand-over-hand self-care (e.g., holding the patient's hand on a toothbrush and lifting their arm to bring their hand to their mouth)

A multimodal approach to addressing cognition for hospitalized patients helps to decrease short- and long-term cognitive impairment while improving overall function, including the ability to actively participate in activities of daily living (ADLs) and instrumental activities of daily living (IADLs). IADLs are activities requiring a higher level of physical and cognitive complexity necessary for independent living and include managing medications and finances, preparing meals, and completing housekeeping and laundry (see Chapter 42 for additional information) [32]. The multimodal approach includes early active engagement in ADL and IADL training, balance activities, sensory stimulation, cognitive reorientation, reminiscence therapy, music therapy, physical activity, cognitive stimulation, cognitive retraining, and cognitive rehabilitation [33]. Multidimensional interventions, such as environmental modification and reorientation, allow for the most benefit from cognitive rehabilitation [8].

A comprehensive multimodal approach to addressing cognition includes engaging patients' loved ones to further enhance cognitive rehabilitation and help mitigate prolonged cognitive impairment. Familiar voices and faces can provide patients with stimuli that can be grounding, comforting, and reassuring. Including family members and loved ones as members of the treatment team, either in person or virtually, both increases the frequency of cognitive stimulation and reorientation and also compounds the salience of the stimulation. The more meaningful the stimulation, the better the opportunity to elicit a response and increase attention. Providing this type of social engagement can also be empowering for loved ones who may feel helpless sitting at the bedside. Social interaction and engagement are associated with improved cognitive abilities [34], and the psychosocial impact of engagement with loved ones at such a critical time in a patient's illness journey is paramount.

Cognitive Rehabilitation Training and Strategies

Cognitive rehabilitation in the ICU and hospital setting is safe and feasible [35]; it should occur early and often during the ICU stay and continue throughout hospitalization [36]. Cognitive rehabilitation interventions focus on many domains of cognition, including arousal, awareness, attention, memory, problem-solving, sequencing, executive functioning, performing daily tasks, and social participation. Cognitive stimulation intervention strategies are geared toward patients with lower levels of arousal and attention. Cognitive training activities are repetitive exercises aimed to remediate specific domains of cognitive impairment, such as memory or attention. Cognitive learning strategies allow patients to accurately practice recalling information or completing tasks. Use of cognitive learning strategies encourages recall of the correct process for task completion and motivates patients when tasks are successfully performed. Specific cognitive rehabilitation integrates cognitive domains in performing ADLs, such as bathing, dressing, and grooming, and IADLs, such as meal preparation, bill paying, and medication management. Compensatory strategies are external tools that can accommodate areas of cognitive impairment. Specific strategies and tools may be used across these areas of cognitive rehabilitation (see Table 13.3) [32,35,37,38,39]. The duration and frequency of interventions varies from 5 minutes twice daily to 30–45 minute sessions thrice weekly [32,38,40]. While the exact frequency and duration of rehabilitation sessions may vary, interventions addressing cognitive impairment should be adapted to the patient's performance, with a gradual increase in difficulty as the patient progresses.

Cognitive training may improve specific test performance, but the overarching goal is to generalize and transfer the skills learned to improve performance with real-life and novel tasks [36]. Professionals, including occupational therapists, speech-language pathologists, and neuropsychologists, can help translate these skills into functional activity. Cognitive rehabilitation training can include traditional pencil-paper tasks, computerized activities, and individual or group interventions. Incorporating compensatory strategies can augment cognitive rehabilitation, and use of tools such as ICU diaries, memory aids, calendars, alarms, and lists can be short- or long-term approaches to aid cognitive functioning. The simple act of a patient being able to recall and demonstrate problem-solving while using a compensatory strategy, such as a memory aid or alarm system, demonstrates active cognitive engagement.

Functional Cognition

Functional cognition is the process of utilizing and integrating thinking and processing skills to overcome the complexity and variability of everyday activities [41,42]. Static tests of cognitive processes often cannot fully predict how a patient will perform cognitively demanding daily activities within real world contexts. Early engagement in functional cognitive activities can prevent or decrease delirium and long-standing cognitive impairments [31,32].

Mirroring the importance of early mobility for critically ill patients (see Chapter 12 for additional information), reinforcement of "early activity," requiring both physical and cognitive skills, has the potential to accelerate recovery throughout the hospital stay and following hospital discharge. Cognitive impairment, even when mild, can result in significant dependencies in ADLs and IADLs [43]; reciprocally, limited activity and mobility can engender cognitive impairment, thereby creating a negative cycle of both cognitive and

Table 13.3 Cognitive intervention techniques and strategies

Type of Cognitive Intervention	Specific Techniques and Strategies
Cognitive Stimulation	Reorientation Sensory stimulation Communication boards Reading to the patient Familiar music Familiar voices and objects
Cognitive Training	Memory games Working memory tasks (such as N-back) Puzzles Mathematic and calculation activities (such as Sudoku) Crossword puzzles Word search Card games Digit span Days of the week/month (forwards and backwards, starting with a specific day/month) Timed tasks Sorting Reading comprehension Computerized cognitive gaming
Cognitive Learning Strategies	Goal-plan-do-review Errorless learning Forward chaining Backward chaining
Cognitive Rehabilitation	ADLs IADLs Wayfinding Dual tasking Family integration
Compensatory Strategies	Memory book (written journal or picture album) ICU diary Alarms (e.g., for medications, appointments, etc.)

physical functional decline [44]. Early mobility and early activity in the hospital setting are commensurate with level of independence in performing ADLs at hospital discharge [45]. In a study by Lavezza and colleagues, greater functional impairments in ADLs during hospitalization were significantly associated with worse outcomes, including longer hospital length of stay, higher risk of injurious falls, higher risk of pressure injuries, and higher likelihood of being discharged to a post-acute care facility [46]. Active engagement in ADLs (much like mobility) throughout the hospital stay, commencing as soon as physiologically possible and continuing until discharge, engages patients' physical and cognitive skills and promotes better outcomes. Focusing on performance-based functional cognition supports continued recovery and return to independence [47].

Functional cognition focuses on the patient's ability to utilize skills through the action of completing an activity [7]. When assessing a patient's ability to perform a meaningful activity, the demands required of the task can be categorized into motor skills (e.g., range of motion and coordination), cognitive skills (e.g., attention and memory), and social participation skills (e.g., orienting one's face toward another person when being spoken to and adapting to another individual's comments). Encouraging patients to increase participation in meaningful activities, such as ADLs and IADLs, requires examining each patient's capabilities in each of these three domains necessary for successful task completion. It is important to match what the patient is capable of with the demands required by the activity [48]. Performance skills are observable, goal-directed actions that result in a patient's successful performance during meaningful tasks [48,49].

Any real-life activity or task, regardless of complexity, can be broken down into the cognitive components required for successful completion (see Figure 13.2): initiation, sequencing, continuation, safety, and termination. One strategy for addressing cognitive impairment during task completion is cuing throughout the activity. Providing the lowest level of cuing required for safe completion of the task allows the patient to be challenged and to engage higher level cognitive processes while completing the activity (see Figure 13.3). Examining the complex interaction between the patient's skills and the activity demands leads to improved awareness of functional cognition. Early engagement in functional mobility and functional activity can help reduce the duration and incidence of delirium while improving overall physical and cognitive functioning and quality of life [50].

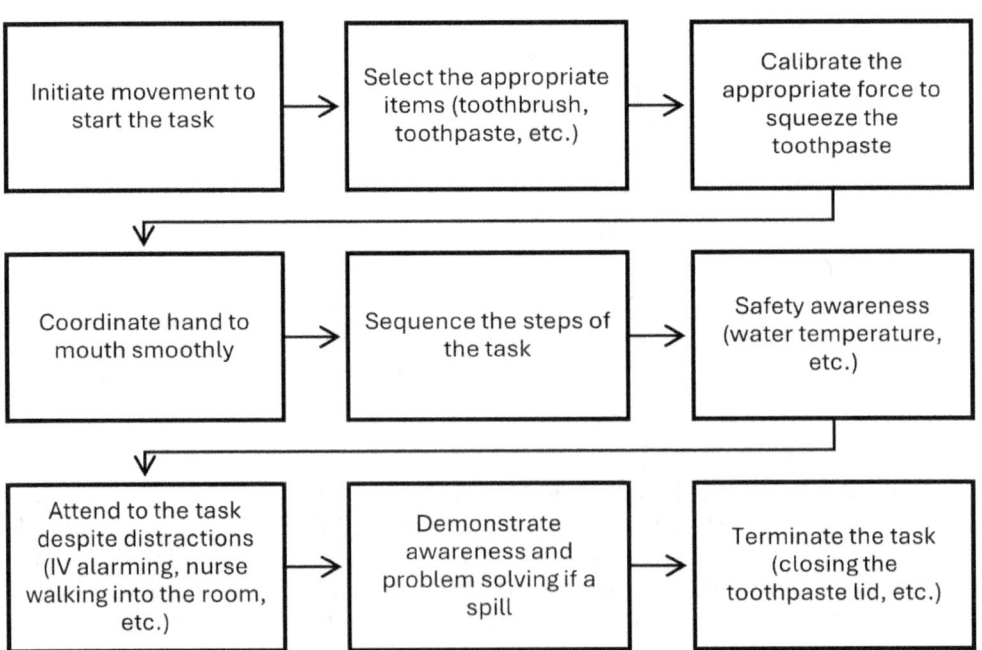

Figure 13.2 Functional cognition during an ADL: the cognitive process of completing oral care.

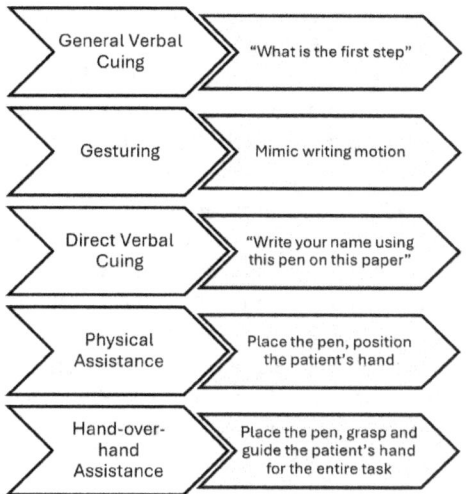

Figure 13.3 Hierarchical levels of cueing to encourage active cognitive engagement in the functional task of name writing. Adapted from the Executive Function Performance Test (EFPT) [15].

Assistive Technology

Assistive technology (AT) can enhance a patient's ability to engage with their environment and ultimately reintegrate into social roles, and it is one strategy to encourage cognitive simulation in the ICU. AT can improve a patient's ability to express thoughts, feelings, and basic medical and emotional needs [51], and it can also be used to address arousal and awareness, enhance communication, and facilitate active engagement in higher demand cognitive tasks. Accordingly, it should be considered for all patients, regardless of level of arousal and apparent cognitive capacity. For patients with impaired arousal and attention, for example, simply handing them a tablet can increase duration of eye opening and sustained attention, even if they fail to demonstrate a more meaningful interaction with the device. Even more simplistic tools, such as a marker and white board, may facilitate initiation of communication and allow for thoughts and emotions to be conveyed.

Communication impairments disrupt a patient's ability to express their needs, symptoms, and pain levels, which can lead to frustration for both the patient and care providers and a decrement in patient-nurse interaction time [52]. Active communication requires sophisticated neural processing: some patients may only have the capacity to provide a simple yes or no response, while others may be able to select responses from a short set of words or phrases. Patients who demonstrate more complex communication skills may be able to express themselves by speaking, spelling, writing, or typing words and phrases, an advanced level of communication known as novel speech or novel communication. Patients who can produce novel speech or written communication are better able to answer open-ended questions and express themselves without restriction. Novel communication can help patients be more cognitively challenged, help them stay engaged in reciprocal communication, and motivate them to participate in conversations.

Picture-based communication using icons on a communication board or a more complex augmentative and alternative communication (AAC) device, such as a dedicated eye-gaze device, may be beneficial for patients with cognitive or linguistic impairments (e.g., aphasia). Tablets can be used to type out novel words or sentences or select from pre-programmed phrases on specific apps. They can also be used for picture-based communication using icons when language expression or processing is a concern; for example, patients with aphasia may be better able to express themselves when choosing from picture-based icons instead of selecting words or phrases. Higher-tech AT may be considered when the patient cannot physically grasp a marker or touch a tablet screen. Eye-gaze technology, for example, allows patients to type letters or select items, words, or phrases on the screen using only their eye movements, removing the physical demands of verbal or written communication. The use of an eye-gaze device with patients in the ICU improves patient-reported self-confidence, psychosocial status, basic communication abilities, and cognitive functioning while decreasing frustration and delirium [53].

Integrating AT can help patients interact with the outside world and feel a sense of control. Providing patients their own personal devices can aid in recovery in the ICU and encourage active cognitive engagement. In patients who have demonstrated limited interaction, providing their personal devices, such as smart phones or tablets, may elicit responses, such as sustained eye opening or reaching and grasping. In patients who are awake, alert, and responsive, access to their personal devices may engage higher level cognitive skills, such as memory, problem solving, and executive functioning. Access to their personal devices can also empower patients to actively engage in conventional daily tasks, including planning and scheduling, setting active reminders (e.g., alarms for medications), making lists (e.g., grocery lists), messaging (e.g., email, texts, and phone calls), managing finances, completing work tasks, and participating in social interactions.

Conclusion

While cognitive impairment is prevalent in the ICU setting, it is often under-diagnosed and unaddressed. Cognitive impairment that develops in the ICU can have durable, life-altering impacts well beyond the hospital stay. Routinely screening for and assessing cognitive impairment recognizes its presence early and allows for initiation of interventions sooner. Cognitive intervention strategies, including stimulation, training, and rehabilitation, collectively decrease the impact of cognitive impairment and improve overall function. Examining patients' performance in real-life functional tasks help to generalize these skills.

Key Points

1. Using standardized tools to systematically screen for and assess cognition in the ICU can help identify cognitive impairment that often goes under-diagnosed in the acute care hospital setting.
2. Patients with disorders of consciousness benefit from early intervention with various modalities of sensory stimulation, including natural light, head of bed elevation, tactile stimulation, and familiar voices.
3. Active cognitive engagement can be encouraged by providing hierarchal levels of cueing during functional tasks, from general verbal cueing to hand-over-hand assistance.
4. Cognitive intervention strategies include reorientation, cognitive stimulation, cognitive gaming, paper-pencil tasks, engagement in ADLs and IADLs, and compensatory strategies.
5. Early activity and engagement in ADLs can demonstrate functional cognition, which is the process of utilizing thinking skills to overcome the complexity of everyday tasks.

References

1. R. Amini, K.H. Chee, J. Swan, et al. The level of cognitive impairment and likelihood of frequent hospital admissions. *J Aging Health* 2019; **31**(6): 967–88.

2. S. Mattke, H. Jun, E. Chen, et al. Expected and diagnosed rates of mild cognitive impairment and dementia in the U.S. Medicare population: observational analysis. *Alzheimers Res Ther* 2023; **15**(1): 128.

3. C. Fogg, P. Meredith, D. Culliford, et al. Cognitive impairment is independently associated with mortality, extended hospital stays and early readmission of older people with emergency hospital admissions: a retrospective cohort study. *Int J Nurs Stud* 2019; **96**: 1–8.

4. T.A. Jackson, A.M.J. MacLullich, J.R. F. Gladman, et al. Undiagnosed long-term cognitive impairment in acutely hospitalised older medical patients with delirium: a prospective cohort study. *Age Ageing* 2016; **45**(4): 493–9.

5. K. Honarmand, R.S. Lalli, F. Priestap, et al. Natural history of cognitive impairment in critical illness survivors: a systematic review. *Am J Respir Crit Care Med* 2020; **202**(2): 193–201.

6. F. Miranda, I. Arevalo-Rodriguez, G. Díaz, et al. Confusion Assessment Method for the intensive care unit (CAM-ICU) for the diagnosis of delirium in adults in critical care settings. *Cochrane Database Syst Rev* 2018; **2018**(9): CD013126.

7. E. Detroyer, A. Timmermans, D. Segers, et al. Psychometric properties of the intensive care delirium screening checklist when used by bedside nurses in clinical practice: a prospective descriptive study. *BMC Nurs* 2020; **19**: 21.

8. J.L. Tingey, N.A. Dasher, A.E. Bunnell, A. J. Starosta. Intensive care-related cognitive impairment: a biopsychosocial overview. *PM R* 2022; **14**(2): 259–72.

9. I. Arevalo-Rodriguez, N. Smailagic, M. R. Figuls, et al. Mini-Mental State Examination (MMSE) for the detection of Alzheimer's disease and other dementias in people with mild cognitive impairment (MCI). *Cochrane Database Syst Rev* 2015; **2015**(3): CD010783.

10. N. Ciesielska, R. Sokołowski, E. Mazur, et al. Is the Montreal Cognitive Assessment (MoCA) test better suited than the Mini-Mental State Examination (MMSE) in mild cognitive impairment (MCI) detection among people aged over 60? Meta-analysis. *Psychiatr Pol* 2016; **50**(5): 1039–52.

11. K. Casey, E. Sim, A. Lavezza, et al. Identifying cognitive impairment in the acute care hospital setting: finding an appropriate screening tool. *Am J Occup Ther* 2023; **77**(1): 7701205010.

12. E. Sim, K. Casey, A. Lavezza, et al. Standardizing identification of cognitive impairment in the acute hospital setting: toward a common language. *Am J Occup Ther* 2024; **78**(6): 7806205090.

13. M.O. Al-Heizan, T.S. Marks, G.M. Giles, D. F. Edwards. Further validation of the menu task: functional cognition screening for older adults. *OTJR Occup Particip Health* 2022; **42**(4): 286–94.

14. K.J. Harper, K. Llewellyn, A. Jacques, et al. Kettle test efficacy in predicting cognitive and functional outcomes in geriatric rehabilitation. *Aust Occup Ther J* 2019; **66**(2): 219–26.

15. C.M. Baum, L.T. Connor, T. Morrison, et al. Reliability, validity, and clinical utility of the executive function performance test: a measure of executive function in a sample of people with stroke. *Am J Occup Ther* 2008; **62**(4): 446–55.

16. S. Ali Saad Al Yaari, N. Almaflehi. Validity and reliability of communication activities of daily living – second edition (CADL-2) and assessment of language-related functional activities (ALFA) tests: evidence from Arab aphasics. *J Study Engl Linguist* 2013; **1**(2): 37-71.

17. M.C. Carlson, L.P. Fried, Q.L. Xue, et al. Validation of the Hopkins medication schedule to identify difficulties in taking medications. *J Gerontol A Biol Sci Med Sci* 2005; **60**(2): 217–23.

18. C. Gong, N. Wang. Validity of the weekly calendar planning activity on measurement

of executive function for adults with stroke. *Am J Occup Ther* 2022; **76** (Supplement 1): 7610500013p1.

19. T. Blyth, A. Scott, A. Bond, E. Paul. A comparison of two assessments of high level cognitive communication disorders in mild traumatic brain injury. *Brain Inj* 2012; **26**(3): 234–40.

20. C. Randolph, M.C. Tierney, E. Mohr, T. N. Chase. The Repeatable Battery for the Assessment of Neuropsychological Status (RBANS): preliminary clinical validity. *J Clin Exp Neuropsychol* 1998; **20**(3): 310–19.

21. L.F. Feliciano, J.C. Baker, S.L. Anderson, et al. Concurrent validity of the cognitive assessment of Minnesota in older adults with and without depressive symptoms. *J Aging Res* 2011; **2011**: 853624.

22. S.T. Meghani, N.S. Punjani. Does communication really a matter of concern in unconscious patients? (accessed 2024 Aug 10); www.imanagerpublications.com/assets/htmlfiles/JNUR4(3)August-October 20142880.html.

23. A.C.G. Puggina, M.J. Paes da Silva, C. Schnakers, S. Laureys. Nursing care of patients with disorders of consciousness. *J Neurosci Nurs* 2012; **44**(5): 260–70.

24. J.T. Giacino, K. Kalmar, J. Whyte. The JFK Coma Recovery Scale – Revised: measurement characteristics and diagnostic utility. *Arch Phys Med Rehabil* 2004; **85**(12): 2020–9.

25. T.G. Fong, S.K. Inouye . The inter-relationship between delirium and dementia: the importance of delirium prevention. *Nat Rev Neurol* 2022; **18**(10): 579–96.

26. S. Lee, J.Y. Sohn, I.E. Hwang, et al. Effect of a repeated verbal reminder of orientation on emergence agitation after general anaesthesia for minimally invasive abdominal surgery: a randomised controlled trial. *Br J Anaesth* 2023; **130**(4): 439–45.

27. P. Tosch. Patients' recollections of their posttraumatic coma. *J Neurosci Nurs J Am Assoc Neurosci Nurses* 1988; **20**(4): 223–8.

28. M. Podurgiel. The unconscious experience: a pilot study. *J Neurosci Nurs* 1990; **22**(1): 51-2.

29. M.M. Lawrence, R.P. Ramirez, P.J. Bauer. Communicating with unconscious patients: an overview. *Dimens Crit Care Nurs DCCN* 2023; **42**(1): 3–11.

30. L. Cheng, D. Cortese, M.M. Monti, et al. Do sensory stimulation programs have an impact on consciousness recovery? *Front Neurol* 2018; **9**: 826.

31. M. Moattari, F. Alizadeh Shirazi, N. Sharifi, N. Zareh. Effects of a sensory stimulation by nurses and families on level of cognitive function, and basic cognitive sensory recovery of comatose patients with severe traumatic brain injury: a randomized control trial. *Trauma Mon* 2016; **21**(4): e23531.

32. K. Deemer, K. Zjadewicz, K. Fiest, et al. Effect of early cognitive interventions on delirium in critically ill patients: a systematic review. *Can J Anaesth* 2020; **67** (8): 1016–34.

33. M.J. Ham, S. Kim, Y.J. Jo, et al. The effect of a multimodal occupational therapy program with cognition-oriented approach on cognitive function and activities of daily living in patients with Alzheimer's disease: a systematic review and meta-analysis of randomized controlled trials. *Biomedicines* 2021; **9** (12): 1951.

34. S. Costa-Cordella, C. Arevalo-Romero, F. J. Parada, A. Rossi. Social support and cognition: a systematic review. *Front Psychol* 2021; **12**: 637060.

35. N.E. Brummel, T.D. Girard, E.W. Ely, et al. Feasibility and safety of early combined cognitive and physical therapy for critically ill medical and surgical patients: the Activity and Cognitive Therapy in ICU (ACT-ICU) trial. *Intensive Care Med* 2014; **40**(3): 370–9.

36. S.F. Herling, I. Egerod, D.G. Bove, et al. Cognitive training for prevention of cognitive impairment in adult intensive care unit (ICU) patients. *Cochrane Database Syst Rev* 2021; **2021**(8): CD014630.

37. S. Wang, J. Hammes, S. Khan, et al. Improving recovery and outcomes every day after the ICU (IMPROVE): study protocol for a randomized controlled trial. *Trials* 2018; **19**: 196.

38. A. Wassenaar, J. de Reus, A.R.T. Donders, et al. Development and validation of an abbreviated questionnaire to easily measure cognitive failure in ICU survivors: a multicenter study. *Crit Care Med* 2018; **46** (1): 79-84.

39. A. Wassenaar, M. van den Boogaard, L. Schoonhoven, et al. Determination of the feasibility of a multicomponent intervention program to prevent delirium in the Intensive Care Unit: A modified RAND Delphi study. *Aust Crit Care Off J Confed Aust Crit Care Nurses* 2017; **30**(6): 321-7.

40. J.M. Garcia. Occupational therapy in a private adult Intensive Care Unit (ICU): an experience report. *Cad Bras Ter Ocupacional* 2023; **31**, e3152.

41. Role of occupational therapy in assessing functional cognition | AOTA [Internet]. 2021 (accessed 2023 Dec 6). Available from: www.aota.org/practice/practice-essentials/payment-policy/medicare1/medicare-role-of-ot-in-assessing-functional-cognition.

42. C.M. Baum, S.C.L. Lau, A.W. Heinemann, L.T. Connor. Functional cognition: distinct from fluid and crystallized cognition? *Am J Occup Ther* 2023; **77**(3): 7703205020.

43. T.R. Gure, K.M. Langa, G.G. Fisher, et al. Functional limitations in older adults who have cognitive impairment without dementia. *J Geriatr Psychiatry Neurol* 2013; **26**(2): 78-85.

44. Y. Minami, I. Tsuji, A. Fukao, et al. Physical status and dementia risk: a three-year prospective study in urban Japan. *Int J Soc Psychiatry* 1995; **41**(1): 47-54.

45. S. Watanabe, J. Hirasawa, Y. Naito, et al. Association between the early mobilization of mechanically ventilated patients and independence in activities of daily living at hospital discharge. *Sci Rep* 2023; **13**: 4265.

46. A. Lavezza, E. Hoyer, L.A. Friedman, et al. Activities of daily living assessment early in hospitalization is associated with key outcomes. *Am J Occup Ther Off Publ Am Occup Ther Assoc* 2023; **77**(5): 7705205100.

47. C.M. Baum, S.C. L. Lau, A. W. Heinemann, L.T. Connor. Functional cognition: distinct from fluid and crystallized cognition? *Am J Occup Ther.* 2023; **77**(3): 7703205020.

48. Occupational Therapy Practice Framework: Domain and Process – Fourth Edition. *Am J Occup Ther* 2020; **74** (Supplement 2): 1–87.

49. A.G. Fisher, A. Marterella. *Powerful Practice: A Model for Authentic Occupational Therapy* [Internet]. Center for Innovative OT Solutions; 2019.

50. C. Pozzi, V.C. Tatzer, E.A. Álvarez, et al. The applicability and feasibility of occupational therapy in delirium care. *Eur Geriatr Med* 2020; **11**(2): 209–16.

51. S. Jansson, T.R.S. Martin, E. Johnson, S. Nilsson. Healthcare professionals' use of augmentative and alternative communication in an intensive care unit: a survey study. *Intensive Crit Care Nurs* 2019; **54**: 64–70.

52. M.B. Happ, S.M. Sereika, M.P. Houze, et al. Quality of care and resource use among mechanically ventilated patients before and after an intervention to assist nurse-nonvocal patient communication. *Heart Lung* 2015; **44**(5): 408–15.

53. J. Garry, K. Casey, T.K. Cole, et al. A pilot study of eye-tracking devices in intensive care. *Surgery* 2016; **159**(3): 938–44.

Chapter 14
Psychological Care in the ICU and Hospital

Erin L. Hall-Melnychuk, Dorothy Wade, and Teresa Deffner

Introduction

Despite the prevalence of adverse psychological outcomes associated with post-intensive care syndrome (PICS), assessment of and interventions for psychological distress experienced by patients in the intensive care unit (ICU) are not routinely performed in most countries. Historically, the use of pharmacologic interventions has been the primary means for addressing psychological distress or agitation in ICU patients; however, medications are frequently ineffective and have adverse side effects, such as the risks of delirium and long-term psychological morbidity associated with benzodiazepine administration [1]. Though non-pharmacologic interventions have become a focus for management of delirium and psychological distress in the ICU, the role of psychological care delivered by psychologists or other mental health clinicians has not yet been fully explored [2].

In the United Kingdom (UK) and parts of Europe, psychologists are incorporated into multidisciplinary ICU teams to recognize and treat adverse psychological experiences in critically ill patients. For example, in the UK, there are more than 120 practitioner psychologists working in approximately one-third of all ICUs in the country, according to their professional network, Psychologists in Intensive Care-UK (PINC-UK). Data for other countries, including the United States and Germany, are scarce, as no representative surveys have been conducted.

Psychologists work alongside physicians, nurses, and other ICU clinicians in the collaborative care of patients. They are highly trained in the recognition and assessment of psychological difficulties and delirium and provide evidence-based care to address acute distress. The intensive care psychologist provides care in three domains: psychological care of ICU patients, psychological care of patients' families, and "indirect" work through consultation and collaboration with nurses, physicians, and other clinicians (see Figure 14.1).

Psychological Care of Patients in the ICU

Indicators of the psychological impact of illness are often not readily apparent and may be more difficult to ascertain than physical manifestations of illness, where vital signs, laboratory values, or imaging studies can be used to identify a problem. This may explain why the psychological impact of critical illness and hospitalization is less often prioritized than the physical and cognitive impairments associated with illness and injury. While ensuring physical health and survival are crucial, psychological recovery is similarly critical for determining overall patient outcomes and quality of life.

The goal of psychological care in the ICU is prevention and alleviation of distress associated with critical illness. Psychologists fulfill an important role in the detection of and early

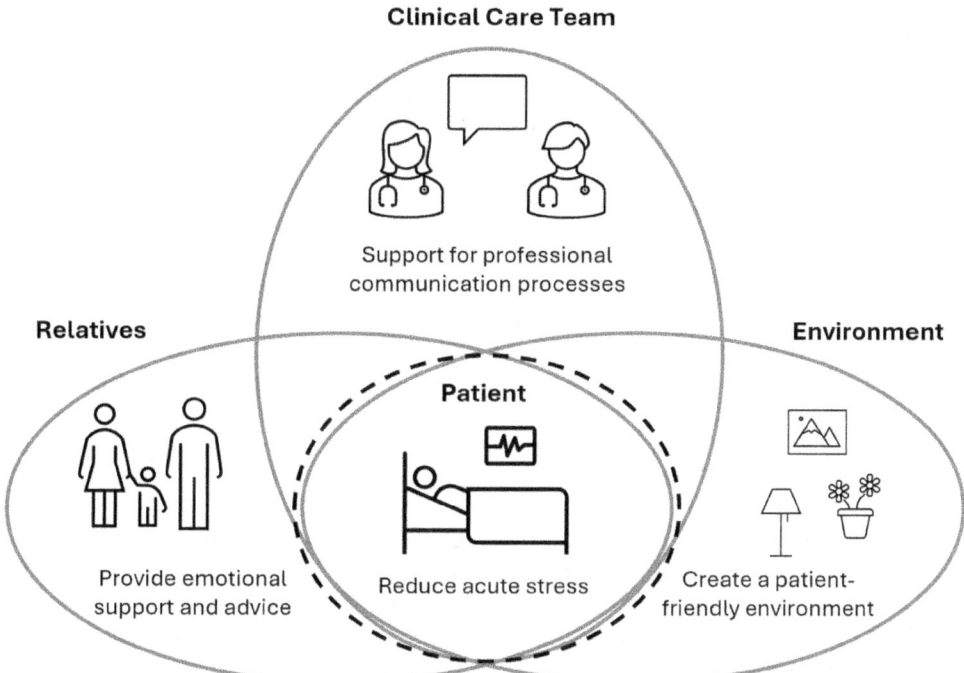

Figure 14.1 Role of the psychologist in intensive care. Psychologists fulfill several roles in the care of critically ill patients, including both direct care of patients and families and indirect care through supporting other members of the critical care team and encouraging a psychologically informed environment.

intervention for patients who are actively experiencing or at risk for developing psychological problems [3]. The ICU psychologist provides a necessary focus of care on the nonphysical impact of critical illness and serves as an educator and advocate for holistic recovery of the patient.

Screening for Psychological Distress in the ICU

The reason for psychological screening and assessment in the ICU is twofold: identification of patients experiencing psychological symptoms and recognition of patients with heightened risk for subsequent psychological morbidity (see Chapter 10 for additional information) [4]. The objective of screening is not to diagnose psychological problems per se but to identify patients who may benefit from psychological care given current distress or risk for greater psychological morbidity. When high-risk patients are identified, psychological interventions can be tailored to lessen distress.

These goals are consistent with the recommendations of several groups, including the Society of Critical Care Medicine [5] and the National Institute for Health and Clinical Excellence [6] in the UK: all critically ill patients should be assessed for a history of psychological problems or distress and should be screened for symptoms and frightening experiences (e.g., intrusive memories, delusions, and nightmares) prior to ICU discharge to assist in determining risk for future psychological morbidity. Despite these recommendations, few effective, evidence-based screening tools exist to serve this purpose.

The Intensive Care Psychological Assessment Tool (IPAT) is a 10-item screening tool that was created to assess acute distress and to predict patients with an increased risk for psychological morbidity [4]. No other tools for ICU patients address both aims. The IPAT can be completed by bedside nurses or non-psychologist staff and demonstrates favorable reliability and validity with adult ICU patients who are alert and oriented. Although several other evidence-based measures have been used for assessment of symptoms in critically ill patients, most have limitations, including prohibitive length, intention for use at the time of ICU discharge or later, and lack of sensitivity to the unique experiences of ICU patients [4]. General symptom screeners for anxiety and depression can be used; however, these measures may overestimate symptoms due to an overlap in common experiences of medically ill patients and symptoms of depression or anxiety (e.g., fatigue or appetite changes). Traditional screening tools for post-traumatic stress disorder (PTSD) are often inappropriate for use during ICU admission, as symptoms of acute stress are commonly experienced in the immediate aftermath of trauma, and a diagnosis of PTSD requires that patients continue to experience symptoms for at least one month following the traumatic event. Communication barriers resulting from delirium, sedating medications, or the inability to speak may impede patients' abilities to be screened appropriately for psychological symptoms.

Psychologists working in intensive care commonly rely on clinical interviews with patients for evaluation of mental status, distress, and psychological symptoms. Screening tools are helpful for identifying patients who might benefit from being seen by a psychologist. They also increase awareness of bedside nurses and other clinicians of the distress patients are experiencing, which is often not readily shared. In settings where psychologists are unavailable to address concerns, however, it is prudent that resources are available to address patient distress, including referrals for follow-up behavioral health. When patients are showing signs of distress, nurses and ICU clinicians should also engage in efforts to address the patient's concerns. This may involve providing education about delirium, its symptoms, and causes; addressing worries related to poor understanding of current medical events; or helping to facilitate conversations with family members or other staff to increase patient social support.

General Approaches to Care

All individuals providing care in the ICU contribute to the patient's outcome, but they may not be aware of the psychological impact of that care. Engaging others in practices geared toward prevention and detection of psychological stress is an important role that psychologists on critical care teams play. Two general approaches should guide the care and communication offered by all clinicians working in intensive care: psychological first aid (PFA) and trauma-informed care (TIC).

Psychological First Aid

PFA is an empirically supported approach to patient care that was initially designed for working with individuals in the aftermath of disaster [7]. It focuses on decreasing distress related to traumatic experiences, supporting adaptive coping, and connecting people with resources by promoting a sense of safety and calm, self- and collective efficacy, connectedness, and hope [7]. This approach is valid for use in intensive care given the ongoing threats, stressors, and traumatic experiences faced by patients and their families. Many interventions utilized by psychologists in the ICU are rooted in PFA, such as leading patients in relaxation strategies [3] and helping mechanically ventilated patients feel more connected by engaging them in a conversation via writing, hand squeezing, or head nodding.

Trauma-Informed Care

TIC is an overarching framework commonly adapted to guide the care of patients at both individual and institutional levels [8]. This approach involves a realization of the widespread prevalence of trauma, its potential impact across all people, and the importance of recognizing its signs and symptoms. TIC focuses on responding with knowledge of trauma and minimizing the potential for re-traumatization. The key principles of TIC, which are core tenets in the care of all patients, include: increasing the sense of safety; recognizing the importance of engaging others in decision-making with transparency to build trust; integrating peer support into patient care; decreasing the power differential between patient and caregiver; empowering patients and recognizing resilience; and responding to biases, stereotypes, and historical trauma with humility [8]. Integration of a TIC approach involves training all ICU staff in and creating policies that are congruent with these principles.

Psychological Interventions in Intensive Care

Psychological intervention studies in intensive care are rare, with few randomized controlled trials (RCTs) investigating the effectiveness of standardized interventions on psychological symptoms with validated assessment measures [9]. A systematic review of 23 studies of non-pharmacologic interventions designed to reduce anxiety, stress, and psychological distress in ICU patients examined a variety of strategies, including music therapy, mind-body interventions (e.g., massage, reflexology, and acupressure), and "psychological interventions" (e.g., talking treatments or patient diaries). Six of 11 studies found a reduction in stress associated with music therapy, and four of five studies demonstrated a reduction in short-term distress with mind-body interventions. Of the studies investigating "psychological interventions" specifically, three out of seven studies showed a measurable improvement. Collectively, a multi-pronged approach combining several of these tested interventions may decrease psychological distress and stress in this patient population [9].

The Psychological Outcomes Following a Nurse-Led Preventive Psychological Intervention for Critical Ill Patients (POPPI) trial is the largest RCT of psychological interventions in the ICU to date [10]. This study utilized a standardized, cognitive behavioral therapy (CBT)-based psychological intervention composed of three one-on-one support sessions provided by specially trained ICU nurses to patients who were alert and oriented. Sessions focused on addressing acute stress symptoms and frightening memories of the ICU; other elements of the complex intervention included promotion of a therapeutic environment and a relaxation and recovery program delivered on tablet computers. At six months following discharge, no significant difference in mean PTSD symptoms as assessed using the PTSD Symptom Scale Self-Report questionnaire was found between hospitals where the intervention was delivered and hospitals where usual care was provided [10]. In patients who received the complete intervention, however, there was a reduction in anxiety symptoms as assessed by the State Trait Anxiety Inventory (6-item version; STAI-6) from baseline to the post-intervention period, although this difference was not statistically significant. The study's process evaluation determined that nurses found these interventions stressful to deliver and that qualified psychological staff should either deliver the interventions themselves or offer closer, in-person supervision to the interventionists [11]. Concerns were also raised regarding the timing of the intervention: nurses suggested earlier, more focused interventions for delirious patients and deferred interventions for patients they deemed to be more receptive to CBT-based sessions.

Only a small number of studies have evaluated outcomes of interventions specifically delivered by psychologists in ICUs. In a paper presenting two patient cases, CBT-based interventions provided by a psychologist resulted in reduced symptoms of anxiety, panic, and depression and faster liberation from mechanical ventilation [12]. Additionally, a multifaceted intervention delivered by clinical psychologists over an average of five sessions, including support, coping strategies, psychoeducation, and stress management, found a significant reduction in symptoms of PTSD in patients admitted to the ICU with traumatic injuries [13]. Those who received the psychological interventions also had lower rates of anxiety and depression and were significantly less likely to be diagnosed with PTSD one year after hospitalization compared to those who received usual care. Of note, interventions were not standardized in these two studies, with patients receiving any combination of the aforementioned strategies depending on their individual needs. In another study, a standardized CBT-based self-management intervention provided by a psychologist to adult ICU patients with acute respiratory failure resulted in reduced anxiety in all eleven patients involved [14]. Although these results are encouraging, because of limited numbers of participants and the absence of control groups, further efforts to study the benefits of psychological interventions on immediate and long-term psychological distress in ICU patients should be prioritized.

ICU diaries have also been suggested as a tool to decrease patient and family distress and later psychological morbidity (see Chapter 18 for additional information). These diaries are completed by ICU clinicians and family members during ICU admission with the goal of reducing the development of anxiety, depression, and PTSD in both patients and their loved ones. Evidence in favor of diaries is mixed; however, the largest RCT of patient diaries to date found no significant difference in reported PTSD symptoms at three months following discharge between patients who received ICU diaries and those who did not [15]. Additionally, in one meta-analysis of studies of ICU diaries, no significant differences in the incidence of depression, anxiety, or PTSD in the relatives of critically ill patients who received ICU diaries were demonstrated [16].

Cognitive Behavioral Therapy

A variety of interventions may be adapted for use by psychologists to address psychological symptoms in the critically ill. Given that CBT interventions are effective in a variety of healthcare settings and have shown promise in some ICU studies, critical care psychologists often use CBT strategies alongside other approaches. The overall goal of these therapeutic techniques is to increase patients' repertoire of coping abilities. Most commonly used CBT-based interventions are effective, evidence-based, and applicable to a variety of challenges associated with an ICU admission, and they can be used individually or paired with relaxation strategies.

Psychoeducation and Normalizing

Psychoeducation involves providing explanations of patient symptoms or experiences to increase understanding and mitigate distress and commonly focuses on deconstructing frightening delusional or hallucinatory experiences associated with delirium. Providing information about why delusions or hallucinations frequently occur can help to lessen fear and anxiety associated with them and increase patients' ability to understand and cope with the experience. Psychoeducation may also be provided for symptoms of panic and anxiety associated with breathlessness or mechanical ventilation and may include teaching coping strategies to help manage psychological distress.

Behavioral Strategies

Patients in intensive care frequently experience muscle weakness, low motivation, and lethargy. They must rely on others to provide basic care and have little influence over their own daily activities. Given the lack of opportunities in the ICU environment for patients to participate in mood-improving activities, several behavioral strategies may be utilized to engage patients. Behavioral activation is a technique based on the influence of behaviors on mood; when mood is low, both motivation and activity tend to decrease, thus reducing opportunities for patients to experience enjoyment or intrinsic reward [3], creating a vicious cycle that perpetuates depressed mood. Scheduling activities with patients to increase engagement, promoting experiences that are pleasurable and meaningful, and assisting in goal setting are used to improve patients' mood and self-efficacy. These behavioral interventions may also be useful to address avoidance behaviors in patients who are experiencing anxiety.

Cognitive Restructuring

Cognitive restructuring involves identifying the relationship between emotional distress (e.g., anxiety) and thoughts and then addressing the thoughts and beliefs that are maladaptive or problematic. For critically ill patients, these thoughts often center around benign physiologic sensations that are perceived as threatening, which may increase sympathetic arousal and anxiety. This appraisal of threat may be associated with prior traumatic experiences, lack of understanding, or physical pain [3]. Through cognitive restructuring, precipitating or perpetuating factors are elicited to better understand and alter the threat response. For example, in the case of ventilator liberation, patients may experience anxiety associated with the weaning process, which may increase sympathetic arousal. These sensations are appraised as harmful or threatening, which further increases arousal and may result in subjective respiratory distress and failure of ventilator weaning [12].

Grounding and Relaxation Skills

Psychologists frequently utilize relaxation strategies to decrease anxiety and physiologic activation. Teaching and engaging patients in relaxation techniques, such as deep breathing, guided imagery, or body scans, can activate a parasympathetic response, thereby decreasing subjective anxiety. It may be difficult for some ICU patients to engage in breathing techniques given certain pathophysiologic and psychological conditions, such as acute respiratory failure and acute psychosis due to schizophrenia, respectively; for this reason, it may be necessary to focus more on relaxation strategies involving imagery or body scans. Instructing patients in relaxation training also results in increasing patients' abilities to cope and to engage in calming behaviors on their own. Grounding techniques are exercises that help a person to focus on the present moment and distract them from distressing thoughts or emotions, often by engaging their five senses (e.g., focusing on sensations such as the soft bed under their legs, listening to music, and using pleasant scents).

Psychological Care of Families in the ICU

The presence of a psychologist as part of ICU care teams is also beneficial to support family members and loved ones of critically ill patients. As part of a multidisciplinary team, psychologists assist patients' families in important ways that enhance the care of the patient and help relatives process and cope with their own emotions associated with the patient's illness. Psychologists provide education to facilitate better communication with and support of the patient while in the ICU and often serve as a liaison between family members and the medical team. They can also prepare and assist families in coping with grief at the end of life.

Dealing with the Critical Illness

During intensive care treatment, relatives often face several concurrent challenges, including coping with their own emotional reactions to their loved one's serious illness. As admission to the ICU often occurs unexpectedly, relatives may feel overwhelmed and paralyzed when confronting the life-threatening situation. A PFA approach is helpful in the care of family members by assisting them in processing their own emotions, engaging their social support systems, and supporting adaptive functioning. The ICU psychologist helps to support family resilience by promoting pre-existing coping skills and teaching additional coping techniques. Psychologists provide a space in which the family can talk openly about their thoughts and feelings regarding their loved one's illness. In addition, the ICU psychologist often acts as an advocate and supporter of relatives' concerns and can share them with the medical team.

Supporting the Patient

Relatives frequently feel insecure when interacting with their loved one in the ICU. Psychologists assist the family in understanding medical information, the ICU environment, and how they can assist in the patient's care. This is especially crucial with respect to delirium, as relatives play an important role in re-orienting and calming patients, thereby reducing delirium risk [17]. Psychologists can help to prepare the family for these interactions by providing information about delirium, why it occurs, and what they can do to help.

Psychologists can also assist families in communicating with a patient who is intubated or has a tracheostomy by providing information about effective communication methods, such as using picture boards or blinking/hand squeezing to letters of the alphabet. Along with this, psychologists can support conversations between patients and relatives to help patients express their wishes; for example, they may assist with moderating discussions about the patient's goals of care, such as consideration of limiting life-sustaining treatment. This is often helpful for families, who may be uncertain how to approach these important conversations.

Decision-Making and Coping with Conflicts

Being responsible for making important medical decisions, often without the input of the patient, can be a source of significant difficulty and confusion for patients' relatives.

Families must make these decisions while simultaneously dealing with their own emotional distress. Psychologists can assist families in decision-making by engaging them in conversation about the patient's values, preferences, and goals; helping to address feelings of self-blame or guilt; and clarifying points of misinformation or misunderstanding. If disagreements arise among family members or between the family and the ICU team, psychologists can moderate discussions to help resolve conflicts [18].

Another common source of family distress in the ICU occurs when patients have young children who may have a difficult time appreciating the gravity of the situation. In this case, psychologists can help plan the involvement of children, which may include providing age-appropriate materials or having discussions with children to prepare them for the ICU environment or to understand the patient's illness or injury. If necessary, psychologists also assist families in finding ways for children to say farewell when death is imminent [19].

End-of-Life and Grief Support

As relatives are often uncertain whether a patient will survive, they may experience distress related to coping with the possibility of death or anticipatory grief. Open discussions about death and dying can be important for the emotional adjustment of relatives and have been identified as protective against prolonged grief [20]. Evidence for bereavement-related interventions in the intensive care setting is limited [21]; however, an RCT using a three-step support intervention lead by physicians caring for patients dying in the ICU found that families of patients in the intervention group, as opposed to usual care, had significantly lower rates of prolonged grief, PTSD-related symptoms, and anxiety following the death of the patient [22]. The intervention involved physicians and nurses communicating with families about the dying process, processing the families' own emotional reactions to this, and encouraging families to ask questions at three time points throughout the dying process. This study underscores the importance of communication and emotional support for patients' families at the end of life.

The integration of psychologists into palliative and end-of-life care processes provides support to assist relatives with medical decision-making and potential transition to comfort-focused care. Psychologists can provide counseling related to grief and loss and help empower family members to feel that they can support the dying patient. Psychologists often play an important role in incorporating patient- and family-specific cultural and religious beliefs and practices related to death and dying to ensure that the patient receives a dignified farewell.

Indirect Work by Practitioner Psychologists in the ICU

As well as working directly with patients and relatives, an embedded practitioner psychologist may intervene indirectly by collaborating with other healthcare team members to create a psychologically informed critical care service [23], which benefits patients by ensuring that their psychological needs to feel safe, calm, informed, reassured, and heard are considered alongside their physical and medical needs. A psychologically-informed service can be promoted by psychologists in at least three key areas: improving communication in the ICU, assisting colleagues in the psychological understanding and care of patients, and creating a more therapeutic environment.

Improving Communication in the ICU

Research has shown that good communication by healthcare professionals improves clinical outcomes in many fields of medicine and is considered an essential component of family-centered care (see Chapter 17 for additional information) and humanizing the ICU experience (see Chapter 16 for additional information) [24]. Communication in the ICU is often challenging because patients may be sedated, delirious, comatose, or unable to speak due to the need for mechanical ventilation. For these and other reasons, many ICU patients have periods where they lack capacity to understand, retain, evaluate, or communicate information. Moreover, when patients awaken from sedation or coma, they are often amnestic to recent events, have inaccurate memories, or have limited understanding of what has happened. Clinicians should make careful efforts to explain to patients their condition, diagnoses, procedures performed or needed, and treatments given or planned. Increasing patients' understanding helps to improve their morale and motivation to engage in rehabilitation activities. In these cases, communication between clinicians, patients, and families is crucial, and psychologists have a role in training clinicians to improve their communication skills [25].

Didactic and experiential communication skills training by psychologists can help clinicians to: address patients in a way that puts them at ease and helps to build rapport; appreciate possible limitations of patients' understanding due to their cognitive state, including memory loss; and deliver information in a way that patients understand. Physicians should avoid medical jargon and provide information in plain language that is easily comprehensible by the lay person. Psychologists can also provide communication skills training in specialized areas, such as delivering bad news (e.g., conveying poor prognoses or imminent death) or talking to delirious or extremely distressed patients.

Psychologists can mediate meetings among doctors, patients, and families by asking clinicians to simplify complicated concepts and by listening for ambivalence, misunderstanding, or resistance by the patient or their loved ones. They can also check in with the patient or family, either during or after the consultation, to explore their understanding and encourage them to ask further questions if necessary. Furthermore, the presence of practitioner psychologists on ICU rounds or in multidisciplinary meetings can also help ICU staff to understand and empathize with patients' mental health or cognitive difficulties. The psychologists can give important background information and use accurate, non-prejudicial language to describe psychological presentations or behaviors of patients or families.

As well as verbal communication, psychologists can help the ICU team to produce written information for patients and families, including general information regarding the ICU environment and interventions, psychological information surrounding delirium and distress in the ICU, and patient-friendly discharge summaries and tailored rehabilitation plans. All of these resources can be given as printed materials or delivered online.

Consultation for Care Team or Individual Staff

Another indirect contribution to the team is to provide consultation to individual staff members or care teams about the psychological aspects of patient care [26]. This can include discussions about an individual patient's stress, mood, feelings, cognition, behavior, or responses related to delirium. As well as helping staff to understand patients' psychological presentations and symptoms, psychologists can also provide simple care plans or protocols to manage and improve mild distress and confusion in patients. ICU psychologists should provide guidelines to help staff understand which patients should be referred to them or to other mental health services in the hospital.

Psychologists can advertise to the ICU team that they are available for psychological consultation or liaison work or can attend rounds and other clinical meetings to offer their input and insights. They can offer training sessions to relevant staff groups on the psychological impact of critical illness and ICU admission, psychological reactions and outcomes in critically ill patients, and techniques to manage mild distress, anxiety, and delirium.

Creating a Therapeutic Environment

Traditionally, an ICU can be a harsh, sterile, and scary environment. Disturbing noises, unnatural bright light, and lack of access to windows may contribute to anxiety, perceptual distortions, and sleep disturbances among patients [27]. Psychologists can be advocates or opinion-formers within the ICU to promote modifications to the challenging physical and social environment. Changes include reducing noise, such as turning off unnecessary alarms; providing more natural light; and enhancing nighttime sleep by providing ear plugs, eye masks, night lights, and devices to play calming music, nature sounds, or meditations [28]. Nurses can be encouraged to cluster care activities at night to avoid waking people unnecessarily and to check patients' bedspaces at bedtime for shapes and items that may look frightening in the night. Items can be moved or removed, or clarification can be given to the patient about the items and their purpose.

The ambience of the ICU can be softened by the introduction of warm or calming colors, decorations such as nature stickers (e.g., birds, flowers, and butterflies), and suitable art on the walls [29]. Psychologists and colleagues may need to be imaginative by making small, inexpensive improvements to the environment that can have a positive impact on patients. Purchasing lightweight boards to display orientation charts, family photographs, and information on what matters to patients can have a significant impact. Programming tablet devices with music, meditations, and other anxiety management materials can also be helpful. In some cases, money has been allocated for larger redesigns or re-builds that aim to create a truly healing environment for patients [30].

Psychologists should also have a role in educating their colleagues about the social stressors of the ICU, including crowding around patients' bedspaces; patients or families witnessing other patients' distress, emergencies, deaths, and grieving; and overhearing upset or angry families. Patients should be shielded, when possible, from disturbing sights and situations. When this is impossible, staff members should talk to the patients later about this experience. Staff may need to be reminded about respecting patients' privacy when discussing their medical conditions in the vicinity of other families.

Psychologists can also advocate for the ICU to provide welcoming, calm areas for families to relax. Waiting areas should include comfortable furniture, relaxing colors and artwork, and displays of helpful information. Psychologists may promote initiatives to improve the environment for patients and families by encouraging quality improvement projects or campaigns to improve the environment, through advocacy and taking part in ICU management meetings, and by providing education for staff about environmental issues such as noise, light, and sleep promotion.

Conclusions

Critically ill or injured patients frequently experience both acute stress and long-term psychological sequelae following hospital discharge. Despite this, incorporating psychologists in the ICU care team to address the psychological impact of critical illness is still uncommon in most parts of the world. Early psychological care of patients by psychologists should be prioritized to decrease psychological distress, and research suggests that the use of psychological interventions delivered during ICU admission are beneficial to patients and their loved ones. Strategies based on CBT, such as psychoeducation, behavioral activation, goal setting, and grounding, and relaxation interventions may offer benefit to patients. Psychological care of ICU patients also involves psychosocial support for their relatives as they cope with the common challenges associated with a relative's critical illness. Finally, ICU psychologists intervene in other important, indirect ways. Psychologists help to improve communication in the ICU, enhance psychological understanding and care from other ICU staff, and foster a more therapeutic environment for patients.

Key Points

1. Psychological care of adult ICU patients aims to identify and treat patients experiencing significant acute psychological distress and those at increased risk for later psychological morbidity.
2. Principles of PFA and TIC provide the basis for psychological care of ICU patients, and CBT techniques can help patients cope with distress associated with ICU admission.
3. Psychological care of relatives in the ICU helps relatives cope with their loved one's illness, supports relatives in optimizing communication to decrease distress and conflicts, and assists in supporting relatives with end-of-life care and grief.
4. Indirect work by psychologists in the ICU involves collaboration with other members of the care team to improve communication in the ICU, increase psychological understanding and care of patients, and enhance the therapeutic environment.

References

1. L Kok, A.J. Slooter, M.H. Hillegers, et al. Benzodiazepine use and neuropsychiatric outcomes in the ICU: a systematic review. *Crit Care Med* 2018; **46**(10): 1673–80.
2. D. Wade, N. Als, V. Bell, et al. Providing psychological support to people in intensive care: development and feasibility study of a nurse-led intervention to prevent acute stress and long-term morbidity. *BMJ Open* 2018; **8**(7): e021083.
3. M. Beadman, M. Carraretto. Key elements of an evidence-based clinical psychology service within adult critical care. *J Intensive Care Soc* 2023; **24**(2): 215–21.
4. D.M. Wade, M. Hankins, D.A. Smyth, et al. Detecting acute distress and risk of future psychological morbidity in critically ill patients: validation of the intensive care psychological assessment tool. *Crit Care* 2014; **18**(5): 519.
5. M.E. Mikkelsen, M. Still, B.J. Anderson, et al. Society of Critical Care Medicine's International Consensus Conference on prediction and identification of long-term impairments after critical illness. *Crit Care Med* 2020; **48**(11): 1670–9.

6. National Institute for Health and Care Excellence (NICE). Rehabilitation After Critical Illness in Adults. Clinical Guideline CG83. 2009. www.nice.org.uk/guidance/cg83.
7. S.E. Hobfoll, P. Watson, C.C. Bell, et al. Five essential elements of immediate and mid-term mass trauma intervention: empirical evidence. *Psychiatry* 2021; **84**(4): 311–46.
8. Substance Abuse and Mental Health Services Administration. SAMHSA's Concept of Trauma and Guidance for a Trauma-Informed Approach. Substance Abuse and Mental Health Services Administration. 2014. https://ncsacw.acf.hhs.gov/userfiles/files/SAMHSA_Trauma.pdf.
9. D.F. Wade, Z. Moon, S.S. Windgassen, et al. Non-pharmacological interventions to reduce ICU-related psychological distress: a systematic review. *Minerva Anestesiol* 2016; **82**(4): 465–78.
10. D.M. Wade, P.R. Mouncey, A. Richards-Belle, et al. Effect of a nurse-led preventive psychological intervention on symptoms of posttraumatic stress disorder among critically ill patients: a randomized clinical trial. *JAMA* 2019; **321**(7): 665–75.
11. P.R. Mouncey, D. Wade, A. Richards-Belle, et al. A nurse-led, preventive, psychological intervention to reduce PTSD symptom severity in critically ill patients: the POPPI feasibility study and cluster RCT. Southampton (UK): NIHR Journals Library; August 2019.
12. J.N. Cohen, A. Gopal, K.J. Roberts, et al. Ventilator-dependent patients successfully weaned with Cognitive-Behavioral Therapy: a case series. *Psychosomatics* 2019; **60**(6): 612–19.
13. A. Peris, M. Bonizzoli, D. Iozzelli, et al. Early intra-intensive care unit psychological intervention promotes recovery from post traumatic stress disorders, anxiety and depression symptoms in critically ill patients. *Crit Care* 2011; **15**(2): 418.
14. M.M. Hosey, S.T. Wegener, C. Hinkle, D.M. Needham. A Cognitive Behavioral Therapy-informed self-management program for acute respiratory failure survivors: a feasibility study. *J Clin Med* 2021; **10**(4): 872.
15. M. Garrouste-Orgeas, C. Flahault, I. Vinatier, et al. Effect of an ICU diary on posttraumatic stress disorder symptoms among patients receiving mechanical ventilation: a randomized clinical trial. *JAMA* 2019; **322**(3): 229–39.
16. B.B. Barreto, M. Luz, M.N.O. Rios, et al. The impact of intensive care unit diaries on patients' and relatives' outcomes: a systematic review and meta-analysis. *Crit Care* 2019; **23**(1): 411.
17. J. Kang, Y.S. Cho, M. Lee, et al. Effects of nonpharmacological interventions on sleep improvement and delirium prevention in critically ill patients: a systematic review and meta-analysis. *Aust Crit Care* 2023; **36**(4): 640–9.
18. J.R. Curtis, P.D. Treece, E.L. Nielsen, et al. Randomized trial of communication facilitators to reduce family distress and intensity of end-of-life care. *Am J Respir Crit Care Med* 2016; **193**(2): 154–62.
19. M. Brauchle, T. Deffner, P. Nydahl. ICU Kids Study Group: ten recommendations for child-friendly visiting policies in critical care. *Intensive Care Med* 2023; **49**(3): 341–4.
20. M.K. Nielsen, M.A. Neergaard, A.B. Jensen, et al. Pre-loss grief in family caregivers during end-of-life cancer care: a nationwide population-based cohort study. *Psychooncology* 2017; **26**(12): 2048–56.
21. S.J. Moss, K. Wollny, T.G. Poulin, et al. Bereavement interventions to support informal caregivers in the intensive care unit: a systematic review. *BMC Palliat Care* 2021; **20**(1): 66.
22. N. Kentish-Barnes, S. Chevret, S. Valade, et al. A three-step support strategy for relatives of patients dying in the intensive care unit: a cluster randomised trial. *Lancet* 2022; **399**(10325): 656–64.
23. D. Wade, J. Highfield. Future directions for psychology in critical care. In Stucky K.J. Stucky and Jutte J.E. (eds.), *Critical Care*

Psychology and Rehabilitation: Principles and Practice. London: Oxford University Press; 2022. pp. 1–16.

24. D. Riedl, G. Schüßler. The influence of doctor-patient communication on health outcomes: a systematic review. *Z Psychosom Med Psychother* 2017; **63**(2): 131–50.
25. L. Fallowfield, V. Jenkins, V. Farewell, I. Solis-Trapala. Enduring impact of communication skills training: Results of a 12-month follow-up. *Br J Cancer* 2003; **89** (8): 1445–9.
26. A.J. Bullock, A. Sorbello, K.L. Gilrain, et al. Patient satisfaction with a psychology consultation-liaison service at an academic medical center. *J Clin Psychol Med Settings* 2022; **29**: 717–26.
27. J. Darbyshire, E. Jeffs, J. Young, L. Hinton. Noises in the intensive care unit: what goes bump in the night. *J Intensive Care Soc* 2015.
28. L.L. Chlan, A. Heiderscheit, D.J. Skaar, M. V. Neidecker. Economic evaluation of a patient-directed music intervention for ICU patients receiving mechanical ventilatory support. *Crit Care Med* 2018; **46** (9): 1430–5.
29. R.L. Rubert. D. Long, M.L. Hutchinson. Creating a healing environment in the ICU. In *Critical Care Nursing: Synergy for optimal outcomes*. Burlington, MA: Jones & Bartlett; 2007, pp. 27–39.
30. O. Tronstad, D. Flaws, S. Patterson, et al. Creating the ICU of the future: patient-centred design to optimise recovery. *Crit Care* 2023; **27**(1): 402.

Chapter 15

The Role of Spirituality throughout the Continuum of Critical Care

Maggie Keogh, Arvind V. Murali, Elizabeth B. Hewett, and Neha S. Dangayach

Introduction

Being admitted to the intensive care unit (ICU) can be a life-altering event for patients and families. In this chapter, "family" and "loved ones" are used interchangeably to be inclusive of everyone who is important to a patient, whether biologically related or not. Admission to an ICU may be associated with emotional turmoil as patients and families are forced to deal with life and death questions and fear of the unknown, and they may seek meaning in their suffering. Critically ill patients are often unable to speak for themselves, and their families are frequently asked to participate in shared decision-making regarding life-prolonging measures that could change their collective future in unexpected ways. The loss of a loved one in the ICU may provoke feelings of complicated grief and guilt [1]. Depending upon patients' and families' religious and spiritual preferences, some may find comfort in specific practices and sacraments, while others may not turn to spirituality as they struggle with uncertainty.

The role of spirituality and religiosity in critical care has been recognized but remains poorly studied. A Dutch survey-based study including intensivists, ICU nurses, and spiritual care providers showed that spiritual care has not been systematically integrated into daily practice despite its importance [2]. Lack of time and dedicated spiritual care education have been identified as barriers to the delivery of spiritual care in the ICU. Despite this, in an integrative review that included 113 studies, spiritual care was shown to improve the quality of care by reducing patient and family distress, offering spiritual comfort, enhancing the spiritual well-being of patients and families, and increasing family satisfaction with care [2]. The American College of Critical Care Medicine (ACCM) has drafted recommendations regarding assessment of spiritual needs in the ICU, spiritual training for doctors and nurses, physician review of interdisciplinary spiritual needs assessments, and honoring requests to pray with patients [3]. A narrative review of 16 studies since the publication of these recommendations found that the terms spirituality and religiosity are used interchangeably in the literature, and describing and measuring these constructs is difficult. In a multi-center, survey-based study of critically ill patients following hospital discharge, a majority reported that they would have wanted a chaplain visit in the ICU, and 80% of those who were visited by a chaplain found it helpful [4]. Most families and surrogate decision-makers for critically ill patients reported that spirituality was important to them when participating in shared decision-making [5].

What Is Spirituality Versus Religiosity?

Spirituality and religiosity are often thought to be synonymous, but they are different. Spirituality involves a personal internal search for meaning in life, which does not necessarily have to include a relationship with a deity. A commonly accepted consensus definition describes spirituality as "a dynamic and intrinsic aspect of humanity through which persons seek ultimate meaning, purpose, and transcendence, and experience a relationship to self, family, others, community, society, nature, and the significant or sacred. Spirituality is expressed through beliefs, values, traditions, and practices" [6]. On the other hand, religiosity is rooted in beliefs in God, the Divine, Sacred, or Transcendent and their role in answering questions about the meaning of life. Religion and religiosity adhere to a system or doctrine that offers answers to existential questions [7]. In the United States, more people describe themselves as spiritual rather than religious. A Pew Research Center survey of 11,201 adults found that 7 in 10 American adults described themselves as spiritual, including 22% who considered themselves spiritual but not religious [8].

Spirituality in Critical Care

Spirituality enhances the quality of life (QOL) for many patients and families. Spiritual care can also improve the quality of care provided in the ICU by relieving distress, diagnosing and addressing spiritual and emotional needs among patients and families, increasing spiritual well-being, and improving family satisfaction with shared decision-making. Spiritual care practices and interventions provided by spiritual care specialists can be grouped into several categories, including religious practices, spiritual practices, counseling, emotional practices, and advocacy, or any combination thereof; the spiritual care interventions are varied, intuitive, and powerful (see Table 15.1). Unfortunately, spiritual care providers are often engaged for the first time near the end of life or at the end of an ICU stay, thereby reducing the benefits of this kind of support [2,9]. The Society of Critical Care Medicine (SCCM) patient- and family-centered guidelines recommend offering routine spiritual care consultation for critically ill patients and families given how consistently patients and families value spiritual care [3]. One of the principal ways that chaplains participate in care is by helping the patient and their loved ones cope with uncertainty and stress while in the ICU.

Spiritual support is critical if the patient or their loved ones have deep questions regarding their lives and their search to find meaning amid suffering and crisis. One of the most important aspects of a chaplain's role is to engage the patient or loved ones in a conversation about how their current situation compares with their life before hospitalization. Listening intently to their words can give a chaplain an understanding of what their struggles may be and the best strategies to provide comfort and strength. Patients and loved ones may engage in deep, existential conversations, and hospital chaplains are trained to listen, to provide a calm and supportive presence, and to offer radical hospitality so that patients and loved ones are comfortable enough to share deeply [6].

A health crisis necessitating ICU admission can bring human fragility and mortality to the forefront of a person's psycho-spiritual framework of living. If the patient or their loved ones are religious, they may rely heavily on their faith and find solace in it; others may question why "God" is doing this to them. Patients who are conscious and cognizant may reflect on their life journey and ask existential questions, such as "Did I live and love well?," as chaplains hold the space and offer empathetic listening during this process. For loved ones, it could be a time of profound reflection with a possible need to reconcile belief systems. A nondenominational hospital chaplain is trained in offering psycho-spiritual support to those of any religious, spiritual, or nonaffiliated belief system [10].

Table 15.1 Spiritual care practices and interventions

Categories of Spiritual Care Practices	Examples of Specific Interventions
Spirituality: The way individuals seek and express meaning and purpose	
Spiritual Care: Attention given to spiritual needs that arise with illness, loss, grief, or pain	
Religious	- Praying - Distributing and discussing religious materials - Encouraging religious development - Discussing patient's relationship to God - Religious witnessing
Spiritual	- Facilitating finding meaning or purpose - Enabling existential empowerment - Guiding spiritual development - Providing end-of-life support
Counseling	- Establishing rapport - Encouraging (self) reflection - Encouraging expression - Enabling hope - Enabling emotion - Negotiating internal/external conflict - Facilitating closure
Emotional	- Communicating empathy - Providing comfort - Consoling patients - Demonstrating care and concern - Providing emotional support
Advocacy	- Cultural brokering - Communicating patient concerns/needs - Referring patients to chaplains or clergy

Spiritual care specialists can provide spiritual support for critically ill patients and families in a variety of ways, such as active listening, addressing spiritual needs, reading scriptures, and praying with patients and families. A single center study that reviewed electronic healthcare record (EHR) notes documented by chaplains found that chaplains addressed many aspects of holistic care for the patient and family: beliefs, practices, coping mechanisms, emotional resources and needs, faith support, medical decision-making, and medical communications [2,11]. The presence of a chaplain to support families during resuscitation events has been found to be helpful [12], and a post-code debrief with a chaplain can provide the staff with an opportunity to honor the patient's life and their teamwork in trying to save it as well as address the spiritual needs of responders [2,13].

Chaplaincy Training and Education

In general, the educational, therapeutic, and clinical foundation for professional hospital chaplains in Europe and North America is guided by the generalist-specialist principle, in which physicians and nurses serve as spiritual care generalists and trained hospital chaplains serve as specialists. The emphasis of research and training for spiritual care has been for care provided in hospital settings; less research and training are available to guide the delivery of spiritual care in the outpatient setting. Assessing the spiritual needs of patients and families in the ICU can help develop strategies for meeting those needs in the outpatient setting using the generalist-specialist model.

Europe

There are no regional professional guidelines for spiritual care providers that provide recommendations on the provision of spiritual care in hospital settings or the ICU; however, when reviewing spiritual care in ICUs across the world, there are similarities in how spiritual care is delivered inclusive of nurses, chaplains, and lay persons. Most European countries have professional associations that are often created by faith communities, groups of chaplains with common interests, or chaplains in a common geographic area; examples in the United Kingdom include the Multi-Faith Group for Healthcare Chaplaincy and the College of Health Care Chaplains. The standards of the European Network for Health Care Chaplains (ENHCC) refer to four requirements for continuous education for chaplains: theological and pastoral education and reflection, awareness of health issues, clinical supervision, and spiritual guidance [14].

In a study from Dutch ICUs, despite the presence of a spiritual care provider, there is no standardized method to assess the spiritual needs of patients and families in the ICU or to guide the delivery of spiritual care [2]. In the Netherlands and Belgium, patients have the legal right to the presence of a chaplain based on the right of freedom of religion [14]. Chaplaincy services are delivered by clergy and lay persons who have been professionally trained in both religious studies and medical education. The Constitution of the Republic of Poland preserves the right to receive religious support in the places where people of faith find themselves; as such, the Patients' Rights Act states that a patient staying in a therapeutic unit has the right to pastoral care. For this reason, hospital chaplains are employed by hospitals to deliver religious services there. Until 2021, pastoral care in Poland was limited to celebrating Mass in patients' rooms, but in recent years, the scope has expanded to include additional spiritual support to patients and families [15].

Muslim Countries

In Muslim countries, spiritual care and education is provided to nurses and includes prayer with patients, turning the bed to Mecca, and reading the Holy Quran [16].

North America

The American Joint Commission on the Accreditation of Healthcare Organizations and the Canadian Counsel on Health Services Accreditation both state that spiritual care is a necessary component of patient and family care in healthcare institutions [17]. The ACCM has published guidelines that include spiritual and religious support in ICUs [3]. The Board of Chaplaincy Certification, Inc. (BCCI), within the Association of Professional

Chaplains (APC), is the main professional association that offers a certification program for hospital chaplaincy. Other American professional chaplaincy organizations are faith-centered, including the National Association of Catholic Chaplains (NACC) and the National Association of Jewish Chaplains (NAJC), both of which require a high standard of education and clinical and ethical training.

Assessing the Spiritual Needs of Patients and Families

In this section, we describe how to assess the spiritual needs of patients and families, how to obtain a spiritual history, and the training medical teams should receive to improve their competency for spiritual care. There are several barriers to the delivery of spiritual care in both the ICU and outpatient settings, including inadequate time, insufficient training to develop the requisite skills, and underutilization of spiritual care services [18]. A Delphi consensus process led by Balboni and colleagues produced several evidence-based statements for addressing spiritual needs in serious illness and health. One of the principal recommendations is that members of the multidisciplinary care team should receive training in addressing spiritual care, especially since clinicians consider themselves poor at the assessment of spiritual distress [18]. Additional recommendations include taking a spiritual history using a generalist-specialist model, providing access to spiritual history resources, and supplementing medical school curricula with lectures on spiritual care, all of which could help improve the competency of medical teams [18].

Obtaining a spiritual history from the patient is preferred, but if their condition precludes such a conversation, obtaining a spiritual history from a family member is acceptable. A spiritual history involves learning the person's life story, elucidating what events and people have helped shape them, learning what things help them cope or feel grounded, and determining how they best feel supported. People may find comfort in the rituals of their faith (e.g., prayer, anointing, sacred texts, and meditation), while others may find comfort in music, art, or nature. A spiritual history should include details of a person's religious beliefs or lack thereof. Taking a spiritual history allows the patient or family to discuss what makes sense to them, what motivates them, and what hinders them. Sharing the information gained from a spiritual history with the medical team can provide important guidance about what matters most to the patient. Although the spiritual history can be taken by any healthcare provider, hospital chaplains are specialists trained in empathic engagement who are skilled in taking a spiritual history. Importantly, as with obtaining goals of care, this conversation with a patient or loved one may require more than one visit.

Spiritual Competency and Training

Increased access to spiritual care services in hospitals in North America and Europe has also improved access to spiritual education, competency, and training for ICU physicians, nurses, and other clinicians. These team members can serve effectively as spiritual care "generalists" as part of a holistic experience for patients and families. If the generalist decides that the patient or family needs more in-depth spiritual care interventions or they are in spiritual distress, they may refer them to a spiritual care provider for specialist consultation. Spiritual distress occurs when any aspect of the human experience is questioned, challenged, nonexistent, or troubling. Oftentimes, a spiritual history taking tool (see Table 15.2) can be used by a nurse or physician without specific training to begin explorations of faith, the importance of religiosity or spirituality, and what aspects of spiritual well-being matter to the patient.

Table 15.2 Spiritual assessment tools

Spiritual Assessment Tool	Developer	Acronym Meaning	Main Focus
FICA (Faith, Importance/Influence, Community, Action/Address in care) [6]	Christina Puchalski, MD	**F. Faith, Belief, Meaning:** Determine whether or not the patient identifies with a particular belief system or spirituality at all. **I. Importance and Influence:** Understand the importance of spirituality in the patient's life and the influence on healthcare decisions. **C. Community:** Find out if the patient is part of a religious or spiritual community or if they rely on their community for support. **A. Address/Action in Care:** Learn how to address spiritual issues while caring for the patient.	Offers a step-by-step guide to elicit a patient's spiritual history and preferences.
HOPE Questions [19]	Dr. Gowri Anandarajah	**H**ope **O**rganized religion **P**ersonal spirituality **E**ffects on medical care and end-of-life issues	Explores patients' sources of hope, connections to organized religion or spirituality, personal spiritual practices or beliefs, and the impact of spirituality on medical care and end-of-life issues.
SPIRITual History [20]	Dr. Maugans	**S**piritual belief system **P**ersonal spirituality **I**ntegration within a spiritual community **R**itualized practices **I**mplications for medical care **T**erminal events planning	Provides a comprehensive assessment covering a patient's spiritual belief system, personal spirituality, involvement in a spiritual community, ritualized practices, and the implications of spirituality for medical care and end-of-life planning.

JAREL Spiritual Well-Being Scale [21]	Dr. Joanne R. McSherry and Dr. Linda Ross	Not applicable	Measures the spiritual well-being of patients, focusing on their sense of meaning and purpose, inner peace, faith, and the strength of their spiritual beliefs.
Spiritual Needs Assessment [22]	Various researchers	Not applicable	Identifies the specific spiritual needs of patients, such as the need for meaning, hope, love, forgiveness, and connection, and explores how these needs can be addressed in the healthcare setting.
FACIT-Sp [23]	Dr. David Cella and colleagues	Functional Assessment of Chronic Illness Therapy – Spiritual Well-being	Measures the spiritual well-being of patients with chronic illnesses, focusing on their sense of meaning, peace, faith, and the impact of spirituality on their quality of life.

Spiritual Crisis and Spiritual Distress in the ICU

Spiritual crisis is defined as a unique form of grieving marked by a profound questioning of life, in which an individual reaches a juncture that leads to a significant alteration in the way one views oneself and life [2,21]. Spiritual distress is an impaired ability to experience and integrate meaning and purpose in life through the individual's connectedness with self, others, art, music, literature, nature, or a power greater than oneself [2,22]. Chaplains may receive questions including: "Why is this happening to me? Did I do something wrong? Why is God punishing me? Can I make sense out of my suffering? What am I to learn from this experience?" In addition, due to the fragility and uncertainty of one's health in the ICU, death is at the forefront of many patients' minds. This could bring up life review questioning: "Have I lived a good life? Has my life had meaning? Did I live the way I wanted? Do I have regrets? What will happen when I die? Are there things still left for me to do?" These types of questions often reflect intense spiritual distress [2,21,23,24]. At the end of a person's life, there is a desire to know that they are loved and that their life had value and still does. Sometimes there is a need for forgiveness and reconciliation – not only from the people whom they love but also from themselves. Professional chaplains can help families and patients have a positive end-of-life experience whenever possible.

Ideally, it is best to have a chaplain or spiritual caregiver work with patients and families early in the ICU stay so that they may address any spiritual concerns or existential pain that arises. Helping families talk with their loved ones and encouraging families to share stories of their loved ones are important [25]. It is also critical to seek forgiveness and to provide forgiveness and reconciliation if this is sought. When caring for unconscious patients, encouraging loved ones to continue speaking to them as if they can hear and understand their words may help in humanizing patients, preventing depersonalization, and processing trauma. It can be challenging to find a calm and quiet space in an ICU, and the chaplain can help facilitate this to address spiritual needs despite the chaotic ICU environment [26].

Spiritual Care Beyond the ICU

Post-intensive care syndrome (PICS) is defined as new or worsened physical, cognitive, or mental health impairments that arise during hospitalization and persist after discharge, and post-intensive care syndrome-family (PICS-F) refers to new or increased mental health or social impairments in family members after a loved one is hospitalized in a critical care setting [27]. Estimates of the prevalence of PICS-F typically range from 14% to 50% (see Chapter 48 for additional information). This wide range may be related to differences in how the syndrome is defined and assessed across settings, the timing of the assessment, and different patient populations; for example, the prevalence of PICS-F is as high as 80% when families must make end-of-life decisions with inadequate support and as high as 65% if the patient dies [27]. Interventions from the healthcare team, including spiritual care, can be helpful in offering education, supportive presence, and spiritual direction. The psycho-spiritual trauma and healing of patients and loved ones in an ICU when they leave (deceased or not) is a wide-reaching aspect of the human experience that should not be ignored when assessments of other PICS and PICS-F domains are performed [3].

Resources for Patients and Families on What to Expect When They Leave the Hospital and How to Navigate Their Spiritual Needs

Symptoms of PICS and PICS-F can last for years, and SCCM has a resource page to help patients and their loved ones understand and manage them [27]. To provide holistic care to survivors of critical illness and their families, it is important that they have tools to address their spiritual well-being in addition to impairments in other PICS and PICS-F domains [27]. Prior to patients being discharged from the ICU, they should be screened for risk factors for developing PICS and should be encouraged to talk with their care team to better understand their risks. A spiritual needs assessment completed by a chaplain or other frontline team members can help guide the need for ongoing spiritual support in the recovery phase.

While spiritual needs should be addressed through all phases of care, they are not routinely discussed in the ICU, on the ward, or following hospital discharge. Irrespective of whether spiritual needs were addressed during the ICU, they should be re-addressed during recovery, as spiritual needs continue to evolve over time. For hospitals that do not have an ICU follow-up program, a patient's primary care physician may also be able to screen for spiritual needs and refer patients and families to spiritual care specialists. While seeing patients in ICU follow-up clinics, spiritual care providers can engage in active listening and prayer with patients and can help patients and families cope with their ongoing struggles, ensure that their spiritual needs are met as their survivorship journey evolves, and help them find meaning and purpose. Unfortunately, few ICU follow-up clinics currently include spiritual care providers as part of the multidisciplinary team [28].

Conclusion

Spiritual needs should be addressed throughout the continuum of critical care. ICU team members should receive training on obtaining a spiritual history and screening for spiritual distress so that they can serve as effective spiritual care generalists and collaborate early with chaplains as specialists for patients with unmet spiritual needs. ICU team members and chaplains should be aware of spiritual care resources for patients and families and how to refer patients and families to these services both in the ICU and beyond. Despite spiritual needs being identified as an important unmet need for survivors of critical illness, spiritual care and the role of the chaplain have not been systematically integrated in care delivery both in the ICU and outpatient settings. Spiritual care presents an important avenue for improving the overall quality of care delivery for critically ill patients and families as well as an important area for ongoing multidisciplinary research throughout the continuum of care. More research is needed to better understand how spiritual needs can be addressed for patients and families beyond the ICU and how hospital chaplains can help reduce PICS and PICS-F symptoms.

Key Points

1. Addressing the roles of spirituality and religiosity in critical care can provide significant support for patients, families, loved ones, and staff.

2. Spirituality involves a personal internal search for meaning in life, which does not necessarily have to include a relationship with a deity, while religiosity is rooted in beliefs in God, the Divine, Sacred, or Transcendent and their role in answering questions about the meaning of life.
3. Hospital staff are considered spiritual care generalists who can receive training to identify spiritual distress; they can consult chaplains, spiritual care specialists, for patients and families who need more in-depth spiritual care interventions or who are in spiritual distress.
4. Literature supports addressing the spiritual needs of patients and loved ones in the ICU as part of providing holistic care; spiritual needs should be assessed throughout the continuum of care, even in outpatient settings, as spiritual needs may change during the course of recovery.
5. Multidisciplinary teams should receive education in addressing spiritual needs.
6. More research is needed to better understand the role of spirituality and how spiritual needs of ICU patients and their loved ones can be addressed throughout the continuum of care.

References

1. W.G. Anderson, R.M. Arnold, D.C. Angus, C.L. Bryce. Posttraumatic stress and complicated grief in family members of patients in the intensive care unit. *J Gen Intern Med* 2008; **23**: 1871–6.
2. S. Willemse, W. Smeets, E. van Leeuwen, et al. Spiritual care in the intensive care unit: an integrative literature research. *J Crit Care* 2020; **57**: 55–78.
3. J.E. Davidson, R.A. Aslakson, A.C. Long, et al. Guidelines for family-centered care in the ICU. *Crit Care Med* 2017; **45**: 103–28.
4. K.M. Piderman, D.V. Marek, S.M. Jenkins, et al. Predicting patients' expectations of hospital chaplains: a multisite survey. *Mayo Clin Proc* 2010; **85**: 1002–10.
5. T.A. Balboni, T.J. VanderWeele, S.D. Doan-Soares, et al. Spirituality in serious illness and health. *JAMA* 2022; **328**: 184–97.
6. C.M. Puchalski, R. Vitillo, S.K. Hull, et al. Improving the quality of spiritual care as a dimension of palliative care: the report of the consensus conference. *J Palliat Med* 2014; **17**: 642–56.
7. H.G. Koenig. Religion, spirituality, and health: the research and clinical implications. *ISRN Psychiatry* 2012; **2012**: 278730.
8. Pew Research Center. The American Trends Panel. Washington, DC: Pew Research Center; 2014. www.pewresearch.org/the-american-trends-panel/ (Accessed October 9, 2023).
9. P.J. Choi, F.A. Curlin, C.E. Cox. "The patient is dying, please call the chaplain": the activities of chaplains in one medical center's intensive care units. *J Pain Symptom Manage* 2015; **50**: 501–6.
10. J.Q. Ho, C.D. Nguyen, R. Lopes, et al. Spiritual care in the intensive care unit: a narrative review. *J Intensive Care Med* 2018; **33**: 279–87.
11. J.R. Johnson, R.A. Engelberg, E.L. Nielsen, et al. The association of spiritual care providers' activities with family members' satisfaction with care after a death in the ICU. *Crit Care Med* 2014; **42**: 1991–2000.
12. D. Clark. Chaplaincy in resuscitation events. *Am J Crit Care* 2005; **14**: 86–9.
13. P. Copeland. Post-code debrief with chaplains: supporting healthcare teams. *J Spiritual Care* 2016; **43**: 83–90.

14. A. Vandenhoeck. Chaplaincy in European healthcare: roles and training. *Euro J Healthcare Chapl* 2013; **5**: 21–9.
15. M.W. Klimasiński. Spiritual care in the intensive care unit. *Anaesthesiol Intensive Ther.* 2021; **53**(4): 350–7.
16. M. Rababa, S. Al-Sabbah. The use of Islamic spiritual care practices among critically ill adult patients: A systematic review. *Heliyon.* 2023; **9**(3): e13862.
17. Association of Professional Chaplains, Association for Clinical Pastoral Education, Canadian Association for Pastoral Practice and Education, National Association of Catholic Chaplains, National Association of Jewish Chaplains. A white paper: professional chaplaincy, its role and importance in healthcare. *J Pastoral Care* 2001; **55**: 81–97.
18. M.J. Balboni, T.J. Van der Weele, S.D. Doan-Soares, et al. Spirituality in serious illness and health. *J Clin Oncol* 2013; **31**: 461–7.
19. G. Anandarajah, E. Hight. Spirituality and medical practice: using the HOPE questions as a practical tool for spiritual assessment. *Am Fam Physician* 2001; **63**: 81–9.
20. T.A. Maugans. The SPIRITual history. *Arch Fam Med* 1996; **5**: 11–16.
21. W. McSherry, L. Ross. Dilemmas of spiritual assessment: considerations for nursing practice. *J Adv Nurs* 2002; **38**: 479–88.
22. M. Best, P. Butow, I. Olver. Spiritual support of cancer patients and the role of the doctor. *J Clin Oncol* 2015; **33**: 101–7.
23. D. Cella, A.H. Peterman, G. Fitchett, et al. Reliability and validity of the Functional Assessment of Chronic Illness Therapy-Spiritual Well-being (FACIT-Sp) instrument. *Psychooncology* 2002; **11**: 349–61.
24. R. Weiland. Spiritual crisis and ICU care. *Psycho-Spiritual Med* 2010; **15**: 14–22.
25. C. Kociszewski. Spiritual care: a phenomenologic study of critical care nurses. *Heart Lung* 2004; **33**: 401–11.
26. R. Gillilan, E. Baxter, E. Manning, et al. The role of chaplaincy in ICU trauma. *Spiritual Health Rev* 2019; **12**: 51–8.
27. S.M. Petrinec, B. Martin. Post-intensive care syndrome and post-intensive care syndrome-family: a review. *Crit Care Med* 2018; **46**: 1620–6.
28. V. Danesh, L.M. Boehm, T.L. Eaton, et al. Characteristics of post-ICU and post-COVID recovery clinics in 29 U.S. health systems. *Crit Care Explor* 2022; **4**: e0658.

Chapter 16

Humanization of the ICU

Gabriel Heras La Calle and José Manuel Velasco Bueno

Humanization of Healthcare

Over the past several years, humanization of healthcare has received increased attention from the medical community. This may seem paradoxical, since it might be considered that there is nothing more human than caring for others,[1] but the collective experience of patients, families, and healthcare professionals over the past decades reveals a concerning shift toward depersonalization and a technology-centered, rather than patient-centered, approach.

Humanization cannot be separated from dignity. According to Bermejo, "To speak of humanisation calls for the intrinsic dignity of every human being and the rights that derive from it. And this makes it a need of vital importance and transcendence" [1]. Similarly, Albert Jovell points out that humanizing "is the way of caring for and curing the patient as a person, based on scientific evidence, incorporating the dimension of the patient's dignity and humanity, establishing care based on trust and empathy, and contributing to the patient's well-being and the best possible health outcomes" [2].

Humanization and technification, the latter of which better characterizes our current healthcare model, might at first seem to be adversarial, but this need not be the case. Patients who are ill and vulnerable want to be cared for by the best-trained professionals using the most advanced technologies and treatments, but they also want to be treated as individuals with dignity, respect, and compassion. Scientific and technological advances have resulted in markedly improved survival rates globally, but this focus on technology, research, and a frequently mercantilist approach to health systems management has left the human beings who make up this complex system behind.

Fragmentation of clinical practice has engendered a depersonalization of care and a reification of patients, forgetting the biography behind them, their feelings and values, and everything that makes them unique. Recently, there has been increasing interest in developing *patient-centered care* [3] or *patient and family-centered care* models [4]. Despite this, these reflections in the literature do not translate into actual practice in a comprehensive and tangible way, although stakeholders perceive it as a necessity.

There are many elements in the complex healthcare ecosystem that have driven this concerning trend of depersonalized care. These include: pressure to provide expeditious care; lack of human and technical resources; often precarious working conditions; super-specialization of professionals; and challenging interpersonal relationships among patients,

---

[1] For anthropologist Margaret Mead, the first sign of human civilization was the finding of a fractured and healed femur; this meant that someone took the time to care for another wounded person and stayed with them until the leg was healed, avoiding a certain death.

relatives, and professionals. Collectively, these factors can leave patients feeling a lack of concern for their problems, inadequate empathy for their pain and suffering, and ultimately a loss of trust in their healthcare providers. Depersonalization, together with emotional fatigue and low personal fulfilment, are the fundamental components of the burnout syndrome common among healthcare providers.

It is possible to humanize clinical practice? To do so, we must begin with the premise that healthcare must be centered on the uniqueness, dignity, and autonomy of the individual.

Reflecting on this premise, we must reject the current model and consider another path that prioritizes better care for patients, their families, and the professionals caring for them. To do this requires undertaking measures that will affect management, the adequacy of structures, clinical practice itself, and training of professionals in "non-technical skills." These skills, which should be taught in the same way as other academic and procedural skills, include communication, active listening, empathy, compassion, respect, and ethics.

Redesigning healthcare delivery through a humanistic lens must include the opinions of patients and family members; those who receive care must be listened to and their voices must be integrated into decision-making. Components that are critical to the "patient experience" [5], which is understood as the sum of the interactions that take place in an organization and that influence the patient's perception during the continuum of care, include frequent and clear communication with providers, continuity of care, a focus on pain management, and attention to the environment of care with respect to cleanliness and ambient noise.

In order to improve humanization in healthcare, three essential points can be agreed upon:

1. Respect for the individual: each person is unique and responds differently to crisis.
2. Recognition of the leading role of patients and family members in healthcare processes: their fundamental right to participate in decision-making and their responsibility to actively participate in their recovery.
3. The need to turn healthcare centers into friendly spaces for healthcare professionals as well: *caring for the caregiver* is an unresolved issue in many healthcare systems.

Humanization of Intensive Care Units

Dehumanization of care is probably most problematic in intensive care units (ICU), where technification, depersonalization, and reification of patients are predominant. While healthcare providers are understandably focused on treating the pathophysiological processes that necessitate critical care, factors that are equally important to patients – and to their experience of illness – are often relegated to second place. Such factors include the inability to communicate, loss of autonomy, impaired mobility, loneliness, a lack of information, and a loss of identity. Although they are the focus of clinical attention, patient's needs are often not taken into account, and those of their relatives are similarly ignored.

Given this, in February 2014, the International Research Project for the Humanisation of Intensive Care Units (HU-CI Project) was developed with the goal of prioritizing the humanization of ICUs, putting the human being at the center of care, and redesigning healthcare with the dignity of the person as a non-negotiable premise [6,7,8]. The HU-CI Project was conceived as a multidisciplinary research group that seeks, through participatory and networked research, to evaluate different components of humanized healthcare and to implement the corresponding improvement actions. Each line of action is always approached from a three-pronged perspective that considers the patients, their families, and the professionals who care for them:

- Critically ill patients are especially vulnerable both physically and emotionally. They need to be listened to and must be involved in their own care, regardless of the outcome.
- Families' emotional needs are generally not met. Despite the fundamental role they play in patient recovery both during admission and after hospital discharge, their emotional and social needs are often unconsidered or underappreciated.
- Critical care professionals are exposed to many factors that can influence their physical and emotional health, which, in addition to having an impact on a personal and professional level, can influence patient outcomes.

The main objective for the humanization of the ICU is to promote tangible and specific measures to help care for all those involved: patients, family members, and professionals. This is not merely a declaration of intent, but a real roadmap for transforming reality and delivering change. The following proposed measures have already been integrated into the humanization plans of the Community of Madrid [9,10] and the Manual of Good Practices for the Humanisation of Intensive Care Units [11] (see Figure 16.1); they serve as a solid foundation for the development of humanization plans for other healthcare systems around the world.

Each of the following components of a comprehensive approach to the humanization of healthcare may have a role in preventing post-intensive care syndrome (PICS). Each is meaningful on its own, but together, their effects are synergistic to achieve the proposed objective. We will now briefly analyze each of them.

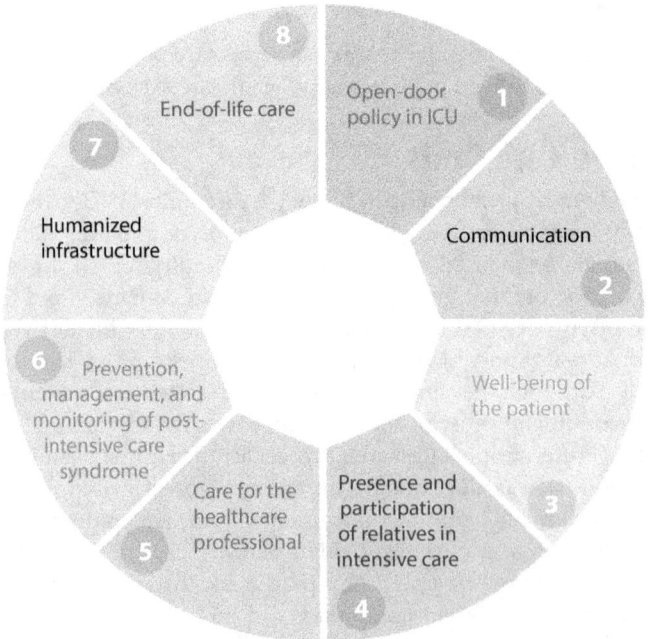

Figure 16.1 Strategic components of the HU-CI Project for the humanization of intensive care units. From: N. Nin Vaeza, M.C. Martin Delgado, G. Heras La Calle. Humanizing intensive care: toward a human-centered care ICU model. *Crit Care Med* 2020; **48**(3): 385–90. Reproduced with permissions from Wolters Kluwer Health, Inc.

Open-Door Visitation Policies and Presence and Participation of Family Members

Conventional visiting policies for ICU patients are restrictive [12,13], and these were intensified by the COVID-19 pandemic, during which visitation of loved ones was often completely prohibited. Restrictive visitation policies are not based on scientific evidence or the needs of patients and their loved ones, but rather on the misguided belief that designated quiet times are necessary for patient recovery and for facilitating delivery of care. In contrast, the unrestricted presence of family members could be beneficial to the patient by providing the comforting presence of a familiar face and hand to hold, frequent orientation, encouragement with occupational and physical therapy exercises, and, in a study performed during the COVID pandemic, a reduction in delirium [14]. Liberal visitation policies also benefit families by minimizing anxiety through unrestricted access to their loved one and reduce stress by allowing them to juggle more effectively the competing responsibilities of work and family life. Indeed, family members would prefer to visit their loved ones, and even assist with basic care, according to their own schedule rather than one set by the hospital [15]. Such flexible or "open-door" models of visitation have been utilized by some ICUs for many years, demonstrating the feasibility of such an approach and confirming its benefits with respect to patients, families, and even healthcare professionals.

Existing barriers to changing visitation policies may be related to the physical structure of the units, but they are more often associated with the mental structure of the professionals. To evolve from the concept of a "visiting family member" to a "partner in care" requires examination of inherited maladaptive ways of thinking, dialogue and consensus among professionals, and openness to learning from the experiences of others. There are several ways in which open visitation policies can be beneficial to healthcare professionals. The ability of family members to assist in basic personal care, such as grooming and feeding, while under the supervision of healthcare professionals, not only allows them to feel directly involved in the patient's recovery but also may ease the task burden that nurses and therapists face. Family participation in daily rounds facilitates improved communication with the healthcare team, presents an opportunity to ask questions or to clarify areas of uncertainty, and provides a venue to re-examine goals of care if necessary. Furthermore, frequent family presence can promote the establishment of a more therapeutic relationship between providers and families and increase family satisfaction with care, particularly when the patient does not survive, which can in turn reduce the emotional stress faced by providers. Family presence could also improve clinicians' attention to privacy, dignity, and pain management while procedures are being performed.

Communication

Communication in the ICU is fundamental, both among healthcare professionals themselves and with patients and family members, and improving it is a major priority in any ICU humanization program. Effective communication and joint decision-making between professionals avoid errors, favor consensus on treatment and care, and improve trust and respect. Communication involves a transfer of both information and responsibilty. The provision of training in communication skills is required to help eliminate or minimize conflict [16] and to improve patient and family satisfaction.

Patients and relatives deserve and require information. When engaging in highly significant conversations regarding goals of care or sharing information that is difficult to hear, specialized communication skills are required. Most professionals have not received dedicated and specific training in this area and learn either by trial and error or by observing how senior colleagues approach such conversations. In addition, variability in communication style and content may increase uncertainty for family members, who are often the only interlocutors given the patient's situation [17]. Effective, clear, and respectful communication allows joint decision-making among all parties and may minimize psychological stress in patients and their loved ones. Ideally, particularly during important conversations, both doctors and nurses should be present, given that nurses, who spend more time in contact with the patients and families, can bring valuable insights and information, leading to a richer conversation and one in which families may feel more comfortable.

Many critically ill patients are unable to communicate, either because of their disease process, interventions such as mechanical ventilation, or isolation from their loved ones, which generates frustration and discomfort. When disease or interventions prevent communication, the use of augmentative and alternative communication technology (e.g., pictograms or eye-tracking technology) may be helpful (see Chapter 13 for additional information). In the case of isolation, the use of technology (e.g., a patient's own devices and organized video calls) may help improve the situation for those patients who are able to communicate and whose loved ones are reachable.

Patient Well-Being

ICUs have been characterized by patients as "a branch of hell" [18]. The patient's well-being should be just as important as the patient's cure, and even more so if a cure is not possible. Patient discomfort has multiple causes, with pain being the most common. In addition to the organic pain caused by the disease itself, many interventions, including intubation, catheterization, tracheal aspiration, placement of thoracic drains, and cannulation of blood vessels, cause pain and exacerbate immobility. Assessments of pain and sedation should occur frequently, and the treatment of pain should be multimodal, including both pharmacological and non-pharmacological approaches. Similarly, approaches to sedation should be thoughtful and dynamic, with particular care to avoid the complications of both undersedation and oversedation [19,20]. Other factors contributing to physical discomfort include hunger and thirst; being too cold or too warm; difficulty in resting because of frequent interruptions, uncomfortable beds, and elevated ambient noise levels; and the use of unnecessary restraints.

Discomfort is not only physical; psychological and spiritual suffering are particularly common in both patients and their families. This is compounded by feelings of loneliness, isolation, fear, dependency, uncertainty, loss of identity, and lack of understanding, among others. The assessment and support of these needs should be considered a key element in the humanization of the ICU. It is necessary to train professionals to heighten their empathy and compassion, so that they may detect the suffering of patients and family members and thus promote measures aimed at resolving these problems.

Caring for the Professionals

Given the high rate of burnout among critical care providers [21] and the desire of many to leave the profession, prioritizing the mental health of healthcare professionals is paramount. Stressful situations in the ICU may have significantly negative impacts on healthcare workers, highlighted by the rise in burnout among critical care nurses and physicians caused by an intellectually, physically, and emotionally demanding work environment. End-of-life issues, ethically complicated decision-making, observation of patients' suffering, futile or disproportionate care, poor communication, and the demands of family members are all factors that impact professionals' emotional health. They also find themselves in an increasingly technical environment that requires developing and renewing skills in new techniques and treatments. All of these factors contribute to burnout syndrome [22].

Burnout is defined by emotional exhaustion, depersonalization, and feelings of low professional self-esteem. This problem affects providers on both personal and professional levels, and it can lead to post-traumatic stress syndrome, other serious psychological disorders, and even suicide. Professional burnout affects quality of care, patient outcomes, and patient satisfaction, and it is related to the lack of involvement of professionals in organizations. Preventing burnout requires promotion of strategies at the individual level, such as training in and acquisition of self-care tools (e.g., resilience, teamwork, emotional self-regulation, mindfulness, and compassion), as well as at institutional and governmental levels, promoting policies that improve working conditions.

Prevention, Detection, and Management of PICS

Given that surviving a critical illness is often a life-changing event for many patients, attention must be paid to survivorship following critical illness. In addition to the illness itself, care provided in the hospital, while necessary to treat the disease, can also have a dramatic and deleterious impact on a patient's physical, cognitive, and emotional health. Immobility, sedating drugs, impaired nutrition and sleep, anxiety induced by a life-threatening illness, and separation from family and loved ones can all contribute to PICS, and therefore, these risk factors must be recognized and addressed during hospitalization (see Section 2 of this book, "The Hazards of Hospitalization," and Section 3 of this book, "Strategies to Prevent PICS," for additional information). The multidisciplinary team caring for the patient in the ICU should be trained in minimizing the risks of PICS, and educating the patient and family about PICS should begin shortly after admission to the ICU provided that survival seems likely. Family members can play a fundamental role in the prevention of PICS by participating in the patient's care as much as feasible, but they are also at risk for developing the psychological and social sequelae of PICS, known as PICS-Family (PICS-F; see Chapter 48 for additional information).

Humanized Architecture and Infrastructure

The physical environment of the ICU is one of the main factors that hinders the provision of humanized care, since the design and space of the ICU often fails to respect the privacy and dignity of individual patients. Open units, with no separation between patients other than screens or curtains, still exist, as do improvised units, such as those required during the COVID-19 pandemic, both of which hinder person-centered care. These spaces do not guarantee the privacy of patients in times of significant vulnerability, nor do they allow for confidential interactions with loved ones.

Similarly, spaces for patient families and healthcare professionals should be designed with the often-competing goals of technical efficiency and comfort in mind. Important factors in designing such spaces include: appropriate location; adaptation to users' workflows; attention to (natural) light, temperature, and ambient noise; suitable materials and finishes; and functional and comfortable furniture and decoration. Patient rooms should have elements that minimize delirium and enhance time-space orientation, such as windows that provide natural light. Modification of existing spaces aimed at improving comfort, privacy, and companionship – without compromising functionality – can positively influence the well-being of patients, families, and professionals [23]. These concepts are equally applicable both to family waiting rooms, which should be redesigned to become more like "living rooms," and to healthcare professionals' work and rest spaces.

End-of-Life Care

For many patients requiring critical care, treatment of the underlying disease process and recovery may not be possible, and death may be unavoidable. Under these circumstances, goals and objectives must be changed from recovery and rehabilitation to alleviation of suffering and provision of comfort during the dying process. Prioritizing symptom management, with an emphasis on the treatment of pain, breathlessness, and anxiety, coupled with respect for ethical, religious, and cultural traditions is paramount for humanizing the end-of-life process. Palliative care and intensive care need not be considered mutually exclusive, rather they should coexist throughout the care of the critically ill patient [24].

Limitation of life support should be carried out following the recommendations and guidelines established by scientific societies [25,26]. It should be included in a comprehensive and multidisciplinary palliative care plan, with the aim of addressing the physical, psychosocial, and spiritual needs of the patient and their family members. Occasionally, decisions surrounding limitation of life support and other end-of-life care may elicit conflict among healthcare professionals or between healthcare professionals and family members. Professionals should have the necessary skills to address and resolve such conflict, with an emphasis on open and constructive communication as one strategy to minimize the emotional burden caused by the conflict.

Key Points

1. Humanization is the pursuit of excellence through person-centered care that translates into real and concrete cultural and structural changes.
2. Families are partners in care, and their presence and participation are critical to improve the patient and family experience. No patient should be left alone unless they wish to be.
3. High-quality communication is essential and often requires education and training.
4. Respecting patients' preferences, values, and needs is crucial to taking care of their physical, psychological, and spiritual well-being.
5. Caring for professionals, who are tools of humanization, is necessary; attention must be paid to contract stability, working conditions, stress management, burnout prevention, teamwork, and psychological and emotional support.
6. Survival is not the only important outcome; prevention, diagnosis, and treatment of PICS is critical.
7. Attention to the physical environment is fundamental in a model that focuses on people's dignity.
8. No one should die alone; palliative care and spiritual care should be seamlessly integrated into critical care at the end of life.

References

1. J.C. Bermejo. *Humanizing health care.* Bilbao: Desclée De Brouwer; 2014.
2. A.J. Jovell. Affectivity-based medicine. *Med Clin (Barc)* 1999; **113**(5): 173–5.
3. M.J. Goldfarb, L. Bibas, V. Bartlett, et al. Outcomes of patient- and family-centered care interventions in the ICU: a systematic review and meta-analysis. *Crit Care Med* 2017; **45**(10): 1751–61.
4. J.E. Davidson, R.A. Aslakson, A.C. Long, et al. Guidelines for family-centered care in the neonatal, pediatric and adult ICU. *Crit Care Med* 2017; **45**(1): 103–28.
5. J.A. Wolf, V. Niederhauser, D. Marshburn, S.L. LaVela. Defining patient experience. *Patient Experience Journal* 2014; **1**(1): 7–19.
6. N. Nin Vaeza, M.C. Martin Delgado, G. Heras La Calle. Humanizing intensive care: toward a human-centered care ICU model. *Crit Care Med* 2020; **48**(3): 385–90.
7. G. Heras and Members of the HU-CI Project. *Humanizing intensive car: present and future centered on people.* Bogotá: Distribuna; 2017.
8. G. Heras, A. Alonso, V. Gómez. A plan for improving the humanisation of intensive care units. *Intensive Care Med* 2017; **43**(4): 547–9.
9. Ministry of Health and Consumer Affairs. INSS. Plan de Humanización de la Asistencia Hospitalaria. https://ingesa.sanidad.gob.es/Publicaciones-y-Documentaci-n/Publicaciones/Descargas-gratuitas/Plan-de-Humanizaci-n-de-la-Asistencia-Hospitalaria.html (last accessed on April 15, 2024).
10. Ministry of Health of the Community of Madrid. Plan de Humanización de la Asistencia Sanitaria 2016–2019. www.comunidad.madrid/transparencia/informacion-institucional/planes-programas/plan-humanizacion-asistencia-sanitaria-2016-2019 (date last accessed April 15, 2024).
11. HU-CI Project Certification Working Group. *Manual of good practices of humanization in Intensive Care Units.* Madrid: HU-CI Project; 2019. https://proyectohuci.com/es/buenas-practicas/ (date last accessed April 15, 2024).
12. D. Escudero, L. Martín, L. Viña, et al. Visiting policy, design and comfort in Spanish intensive care units. *Rev Calid Asist* 2015; **30**(5): 243–50.
13. B.H. Riley, J. White, S. Graham, A. Alexandrov. Traditional/restrictive vs patient-centered intensive care unit visitation: perceptions of patients' family members, physicians, and nurses. *Am J Crit Care* 2014; **23**(4): 316–24.
14. B.T. Pun, R. Badenes, G. Heras La Calle, et al. Prevalence and risk factors for delirium in critically ill patients with COVID-19 (COVID-D): a multicentre cohort study. *Lancet Respir Med* 2021; **9**(3): 239–50.
15. M. Imanipour, F. Kiwanuka, S. Akhavan Rad, et al. Family members' experiences in adult intensive care units: a systematic review. *Scand J Caring Sci* 2019; **33**(3): 569–81.
16. E. Azoulay, J.F. Timsit, C.L. Sprung, et al. Prevalence and factors of intensive care unit conflicts: the conflicus study. *Am J Respir Crit Care Med* 2009; **180**(9): 853–60.
17. A. Alonso-Ovies, J. Álvarez, C. Velayos, et al. Expectations of critically ill patients' relatives regarding medical information: a qualitative research study. *Rev Calidad Asistencial* 2014; **29**(6): 325–33.
18. Á. Alonso-Ovies, G. Heras La Calle. ICU: a branch of hell? *Intensive Care Med* 2016; **42**(4): 591–2.
19. J. Barr, G.L. Fraser, K. Puntillo, et al. Clinical practice guidelines for the management of pain, agitation, and delirium in adult patients in the Intensive Care Unit: executive summary. *Am J Health Syst Pharm* 2013; **70**(1): 53–8.
20. J.L. Vincent, Y. Shehabi, T.S. Walsh, et al. Comfort and patient-centred care without excessive sedation: the eCASH concept. *Intensive Care Med* 2016; **42**(6): 962–71.
21. M. Moss, V.S. Good, D. Gozal, et al. A critical care societies collaborative

statement: burnout syndrome in critical care health-care professionals. A call for action. *Am J Respir Crit Care Med* 2016; **194** (1): 106–13.

22. M.M. van Mol, E.J. Kompanje, D.D. Benoit, et al. The prevalence of compassion fatigue and burnout among healthcare professionals in intensive care units: a systematic review. *PLoS One* 2015; **10**(8): e0136955.

23. S. Saha, H. Noble, A. Xyrichis, et al. Mapping the impact of ICU design on patients, families and the ICU team: a scoping review. *J Crit Care* 2022; **67**: 3–13.

24. R.A. Aslakson, J.R. Curtis, J.E. Nelson. The changing role of palliative care in the ICU. *Crit Care Med* 2014; **42**(11): 2418–28.

25. J.L. Monzón Marín, I. Saralegui Reta, R. Abizanda Campos, et al. Recommendations for treatment at the end of life of the critically ill patient. *Med Intensiva* 2008; **32**(3): 121–33.

26. R.D. Truog, M.L. Campbell, J.R. Curtis, et al. Recommendations for end-of-life care in the intensive care unit: a consensus statement by the American College of Critical Care Medicine. *Crit Care Med* 2008; **36**(3): 953–63.

Chapter 17

Family-Centered Care in the ICU and Hospital

Cassiano Teixeira and Regis Goulart Rosa

Introduction

The intensive care unit (ICU) is designed to utilize life-sustaining technology, and ICU clinicians are adept at preserving lives amidst rapid decision-making with limited information. The inherent nature of the ICU gives rise to a mandate to use life-sustaining technology (when consistent with patient values and preferences), characterized by medical social scientists as "providing the optimal care that is technically feasible; the only acknowledged constraint is the state of the art" [1]. Although technological advancements have undeniably decreased mortality in critical illness, there is increasing awareness that an exclusive focus on technology may overshadow the human dimensions of care [2], transforming the patient into a body requiring organ maintenance, obscured behind the machinery (see Chapter 16 for additional information) [1]. Moreover, critically ill patients often have communication challenges, posing difficulties for the ICU team in understanding and upholding individual values, goals, and preferences [3]. Additionally, when surrogate decision-makers assume the responsibility of making treatment decisions for critically ill patients, accurately representing the patient's preferences is often challenging [4,5].

In this chapter, we explore the history and definition of Patient and Family-Centered Care (PFCC), elucidate interventions to foster PFCC, spotlight the shortcomings of the current model, and suggest future directions. Increasing evidence underscores the profound impact of critical illness on family members of the critically ill and the need for care that appreciates their value. Family members often endure much of the decision-making burden when critically ill patients are unable to participate due to their illness [6]. Moreover, more than 50% of survivors of critical illness develop disabilities that require assistance by a caregiver once they return home, which can place a substantial burden on family members [7,8]. Approximately 25% to 50% of family members of the critically ill and survivors of critical illness experience psychological symptoms, including acute stress, post-traumatic stress disorder (PTSD), generalized anxiety, depression, and caregiver burden [9,10], a constellation of symptoms referred to as "Post-Intensive Care Syndrome-Family" (PICS-F; see Chapter 48 for additional information) [10,11]. Awareness of the need to enhance outcomes for family caregivers has been increasing with the recognition that their support in the ICU can positively affect patient outcomes [12,13]. Structured interventions and approaches to aid family members of critically ill patients are imperative to alleviate the strain of the critical illness crisis and to prepare family members for the challenges of decision-making and caregiving.

PFCC acknowledges the paramount role of the family in a critically ill patient's recovery and outlines the healthcare team's responsibilities to support families of seriously ill patients. PFCC, which is centered on the needs, values, and preferences of patients and their families, is widely acknowledged as an integral aspect of healthcare delivery [14]. Although the concept is theoretically simple, evidence indicates that the implementation of PFCC is challenging, particularly in the technical environment of the ICU [1,10].

Definitions

The definitions of "family" and "family-centered care" were formulated based on input from the PFCC-guideline writing committee, composed in part by previous ICU patients and their family members [10]. *Family* is determined by the patient or, in the case of minors or those lacking decision-making capacity, by their surrogate decision-makers, who may or may not have a personal connection with the patient. Family generally includes individuals who offer support and share a substantial relationship with the patient. *Family-centered care* involves an approach to healthcare that respects and addresses the unique needs and values of individual families. Practicing PFCC in the ICU focuses on addressing the needs, values, and preferences of both patients and their families by actively involving them in the care process, particularly when patients are unable to communicate on their own. Effective PFCC may include allowing families to visit more freely, bringing them into daily care routines and medical rounds, and offering emotional support through tools like ICU diaries and better communication strategies.

Quantifying the Problem

Approximately 30% of critically ill patients and their families experience disrespect during their ICU stay, which can harm relationships with the care team, cause enduring adverse effects, and even risk physical harm [15,16]. Over one-third of ICUs have a poor "climate of mutual respect," potentially fostering such inappropriate behaviors and contributing to deficiencies in patient care [17]. ICU clinician burnout may result in part from witnessing or participating in acts of dehumanization and disrespect [18].

Dignity refers to the inherent worth of every human being, while respect involves the behavioral or social norms that appropriately recognize and honor this dignity [1]. Executing respectful care entails recognizing fundamental human needs, acknowledging patient uniqueness, and attending to vulnerability [19]. Providing respectful care should be recognized as a system-level outcome, and it should be measured using validated tools that evaluate specific clinician behaviors, including providing greetings and introductions, demonstrating good bedside manner, listening, sharing information, attending to modesty, honoring preferences, and responding to needs and requests, all of which are simple yet powerful actions that promote humanization [20,21]. The Ethical Decision-Making Climate Questionnaire is a tool used to assess the decision-making climate by examining four domains: interdisciplinary collaboration, communication, physician leadership, and ethical environment [1]. Addressing disrespectful interactions as patient safety events and applying quality and safety frameworks, such as root cause analysis, can be important steps in leading to more respectful care delivery [22].

Interventions to Promote Patient-Centered and Family-Centered Care

Promote Family Presence in the ICU

Active collaboration between healthcare team members and patient families in the ICU is crucial for PFCC [23]. Family presence interventions include unrestricted family visitation,

Box 17.1 Adult ICU family-centered care recommendations [10]

Promote family presence in the ICU

- Provide family members with the choice of an open or flexible presence at the bedside tailored to their needs. This approach should offer support for staff and encourage positive collaboration with families to enhance family satisfaction.
- Offer family members of critically ill patients the opportunity to engage in interdisciplinary team rounds, aiming to improve communication satisfaction and foster increased family engagement.
- Extend the option for family members of critically ill patients to be present during resuscitation efforts, ensuring the assignment of a staff member to support the family throughout the process.

Provide support to family members

- Incorporate family education programs into clinical care, as these programs have proven to be beneficial in the ICU setting. They contribute to the reduction of anxiety, depression, post-traumatic stress, and generalized stress among family members while simultaneously enhancing family satisfaction with care.
- Provide families in ICUs with informational leaflets detailing the ICU environment to mitigate family member anxiety and stress.
- Implement ICU diaries as a strategy to alleviate family member anxiety, depression, and post-traumatic stress.
- Introduce validated decision support tools for family members in the ICU setting when applicable, utilizing existing validated tools to optimize the quality of communication, enhance medical comprehension, and decrease family decisional conflict.
- For surrogates of ICU patients deemed by clinicians to have a poor prognosis, employ a communication approach such as the "VALUE" mnemonic (Value family statements, Acknowledge emotions, Listen, Understand the patient as a person, Elicit Questions) during family conferences. This facilitates effective clinician-family communication.

Improve communication with family members

- Implement routine interdisciplinary family conferences within the ICU to enhance family satisfaction with communication, build trust in clinicians, and mitigate conflicts between clinicians and family members.
- Include family-centered communication training for ICU clinicians as a component of critical care training. This initiative is designed to improve clinician self-efficacy and enhance family satisfaction.
- Advocate for healthcare clinicians in the ICU to adopt structured communication approaches, such as the "VALUE" mnemonic. This involves incorporating active listening, expressing empathy, and making supportive statements regarding non-abandonment and decision-making, especially when communicating with family members. Additionally, offer a written bereavement brochure to family members of critically ill patients nearing the end of life. This strategy aims to decrease family anxiety, depression, and post-traumatic stress while enhancing family satisfaction with communication.

Implementation of specific consultations and ICU team members

- Provide proactive palliative care consultation to decrease ICU and hospital lengths of stay among selected critically ill patients (e.g., advanced dementia, global cerebral ischemia after cardiac arrest, patients with prolonged ICU stay, and patients with subarachnoid hemorrhage requiring mechanical ventilation).

- Provide ethics consultation to decrease ICU and hospital lengths of stay among critically ill patients for whom there is a value-related conflict between clinicians and family.
- Include social workers in the interdisciplinary team to participate in family meetings to improve family satisfaction.
- Assign family navigators (care coordinators or communication facilitators) to families throughout the ICU stay to improve family satisfaction with physician communication, decrease psychological symptoms, and reduce costs of care and ICU and hospital lengths of stay.
- Offer spiritual support from a spiritual advisor or chaplain to families of ICU patients to meet their expressed desire for spiritual care and accreditation standard requirements.

Enhance operational and environmental factors

- Enact protocols to ensure the appropriate and standardized application of sedation and analgesia during the withdrawal of life support.
- Engage nurses in decision-making processes regarding care goals and equip them with training to offer support to family members. This is part of a comprehensive program aimed at reducing ICU and hospital lengths of stay and enhancing communication quality in the ICU.
- Institute hospital policies that endorse family-centered care in the ICU, contributing to the enhancement of the family experience.
- Acknowledge the documented harm associated with noise and implement practices for noise reduction and environmental hygiene in ICUs. Additionally, utilize private rooms, when possible, to heighten patient and family satisfaction.
- Prioritize family sleep considerations and furnish families with sleep surfaces to alleviate the impact of sleep deprivation.

participation in daily rounds with the ICU team, and the option to be present during cardiopulmonary resuscitation (CPR) and other procedures (see Box 17.1) [24,25]. Such interventions are linked to reduced anxiety among family members, improved patient and family satisfaction with care [26,27], shorter ICU length of stay, and decreased risk of delirium in the patient [28,29]. The stress of having a loved one in the ICU often translates into clinically significant symptoms of depression, anxiety, and PTSD. The RECOVER study highlighted that 67% of family members experienced depressive symptoms during the ICU stay, which persisted in 43% of family members one year following discharge [30]. This psychological stress, which can significantly impact caregivers' quality of life, can be mitigated through family engagement in care. Actively engaging family members in patient care activities, such as bathing the patient or providing massage, results in the perception of increased respect, collaboration, and support, and in turn, reduces symptoms of PTSD after patient discharge or death [31]. Consequently, family engagement policies and practices are integral components of the recommended ABCDEF care bundle proposed by the Society of Critical Care Medicine, where "F" represents family engagement and empowerment (see Chapter 11 for additional information) [32].

In a meta-analysis of 52 randomized controlled trials (RCTs) that primarily focused on communication, providing information, delivering care, and addressing the needs of family members, family-centered interventions improved several outcomes in the adult ICU, benefiting both patients and healthcare workers [33]. About two-thirds of these interventions were beneficial to family members, with improved mental health outcomes, including reduced incidence of anxiety and depression, and increased satisfaction with patient care.

The COVID-19 pandemic led to the de-implementation of many family-centered care practices, resulting in compromised PFCC [34]. Bereaved family members of COVID-19 patients reported poor communication, inadequate support, feelings of abandonment and powerlessness, and disruptions in typical end-of-life rituals, contributing to complicated grief. Restricted family presence correlated with delayed decisions to limit life-sustaining treatments, prolonged ICU stays, and a higher risk of delirium for ICU patients with COVID-19 [35]. These restrictions also negatively affected healthcare workers, contributing to moral distress and burnout in critical care providers.

Provide Support to Family Members

PFCC necessitates recognizing family members as unique individuals. Various interventions prioritize learning about patients, redirecting attention to personhood, preventing dehumanization, and fostering deeper connections among patients, families, and clinicians.

To enhance the experience of families in the ICU setting, several strategies can be employed. First, incorporating family education programs, including nurse-led family interventions, psychological support for family members, family participation in daily rounds, and multidisciplinary approaches, into clinical care is essential [36,37,38,39]. Additionally, providing families with informational leaflets or access to web-based resources about the ICU environment can be valuable [40]. These strategies collectively contribute to reducing anxiety, depression, PTSD, and generalized stress among family members, while also increasing their satisfaction with the care provided [41].

Furthermore, implementing ICU diaries can be an effective strategy for family engagement. ICU diaries further affirm personhood and provide support for patients and families (see Chapter 18 for additional information). Both family members and clinicians can write in ICU diaries, documenting words of encouragement and meaningful moments in the ICU stay, which in turn enables patients to reconstruct their illness narrative, counteract distressing memories, and regain a sense of reality following resolution of their critical illness [41]. In a study by Parker and colleagues [42], ICU diaries were found to alleviate symptoms of PTSD, anxiety, and depression in ICU patients and potentially improve family outcomes, including improved sense of well-being, improved coping mechanisms, enhanced communication, and reduced levels of PTSD, anxiety, and depression [43]. Family members appreciate ICU diaries for aiding in the comprehension of medical information, facilitating communication with clinicians, and humanizing the relationship with both the patient and the ICU team [44].

Improve Communication with Family Members

A fundamental principle of PFCC lies in elucidating and providing care that is consistent with a patient's values, goals, and preferences. Because family members often assume the role of surrogate decision-makers when patients are no longer capable of making their own decisions, engaging in regular, structured communication with the healthcare team is widely advocated, with a focus on meeting surrogates' informational needs. International guidelines and meta-analyses emphasize communication interventions as integral to comprehensive family support strategies [10,45,46]. These guidelines highlight key skills, such as explaining the patient's medical condition, establishing a trusting partnership, providing emotional support, assessing patient or surrogate understanding of the information presented, and clarifying the role of surrogate decision-makers. They also stress the importance of ensuring patients and surrogates recognize available choices and their preferred roles in decision-making. Additionally, the guidelines recommend explaining treatment options, eliciting patient values and goals, deliberating with surrogates, and ultimately making a well-informed decision together through the process of shared decision-making [10,45]. Higher quality family communication is associated with fewer reported conflicts between families and physicians and greater family satisfaction with the care provided [10,45].

It is always recommended to use proven communication strategies in family conferences in the ICU. One such example is the VALUE communication strategy, which aims to cultivate effective and empathetic interactions between healthcare clinicians and families of critically ill patients [47]. The essential components of the VALUE communication strategy are: valuing family statements (recognizing and appreciating contributions from family members), acknowledging emotions (validating and addressing emotional experiences), listening (prioritizing active listening to comprehend family concerns), understanding the patient as a person (considering patients holistically), and eliciting questions (encouraging family involvement and inquiries). By integrating these principles, the VALUE strategy strives to enrich communication, enhance family satisfaction, and establish a compassionate healthcare environment within the ICU. Moreover, enhancing communication with nonverbal patients is crucial to enable their participation in decision-making and to express their needs. Strategies aimed at improving nonverbal patients' communication abilities include the use of communication boards, speaking valves, and leak speech for mechanically ventilated patients [48].

Implementation of Specific Consultations and ICU Team Members

The use of targeted consultations and ICU team members can enhance patient management by providing proactive palliative care consultations to reduce ICU and hospital lengths of stay among critically ill patients [4,7,11,49]. Ethics consultations should be offered to address value-related conflicts between clinicians and families, which can also decrease ICU and hospital lengths of stay and increase both family and healthcare provider satisfaction. Incorporating social workers into the interdisciplinary team to engage in family meetings also improves family satisfaction [50]. Assigning family navigators (care coordinators or communication facilitators) throughout the ICU stay can enhance family satisfaction with physician communication, mitigate psychological symptoms, and reduce care costs and length of stay [10]. Additionally, providing spiritual support from a spiritual advisor or chaplain can address the expressed needs for spiritual care; enhance spiritual well-being, hope, and satisfaction with life; and help alleviate feelings of loneliness among critically ill patients while also meeting accreditation standards (see Chapter 15 for additional information) [10,51].

Enhance Operational and Environmental Factors

To enhance operational and environmental factors in the ICU, it is crucial to implement standardized protocols for the appropriate use of sedation and analgesia during mechanical ventilation and the withdrawal of life support [52,53]. Additionally, involving nurses in decision-making processes related to goals of care and providing them with specialized training to support family members effectively can help reduce ICU and hospital lengths of stay and improve communication quality within the ICU [54].

Optimally designed ICUs establish a healing environment that also humanizes the medical setting, alleviates environmental stressors, supports patients and families, and mitigates staff stress [55,56,57,58]. ICU design guidelines, derived from both ICU-specific and non-ICU-specific evidence, now guide the planning of ICU spaces [59]. Recommendations include considering maximum bed capacity, using noise-absorbing materials and natural lighting, and optimizing storage unit placement. Certain design features within the ICU may enhance patient and family outcomes, particularly those related to psychological well-being, stress reduction, and overall satisfaction [57]. These features include elements that facilitate noise reduction, such as sound-absorbing ceiling tiles; windows for exposure to natural light; private individual rooms; access to outdoor spaces or views connecting with nature (see Chapter 21 for additional information); and ventilation and filtration systems ensuring high air quality [57].

Understanding the literature regarding ICU design is challenging. Heterogeneity in design features, participant groups, and the outcomes measured complicates the understanding of the impact of specific ICU design characteristics on patient-, family-, and healthcare professional-related outcomes. Implementing protocols to promote sleep hygiene, noise reduction, and respect for others requires a cultural shift that is tailored to accommodate the workflows of individual institutions and critical care settings; this requires educating ICU physicians, nurses, and ancillary staff in addition to ongoing measurement of performance and protocol compliance.

The Future of Patient- and Family-Centered Care

Considerable progress in promoting PFCC within the ICU has been observed in recent years; however, three key areas require additional focus: addressing healthcare delivery disparities, enhancing PFCC, and deliberately fostering a humanized work environment in the ICU for the benefit of patients, families, and staff.

Addressing Health Disparities Through Patient-Centered and Family-Centered Care

Racial, ethnic, and socioeconomic disparities are key risk factors in the development of acute illness, chronic disease, and death, irrespective of country (see Chapter 25 for additional information). Discrepancies in the incidence and outcomes of critical illness include factors at the individual, hospital, and community levels [60]. Noteworthy variations surface in PFCC-centric practices, particularly with respect to communication regarding serious illness and end-of-life care [61,62]. Multiple factors, including impaired and inconsistent access to care, provider implicit biases, healthcare literacy, and patient and family preferences, contribute to the observed disparities in end-of-life care [63].

PFCC, attuned to the preferences, needs, values, and cultural traditions of patients and families, has the potential to mitigate inequities in the delivery of critical care. Specialized palliative care consultation and a focus on enhanced and culturally-competent communication around serious illness can help improve care disparities [64]. Hospitals are urged to categorize clinical, quality, and patient experience data based on race, ethnicity, language, and socioeconomic status to effectively identify and address disparities [65]. Health systems should equip clinicians with evidence-based training in racial and cultural sensitivity and implicit and explicit bias. Patients and families from diverse cultures and linguistic backgrounds should be included in research studies to better inform the best practices of PFCC.

Fostering Meaningful Engagement of Patients and Families

PFCC positions healthcare delivery to revolve around the experiences and priorities of patients and families [39]. Three critical aspects define PFCC: engagement unfolds along a continuum, engagement manifests at various levels, and numerous factors influence patients' willingness and ability to engage. Healthcare systems primarily incorporate patient and family opinions and feedback through participation in Patient and Family Advisory Councils (PFACs), which are comprised of current and former patients, family members, and caregivers in collaboration with clinicians and hospital leadership. PFACs aim to enhance the patient and family experience, provide advice on patient care practices, shape organizational policies and procedures, and recommend improved measurement and evaluation of PFCC [1]. Genuine PFCC avoids tokenism, wherein unequal power relations limit the roles of patients and families within the healthcare system [66]. Organizations are encouraged to empower PFACs for meaningful projects, integrate patient and family advisors into governance bodies, ensure participation in community health activities, and foster diverse representation through recruitment and sustained engagement.

Similarly, patient engagement in research demands a shift from mere participation to active partnership [67]. The benefits of PFCC in the research process are manifold, including lived experiences shaping research questions and priorities, pinpointing patient- and family-centered outcomes, and guiding researchers in refining enrollment and consent processes [68].

Promoting Humanism Among Healthcare Providers

Healthcare providers (HCPs) in critical care often experience high rates of burnout syndrome (BOS), characterized by exhaustion, depersonalization, and diminished personal accomplishment [18]. BOS correlates with adverse mental health outcomes for healthcare workers, elevated job turnover, decreased patient satisfaction, and compromised quality of care. Addressing BOS among ICU clinicians is crucial for advancing PFCC. Effectively mitigating BOS demands a comprehensive approach, which aligns with the broader theme of humanizing the ICU for patients, families, and clinicians (see Chapter 16 for additional information). Recognizing and appreciating the humanity of HCPs is paramount to fostering a humanized environment for patients and families; however, implementing programs to monitor and enhance respectful practices may inadvertently increase clinician workload, potentially heightening the risk of burnout. Therefore, interventions aimed at humanizing the ICU must be meticulously crafted and evaluated to ensure the intended outcome of enhancing the ICU environment for all stakeholders.

Conclusions

PFCC is a cornerstone of high-quality health care, with advantages for patients, families, and clinicians. The intricate landscape of critical care, with its highly technical aspects, exposes patients and families to the risk of dehumanization, making PFCC implementation a complicated but essential endeavor. To succeed in PFCC within the ICU, intentionally fostering respectful and humanizing interactions among patients, families, and clinicians is crucial [69]. Current initiatives in PFCC concentrate on recognizing the personhood of patients, fostering patient-centered and family-centered communication, and implementing interventions to enhance family presence, support, and participation. The impact of healthcare disparities on PFCC and how PFCC can act as a catalyst for promoting health equity require further investigation. Achieving optimal PFCC necessitates genuine engagement with patients and families from diverse backgrounds and experiences, offering invaluable insights for enhancing both quality improvement initiatives and research efforts.

As we strive for these advancements, creating a humanistic ICU environment is not only beneficial for our patients but also a collective responsibility for our well-being. In fostering a humanistic ICU, we embrace a path that transcends the technicalities, affirming the shared humanity that binds patients, families, and clinicians in the journey toward comprehensive and compassionate critical care (see Figure 17.1).

Family-Centered Care

Family Presence
Flexible Visits
Comfortable ICU Design

Environmental Factors
A to F Bundle
ICU-noise Reduction
Sleep Protocol

Support to Family
Education Program
Information Leaflets
ICU Diaries
Decision Support Tools Use

Medical Leadership
Mentorship
Decision-Making

Communication
Interdisciplinary Conferences
Nurse Engagement
Structured Communication Approaches

Specific Consultations
Palliative Support
Ethics Support
Social Worker Support
Communication Facilitators
Spiritual Support

Figure 17.1 ICU family-centered care strategies.

Key Points

1. The technical demands of critical care can lead to dehumanization, making the implementation of PFCC in the ICU both challenging and essential.
2. PFCC in ICU focuses on meeting the needs, values, and preferences of patients and their families by actively involving them in decision-making and care, especially when patients cannot communicate on their own. Effective PFCC might involve encouraging family presence through open visitation policies, bringing them into daily care routines and medical rounds, and supporting their emotional well-being with tools like ICU diaries and improved communication methods.
3. PFCC practices have been linked to lower anxiety levels, increased satisfaction for both patients and families, and a reduced risk of delirium and post-traumatic stress disorder.
4. Implementing PFCC comes with challenges, such as ensuring staff are well-trained and have the resources to genuinely involve families, all while managing the stress healthcare providers face.
5. Fostering a humanistic ICU environment through PFCC promotes compassion and reinforces the shared humanity between patients, families, and clinicians.

References

1. K.E. Secunda, J.M. Kruser. Patient-centered and family-centered care in the intensive care unit. *Clin Chest Med* 2022; **43**: 539–50.
2. L. Todres, K.T. Galvin, I. Holloway. The humanization of healthcare: a value framework for qualitative research. *Int J Qual Stud Health Well-Being* 2009; **4**: 68–77.
3. C.L. Auriemma, C.A. Nguyen, R. Bronheim, et al. Stability of end-of-life preferences: a systematic review of the evidence. *JAMA Intern Med* 2014; **174**: 1085–92.
4. H. Kim, J. Cho, S. Shin, S.S. Kim. Uncertainty in surrogate decision-making about end-of-life care for people with dementia: An integrative review. *J Adv Nurs* 2024; 1–16.
5. R. Spalding. Accuracy in surrogate end-of-life medical decision-making: a critical review. *Appl Psychol Heal Well-Being* 2021; **13**: 3–33.
6. J.M. Luce. A history of resolving conflicts over end-of-life care in intensive care units in the United States. *Crit Care Med* 2010; **38**: 1623–9.
7. S.L. Hiser, A. Fatima, M. Ali, D.M. Needham. Post-intensive care syndrome (PICS): recent updates. *J Intensive Care* 2023; **11**: 1–10.
8. M.S. Herridge, É. Azoulay. Outcomes after critical illness. *N Engl J Med* 2023; **388**: 913–24.
9. R.D. Adelman, L.L. Tmanova, D. Delgado, et al. Caregiver burden: a clinical review. *JAMA* 2014; **311**: 1052–9.
10. J.E. Davidson, R.A. Aslakson, A.C. Long, et al. Guidelines for family-centered care in the neonatal, pediatric, and adult ICU. *Crit Care Med* 2017; **45**: 103–28.
11. S.E. Bryant, K. McNabb. Postintensive care syndrome. *Crit Care Nurs Clin North Am* 2019; **31**: 507–16.
12. J. Lynn. Strategies to ease the burden of family caregivers. *JAMA* 2014; **311**: 1021–2.
13. A. Heydari, M. Sharifi, A.B. Moghaddam. Family participation in the care of older adult patients admitted to the intensive care unit: a scoping review. *Geriatr Nurs* 2020; **41**: 474–84.

14. A.C.K.B. Amaral, G.D. Rubenfeld. The future of critical care. *Curr Opin Crit Care* 2009; **15**: 308–13.
15. W.O. Cooper, O. Guillamondegui, O. J. Hines, et al. Use of unsolicited patient observations to identify surgeons with increased risk for postoperative complications. *JAMA Surg* 2017; **152**: 522–9.
16. V.A. Entwistle. Hurtful comments are harmful comments: respectful communication is not just an optional extra in healthcare. *Heal Expect* 2008; **11**: 319–20.
17. N. Duma, S. Maingi, W.D. Tap, et al. Establishing a mutually respectful environment in the workplace: a toolbox for performance excellence. *Am Soc Clin Oncol Educ B* 2019; **39**: e219–26.
18. M. Moss, V.S. Good, D. Gozal, et al. A critical care societies collaborative statement: Burnout syndrome in critical care health-care professionals a call for action. *Am J Respir Crit Care Med* 2016; **194**: 106–13.
19. S.M. Brown, É. Azoulay, D. Benoit, et al. The practice of respect in the ICU. *Am J Respir Crit Care Med* 2018; **197**: 1389–95.
20. S.C. Handley, S. Bell, I.M. Nembhard. A systematic review of surveys for measuring patient-centered care in the hospital setting. *Med Care* 2021; **59**: 228–37.
21. G. Geller, E.D. Branyon, L.K. Forbes, et al. ICU-RESPECT: An index to assess patient and family experiences of respect in the intensive care unit. *J Crit Care* 2016; **36**: 54–9.
22. L. Sokol-Hessner, G.J. Kane, C.L. Annas, et al. Development of a framework to describe patient and family harm from disrespect and promote improvements in quality and safety: a scoping review. *Int J Qual Heal Care* 2019; **31**: 657–68.
23. R.G. Rosa and C. Teixeira. Flexible ICU visiting policies. In: Haines K.J., McPeake J., Sevin C.M., eds. *Improving Critical Care Survivorship*. Springer International Publishing, 2021; 103–9.
24. K.A. Milner. Evolution of visiting the intensive care unit. *Crit Care Clin* 2023; **39**: 541–58.
25. S.J. Beesley, R.O. Hopkins, L. Francis, et al. Let them in: family presence during intensive care unit procedures. *Ann Am Thorac Soc* 2016; **13**: 1155–9.
26. R.G. Rosa, M. Falavigna, D.B. da Silva, et al. Effect of flexible family visitation on delirium among patients in the intensive care unit: the ICU visits randomized clinical trial. *JAMA* 2019; **322**: 215–28.
27. R.G. Rosa, J.A.S. Pellegrini, R.B. Moraes, et al. Mechanism of a flexible ICU visiting policy for anxiety symptoms among family members in Brazil: a path mediation analysis in a cluster-randomized clinical trial. *Crit Care Med* 2021; **49**: 1504–12.
28. A.P. Nassar-Junior, B.A.M.P. Besen, C.C. Robinson, et al. Flexible versus restrictive visiting policies in ICUs. *Crit Care Med* 2018; **46**: 1175–80.
29. Y. Wu, G. Wang, Z. Zhang, et al. Efficacy and safety of unrestricted visiting policy for critically ill patients: a meta-analysis. *Crit Care* 2022; **26**: 1–15.
30. J.I. Cameron, L.M. Chu, A. Matte, et al. One-year outcomes in caregivers of Critically Ill Patients. *N Engl J Med* 2016; **374**: 1831–41.
31. Y. Ito, M. Tsubaki, M. Kobayashi, et al. Effect size estimates of risk factors for post-intensive care syndrome-family: a systematic review and meta-analysis. *Hear Lung*. 2023; **59**: 1–7.
32. A. Marra, E.W. Ely, P.P. Pandharipande, M.B. Patel. The ABCDEF bundle in critical care. *Crit Care Clin* 2017; **33**: 225–43.
33. G. Wang, R. Antel, M. Goldfarb. The impact of randomized family-centered interventions on family-centered outcomes in the adult intensive care unit: a systematic review. *J Intensive Care Med* 2023; **38**: 690–701.
34. J. Mailer, K. Ward, C. Aspinall. The impact of visiting restrictions in intensive care units for families during the COVID-19 pandemic: an integrative review. *J Adv Nurs*. 2023; **11**: 1–15.

35. C. Kanaris. Moral distress in the intensive care unit during the pandemic: the burden of dying alone. *Intensive Care Med* 2021; **47**: 141–3.

36. K. Kydonaki, M. Takashima, M. Mitchell. Family ward rounds in intensive care: an integrative review of the literature. *Int J Nurs Stud* 2021; **113**: 103771.

37. L. Rose, L. Istanboulian, A.C.K.B. Amaral, et al. Co-designed and consensus based development of a quality improvement checklist of patient and family-centered actionable processes of care for adults with persistent critical illness. *J Crit Care* 2022; **72**: 154153.

38. F. Kiwanuka, N. Sak-Dankosky, Y. Hagos. The evidence base of nurse-led family interventions for improving family outcomes in adult critical care settings: a mixed method systematic review. *Int J Nurs Stud* 2020; **125**: 104100.

39. A. Klimesch, A. Martinez-Pereira, C. Topf, et al. Conceptualization of patient-centered care in Latin America: a scoping review. *Heal Expect* 2023; **26**: 1820–31.

40. T.S.R. Haack, R.G. Rosa, C. Teixeira, et al. Does an educational website improve psychological outcomes and satisfaction among family members of intensive care unit patients? *Crit Care Sci* 2023; **35**: 31–6.

41. C. Teixeira, R.G. Rosa. Unmasking the hidden aftermath: postintensive care unit sequelae, discharge preparedness, and long-term follow-up. *Crit Care Sci* 2024; **36**: e20240265.

42. A.M. Parker, T. Sricharoenchai, S. Raparla, et al. Posttraumatic stress disorder in critical illness survivors: a metaanalysis. *Crit Care Med* 2015; **43**: 1121–9.

43. Y. Zheng, L. Zhang, S. Ma, et al. Care intervention on psychological outcomes among patients admitted to intensive care unit: an umbrella review of systematic reviews and meta-analyses. *Syst Rev* 2023; **12**: 1–12.

44. M. Garrouste-Orgeas, A. Périer, P. Mouricou, et al. Writing in and reading ICU diaries: qualitative study of families' experience in the ICU. *PLoS One* 2014; **9**: 1–10.

45. A.A. Kon, J.E. Davidson, W. Morrison, et al. Shared decision making in ICUs: an American college of critical care medicine and American thoracic society policy statement. *Crit Care Med* 2016; **44**: 188–201.

46. H. Lee, Y. Park, E.J. Jang, Y.J. Lee. Intensive care unit length of stay is reduced by protocolized family support intervention: a systematic review and meta-analysis. *Intensive Care Med* 2019; **45**: 1072–81.

47. S. Warrillow, K.J. Farley, D. Jones. Ten practical strategies for effective communication with relatives of ICU patients. *Intensive Care Med* 2015; **41**: 2173–6.

48. N.R. Kuruppu, W. Chaboyer, A. Abayadeera, K. Ranse. Augmentative and alternative communication tools for mechanically ventilated patients in intensive care units: a scoping review. *Aust Crit Care* 2023; **36**: 1095–109.

49. N. Nakanishi, K. Liu, J. Hatakeyama, et al. Post-intensive care syndrome follow-up system after hospital discharge: a narrative review. *J Intensive Care* 2024; **12**: 1–16.

50. S.S. Au, P. Couillard, A. Roze-Des-Ordons, et al. Outcomes of ethics consultations in adult ICUs: a systematic review and meta-analysis. *Crit Care Med* 2018; **46**: 799–808.

51. T.Y. Bulut, Y. Çekiç, B. Altay. The effects of spiritual care intervention on spiritual well-being, loneliness, hope and life satisfaction of intensive care unit patients. *Intensive Crit Care Nurs* 2023; **77**: 103438.

52. R.G. Rosa, C. Teixeira, M. Sjoding. Novel approaches to facilitate the implementation of guidelines in the ICU. *J Crit Care* 2020; **60**: 1–5.

53. C. Teixeira. High mortality in Brazilian intensive care units can be a problem of laws rather than a technical one: focus on sedation practices. *Crit Care Sci* 2023; **35**: 230–2.

54. R.G. Rosa, C. Teixeira, S. Piva, A. Morandi. Anticipating ICU discharge and long-term follow-up. *Curr Opin Crit Care* 2024; **30**: 157–64.
55. N.A. Halpern, E. Scruth, M. Rausen, D. Anderson. Four decades of intensive care unit design evolution and thoughts for the future. *Crit Care Clin* 2023; **39**: 577–602.
56. D.K. Hamilton, J. Kisacky, F. Zilm. Critical care 1950 to 2022: evolution of medicine, nursing, technology, and design. *Crit Care Clin* 2023; **39**: 603–25.
57. S. Saha, H. Noble, A. Xyrichis, et al. Mapping the impact of ICU design on patients, families and the ICU team: a scoping review. *J Crit Care* 2022; **67**: 3–13.
58. R.J. Branaghan. Human factors in medical device design: methods, principles, and guidelines. *Crit Care Nurs Clin North Am* 2018; **30**: 225–36.
59. D.R. Thompson, D.K. Hamilton, C.D. Cadenhead, et al. Guidelines for intensive care unit design. *Crit Care Med* 2012; **40**: 1586–600.
60. G.J. Soto, G.S. Martin, M.N. Gong. Healthcare disparities in critical illness. *Crit Care Med* 2013; **41**: 2784–93.
61. J. Yang. The effects of race and racial concordance on patient-physician communication: a systematic review of the literature. *J Racial Ethn Heal Disparities* 2018; **5**: 117–40.
62. J.D. Thornton, K. Pham, R.A. Engelberg, et al. Families with limited English proficiency receive less information and support in interpreted intensive care unit family conferences. *Crit Care Med* 2009; **37**: 89–95.
63. M. Bazargan, S. Bazargan-Hejazi. Disparities in palliative and hospice care and completion of advance care planning and directives among non-Hispanic Blacks: a scoping review of recent literature. *Am J Hosp Palliat Med* 2021; **38**: 688–718.
64. L.T. Starr, N.R. O'Connor, S.H. Meghani. Improved serious illness communication may help mitigate racial disparities in care among Black Americans with COVID-19. *J Gen Intern Med* 2021; **36**: 1071–6.
65. I.W. Maina, T.D. Belton, S. Ginzberg, et al. A decade of studying implicit racial/ethnic bias in healthcare providers using the implicit association test. *Soc Sci Med* 2018; **199**: 219–29.
66. U. Majid. The dimensions of tokenism in patient and family engagement: a concept analysis of the literature. *J Patient Exp* 2020; **7**: 1610–20.
67. K.M. Fiest, B.G. Sept, H.T. Stelfox. Patients as researchers in adult critical care medicine: fantasy or reality? *Ann Am Thorac Soc* 2020; **17**: 1047–51.
68. J.V. Selby, L. Forsythe, H.C. Sox. Stakeholder-driven comparative effectiveness research an update from PCORI. *JAMA* 2015; **314**: 2235–6.
69. M. Ostermann, J.L. Vincent. ICU without borders. *Crit Care* 2023; **27**: 1–5.

Chapter 18

ICU Diaries

Peter Nydahl, Brigitte Teigeler, and Teresa Deffner

Introduction

Patients in critical care often experience extreme situations that can have profound implications for their future cognitive and emotional health. Severe infections, neurological insults, medications, sedation, delirium, and other conditions can lead to disturbances in consciousness and fragmented and distorted memories. Many survivors of critical illness do not have memories of their time in the intensive care unit (ICU), often reporting memory gaps of days to weeks covering one of the most important periods of their life. Other survivors cannot distinguish real experiences from dreams and hallucinations that occurred while they were critically ill. Family members and friends may struggle managing their emotions and experience feelings of helplessness as they watch their loved ones endure critical illness and its attendant complications. Coping with these experiences can be challenging. A diary for critically ill patients and their families, the "ICU diary," is one solution to improve understanding of the ICU experience, to fill in memory gaps, and to process the complex emotions experienced by patients and their loved ones.

The ICU Diary

Definition

ICU diaries, also referred to as journals, narratives, or books, are defined as personalized narratives written *for* and *to* critically ill patients [1] and are different than diaries that report specific medical information, such as blood pressure and blood sugar. ICU diaries are written *for* patients by families and clinicians in plain language and include significant medical events, personal perceptions and reflections, and interpersonal interactions. Diaries can also written *to* patients, with entries starting with greetings (e.g., "Hello Mr. Smith, today is … "), and concluding with a signature (e.g., "Your nurse, Betty") [2]. Following discharge or death, these diaries are given to surviving patients or their bereaved families to improve their understanding of and coping with their experiences in the ICU.

Development

The development of ICU diaries can be traced back to the early 1990s, primarily in Scandinavian countries such as Sweden and Denmark. Initially conceptualized as a tool to build a coherent story and to reduce the psychological trauma experienced by patients and their families following ICU discharge, the idea swiftly gained traction within critical care settings [3]. Over the years, the concept has progressed via a grassroots movement from an empirically practical instrument to a scientifically grounded intervention [4].

This progression mirrors a broader shift toward patient-centered care paradigms, where holistic well-being encompasses not only physical, but also psychological, emotional, and social aspects. Following the identification and description of post-intensive care syndrome (PICS) and post-intensive care syndrome family (PICS-F), early interventions to improve long-term outcomes in survivors of critical illness and their loved ones, including ICU diaries, have become an increasingly important focus of research [5].

Purpose

ICU diaries serve several purposes, addressing the needs of patients, families, and the clinicians caring for them. ICU diaries function as memory aids for patients who may experience PICS, a cluster of physical, cognitive, and psychological challenges following critical illness. Through the reconstruction of their ICU experiences by reading diary entries, patients acquire a sense of coherence and affirmation, fostering a feeling of empowerment in their journey toward recovery [6]. Moreover, ICU diaries facilitate communication and closure for families grappling with the trauma of witnessing a loved one's critical illness. They also offer insights into daily care routines, medical interventions, and emotional support provided by healthcare teams, thereby promoting transparency and trust within the patient-family-caregiver relationship [7]. From the clinician's perspective, ICU diaries serve as invaluable documentation tools, allowing healthcare providers to retrospectively assess a patient's progress and to identify areas for enhancement in care delivery. Additionally, they provide a platform for reflection and debriefing among ICU personnel, creating a culture of ongoing learning and quality advancement [8]. ICU diaries may be helpful for parents and families of premature babies during the acute hospital stay and may be beneficial in the long-term for the grown-up children for whom they were written [9]. Due to the increased risk of disturbing experiences and memories, diaries can also be used for hospitalized patients with delirium outside of the ICU [10]. Finally, diaries can be used for, with, and by dying patients, who may use the diaries to write farewell letters to others [11,12], and by their bereaved families to cope with the loss of their loved one [13].

Format

ICU diaries are most commonly paper diaries, often including a cover picture and blank pages for entries. There are no evidence-based recommendations for a specific format or size. Diaries can range from simple spiral notebooks to professionally printed books with the hospital's logo. Additionally, diaries may include (see Figures 18.1, 18.2, and 18.3):

- A get-to-know-me page with personal information and photos of the patient, including their preferred name; profession; religion; favorite foods, music, and television shows; and pets
- A brief introduction on the purpose of the diary and how to write and read diary entries
- A disclaimer that the diary is not part of the medical record and includes personal views only
- Photos of the patients, visitors, and staff [14]
- A glossary with medical terms, procedures, and personnel written in plain language
- Contact information for questions after discharge
- A description of PICS and recommendations for further rehabilitation

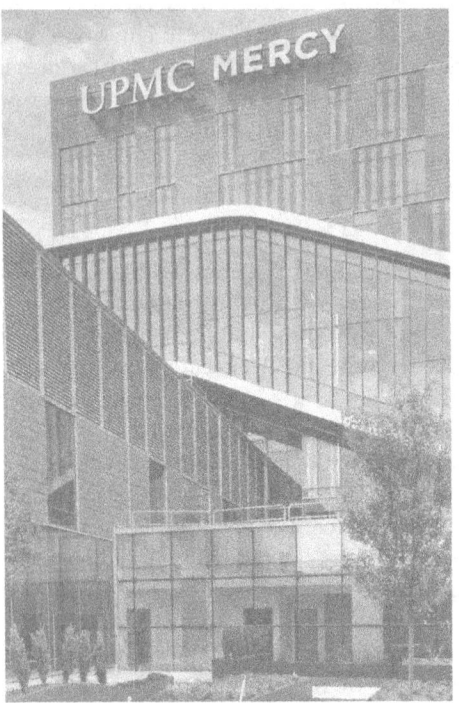

Figure 18.1 Table of contents of an ICU diary.

Due to technological advancement, digital ICU diaries, which can be internet-based, app-based, or written by artificial intelligence [1,2,15], are becoming increasingly popular. Although feasible and convenient, digital diaries raise several ethical concerns, including data security, misuse in social media, and privacy.

Psychological Concepts

Memory Building

Critical illness itself, treatment in the ICU, and disturbing experiences of disorientation and delirium can all be traumatizing events, unified by the core criterion of the real or perceived threat to life experienced directly by patients and indirectly by their relatives [16]. Such situations of extreme psychological stress frequently result in impaired memory formation [20,21], and survivors of critical illness often suffer from fragmented factual and non-factual memories [17]. Consequently, the ICU experience is frequently not remembered in a linear, unified, and coherent manner, irrespective of sedation strategies utilized during treatment or cognitive impairment caused by the illness. By reconstructing the fragmented narrative of critical illness, ICU diaries support memory formation and reconciliation by facilitating coherence and meaning-making and by enhancing patients' and families' sense of control [10,18]. Three main mechanisms can be assumed here. First, diaries facilitate communication between patients and relatives; reading the diary together, for example, helps to

GET TO KNOW ME

Please share information you would like us to know about you as a person.

- Important people to you
- Music you enjoy
- Pets
- Shows you like to watch on TV
- Things that cheer you up
- Things that help you relax
- How you spend your free time

Figure 18.2 Example of a get-to-know-me page from an ICU diary.

verbalize the experience of illness [19], which contributes to coherent memory formation. Second, diaries can help differentiate fragmented memories into factual and nonfactual memories, which supports the formation of a coherent illness story [20]. Third, from a psycho-traumatological perspective, by reading an ICU diary, memories can be better differentiated into real and unreal experiences. Furthermore, the memory building process is enriched through the information added by the ICU diary.

Coping and Grief Support

For relatives, writing in the ICU diary is a component of active, emotion-focused coping to reduce stressful experiences, and writing provides a sense of agency and purpose [19]. It also enables relatives to stay connected to and communicate with patients who temporarily may not be able to meaningfully interact with their environment [21]. Even bereaved relatives of dying patients have found ICU diaries helpful both during and after the ICU stay [13] by helping them recognize the severity of the patient's illness and reminding them how the patient was provided comfort during the dying process. Through these mechanisms, ICU

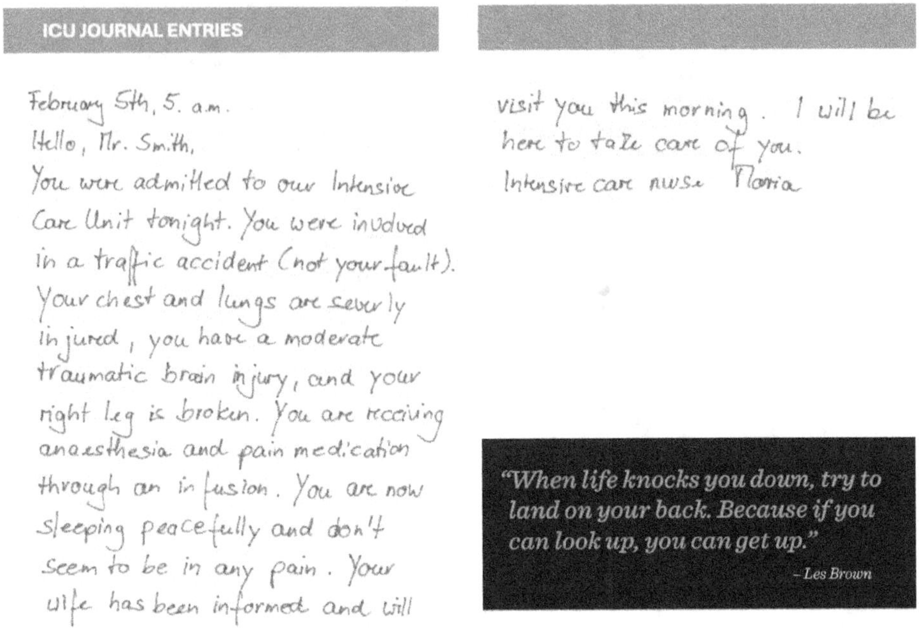

ICU JOURNAL ENTRIES

February 5th, 5 a.m.
Hello, Mr. Smith,
You were admitted to our Intensive Care Unit tonight. You were involved in a traffic accident (not your fault). Your chest and lungs are severly injured, you have a moderate traumatic brain injury, and your right leg is broken. You are receiving anaesthesia and pain medication through an infusion. You are now sleeping peacefully and don't seem to be in any pain. Your wife has been informed and will visit you this morning. I will be here to take care of you.
Intensive care nurse Maria

> "When life knocks you down, try to land on your back. Because if you can look up, you can get up."
> – Les Brown

Figure 18.3 Example of an ICU diary entry.

diaries can help reduce both the acute and long-term emotional burden that relatives of critically ill patients often experience. Furthermore, ICU diaries are a component of holistic care. Writing can be understood as part of humanized intensive care (see Chapter 16 for additional information) [22], with personalized entries in ICU diaries showing patients that they are respected and cared for uniquely and individually.

Evidence for ICU Diaries

Impact on Psychological Symptoms in Patients

Numerous studies have demonstrated the beneficial effects of ICU diaries on patients' psychological well-being following hospital discharge. In general, patients appreciate the diaries and perceive them as a valuable tool for understanding critical illness and challenges in recovery [23], but reading them can be challenging and may elicit strong emotions as patients recount the trauma that they and their loved ones experienced [24]. A meta-analysis of 10 studies including 1,210 patients showed with moderate confidence a decreased risk for psychological symptoms in survivors of critical illness. The odds ratio (OR) for development of post-traumatic stress disorder (PTSD), as assessed by the PTSS-14 or IES-R, was reduced by nearly one-third in 9 studies totaling 1,174 patients (OR 0.69, 95% confidence interval CI 0.51–0.93, p=0.01), with no heterogeneity. The risk for development of depression was reduced by nearly half in 6 studies totaling 622 patients (OR 0.56, CI 0.37–0.85, p=0.006), with no heterogeneity. The risk of developing anxiety was not significantly reduced in 6 studies including 622 patients (OR 0.45, CI 0.19–1.06, p=0.07), with moderate heterogeneity ($I2 = 66\%$, p=0.01) [25].

Synthesis of 17 qualitative studies showed that many patients expressed positive experiences with the ICU diary. They found it beneficial for comprehending the challenges they faced during critical illness, gaining insight into the recovery journey, reconciling disturbing memories like nightmares and delusions, recognizing the significance of family and loved ones' presence during their ICU stay, and fostering a human connection with healthcare professionals who aided them in overcoming their critical condition [22].

Impact on Psychological Symptoms in Family Members

Although ICU diaries intuitively help family members manage the uncertainty and distress of the ICU environment, somewhat surprisingly, studies suggest that ICU diaries do not meaningfully decrease rates of PTSD, depression, or anxiety among family members of critically ill patients [26,27]. Qualitative data indicate that ICU diaries may improve coping mechanisms within families, offering a tangible tool to navigate the complexities of their loved one's illness journey [28]. By providing a documented narrative of the patient's ICU experience, these diaries facilitate a deeper understanding and acceptance of the emotional challenges such as stress, hope, and (potential) grief, aiding in the family's ability to cope with the emotional turmoil. Moreover, they serve as a catalyst for the development and maintenance of relationships, encouraging open communication with survivors of critical illness and empathy among family members [28]. Perhaps most notably, ICU diaries have been associated with post-traumatic growth among families, enabling them to find meaning and resilience in the face of adversity [19].

Outcome on Healthcare Workers

The psychological well-being of the ICU staff is often overlooked, and the emotional demands of critical care can be a challenging burden for clinicians, resulting in high rates of burnout syndrome among providers of critical care [29]. There is limited evidence for the effects of implementing ICU diaries on clinicians' emotional health and job satisfaction. Clinicians report increased reflection skills, awareness of the needs of patients and families, and recognition of the importance of PICS [30]. Writing diaries is perceived as beneficial for clinicians by enhancing relationships with patients and families, improving the quality of care delivered, and enabling humanization of critical care [28]. Writing diaries requires empathy, but not emotional closeness, and clinicians might need to be educated regarding this difference [31]. The impact of writing in ICU diaries on clinician burnout rates and other symptoms of emotional stress has not yet been examined.

Practical Aspects

The implementation of ICU diaries into daily practice represents a fusion of critical care and compassionate storytelling. As clinicians strive to deliver patient-centered care amidst the demands of patients with critical illness, understanding the practical aspects of ICU diaries becomes crucial for successful implementation.

Indication

ICU diaries are typically indicated for patients with, or at high risk for, prolonged ($\geq$ 48 hours) disturbances in consciousness due to sedation, delirium, coma, or other reasons, where gaps in memory formation are likely to occur. The decision to initiate ICU diaries is predicated upon a nuanced assessment of patient needs, family dynamics, clinical context, and culture [2]. Challenges may include language barriers or difficulties with writing, but these can be overcome with smartphones, translators, and other technological support. There are no strong contraindications for initiating ICU diaries. In patients with difficulties in understanding language (severe and persistent aphasia or severe dementia, for example), a diary may be less beneficial for the patient but still helpful for the family; in such cases, individualized decisions are required [2].

Writing Style

The writing style of ICU diaries is different from that of medical records [32]. Diaries should be written in plain language with a style that is appreciative, honest, and descriptive, as if addressing the patient directly. Each entry should include a salutation, date, and signature and should consider cultural aspects, such as the use of local dialects. Entries should be written in a polite and respectful manner, and offending phrases should be avoided (see the Case Report below). Due to data protection, including specific medical diagnoses should be avoided, but a general description such as "pneumonia" instead of ARDS can be used. Any potentially sensitive information (such as a new diagnosis of HIV or information regarding substance abuse, for example) should be avoided.

Content may vary during the course of critical illness. During the first days, the reasons for admission and initial treatments may be reported, while during the stabilization and recovery phases, attention may turn to major events (such as extubation) and the initiation of rehabilitation therapies. While clinicians often report medical stories, families more commonly write about their feelings and impressions. Patients are interested in not only the story, but also in how they behaved in different phases of their illness and how they interacted with the staff and family members [33]. Importantly, diaries should be tailored to individual preferences and cultural sensitivities, fostering a sense of ownership and authenticity in the narrative construction process [34].

Handing Over and Reading Diaries

In most studies, diaries were given to patients after a defined time frame, ranging between three weeks and three months. The handover of the ICU diary can potentially evoke traumatic recollections, and perhaps unsurprisingly, an estimated 10–15% of patients refuse to read their diary. Accordingly, it is imperative to adhere to specific recommendations during this process. The patient should be fully alert and engaged in their journey of illness and recovery. Based on expert opinion, the optimal timepoint would be when patients are raising concerns about persistent weakness, helplessness, and impaired memory. They should also be prepared for the possibility of encountering intense emotions while reading the diary. Additionally, it is essential for relatives to feel capable accompanying the patient during the initial reading. Should both the patient and their relatives struggle with intense symptoms, it is advisable to have psychosocial professionals oversee the reading session. There is no one-size-fits-all recommendation regarding when to start reading the diary, as patients hold varying perspectives on the matter [10]. In the event that the patient died and the family was not given the diary at the time of death, it should be stored for one year in case the family asks for it later.

Implementation

ICU diaries have emerged as a promising intervention to support the psychological well-being of patients, families, and healthcare professionals. Successful implementation of ICU diaries hinges upon robust infrastructure, interdisciplinary collaboration, and stakeholder engagement [35]. Dedicated diary coordinators or champions play a crucial role in diary initiation, maintenance, and quality assurance. Standardized templates, training modules, and periodic audits ensure consistency and fidelity to diary objectives. Furthermore, fostering a culture of openness and transparency within ICU teams cultivates sustainability of diary projects over time [36].

The integration of ICU diaries into clinical care pathways represents a paradigm shift toward patient-centered and trauma-informed approaches within critical care settings. Despite their potential benefits, the implementation of ICU diaries is fraught with challenges stemming from organizational, cultural, and logistical barriers. Understanding the interplay between these barriers and facilitators is essential for fostering successful adoption and dissemination of diary initiatives [37].

Several key barriers and facilitators have emerged from the synthesis of literature on ICU diary implementation (see Table 18.1) [2].

Barriers

- Organizational culture: Resistance to change, hierarchical structures, and competing priorities within healthcare organizations impede the adoption of ICU diaries.
- Resource constraints: Limited staffing, time constraints, and financial resources hinder the sustainability of diary initiatives.
- Staff training and education: Inadequate training in diary maintenance and lack of awareness regarding the rationale and benefits of diaries contribute to implementation challenges.
- Patient and family engagement: Variability in patient and family preferences, language barriers, and cultural differences pose challenges in engaging stakeholders in diary usage.
- Data security and confidentiality: Concerns regarding privacy breaches, data protection regulations, and medico-legal implications deter healthcare professionals from incorporating diaries into routine practice.

Facilitators

- Leadership support: Strong leadership commitment, vision, and advocacy for diary initiatives promote organizational buy-in and facilitate culture change.
- Interdisciplinary collaboration: Multidisciplinary teamwork, communication, and collaboration enhance the feasibility and acceptability of diary implementation.
- Standardized protocols: Development of clear guidelines, protocols, and templates streamlines diary maintenance and ensures consistency in documentation.
- Patient and family involvement: Empowering patients and families as partners in decision-making and diary documentation fosters engagement and ownership.
- Technology integration: Utilization of electronic platforms, mobile applications, and telehealth technologies facilitates remote access to diaries and enhances communication between stakeholders.

Table 18.1 Barriers and solutions for implementing ICU diaries

Barrier	Potential Solutions
Organizational Culture	
Resistance to change	• Prioritize ICU diaries as an important project for the healthcare team • Find support from other medical or psychological professions • Communicate feedback from patients and families to staff about their experiences with critical care and ICU diaries • Seek out and address concerns raised by team members • Share evidence regarding efficacy of diaries • Communicate timeline for change • Ensure frequent meetings for feedback • Implementing ICU diaries is generally feasible if 50% of the nursing staff supports the project
Hierarchical structures	• Build a multidisciplinary team with frontline staff and leaders • Include patient and family representatives on the team • Cooperate with local self-help groups such as ICUsteps.org
Competing priorities within healthcare organizations	• Emphasize the importance of patient-centered care • Highlight potential for public awareness by reporting the project in local newspapers, TV, and social media
Resource Constraints	
Limited staffing	• Communicate that ICU diaries are written primarily for patients with long stays, representing 10–20% of all patients • Provide a brief tutorial for writing in diaries • Provide information in native languages if nurses with different languages are supporting
Time constraints	• Spend ~3–5 minutes writing the diary entry, which is generally feasible • Consider writing entries the following day or during handover to next shift

Staff Training and Education

Inadequate training in diary maintenance
- Provide training sessions for writing diary entries with staff
- Provide written examples of diary entries and guidelines for writing entries (see www.icu-diary.org for templates)

Lack of awareness regarding the rationale and benefits of diaries
- Provide literature about diaries, including scientific studies
- Share interviews and quotes from patients and families or videos on social media

Patient and Family Engagement

Variability in patient and family preferences
- Ask patients and families for their preferences
- Include a get-to-know-me page to learn more about patients' preferences
- Consider including photos of the patient and family members
- Place an example diary in the waiting area for families to review
- Provide information in plain language via flyers or the hospital's website

Language barriers and cultural differences pose challenges
- Provide diary templates in different languages
- Consider use of electronic or web-based diaries with translation apps
- Consider use of voice messages or dictation into electronic diaries by voice for those with difficulties reading and writing

Data Security and Confidentiality

Concerns regarding privacy breaches and data protection regulations
- Establish local standard operating procedures with rules for the use of ICU diaries
- Determine if consent from patients or representatives is required in your country
- Provide a declaration that the diary is not part of the hospital's medical record but property of the patient
- Develop policies for data protection and privacy specific for your ICU or institution

The identification of barriers and facilitators in ICU diary implementation underscores the complexity of integrating novel interventions into clinical practice. Addressing organizational, cultural, and logistical barriers requires multifaceted strategies encompassing leadership engagement, staff training, resource allocation, and patient involvement. Moreover, leveraging facilitators such as interdisciplinary collaboration, standardized protocols, and technological innovations can optimize the feasibility and sustainability of diary projects. Furthermore, specific countries may have their own cultures and barriers, requiring specific facilitators [2].

Conclusion

In conclusion, the successful implementation of ICU diaries hinges upon a holistic understanding of the barriers and facilitators encountered in clinical practice. By addressing systemic challenges and capitalizing on facilitative factors, healthcare organizations can foster a culture of narrative-based care that promotes resilience, empathy, and healing for patients, families, and healthcare professionals within critical care.

Case Report

This following case report is a fictitious extract from an ICU diary. The example is compiled from various case histories, but all personal information has been deidentified. The diary entries may look different in practice; they may be shorter or more simply written. It is not important to write texts that are as "nice" as possible but to find the words that suit you and that can help the patient to understand their ICU stay later.

Brief History

Peter Smith, a 57-year-old teacher, was admitted to the Accident & Emergency (A&E) department approximately one hour following a road traffic accident. He presented with loss of consciousness and multiple limb injuries, including a fractured right femur. Subsequent X-rays and a CT scan revealed a moderate traumatic brain injury with a Glasgow Coma Scale score of 11. Consequently, the medical team initiated a pharmacological-induced coma and intracranial pressure monitoring. Mr. Smith was transferred to the ICU that night. On the fifth day of hospitalization, Mr. Smith developed pneumonia, which was effectively treated with antibiotics. Following this complication, his recovery progressed smoothly, and he was transferred to the general ward on the tenth day post-admission, free from further complications.

Diary Entries

February 5th, 5 a.m.

Hello, Mr. Smith,

You were admitted to our Intensive Care Unit tonight. You were involved in a traffic accident (not your fault). Your chest and lungs are severely injured, you have a moderate traumatic brain injury, and your right leg is broken. You are receiving anesthesia and pain medication through an infusion. You are now sleeping peacefully and don't seem to be in any pain. Your wife has been informed and will visit you this morning. I will be here to take care of you.

Intensive care nurse Maria

February 5th, 11 a.m.

My sweetheart, I'm so relieved to finally be with you! I couldn't sleep all night long after the police called me in the evening! But since I'm here with you, I've been feeling calmer. The doctors seem optimistic that you'll fully recover! You do look quite battered with all those bruises, but you seem to be sleeping soundly. They've placed you in an induced coma. The young doctor explained to me that this way, you won't feel any pain, and your body can recover faster. The nurses have been very kind and showed me everything: the ventilator assisting your breathing, the chest drainage to remove blood and air from your lungs, the intracranial pressure probe, and the IV drips you're receiving. They also gave me this intensive care diary. When you wake up from the coma it can help you to understand and process the time you've lost. I think it's a wonderful idea!

Now, I'm going to head home and call Sophie right away. She had her final exam this morning, and I didn't want her to worry about her dad while she was taking it. I love you. See you this evening, Katrin

February 6th, 2 p.m.

Hello, Mr. Smith,

Today has been quite hectic in your room. A new patient arrived, and we had to resuscitate him. It was very hectic and involved a lot of running around. Thankfully, your roommate made it. It seemed as if you hadn't noticed any of the excitement. But what do we know? Some patients say after waking up that they can remember things and situations during the coma. Others incorporate their experiences into their dreams. This can be very disturbing, as can all the noises you hear. There is a lot of equipment here that makes a lot of noise: the ventilator, the chest tube, etc. In any case, if you are dreaming, I hope you have nice dreams and remain as stable as you are right now.

Best wishes, Intensive care nurse Tim

February 6th, 8 p.m.

Dad, what are you doing?! I was so scared when Mum called me yesterday after the exam! Instead of celebrating, I dropped everything and got the next train home right away! We'll do the celebrating later – together! And until you're well again, we'll visit you often. The people here are so nice. They look after you very well and tell us what we can do for you. We talk to you a lot and have brought your favorite Bach piano concerto with us. Maybe you'll listen to it! I'll be back tomorrow; I have a lot of time now that the exams are over. Please get well again very quickly, Dad! Love, Sophie

February 9th, 8 p.m.

Hello, Mr. Smith,

You've remained stable over the past few days. We were able to remove the chest tube and the intracranial pressure probe. The MRI showed no bleeding – that was good news for all of us, especially for your wife and daughter. They were so happy. Unfortunately, you have had a fever since this afternoon, and we suspect pneumonia. Your breathing is fast and shallow, and your sleep is restless. You are on antibiotics now. Hopefully, they will work quickly!

Take care, Intensive care nurse Tim

February 10th, 5 p.m.

If only I knew what I could do for you, my sweetheart! I feel so helpless. I'm really scared: What if the fever doesn't go down? I hope so much that the antibiotics will work soon. The nurses told me that it may take a while. I don't want to go home while you're so sick. I'm sitting here, talking to you, holding your hand and playing the music Sophie brought for you over and over again. The nurses have told me that you are aware of many things even in an induced coma, even if you don't react to them. I want you to feel me so much. I am always there for you. Your Katrin

February 11th, 1 p.m.

Hello, Mr. Smith,

You were very restless all night, the night shift said. Your temperature has risen again to over 40 degrees. You were moaning and tossing and turning as if you were having a nightmare. Fortunately, the fever is down now, and you are sleeping peacefully. The antibiotics seem finally to be working. You are breathing calmly, and I haven't had to suction you as often as yesterday. Your wife sat next to your bed all morning and held your hand. Your daughter was also here. Now the two of them are off to the canteen. When the fever has been down for 24 hours and you are stable, we can bring you out of the induced coma. I do hope that works out.

Intensive care nurse Maria

February 11th, 8 p.m.

Finally, finally! The fever is gone. I am so relieved! The doctor came this evening and said that everything looks fine. I'll be so happy when you can finally wake up and I can talk to you again. Your boss called me yesterday. He wanted to hear how you were doing. He said that all your colleagues are thinking of you and sending their regards. And last night the woman who caused the accident got in touch. She wanted to know how you are and would like to visit you. But we can discuss that later when you're feeling better. I'm so glad when you're back with me! Now I'm going home and I'm sure I'll get a good night's sleep. I'll be back with you tomorrow morning. Your Katrin

February 12th, 10 a.m.

Hello sweetheart! Unfortunately, the wake-up attempt won't start before midday. However, the doctors and nurses have already explained everything to me. First, you will be given less anesthetic to see how you react. If this works well and you become more alert, the anesthetic can be stopped completely. However, these drugs are still stored in your body, so it can take a while for you to wake up properly. Nurse Tim explained it yesterday to me. Once you're fully awake, the breathing tube can be removed. I'm so excited! Love, Katrin

February 12th, 7 p.m.

Hello Mr. Smith,

That went so well! We started to stop the anesthetic at midday today. You opened your eyes shortly afterwards and showed signs of thirst. We then moistened your lips and mouth, and you raised your hand briefly as if to say thank you. Then you went back to sleep. This afternoon you sweated a lot. Your blood pressure was high, and you were quite upset. But that's all normal. You recognized your wife with a smile. Your wife was overjoyed. Some patients don't recognize their relatives straight away, and some have delusions. It went very well, and we can now start to wean you off the ventilator. You'll be fine!

Intensive care nurse Tim

February 13th, 1 p.m.

When I came into your room this morning, you smiled at me and looked very relaxed. The doctors removed the artificial respiration at 10 a.m. You managed to breathe on your own again the first time. That doesn't always work so well, nurse Maria told me. Later, the physiotherapist came and put you on the edge of the bed with Maria for the first time. Sophie took a photo of it – you look very proud and are holding your thumb up! I am so grateful! If everything continues to go so well, the doctors have just told me that we can go to the general ward tomorrow or the day after. I'm so happy! Even if it's a shame because the people here are taking such good care of you. I'll take the intensive care diary with me. Maybe we can read it together at home and I can tell you what you've missed. I am so incredibly happy and relieved! Love, Katrin

Key Points

1. Many patients requiring critical care experience stressful and traumatic situations, which often result in fractured and delusional memories. These patients are at increased risk of developing depression, anxiety, and PTSD, which comprise the psychological sequelae of PICS.
2. Family members of loved ones requiring critical care are similarly traumatized and may find coping with their loved one's illness challenging. They, too, are at risk for developing depression, anxiety, and PTSD, which comprise PICS-F.
3. ICU diaries are written for and to critically ill patients by families and staff. They can be read by patients during rehabilitation to reconstruct their illness narrative, fill memory gaps, and reframe delusional memories; can be used by families to establish communication with their loved one, cope with their illness, and build resilience; and can be used by healthcare team members to enhance relationships with patients and their families, reflect on the care provided, and humanize critical care.
4. Diaries contain daily entries written in plain language that recount the crisis, stabilization, and recovery of patients. They may also include a get-to-know-me page, photos, and glossaries of medical terms, procedures, and personnel.
5. ICU diaries have been shown to decrease PTSD and depression in survivors of critical illness; qualitatively, they have been shown to be helpful to families as they process and cope with their loved one's critical illness.
6. Numerous barriers to building an ICU diary program exist, but these can be overcome with strong leadership, interdisciplinary collaboration, standardized protocols, and patient and family involvement.

References

1. E. Peschel, S. Krotsetis, A.-H. Seidlein, P. Nydahl. Opening Pandora's box by generating ICU diaries through artificial intelligence: a hypothetical study protocol. *Intensive Crit Care Nurs* 2024; **82**: 103661.
2. P. Nydahl, I. Egerod, M.M. Hosey, et al. Report on the Third International Intensive Care Unit Diary Conference. *Crit Care Nurse* 2020; **40**: e18–e25.
3. C.G. Backman, S.M. Walther. Use of a personal diary written on the ICU during critical illness. *Intensive Care Med* 2001; **27**: 426–9.
4. I. Egerod, S.L. Storli, E. Akerman. Intensive care patient diaries in Scandinavia: a comparative study of emergence and evolution. *Nurs Inq* 2011; **18**: 235–46.
5. D.M. Needham, J. Davidson, H. Cohen, et al. Improving long-term outcomes after discharge from intensive care unit: report from a stakeholders' conference. *Crit Care Med* 2012; **40**: 502–9.
6. I. Egerod, K.H. Schwartz-Nielsen, G.M. Hansen, E. Laerkner. The extent and application of patient diaries in Danish ICUs in 2006. *Nurs Crit Care* 2007; **12**: 159–67.
7. P. Heindl, A. Bachlechner, P. Nydahl, I. Egerod. Extent and application of patient diaries in Austria: process of continuing adaptation. *Nurs Crit Care* 2019; **24(6)**: 343–8.
8. P. Nydahl, D. Knueck, I. Egerod. Extent and application of ICU diaries in Germany in 2014. *Nurs Crit Care* 2015; **20**: 155–62.
9. S.H. Wang, T. Owens, A. Johnson, E.A. Duffy. Evaluating the feasibility and efficacy of a pediatric intensive care unit diary. *Crit Care Nurs Q* 2022; **45**: 88–97.
10. P. Nydahl, T. Deffner. Use of diaries in intensive care unit delirium patients: German nursing perspectives. *Crit Care Nurs Clin North Am* 2021; **33**: 37–46.
11. C.B. Willis. *Lasting words*. Brattleboro, Vermont: Green Writers Press; 2013.
12. L.M. Högvall, I. Egerod, S.F. Herling, et al. Finding the right words: a focus group investigation of nurses' experiences of writing diaries for intensive care patients with a poor prognosis. *Aust Crit Care* 2023; **36**: 1011–18.
13. A. Galazzi, I. Adamini, G. Bazzano, et al. Intensive care unit diaries to help bereaved family members in their grieving process: a systematic review. *Intensive Crit Care Nurs* 2022; **68**: 103121.
14. S. Daltveit, L. Kleppe, M.O. Petterteig, A.L. Moi. Photographs in burn patient diaries: a qualitative study of patients' and nurses' experiences. *Intensive Crit Care Nurs* 2024; **82**: 103619.
15. M.M.C. van Mol, N. Tummers, C. Leerentveld, et al. The usability of a digital diary from the perspectives of intensive care patients' relatives: a pilot study. *Nurs Crit Care* 2024: **29(6)**: 1280-9.
16. B.P. Marx, B. Hall-Clark, M.J. Friedman, et al. The PTSD criterion a debate: a brief history, current status, and recommendations for moving forward. *J Trauma Stress* 2024; **37**: 5–15.
17. D.M. Wade, C.R. Brewin, D.C. Howell, et al. Intrusive memories of hallucinations and delusions in traumatized intensive care patients: an interview study. *Br J Health Psychol* 2015; **20**: 613–31.
18. T. Deffner, H. Skupin, F. Rauchfuß. The war in my head: a psychotraumatological case report after a prolonged intensive care unit stay. *Medizinische Klinik, Intensivmedizin und Notfallmedizin* 2020; **115**: 372–9.
19. R. Schofield, B. Dibb, R. Coles-Gale, C.J. Jones. The experience of relatives using intensive care diaries: a systematic review and qualitative synthesis. *Int J Nurs Stud* 2021; **119**: 103927.
20. N. Pattison, G. O'Gara, C. Lucas, et al. Filling the gaps: a mixed-methods study exploring the use of patient diaries in the critical care unit. *Intensive Crit Care Nurs* 2019; **51**: 27–34.
21. M. Garrouste-Orgeas, A. Perier, P. Mouricou, et al. Writing in and reading ICU diaries: qualitative study of families' experience in the ICU. *PLoS One* 2014; **9**: e110146.

22. B. Brandao Barreto, M. Luz, S. Alves Valente do Amaral Lopes, et al. Exploring patients' perceptions on ICU diaries: a systematic review and qualitative data synthesis. *Crit Care Med* 2021; **49**: e707–e18.

23. S. Calzari, M. Villa, S. Mauro, et al. The intensive care unit diary as a valuable care tool: a qualitative study of patients' experiences. *Intensive Crit Care Nurs* 2024; **80**: 103558.

24. A. Engstrom, K. Grip, M. Hamren. Experiences of intensive care unit diaries: 'touching a tender wound'. *Nurs Crit Care* 2009; **14**: 61–7.

25. X. Sun, D. Huang, F. Zeng, et al. Effect of intensive care unit diary on incidence of posttraumatic stress disorder, anxiety, and depression of adult intensive care unit survivors: a systematic review and meta-analysis. *J Adv Nurs* 2021; **77**: 2929–41.

26. P.A. McIlroy, R.S. King, M. Garrouste-Orgeas, et al. The effect of ICU diaries on psychological outcomes and quality of life of survivors of critical illness and their relatives: a systematic review and meta-analysis. *Crit Care Med* 2019; **47**: 273–9.

27. B.B. Barreto, M. Luz, M.N.O. Rios, et al. The impact of intensive care unit diaries on patients' and relatives' outcomes: a systematic review and meta-analysis. *Crit Care* 2019; **23**: 411.

28. B. Brandao Barreto, M. Luz, S.A.V. do Amaral Lopes, et al. Exploring family members' and health care professionals' perceptions on ICU diaries: a systematic review and qualitative data synthesis. *Intensive Care Med* 2021; **47**: 737–49.

29. L. Papazian, S. Hraiech, A. Loundou, et al. High-level burnout in physicians and nurses working in adult ICUs: a systematic review and meta-analysis. *Intensive Care Med* 2023; **49**: 387–400.

30. A.N. Holme, K. Halvorsen, R.S. Eskerud, et al. Nurses' experiences of ICU diaries following implementation of national recommendations for diaries in intensive care units: a quality improvement project. *Intensive Crit Care Nurs* 2020; **59**: 102828.

31. A. Perier, A. Revah-Levy, C. Bruel, et al. Phenomenologic analysis of healthcare worker perceptions of intensive care unit diaries. *Crit Care* 2013; **17**: R13.

32. I. Egerod, D. Christensen. A comparative study of ICU patient diaries vs. hospital charts. *Qual Health Res* 2010; **20**: 1446–56.

33. I. Egerod, D. Christensen. Analysis of patient diaries in Danish ICUs: a narrative approach. *Intensive Crit Care Nurs* 2009; **25**: 268–77.

34. A.H. Nielsen, I. Egerod, T.B. Hansen, S. Angel. Intensive care unit diaries: developing a shared story strengthens relationships between critically ill patients and their relatives: a hermeneutic-phenomenological study. *Int J Nurs Stud* 2019; **92**: 90–6.

35. A. Veloso Costa, O. Padfield, S. Elliott, P. Hayden. Improving patient diary use in intensive care: a quality improvement report. *J Intensive Care Soc* 2021; **22**: 27–33.

36. J. Rogan, M. Zielke, K. Drumright, L.M. Boehm. Institutional challenges and solutions to evidence-based, patient-centered practice: implementing ICU diaries. *Crit Care Nurse* 2020; **40**: 47–56.

37. T.-G. Huynh, M. Covalesky, S. Sinclair, et al. Measuring outcomes of an intensive care unit family diary program. *AACN Adv Crit Care* 2017; **28**: 179–90.

Chapter 19

Music as Therapy in the ICU

Sikandar H. Khan, Sophia Wang, and Babar Khan

Introduction

Delirium is highly prevalent in the intensive care unit (ICU), and prevalence increases with age, with up to 80% of mechanically ventilated older adults experiencing delirium during their ICU stay (see Chapter 8 for additional information) [1,2,3,4,5]. The development of delirium predisposes adults to both in-hospital and long-term complications, including longer ICU and hospital lengths of stay, higher rates of institutionalization following discharge, increased mortality, and newly acquired cognitive impairments or acceleration of dementia [6,7,8,9,10]. In addition to the presence of delirium, its duration and severity also correlate with cognitive impairments and worsened mortality [11,12,13]. Delirium management has conventionally relied on the use of pharmacological agents, commonly typical and atypical antipsychotics, but the recent publication of multiple, well-designed randomized controlled trials (RCTs) have demonstrated no benefit of antipsychotics for delirium prevention or treatment in the ICU [14,15,16,17]. Although other pharmacological agents for the management of delirium show promise, such as the α_2-agonist dexmedetomidine, their use may be limited by untoward side effects, particularly in elderly populations [18,19].

The limitations of pharmacologic management for delirium were acknowledged in the 2018 Society of Critical Care Medicine (SCCM) Pain, Agitation/Sedation, Delirium, Immobility, and Sleep Disruption (PADIS) guidelines [20]. In these guidelines, SCCM recommends managing delirium with the use of multi-component, non-pharmacologic interventions, such as the ABCDEF bundle (see Chapter 11 for additional information), despite low quality of evidence [20]. A pre-post implementation study showed that ABCDEF bundle implementation decreased the odds of developing delirium the next day (AOR 0.60, 95% CI 0.49–0.72), but full adherence to the complete bundle was achieved on only 8% of all ICU days, reflecting the challenges of implementing multicomponent interventions [21]. In the absence of high-quality pharmacological and non-pharmacological options for the prevention and management of ICU delirium, a novel approach integrated in routine care is desirable [22].

Given its calming effects, scalability, and low-risk nature, music may be an ideal non-pharmacological intervention for ICU patients at risk for delirium. As an intervention, music offers generalizable and low-cost delivery to the bedside or within the homes of survivors, expanding beyond the reach of traditional services such as music therapy. If music decreases the incidence of delirium and its attendant long-term adverse outcomes, then music could also potentially reduce the burden of post-intensive care syndrome (PICS). As we describe in this chapter, the multiple effects of music on various symptoms prevalent among critically ill patients and survivors of critical illness offer further insights into its potential mechanistic benefits.

Effects of Music on Pain, Anxiety, Stress, and Sedative Exposure

Music is associated with reduced pain, anxiety, physiologic stress, and sedative exposure in ICU and perioperative patients [23,24]. The beneficial effects of music on pain are presumed to be modulated through changes in circulating levels of β-endorphin [25]. A systematic review and meta-analysis of clinical trials examining the effects of music in ICU patients found that music significantly decreased pain scores by a standardized mean difference of -0.63, translating to a difference of 0.74 points for pain reported on a numerical scale from 0 to 10 [26]. Music was also more efficacious at reducing pain than noise reduction alone (standardized mean difference -0.57). The minimum duration of music listening associated with decreased pain was as brief as 20 to 30 minutes, resulting in a nearly 2-point decrease in self-reported pain scores (on a 0 to 10 scale). Among the 18 randomized trials included in the review, there were no reported adverse effects, highlighting the low-risk nature of music interventions in critically ill patients [26].

A Cochrane review of both critically ill and non-critically ill patients demonstrated that music also has an anxiolytic effect [27]. A subsequent systematic review limited to critically ill patients found that music reduced anxiety measured using a visual analog scale by a standardized mean difference of 1.81, which did not differ significantly from patients who received noise cancellation headphones [28]. While some studies have suggested music may also entrain the autonomic nervous system, thereby leading to reduced blood pressure, respiratory rate, and heart rate, recent evidence in critically ill patients suggests an alternative hypothesis: music's effects on pain and anxiety may instead be synergistically related to its stress-reducing and neurohormonal properties [28,29]. A systematic review found music to be associated with reduced serum cortisol levels in ICU patients; an elevated serum cortisol level is considered a major driver of stress and anxiety and has been implicated in the pathophysiology of delirium [29,30,31]. In a trial of 56 mechanically ventilated patients, listening to preferred, slow-tempo (60–80 beats/minute) music chosen by the research team for one hour twice daily reduced anxiety and lowered sedation frequency and intensity compared with controls [32]. By managing pain and anxiety symptoms, music can potentially reduce exposure to opioid analgesics and sedatives, thereby effectively reducing two risk factors directly implicated in the development of delirium [33,34].

The Effects of Music on Sleep

Sleep is highly disrupted during critical illness (see Chapter 9 for additional information). Music is associated with improvements in sleep quality and mood symptoms that frequently disrupt sleep (e.g., depression and anxiety) [35,36]. In the majority of published studies investigating the impact of music on sleep, researchers tested relaxing music that was played for at least 30 minutes in the evenings. In nonsurgical ICU populations, longer duration of music listening may have more benefit: in one study, for example, listening to music for more than 45 minutes was associated with improved sleep quality (standardized mean difference of 0.93) and less depressive symptoms (standardized mean difference of -1.08). In this study, music was also associated with more non-rapid eye movement stage 3 sleep (N3) and less N2 sleep [36].

Immunomodulatory, Neurohormonal, and Catecholamine Effects of Music

Music exerts a salutary neuromodulatory role on immune regulation via stress-related cytokine production. Stressful events that are severe, prolonged, or have an uncertain duration (e.g., critical illness requiring mechanical ventilation) result in persistent activation of the stress-response system and increased production of pro-inflammatory cytokines [37]. There is growing evidence that playing relaxing music for patients can ameliorate the stress response and reduce inflammation by virtue of decreasing the concentration of circulating cytokines [38,39]. A small study of 10 mechanically ventilated patients in a surgical ICU, for example, showed a reduction in interleukin (IL)-6 concentration after only 60 minutes of investigator-initiated, slow-tempo music composed by Mozart [38]. The investigators concluded that music's ability to modulate IL-6 is a central pathway for stress reduction and may reduce the concentration of circulating cortisol and its pathologic effects on systemic inflammation in critically ill patients [38,39].

In a three-arm pilot trial of 60 patients undergoing non-cardiac surgery, music delivered via headphones was associated with lower circulating levels of natural killer cells, suggesting music may have beneficial immune modulating functions [40]. Given the role of neuroinflammation in the pathophysiology of delirium and the effects of music noted on neuroimmune biology, music may help modulate chemotactic activity implicated in processes upstream of delirium [29].

Delirium pathophysiology is not completely understood, but inflammation and glucocorticoids are implicated as inciting factors in its development [41]. Using a neuroinflammatory lens, delirium can be considered a cytokine-mediated inflammatory syndrome, with pro-inflammatory cytokines, including IL-1, IL-6, IL-8, and tumor necrosis factor (TNF)-α, disrupting the blood brain barrier and recruiting peripheral leukocytes to the central nervous system [41,42,43,44]. The resultant microglial activation produces local pro-inflammatory cytokines (IL-1, TNF-α), reactive oxygen species, expansion of the microglial population, activation of astrocytes, and cholinergic failure, all of which contribute to the development of delirium [45,46,47]. The complementary neuroendocrine hypothesis posits that delirium represents an exaggerated physiologic reaction to acute or chronic stress mediated by high glucocorticoids levels, which impair the ability of neurons to survive metabolic insults [48,49]. Given its potential beneficial effects on modulation of stress pathways mediated by inflammatory cytokines, cortisol, and catecholamines, music may mitigate delirium duration and severity, and accordingly, lessen the risk of developing PICS.

Music and Cognition

Delirium is a complex neuropsychiatric syndrome characterized by acute and fluctuating changes in cognition and consciousness [11,12] and is associated with accelerated cognitive decline (see Chapter 43 for additional information) [12,13,15,18,20]. Patients who experience delirium are at a higher risk of developing Alzheimer's disease and related dementias (ADRD); indeed, up to 71% of survivors of critical illness have mild cognitive impairment (MCI) or ADRD at one year after hospital discharge, and close to 18% are diagnosed with new ADRD within three years following critical illness [2,4,5,6]. Delirium and dementia are likely connected through overlapping neuroinflammatory mechanisms, and music, by reducing neuroinflammation and physiologic stress, has biological plausibility to ameliorate both delirium and subsequent ADRD [50].

Effects of Music on Brain Functional Networks

Music has been shown to have positive effects on attention, cognition, and improving the function of cortical networks, all of which are disrupted in delirium [51,52,53,54,55]. Studies have identified decreased functional connectivity in the posterior cingulate cortex, dorsal anterior cingulate cortex, thalamus, and dorsolateral prefrontal cortex during delirium [51,52]. These brain regions, in association with the limbic system, include networks critical for processing incoming auditory and visual stimuli, as well as focusing, shifting, and sustaining attention [56]. The networks involved in these tasks include the salience and default mode networks; each of these regions has shown increased activation with music [55,57,58,59]. The neurocognitive processing of music involves signal transduction from the cochlea in the inner ear to the auditory brainstem, the thalamus, and ultimately the auditory cortex for perceptual analysis; centers related to emotion, perception, cognition, and the autonomic nervous system are therefore activated during music listening [60]. This leads to positive cortical, subcortical, and limbic system effects on memory, emotion, and stress-related pathways through the autonomic nervous system [60].

As described above, music engages with functional cortical networks, which may enhance its ability to distract patients from auditory and tactile stimuli in the stressful ICU environment [55,59,61,62,63]. In functional MRI studies, numerous cortical and cerebellar areas (e.g., parietal cortex, ventrolateral prefrontal cortex, cerebellum, basal ganglia, thalamus, and premotor areas) were noted to be metabolically active during music listening, and in EEG studies, music increased neural networks and bi-hemispheric communication [54,59,62,63]. Thus, one possible pathway for how music intervention may decrease delirium is through activation and amplification of neural connectivity.

Effects of Music on Cognitive Performance

A variety of studies have tested the effect of music on cognitive performance among healthy older adults and patients with mild cognitive impairment or dementia, but there are few studies testing the effect of music on cognition in survivors of critical illness [64]. In older adults passively listening to music (Mozart and Mahler versus white noise or no music), those listening to Mozart versus no music had improved episodic memory, semantic memory, and processing speed [53].

In non-ICU settings, a variety of approaches have been used in the delivery of music to treat memory disorders. In a recent systematic review, the effects of passive listening, reminiscence listening (listening to familiar music to jog memories), and music therapy were compared in patients with mild cognitive impairment [65,66]. Cognitive performance significantly improved with music therapy (which required music making by patients under the supervision of a highly trained music therapist). In that group, performance on specific items of the Montreal Cognitive Assessment (MoCA) tool suggested that music therapy may have beneficial effects on frontal lobe and executive function. As executive function is predominantly impaired in survivors of critical illness, this raises the possibility that music may similarly provide an effective and low-risk intervention for ICU delirium and survivors of critical illness. Similarly, passive music listening was also associated with improved memory, while reminiscence listening was not. Whether these results translate to ICU patients is not known and needs further study.

In patients with dementia, a systematic review of eight studies identified music therapy as beneficial for cognitive function, although the analysis was limited by varying methodological rigor and high heterogeneity among studies [65]. Nevertheless, the systematic review found that shorter duration of music therapy (less than 20 weeks) and passive listening was associated with improved cognitive performance compared with longer intervention periods or combining activities (including singing or dancing) with music [65].

Implications for the Future: Music as a Scalable Non-pharmacological Intervention for PICS

Music is a highly promising, scalable, non-pharmacological intervention which may help prevent and treat delirium in the ICU, which, in turn, may mitigate the subsequent development of mild cognitive impairment, ADRD, and potentially PICS in a subset of vulnerable patients. Clinical trials, including the NIA-funded Decreasing Delirium through Music (DDM) RCT, will lay the groundwork to identify the neuroprotective mechanisms by which music interventions can reduce the risk of ICU delirium and long-term cognitive impairments [67]. Results from this and other studies will also provide guidance on how music interventions can be designed, customized, delivered, and monitored in pragmatic ways [32,68]. Feasibility studies have provided lessons for the implementation of music interventions so they may achieve high acceptability. These include providing choice of playlists for patients or their families to tailor the listening experience and reduce drop-out from studies. Longer durations of music intervention may also provide more benefit for pain and stress, but sessions as short as 15 minutes were found beneficial in preoperative and postoperative environments. For critically ill patients unable to communicate due to invasive mechanical ventilation or their clinical condition, family members may be a valuable resource to provide culturally suitable and patient-preferred music playlists.

Development and testing of "ready access" interventions like those being tested in the DDM trial to reduce the risk of ADRD may represent a novel advancement in the field of ADRD therapeutics, particularly for at-risk, older adult populations who may not have access to academic tertiary ICU care or who reside in lower- and middle-income areas with limited resources.

Suggestions for Implementing Music in the ICU

These are some important considerations when developing and implementing a "music as medicine" program for critically ill patients.

1. Identify stakeholders (patients, informal caregivers, bedside clinicians, and music therapists) to co-develop a music program that meets the needs of ICU patients. This may personalize a music program to the local clinical environment.
2. Consider providing choice of music and delivery methods (types of music offered, delivery through headphones versus speakers, live or prerecorded music guided by a music therapist, ability to control devices [e.g., to adjust volume], and duration and timing of music programs).
3. While patient-preferred music may have greater acceptability, slow-tempo music may offer more stress-relieving effects.
4. If possible, consider integration of a music as medicine program into the workflow of the busy ICU. This may allow clinicians to harness the pain, anxiety, and stress mitigation properties of music, thereby helping patients better tolerate components of delirium-management protocols (e.g., ABCDEF bundle). In particular, this may offer advantages for spontaneous awakening and breathing trials or mobilization in the ICU.

Key Points

1. Music is associated with reduced pain, anxiety, physiologic stress, and sedative exposure in ICU patients.
2. Music may also offer positive effects on attention and cognition and improve the function of cortical networks, all of which are disrupted in delirium.
3. Compared to playlists personalized to each patient, slow-tempo music may offer greater benefits for pain, anxiety, and sleep in the ICU and be easier to implement and scale within health systems.

References

1. American Psychiatric Association. *Diagnostic and Statistical Manual of Mental Disorders.* 5th ed. American Psychiatric Association; 2013.
2. S.-M. Lin, C.-Y. Liu, C.-H. Wang, et al. The impact of delirium on the survival of mechanically ventilated patients. *Crit Care Med* 2004; **32**: 2254–9.
3. P.P. Pandharipande, T.D. Girard, J. C. Jackson, et al. Long-term cognitive impairment after critical illness. *N Engl J Med* 2013; **369**: 1306–16.
4. T.D. Girard, J.C. Jackson, P. P. Pandharipande, et al. Delirium as a predictor of long-term cognitive impairment in survivors of critical illness. *Crit Care Med* 2010; **38**: 1513–20.
5. E.W. Ely. Delirium as a predictor of mortality in mechanically ventilated patients in the intensive care unit. *JAMA* 2004; **291**: 1753–62.
6. J.C. Jackson, S.M. Gordon, R.P. Hart, et al. The association between delirium and cognitive decline: a review of the empirical literature. *Neuropsychol Rev* 2004; **14**: 87–98.
7. B.A. Khan, M. Zawahiri, N.L. Campbell, et al. Delirium in hospitalized patients: Implications of current evidence on clinical practice and future avenues for research – a systematic evidence review. *J Hosp Med* 2012; **7**: 580–9.
8. E.B. Milbrandt, S. Deppen, P.L. Harrison, et al. Costs associated with delirium in mechanically ventilated patients. *Crit Care Med* 2004; **32**: 955–62.
9. M.A. Pisani, S.Y.J. Kong, S.V. Kasl, et al. Days of delirium are associated with 1-year mortality in an older intensive care unit population. *Am J Respir Crit Care Med* 2009; **180**: 1092–7.
10. P.P. Pandharipande, B.T. Pun, D.L. Herr, et al. Effect of sedation with dexmedetomidine vs lorazepam on acute brain dysfunction in mechanically ventilated patients: the MENDS randomized controlled trial. *JAMA* 2007; **298**: 2644–53.
11. K.G. Kelly, M. Zisselman, T. Cutillo-Schmitter, et al. Severity and course of delirium in medically hospitalized nursing facility residents. *Am J Geriatr Psychiatry* 2001; **9**: 72–7.
12. E. Marcantonio, T. Ta, E. Duthie, N. M. Resnick. Delirium severity and psychomotor types: their relationship with outcomes after hip fracture repair. *J Am Geriatr Soc* 2002; **50**: 850–7.
13. Y. Shehabi, R.R. Riker, P.M. Bokesch, et al. Delirium duration and mortality in lightly sedated, mechanically ventilated intensive care patients. *Crit Care Med* 2010; **38**: 2311–18.
14. T.D. Girard, M.C. Exline, S.S. Carson, et al. Haloperidol and ziprasidone for treatment of delirium in critical illness. *N Engl J Med* 2018; **379**: 2506–16.
15. B.A. Khan, A.J. Perkins, N.L. Campbell, et al. Pharmacological management of delirium in the intensive care unit: a randomized pragmatic clinical trial. *J Am Geriatr Soc* 2019; **67**: 1057–65.

16. V.J. Page, E.W. Ely, S. Gates, et al. Effect of intravenous haloperidol on the duration of delirium and coma in critically ill patients (Hope-ICU): a randomised, double-blind, placebo-controlled trial. *The Lancet Respir Med* 2013; **1**: 515–23.

17. M. Van Den Boogaard, A.J.C. Slooter, R.J. M. Brüggemann, et al. Effect of haloperidol on survival among critically ill adults with a high risk of delirium: the REDUCE randomized clinical trial. *JAMA* 2018; **319**: 680-90.

18. R. Cavallazzi, M. Saad, P.E. Marik. Delirium in the ICU: an overview. *Ann Intensive Care* 2012; **2**: 49.

19. M.F. Mart, S. Williams Roberson, B. Salas, et al. Prevention and management of delirium in the intensive care unit. *Semin Respir Crit Care Med* 2021; **42**: 112–26.

20. J.W. Devlin, Y. Skrobik, B. Rochwerg, et al. Methodologic innovation in creating clinical practice guidelines: insights from the 2018 society of critical care medicine pain, agitation/sedation, delirium, immobility, and sleep disruption guideline effort. *Crit Care Med* 2018; **46**: 1457–63.

21. B.T. Pun, M.C. Balas, M.A. Barnes-Daly, et al. Caring for critically ill patients with the ABCDEF bundle: results of the ICU liberation collaborative in over 15,000 adults. *Crit Care Med* 2019; **47**: 3–14.

22. J.A. Palakshappa, C.L. Hough. How we prevent and treat delirium in the ICU. *Chest* 2021; **160**: 1326–34.

23. J. Hole, M. Hirsch, E. Ball, C. Meads. Music as an aid for postoperative recovery in adults: a systematic review and meta-analysis. *Lancet* 2015; **386**: 1659–71.

24. J.H. Lee. The effects of music on pain: a meta-analysis. *J Music Ther* 2016; **53**: 430–77.

25. C.H. McKinney, F.C. Tims, A.M. Kumar, M. Kumar. Effects of guided imagery and music therapy on mood and cortisol in healthy adults. *J Behav Med* 1997; **20**: 85–99.

26. M. Richard-Lalonde, C. Gélinas, M. Boitor, et al. The effect of music on pain in the adult intensive care unit: a systematic review of randomized controlled trials. *J Pain Symptom Manage* 2020; **59**: 1304–19.

27. J. Bradt, C. Dileo. Music interventions for mechanically ventilated patients. *Cochrane Database of Syst Rev* 2014; **2014**(12): CD006902.

28. Ö. Erbay Dalli, C. Bozkurt, Y. Yildirim. The effectiveness of music interventions on stress response in intensive care patients: a systematic review and meta-analysis. *J Clin Nurs* 2023; **32**: 2827–45.

29. S.H. Khan, M. Kitsis, D. Golovyan, et al. Effects of music intervention on inflammatory markers in critically ill and post-operative patients: a systematic review of the literature. *Heart & Lung* 2018; **47**: 489–96.

30. Y. Colkesen, S. Giray, Y. Ozenli, et al. Relation of serum cortisol to delirium occurring after acute coronary syndromes. *Am J Emerg Med* 2013; **31**: 161–5.

31. D.-L. Mu, D.-X. Wang, L.-H. Li, et al. High serum cortisol level is associated with increased risk of delirium after coronary artery bypass graft surgery: a prospective cohort study. *Crit Care* 2010; **14**: R238.

32. S.H. Khan, C. Xu, R. Purpura, et al. Decreasing delirium through music: a randomized pilot trial. *Am J Crit Care* 2020; **29**: e31–e8.

33. J.L. Stollings, J.L. Thompson, B.A. Ferrell, et al. Sedative plasma concentrations and delirium risk in critical illness. *Ann Pharmacother* 2018; **52**: 513–21.

34. S.M. Weinstein, L. Poultsides, L. R. Baaklini, et al. Postoperative delirium in total knee and hip arthroplasty patients: a study of perioperative modifiable risk factors. *Br J Anaesth* 2018; **120**: 999–1008.

35. L. Chen, J. Yin, Y. Zheng, et al. The effectiveness of music listening for critically ill patients: a systematic review. *Nurs Crit Care* 2023; **28**: 1132–42.

36. K.V. Jespersen, M.H. Hansen, P. Vuust. The effect of music on sleep in hospitalized patients: a systematic review and meta-analysis. *Sleep Health* 2023; **9**: 441–8.

37. S.C. Segerstrom. Resources, stress, and immunity: an ecological perspective on

human psychoneuroimmunology. *Ann Behav Med* 2010; **40**: 114–25.

38. C. Conrad, H. Niess, K.-W. Jauch, et al. Overture for growth hormone: requiem for interleukin-6?. *Crit Care Med* 2007; **35**: 2709–13.

39. A. Nelson, W. Hartl, K.-W. Jauch, et al. The impact of music on hypermetabolism in critical illness. *Curr Opin Clin Nutr Metab Care* 2008; **11**: 790–4.

40. S. Leardi, R. Pietroletti, G. Angeloni, et al. Randomized clinical trial examining the effect of music therapy in stress response to day surgery. *Br J Surg* 2007; **94**: 943–7.

41. J.R. Maldonado. Neuropathogenesis of delirium: review of current etiologic theories and common pathways. *Am J Geriatr Psych* 2013; **21**: 1190–222.

42. S. Hofer, C. Bopp, C. Hoerner, et al. Injury of the blood brain barrier and up-regulation of ICAM-1 in polymicrobial sepsis. *J Surg Res* 2008; **146**: 276–81.

43. T. Nishioku, S. Dohgu, F. Takata, et al. Detachment of brain pericytes from the basal lamina is involved in disruption of the blood–brain barrier caused by lipopolysaccharide-induced sepsis in mice. *Cell Mol Neurobiol* 2009; **29**: 309–16.

44. A. Semmler, T. Okulla, M. Sastre, et al. Systemic inflammation induces apoptosis with variable vulnerability of different brain regions. *J Chem Neuroanat* 2005; **30**: 144–57.

45. M.L. Block, L. Zecca, J.-S. Hong. Microglia-mediated neurotoxicity: uncovering the molecular mechanisms. *Nat Rev Neurosci* 2007; **8**: 57–69.

46. A.E. Cardona, M. Li, L. Liu, et al. Chemokines in and out of the central nervous system: much more than chemotaxis and inflammation. *J Leukoc Biol* 2008; **84**: 587–94.

47. T.T. Hshieh, T.G. Fong, E.R. Marcantonio, S.K. Inouye. Cholinergic deficiency hypothesis in delirium: a synthesis of current evidence. *The Journals of Gerontology Series A: Biological Sciences and Medical Sciences* 2008; **63**: 764–72.

48. A.M.J. MacLullich, K.J. Ferguson, T. Miller, et al. Unravelling the pathophysiology of delirium: A focus on the role of aberrant stress responses. *J Psychosom Res* 2008; **65**: 229–38.

49. S.T. O'Keeffe, J.G. Devlin. Delirium and the dexamethasone suppression test in the elderly. *Neuropsychobiology* 1994; **30**: 153–6.

50. T.G. Fong, S.K. Inouye. The inter-relationship between delirium and dementia: the importance of delirium prevention. *Nat Rev Neurol* 2022; **18**: 579–96.

51. S.-H. Choi, H. Lee, T.-S. Chung, et al. Neural network functional connectivity during and after an episode of delirium. *AJP* 2012; **169**: 498–507.

52. S. Kyeong, S.-H. Choi, J. Eun Shin, et al. Functional connectivity of the circadian clock and neural substrates of sleep-wake disturbance in delirium. *Psychiatry Res Neuroimaging* 2017; **264**: 10–12.

53. S. Bottiroli, A. Rosi, R. Russo, et al. The cognitive effects of listening to background music on older adults: processing speed improves with upbeat music, while memory seems to benefit from both upbeat and downbeat music. *Front Aging Neurosci* 2014; **6**.: 284.

54. A. Gupta, B. Bhushan, L. Behera. Short-term enhancement of cognitive functions and music: a three-channel model. *Sci Rep* 2018; **8**: 15528.

55. J.B. King, K.G. Jones, E. Goldberg, et al. Increased functional connectivity after listening to favored music in adults with Alzheimer dementia. *J Prev Alz Dis* 2018: 1–7.

56. S.J.T. van Montfort, E. van Dellen, C.J. Stam, et al. Brain network disintegration as a final common pathway for delirium: a systematic review and qualitative meta-analysis. *Neuroimage Clin* 2019; **23**: 101809.

57. V. Menon. *Salience Network. Brain Mapping.* Elsevier; 2015. pp. 597–611.

58. I. Peretz, D. Vuvan, M.-É. Lagrois, J. L. Armony. Neural overlap in processing

music and speech. *Phil Trans R Soc B* 2015; **370**: 20140090.

59. M. Reybrouck, P. Vuust, E. Brattico. Brain connectivity networks and the aesthetic experience of music. *Brain Sciences* 2018; **8**: 107.

60. I. Peretz, R. Zatorre (eds), *The Cognitive Neuroscience of Music*. Oxford: Oxford University Press.

61. M.H. Thaut, W.B. Davis. The influence of subject-selected versus experimenter-chosen music on affect, anxiety, and relaxation. *J Music Ther* 1993; **30**: 210–23.

62. V.J. Schmithorst. Separate cortical networks involved in music perception: preliminary functional MRI evidence for modularity of music processing. *NeuroImage* 2005; **25**: 444–51.

63. J. Wu, J. Zhang, X. Ding, et al. The effects of music on brain functional networks: a network analysis. *Neuroscience* 2013; **250**: 49–59.

64. H.-C. Li, H.-H. Wang, F.-H. Chou, K.-M. Chen. The effect of music therapy on cognitive functioning among older adults: a systematic review and meta-analysis. *J Am Med Dir Assoc* 2015; **16**: 71–7.

65. C. Moreno-Morales, R. Calero, P. Moreno-Morales, C. Pintado. Music therapy in the treatment of dementia: a systematic review and meta-analysis. *Front Med* 2020; **7**: 160.

66. C. Jordan, B. Lawlor, D. Loughrey. A systematic review of music interventions for the cognitive and behavioural symptoms of mild cognitive impairment (non-dementia). *J Psychiatr Res* 2022; **151**: 382–90.

67. S. Seyffert, S. Moiz, M. Coghlan, et al. Decreasing delirium through music listening (DDM) in critically ill, mechanically ventilated older adults in the intensive care unit: a two-arm, parallel-group, randomized clinical trial. *Trials* 2022; **23**: 576.

68. L.L. Chlan, C.R. Weinert, A. Heiderscheit, et al. Effects of patient-directed music intervention on anxiety and sedative exposure in critically ill patients receiving mechanical ventilatory support: a randomized clinical trial. *JAMA* 2013; **309**: 2335.

Chapter 20

Animal-Assisted Interventions in the ICU

Kate Tantam, Tania Lovell, and Lyndsey Uglow

Introduction

Animal-assisted intervention (AAI) is the umbrella term used for a field that encompasses many types of interventions across multiple sectors of society; the interventions most closely related to healthcare are animal-assisted activity (AAA) and animal-assisted therapy (AAT). AAA includes general activities in which a handler presents an animal to engage with a patient for the patient's pleasure, while AAT is a structured, goal-directed activity in which an animal is used to help a patient achieve specific objective outcomes with documentation of the results.

The understanding that animal companionship enriches the human experience and improves physical, emotional, and social well-being has inspired research into the benefits of animal visitations in hospital settings, including intensive care units (ICUs). Several mechanisms have been hypothesized to explain the benefits of animal interaction to the human experience [1]. The biophilia theory suggests that humans have an innate affinity to nature, and fulfilling this desire through interaction with animals can have positive effects [2]. This idea is complemented by physiological models, which posit that interaction with animals reduces stress hormones and increases oxytocin, promoting a state that is conducive to healing [1].

In addition to its salutary impact on the endocrine system, there is increasing empirical evidence to suggest that AAI supports a healing environment [1,3,4,5]. Aubrey Fine, one of the founders of the field, describes the animal in AAI as 'social lubricant'. This may be particularly impactful in intensive care environments, where strangers are brought together in a challenging situation yet can be connected by the power of the human-animal bond [6]. For patients who are receptive to animal engagement, AAIs can create positive memories for them, their families, and the staff caring for them during an otherwise chaotic and frightening time.

AAAs, in which a handler and animal visit to provide comfort, can have a profoundly positive effect on a patient's psyche, but animals can also be incorporated into early rehabilitation programs to help patients improve physical health as well. Indeed, AAT can motivate patients in an innovative way to achieve specific physical and functional goals, and their progress can be documented and shared with loved ones as milestones of recovery.

This chapter aims to support clinical teams that already have AAI handlers and animals as well as teams who are yet to welcome animals into their clinical environments. We do this by exploring the evidence base, offering relevant case studies of AAI in intensive care, and providing clear guidance and recommendations to support the incorporation of AAI across the trajectory of recovery after critical illness.

Evidence of AAI in ICUs

There is significant evidence to support the use of AAI in acute care settings, including oncology units, burn units, and general surgical and medical wards [5,6,7,8,9]. Numerous studies have demonstrated that AAIs for hospitalized patients are associated with salutary physiological changes [7,9,10], enhanced mood [5,7,9], reduced pain [5,7,9,11], and increased engagement with care [12]. A meta-analysis of 22 studies of AAIs in pediatric (n=13) and adult (n=9) medical settings also demonstrated that AAIs are an effective intervention to reduce pain, distress, and anxiety [6]. Cole and colleagues found that a combined dog-human volunteer intervention for patients hospitalized with heart failure resulted in significant decreases in both systolic pulmonary artery pressures (mean difference, -5.34 mmHg; p=0.002) and neurohormone levels (e.g., epinephrine and norepinephrine levels) compared to human volunteers alone [10]. Inpatient studies also indicate that AAIs may increase patient engagement with care; in another trial of hospitalized patients with heart failure, AAIs significantly reduced patient refusal to participate in mobilization therapies and increased the distance mobilized compared with patients who did not receive the intervention [12].

The use of AAI in acute care settings is well supported by research, but its use in ICU settings is considered novel, and the evidence base is limited [4,13,14,15]. Researching AAIs in the intensive care environment is challenging, and significant limitations in the evidence base include small sample sizes and lack of control groups, randomized allocation of interventions, and objective measures of effectiveness [14,15]. A scoping review by Lovell and colleagues [15] identified only six studies exploring the use of AAA in intensive care, with half being conducted in pediatric settings [16,17,18] and half in adult settings [19,20,21]. All studies were designed as either feasibility or observational studies, and only two [16,19] were conducted exclusively in ICUs; the other four studies [17,18,20,21] were performed across ICUs, general wards, and emergency departments (see Table 20.1).

Results of the scoping review demonstrated that AAA interventions were associated with positive outcomes for both staff and patients in ICU settings, with patients experiencing reductions in pain, anxiety, and stress after receiving an AAA [15]. AAAs received overwhelmingly positive feedback from patients, family members, and clinicians, with satisfaction rates ranging from 93% to 100% across studies, and a similar percentage of clinicians and families agreed that AAA visitations should be continued or expanded. Evidence of the benefits of AAAs was mostly limited to self-reported outcome measures (e.g., stress, pain, anxiety, and patient satisfaction) and qualitative findings [15]; only two studies measured biophysical outcomes. Branson and colleagues measured biomarkers of stress, including salivary C-reactive protein, salivary cortisol, and interleukin-1B [19], while Walden and colleagues assessed pre- and post-intervention blood pressure and respiratory rate, distance ambulated, and duration of ambulation while the patient walked with a dog [16]. Results from both studies were inconclusive, as the sample sizes were insufficiently powered due to recruitment challenges [15,16,19].

In a randomized controlled trial conducted in pediatric intensive care and ward settings, Jennings and colleagues demonstrated that a 5 to 10 minute AAA intervention compared with a delayed intervention control group (i.e., patients received the intervention 4–5 hours after data collection) was associated with significantly higher activity levels and improved

Table 20.1 Summary of AAI evidence in an intensive care setting

Authors (year) Country	Design	Setting and Participants	Intervention	Findings	Limitations
Branson et al. (2020) USA	Randomized pilot and feasibility trial	Setting: ICU Sample: ICU patient >60 years Intervention n = 9 Control = 6	Intervention: Ten-minute AAA with dog and handler Control: Usual care	Decreased stress and anxiety in intervention group (median change of −2.5 on 10-point scale and −1.0 on 4-point scale, respectively) compared to no change in control. Biomarker results inconclusive.	Insufficiently powered sample size due to recruitment challenges Standard care control didn't control for volunteer visit.
Caton et al. (2021) Canada	Two phase mixed methods study	Setting: Emergency department (ED) and ICU Sample: Phase 1 – ED and ICU staff (n = 98), dog handler (n = 1) Phase 2: ED and ICU staff (n = 93), dog handler (n = 4)	Phase 1: Single dog handler team biweekly AAA 30–60-minute visits including a walk around ED and ICU and then static time in a private room where staff could visit the dog. Phase 2: 4 certified therapy dog-handler teams conducted 90-minute walk arounds in ICU, ED, and burns and trauma units.	Staff agreed/strongly agreed that they were satisfied with the intervention (Phase 1 = 93%, Phase 2 = 94%). > 85% of staff agreed the intervention reduced stress, improved morale, and the intervention should continue. Qualitative themes: (1) feelings of being cared for by the organization, (2) improved unit environment, (3) increased staff wellness.	Potential for participation bias. Results were aggregated so could not be specifically attributed to ICU setting. Adverse advents not measured.

Table 20.1 (cont.)

Authors (year) Country	Design	Setting and Participants	Intervention	Findings	Limitations
Hastings et al. (2008) USA	Observational Case study	Setting: Burn PICU and acute care burns unit. Sample: 611 patients received AAT over 3.5 years.	AAT dog visited pre-approved patients twice weekly.	614 patient/family visited. Observed experiences of patients, families, and staff were overwhelmingly positive. No reported infection control issues.	Limited outcomes reported, evidence largely anecdotal. Results were aggregated and therefore cannot be solely attributed to ICU setting.
Pruskowski et al. (2020) USA	Observational feasibility study.	Setting: Burn Center outpatients, wards, and ICU Sample: Survey completed by patients (n = 14) and staff (n = 23)	Dog handler teams visited patients in ICU and ward (AAA) and inpatient gym (AAT).	All patients and staff were satisfied or very satisfied with AAA/AAT and agreed that they would like more sessions with a therapy dog. > 85% of patients agreed or strongly agreed that the visit reduced pain, improved anxiety levels and mood. > 95% of staff enjoyed the dog's presence, reported improved mood and supported another visit	Low response rate and potential participation bias. Results were aggregated and therefore cannot be solely attributed to the ICU setting.

Uglow et al. (2019) UK	Observational	Setting: Pediatric day surgical, medical, oncology wards, and PICU Participants: Staff (n = 82) and parents (n = 118). 11% of participant ICU visit (n = 13)	Sessions included walking the dog, around the ward, providing meet and greet, as well as more targeted individual interventions.	All staff reported that there was either "a great benefit" or "quite a lot of benefit" from the intervention. All staff and 96% of parents reported no concerns of seeing therapy dogs in hospital. All staff reported no/hardly any disruption to care.	Results were aggregated and therefore cannot be solely attributed to the ICU setting. Lack of objective outcome measures.
Walden et al. (2020) USA	Pilot study using a two-period, two-sequence cross-over design	Setting: Cardiovascular PICU Participants: pediatric heart transplant patients (n = 5)	Each participant completed one AAI and one non-AAI 30-minute session. Each session included a walk with/without a dog and play session with/without a dog.	Mean distance/time walked was 1906 ft /17 min in AAI session compared to 1933 ft / 15 min in the non-AAI session. No hemodynamically significant differences noted in blood pressure or respiratory rate. No adverse events reported. All participants agreed they would like another dog visit	Small sample size related to recruiting specific target population and number of required sessions.

Table 20.1 (cont.)

Authors (year) Country	Design	Setting and Participants	Intervention	Findings	Limitations
Jennings et al. (2021) USA	Randomized control trial	Setting: PICU, Cardiac ICU, hematology and oncology wards Sample: Control n = 36 Intervention n = 44 *Vent patients excluded	Intervention: 5 –10 min AAA with dog and handler Control: Delayed intervention. Control participants received intervention >5hrs post recruitment. All study measures were collected before AAA session.	Activity level: AAA group had significantly higher activity and positive mood score post-intervention. Cortisol levels: Significant differences in cortisol recovery score in AAA group compared to control. No significant difference between mean cortisol levels at each time point.	Controls delayed intervention may have confounded cortisol recovery results. Recruitment challenges, 4-year study period. Results were not aggregated and therefore cannot be solely attributed to ICU
López-Fernández (2024) Spain	Quasi-experimental study, feasibility	Setting: PICU Sample: Patients > 3 years, n = 61 Family surveys, n = 47 Animal therapy technicians, n = 67	Intervention: AAT session averaged 38 minutes in length and incorporated an occupational therapist and a psychologist. The sessions were guided by pre-existing objectives decided by healthcare team.	No difference in physiological measures. Significant decrease in pain, fear, and anxiety levels (p<0.01) pre- and post-session No adverse events	Lack of control

mood up to three hours post-intervention [22]. They also found that participants who received AAA showed a decrease in salivary cortisol levels with time, while participants in the control group had an increase in salivary cortisol levels. Although promising, further research is required to better understand the physiological impact of AAI in critically ill populations [22].

Although research of AAI in intensive care is growing, few studies have investigated the use of animals in goal-oriented, therapy-driven interventions [23]. López-Fernández and colleagues investigated the feasibility and safety of conducting AAT sessions incorporating occupational therapists and psychologists in a level three pediatric intenisve care unit (PICU). They found a significant decrease in pain, fear, and anxiety levels following AAT sessions compared with before (p<0.01). Patients, caregivers, and staff expressed high levels of satisfaction with the AAT sessions, and surveys demonstrated that staff perceived improvement in patient comfort with no additional burden to daily routine. During the 74 AAT sessions, there were no adverse events observed, including medication extravasation, dislodgement of drains or probes, falls, oxygen desaturations, or delays in medication administration, demonstrating that implementation of AAT in a PICU is feasible and safe [23]. More research is required to understand how AAT may be used to facilitate recovery in ICUs and how this might impact the development of post-intensive care syndrome (PICS).

Across several hospital settings and participant groups (i.e., patients, staff, and family members), AAIs are associated with a high level of measured satisfaction and substantial qualitative reports of improved experiences [7,9,11,15,22,23]. Evidence that AAI reduces pain, anxiety, and stress highlights the potential usefulness of AAI interventions in ICUs, in which all three are prominent features of the patient experience [5,6,7,8,9,10,11,15,23]. There are challenges, however, in quantifying the "power of puppies," as most of the evidence in ICUs is limited to self-reported measures [4,14,15]. Further research into AAI in ICUs is required to establish its effectiveness, to reduce barriers to implementation, and to address the limitations of current research [14,15].

AAIs in Intensive Care: Practical and Clinical Implications for Practice

Clinical Guidance and Risk Assessment

There are published guidelines in the United Kingdom from both the Royal College of Nursing [24] and Intensive Care Society [25] offering guidance to teams wishing to establish AAI programs. These guidelines should be discussed with the clinical, managerial, and infection prevention and control teams at the hospital where an AAI program will be introduced. Every hospital has different parameters for permitting this type of work, and local issues must be considered in conjunction with these guidelines to ensure safe and effective incorporation of AAI programs. Like every aspect of healthcare provision, nothing is appropriate for every setting, and clear local risk assessments and patient-centered decisions must be made. Table 20.2 details the most common clinical factors to consider for patients, loved ones, and staff, and Figure 20.1 additionally addresses considerations for handlers and their therapy animal.

Table 20.2 Key things to consider in clinical environments

Patient	Loved Ones/Visitors	Clinical team
- Infection control measures (including hand hygiene) - Allergies - Phobias - Consent - Capacity to participate (e.g., presence of delirium) - Clinical stability - Accessibility to bed space for animal to visit (e.g., height of bed, chair, use of aids to support contact) - All lines/wounds covered and secured with waterproof clear, adhesive dressing	- Infection control measures (including hand hygiene) - Allergies - Phobias - Hazards associated with animal visit (e.g., trips/falls/over reaching - Respiratory risk factors (e.g., asthma) - Access to animal (i.e., will the loved one want to touch the animal or simply watch)	- Infection control measures (including hand hygiene) - Allergies - Phobias - Clinical workload - Requirement for extra staff for support visit - Cleaning regime for bedspace, patient, staff, and loved ones

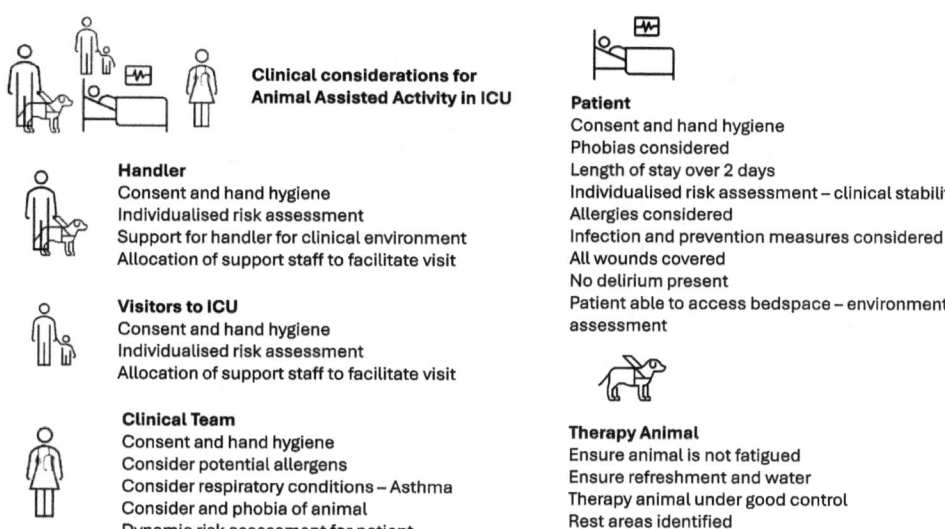

Figure 20.1 Clinical considerations for animal assisted activity in ICU.

Care of Animal and Handler

Even if the handler has a healthcare background, AAI in intensive care is best done in a diamond model [26], which describes the positioning of the animal, handler, patient, and healthcare team member. Utilizing this model, the handler advocates for the animal, and the healthcare team member advocates for the patient. There are many types of handlers involved in AAI in healthcare, some of whom are employed with their animal, while others are volunteers from charities supporting AAI, who may or may not have a medical background. Irrespective of their background, every handler must have appropriate indemnity insurance, a qualified animal, and a passion to work with their animal partner to provide a service.

A rigorous assessment of the animal should be performed, both in the general areas of the hospital and the highly stimulatory environment of the ICU. Prior to commencement of ICU visiting, simulation training is recommended to ensure both the handler and dog are properly prepared for and suited to the environment [25]. This should be conducted at a time after the general hospital assessment and should adequately mimic the full range of noises, stressors, and equipment that the handler and animal might encounter. Although many handlers may want to work in an intensive care environment, not all handlers or animals will be suited to it; indeed, handler desire may not always equate to canine ability [27]. Responsibility for the handler and their safety in the clinical environment sits with the member of staff accompanying the AAA team.

Therapy dogs that excel in general wards and school rooms in inpatient settings may not be suited to the intensive care environment; each dog has its personality and preferences, and not all animals have the same capacity to engage in acute environments. A handler must ensure that their animal is suited to the environment and activity they are being asked to do and must be able to identify stress signals in their animal. It is important to develop strong relationships between the handlers and the clinical team so that they feel empowered to end a session when their dog is showing signs of stress or fatigue. An animal that struggles to communicate their desire to end the session will not wish to return in the future. Handlers should be encouraged to advocate for their animal, interpret their body language, and centralize the session around the animal's capacity to engage. It should always be remembered that AAI handlers "partner" with animals rather than "use" them.

Handlers working in the ICU must understand that the environment is at times chaotic and unpredictable. When considering the need for occupational health support, handlers should be considered staff and should have access to the same support when exposed to challenging clinical situations.

Utilization of Other Animals

Dogs are the animal most commonly used for AAIs [28], but research exists supporting the use of other animals as therapy animals, including horses, cats, birds, rabbits, guinea pigs, and farm animals. Horses and ponies can be trained to observe and respond to nonverbal cues, allowing them to bond with humans for the purpose of therapy and recovery from trauma [29]. Domesticated cats and rabbits are useful in rehabilitating fine motor skills as patients stroke them, and they have been shown to improve blood pressure and reduce risks for cerebrovascular events and myocardial infarction [30].

Special considerations and guidance must be sought from infection prevention and control teams within clinical settings for any AAIs that are outside normal practice within the center. Different animals present different clinical considerations, phobias, zoonotic risk factors, and behavioral presentations.

Humanization of Intensive Care

Intensive care can be an intimidating and highly impersonal environment for patients and their loved ones. Patients and relatives report that when they experienced a humanized ICU, they felt that healthcare professionals expressed genuine attention and support by providing opportunities to stay connected despite the disruption caused by critical illness (see Chapter 16 for additional information) [3]. AAI is an example of a shared connection between patients and relatives, and patients report that this helps to re-establish relationships after periods of time apart [31].

Memories of AAI are often treasured and can be captured photographically. Many relatives may be reluctant to take pictures of their loved ones, but the addition of an animal often helps them overcome their reluctance. Clear consent, capacity, and appropriateness of position and location for photography of the animal, handler, patient, and loved one must be considered. Images as a supplement to patient diaries can be a useful adjunct to reconstructing the narrative of intensive care experiences but need to be locally managed by the clinical team (see Chapter 18 for additional information) [32].

Case Study: Barry and Hospital Therapy Dog Leo (see Figures 20.2 and 20.3)

Handler

"Once we had the consent of the team looking after him, I positioned Leo as close as I could to Barry as he lay there, and although I did not expect any response, it was amazing to see Barry's hand move slowly when we put it on Leo's paw!"

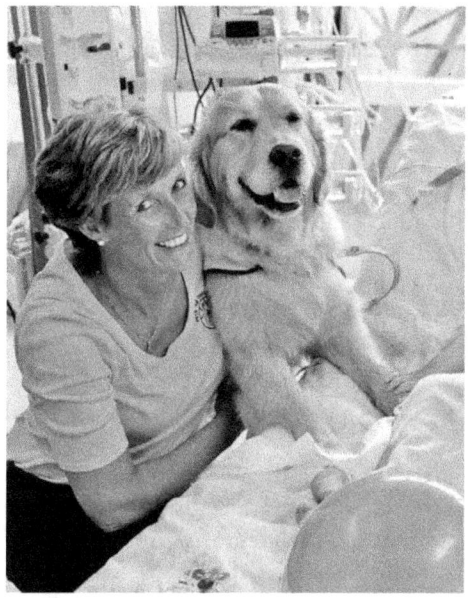

Figure 20.2 Handler Lyndsey and therapy dog Leo.

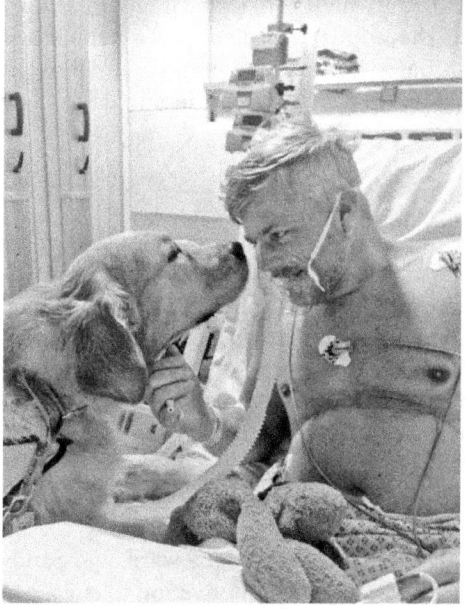

Figure 20.3 Therapy dog Leo and Barry.

Sophie (Barry's wife)

It was like seeing a snippet of Barry, not just a patient linked to a machine in a hospital bed. And, having two young children at home who were unable to visit their dad in hospital, it was so comforting to be able to tell them about Leo's visit, and that made them smile and cry happy tears to know Leo made their dad's hand move. Leo took the scary out of a scary situation, and I don't think anyone else could have done that for us at that horrible time.

Handler

A few months later, I was so surprised to run into Sophie again on the same hospital corridor. I recognized her straight away and, I'll admit, that my heart sank for a second wondering what had brought her back to the hospital. Barry had been re-admitted and once again was in an induced coma. She asked me if I could take Leo in again, as having him there before was such a wonderful thing, and of course I agreed on the spot. Our visit couldn't not have been timed more perfectly – we stepped into the room just a few minutes after Barry had been woken up from the coma. His breathing tube had just been taken out, and he was still on oxygen, but as soon as he saw Leo, he pulled off his mask and moved his face toward the dog . . . and he cried.

It was quite a moment to witness. To be there with a family going through hell on earth and being able to bring some comfort through Leo was an absolute privilege. A long time later, talking to his family, Barry said that he had memories of a dog being with him during his first coma and felt calm and comforted, as if he were home with their own dog. Sophie wrote to say how Leo gave that comfort to Barry in hospital and how that relationship had comforted them all in different ways. He was the perfect distraction for their children, who came to see Leo as their dad's guardian while they couldn't visit him, and his presence connected the adults, too. Leo was a vehicle for communication while they were apart and at Barry's bedside. I'm not sure how it works, but I know that it does, and I was convinced that I had seen therapy dog magic in action with their family, and I still believe it now.

Case Study: Motivation to Move

Sheila had been in hospital for three months after a prolonged admission to intensive care with intra-abdominal sepsis. She had a poodle named Sandy, and reuniting with Sandy was a key motivating factor for her to engage in therapy and return home. Sandy was staying with a neighbor while Sheila was unwell, and she had not been in to see her since admission, the longest period that Sheila had ever gone without seeing her beloved pet. The clinical team knew that Sheila was finding the separation challenging, so they arranged for Sandy to visit her, with clear agreement and risk assessment performed by the clinical team caring for her.

On a warm spring afternoon, the clinical team was able to reunite Sandy with Sheila, who was profoundly emotional at the sight of her dog. Sandy, an elderly dog, enjoyed the visit but largely stayed sitting on Sheila's lap. After an hour, Sheila returned to the ward, and Sandy returned home. This intervention had a profound effect on Sheila's motivation to engage in rehabilitation. After Sandy's visit, Sheila was reinvigorated with a desire to return home to see Sandy again and to get back to walking. AAAs can be very useful in helping patients visualize their goals and realize that prolonged hospitalization can impact their perception of their recovery trajectory.

For the rest of her hospital stay, the photograph that was taken of Sheila and Sandy that spring afternoon was permanently pinned to the wall as a clear reminder of her goal.

Conclusion

Through creating humanized ICU environments, patients must no longer wait for hospital discharge before they begin to live again. Non-pharmacological intervention programs, such as AAI, may reduce suffering and help patients take an active role in their recovery. The benefits of AAI are not limited to the patients receiving care and their families but also extend to those providing care as well [3].

Key Points

1. AAI offers opportunities to humanize a clinical environment and optimize a patient and their loved one's experience.
2. The health benefits of AAI in intensive care are not well established, and further research is needed.
3. Infection prevention and control measures and appropriate risk assessment for the environment, patient, animal, handler, staff, and visitors are fundamental.

References

1. D.A. Marcus. The science behind animal-assisted therapy. *Curr Pain Headache R* 2013; **17**: 322.
2. S. Burres, N.E. Edwards, A. M. Beck, et al. Incorporating pets into acute inpatient rehabilitation: a case study. *Rehabil Nurse* 2016; **41**: 336–41.
3. M.M. Hosey, J. Jaskulski, S.T. Wegener, et al. Animal-assisted intervention in the ICU: a tool for humanization. *Crit Care* 2018; **22**: 22.
4. J. Malik. Animal-assisted interventions in intensive care delirium: a literature review. *AACN Adv Crit Care* 2021; **32**: 391–7.
5. A.B. Coakley, C.D. Annese, J.H. Empoliti, J. M. Flanagan. The experience of animal assisted therapy on patients in an acute care setting. *Clin Nurs Res* 2021; **30**: 401–5.
6. T.C. Waite, L. Hamilton, W. O'Brien. A meta-analysis of animal assisted interventions targeting pain, anxiety and distress in medical settings. *Complement Ther Clin Prac* 2018; **33**: 49–55.
7. T.R. Holder, M.E. Gruen, D.L. Roberts, et al. A systematic literature review of animal assisted interventions in oncology (part I): methods and results. *Integr Cancer Ther* 2020; **19**: 1534735420943278.
8. B. Hetland, T. Bailey, M. Prince-Paul. Animal-assisted interactions to alleviate psychological symptoms in patients receiving mechanical ventilation. *J Hosp Palliat Nurs* 2017; **19**: 516–23.
9. M. Lundqvist, P. Carlsson, R. Sjödahl, et al. Patient benefit of dog-assisted interventions in health care: a systematic review. *BMC Complement Altern Med* 2017; **17**: 358.
10. K.M. Cole, A. Gawlinski, N. Steers, J. Kotlerman. Animal-assisted therapy in patients hospitalized with heart failure. *Am J Crit Care* 2007; **16**: 575–85.
11. C.M. Harper, Y. Dong, T.S. Thornhill, et al. Can therapy dogs improve pain and satisfaction after total joint arthroplasty? A randomized controlled trial. *Clin Orthop Relat Res* 2015; **473**: 372–9.
12. S.V. Abate, M. Zucconi, B.A. Boxer. Impact of canine-assisted ambulation on hospitalized chronic heart failure patients' ambulation outcomes and satisfaction: a pilot study. *J Cardiovasc Nurs* 2011; **26**: 224–30.
13. A. Phung, C. Joyce, S. Ambutas, et al. Animal-assisted therapy for inpatient adults. *Nursing* 2017; **47**: 63–6.
14. M. Fiore, A. Cortegiani, G. Friolo, et al. Risks and benefits of animal-assisted

interventions for critically ill patients admitted to intensive care units. *J Anaesth Crit Care* 2023; **31**: 15–20.

15. T. Lovell, K. Ranse. Animal-assisted activities in the intensive care unit: a scoping review. *Intensive Crit Care Nurs* 2022; **73**: 103304.

16. M. Walden, A. Lovenstein, A. Randag, et al. Methodological challenges encountered in a study of the impact of animal-assisted intervention in pediatric heart transplant patients. *J Pediatr Nurs* 2020; **53**: 67–73.

17. T. Hastings, A. Burris, J. Hunt, et al. (2008). Pet therapy: a healing solution. *J Burn Care Res* 2008; **29**: 874–6.

18. L.S. Uglow. The benefits of an animal-assisted intervention service to patients and staff at a children's hospital. *Br J Nurs* 2019; **28**: 509–15.

19. S. Branson, L. Boss, S. Hamlin, N. S. Padhye. Animal-assisted activity in critically ill older adults: a randomized pilot and feasibility trial. *Biol Res Nurs* 2020; **22**: 412–17.

20. N. Caton, K. Campbell, T. Brumwell, et al. Pups assisting wellness for staff (P.A.W.S.): evaluating the impact of canine-assisted interventions on critical care staff wellness. *Healthc Manage Forum* 2021; **34**: 119–22.

21. K.A. Pruskowski, J.M. Gurney, L. C. Cancio. Impact of the implementation of a therapy dog program on burn center patients and staff. *Burns* 2020; **46**: 293–7.

22. M.L. Jennings, D.A. Granger, C.I. Bryce, et al. Effect of animal assisted interactions on activity and stress response in children in acute care settings. *Compr Psychoneuroendocrinol* 2021; **8**: 100076.

23. E. López-Fernández, A. Palacios-Cuesta, A. Rodríguez-Martínez, et al. Implementation feasibility of animal-assisted therapy in a pediatric intensive care unit: effectiveness on reduction of pain, fear, and anxiety. *Eur J Pediatr* 2024; **183**: 843–51.

24. Nursing RCo. *Working with Dogs in Healthcare Settings*. London: RCN; 2019.

25. Society IC. *Animal assisted intervention guidance*. London: Intensive Care Society; 2020.

26. A.H. Fine. *Handbook on animal assisted therapy: foundations and guidelines for animal-assisted interventions*. 4th ed. San Diego: Elsevier; 2019.

27. L. Uglow. *Leo and Friends, the Extraordinary Dogs with the Healing Touch*. London: HarperCollins; 2021.

28. J.D. Charry-Sanchez, I. Pradilla, C. Talero-Gutierrez. Animal-assisted therapy in adults: a systematic review. *Complement Ther Clin Pract* 2018; **32**: 169–80.

29. J. Yorke, C. Adams, N. Coady. Therapeutic value of equine-human bonding in recovery from trauma. *Anthrozoos* 2008; **21**: 17–30.

30. A.I. Qureshi, M.Z. Memon, G. Vazquez, M.F. Suri. Cat ownership and the risk of fatal cardiovascular diseases: results from the second national health and nutrition examination study mortality follow-up study. *J Vasc Interv Neurol* 2009; **2**: 132–5.

31. A.H. Nielsen, M.E. Kvande, S. Angel. Humanizing and dehumanizing intensive care: thematic synthesis (HumanIC). *J Adv Nurs* 2023; **79**: 385–401.

32. C. Jones. Introducing photo diaries for ICU patients. *J Intensive Care Soc* 2009; **10**: 183–5.

Chapter 21

The Importance of Fresh Air in Intensive Care

Kate Tantam, Louise Rose, and Natalie Pattison

Introduction

Across all health care environments, views of nature are reported to inspire positive feelings, with access to outside spaces deemed to be valuable to patients and their loved ones [1,2]. Studying the impact of the intensive care unit (ICU) environment on patient recovery is in its infancy, but it is increasingly gaining serious attention. An ideal ICU design creates a "healing environment" that humanizes the medical setting and minimizes environmental stressors to patients, their family members, and the staff caring for them [3,4]. Biophilia, or contact with nature through access to outdoor spaces or views, is an important element of ICU design that may positively impact patient recovery and staff well-being [5]. The US-based Facilities Guidelines Institute recommends that therapeutic gardens with access to sunlight, shade, and vegetation be included in the design and construction of all new and refurbished hospitals [2]. Some ICU health facility guidance documents recommend equipping an outdoor space for ICU patients [1], although this is not currently stated in professional standards [6].

Examples of ICU Access to an Outdoor Space

Many ICUs around the world provide access to a garden space, such as the "Balcony of Hope" at the Virgen Macarena University Hospital in Seville, Spain [7], which is composed of an indoor "living" space and an accompanying outdoor terrace. The ICU rehabilitation program of the Hospital San Juan de Dios, also in Spain, includes a "healing walk" protocol and a checklist for access to the outdoors [8]. More recently, dedicated outside facilities fitted with medical gas supply, monitoring devices, and other technology required to care for ICU patients have been developed, such as at the Rijnstate Hospital in the Netherlands, which has two outdoor ICU bedspaces [9]. In the United Kingdom (UK), University Hospitals Plymouth has dedicated ICU bedspace in a garden, and King's College Hospital in London is currently building a dedicated ICU rooftop garden with five level three-dedicated ICU bedspaces (see Figures 21.1 and 21.2 for examples) [10]. An interprofessional team representing intensive care clinicians from the UK developed the UK Intensive Care Guidance on Transfer of Critically Ill Patients to the Outdoors to enable ICU teams to provide patient access to nature (see below for further details and recommendations) [11].

The Evidence for "Fresh Air Therapy" for ICU Patients and Their Families

The current evidence on exposure to "fresh air therapy" for ICU patients is largely restricted to single-center descriptions of access to an outdoor space [7,9], recommendations for

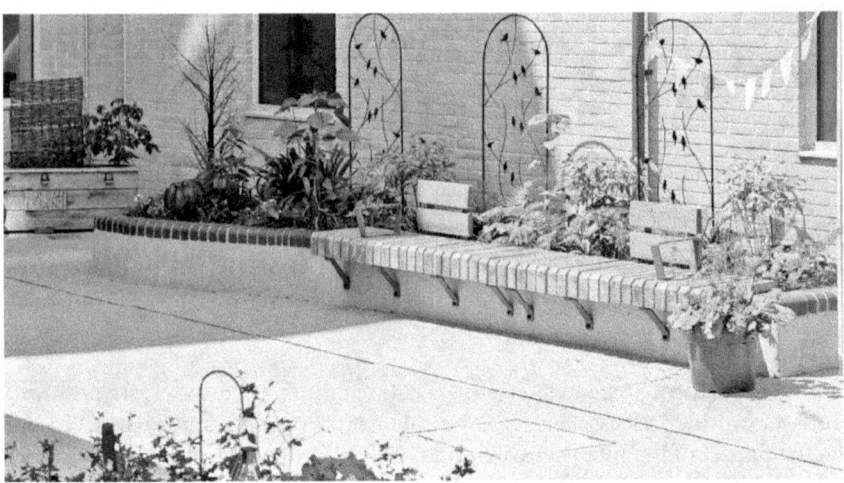

Figure 21.1 A sunlit seating area in an urban ICU garden at University Hospitals Plymouth NHS Trust, UK.

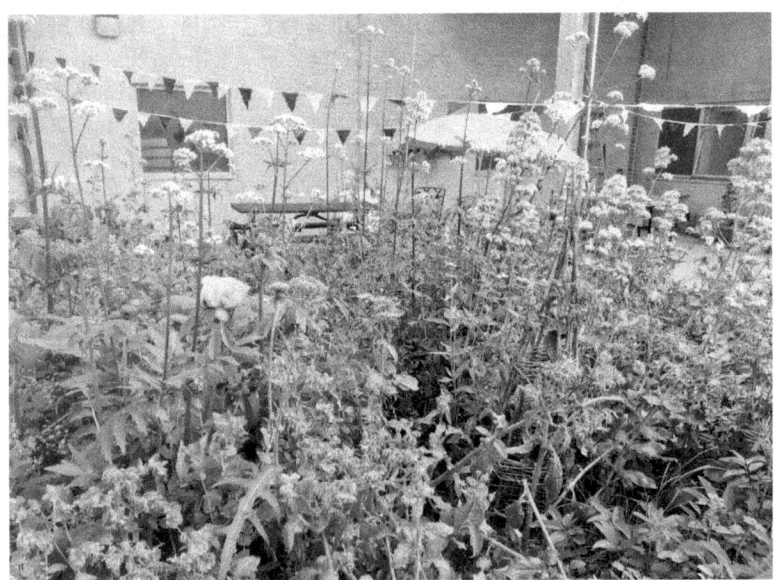

Figure 21.2 Flowers donated during the COVID-19 pandemic to a hospital garden for patients and staff to enjoy.

designing a therapeutic garden [5], guidance documents and checklists [8,11], and case reports [12]. In a retrospective cohort study of 423 out-of-ICU mobilization sessions at the Nagoya City University West Medical Center in Japan, 65% of sessions were to visit the hospital garden, while the remainder were within the hospital building [13]. During the 423 mobilization sessions, only 24 potential safety events were identified, and none required additional treatment, indicating that mobilization outside the ICU is both feasible and safe if planned for and managed by experienced staff. More recently, Maiden and colleagues conducted a prospective, one-day point prevalence survey of "fresh air therapy" in 49 ICUs across Australia and New Zealand [14]. Of the 649 patients admitted to an ICU on the day of data collection, 24% were believed by their ICU team to potentially benefit from "fresh air therapy." Despite this belief, only 1.1% (7 patients) actually spent time outdoors, even though 19 ICUs in the study had a dedicated outdoor area for patients and 8 ICUs had guidelines for providing such an experience [14].

Greenspace exposure has been associated with a wide range of health benefits, including positive effects on psychological, cognitive, social, and physical health in general patient populations [15,16,17] and various non-ICU patient populations, including patients with long-term conditions [18]. With respect to impacts on physical health, greenspace exposure has been associated with decreased heart rate, diastolic blood pressure, and salivary cortisol levels [17] and improvements in obesity and cardiovascular-related mortality [16,19]. Meanwhile, insufficient sunlight exposure is associated with increased mortality and rates of cancer in the general population due to diminished vitamin D synthesis and other hypothetical mechanisms, such as release of nitric oxide from the skin [20]. The impact of exposure to nature on anxiety and depression is well documented [15], but the quality and rigor of the evidence base is often criticized [17].

In addition to providing benefit to critically ill patients, "fresh air therapy" may also benefit family members of critically ill patients. For example, using convenience sampling, Ulrich and colleagues demonstrated a reduction in both the stress and sadness subscales of the Present Functioning Visual Analogue Scales after visiting an ICU garden in 42 family members of ICU patients [21].

The Impact of Fresh Air Spaces on Staff

The benefit of exposure to greenspaces extends beyond patients and their families to the healthcare workers who care for them. To study the impact of a garden space on ICU healthcare workers, 29 nurses were assigned to 6 weeks of a daily outdoor work break in the hospital garden and 6 weeks of indoor-only breaks in random order using a crossover trial design. When randomized to garden breaks, nurses reported less emotional exhaustion and depersonalization on the Maslach Burnout Inventory subscales than they did during the weeks when indoor-only breaks were taken [22].

Numerous systematic reviews and qualitative studies suggest that, in comparison to nurses in other disciplines and other colleagues working in the critical care setting, ICU nurses experience the highest level of burnout syndrome, and greenspace exposure may be one tool to combat its development [23,24,25,26,27]. There are numerous reasons for this, such as caring for patients at the end-of-life, witnessing intense grief and suffering, interacting with distressed families, and working in a dynamic, stressful environment [23,24,25,26,27]. Critical care nurses rarely take fully restorative breaks, if any at all, which is directly linked to both patient safety [28,29] and to professional outcomes, such as the intention to leave nursing [29] and development of burnout syndrome [30]. In addition to the lack of opportunity for a break, in recent years, there has been a decrease in the number of available break areas, both in the UK and globally [31]. Although rest areas were often created during the COVID-19 pandemic, these have largely been assimilated into wider hospital use and no longer accommodate breaks.

Staff are more likely to take breaks if there are attractive areas for them to do so, particularly in gardens and other outdoor spaces [32,33,34]. The value of fresh air spaces for healthcare staff has been demonstrated in several studies, with beneficial impacts on mood, stress levels, and emotional well-being [34,35,36,37,38,39,40]. Moreover, during the COVID-19 pandemic, one study suggested that even 20 to 30 minutes of rest in a nature space could improve healthcare workers' moods [39]. In addition to the psychological benefits, exposure to nature for hospital staff is linked to a range of salutary physiological changes, including decreased stress hormones, cortisol, and blood pressure [19].

Common barriers to utilizing fresh air spaces include limited awareness of such spaces, limited accessibility to the spaces (e.g., too distant from the ICU), and insufficient safety considerations (e.g., isolated spaces may increase staff vulnerability). Staff deem the following qualities to be important when designing an outdoor space: adequate comfort (including seating and tables for eating), the presence of a water feature, a variety of flora and fauna, use of natural rather than artificial materials, absence of hard paving [41], and aesthetic views from and within the area [34]. The type of space is also important in terms of intended garden function (e.g., healing, sensory, or therapeutic garden), but evidence on how the intent of different spaces might impact staff is not yet available [42]. Studies also suggest that other hospital staff are willing to help maintain these outdoor spaces to benefit both staff and patients [43].

Aside from the issues of staff rest, staff also feel able to provide more holistic care when taking critically ill patients and their families to outdoor spaces [44]. This is even more crucial at the end of life, when feeling fulfilled while providing care at a distressing time is highly important for staff [45].

Case Study

Susie, a senior staff ICU nurse with seven years of experience, developed post-traumatic stress disorder as a result of caring for medically and emotionally complex patients in a high-stress environment. The unit was often under-staffed, and Susie frequently had to take charge, alongside caring for her own patients, meaning that she was rarely able to take breaks. At home, she was an unpaid carer to elderly relatives and struggling financially. A particularly difficult end-of-life case, in which Susie felt disempowered and unsupported, left her traumatized. Susie felt that she could no longer cope, and she was often seen crying at work. Her managers finally recognized her distress and recommended an extended leave. On her phased return, Susie appreciated that the absence of a restful space away from the ICU contributed to her condition, prompting her to lobby her managers for an outdoor space that both staff and patients could use. Susie was given one paid day a month to realize her vision of an ICU garden, raising funds via the hospital charity and developing a design group composed of former patients and families. The ICU team redesigned staff breaks to ensure that nurses received a break on each shift. Under Susie's leadership, the ICU garden opened after 18 months, with several staff asking to participate in its ongoing design and upkeep. Staff reported significant benefits in having a peaceful outdoor space in which to decompress during stressful shifts.

Clinical Impact and Value of Fresh Air Spaces in Intensive Care

Although examples from the evidence base are limited, access to a fresh air space can meaningfully impact the quality and dignity of care provided to the critically ill by supporting the humanization of intensive care, providing a meaningful experience for patients at the end of life, and enabling functional rehabilitation tailored to optimize the patient experience.

Humanization of Intensive Care

Humanization of intensive care is now a cornerstone of practice (see Chapter 16 for additional information), and the utilization of fresh air spaces and natural light can be considered an important component to optimizing the experiences of patients, their loved ones, and the staff caring for them. Patients and loved ones report that ICU environments can be detrimental to recovery and can feel isolating [46], dark, loud, intimidating, and challenging [47,48]. The oftentimes chaotic environment of the ICU can disturb restorative sleep and circadian rhythms, disruptions of which are a potentially modifiable cause of delirium among critically ill patients [49]. Fresh air spaces could be useful as part of a multi-component delirium management program [50], an approach that has been validated in older adults [51] but not rigorously studied in the critically ill. Patients also report the value of rehabilitation and functional activity and the ability to visit with their loved ones in fresh air spaces (see Figure 21.3) [52]. The capacity for teams to provide such opportunities in a safe, flexible, and innovative manner enables patients and loved ones to achieve goals that matter to them. Sometimes in the ICU, having an ice cream in the sun with loved ones is absolutely the key priority. Moreover, it can be highly stressful for loved ones and family members to visit ICU environments due to previous negative experiences and hospital-associated trauma [53]. Fresh air spaces can offer a more private and peaceful space for loved ones to be reunited and for children and young people to see loved ones in a less intimidating clinical setting [21].

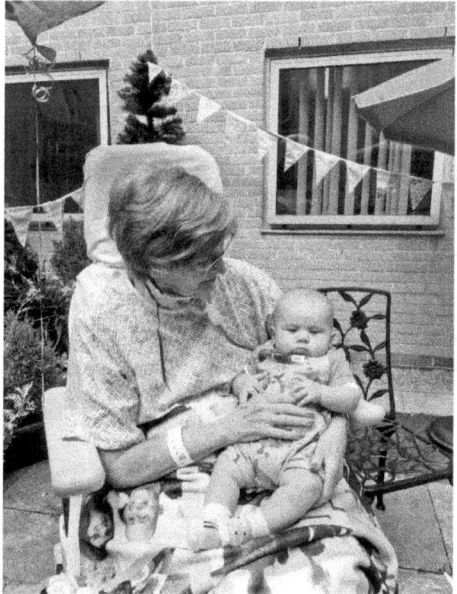

Figure 21.3 A family reunion in the ICU Secret Garden, University Hospitals Plymouth NHS Trust, UK.

End-of-Life Care in Fresh Air Spaces

End-of-life care in a fresh air space can offer privacy for the patient and their loved ones away from the less intimate environment of the ICU. End-of-life care provided in inpatient settings should be patient-centered, holistic, and extend beyond managing physical symptoms alone. Supporting end-of-life care outside the confines of a hospital room may be challenging, but recent guidance from the UK Intensive Care Society offers suggestions to support the provision of palliative care in garden spaces [45]. Although there is currently no data investigating the impact of fresh air spaces on patient and family experiences at the end of life, there is no doubt that for some patients and families, the opportunity to commune with nature before death would be cherished.

Case Study

Mr. G. was an elderly gentleman admitted to the ICU after cardiac arrest. In his last hours of life, the ICU garden offered a private space for the family to be reunited with him in a nonclinical environment. Clinical teams were able to provide comfort-focused care, optimize his and his family's experience, and offer space for more visitors than a conventional hospital room allows. The family reported that the environment created by the clinical team provided an increased sense of peace, privacy, and dignity.

Optimization of the Care of Patients with Multi-Drug-Resistant Organisms

Patients in critical care are at especially high risk of multi-drug-resistant organism (MDRO) colonization and infection due to comorbidities, frailty, immunological compromise, presence of indwelling care devices, and exposure to antimicrobial therapy [54]. The standard treatment for MDROs includes clinical isolation and strict infection prevention and control measures. In some countries, infection prevention and control teams mandate that MDRO patients must be treated when possible at the end of the clinical day to reduce transmission risk to other patients. This can lead to lost rehabilitation sessions and time lost due to operational pressures.

Rehabilitation gym environments present significant challenges to infection prevention and control measures, with increased risk of transmission due to shared equipment use and environmental contamination, and many hospitals limit the utilization of these facilities by patients colonized or infected with MDROs [55]. In this context, fresh air spaces can offer a novel infection prevention and control compliant rehabilitation space that can optimize patients' experience of rehabilitation and equipment utilization. Fresh air spaces are typically larger than patient bed spaces, facilitating the ability to mobilize patients over longer distances. Clinical teams report that the provision of therapy in a fresh air space allows for greater functional engagement in rehabilitation activities, such as walking longer distances, improving balance skills, applying sun cream, washing hands, and playing games, in an environment that optimizes the rehabilitation experience for all.

Safety Concerns When Accessing Fresh Air Spaces

Supporting critically ill patients to engage in functional activity while in fresh air spaces is a new endeavor, and the operational and clinical challenges of accessing fresh air spaces

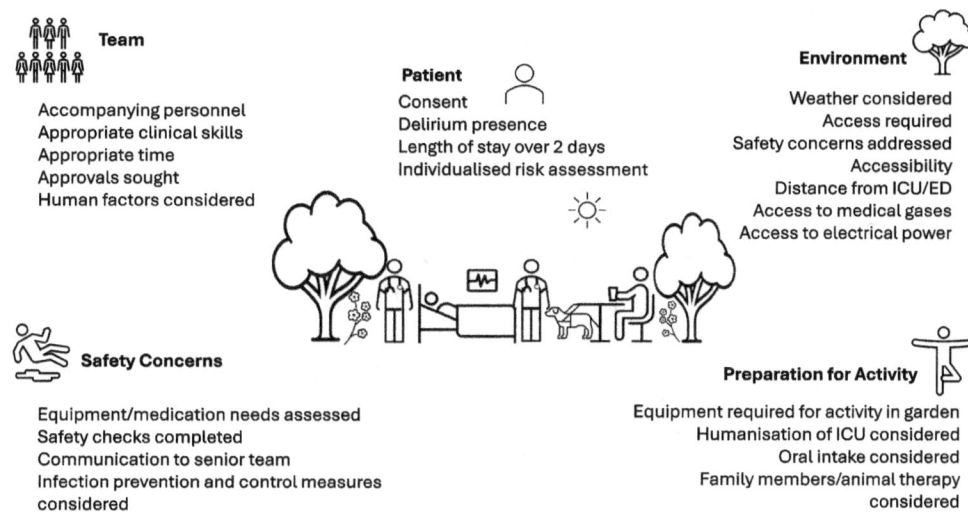

Figure 21.4 Considerations for safe transport to fresh air spaces.

for critically ill patients and their loved ones can make using them difficult for many clinical teams. Accessibility, safety concerns, and infection prevention and control measures are core considerations to all risk assessments prior to transferring patients to fresh air spaces. The UK-based Intensive Care Society has recently published two clinical guidelines that outline these issues and offer clinical solutions for routine transfer and end-of-life care (see Figure 21.4) [11,45].

When transferring a patient away from the intensive care environment, due diligence and consideration must be given to proactively plan and prepare for potential changes in the patient's clinical condition, and extra clinical supervision may be required from the interprofessional team. Preparation is key, both for the clinical staff accompanying the patient and for all the equipment, monitoring devices, and medications that may be required. Access to medical gases, power, shade, and cover in case of inclement weather are essential considerations that allow patients and their loved ones to spend longer times in fresh air spaces while reducing risks related to power failure and the transportation of medical gas cylinders. It is important to consider the durability of floor surfaces related to falls risk, the capacity to call for assistance, and the space available for moving and handling in case of falls.

Considerations for Designing a Fresh Air Space

Since 2006, the American Institute of Architects and the Facilities Guidelines Institute have recommended the development of greenspaces in hospitals to promote interaction with nature [2]. Greenspaces in hospitals, predominately composed of plants and trees, offer a change in environment for patients, loved ones, and staff to enjoy. Healing gardens in different specialties can have a different design brief; for example, patients with neurological injuries may require gardens with design features that optimize use of

Table 21.1 Considerations for planning and building an ICU garden

Factor	Considerations
Location	Proximity to support in case of clinical emergencies
	Consideration of bed/chair accessibility (patient and family)
Design	Must meet relevant building regulations
	Service user involvement is fundamental
	Consider infection prevention and control measures
	Sustainability and environmental considerations
Planting	Consider low allergy planting
	Location of shade and water sources
	Raised beds for planting for visibility for garden users
	Height and seasonal color
	Consider care requirements for planting
	Consider hazards related to accidental ingestion
External structures	Can be useful to provide respite from inclement weather (heat/wind/rain)
	Must be compliant with fire and infection and prevention control measures
Electricity and medical gases	Useful for gardens related to critical care areas
	Consider safety and fire risk
	Lighting useful as it extends duration of utilization in months with less natural light
Environmental infection and prevention control measures	Consider water
	Consider animals
	Consider potential pests (birds, rats, insects)
	Consider environmental pollutants
Ongoing maintenance	Cost associated with care for greenspaces to ensure their longevity

mobilization equipment, including motorized wheelchairs, and that include embedded power supplies for battery-operated equipment. All greenspace design should include a service user co-design process to ensure that the space meets the needs of the people it serves (see Table 21.1).

Conclusions

The Society of Critical Care Medicine guidelines for ICU design and the recent Guidelines for the Provision of Intensive Care Services in the UK consider access to natural light essential to the well-being of ICU patients and visitors [6,56]. Despite limited research in this field, greenspaces have been shown to have salutary impact on the physical health of patients and the mental health of patients, families, and staff. The risks associated with facilitating fresh air therapy are not insignificant, but the optimization of the environment and humanization of the ICU experience clearly positively impacts patients and their recovery trajectories, their loved ones, and the staff caring for them.

Key Points

1. It is recommended that therapeutic gardens with access to sunlight, shade, and vegetation be included in the design and construction of all new and refurbished hospitals.
2. The opportunity to interact with nature in an outdoor space can have a salutary impact on the physical, cognitive, and emotional health of critically ill patients and on the emotional health of their families and healthcare providers.
3. Fresh air spaces can be useful for some intensive care staff as a place to rest and take breaks, ideally mitigating the development of burnout syndrome.
4. Transfer to a fresh air space for ICU patients is safe and feasible and, with appropriate planning and risk assessment, is an intervention that can optimize the patient experience.
5. More evidence is required to fully explore the impact of fresh air spaces for ICU patients, their loved ones, and the staff caring for them.

References

1. Australasian Health Infrastructure Alliance. Australasian health facility guidelines part B – health facility briefing and planning HPU 360 intensive care unit. Australasian Health Infrastructure Alliance; 2019. https://healthfacilityguidelines.com.au/part/part-b-health-facility-briefing-and-planning-0. Accessed December 2023.
2. Australasian Health Infrastructure Alliance. Health Facility Briefing and Planning: HPU 360 Intensive Care Unit. 2015. https://healthfacilityguidelines.com.au/health-planning-units. Accessed December 2023.
3. S. Verderber, S. Gray, S. Suresh-Kumar, et al. Intensive care unit built environments: a comprehensive literature review (2005–2020). *HERD* 2021; **14**: 368–415.
4. S. Saha, H. Noble, A. Xyrichis, et al. Mapping the impact of ICU design on patients, families and the ICU team: a scoping review. *J Crit Care* 2022; **67**: 3–13.
5. I. van Iperen, J. Maas, P. Spronk. Greenery and outdoor facilities to improve the wellbeing of critically ill patients, their families and caregivers: things to consider. *Intensive Care Med* 2023; **49**: 1229–31.
6. FICM/ICS. Guidelines for the provision of intensive care services. London; 2022.
7. D. González-Caro, V. Blázquez-Romero, J. Garnacho-Montero. "Balcony of Hope": a key element of new intensive care units. *Intensive Care Med* 2023; **49**: 379–80.
8. J. Igeño-Cano. Benefits of walks in the outdoor gardens of the hospital in critically ill patients, relatives and professionals. #healingwalks. *Med Intensiva (Engl Ed)* 2020; **44**: 446–8.
9. M. Blans, A. Strang. Fresh air for intensive care patients in the Netherlands: an example to be followed? *Intensive Care Med* 2023; **49**: 1411–12.
10. K. Johnston. King's College Hospital is planning roof garden for patients on life-support. Southwark News; 2018.
11. K. Tantam, E. Jackson, N. Pattison, et al. Guidance on transfer of critically ill patients to the outdoors. London: UK Intensive Care Society; 2021.
12. B. Fazzini, G. Sim. Time outside for a long-term ventilated ICU patient. *Intensive Care Med* 2021; **47**: 1167–8.
13. N. Sasano, Y. Kato, A. Tanaka, N. Kusama. Out-of-the-ICU mobilization in critically ill patients: the safety of a new model of rehabilitation. *Crit Care Explor* 2022; **4**: e0604.

14. M. Maiden, M. Horton, P. Power, et al. Critically ill patients having time outdoors: prevalence and resources in Australia and New Zealand. *Intensive Care Med* 2024; **50**: 475–7.
15. M. Howarth, A. Brettle, M. Hardman, M. Maden. What is the evidence for the impact of gardens and gardening on health and well-being: a scoping review and evidence-based logic model to guide healthcare strategy decision making on the use of gardening approaches as a social prescription. *BMJ Open* 2020; **10**: e036923.
16. N. Blas-Miranda, A. Lozada-Tequeanes, J. Miranda-Zuñiga, M. Jimenez. Green space exposure and obesity in the Mexican adult population. *Int J Environ Res Public Health* 2022; **19**: 15072.
17. M. Jimenez, E. Elliott, N. DeVille, et al. Residential green space and cognitive function in a large cohort of middle-aged women. *JAMA Netw Open* 2022; **5**: e229306.
18. J. Klompmaker, F. Laden, M. Browning, et al. Associations of greenness, parks, and blue space with neurodegenerative disease hospitalizations among older US adults. *JAMA Netw Open* 2022: e2247664.
19. C. Twohig-Bennett, A. Jones. The health benefits of the great outdoors: a systematic review and meta-analysis of greenspace exposure and health outcomes. *Environ Res* 2018; **166**: 628–37.
20. L. Alfredsson, B. Armstrong, D. Butterfield, et al. Insufficient sun exposure has become a real public health problem. *Int J Environ Res Public Health* 2020; **17**: 5014.
21. R. Ulrich, M. Cordoza, S. Gardiner, et al. ICU patient family stress recovery during breaks in a hospital garden and indoor environments. *HERD* 2020; **13**: 83–102.
22. M. Cordoza, R.S. Ulrich, B.J. Manulik, et al. Impact of nurses taking daily work breaks in a hospital garden on burnout. *Am J Crit Care* 2018; **27**: 508–12.
23. L. Papazian, S. Hraiech, A. Loundou, et al. High-level burnout in physicians and nurses working in adult ICUs: a systematic review and meta-analysis. *Intensive Care Med* 2023; **49**: 387–400.
24. S.H. Bae. Intensive care nurse staffing and nurse outcomes: a systematic review. *Nurs Crit Care* 2021; **26**: 457–66.
25. L. McCallum, J. Rattray, B. Pollard, et al. The CANDID Study: impact of COVID-19 on critical care nurses and organisational outcomes: implications for the delivery of critical care services. A questionnaire study before and during the pandemic. *medRxiv* 2022: 2022.11.16.22282346.
26. J. Miller, B. Young, L. Mccallum, et al. "Like fighting a fire with a water pistol": a qualitative study of the work experiences of critical care nurses during the COVID-19 pandemic. *J Adv Nurs* 2024; **80**: 237–51.
27. T. Woo, R. Ho, A. Tang, W. Tam. Global prevalence of burnout symptoms among nurses: a systematic review and meta-analysis. *J Psychiatr Res* 2020; **123**: 9–20.
28. O.S. Daouda, M.N. Hocine, L. Temime. Determinants of healthcare worker turnover in intensive care units: a micro-macro multilevel analysis. *PLOS ONE* 2021; **16**: e0251779.
29. A. Min, Y.S. Yoon, H.C. Hong, Y.M. Kim. Association between nurses' breaks, missed nursing care and patient safety in Korean hospitals. *J Nurs Manag* 2020; **28**: 2266–74.
30. H.L. Stutting. The relationship between rest breaks and professional burnout among nurses. *Crit Care Nurse* 2023; **43**: 48–56.
31. J. Maben, C. Taylor, J. Jagosh, et al. Causes and solutions to workplace psychological ill-health for nurses, midwives and paramedics: the Care Under Pressure 2 realist review. *Health Soc Care Deliv Res* 2024; **12**: 1–171.
32. S. Valipoor, S.J. Bosch, L.Y.T. Chiu. From stressful to mindful: reactions to a proposed emergency department design for enhancing mindfulness and stress reduction among healthcare clinical staff. *HERD* 2023; **16**: 82–102.
33. E. Dore, D. Guerero, T. Wallbridge, et al. Sleep is the best medicine: how rest facilities and EnergyPods can improve staff wellbeing. *Future Healthc J* 2021; **8**: e625–e8.

34. R. Weerasuriya, C. Henderson-Wilson, M. Townsend. Accessing green spaces within a healthcare setting: a mixed studies review of barriers and facilitators. *HERD* 2019; **12**: 119–40.

35. A. Brambilla, M. Del Pio, R. Ravegnani Morosini, S. Capolongo. Green space in hospital built environment: a literature review about therapeutic gardens in acute care healthcare settings before Covid-19. *Acta Biomed* 2023; **94**: e2023137.

36. A. Brambilla, A. Morganti, G. Lindahl, et al. Complex Projects Assessment. The Impact of Built Environment on Healthcare Staff Wellbeing. In *Computational Science and Its Applications – ICCSA 2020. 20th international conference, Cagliari, Italy*. Berlin: Springer; 2020, pp. 345–54.

37. M. Cordoza, R. Ulrich, B. Manulik, et al. Impact of nurses taking daily work breaks in a hospital garden on burnout. *Am J Crit Care* 2018; **27**: 508–12.

38. K. Nieberler-Walker, C. Desha, C. Bosman, et al. Therapeutic hospital gardens: literature review and working definition. *HERD* 2023; **16**: 260–95.

39. M. Gola, M. Botta, A.L. D'Aniello, S. Capolongo. Influence of nature at the time of the pandemic: an experience-based survey at the time of SARS-CoV-2 to demonstrate how even a short break in nature can reduce stress for healthcare staff. *HERD* 2021; **14**: 49–65.

40. S.A. Iqbal, I.R. Abubakar. Hospital outdoor spaces as respite areas for healthcare staff during the COVID-19 pandemic. *HERD* 2022; **15**: 343–53.

41. W. Cui, Z. Li, X. Xuan, et al. Influence of hospital outdoor space on physiological electroencephalography (EEG) feedback of staff. *HERD* 2021; **15**: 239–55.

42. C. Carroll, J. Higgs, S. McCray, J. Utter. Implementation and impact of health care gardens: a systematic scoping review. *J Integr Complement Med* 2024; **30(5)**: 431-49.

43. C. Carroll, S. McCray, J. Utter. Acceptability and feasibility of a hospital-based herb and vegetable garden for health care workers. *J Nutr Educ Behav* 2023; **55**: 877–83.

44. Intensive Care Society. Guidance On: Transfer of Critically Ill Patients to the Outdoors. 2021. www.baccn.org/static/uploads/resources/Transfer_outdoors_guidance_final.pdf. Accessed December 2023.

45. S. Clark, K. Williams, E. Jackson, et al. *Guidance for: the transfer of critically ill adults to an outdoor space during end of life care*. London: Intensive Care Society; 2022.

46. R. Baron, R. Eilers, M.R. Haverkate, et al. A qualitative study examining the impact of multidrug-resistant organism (MDRO) carriage on the daily lives of carriers and parents of carriers with experiences of hospital precautionary measures. *Antimicrob Resist Infect Control* 2022; **11**: 103.

47. J.A. Alasad, N. Abu Tabar, M.M. Ahmad. Patients' experience of being in intensive care units. *J Crit Care* 2015; **30**: 859. e7–.e11.

48. H. Krampe, C. Denke, J. Gülden, et al. Perceived severity of stressors in the intensive care unit: a systematic review and semi-quantitative analysis of the literature on the perspectives of patients, health care providers and relatives. *J Clin Med* 2021; **10(17)**.

49. M.A. Pisani, C. D'Ambrosio. Sleep and delirium in adults who are critically ill: a contemporary review. *Chest* 2020; **157**: 977–84.

50. K. Kotfis, I. van Diem-Zaal, S. Williams Roberson, et al. The future of intensive care: delirium should no longer be an issue. *Crit Care* 2022; **26**: 200.

51. K. Wang, Y. Li, X. Chen, et al. Gardening and subjective cognitive decline: a cross-sectional study and mediation analyses of 136,748 adults aged 45+ years. *Nutr J* 2024; **23(1)**: 59.

52. R. Berto. Exposure to restorative environments helps restore attentional capacity. *J Environ Psychol* 2005; **25**: 249–59.

53. H.A. Abdul, L. Tang, M. Chong, et al. Psychological distress among the family members of Intensive Care Unit (ICU) patients: a scoping review. *J Clin Nurs* 2022; **31**: 497–507.
54. L.J. Strausbaugh, C.L. Joseph. The burden of infection in long-term care. *Infect Control Hosp Epidemiol* 2000; **21**: 674–9.
55. J.M. Boyce. Environmental contamination makes an important contribution to hospital infection. *J Hosp Infect* 2007; **65 Suppl 2**: 50–4.
56. D. Thompson, D. Hamilton, C. Cadenhead, et al. Guidelines for intensive care unit design. *Crit Care Med* 2012; **40**: 1586–600.

Chapter 22

Transitioning from the ICU to Home

Anna G. Kalema, Ashley A. Montgomery, Brad W. Butcher, and Melissa Soper

Introduction

The Society of Critical Care Medicine (SCCM) THRIVE post-intensive care unit (ICU) clinic and peer support collaboratives performed a qualitative study of 66 survivors of critical illness and 20 of their caregivers to better understand their thoughts, feelings, and perspectives as they progressed through the continuum of care from the ICU to home [1]. In the study, 79% of the patients and 55% of the caregivers had participated in an ICU follow-up program, either in the United States, the United Kingdom, or Australia. They found that, perhaps unsurprisingly, most patients recalled their illness as a profound shock that ultimately resulted in a loss of their former identity, including changes in their physical appearance, in their ability to care for themselves, in their social networks, and in their general independence. The study highlighted that as recovery in the hospital began, patients were often overwhelmed with the magnitude of their disabilities, and adaptation to them was slow, challenging, and often frustrating. As they left the hospital, patients feared the transition from a supportive environment where help was constantly available to one in which help was limited and adaptation to their new disabilities frequently occurred in the absence of guidance and support. In the long term, many patients described a pervasive psychological burden created by continued interactions with the healthcare system, where they felt retraumatized and unable to sustain a psychological recovery. Similarly, on leaving the hospital, the loved ones of survivors feared adopting the role of caregiver with no professional support available. As patients began to recover, caregivers noted that they had to accommodate new roles, such as medical decision-maker and patient advocate, while simultaneously maintaining their usual roles and activities; these competing demands often resulted in caregiver burden [1].

A companion study also sought to clarify the challenges that survivors of critical illness and their caregivers faced with the healthcare system as they transitioned from the ICU to the community [2]. Patients described a general lack of empathetic care from inpatient and outpatient clinicians and inadequate communication throughout their hospitalization, with declines in support at each transition to a lower intensity of care. Specific examples included lack of phone calls following discharge to check in, difficulty in obtaining outpatient rehabilitation services, and lack of understanding of post-intensive care syndrome (PICS) by primary care physicians and outpatient specialists. Patients also found it frustrating to manage how others regarded their post-ICU disabilities, including their family, employers, colleagues, and people in their social networks. The inability for others to understand – or even believe – their struggles led to feelings of loneliness and isolation and an active avoidance of social situations. Caregivers also described inadequacies in care that were most noticeable at times of transition, including insufficient communication and a failure to manage expectations, particularly at the time of hospital discharge. Loved ones also lamented a lack of support and resources for them as the role of caregiver was thrust upon them; as with patients, this lack of support also led to feelings of loneliness and isolation [2].

Aside from these studies, limited research exists regarding best practices for management of care transitions from the ICU to the hospital wards and from the hospital wards to rehabilitation centers or home. ICU follow-up clinics are the most sophisticated solution to facilitate patient recovery and rehabilitation efforts once patients return home (see Chapter 28 for additional information). Successful recruitment and patient participation in these clinics remain challenging but may be facilitated by the presence of a "post-ICU team" to engage with the patient and family prior to hospital discharge [1,2,3]. A post-ICU team can facilitate care transitions and assuage many of the concerns highlighted by the aforementioned studies; through early and consistent communication, the team can alleviate care- and recovery-related worries and improve patient and family satisfaction with their care. More importantly, developing rapport during these transitions increases the likelihood of patient engagement with ICU follow-up programs and the earlier delivery of PICS-related interventions for the patient and their family. Engagement with the post-ICU team allows identification of patient barriers to follow up, streamlines referral processes, and stresses the importance of effective care team communication across the patient recovery continuum.

Identification of Barriers to ICU Clinic Follow-Up

As new ICU follow-up clinics are being developed, early identification of barriers to recruitment and clinic attendance is key to developing standard operating procedures that overcome these hurdles and enhance clinic success. Seasoned clinics engage in repeated assessments to evaluate the effectiveness of process improvement measures designed to address these challenges, incorporating feedback from patients and staff. Many barriers to patient recruitment and follow-up fall into the following categories: staff-related, patient-related, insufficient organizational support, failure to appreciate the importance of ICU follow-up, and social determinants of health (SDOH).

Staff barriers include knowledge deficits and biases related to PICS. Early conversations during formation and socialization of the clinic may uncover knowledge gaps related to resource availability and flawed perceptions about survivorship following critical illness. Even at institutions with an existing ICU follow-up clinic, the availability of the clinic and the clinic referral process may not be well known. By increasing staff knowledge of the clinic's referral process and services, the team can promote expedited patient referrals from within the organization.

The patient's clinical course and the varied discharge destinations available can make arranging follow-up difficult [4,5]. Figure 22.1 outlines potential patient paths through the phases of care. Patient transitions during the hospital course, including transfers to other service lines or other ICUs, frequently lead to patients being lost to follow-up in the absence of a centralized screening process to track them throughout hospitalization. Frequently, payors in the United States require prior authorization to approve discharge to a rehabilitation hospital or a long-term acute care hospital, which may delay discharge for several days. On occasion, the patient's medical condition changes significantly enough that they either remain admitted to the hospital or their discharge disposition changes, which proves problematic when trying to establish a follow-up timeline to achieve a true transitional care appointment [4]. Conversely, sufficient patient recovery to allow them to be

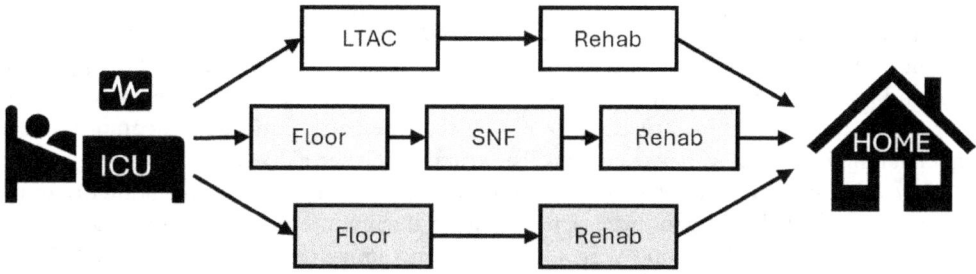

Figure 22.1 Patient recovery pathways.

discharged home can expedite their access to an ICU follow-up clinic. The unpredictable patient clinical course and the fragmentation of the healthcare system necessitate that ICU follow-up clinics have a system to track patients throughout the hospital and rehabilitation sectors. Consistently assigning this role to one team member and harnessing the power of the electronic health record (EHR), if possible, can make this often arduous task easier.

Organizational education efforts can help bridge these gaps as well. Outreach by clinic staff should include networking with regional rehabilitation facilities and establishing points of contact outside of the organization to open lines of communication and referral to the ICU follow-up clinic. Increasing rehabilitation centers' awareness of PICS and the ICU follow-up clinic's services enhances interfacility communication and coordination of care. Increasing the general public's knowledge about the function of the clinic and the services that it offers is equally important. Appearances in online or written editorials, presentations at professional organization meetings, and advertisements are all important to increase knowledge of PICS and the clinical and social resources that are available to aid patient recovery.

ICU follow-up clinics located in "healthcare deserts" with limited primary and tertiary healthcare services must consider geographical barriers and SDOH that drive patient comorbid conditions and prevent access to care (see Chapter 25 for additional information). The financial hardships of travel, the potential need for supplemental oxygen during travel, and ongoing physical debility may be prohibitive to some patients [5,6,7]. Even with clinics using telemedicine platforms to overcome some of these barriers, the inability of patients to afford or access the requisite technology, internet, or phone services may prevent them from accessing ICU follow-up clinics via telehealth [6,8,9]. In many states, legislation that once allowed reimbursement for voice-only telehealth appointments was repealed following the easing of the COVID-19 pandemic. Collectively, these factors serve to limit a clinic's outreach opportunities and financial feasibility to serve patients that may not otherwise have access to care. ICU follow-up clinics must consistently evaluate their effort to address such barriers to care and to enhance equity in care delivery.

Proposed Solutions

Addressing Recruitment Challenges and Low Clinic Attendance

There are several solutions to address recruitment challenges and remove barriers to attendance in ICU follow-up clinics. One solution is to increase awareness of PICS by formally incorporating it into the training programs for medical students, residents, fellows, nurses, and other members of the multidisciplinary team caring for patients at risk. Successful implementation of this intervention requires collaboration between the ICU follow-up clinic and the relevant training programs and may include didactic lectures, shadowing opportunities, and more immersive clinical rotations in the ICU follow-up clinic. The content of the training sessions should be structured to ensure that the participants gain a comprehensive understanding of PICS, who is at greatest risk, criteria for referral to the ICU follow-up clinic, and processes used to refer patients to the clinic. Some graduate medical education programs for residents and fellows introduce learners to PICS during orientation sessions and lectures given throughout the academic year, along with encouragement to participate in clinical rotations with exposure to this patient population. It is similarly essential to educate healthcare staff who are integral to discharging patients from the hospital, such as non-ICU attending physicians, advanced practice providers, social workers, and case managers, who can collectively ensure that patients meeting criteria have a referral to the ICU follow-up clinic or an appointment made prior to discharge. This education can be provided during hospital-wide seminars or conferences such as grand rounds.

A second solution is to enhance communication between survivors of critical illness and care providers following hospital discharge, which can be challenging, particularly when the patient is discharged to a rehabilitation facility or skilled nursing facility. Establishing a transitions of care facilitator to optimize the coordination of patient care and facilitate communication between patients or their loved ones and the ICU follow-up clinic during this critical transition phase is important. This role ensures that care and support are provided to patients as they move from hospital to home and addresses potential barriers to patient follow-up, thereby increasing the likelihood of clinic attendance.

Several solutions can address patients' impaired access to care and inability to travel to clinic appointments. These include conducting follow-up visits virtually using telemedicine (see Chapter 29 for additional information), offering follow-up outside of standard business hours, providing in-home visits, and clustering clinic visits on the same day as follow-up appointments with other healthcare providers. Implementing such strategies improves access to care and promotes better health outcomes for patients with otherwise limited access to healthcare services. Furthermore, partnering with existing services at an institution, such as high-risk discharge clinics, transition of care clinics, primary care physician offices, and outpatient scheduling centers can help share resources and expand the reach of the ICU follow-up clinic.

The ICU Follow-Up Clinic Inpatient Screening Process

Eligibility criteria for participation in ICU follow-up clinics differ among institutions based on personnel, financial, and other available resources. Over time, these criteria may require modification based on resource availability, clinic attendance, or significant changes in patient care needs, such as following the COVID-19 pandemic (see Chapter 53 for additional information). In general, patient eligibility criteria and screening paradigms are focused on identifying patients at high risk for developing PICS (see Box 22.1) [3,10,11,12,13,14,15,16,17,18]. Table 22.1 outlines various inclusion and exclusion criteria that can be used to identify patients appropriate for ICU follow-up clinic referral; if sufficient resources are available, using broad inclusion criteria can drive clinic attendance and expand its reach.

Box 22.1 PICS risk factors identified during literature review [14]

Advanced age
Delirium
Disease severity
Female gender
Glucose dysregulation
Immobility
Multiple organ failures (>2 organ systems)
Pharmacologic exposures (e.g., benzodiazepines)
Preexisting comorbid conditions
Preexisting mood disorder
Prolonged ICU stay (>7 days)
Prolonged mechanical ventilation
Sepsis with or without shock
Sleep disruption

Table 22.1 Sample ICU follow-up clinic patient recruitment inclusion and exclusion criteria

Inclusion	Exclusion
Acute hypoxic respiratory failure • Mechanical ventilation • Noninvasive positive pressure ventilation • High-flow nasal cannula	Imminent death or limited life expectancy (likely death within 6 months)
Acute respiratory distress syndrome	Limited rehabilitation potential (e.g., preexisting long-term dependencies in activities of daily living)
Cognitive dysfunction or delirium during hospitalization	Neurologic injury affecting level of consciousness and awareness
Need for ECMO	Residence outside of state and inability to drive
ICU-acquired weakness	Patient or stakeholder decline follow up
New tracheostomy or surgical feeding tube placement	Ventilator dependence at a facility
Acute organ failure during ICU admission	Severe psychiatric disease or substance use disorder
Prolonged ICU course (>72 hours)	Incarceration
Prolonged hospital course	
Recent surgery • Urgent • Emergent • Peri-operative complications	
Shock requiring vasopressor or inotropic support	

Minimizing the number of patients who fail to attend an ICU follow-up clinic appointment or who are lost to follow-up is similarly important. Decreased likelihood of clinic attendance is strongly associated with geographical location, reduced socioeconomic status, alcohol and illicit substance use, male gender, and significant disability and weakness following discharge [19]. Some clinics employ exclusion criteria to enrich the clinic population with those most likely to benefit and to minimize the risk of attrition and loss to follow-up. Examples of such exclusion criteria include limited life expectancy (e.g., patients discharged to hospice services), limited rehabilitation potential (e.g., patients dependent for care prior to hospitalization), patients with severe psychiatric illness or substance abuse disorders, and incarceration.

Screening for clinic eligibility can be performed in many ways and is dependent on the personnel, EHR, and time resources available. Candidate patients may be identified by tools embedded in the EHR or by routine screening of critically ill patients, which can be performed by intensivists, advanced practice providers, nurses, pharmacists, therapists, research coordinators, or social workers. The screening process commonly includes review of the patient's demographic characteristics, pre-morbid function, reason for admission, progress notes, SDOH, and familial support. As patients approach readiness for discharge, referral to the clinic can be initiated to prompt scheduling at the appropriate follow-up interval, or an appointment can be made and placed in the discharge paperwork. In addition to screening hospitalized patients, referrals may be placed by other inpatient physicians, primary care physicians, and other outpatient specialists via the EHR, with an order set outlining the appropriate patient population for referral and the steps to secure an appointment. Developing a clinic website that includes a referral portal is another potential platform for patients or their providers to seek an appointment; ideally, the referrals should be internally reviewed to ensure appropriateness.

Early Patient Education on PICS While in the Hospital

According to patients and loved ones who participated in an ICU follow-up program, successful programs have five key components: providing continuity of care, improving symptom status, normalizing the recovery process and managing expectations, providing internal and external validation of progress, and reducing feelings of guilt and helplessness [20]. Meeting the patient and family in the ICU and continuing the relationship throughout hospitalization builds rapport and solidifies the post-ICU team as a vital part of the recovery process. Involving the ICU nurses, respiratory therapists, physical therapists, and other providers to educate patients and families about the challenges faced following critical illness and to emphasize the importance of follow-up is key. Early education about PICS helps the patient and family understand that impairments may be long-lasting and that the ICU follow-up clinic provides care that is frequently overlooked in the current healthcare model. For example, symptoms that create significant patient burden, such as weakness, are often viewed as insignificant by many outpatient providers and may go unassessed or unaddressed during specialist clinic visits. Normalizing these symptoms and discussing how the ICU follow-up clinic can support the patient and their caregivers holistically gives the clinic an important space in the care continuum (see Chapter 23 for additional information).

Early Engagement with the Family and Expectation Management

During the hospitalization, it is important to identify who will be the patient's surrogate decision-maker(s) and caretaker(s) following discharge, ideally in the presence of both the patient and their family members [21]. This allows for important questions to be asked directly, normalizes the dependence that often occurs after hospital discharge, and manages expectations about the pace of recovery. Questions to consider asking the patient and their loved ones include:

1. Do you have any questions about what happened to you in the ICU?
2. Who will being staying with you when you first go home?
3. Who will be driving you to your appointments?
4. Who will help you get groceries and medications? Who will prepare your meals for you?
5. Who is your primary care provider? Have you seen them in the last year?
6. How will you pay your bills for the next several months?
7. What are the things you are worried about at home?

Establishing a relationship with the patient and their family early in the hospitalization, with an emphasis on normalizing the recovery process, helps the family plan for the support needed during this transitional period. It is important that contact information for the patient and their surrogates are properly recorded in the EHR and confirmed with the family, case management team, and discharge planners. Providing the patient's loved ones a binder or notebook early in the ICU course allows them to create a repository of information about the hospital stay, the names of clinical teams and care providers, resources for support after discharge, and information about PICS [22]. PICS-related education should manage expectations about the pace and breadth of recovery and normalize the likelihood of new physical, functional, cognitive, psychiatric, and social dependencies, concepts that are crucial to convey prior to hospital discharge. Education for family about the patient's functional limitations can help them prepare to assist with activities of daily living (ADLs). The post-ICU team can help caregivers visualize the patient's potential barriers to performing these ADLs in the home environment and identify the modifications that could make such tasks easier and promote independence [23,24].

Enhancing Contact with Transition-Related Phone Calls

Scheduling should be accompanied by a "pre-discharge, post-ICU" phone call by an ICU clinician, which is an ideal time to re-explain the clinic's purpose and to ensure that stakeholders are aware of the clinic appointment [25]. Typically, these calls are scripted, and an example is presented in Box 22.2.

Once patients leave the hospital, a "transitional" phone call, made within the first 24 to 48 hours by a clinic team member, a transitions-of-care team, or a case manager, is a useful tool. It reinforces the information provided in discharge instructions, identifies patient struggles at home, and remedies potential barriers to making follow-up appointments. Early contact during this important transition may reduce clinic attrition and reinforces that the post-ICU team is invested in the patient's recovery [26]. Additionally, this phone call may help decrease hospital readmissions and unnecessary emergency department visits caused by a lack of understanding of the home treatment plan. An example of a script used during this phone call is presented in Box 22.3.

Disposition Locations for Patients Transitioning from the ICU

ICU patients are typically discharged to one of four locations, and each location has a different set of variables for both the family and the follow-up team to take into

Box 22.2 Script for pre-discharge, post-ICU phone call

Hello, Mr./Mrs./Miss_____, my name is _____ and I am a _____ with the ICU team and the ICU follow-up clinic at _____. You are listed as a point of contact for patient _____. May I ask how you are related?

    The purpose for my call is to discuss a discharge follow-up with the _____ ICU follow-up clinic for your loved one. I typically contact the care stakeholders before the patient is discharged because the majority of critically ill patients have memory loss related to their hospital stay. I have a couple of questions for you. Will you be the person bringing them to their appointments? Would you or your loved one be comfortable with me discussing their care with you?

    I would like to tell you about our team and what we do in our clinic to assist your loved-one's recovery. I would also like to answer any questions you have and to prepare you for what to expect when _____ leaves the hospital and rehabilitation facility.

    It's been so nice speaking with you today, and I look forward to seeing you at the upcoming appointment scheduled for 1–2 weeks post discharge from the hospital or the rehabilitation facility. If you have any questions or need anything before the follow up, please message me via the electronic health record or call me at: _____.

Box 22.3 Script for the care transition phone call performed 24–48 hours following discharge

Hello, Mr./Mrs./Miss_____, my name is _____ and I am a _____ with the transition of care team and ICU follow-up clinic at _____. I wanted to check on you following your recent critical illness and see how you are doing now that you've been at home for a couple of days. I would like to ask you a few questions if you have the time. This is important because it allows the ICU follow-up clinic team to be prepared for your upcoming appointment on _____ and can also help us ensure everything you need to be successful after discharge.

- I am going to review and confirm the patient's/your medications and supplements with you. Have there been any changes in your medications since you were discharged from _____?
- I am going to review the patient's/your health history. Have there been any changes in the health history or new surgeries since the discharge from _____?
- Were they/you discharged home with durable medical equipment? Is there any equipment you haven't received or could not afford? Do you have questions on how to use the equipment? What medical equipment company are you working with?
- Do they/you require supplemental oxygen at home? If so, how much and who is the supplier? Have you received it?
- Do they/you have home health services prescribed? This would include physical therapy, occupational therapy, respiratory therapy, and/or nursing. What agency is following you and have they set up the first appointment?
- Do they/you have a list of all of your upcoming appointments? I would like to review these with you.
- Is there any reason that you wouldn't be able to make your upcoming appointments? If so, what is the reason?
- Are they/you having difficulty with any of the "Social Determinants of Health"? If so, are you aware of or have you been referred to any programs to help you with this? Would it be okay if I have our social worker reach out to you?

> It's been so nice speaking with you today, and we look forward to seeing you at your upcoming appointment on _____. Do you know where the clinic is located and where to park?
>
> I will notify the members of our team of our conversation today, and the appropriate people will be in touch to help you. If you need anything prior to your clinic appointment, please call us at _____.

consideration. These locations can be a continuum or a single step between the hospital and home environments. These facilities are termed long-term acute care hospitals (LTACHs), acute (or inpatient) rehabilitation facilities, sub-acute rehabilitation facilities (or skilled nursing facilities [SNFs]), and home. The destination of the patient at discharge is typically based on the degree of physical rehabilitation that they will need, their ability to participate in that rehabilitation, and the insurance company's willingness to pay for it.

An LTACH is an appropriate discharge destination if the patient has significant ongoing medical needs, which may include: specialized wound care, weaning from mechanical ventilation, chronic critical illness, new initiation of hemodialysis, new tracheotomy, and/or the need for multiple intravenous medications. LTACH stays are typically billed to private insurance or Medicare with an anticipated length of stay of approximately 21 to 28 days. From this facility, patients may be discharged home or to another rehabilitation or nursing facility.

Acute rehabilitation services are provided in free-standing rehabilitation centers or facilities that are partnered with a local hospital. Patients are typically discharged to an acute rehabilitation facility, either from the hospital or LTACH, when they are deemed able to complete at least three hours per day of physical, occupational, and cognitive therapy. Patients eligible for acute rehabilitation generally require significantly less medical care and no longer require ventilator support, and a typical length of stay is 14 to 21 days. Obtaining insurance or payor authorization for these visits can be challenging despite patients having significant rehabilitation needs. Certain diagnoses, including stroke, traumatic brain injury, and spinal cord injury, are commonly admitted to rehabilitation hospitals, while survivors of non-neurological critical illness may find it more challenging to win insurance approval despite the ongoing physical and cognitive deficits related to their hospitalization.

Sub-acute rehabilitation is typically performed at a SNF, and patients are admitted to this location from the hospital and less frequently from LTACHs. Private or public insurance is billed for this admission, which typically lasts four to six weeks. Patients in these settings generally have few medical needs, require variable assistance with ADLs, and may be able to complete short sessions of rehabilitation, but less than three hours per day. If the patient is unable to be discharged home based on the inability to independently perform ADLs, remain safe, or have social support, the patient may be admitted as a long-term resident of the facility.

The last option for patient discharge is home with or without assistance of home healthcare services, a decision typically made in consultation with hospital-based physical and occupational therapists. Patients discharged home may still require a significant amount of assistance with ADLs and mobility, and the burden of care is placed on the family and the patient's primary care provider. The patient may or may not have a home healthcare agency that will provide physical and cognitive rehabilitation, nursing care, infusion care, nutrition support, tracheotomy care, medication management, and/or wound care services. If available, these services are typically provided one to two days per week for an hour at a time, and the remaining care needs are the family's responsibility. The care providers for these patients are at the highest risk for PICS-Family, and they should be assessed alongside the patient during the ICU follow-up clinic visit.

Conclusion

Referral to ICU follow-up clinics is not currently embedded in the United States healthcare system and, given the limited number of ICU follow-up clinics available, may not be for the foreseeable future. The goal of recruiting and ensuring patient attendance in ICU follow-up clinics is overshadowed by many potential barriers within the healthcare system. Despite the best efforts of those hospitals that do offer ICU follow-up services, getting patients to clinic appointments can be challenging, particularly within the first months after hospital discharge, when the potential for rehabilitation is at its greatest. In addition to navigating a series of appointments with providers in other specialties, which are often considered by patients to be of greater importance, the very impairments associated with PICS make attending an ICU follow-up clinic appointment difficult. Patients may be too weak to come, they may fail to remember their appointment, they may prefer to avoid the location of their recent trauma, or they may not have transportation or financial resources to attend the appointment.

Transitional care points of contact with the post-ICU team prior to both hospital discharge and the first ICU follow-up clinic appointment can help bridge these gaps and allow for early recognition and mitigation of patient barriers to attendance and identification of new health problems. More importantly, it conveys a community of support with an entire multidisciplinary team checking in with the patient and their caregivers, which, as qualitative studies tell us, is desperately wanted.

Key Points

1. Transitions of care are frequently the source of miscommunication, missed follow-up, and reduced opportunities to ensure that ICU patients and their care providers have the resources to be successful in the next phase of the patient's care.
2. Resources are defined as medications, supplies, teaching, and continued interdisciplinary team interventions to support the patient's recovery over the next several months.
3. Incorporation of a strong recruiting process while patients are in the ICU and hospital with early contact from the ICU team, follow-up phone calls before and after discharge to care stakeholders, and creation of a transition of care network can serve to prevent clinic attrition, increase patient and caregiver satisfaction, and prevent hospital readmissions.
4. An interdisciplinary approach is key and should involve all members of the healthcare team to focus on all facets of the patient's recovery from critical illness.

References

1. K.J. Haines, N. Leggett, E. Hibbert, et al. Patient and caregiver-derived health service improvements for better critical care recovery. *Crit Care Med* 2022; **50**(12): 1778–87.

2. K.J. Haines, E. Hibbert, N. Leggett, et al. Transitions of care after critical illness: challenges to recovery and adaptive problem solving. *Crit Care Med* 2021; **49**(11): 1923–31.

3. T.J. Iwashyna. Trajectories of recovery and dysfunction after acute illness, with implications for clinical trial design. *Am J Resp Crit Care Med* 2012; **186**: 302–4.

4. N.H. Merbitz, K. Westie, J.A. Dammeyer, et al. After critical care: challenges in the transition to inpatient rehabilitation. *Rehabil Psychol* 2016; **61**(2): 186–200.

5. R. Zbar. Socio-ecologic perspective: barriers complicating post-intensive care syndrome mitigation. *J Patient Exp* 2022; **9**: 23743735211074434.

6. K.M. Potter, L.P. Scheunemann, T.D. Girard. Health equity and critical care survivorship: where do we go from here? *Ann Intern Med* 2022; **175**: 749–50.

7. M. Tackett, L. Jubina, A. Kalema, et al. 947: Social determinants of health influence attendance at an ICU recovery clinic. *Crit Care Med* 2023; **51**: 466.

8. T.L. Eaton, C.M. Sevin, A.A. Hope, et al. Evolution in care delivery within critical illness recovery programs during the COVID-19 pandemic: a qualitative study. *Ann Am Thorac Soc* 2022; **19**(11): 1900–6.

9. L.A. Zughni, A.I. Gillespie, J.L. Hatcher, et al. Telemedicine and the interdisciplinary clinic model: during the COVID-19 pandemic and beyond. *Otolaryngo Head Neck Surg* 2020; **163**: 673–5.

10. J.W. Devlin, Y. Skrobik, C. Gélinas, et al. Executive summary: clinical practice guidelines for the prevention and management of pain, agitation/sedation, delirium, immobility, and sleep disruption in adult patients in the ICU. *Crit Care Med* 2018; **46**: 1532–48.

11. E.W. Ely, S.K. Inouye, G.R. Bernard, et al. Delirium in mechanically ventilated patients: validity and reliability of the confusion assessment method for the intensive care unit (CAM-ICU). *JAMA* 2001; **286**: 2703–10.

12. E.W. Ely, A. Shintani, B. Truman, et al. Delirium as a predictor of mortality in mechanically ventilated patients in the intensive care unit. *JAMA* 2004; **291**: 1753–62.

13. S. Inoue, J. Hatakeyama, Y. Kondo, et al. Post-intensive care syndrome: its pathophysiology, prevention, and future directions. *Acute Med Surg* 2019; **6**: 233–46.

14. M. Lee, J. Kang, Y. J. Jeong. Risk factors for post–intensive care syndrome: a systematic review and meta-analysis. *Aust Crit Care* 2020; **33**: 287–94.

15. Y. Lee, K. Kim, C. Lim, J.S. Kim. Effects of the ABCDE bundle on the prevention of post-intensive care syndrome: a retrospective study. *J Adv Nurs* 2020; **76**: 588–99.

16. A. Montgomery-Yates, A. Kelly, E. Cassity, et al. 1063: International challenge to develop uniform criteria for outpatient ICU survivors clinic. *Crit Care Med* 2016; **44**: 342.

17. A. Montgomery-Yates, A. Kelly, A. Kalema, et al. D22: The course of critical illness: admission to follow-up: anticipating need for a survivors clinic appointment by examining ICU survivors' trajectories of healthcare utilization in the year preceding critical illness. *Am J Resp Crit Care Med* 2017; **195**.

18. G. Rawal, S. Yadav, R. Kumar. Post-intensive care syndrome: an overview. *J Transl Int Med* 2017; **5**: 90–2.

19. K.P. Mayer, H. Boustany, E.P. Cassity, et al. ICU recovery clinic attendance, attrition, and patient outcomes: the impact of severity of illness, gender, and rurality. *Crit Care Explor* 2020; **2**: e0206.

20. J. McPeake, L.M. Boehm, E. Hibbert, et al. Key components of ICU recovery programs: what did patients report

provided benefit? *Crit Care Explor* 2020; **2**: e0088.

21. D. Elliott, J.E. Davidson, M.A. Harvey, et al. Exploring the scope of post–intensive care syndrome therapy and care: engagement of non-critical care providers and survivors in a second stakeholders meeting. *Crit Care Med* 2014; **42**: 2518–26.

22. J.L. Stollings, J.W. Devlin, J.C. Lin, et al. Best practices for conducting interprofessional team rounds to facilitate performance of the ICU liberation (ABCDEF) bundle. *Crit Care Med* 2020; **48**: 562.

23. C.M. Sevin, L.M. Boehm, E. Hibbert, et al. Optimizing critical illness recovery: perspectives and solutions from the caregivers of ICU survivors. *Crit Care Explor* 2021; **12**: e0420.

24. A.A.M. Hope, J. McPeake. Healthcare delivery and recovery after critical illness. *Curr Opin Crit Care* 2022; **28**: 566–71.

25. L.M. Boehm, V. Danesh, T. Eaton, et al. Multidisciplinary ICU recovery clinic visits: a qualitative analysis of patient-provider dialogues. *Chest* 2023; **163**: 843–54.

26. U. Pant, K. Vyas, S. Meghani, et al. Screening tools for post–intensive care syndrome and post-traumatic symptoms in intensive care unit survivors: a scoping review. *Aust Crit Care* 2023; **36**(5): 863–71.

Section 4 General Principles of Critical Illness Survivorship and Follow-Up Care

Chapter 23

A Holistic Approach to Care

Kehllee L. Popovich and Janet A. Kloos

We come together to develop a plan for the patient, with the patient, working together to address the complex physical, cognitive, and emotional challenges of post-intensive care syndrome (PICS). This interprofessional teamwork ensures that care is holistic, tailored to each patient's unique needs, and aimed at maximizing recovery, enhancing quality of life, and preventing long-term complications.

PICS provider, University Hospitals, Cleveland Medical Center

Introduction

Post-intensive care syndrome (PICS) is a complex condition affecting many survivors of critical illness that is characterized by physical, cognitive, and psychological impairments that persist long after discharge from the intensive care unit (ICU) [1,2]. Impairments in these three domains often overlap and impact one another, leading to significant functional limitations; difficulties reintegrating into familial, occupational, and social roles; and consequently, a decline in quality of life [3,4]. Developing and enacting a comprehensive recovery plan for patients with PICS requires a coordinated, interprofessional team that approaches the patient holistically. By working together, healthcare professionals from various disciplines – physicians, therapists, mental health specialists, dietitians, and nurses – provide a holistic plan of care that supports optimal healing and enables patients to achieve the highest possible quality of life in their recovery journey. The importance of interdisciplinary cooperation and multidisciplinary interventions cannot be overstated, as managing the interplay between physical disability, cognitive dysfunction, and psychological disorders is essential for optimizing patient outcomes.

By utilizing a multidisciplinary, interprofessional approach, ICU follow-up clinics offer significant advantages for managing complex patients who have survived intensive care but are facing chronic, complicated, and interrelated impairments. This holistic model for providing care emphasizes the "whole person," recognizing the interconnection of physical, cognitive, emotional, and spiritual health, while also considering the potential for disrupted social relationships and financial toxicity as a consequence of lost employment and ongoing healthcare costs [3,5].

Interrelatedness of Impairments

Impairments in the three classically defined PICS domains are not mutually exclusive and frequently impact one another (see Figure 23.1). This idea is supported by a nested study of the BRAIN-ICU cohort, in which survivors of critical illness were assessed at 3 and 12

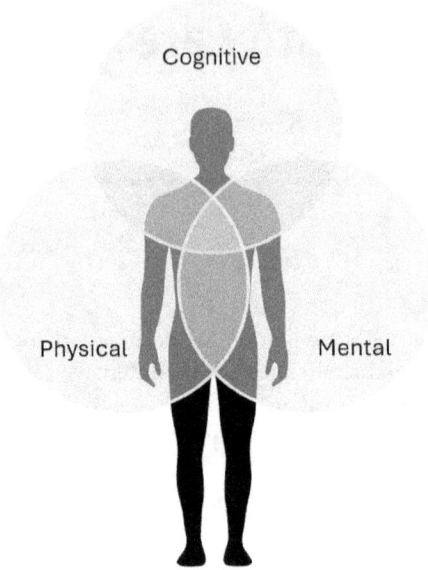

Figure 23.1 The overlap between physical, cognitive, and psychological impairments in PICS presents unique challenges that must be addressed through coordinated care. (Silhouette image credit Seamartini/iStock/Getty Images Plus).

months for combinations of cognitive impairment, depression, and dependencies in performing activities of daily living (ADLs) [1]. One manifestation of PICS was present in 64% and 56% of the patients at 3 and 12 months, respectively, and problems in two or more PICS domains were present in 25% and 21% of the patients at 3 and 12 months, respectively. This frequent co-occurrence of PICS impairments was emphasized in a more recent analysis of data from 289 survivors of sepsis who required intensive care, in which three classification models were utilized to report the prevalence of impairments consistent with PICS [6]:

- Model 1 (low threshold): an impairment in any domain (mental, cognitive, or physical).
- Model 2 (conservative threshold): an impairment in both a combined neuropsychiatric domain (e.g., presence of depression, post-traumatic stress disorder [PTSD], or cognitive impairment) and physical domain (e.g., presence of chronic pain, neuropathic symptoms, or dysphagia).
- Model 3 (strict threshold): an impairment in each of the three domains: mental, cognitive, and physical.

Perhaps unsurprisingly, the prevalence of PICS varied widely depending on the model considered: over a follow-up period of 24 months, 98.6%, 81.7%, and 32.9% of patients had impairments consistent with PICS when Models 1, 2, and 3 were applied, respectively.

Impairments in multiple domains are common, and the presence of an impairment in one domain often results in or intensifies an impairment in another. For example, in a study of 186 survivors of acute lung injury by Bienvenu and colleagues, symptoms of depression were significantly associated with impaired physical function (OR 2.7; 95% CI, 1.2–6.0) [7]. The ability to independently perform ADLs was also positively correlated with scores of cognitive function (as determined by the Montreal Cognitive Assessment tool) at both ICU discharge and one month later, suggesting a relationship between physical and cognitive performance [7]. Complementary findings confirmed an association between higher physical function measures and lower anxiety and depression symptom scores, further emphasizing the correlation between physical and mental health [8]. Furthermore, treatment for impairments in one domain may have a salutary impact on impairments in another domain as demonstrated by a meta-analysis of four randomized controlled trials, which suggested that the provision of physical therapy reduced the severity of depression (mean difference [MD] = -1.21; 95% CI, -2.31 to -0.11, $I^2 = 0\%$) [9].

A Theoretical Model for Recovery Following Critical Illness

Facilitated sensemaking, a middle-range theory developed by Davidson, provides a framework for understanding the ICU experience and the adaptation to new impairments following critical illness [10]. This theory builds upon Roy's Adaptation Model and Weick's Organizational Sensemaking Model to guide patients and their families through the recovery process by helping individuals make sense of the changes they are experiencing and by supporting them in the development of strategies to cope with new limitations. The facilitated sensemaking theory views illness as a significant disruption that requires individuals to engage in coping processes and to develop adaptive responses [10]. Weick's model emphasizes the need for an iterative process to make sense of cues, such as information provided by healthcare providers, so that patients and their families can form a coherent, consistent understanding of their situation [11]. Facilitated sensemaking extends these ideas by incorporating practical interventions, such as home-based exercise regimens or electronic reminders, to help patients and families cope with physical and cognitive challenges. By supporting the understanding of these changes, facilitated sensemaking is thought to reduce the risk of PTSD in patients and families through activation of the prefrontal cortex, which can mitigate the release of stress hormones and improve emotional regulation during recovery [10,11].

Benefits of Multidisciplinary Clinics in Chronic Disease

Multidisciplinary teams in healthcare settings have been shown to be effective in the management of numerous conditions, including heart disease and cancer, and they improve patient outcomes by ensuring the simultaneous management of all facets of a patient's condition, leading to more comprehensive and effective treatment strategies [12,13,14]. For example, in patients with complex coronary disease, a multidisciplinary heart team (MDHT) consisting of a cardiac surgeon, interventional cardiologist, and interventional imaging physician, composed to discuss the risks and benefits of percutaneous and surgical interventions when complex decision-making is required, became a class 1C recommendation in guidelines produced by the European Society of Cardiothoracic Surgery [13]. Other core members of the MDHT could include advanced practice providers, pharmacists, cardiac catheterization laboratory and operating room staff, referring physicians, nurses, social workers, clinical research coordinators, and other specialists related to the patient's health problems.

Similarly, oncology clinics have utilized multidisciplinary teams for many years to address the physical, psychological, social, financial, and spiritual symptoms affecting those with cancer [14]. Managing treatment with a multidisciplinary team that includes a medical oncologist, surgical oncologist, radiation oncologist, a nurse coordinator, pharmacist, dietician, psychologist, social worker, geriatrician (for older patients), physical therapist, and speech-language therapist is recommended to improve patient outcomes [14]. Given the complexity and chronicity of PICS, its management is well-suited to similar multidisciplinary, interprofessional clinics that approach management with a patient-centered and holistic paradigm.

ICU Follow-Up Clinics

Qualitative studies have highlighted that patients recovering from critical illness often face fragmented follow-up care, and they desire better coordination between healthcare providers, including acute, social, and community practitioners [2,9]. By employing a multidisciplinary team of diverse specialties and services to develop one unifying, patient-centered plan, ICU follow-up clinics address this gap, offering a cohesive and well-coordinated approach that spans the continuum of recovery (see Chapter 28 for additional information) [15]. Moreover, this model ensures that all aspects of a patient's well-being – physical, cognitive, psychological, social, and spiritual – are addressed holistically. Such an ICU follow-up clinic model offers a powerful, integrated framework for addressing the complex needs of patients and families with PICS, helping them navigate the challenges of recovery with greater support and understanding [15].

An essential part of caring for survivors of critical illness involves processing and normalizing the ICU experience and managing expectations regarding the pace, breadth, and depth of recovery. Patients benefit from discussing their ICU stay, reviewing their ICU diary (if available; see Chapter 18 for additional information), and recounting events, such as frightening dreams and hallucinations [2,9,10]. This approach, either with clinic staff during an appointment or with other survivors of critical illness during peer support groups or more informal conversations, helps patients make sense of their ICU experience and fosters emotional and psychological recovery.

Effective coordination and communication are essential for the success of multidisciplinary teams, especially in the context of PICS (see Chapter 31 for additional information). Multidisciplinary teams improve coordination of care by facilitating communication between specialists, which is crucial for managing complex medical conditions effectively [13,14,15]. Coordination among various healthcare providers and specialists reduces duplication of efforts and conflicting treatments, and such integration creates a unified care plan tailored to the patient's specific needs, while avoiding gaps in care. Multidisciplinary meetings and shared patient care plans are essential tools for maintaining clear communication and ensuring that interventions are coordinated. Regular meetings allow team members to discuss progress, adapt treatment plans, and make collaborative decisions that consider the patient's overall well-being, personal goals, and progress toward recovery. Many ICU follow-ups clinics utilize shared appointments, where team members rotate through the patient's room rather than having patients move to several locations, enhancing efficiency and coordination of care and minimizing patient inconvenience and effort [12,16]. Multidisciplinary teamwork and interprofessional planning not only improve the quality of life in patients with PICS and reduce feelings of depersonalization but also increase feelings of accomplishment and job satisfaction in members of the interprofessional team, key tools to prevent burnout syndrome.

Addressing the Four Pillars of Health

One approach that some ICU follow-up clinics take to provide a holistic or whole-person approach to the patient's recovery is to focus on what is referred to as the "four pillars of health": mental wellness and stress management, nutrition, sleep, and movement [17]. A comprehensive approach that addresses these four pillars through physical rehabilitation, cognitive therapy, psychological support, and social reintegration can significantly improve outcomes for patients with PICS and is supported by guidelines recommending tailored interventions to address the diverse impairments associated with PICS [16,17,18]. This holistic approach recognizes the immutable integration of the body, mind, spirit, and soul.

Nutrition

Nutrition plays a pivotal role in the recovery of patients experiencing PICS, and malnutrition, sarcopenia, and dysphagia are common concerns in survivors of critical illness (see Chapters 38 and 40 for additional information). Targeted nutrition support provided in the ICU significantly improves key recovery metrics, including immune function, muscle preservation, and overall physical strength, all of which are important in reducing complications and promoting functional recovery following discharge [19]. Integrating discussion of nutrition rehabilitation in the outpatient setting is essential to formulating an effective recovery plan given the impact of nutrition on immune function, cognitive recovery, and physical rehabilitation [19].

Movement

Physical impairments can limit a patient's ability to perform daily activities, which can lead to feelings of frustration and helplessness and ultimately contribute to depression. Prolonged disability also increases the risk of social isolation, which may further contribute to psychological distress [18]. Physical activity, which is decidedly important for regaining physical function, rebuilding muscle strength, improving cardiovascular health, and enhancing psychological well-being, is an essential component of a treatment plan for the management of PICS (see Chapter 41 for additional information). Improved cardiovascular health through structured movement activities aids in overall endurance, supports immune function, and reduces inflammation, all of which contribute to faster recovery and lower risks of complications following critical illness [18]. Furthermore, physical activity has been associated with improved mood; reduced symptoms of depression, anxiety, and PTSD; and better cognitive function, and treatment plans incorporating both physical rehabilitation and psychological counseling can address these interrelated issues simultaneously [7,8,15]. Additionally, promoting physical rehabilitation and cognitive recovery can help address the physical and cognitive aspects of PICS, potentially supporting the broader process of recovery and growth [20,21].

Sleep

Sleep is essential for the repair and maintenance of the immune, muscular, and cardiovascular systems, all of which may be compromised following critical illness [22], and sleep impairments are particularly common, both during critical illness and the recovery phase (see Chapters 9 and 37 for additional information). Cognitive impairment following critical illness is similarly common, affecting up to 70% of patients following discharge (see Chapter 43 for additional information), and sleep plays a key role in consolidating memory and improving attention, which are important for cognitive recovery. Sleep can also foster neuroplasticity, the ability of the brain to reorganize itself and form new neural connections, which may help contribute to management of cognitive impairments in survivors of critical illness [22,23]. Sleep may also contribute to psychological recovery, as sleep disturbances, such as insomnia and fragmented sleep, may be both a symptom of and contributor to depression, anxiety, and PTSD. Indeed, patients with poor sleep quality following critical illness are more likely to develop depression and anxiety [24], and improving sleep in this patient population can reduce the severity of PTSD symptoms and help in emotional recovery [25].

Stress Management and Mental Wellness

Patients with PICS often experience high levels of stress, along with clinically significant anxiety and PTSD, all of which can hinder recovery and worsen other impairments associated with PICS (see Chapter 46 for additional information); managing stress can reduce the burden of psychological symptoms and support more effective recovery [26]. Addressing stress through psychological interventions, including cognitive-behavioral therapy (CBT), mindfulness-based stress reduction (MBSR), and relaxation techniques, can reduce symptoms of PTSD and anxiety, thereby improving quality of life and mental resilience [27]. High stress levels are associated with impaired cognitive function, and stress management techniques can help reduce cognitive strain and promote cognitive recovery by reducing inflammation and cortisol levels, which have been associated with cognitive impairments [27]. Chronic stress can also have adverse effects on physical health, including a weakened immune response and increased inflammation, both of which can delay recovery [28]. By integrating stress management techniques into the recovery plan, patients may experience improvements in immune function, reduced inflammation, and enhanced physical recovery. Stress management not only reduces specific symptoms of PICS but also empowers patients to take an active role in their recovery. Approaches like stress-reduction counseling, group therapy, and self-help strategies foster resilience, helping patients cope with the challenges of recovery and adjust to new physical and mental health baselines [27,28].

Integrative and Complementary Therapies

Spiritual Care

Including services such as social work and spiritual care in a multidisciplinary clinic provides additional holistic support, addressing not just medical needs, but also the emotional, psychological, and spiritual needs of patients. Integrating spiritual care into multidisciplinary teams enhances patient satisfaction and well-being by addressing the psychological and emotional needs of patients with PICS, especially considering the existential and life-altering impact of critical illness (see Chapter 15 for additional information) [29]. Attending to spiritual needs may alleviate suffering and foster resilience, as spirituality often helps patients find meaning, peace, and connection; this type of care may include interventions such as guided spiritual discussions, prayer, or involvement of pastoral staff. The emphasis on spiritual well-being may further empower patients, granting them a sense of control over their recovery and promoting a more comprehensive healing experience [29].

Social Determinants of Health

The influence of social determinants of health, including economic stability, social support, and access to healthcare, is increasingly recognized as pivotal to the outcomes of survivors of critical illness (see Chapter 25 for additional information) [30]. Factors such as socioeconomic status, educational achievement, and neighborhood environments can significantly impact a patient's ability to manage PICS, as they affect access to resources, rehabilitation services, and post-hospitalization support. Social determinants play a major role in shaping disparities in health outcomes among survivors of critical illness, with those in lower socioeconomic brackets often facing more barriers to achieving full recovery [30]. Addressing these disparities requires healthcare providers to consider socioeconomic challenges and connect patients to resources that address these barriers, ensuring equitable access to recovery services and overall health maintenance.

Conventional and Alternative Therapies

Survivors of critical illness may benefit from a combination of conventional medical treatments, rehabilitative therapies, nutritional interventions, mind-body practices, and complementary modalities, including acupuncture, massage therapy, and herbal medicine. Integration of these alternative approaches has gained momentum, complementing conventional treatments to address the multifaceted needs of survivors of critical illness. Studies have shown that complementary therapies can alleviate symptoms, such as chronic pain, fatigue, and anxiety, which are commonly experienced in patients with PICS. For example, acupuncture has demonstrated efficacy in reducing pain and promoting relaxation, massage therapy can support physical and emotional relief from stress, and chiropractic adjustments may address musculoskeletal discomfort stemming from prolonged bed rest [31]. An integrative approach that combines these alternative therapies with standard medical and rehabilitation therapies provides a more patient-centered strategy, fostering self-directed healing and empowering patients to engage actively in their own recovery [32,33]. This synergy between conventional and alternative treatments not only enhances the overall experience but also aligns with the goal of comprehensive, individualized care.

Post-Traumatic Growth

Post-traumatic growth (PTG) as defined by Tedeschi is a "positive change experienced as a result of the struggle with a major life crisis or a traumatic event" [34]. Qualitative studies have reported that survivors of critical illness describe having to find the "new me" [2,9,10]. There are five domains of PTG: warmer, more intimate relationships with others, a greater sense of personal strengths, a greater appreciation of life and a changed sense of priorities, recognition of new possibilities or paths for one's life, and spiritual development [34]. The multidisciplinary ICU follow-up clinic can play a crucial role in fostering PTG in survivors of critical illness by incorporating interventions that validate and address the psychological and emotional needs of patients, such as psychological counseling, support groups, or trauma-informed care, which can collectively help people process their experiences in a way that promotes positive outcomes [34,35,36].

Conclusion

Building a collaborative, multidisciplinary team around patients with PICS can enhance their sense of completeness and empowerment, providing essential support for this medically fragile population. Managing these complex cases with holistic, coordinated, and personalized care offers the most promising chance for positive outcomes, potentially reducing healthcare resource utilization and the overall cost of care for survivors of critical illness. The integration of diverse disciplines – such as physical, occupational, and cognitive therapy; nutrition; spiritual care; and social support – ensures that all aspects of recovery are addressed and leads to improved outcomes, more efficient care delivery, and enhanced patient satisfaction.

One approach to an effective recovery plan for patients with PICS rests on an interprofessional framework that addresses the four foundational pillars of health: nutrition, sleep, mental health, and movement. By collaborating closely, diverse healthcare professionals unite to deliver an individualized recovery strategy that promotes balanced nutrition, quality sleep, stress management, and physical activity, all of which are essential to restoring physical, cognitive, and psychological health. Such interdisciplinary teamwork not only fosters recovery but also offers patients the potential for PTG, transforming their recovery journey into one of healing and empowerment.

Key Points

1. Holistic, multidisciplinary care: A coordinated, interprofessional approach is essential for managing the complex, interconnected impairments in physical, cognitive, and psychological health that survivors of critical illness face, ensuring comprehensive recovery and improved quality of life.
2. Interrelationship of PICS domains: Physical, cognitive, and emotional impairments in PICS often overlap, and addressing one domain can improve outcomes in others, reinforcing the need for integrated care strategies.
3. Four pillars of health: Effective recovery for PICS patients is supported by focusing on the four pillars of health: nutrition, sleep, mental wellness, and physical movement, all of which are crucial for restoring balance and promoting long-term recovery.
4. Post-traumatic growth: Multidisciplinary follow-up clinics not only aid in managing impairments but also foster PTG, helping patients find new strengths, deeper relationships, and a renewed sense of life purpose following their ICU experience.

References

1. A. Marra, P.P. Pandharipande, T.D. Girard, et al. Co-occurrence of Post-Intensive Care Syndrome problems among 406 survivors of critical illness. *Crit Care Med* 2018; **46**(9): 1393–401.
2. J. McPeake, L.M. Boehm, E. Hibbert, et al. Key components of ICU recovery programs: what did patients report provided benefit? *Crit Care Explor* 2020; **2**(4): e0088.
3. J. Griffiths, R.A. Hatch, K. Morgan, et al. An exploration of social and economic outcome and associated health-related quality of life after critical illness in general intensive care unit survivors: a 12-month follow-up study. *Crit Care* 2013; **17**(3): R100.

4. J.H. Maley, I. Brewster, I. Mayoral, et al. Resilience in survivors of critical illness in the context of survivors' experience and recovery. *Ann Am Thorac Soc* 2016; **13**(8): 1351–60.

5. E. Schwitzer, K.S. Jensen, L. Brinkman, et al. Survival ≠ Recovery: a narrative review of post-intensive care syndrome. *Chest Crit Care* 2023; **1**(1): 1–14.

6. R.P. Kosilek, K. Schmidt, S.E. Baumeister, et al. Frequency and risk factors of post-intensive care syndrome components in a multicenter randomized controlled trial of German sepsis survivors. *J Crit Care* 2021; **65**: 268–75.

7. O.J. Bienvenu, E. Colantuoni, P. Mendez-Tellex, et al. Depressive symptoms and impaired physical function after acute lung injury. *Am J Respir Crit Care Med* 2012; **185**: 517–24.

8. T. Proffitt, V. Menzies, M.J. Grap, et al. Cognitive impairment, physical impairment, and psychological symptoms in intensive care unit survivors. *Am J Crit Care* 2023; **32**(6): 410–20.

9. R.G. Rosa, G.E. Ferreira, T.W. Viola, et al. Effects of post-ICU follow-up on subject outcomes: a systematic review and meta-analysis. *J Crit Care* 2019; **52**: 115–25.

10. J. E. Davidson. Facilitated sensemaking: a strategy and new middle-range theory to support families of intensive care unit patients. *Crit Care Nurse* 2010; **30**(6): 28–39.

11. A. Callis. Application of the Roy Adaptation Theory to a care program for nurses. *Appl Nurs Res* 2020; **56**: 151340.

12. K.P. Snell, C.L. Beiter, E.L. Hall, et al. A novel approach to ICU survivor care: a population health quality improvement project. *Crit Care Med* 2020; **48**(12): e1164–e1170.

13. W.B. Batchelor, S. Anwaruddin, D.D. Wang, et al. The multidisciplinary heart team in cardiovascular medicine: current role and future challenges. *JACC Adv* 2023; **2**(1): 100160.

14. M. Taberna, F. Gil-Moncayo, E. Jane-Salas, et al. The multidisciplinary team (MDT) approach and quality of care. *Front Oncol* 2020; **10**: 85.

15. K.J. Haines, E. Hibbert, N. Leggett, et al. Transition of care after critical illness: challenges to recovery and adaptive problem solving. *Crit Care Med* 2021; **49**(11): 1923–31.

16. S.S. Daundasekara, K.R. Arlinghaus, C.A. Johnston. Quality of life: the primary goal of lifestyle intervention. *Am J Lifestyle Med* 2020; **14**(3): 267–70.

17. National Center for Complementary and Integrative Health. NCCIH Strategic Plan FY 2021–2025: Mapping the Pathway to Research on Whole Person Health [Internet]. National Center for Complementary and Integrative Health. https://nccih.nih.gov/about/nccih-strategic-plan-2021-2025. Accessed September 5, 2024.

18. W. Jonas, E. Rosenbaum. The case for whole-person integrative care. *Medicina* 2021; **57**(7): 677.

19. E. Ridley, D. Gantner, V. Pellegrino. Nutrition therapy in critically ill patients: a review of current evidence for clinicians. *Clin Nutr* 2015; **34**(4): 565–71.

20. J.C. Jackson, P.P. Pandharipande, T.D. Girard, et al. Depression, post-traumatic stress disorder, and functional disability in survivors of critical illness: results from the BRAIN-ICU Study. *Am J Respir Crit Care Med* 2014; **190**(3): 340–7.

21. B. Connolly, L. Salisbury, B. O'Neill, et al. Exercise rehabilitation following intensive care unit discharge for recovery from critical illness. *Cochrane Database of Syst Rev* 2015; **2015**(6): CD008632.

22. R. Elliott, S. McKinley, M. Fien, et al. Posttraumatic stress symptoms in intensive care patients: an exploration of associated factors. *Rehabil Psychol* 2016; **61**(2): 141–50.

23. D.M. Wade, D.C. Howell, J.A. Weinman, et al. Investigating risk factors for psychological morbidity three months after intensive care: a prospective cohort study. *Crit Care* 2012; **16**(5): R192.

24. N. Gujar, S.S. Yoo, M.P. Walker. Sleep deprivation amplifies the temporal focus of

the human brain. *Nature* 2011; **474**(7351): 128–31.

25. M. Henríquez-Beltrán, R. Vaca, I. Benítez, et al. Sleep and circadian health of critical survivors: a 12-month follow-up study. *Crit Care Med* 2024; **52**(8): 1206–17.

26. M. Wallace, P. Lieu, D. Marshall. Sleep and depression in critical illness survivors: a review of the literature. *J Clin Sleep Med* 2017; **13**(8): 951–7.

27. R. Elliott, S. McKinley, M. Fien, et al. Posttraumatic stress symptoms in intensive care patients: an exploration of associated factors. *Rehabil Psychol* 2016; **61**(2): 141–50.

28. D.M. Wade, D.C. Howell, J.A. Weinman, et al. Investigating risk factors for psychological morbidity three months after intensive care: a prospective cohort study. *Crit Care* 2012; **16**(5): R192.

29. C.M. Puchalski. The role of spirituality in health care. *Proc (Bayl Univ Med Cent)* 2001; **14**(4): 352–7.

30. H. Su, A.L. Fuentes, H. Chen, et al. The financial impact of post intensive care syndrome. *Crit Care Clin* 2025; **41**(1): 103–19.

31. P. Formenti, G. Piuri, R. Bisatti, et al. Role of acupuncture in critically ill patients: a systematic review. *J Tradit Complement Med* 2022; **13**(1): 62–71.

32. P.J. Ohatake, D.C Strasser, D.M. Strasser. Rehabilitation for people with critical illness: taking the next steps. *Phys Ther* 2018; **98**(12): 913–17.

33. D.M. Needham, R. Korupolu, J.M. Zanni, et al. Early physical medicine and rehabilitation for patients with acute respiratory failure: a quality improvement project. *Arch Phys Med Rehabil* 2010; **91**(4): 536–42.

34. R.G. Tedeschi, L.G. Calhoun. The Posttraumatic Growth Inventory: measuring the positive legacy of trauma. *J Trauma Stress* 1996; **9**(3): 455–71.

35. A.C. Jones, R. Hilton, B. Ely, et al. Facilitating posttraumatic growth after critical illness. *Am J Crit Care* 2020; **29**(6): e108–e115.

36. K.E. Weick, K.M. Sutcliffe, D. Obstfeld. Organizing and the process of sensemaking. *Organ Sci* 2005; **16**(4): 409–21.

Chapter 24

Health Equity and the Social Model of Disability

Leslie P. Scheunemann, Hiam Naiditch, and Gitouf Elnema

Introduction

The World Health Organization (WHO) recognizes that disability is part of being human [1]; significant disability affects 16% of the global population and 27% of the United States population [1,2]. This difference in disability prevalence reflects complex issues, including who experiences an acute event and survives with disability instead of dying, who is exposed to disabling working or living conditions, who gets counted as experiencing disability, and what kinds of support are provided to those with disabilities, all of which vary by region and culture.

An increasing number of people are surviving critical illness, and at least half of those who survive have new and long-lasting physical, functional, cognitive, psychiatric, and social impairments, collectively known as the post-intensive care syndrome (PICS). Perhaps unsurprisingly, much of the research into post-ICU disability to date has involved characterizing the pathophysiology and epidemiology of PICS; more recently, research has demonstrated that gender, race, and socioeconomic status are risk factors for PICS and PICS-Family [3,4,5,6], which are in turn risk factors for financial strain, unemployment, and institutionalization (see Chapter 25 for additional information) [3,7,8,9]. What remains underrecognized is that the patterns of health disparities in patients with PICS replicate societal patterns of disparities related to *disability itself* [10]. Compared to people without disabilities, people with disabilities have more problems functioning, more chronic health conditions, and earlier deaths [11], the implications of which are twofold: first, people with PICS are part of a global disabled population at high risk of disparities, and second, among people with PICS, those with additional sources of marginalization are at even higher risk.

To better explore PICS as a subgroup within a larger disabled community, this chapter reviews international consensus statements on human rights and disability, the difference between equality and equity, the Biomedical and Social Models of Disability, application of the Social Model of Disability to the lived experiences of people with PICS, and practical strategies to make care more just and inclusive for people with PICS.

Human Rights and Disability

The International Classification of Functioning, Disability, and Health (ICF) defines disability as "an umbrella term for impairments, activity limitations, and participation restrictions. It denotes the negative aspects of the interaction between an individual (with a health condition) and that individual's contextual factors (environmental and personal factors)" [12]. Thus, the ICF does not dictate who is "disabled" but instead identifies persons or groups who have a disability within a particular context.

In the context of that definition, the United Nations Convention on the Rights of Persons with Disabilities (CRPD) elucidates eight guiding principles [13]:
1. Respect for inherent dignity; individual autonomy, including the freedom to make one's own choices; and independence of persons
2. Nondiscrimination
3. Full and effective participation and inclusion in society
4. Respect for difference and acceptance of persons with disabilities as part of human diversity and humanity
5. Equality of opportunity
6. Accessibility
7. Equality between men and women
8. Respect for the evolving capacities of children with disabilities and respect for the right of children with disabilities to preserve their identities.

This amounts to a declaration that all persons with disabilities have the rights to pursue their highest potential, to participate fully in society, and to have equality of opportunity regardless of identity. Honoring those principles requires a deep understanding of equality and equity.

Equality and Equity

Equality is about sameness, while equity is about fairness. Understanding how they work together is fundamental to make progress toward a just society. The CRPD recognizes that *all persons have equal rights*, meaning that all people are "equal before and under the law and are entitled without any discrimination to the equal protection and equal benefit of the law" [13]. The CRPD's specific insistence on equality of opportunity for disabled people both sets a standard in stark opposition to the history of reduced opportunity experienced by disabled people and prohibits discrimination on the basis of disability.

Promoting equality and eliminating discrimination requires the provision of reasonable accommodation and attention to equity. Equity involves the specific measures that accelerate or achieve equality of persons with disabilities and that recognize their rights to freedom, respect, dignity, and belonging [14]. In an equitable society, resource allocation ensures that everyone has the same opportunity to participate. This frequently means that resource allocation is unequal because everyone does not start from the same place; some people face barriers to participation that are not present for others. Equity aims to reduce such barriers to facilitate participation among those who would otherwise be excluded.

The Biomedical and the Social Models of Disability

The WHO insists on the universal right to the highest attainable standard of health, which, under the CRPD, obligates governments to work to eliminate health disparities. Health disparities are "health differences that adversely affect disadvantaged populations in comparison to a reference population, based on one or more health outcomes" [15]. When the disadvantage at issue is a disability, questions immediately arise about the origin of the disadvantage: is it due to the person's health condition or due to the person's environment? These questions highlight the contrast between the two dominant models of disability: the Biomedical Model and the Social Model.

The Biomedical Model emphasizes the pathophysiological basis of disease, stating that disability arises from impairments due to a health condition (see Figure 24.1), and

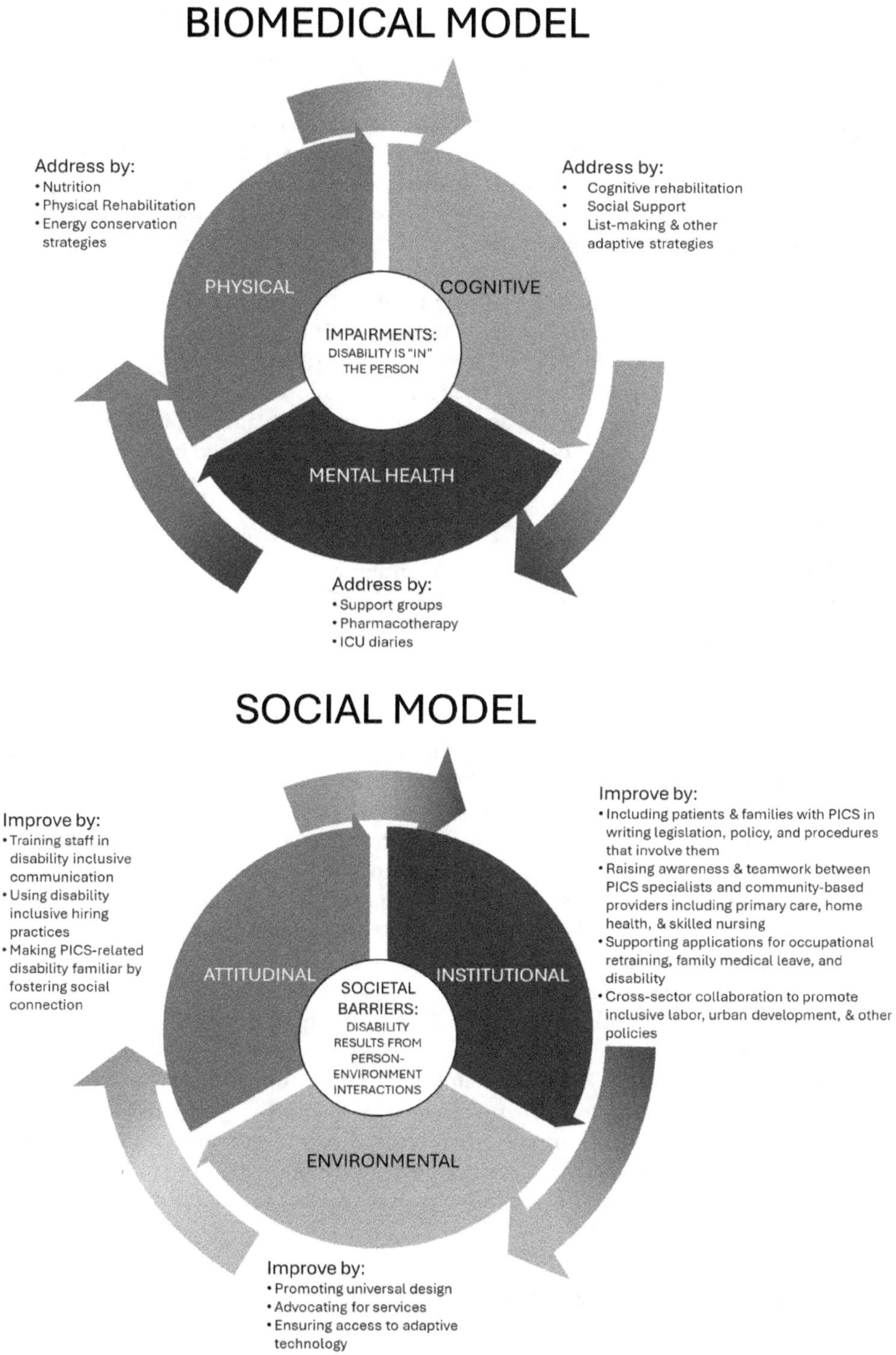

BIOMEDICAL MODEL

Address by:
- Nutrition
- Physical Rehabilitation
- Energy conservation strategies

Address by:
- Cognitive rehabilitation
- Social Support
- List-making & other adaptive strategies

PHYSICAL

COGNITIVE

IMPAIRMENTS: DISABILITY IS "IN" THE PERSON

MENTAL HEALTH

Address by:
- Support groups
- Pharmacotherapy
- ICU diaries

SOCIAL MODEL

Improve by:
- Training staff in disability inclusive communication
- Using disability inclusive hiring practices
- Making PICS-related disability familiar by fostering social connection

Improve by:
- Including patients & families with PICS in writing legislation, policy, and procedures that involve them
- Raising awareness & teamwork between PICS specialists and community-based providers including primary care, home health, & skilled nursing
- Supporting applications for occupational retraining, family medical leave, and disability
- Cross-sector collaboration to promote inclusive labor, urban development, & other policies

ATTITUDINAL

INSTITUTIONAL

SOCIETAL BARRIERS: DISABILITY RESULTS FROM PERSON-ENVIRONMENT INTERACTIONS

ENVIRONMENTAL

Improve by:
- Promoting universal design
- Advocating for services
- Ensuring access to adaptive technology

Figure 24.1 Contrasting the biomedical model and the social model of disability.

its solutions focus on identifying and remediating the underlying impairments. Examples in PICS include research to identify the biological mechanisms of delirium and prescribing physical therapy to address ICU-acquired weakness [16,17]. In contrast, the Social Model emphasizes person-environment interactions, stating that impairments related to a health condition become disabilities due to insurmountable barriers in the physical and social environment [18,19], and its solutions focus on reducing barriers and providing adaptations that enable physical and social participation. Examples in PICS include inadequate accommodations to return to work, high rates of social isolation, and experiences of ableism [5,9].

While some scholars and activists have treated the Biomedical Model and Social Model as mutually exclusive, they need not be [20]. Some disability-related outcome disparities are explained, at least to some extent, by both the underlying health condition (Biomedical Model) *and* concomitant unjust and avoidable inequities (Social Model) [11]. Confronting health disparities and promoting human rights involves addressing both; however, emphasizing the Biomedical Model over the Social Model represents a major ongoing source of stigma and health inequity. The Social Model of Disability is enshrined in international law: the CRPD has 164 signatories and 191 parties (190 states plus the European Union), signaling broad global support for addressing the human rights of persons with disabilities [20]. The ICF insists that disability *always* involves person-environment interaction and *cannot* be decontextualized [12]; despite this, translation of the Social Model of Disability into healthcare practice has been slow. Indeed, scholars have argued that ableism (discrimination against people with disabilities) is structural within healthcare systems and a major ongoing source of health inequity [10].

Disability activists have long promoted the Social Model of Disability [21,22]. Communities often prioritize certain skills and strengths, benefiting those with the relevant capabilities and disadvantaging those without, creating inequities related to (dis)ability. One inequity arises from a reliance on the Biomedical Model, which generates an imperative to "fix" the disability. When medical science is insufficiently advanced to heal damaged tissue or when a disabled person is deemed nonadherent or nonresponsive to rehabilitation, the Biomedical Model considers the disability "unfixable" and uses that to deny people access to resources that could enable participation *with* their ongoing impairments [23]. This not only de facto disables them but also fundamentally undermines their well-being and personhood.

Well-being and serious health conditions are not mutually exclusive [24,25]. Well-being is grounded in security (i.e., safety, connection, and self-esteem) and requires growth (i.e., exploration, love, and purpose) for people to reach their highest potential. Disability studies, human rights tenets, and international law hold that well-being is possible for everyone regardless of disability status. Models of healing after trauma further demonstrate that people who have experienced life-threatening harm can reestablish security, grow, and flourish [26,27]. These models show that quality of life – that well-being – is not written in our personal limitations, rather that well-being occurs when people make meaning out of their experiences and utilize their strengths to live lives of purpose. Society needs to reduce barriers to meaning and purpose for people with PICS.

The Social Model of Disability in PICS

Critical illness is, by definition, a trauma. Although people can heal, trauma may change them in subtle and dramatic ways [24]. The lived experiences around these long-term changes are at odds with a false but culturally prevalent belief that being healthy is normal and being ill is an abnormal and temporary event from which people rapidly and spontaneously recover [28]. Current models of care delivery are built on this false belief without any of the following disability-inclusive considerations [25]: (a) accountability for disability prevention strategies in the hospital [26,27]; (b) routine screening for PICS symptoms or referral for relevant therapies [17,28]; (c) insurance coverage of long-term therapy to match the long course of PICS [29]; (d) support for adaptation regardless of ongoing impairment; (e) addressing disability-related social isolation, which is itself morbid [5]; and (f) involving community-based providers in recognizing and managing PICS [30]. It is clear that PICS-related disability is associated with inequities both in healthcare utilization (e.g., lower rates of referral to home health and higher rates of institutionalization) and in health outcomes (e.g., higher mortality), but the healthcare system has not held itself accountable for its contributions to these outcomes [5,6,31,32].

Indeed, the Biomedical Model has implicitly permeated the study of and care for patients with PICS. Most of the literature focuses on the underlying biological impairments with little understanding of how patients' physical and social environments impact their ability to adapt to new or worsened impairments. Most current interventions target remediation of deficits, such as weakness, exhaustion, and inabilities to perform activities of daily living (ADLs) and instrumental activities of daily living (IADLs), and often lower expectations for recovery because we do not yet have definitively proven therapies to address any of these common challenges.

Survivors of critical illness themselves typically approach their own care with a focus on identifying and reducing impairments [33]. In many ways, that is not surprising: the context in which they are receiving care is largely not inclusive for people with disabilities and constantly reminds them of their impairments. While lack of an International Classification of Diseases, tenth edition (ICD-10) code adds barriers to services that are specific to PICS [29], people with PICS experience patterns of discrimination and exclusion that replicate the broader disability literature. For example, across the United States, primary care settings typically lack height-adjustable examination tables or accessible weight scales [34,35]. Physicians have poor understanding of their responsibilities under the Americans with Disabilities Act (ADA), and many express significant bias, either explicit or implicit, against people with disabilities [36,37]. Applicants for Social Security Disability Insurance (SSDI), most of whom experience poverty or financial insecurity, often wait months for an initial determination, and only half ultimately receive benefits [38,39]. Few clinicians know how to support patients seeking SSDI or workplace accommodations. The United States Supreme Court has consistently sided with employers claiming compliance with the ADA when employees have sued seeking reasonable accommodations [22]. These physical and institutional barriers both create and reinforce attitudinal barriers, including stigma related to ableism [10], which can deeply undermine safety, belonging, and self-esteem.

International perspectives differ. Importantly, a randomized control trial of an integrated health and social care intervention conducted in Scotland improved mental health and caregiver strain [40], suggesting that attending to inequities improves outcomes. Further, Germany has a national policy requiring larger employers to hire people with disabilities, which likely favorably impacts return to work after critical illness [9,10]. PICS communities in countries with more disability-inclusive health and social policies can and should share strategies that could be adapted to countries that are less inclusive. The Global Action on Disability Network could support such efforts.

More recently, PICS scholars have begun to integrate the Social Model of Disability in three key ways: characterizing environmental and social factors in disability [5,33,41], utilizing strengths-based models to characterize adaptive coping [36,37,38,39,42], and using measures, like the Patient-Reported Outcomes Measurement Information System (PROMIS), which capture a spectrum of well-being [43]. PICS clinicians and scholars need to capitalize on this shift. To date, no available therapies definitively improve PICS-related impairments, and progress using the Biomedical Model requires unpredictable scientific breakthroughs. In contrast, the physical and social environment are inherently modifiable; progress using the Social Model is not only within our control but also required for a just and inclusive society. The next section provides practical strategies for advancing that work for people with PICS.

Practical Strategies to Make Care More Just and Inclusive for People with PICS

A well-known disability rights slogan is "Nothing about us without us" [21]. While patients and family members are increasingly represented in PICS research and clinical care, we cannot achieve the highest standards of just and inclusive care unless patients and families with PICS are active members of the global community working on disability inclusion and have full partnership in co-design of research and care delivery related to PICS. No one with PICS was involved in writing this chapter; refer to Chapter 57 to read the experiences of people with PICS. We should aim to make our future work more inclusive of patient and family voices in order to better represent their perspectives and make our writing more accessible. For now, PICS clinicians and researchers should begin to consider their work as part of applied disability studies, learning its history and methods in order to rapidly integrate and build on its approaches to enablement and inclusion.

Co-design can make care more just and inclusive for people with PICS at the interpersonal, organizational, and societal levels. At the societal level, it needs to simultaneously operate within the healthcare sector and across all other sectors that impact patients and families with PICS (e.g., urban planning, transportation, and employment). The remainder of this section will sketch practical approaches for each level.

Three strategies for individual clinicians are: recognizing the diversity of disability identities, valuing and validating peoples' capabilities, and operationalizing social access (see Table 24.1). All three are lifelong practices at which everyone can constantly improve; part of the work is having the disability humility to keep practicing. Some people with PICS do not identify as disabled, some do, and some have the identity imposed on them by others. These are very different experiences. Inclusion means respecting their own self-identification and making space for them to participate in the ways that matter to them. Further, people with long-standing disabilities are typically experts in their capabilities and can coach others on their access needs, while newly disabled people may need help finding adaptive strategies that work for them and may need their strengths recognized and reinforced. Finally, clinicians should educate themselves in disability inclusion in collaboration with their organizations (see below) and work to operationalize access.

ICU follow-up clinics and other organizations caring for people with PICS can assume key leadership roles to make care more just and inclusive by promoting:

Table 24.1 Strategies clinicians can use to practice disability inclusion

Disability Construct	Principles	Actions	Examples
Identity	Recognize diversity	• Be curious. Notice the words people use to describe themselves • Ask about what helps them participate the way they want	• A person with PICS identifies as DeafDisabled (deaf with an additional disability). Use that term for them, too. Offer interpreter services and ask what else will help them manage their health. • A person with PICS has hearing impairment but does not identify as deaf, sign, or use hearing aids. Ask what helps them participate in the ways they want. If they describe participation barriers, ask if they'd like to discuss strategies to enable fuller participation.
Capability	Validate and value	• Believe what people say about their experiences and perspectives • Actively look for and name strengths • Facilitate healthy adaptation in context	• A person with PICS sets a goal that the home health team thinks is overambitious for the rehabilitation period. Align with their goal. Problem-solve with them to address barriers to achieving their goal, including how to keep practicing after the rehabilitation period ends. • A person with PICS focuses on their exhaustion and memory problems. Reflect their progress back to them, help them conserve energy for the activities that matter most to them, and use their own creativity, humor, organizational skills, and social supports to work around memory challenges.
Environment	Operationalize access	• Make it safe to disclose disability • Offer choice and agency • Identify and eliminate barriers to participation	• A person with PICS is having difficulty managing at home but does not disclose. Instead, their family care partner raises concerns. Recognize that there are many reasons for nondisclosure, including lack of awareness due to cognitive impairment as well as fear of losing independence. Explore what is going on. Align with the

Table 24.1 (cont.)

Disability Construct	Principles	Actions	Examples
		• Encourage representation of disability everywhere • Call out patronization and infantilization	patient's values. Let the patient choose what kinds of support are feasible and acceptable whenever possible. • Assess social networks and participation in meaningful activities as part of the health of people with PICS. Avoid medicalizing these needs. Instead, build bridges to social services and community organizations to meet them. Consume books, journalism, and other forms of media created by disabled people for disabled people. Make them accessible to people with PICS. • Avoid binary thinking that says people with PICS need help or protection on the one hand, or are inspiring on the other. Practice seeing them as people with the same kinds of dreams and aspirations as other people, but without the same environmental supports to pursue them.

- Attitudinal inclusivity:
    - Advancing practices for co-design and implementation of all clinic initiatives in equal partnership with patients and families.
    - Making it the mission of the practice to leave no one behind.
    - Developing respectful practices for asking and honoring what people need in order to participate in the ways that matter to them during all interactions.
        - Training staff in disability inclusion.
        - Addressing common barriers to communication:
            - Providing interpreters, including sign language, as needed
            - Using hearing aids with patients with hearing impairment who do not sign; only 30–40% of spoken English can be understood through lip-reading.
            - Targeting a 4th–5th grade reading level and using visual aids in all written communications [44].
            - Using large font reading materials and offering Braille and/or electronic materials that can be read aloud by an app [44].
            - Recognizing that everyone has the right to decision-making regardless of cognitive ability.
            - Speaking to patients directly as much as possible and working with care partners as "resource[s] available to support the patient's preferences" [44].
            - Using visual aids, especially with patients with cognitive limitations.
            - Using strategies for inclusive communication developed by people in the disabled community (e.g., Anti-Ableism Action Steps for Health Care Provision) [45].
- Institutional inclusivity:
    - Integrating social workers into the multidisciplinary team to model and coach team members in trauma-informed practices; measure resource gaps and disparities; and recognize and respond to patients' experiences of stigma, whether internalized or occurring in healthcare settings or other communities.
    - Sending primary and home care providers clear, well-formatted documentation of the ICU hospitalization and current PICS-related needs. Empower them to recognize PICS and identify community resources that can help.
    - Offering affordable support to patients and families seeking access to occupational retraining, employment accommodations, disability coverage, and family medical leave.
- Environmental accessibility:
    - Keep innovating until quality PICS care is equally accessible in rural and urban communities. This will require advocacy for changes in policy related to transportation, broadband, and insurance coverage for telehealth [46].
    - Promoting use of universal design and ensuring physical accessibility of brick-and-mortar clinics [47].

At the societal level, the WHO's global report on health equity articulates health sector strategies to advance health equity for persons with disabilities, all of which focus on "integration" and "inclusion" in some way [1]. The remainder of this section highlights four related topics not addressed elsewhere in this chapter that are of immediate relevance to PICS.

First, integrating disability inclusion in the accountability mechanisms of the health sector requires a different approach to measuring both processes and outcomes for people with PICS. Inclusive processes promote people's opportunities to pursue their highest potential by addressing barriers identified in the Social Model of Disability; process measurement should focus on identifying relevant barriers. In the attitudinal domain, there are scales to assess experiences of ableism, inclusion, and social connection. In the institutional domain, measures should assess gaps in access to healthcare, employment, transportation, and other resources. In the environmental domain, measures should assess gaps in physical accessibility at home and in the community. Similarly, inclusive outcome measures assess whether people with disabilities achieve equal sense of well-being and community participation compared with other nondisabled community members. While it is valuable to assess whether interventions designed to improve strength or stamina can do that, those are intermediate outcomes. The vision of the CRPD and WHO includes multi-dimensional quality of life, satisfaction with life, the ability to participate in meaningful activities and roles, life space, and community participation. When co-designing approaches with patients who have PICS, it is important to ask questions that are safe and appropriate to the stage of recovery. For example, measurement early in the course of recovery could assess whether gaps in caregiver training and adaptive strategies (process measures) impact safe discharge (an outcome measure), while measurement later in the course of recovery could assess whether return to work or gaps in transportation (process measures) impact their role satisfaction, community participation, and well-being (outcome measures).

Second, people with PICS may experience additional sources of stigma (e.g., age, race, gender, sexual identity, non-PICS disability), which can compound care inequities. The scope of systemic change required is large. Generating such change will take sustained advocacy and activism that is only imaginable if the PICS community can effectively partner with other disability communities with shared interests. The power in creating disability networks, partnerships, and alliances is in working together toward integrative solutions for how to make inclusion, belonging, and access possible for everyone. Pooling values and resources is the way to make cultural changes that can translate to lasting systems changes [48,49].

Third, adopting progressive universalism as a core principle and driver of health financing is a key consideration. "Progressive universalism" means putting the needs of the most vulnerable first. In PICS, that likely means focusing budgeting and intervention development on people from low-income, minoritized populations with cognitive and mental health impairments, especially those in rural communities. Economic modeling tends to project substantial returns on investment for the provision of disability-inclusive care, especially for minoritized disabled populations at highest risk for poor access to care coordination services [11,50]. Further, because PICS is a common consequence of surviving critical illness, PICS care should be included in economic modeling for critical illness. Such modeling has been insufficiently inclusive of both upstream factors that increase the risk of becoming critically ill (e.g., poor access to mental health, substance use, and chronic disease management services) and downstream factors that are not part of medical billing (e.g., family caregiving and lost work). Each year in the United States, family caregivers provide an estimated US $470 billion of unpaid care and lose an estimated $522 billion in wages [50], while employers lose an estimated $33 billion per year due to employees' caregiving responsibilities. And so, for both humanitarian and fiscal reasons, we must develop and implement fiscal policies focused on prevention and holistic care.

Fourth, healthcare finance and models of care are interrelated. All current models of PICS care delivery – even ICU follow-up clinics – replicate fragmentation inherent to health systems that were not designed to provide efficient, holistic care for people with disabilities. People experiencing serious illness need care that addresses a range of health, functional, and social needs, including personal care assistance, transportation, food services, employment accommodations, and iterative courses of rehabilitation as functional adaptation needs change across the illness trajectory. "Integration" and "inclusion" ultimately mean that people with PICS would receive care in a health system designed to attend to their health and rehabilitation needs while seamlessly linking to other sectors (e.g., urban planning, employment, and social services) to address needs outside the scope of healthcare. Practical steps toward that vision include: (1) promoting adherence to national accessibility mandates (e.g., the ADA in the United States) through a combination of accreditation requirements, financial penalties for nonadherence, and government accountability for system-wide failures [47]; (2) ensuring health professional curricula and ongoing training requirements provide rigorous education and training on disability inclusion; (3) increasing representation of people with disabilities, including PICS, in all sectors, especially media and governance; and (4) building mechanisms for coordination between healthcare service providers and other sectors (e.g., social services, employment, and transportation) that attend to nonmedical needs of people with PICS.

Ultimately, healthcare alone is insufficient to provide patients with PICS security and opportunities for growth and purpose – the substance of well-being. What we can do is provide patients supportive and empowering infrastructure for adapting to the ways critical illness has changed their lives, including better preparing society to include and center disability. The central message is that stewardship of the healthcare system is a global imperative to which everyone can contribute, and clinicians and administrators can take action in daily practice to improve care.

Below is a list of WHO targeted actions and recommendations for disability inclusion applied to PICS accompanied by specific examples of actions that clinicians, researchers, and administrators can take. Many terms in this list are integral to WHO policy. Please refer to its website for additional resources.

Political Commitment, Leadership, and Governance

1. Prioritize health equity for persons with disabilities.

- Conceptualize unmet social needs in PICS as responsibilities of communities and governments; measure them to drive policy.
- Advocate for incorporating adherence to disability inclusion policies as a focus of accreditation for healthcare organizations and educational institutions along the entire pre-, intra-, and post-ICU trajectory.
- Design all new PICS initiatives to monitor equity of implementation related to disability status.

2. Establish a human rights-based approach to health.

- The right to health is indivisible from other human rights, including education, participation, food, housing, work, and information. Champion these rights alongside the right to health for people with PICS.

- Ensure all people with PICS have affordable, equitable access to health services by becoming advocates for Universal Health Coverage grounded in primary health care.
- Engage people with PICS to develop a set of "minimum requirements" for access to PICS-related services and supports. Monitor their implementation.
- Protect persons with PICS against violations of human rights laws by revising policies and laws that discriminate against them.

3. Assume a stewardship role for disability inclusion in the health sector.
- The WHO defines stewardship as "the careful and responsible management of the well-being of the population." It requires multisectoral coordination to ensure social protection, education, food, housing, and other policies are disability inclusive. We can and should ask how any new policy in any sector will affect people with disabilities, including those with PICS, and suggest that disability advocacy groups review the policy for disability inclusion, especially monitoring of implementation.

4. Make international cooperation more effective by increasing funding to address health inequities for persons with disabilities.
- Establish international networks to monitor PICS outcomes. Countries with better performance can share knowledge, training platforms, and policies tied to better outcomes.
- International cooperation can work in two main ways:
  - Helping countries with developing critical care infrastructure to design policies and practices to be inclusive of PICS from the beginning.
  - Helping countries with established critical care infrastructure to reverse engineer or retrofit policies and practices that can improve disability inclusion for people with PICS.
- Promoting universal design to address environmental factors.

5. Integrate disability inclusion in national health strategies, including preparedness and response plans for health emergencies.
- Work with people with disabilities, including those with PICS, on:
  - Individual response plans for various emergencies.
  - Ethical triage guidelines for emergency services during future disasters.
  - Multisectorial collaboration in planning the wider response to disasters, including data collection and analysis.

6. Set actions that are specific to the health sector in national disability strategies or plans.
- People with disabilities, including PICS, should inform the ways that the health sector interacts with national disability policies, including assigning responsibility for leaders within the health sector to implement those policies.

7. Establish a committee or a focal point in the Ministry of Health for disability inclusion.
- Advocate for National and Regional Committees on Disability Inclusion that include people disabled after acute illness hospitalizations with roles and functions including:

- Review of all national and regional legislation to optimize consideration of disability inclusion.
- Support the implementation of multi-sectorial policies related to disability inclusion, including educating, advising, and participating in oversight.

8. Integrate disability inclusion in the accountability mechanisms of the health sector.
   - Instead of measuring needs, measure gaps in addressing needs (shifts the problem from the person to the community). For example, measure the percentage of people with PICS who have:
     - Unmet transportation needs that affected their ability to access healthcare in the two years after a critical illness hospitalization.
     - Unmet instrumental and relational needs in the two years following a critical illness hospitalization.
   - Inclusion of persons with PICS and their organizations in setting accountability mechanism.

9. Create disability networks, partnerships, and alliances.
   - Establish active collaborations with existing groups focused on disability inclusion. For example:
     - Administration for Community Living (United States).
     - Organizations that advocate for groups with high rates of disability (e.g., veterans, people with cancer, people living with HIV, and people living with diabetes).
     - Organizations representing paid and unpaid caregivers for people with disabilities.
   - Join the Global Action on Disability (GLAD) Network.
   - Work with the United Nations Partnership on the Rights of Persons with Disabilities (UNPRPD) Multi-Partner Trust Fund.
   - Attend the Global Disability Summit.

10. Ensure the existing mechanisms for social protection support the diverse health needs of persons with disabilities.
    - Advocate for improved social protections for the diverse health needs of persons with disabilities.
      - Start by attending to the needs of women with disabilities and women who are caregivers, who experience among the highest rates of inequitable access to social protections.
      - Promote equitable disability assessment, determination, and eligibility. These processes should not only identify who requires benefits, services, products, or protection, but also barriers and facilitators of equal opportunity, accessibility, and inclusion.
      - Dependence on an ICD code linked to a disability diagnosis restricts disability inclusion for people with PICS. This should be a specific area of advocacy.

Health Financing

11. Adopt progressive universalism as a core principle and as a driver of health financing, putting persons with disabilities at the center.
    - "Progressive universalism" means putting the needs of the most vulnerable first. In PICS, that likely means focusing intervention development on people from low-income, minoritized populations with cognitive and mental health impairments, especially those in rural communities and residential settings.

12. Consider health services for specific impairments and health conditions in packages of care for Universal Health Care.
    - Critical care services should not be conceptualized simply as physiologic rescue but as whole-person care across the post-ICU trajectory.
    - PICS services should include a bundle of physical, cognitive, and mental health support services that individuals can tailor to their needs.

13. Include into healthcare budgets the costs of making facilities and services accessible.
    - Budget for universal design of healthcare facilities and disability inclusive health services, including education and training for staff; provision of interpreter services; designing educational materials for a range of sensory needs and cognitive capabilities; accessible transportation; telehealth; and accessible rehabilitation services that meet the needs of people with changing functional capabilities like those with PICS.

Engagement of Stakeholders and Private Sector Providers

14. Engage persons with disabilities and their representative organizations in health sector processes.
    - Ensure people with PICS are part of strategic decision-making, as well as the design, planning, development, and delivery of health services relevant to PICS care.
    - Ensure people with PICS from low-income, minoritized, rural, and residential care populations have active representation/roles.
    - Engage in cross-sectoral collaboration with private sector providers, civil society, and other government departments as part of a comprehensive strategy to provide disability inclusive services.

15. Include gender-sensitive actions that target persons with disabilities in the strategies to empower people in their communities.
    - Provide accessible health and legal information and tools about the rights of persons with disabilities to people with PICS, with a specific focus on women and non-cisgender persons with disabilities.
    - Enable informed decisions for persons with disabilities, such as women, regarding all aspects of their health.

16. Engage the providers of informal support for persons with disabilities.
    - Develop and implement pathways of care that ensure family care partners for people with PICS receive relevant education and training to support the patient's health,

function, and care coordination needs. An ICU Family Workbook to provide self-screening and education is available at https://picturethis.pitt.edu.
- Advocate for flexible working arrangements, training programs, and self-care to care partners supporting people with PICS.

17. Engage persons with disabilities in research and include them in the health research workforce.
    - Involve people with PICS and their care partners in co-design of research.
    - Develop communities in which people with PICS can develop expertise in disability inclusion, shared identity, and skills for collaborating with researchers.

18. Request that providers in the private sector support the delivery of disability-inclusive health services.
    - Provide publicly accessible tools for nonstate actors to make their organizations more disability inclusive.
    - Make disability inclusion a category in rankings of best healthcare organizations.
    - Promote universal health records.
    - Disseminate PICS information in a range of accessible formats (e.g., Braille, Easy-Read, captioning, and sign language).

Models of Care

19. Enable the provision of integrated people-centered care that is accessible and close to where people live.
    - Concentrate planning resources in addressing the needs of hard-to-reach populations, such as those in rural communities.
    - Provide both essential health services (e.g., primary care) and specialized services (e.g., rehabilitation services, mental health services, and social services) to people with PICS within their communities.

20. Ensure universal access to assistive products.
    - Advocate to increase political will, legislation, and effective financing for assistive products.
    - Coordinate between the health sector and other sectors to assure people with PICS have universal access to assistive technology by improving the range, quality, affordability, procurement, and supply of assistive products relevant to PICS (e.g., mobility equipment, housing adaptations, cognitive support tools, portable oxygen, and apps that address mood, cognition, and sleep).
    - Address issues of equity in service provision for people with financial and geographic access barriers.

21. Invest more finances in support persons, interpreters, and assistants to meet the health needs of persons with disabilities.
    - Promote collaboration between the health and social support sectors to ensure support is available in all spheres of life.

- Improve the ability to identify and plan for gaps in equity.
  - Increase workforce training to improve effective identification, referral, and provision of services.
  - Budget to address gaps in access to needed services.
22. Consider the full spectrum of health services along a continuum of care for persons with disabilities.
    - Reconceptualize PICS care as an integral part of critical care delivery.
      - Design longitudinal services to address PICS-related needs starting in the ICU and continuing into the community.
      - Align payment models and financing to follow this design.
    - Coordinate between health services and other sectors (e.g., social services, housing, and employment) to ensure persons with PICS have appropriate access to a wide spectrum of services.
23. Strengthen models of care for children with disabilities.
    - Develop healthcare delivery models that are age- and developmentally appropriate to address common functional consequences of critical illness among children and families.
    - Provide home visits and parent groups facilitated by skilled providers.
    - Provide interdisciplinary services that target mental, physical, and social needs for children with PICS.
24. Promote deinstitutionalization.
    - Build coordinated community-based resources and supports to increase capacity to provide most PICS-related care in people's homes and communities instead of healthcare facilities, especially long-term care facilities.

Health and Care Workforce

25. Develop competencies for disability inclusion in the education of all health and care workers.
    - Coordinate between the health sector and professional and academic accreditation bodies to help build disability educational curricula.
    - Engage people with PICS to review health professional curricula to ensure that they address their needs.
    - Ask critical care and primary care professional accreditation bodies to mandate continuing education and training for disability inclusion that is relevant to PICS care.
26. Provide training in disability inclusion for all health service providers.
    - Involve people with PICS in designing and delivering trainings whenever possible.

27. Ensure the availability of a skilled health and care workforce.
    - Use task-sharing to involve nonspecialists, such as community health workers, health aides, and technicians, in providing services.
    - Upskill existing health aides in disability inclusion.
28. Include persons with disabilities in the health and care workforce.
    - Promote disability-inclusive hiring practices in healthcare.
    - Encourage healthcare organizations to hire and retain people with disabilities, including PICS.
29. Train all nonmedical staff working in the health sector on issues relating to accessibility and respectful communication.
    - Mandate disability inclusion training as a part of annual competencies to nonmedical staff.
    - Include training on accessibility, proper use of language, and communication skills with people with disabilities.
    - Amplify communication strategies advocated by people with disabilities (e.g., https://eliclare.com/wpcontent/uploads/2023/02/Action_Steps_for_Medical_Providers-12pt.pdf).
30. Guarantee free and informed consent for persons with disabilities.
    - Provide clear, understandable information that respects people's sensory and cognitive needs (e.g., large print, pictural or simple written language, and interpretative services).
    - Support people's right to choose, including refusing treatment.
    - Monitor for coercion from family, support persons, or service providers.

Physical Infrastructure

31. Incorporate a universal design-based approach to the development or refurbishment of health facilities and services.
    - Continue to optimize ICU and hospital design to promote circadian rhythms, family availability at bedside, noise reduction, and management of other sensory stimuli.
    - Ensure PICS clinics are physically accessible.
    - Incorporate common principles of equitable use, flexibility, simplicity, perceptible information, tolerance for error, low physical effort, and appropriate size and space.
32. Provide appropriate, reasonable accommodation for persons with disabilities.
    - Conceptualize use of restraints as a suboptimal ability to make accommodations.
    - Ensure discharge planning includes home adaptations for accessibility and planning to maintain social connections regardless of PICS symptoms.
    - Identify needs for physical modifications at home, in transportation, and in the community to enable people with PICS to reestablish routines and participate in their communities.

Digital Technologies for Health

33. Adopt a systems-approach to the digital delivery of health services with health equity as a key principle.
    - Promote policy for universal broadband and telehealth access.
    - Adopt universal Electronic Health Records that communicate between hospitals, rehabilitation facilities, primary and home-based care, and long-term care facilities.

34. Adopt international standards for accessibility of digital health technologies.
    - Promote the development and use of international standards, such as the Web Content Accessibility Guidelines (WCAG) or the WHO-ITU global standard on accessibility of telehealth services.
    - Share effective strategies in international disability forums like GLAD.

Quality of Care

35. Integrate the specific needs and priorities of persons with disabilities into existing health safety protocols.
    - Have people with PICS and their families review health safety protocols in hospitals and community-based care settings to ensure they address their needs, and revise them in response to their feedback.
    - Include patients and families on the Quality and Safety Committees of healthcare organizations.
    - Integrate asking about access needs at the beginning of health encounters (e.g., clinic visits and hospitalizations).

36. Ensure disability-inclusive feedback mechanisms for quality of health services.
    - Integrate questions about whether access needs were met into satisfaction surveys after health encounters.

37. Consider the specific needs of persons with disabilities in systems to monitor care pathways.
    - Establish good referral systems to meet the health and social needs of people with PICS:
        - Employment and legal services.
        - Transportation, utility, housing services.
        - Personal care and social services.
        - Care coordination services, caregiver support.

Monitoring and Evaluation

38. Create a monitoring and evaluation plan for disability inclusion.
    - Develop an evaluation framework for PICS inclusion across sectors (e.g., employment, transportation, housing, social services, and healthcare).
    - Identify measures and benchmarks.
    - Work with regional and national leaders to develop and implement monitoring.

39. Integrate indicators for disability inclusion into the monitoring and evaluation frameworks of country health systems.
    - Champion PICS-relevant measures, such as:
        - Percentage of previously community-dwelling people who remain home-bound or institutionalized three months after an acute illness hospitalization.
        - Percentage of previously employed people who have reduced hours/income, unaccommodated adaptive needs, or who have become unemployed six months and one year after a critical illness hospitalization.
        - Percentage of people reporting timely, affordable access to needed adaptive or rehabilitative services in their homes or communities after an acute illness hospitalization.
        - Percentage of families reporting caregiver stress or financial toxicity in the 12 months after an acute illness hospitalization.
    - Link such measures not just to PICS, but to other sources of disadvantage, such as geography, gender, and minoritized race or sexual identity to monitor intersectional equity.

Health Policy and Systems Research

40. Develop a national health policy and systems research agenda on disability.
    - Lobby critical care professional organizations to partner with affinity groups across sectors (e.g., interprofessional healthcare networks, labor unions, employers, organizers, and activities) to work toward these policies.

Conclusions

In this chapter, we contextualize PICS within a broader international disability community, introduce international policy on disability rights and inclusion, and argue to integrate the Social Model of Disability into the study and care of patients with PICS. A core goal of the Social Model of Disability is to recognize that inability to remediate impairments does not inevitably limit meaningful participation in activities if social barriers to participation are addressed. Identifying social concerns among survivors of critical illness, improving community accessibility for patients with PICS regardless of access to ICU follow-up clinics, and advocating for just healthcare for this important patient population can lead to key improvements in the care of patients with PICS.

Key Points

1. To address health equity and care delivery for people with PICS, it is essential to contextualize PICS within the international disability community, review international consensus statements on human rights and disability, and appreciate the distinction between equality and equity.
2. Contrasting the Biomedical and Social Models of Disability as frameworks to study and care for people with disabilities, including people with PICS, is crucial for

shifting the focus from merely addressing the biological impairments to tackling the societal barriers stemming from person-environment interactions.
3. Integrating the Social Model of Disability into the study and care of people with PICS will make care delivery more just and inclusive.
4. Attitudinal, institutional, and environmental inclusivity must be promoted as key practical strategies to achieve disability inclusion for patients with PICS.
5. Applying the WHO's global report on health equity, which outlines health sector strategies for advancing health equity and inclusion for persons with disabilities, is relevant for people with PICS.

References

1. G. Zhao, C.A. Okoro, J. Hsia, et al. Prevalence of disability and disability types by urban-rural county classification-U.S., 2016. *Am J Prev Med* 2019; **57**: 749–56.
2. C.A. Okoro, N.D. Hollis, A.C. Cyrus, et al. Prevalence of disabilities and health care access by disability status and type among adults: United States, 2016. *MMWR Morb Mortal Wkly Rep* 2018; **67**: 882–7.
3. L.P. Scheunemann, N.E. Leland, S. Perera, et al. Sex disparities and functional outcomes after a critical illness. *Am J Respir Crit Care Med* 2020; **201**: 869–72.
4. S. Jain, T.E. Murphy, J.R. O'Leary, et al. Association between socioeconomic disadvantage and decline in function, cognition, and mental health after critical illness among older adults: a cohort study. *Ann Intern Med* 2022; **175**: 644–55.
5. J.R. Falvey, T.E. Murphy, L. Leo-Summers, et al. Neighborhood socioeconomic disadvantage and disability after critical illness. *Crit Care Med* 2022; **50**: 733–41.
6. J.R. Falvey, A.B. Cohen, J.R. O'Leary, et al. Association of social isolation with disability burden and 1-year mortality among older adults with critical illness. *JAMA Intern Med* 2021; **181**: 1433–9.
7. K.E. Hauschildt, C. Seigworth, L. A. Kamphuis, et al. Financial toxicity after acute respiratory distress syndrome: a national qualitative cohort study. *Crit Care Med* 2020; **48**: 1103–10.
8. N. Khandelwal, R.A. Engelberg, C.L. Hough, et al. The patient and family member experience of financial stress related to critical illness. *J Palliat Med* 2020; **23**: 972–6.
9. H. Su, N.J. Dreesmann, C.L. Hough, et al. Factors associated with employment outcome after critical illness: systematic review, meta-analysis, and meta-regression. *J Adv Nurs* 2021; **77**: 653–63.
10. D.J. Lundberg, J.A. Chen. Structural ableism in public health and healthcare: a definition and conceptual framework. *Lancet Reg Health Am* 2024; **30**: 100650.
11. Global report on health equity for persons with disabilities 2022, www.who.int/publications/i/item/9789240063600 (accessed October 11, 2024).
12. G. Stucki. International classification of functioning, disability, and health (ICF). *Am J Phys Med Rehabil* 2005; **84**: 733–40.
13. Convention on the Rights of Persons with Disabilities | OHCHR, www.ohchr.org/en/instruments-mechanisms/instruments/convention-rights-persons-disabilities (accessed October 12, 2024).
14. The United Nations Convention on the Rights of People with Disabilities Equality and Human Rights Commission Guidance: What Does It Mean for You? A Guide for Disabled People and Disabled People's Organisations. www.equalityhumanrights.com/sites/default/files/uncrpdguide_0.pdf (accessed October 10, 2024).
15. Minority Health and Health Disparities Definitions, www.nimhd.nih.gov/resources/understanding-health-disparities/minority-health-and-health-disparities-definitions.html (accessed October 12, 2024).

16. T.D. Girard, J.L. Thompson, P. P. Pandharipande, et al. Clinical phenotypes of delirium during critical illness and severity of subsequent long-term cognitive impairment: a prospective cohort study. *Lancet Respir Med* 2018; **6**: 213–22.

17. M.E. Major, R. Kwakman, M.E. Kho, et al. Surviving critical illness: what is next? An expert consensus statement on physical rehabilitation after hospital discharge. *Crit Care* 2016; **20**: 354.

18. M. Oliver. The social model of disability: thirty years on. *Disabil Soc* 2013; **28**: 1024–6.

19. J.M. Levitt. Exploring how the social model of disability can be re-invigorated: in response to Mike Oliver. *Disabil Soc* 2017; **32**: 589–94.

20. United Nations. Status of Treaties: Convention on the Rights of Persons with Disabilities. United Nations Treaty Collection. United Nations Treaty Collection. Published May 2008, https://treaties.un.org/pages/viewdetails.aspx?src=treaty&mtdsg_no=iv-15&chapter=4&clang=_en (accessed October 12, 2024).

21. J.I. Charlton. *Nothing about us without us: disability oppression and empowerment.* Berkley, CA: University of California Press; 1989.

22. M. Russell. *Beyond ramps: disability at the end of the social contract: a warning from an Uppity Crip.* Monroe, ME: Common Courage Press, 1998.

23. J.A. Haegele, S. Hodge. Disability discourse: overview and critiques of the medical and social models. *Quest* 2016; **68**: 193–206.

24. J. Herman. *Trauma and recovery: the aftermath of violence – from domestic abuse to political terror.* 4th ed. New York: Basic Books, Hachette Book Group; 2022, www.literatibookstore.com/book/9781541602953 (accessed October 12, 2024).

25. Becoming Anti-Ableist: A Disability Justice-Informed Approach to Supporting the Disability Community; 2022.

26. B.T. Pun, M.C. Balas, M.A. Barnes-Daly, et al. Caring for critically ill patients with the ABCDEF bundle: results of the ICU liberation collaborative in over 15,000 adults. *Crit Care Med* 2019; **47**: 3–14.

27. L.P. Scheunemann, T.D. Girard, E. R. Skidmore, et al. The hospital elder life program: past and future. *Am J Geriatr Psychiatry* 2018; **26**: 1034–5.

28. National Institute for Health and Care Excellence. Rehabilitation after critical illness in adults: Clinical guidelines. www.nice.org.uk/guidance/qs158. Published 2009.

29. B.C. Peach, M. Valenti, M.L. Sole. A call for the World Health Organization to create international classification of disease diagnostic codes for post-intensive care syndrome in the age of COVID-19. *World Med Health Policy* 2021; **13**: 373–82.

30. K.E. Hauschildt, R.K. Hechtman, H. C. Prescott, et al. Hospital discharge summaries are insufficient following ICU stays: a qualitative study. *Crit Care Explor* 2022; **4**: e0715.

31. J.R. Falvey, T.E. Murphy, T.M. Gill, et al. Home health rehabilitation utilization among Medicare beneficiaries following critical illness. *J Am Geriatr Soc* 2020; **68**: 1512–19.

32. S. Jain, T.E. Murphy, J.R. Falvey, et al. Social determinants of health and delivery of rehabilitation to older adults during ICU hospitalization. *JAMA Netw Open* 2024; **7**: e2410713.

33. J.M. McPeake, P. Henderson, G. Darroch, et al. Social and economic problems of ICU survivors identified by a structured social welfare consultation. *Crit Care* 2019; **23**: 153.

34. T. Lagu, N.S. Hannon, M.B. Rothberg, et al. Access to subspecialty care for patients with mobility impairment: a survey. *Ann Intern Med* 2013; **158**: 441–6.

35. N.R. Mudrick, M.L. Breslin, M. Liang, et al. Physical accessibility in primary health care settings: results from California on-site reviews. *Disabil Health J* 2012; **5**: 159–67.

36. K.E. Hauschildt, C. Seigworth, L. A. Kamphuis, et al. Patients' adaptations after acute respiratory distress syndrome: a qualitative study. *Am J Crit Care* 2021; **30**: 221–9.

37. J. McPeake, T.J. Iwashyna, L.M. Boehm, et al. Benefits of peer support for intensive care unit survivors: sharing experiences, care debriefing, and altruism. *Am J Crit Care* 2021; **30**: 145–9.

38. K.J. Haines, E. Hibbert, N. Leggett, et al. Transitions of care after critical illness: challenges to recovery and adaptive problem solving. *Crit Care Med* 2021; **49**: 1923–31.

39. L. Scheunemann, J.S. White, S. Prinjha, et al. Barriers and facilitators to resuming meaningful daily activities among critical illness survivors in the UK: a qualitative content analysis. *BMJ Open* 2022; **12**: e050592.

40. P. Henderson, T. Quasim, M. Shaw, et al. Evaluation of a health and social care programme to improve outcomes following critical illness: a multicentre study. *Thorax* 2023; **78**: 160–8.

41. K. Potter, S. Miller, S. Newman. Environmental factors affecting early mobilization and physical disability post-intensive care: an integrative review through the lens of the World Health Organization International Classification of Functioning. *Dimens Crit Care Nurs* 2021; **40**(2): 92–117.

42. Post-Intensive Care Transitional Care, Rehabilitation, and Family-Support | MedPath, https://trial.medpath.com/clinical-trial/223f3d9811a6b9a6/nct06501365-post-intensive-care-transitional-care (accessed October 13, 2024).

43. The Recognize Assist Include Support and Engage (RAISE) Act Family Caregiving Advisory Council, The Advisory Council to Support Grandparents Raising Grandchildren. 2022 National Strategy to Support Family Caregivers; 2022, www.gksnetwork.org/resources/2022-national-strategy-to-support-family-caregivers/ (accessed October 12, 2024).

44. N. Agaronnik, E.G. Campbell, J. Ressalam, et al. Communicating with patients with disability: perspectives of practicing physicians. *J Gen Intern Med* 2019; **34**: 1139–45.

45. Anti-Ableism Action Steps for Health Care Provision. https://eliclare.com/wp-content/uploads/2023/02/Action_Steps_for_Medical_Providers-12pt.pdf. Accessed June 2025.

46. K.P. Mayer, H. Boustany, E.P. Cassity, et al. ICU recovery clinic attendance, attrition, and patient outcomes: the impact of severity of illness, gender, and rurality. *Crit Care Explor* 2020; **2**: e0206.

47. T. Lagu, C. Griffin, P.K. Lindenauer. Ensuring access to health care for patients with disabilities. *JAMA Intern Med* 2015; **175**: 157–8.

48. D. Dawes. *The political determinants of health.* Baltimore, MD: Johns Hopkins University Press; 2020.

49. D. Meadows. *Thinking in systems: a primer.* (Wright D, ed.). White River Junction, Vermont: Chelsea Green Publishing; 2008.

50. J. Chen, M.R.T. Spencer, P. Buchongo, et al. Hospital-based health information technology infrastructure: evidence of reduced Medicare payments and racial disparities among patients with ADRD. *Med Care* 2023; **61**: 27–35.

Chapter 25

Social Determinants of Health and Their Relationship with Critical Illness

Jessica Nobile, J. Lloyd Allen, and Jared W. Magnani

Introduction

Social determinants of health (SDOH), the array of nonmedical factors that influence health outcomes, have been formally defined as the conditions and environments in which people are born, live, learn, work, play, worship, and age [1]. A rich literature documents the relationship between SDOH and overall health, well-being, and access to healthcare services [2,3,4,5].

Screening for SDOH in the intensive care unit (ICU) is imperative because of their considerable potential to influence both the presentation and course of critical illness as well as the short- and long-term recovery trajectories from critical illness. This chapter presents an overview of the theoretical framework that highlights the central importance of SDOH and their bidirectional relationship with critical illness, illustrated with examples. This chapter also describes the role of the social worker, both in the ICU and outpatient settings, to identify and address SDOH to promote optimal recovery. Lastly, it explores implications for social work research, policy, and practice, given the critical role that social work plays as part of multidisciplinary ICU and outpatient care teams.

Social Determinants of Health

SDOH constitute numerous, heterogeneous, nonmedical factors that influence daily life. SDOH may be conceptually categorized into three different tiers that are differentiated by their relative proximity to the individual(s) that they impact: the individual tier, which describes innate and acquired qualities of the person, including their race, ethnicity, educational level, and income; the neighborhood/community tier, which includes access to adequate housing, availability of clean air and water, and proximity to healthcare; and the societal/policy tier, which includes the impact of municipal, state, and federal policies on the individual- and neighborhood-level factors that in turn shape daily life (see Table 25.1). This classification schema of SDOH is complemented by a similar model put forth by the Centers for Disease Control and Prevention (CDC) that describes five domains central to SDOH: economic stability, education access and quality, health care access and quality, neighborhood and the built environment, and social and community context [6].

SDOH are inextricably linked to both the development of and the recovery from critical illness, and this relationship along the continuum of care results from multiple factors. First, more generally, SDOH impact one's health from the prenatal state through death, thereby preceding the development of any critical illness [7,8,9,10]; the propensity to develop a critical illness may result in part from the accumulation of social insults that occur throughout life, such as deficits that result from poverty, limited educational attainment, and social

Table 25.1 A three-tiered model of social determinants of health

Individual	Neighborhood/Community	Societal/Policy
Education	Housing	Legislation
General literacy	Transportation	Federal Policy
Health literacy	Opportunity for physical activity	State Policy
Employment and job opportunities	Neighborhood safety	Municipal Policy
Individual and household income	Exposure to industrial waste	-
Racism and discrimination	Access to nutritious food	-
Food insecurity	Housing discrimination Redlining and zoning	-
Housing costs	Neighborhood violence	-
Debt	School funding and quality	-
Access to health insurance	Access to healthcare facilities	-

deprivation, many of which are potentially long-term exposures. Second, compelling data exist demonstrating that SDOH are associated with increased severity of chronic medical conditions, such as diabetes and cardiovascular disease, which, in turn, increase the likelihood of incident critical illness [11,12,13,14,15,16,17,18]. Third, there is often limited access to primordial, primary, and secondary disease prevention in populations that experience adverse SDOH, thereby increasing the burden of risk factors for the development of acute or chronic conditions [19,20]. Fourth, adverse social exposures, such as a lack of sufficiently clean air and water, compromised housing, or absent transportation, may further exacerbate the associations previously described [21,22,23,24,25]. Lastly, returning to a home environment where adverse SDOH persist impairs recovery from critical illness and further increases the risk for the development of the post-intensive care syndrome (PICS) and its attendant morbidities and mortality (see Chapter 33 for additional information) [26].

The array of factors presented here are inherently associated, such that an individual may experience multiple, intersectional SDOH, whose collective impact meaningfully increases the risk of developing critical illness [27]. Populations at particular risk for myriad adverse SDOH include racial and ethnic minorities, sexual and gender minorities, the poor, the chronically ill, the disabled, and youth, particularly those with developmental challenges. One may consequently consider SDOH – multiple, heterogeneous, and long-term – as modifying the associations of proximal exposures to presentation with critical illness, its prognosis, and the development of PICS.

The County Health Rankings and Roadmaps is a program from the University of Wisconsin Population Health Institute to collect and evaluate health data across the 3,000 counties in the United States. The goal in collecting and disseminating this data is to promote health equity and encourage community participation to achieve that goal [28]. Based on this data, Remington and colleagues created a model to demonstrate the relationship between SDOH and health outcomes as shown in Figure 25.1, which also illustrates the

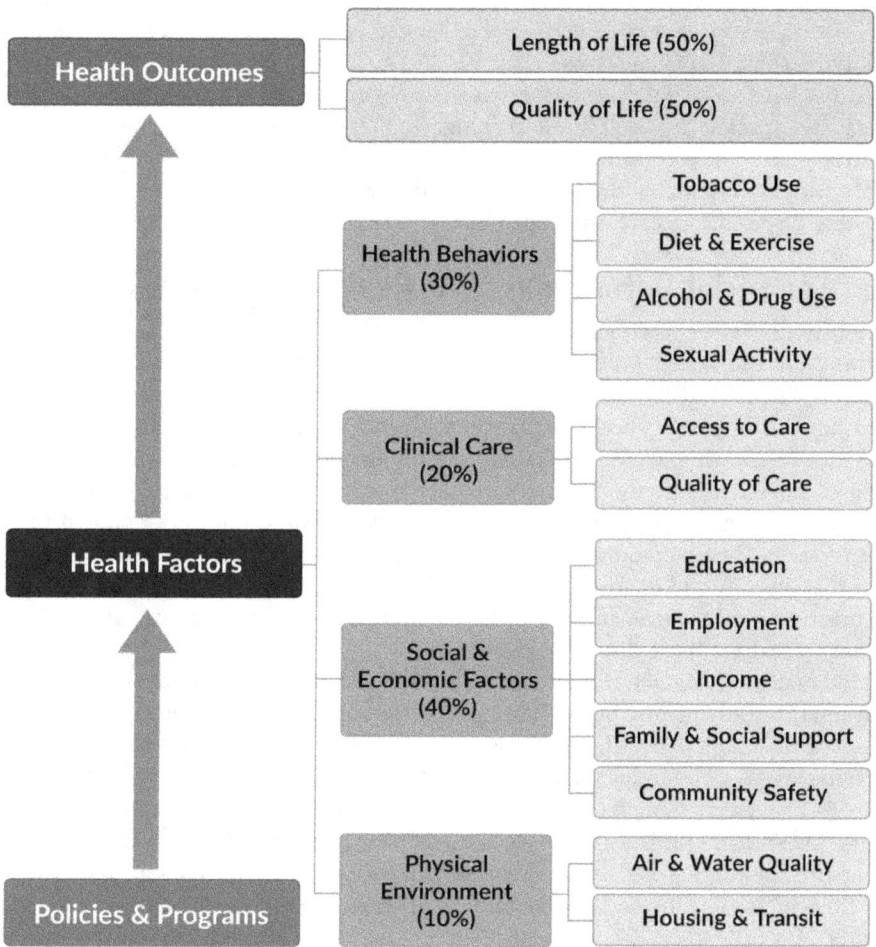

Figure 25.1 The County Health Rankings Model. Reproduced with permissions from The University of Wisconsin Population Health Institute, County Health Rankings & Roadmaps, 2014–2024 [70].

relationships between SDOH and length of life and quality of life, two key patient-centered health outcomes following critical illness. Health behaviors, access to and quality of clinical care, numerous social and economic factors, and the physical environment all play a significant role in health outcomes throughout the continuum of care.

The current understanding of SDOH is influenced by the socioecological theory, which suggests that human physical, emotional, and interpersonal experiences and health are embedded in interactions with the immediate environment and larger social context [29]. The environment, composed of a network of interconnected systems at the individual, interpersonal, organizational, community, and societal levels, influences human development and behaviors throughout life [30]. Some of these connections include home, work, school, family, friends, government, media, and healthcare. The principal framework for incorporating SDOH into the illness experience shifts the focus from the individual's presentation with disease to the individual's environmental context [31,32], centralizing SDOH within the biopsychosocial model advanced by social work and the social model of disability presented in Chapter 24.

Diseases have social patterns that are inextricably influenced by SDOH; as such, healthcare workers have specific responsibilities to recognize SDOH, articulate how they may influence or obstruct care, tailor communication strategies to both survivors and their families, and develop plans of care that address or accommodate SDOH. Ignoring SDOH may perpetuate preexisting disparities in care due to profound barriers to care implementation.

Impact of Social Determinants of Health on Critical Illness

An extensive literature has documented the associations between SDOH and critical illness, describing the individual-, neighborhood-, and society-level social and structural factors associated with critical illness severity and outcomes [33]. Likewise, there is evidence that critical illness has a reciprocal association with SDOH, worsening individual-level social factors due to the impact of critical illness on finances, functional independence, and vocational capacity. Here we summarize selected associations between SDOH and critical illness with further characterization using the generational framework adapted for health equity research. The generational framework classifies the first generation of research as studies that identify and quantify disparities, the second generation as studies that ascertain mechanisms for disparities, and the third generation as studies that evaluate and promote solutions to address these disparities [34,35].

Individual-level SDOH relevant to critical illness span race and ethnicity, income, educational attainment, and health literacy. A large administrative analysis confirmed racial differences in hospital length of stay among patients hospitalized with sepsis; patients identifying as Black race had a 1.3-day greater length of stay (95% confidence interval [CI] 0.68–1.84 days) than referents identifying as White race matched for patient- and hospital-level factors [36]. An analysis of the National Inpatient Sample database reported that patients identifying as Black race had increased risk of in-hospital mortality (odds ratio [OR] 1.09; 95% CI 1.08–1.11) following hospitalization for cardiac arrest compared to referents of White race [37]; one caution in the interpretation of this finding is that National Inpatient Sample data are constrained to hospitalization events and covariates, such as medical history and socioeconomic factors. As a final example, a large, single-center analysis of pediatric critical illness identified that Latinx children scored significantly higher on an index of mortality prediction compared to those of other races and ethnicities [38]; parental income and possession of government health insurance were also related to the index of mortality. This literature spans the first and second generations of the health equity framework [34], identifying distinct racial and ethnic disparities that are attenuated with adjustment for other social and economic factors.

The neighborhood in which one lives and neighborhood-level socioeconomic assets are also prominent SDOH. Neighborhoods shape environmental exposures and access to health-related assets (e.g., greenspaces and healthy food) and additionally reflect historical legacies of redlining and inequitable distribution of resources [39,40]. The critical care literature demonstrates the contribution of neighborhood residence as a SDOH with respect to health outcomes and, importantly, the attenuation of the associations of individual-level factors (e.g., race and ethnicity) on outcomes. In a large administrative analysis of the Pediatric Health Information System Registry, very low Childhood Opportunity Index

(COI; a composite of neighborhood characteristics and severity of presentation) was associated with a 35% increased likelihood of in-hospital mortality (adjusted OR [aOR] 1.35; 95% CI 1.05–1.74) [41]. The COI was additionally associated with need for pediatric ICU admission (aOR 1.06; 95% CI 1.02–1.11) and need for mechanical ventilation (aOR 1.12; 95% CI 1.04–1.21). In a separate study restricted to 15 pediatric ICUs, higher category of COI (i.e., greater socioeconomic advantage) was related to reduced mortality [42]. While children with a very low COI experienced higher mortality than those with a greater COI, those with very low COI did not experience increased mortality risk compared to those with higher COI in multivariable-adjusted analysis (OR 1.30; 95% CI 0.94–1.79).

An administrative analysis of individual-level data from 35 California hospitals identified racial differences in ICU length of stay, severity of physiologic derangement, and mortality [43]; odds of hospital mortality were higher in individuals categorized as Hispanic (OR 1.40; 95% CI 1.20–1.62) and Asian/Pacific Islander (OR 1.37; 95% CI 1.09–1.72) compared to those categorized as White race. Importantly, however, these differences were no longer significant following adjustment for social variables obtained at the census-block level (e.g., median household income and percentage of persons aged 25 years with fewer than 12 years of education). In summary, these studies collectively reinforce the importance of neighborhood-level socioeconomic characteristics on outcomes in the critically ill and furthermore demonstrate the importance of adjusting for such variables when examining the impact of individual-level data, particularly race and ethnicity, on patient outcomes. Further, they demonstrate the relevance of adjustment for such variables when examining other individual-level variables, particularly race and ethnicity, in relation to critical illness.

A comprehensive summary of the literature on the associations between neighborhood-level factors and critical illness is beyond the scope of this chapter, but a rich literature exists that summarizes the relationship between neighborhood industrial exposures and health [39,44]. Pollution is more prevalent in neighborhoods that have historically experienced social and economic disadvantage. A multi-generational, longitudinal study of the Panel Study of Income Dynamics determined that early life exposure to industrial pollutants was significantly associated with the subsequent development of childhood asthma [45]. Census-tract level pollution estimates plausibly explained racial differences in emergency room visits for asthma, suggesting a putative mechanism for racial disparities in acute asthma presentations [46]. Addressing pollution constitutes an evident "third generation intervention" to promote equity and reduce acute and critical illness in populations that heretofore have experienced social and economic deprivation.

Notably, financial stress is common in survivors of critical illness, with one study reporting an incidence of 42.5% in survivors and 48.5% in their family members [47]. It is therefore important for healthcare professionals to ask patients and their loved ones about financial concerns, as financial insecurity can lead to compromised nutrition and housing and prevent necessary medical follow-up. Between 44% and 70% of survivors of critical illness are incapable of returning to work within a year following hospital discharge (see Chapter 44 for additional information), yet they remain responsible for expensive medical bills associated with their ICU care and the recovery process. This bi-directional relationship between SDOH and critical illness leads to material and social hardships [48].

Social Work, Social Determinants of Health, and Critical Illness

Although screening for and appreciating the impact of SDOH are the responsibility of all healthcare providers, social workers are uniquely positioned to address SDOH for survivors of critical illness, both during preparations for hospital discharge and the outpatient recovery period. One example of a screening tool used by the Critical Illness Recovery Center (CIRC) at the University of Pittsburgh Medical Center, created by one of the authors, is provided in Box 25.1. This tool helps the team identify any social, economic, or financial

---

Box 25.1 A screening tool for social determinants of health

1. On average, how many days per week do you engage in moderate exercise?
2. On average, how many minutes do you engage in exercise at this level?
3. How hard is it for you to pay for the very basics, such as food and housing?
4. In the past 12 months, was there a time you could not pay your rent or mortgage?
5. How many times have you moved in the past year?
6. In the past 12 months, were you homeless or living in a shelter?
7. In the past 12 months, has lack of transportation kept you from medical appointments or getting medications?
8. In the past 12 months, has lack of transportation kept you from meetings, work, or from getting things needed for daily living?
9. Within the past 12 months, have you been that food would run out before you had money to buy more?
10. Do you feel stressed, tense, restless, nervous, anxious, or unable to sleep at night because your mind is troubled?
11. In a typical week, how many times do you talk on the phone with family, friends, and neighbors?
12. In a typical week, how often do you get together with relatives and friends?
13. How often do you attend religious services?
14. Do you belong to any clubs or organizations?
15. What is your marital status?
16. Within the last year, have you been afraid of anyone, including family and friends?
17. Within the last year, have you been humiliated or emotionally abused by anyone?
18. Within the last year, have you been physically harmed by anyone?
19. Within the last year, have you been sexually harmed by anyone?
20. How often do you need to have someone help you read instructions, pamphlets, and other written materials from your doctor or pharmacy?
21. How often do you have a drink containing alcohol?
22. How many drinks containing alcohol do you have on a typical day of drinking?
23. How often do you have six or more drinks containing alcohol on one occasion?
24. How many times in the past year have you used an illegal drug?
25. In the past two weeks, have you had little interest or pleasure in doing things?
26. In the past two weeks, have you felt down, depressed, or hopeless?

Note: This screening tool was created by the Critical Illness Recovery Center at UPMC Mercy Hospital, Pittsburgh, PA, USA

needs patients may have and ensures that a plan is created to remediate any concerns identified. This may include connecting patients with post-acute care resources, such as home health or rehabilitative services; helping patients apply for disability; and providing information on how to obtain financial resources. Lastly, patients may be linked to ICU follow-up clinics or primary care physicians that employ social workers to holistically address the needs of patients.

Using a SDOH lens, social workers must be aware of each patient's neighborhood assets to facilitate individual engagement with agencies and neighborhood-based resources. Alternatively, social workers may be informed of and address neighborhood deficits, such as violence, industrial exposures, lack of transportation, and significant distances to access care, which may be barriers to recovery following critical illness. To better assist survivors of critical illness, social workers must engage in research, policy, and practice efforts that support recovery and healing.

Research Implications

Research on SDOH and critical illness must utilize timely and client- or patient-centered approaches to design interventions geared toward reducing the social risks negatively affecting an individual's health and well-being. It must first be recognized that the data described above underscore the fact that healthcare – and access to adequate healthcare – is often unevenly distributed [49]. As such, analyses of multilevel and multidimensional factors using research designs (e.g., experimental, quasi-experimental, and randomized controlled trials) geared toward increasing health equity provide opportunities to invest in both the social and economic well-being of the whole person and their respective communities [49]. A socioecological lens also necessitates integration of multiple sources of complementary data, including demographic, social, and residential characteristics; census-tract or block data describing the neighborhood and residential environment; and the electronic health record to document prior diagnoses and treatments. Such data require appropriate statistical approaches that include multilevel and hierarchical modeling [50,51].

Qualitative research is interested in understanding and interpreting specific phenomena as it relates to the subjective meanings people attribute to them in their natural environments [52]. Qualitative approaches therefore provide opportunities for researchers and healthcare providers to capture individual and group lived experiences describing the reciprocal relationship between SDOH and critical illness, while also empowering individuals to voice in their own words methods that they believe would help. Through the application of qualitative methods that focus on SDOH and critical illness, we can develop a deeper understanding of what it feels like to be a survivor, including the barriers they encounter, the strengths they employ, and their identity formation after medical trauma [48,53,54,55].

Mixed methods that combine both quantitative and qualitative strategies can be used to challenge society's reactive approach to medicine, healthcare, social justice, and social equality [56]. Objective data coupled with subjective data tells a story through both numbers and words that can encourage people to carefully consider how to change the social environment so that the disparities that exist due to SDOH can be alleviated. The intersectionality of social determinants, critical illness, and individual identity present an urgent need to create inter-sectoral partnerships between individuals, healthcare systems, and their communities [57]. Mixed research methods can be utilized to set priorities, monitor progress, and allocate resources following critical illness [58,59]; they can also better inform the creation of tools that will assess SDOH for survivors of critical illness [60].

Policy Implications

Historically, the field of social work has been dedicated to advocating for the most vulnerable and oppressed in hopes of improving their social conditions; indeed, social justice is identified as one of social work's six core values. Political advocacy and community organizing are essential components to meeting the goal of promoting equal treatment of all groups. Social workers intervene at the local, state, and national levels to encourage welfare reform and social equality and to ensure that funding is directed toward physical and mental health parity. Social workers write social policies, disseminate information to the masses, and lobby for policy changes that are geared toward establishing justice and equality for all [61].

With respect to critical illness, social workers must consider policies that emphasize SDOH to recognize the importance of identifying and addressing social factors that lead to health inequity. Many survivors of critical illness become disabled, are unable to work, and are in need of Social Security Disability Insurance (SSDI); however, the process for obtaining health insurance or supplemental income can take up to six months for an initial decision, and oftentimes applicants are denied on their first try. During the decision-making process, survivors are ineligible for benefits and often go without financial resources. The resultant lack of funds may prohibit a person's access to healthcare, endanger their living arrangements, and negatively affect their daily functioning [62]. Advocacy to change policies affecting SSDI and other similar programs is needed to ensure that survivors of critical illness can pay for food, housing, and medical costs.

Furthermore, creation of social policies and health policies that seek to reduce disparities across groups is needed to ensure that social conditions do not disadvantage groups (see Chapter 24 for additional information). The sociopolitical environment in which we live directly influences our ability to be healthy, as public policies assign financial and social resources at the local, state, and federal levels. Despite a growing body of research encouraging governments to consider policies that will alleviate long-standing disparities, very little has been done [63].

Practice Implications

The study of SDOH heavily informs social work practice. Prior research has suggested that the clinical practice of social work should be directed toward adaptation and health promotion, including an appreciation of client experiences with life-long trauma [61,64,65]. Many members of society experience racism and other forms of discrimination due to age, gender or gender identity, sexual orientation, disability status, financial status, and substance abuse, which is often an unrecognized form of trauma that may cause distrust in healthcare providers. Social workers, with their commitment to social justice and person-centered practices, can act as a bridge between consumers and providers of care [61]. Social workers approach survivors from a place of listening and empowerment, which builds trust in both the relationship and the profession and facilitates a survivor's engagement in treatment.

Interventions grounded in addressing social factors that impede overall health can help survivors of critical illness achieve optimal recovery while also having their basic needs met [64,65]. As members of a multidisciplinary team, social workers can inform other healthcare providers about how a patient's SDOH may have affected their medical history and how they may impact the current and future clinical course, important information that should be addressed as part of the patient's plan of care. Furthermore, many survivors of critical illness experience a change in their SDOH as a consequence of their illness. Social workers must carefully consider these changes and help to alleviate financial stress caused by loss of income in both the patient and their family members, who must often reduce or eliminate employment to fulfill the role of caregiver. Social workers can connect survivors and their loved ones with resources that aid in the obtainment of food, housing, transportation, and other essential resources. Additionally, social workers provide ongoing assistance with the application process for SSDI or supplemental security income (SSI), which may include connecting patients with a lawyer.

Social workers providing case management set up a variety of services, such as transportation for medical appointments, including ride shares and medical assistance transportation, for those without vehicles or who are unable to navigate public transportation. Social workers also connect patients with food assistance by assisting them in applying for the Supplemental Nutrition Assistance Program (SNAP), providing a list of local food banks, and setting up Meals on Wheels or other similar programs for those with food and financial insecurity or whose physical and cognitive impairments prevent them from shopping and cooking. Social workers also refer patients to other providers to ensure that they are connected with long-term mental health providers, drug and alcohol counseling services, and/or extensive case management.

In addition to case management, social workers participating in ICU follow-up clinics can provide both individual and group therapy to help survivors suffering from depression, anxiety, post-traumatic stress disorder, and the many additional stressors associated with recovery from critical illness. Therapeutically, social workers can assist patients coming to terms with the many changes caused by their critical illness and support survivors as they navigate a new way of living, filled with obstacles, to facilitate capacity building. For those who develop PICS, social workers can provide individual counseling employing a variety of different modalities geared at acceptance and adaption, such as dialectical behavioral therapy (DBT). DBT is a combination of cognitive and behavioral therapies that increases distress tolerance, strengthens healthy responses to stressors, and reinforces mindfulness techniques [66]. DBT encourages survivors to make meaning of their illness by finding ways to adapt and appreciate their lived experiences. Another approach to providing therapy with survivors of critical illness is person-centered therapy. Survivors of critical illness set both medical and nonmedical goals with respect to their physical, cognitive, emotional, and social health recovery. Approaching these goals from a holistic perspective allows patients to prioritize their needs while working toward a sense of hope and healing despite an intervening decline in their physical, cognitive, or mental health. This is done by allowing survivors to lead their therapeutic treatment, to grieve what once was, and to focus their attention on areas where their abilities shine [67].

Support groups are another platform where social workers can assist survivors in their recovery (see Chapter 49 for additional information). By fostering social relationships that have a reciprocal influence on health and well-being, peer support programs help survivors of critical illness feel validated and less alone. A qualitative study examining the experiences of survivors of critical illness with a peer support group found that being surrounded by others with similar lived experiences assisted survivors in gaining insight into their illness and recovery [68]. Speaking with other survivors further along the recovery trajectory can mitigate social isolation and loneliness, increase hope and motivation, and can lead to a more sophisticated understanding of how to navigate complex healthcare systems, set realistic goals, and manage expectations about the pace and breadth of recovery. Peer support groups can also foster a sense of altruism, giving people a sense of purpose and allowing them to give back to other survivors and their caregivers [69]. Through strengthening coping skills, fostering hope for the future, and motivating survivors in their recovery endeavors, peer support groups are a low-cost intervention that provides important psychosocial benefits and potentially even life-saving ones.

Conclusion

Many survivors of critical illness face overwhelming challenges on their road to recovery, including impaired access to care; a reduction in overall health and quality of life; new or worsened physical, cognitive, and psychiatric impairments; financial, housing, and food insecurity; and an inability to reintegrate into former familial, vocational, and social roles. SDOH play a bidirectional role in people's health and well-being and consequently merit significant attention; they increase the risk of developing critical illness in many, and survivors of critical illness may experience worsened SDOH, which can significantly impact their recovery potential. Given the underappreciated role that social factors play in health and recovery after critical illness, social workers can be invaluable members of multidisciplinary teams caring for survivors of critical illness. Social workers can also engage in research, policy, and practice efforts that can facilitate the recovery journey for future survivors of critical illness.

Key Points

1. SDOH are nonmedical factors that influence health outcomes and include educational attainment, income, access to resources, residential and neighborhood-level factors, legislation, and more.
2. People who experience challenges with SDOH tend to be in poorer health and more likely to suffer critical illness than those who are successful at the individual, community, and policy levels.
3. Following critical illness, patients are more likely to develop worsening SDOH, as they often lose employment, gain medical debt, and experience social isolation.
4. Social workers are uniquely positioned to assess, consider, and address SDOH in survivors of critical illness to promote positive health outcomes.
5. Social workers have the opportunity to intervene with individuals, healthcare providers, communities, and legislators to encourage the improvement of SDOH for survivors through research, policy, and practice.

References

1. M. Marmot, R. Bell. Fair society, healthy lives. *Public Health* 2012; **126**(Suppl 1): S4–10.
2. T.M. Powell-Wiley, Y. Baumer, F.O. Baah, et al. Social determinants of cardiovascular disease. *Circ Res* 2022; **130**: 782–99.
3. R.L. Thornton, C.M. Glover, C.W. Cené, et al. Evaluating strategies for reducing health disparities by addressing the social determinants of health. *Health Aff (Millwood)* 2016; **35**: 1416–23.
4. P.A. Braveman, S.A. Egerter, S.H. Woolf, J.S. Marks. When do we know enough to recommend action on the social

determinants of health? *Am J Prev Med* 2011; **40**: S58–66.

5. P. Braveman, L. Gottlieb. The social determinants of health: it's time to consider the causes of the causes. *Public Health Rep* 2014; **129**(Suppl 2): 19–31.

6. U. S. D. o. H. a. H. Services. Healthy People 2030 [Available from: https://health.gov/healthypeople.

7. R. Chetty, M. Stepner, S. Abraham, et al. The association between income and life expectancy in the United States, 2001–2014. *JAMA* 2016; **315**: 1750–66.

8. N.L. Jones, S.E. Gilman, T.L. Cheng, et al. Life course approaches to the causes of health disparities. *Am J Public Health* 2019; **109**: S48–s55.

9. L.M. Glover, L.R. Cain-Shields, S.B. Wyatt, et al. Life course socioeconomic status and hypertension in African American adults: the Jackson Heart study. *Am J Hypertens* 2020; **33**: 84–91.

10. Z.A. Bhutta, S. Bhavnani, T.S. Betancourt, et al. Adverse childhood experiences and lifelong health. *Nat Med* 2023; **29**: 1639–48.

11. M. Odlum, N. Moise, I.M. Kronish, et al. Trends in poor health indicators among Black and Hispanic middle-aged and older adults in the United States, 1999–2018. *JAMA Netw Open* 2020; **3**: e2025134.

12. O. Akinyelure, B. Jaeger, S. Oparil, et al. Social determinants of health and uncontrolled blood pressure in a national cohort of Black and White US adults: the REGARDS study. *Hypertension* 2023; **80** (7): 1403-13.

13. D. Bann, M. Fluharty, R. Hardy, S. Scholes. Socioeconomic inequalities in blood pressure: co-ordinated analysis of 147,775 participants from repeated birth cohort and cross-sectional datasets, 1989 to 2016. *BMC Med* 2020; **18**: 338.

14. Y. Commodore-Mensah, R.A. Turkson-Ocran, K. Foti, et al. Associations between social determinants and hypertension, stage 2 hypertension, and controlled blood pressure among men and women in the United States. *Am J Hypertens* 2021; **34**: 707–17.

15. R. Hamad, T.T. Nguyen, J. Bhattacharya, et al. Educational attainment and cardiovascular disease in the United States: a quasi-experimental instrumental variables analysis. *PLoS Med* 2019; **16**: e1002834.

16. W. Khaing, S.A. Vallibhakara, J. Attia, et al. Effects of education and income on cardiovascular outcomes: a systematic review and meta-analysis. *Eur J Prev Cardiol* 2017; **24**: 1032–42.

17. J.B. King, L.C. Pinheiro, J. Bryan Ringel, et al. Multiple social vulnerabilities to health disparities and hypertension and death in the REGARDS study. *Hypertension* 2022; **79**: 196–206.

18. J.M. Ochieng, J.D. Crist. Social determinants of health and health care delivery: African American women's T2DM self-management. *Clin Nurs Res* 2021; **30**: 263–72.

19. H. Angier, B.B. Green, K. Frankhauser, et al. Role of health insurance and neighborhood-level social deprivation on hypertension control following the affordable care act health insurance opportunities. *Soc Sci Med* 2020; **265**: 113439.

20. M. Sims, K.N. Kershaw, K. Breathett, et al. Importance of housing and cardiovascular health and well-being: a scientific statement from the American Heart Association. *Circ Cardiovasc Qual Outcomes* 2020; **13**: e000089.

21. J.E. Bennett, H. Tamura-Wicks, R. M. Parks, et al. Particulate matter air pollution and national and county life expectancy loss in the USA: a spatiotemporal analysis. *PLoS Med* 2019; **16**: e1002856.

22. L.M. Besser, O.L. Meyer, M.R. Jones, et al. Neighborhood segregation and cognitive change: multi-ethnic study of atherosclerosis. *Alzheimers Dement* 2023; **19**: 1143–51.

23. L.M. Besser, O.L. Meyer, M. Streitz, et al. Perceptions of greenspace and social determinants of health across the life course: the Life Course Sociodemographics and Neighborhood Questionnaire (LSNEQ). *Health Place* 2023; **81**: 103008.

24. A.V. Diez Roux, M.S. Mujahid, J.A. Hirsch, et al. The impact of neighborhoods on CV risk. *Glob Heart* 2016; **11**: 353–63.
25. M. Kolak, J. Bhatt, Y.H. Park, et al. Quantification of neighborhood-level social determinants of health in the continental United States. *JAMA Netw Open* 2020; **3**: e1919928.
26. P. Charkhchi, S. Fazeli Dehkordy, R. C. Carlos. Housing and food insecurity, care access, and health status among the chronically ill: an analysis of the behavioral risk factor surveillance system. *J Gen Intern Med* 2018; **33**: 644–50.
27. N. Lopez, V.L. Gadsden. Health inequities, social determinants, and intersectionality. In C. Alexander, V. McBride Murray, K. Bogard (eds), *Perspectives on Health Equity and Social Determinants of Health*. Washington, DC: NAM Perspectives, 2017.
28. P.L. Remington, B.B. Catlin, K.P. Gennuso. The County Health Rankings: rationale and methods. *Popul Health Metr* 2015; **13**: 11.
29. U. Bronfenbrenner. Toward an experimental ecology of human development. *Am Psychol* 1977; **32**: 513.
30. B.G. Link, J. Phelan. Social conditions as fundamental causes of disease. *J Health Soc Behav* 1995; **Spec No**: 80–94.
31. K. Froehlich-Grobe, M. Douglas, C. Ochoa, A. Betts. Social determinants of health and disability. *Public Health Perspectives on Disability: Science, Social Justice, Ethics, and Beyond*. 2021: 53–89.
32. B. Wold, M.B. Mittelmark. Health-promotion research over three decades: the social-ecological model and challenges in implementation of interventions. *Scand J Public Health* 2018; **46**: 20–6.
33. D. Ramadurai, H. Patel, S. Peace, et al. Integrating social determinants of health in critical care. *CHEST Critical Care* 2024; **2**: 100057.
34. A.M. Kilbourne, G. Switzer, K. Hyman, et al. Advancing health disparities research within the health care system: a conceptual framework. *Am J Public Health* 2006; **96**: 2113–21.
35. S.B. Thomas, S.C. Quinn, J. Butler, et al. Toward a fourth generation of disparities research to achieve health equity. *Annu Rev Public Health* 2011; **32**: 399–416.
36. C.F. Chesley, M. Chowdhury, D.S. Small, et al. Racial disparities in length of stay among severely ill patients presenting with sepsis and acute respiratory failure. *JAMA Netw Open* 2023; **6**: e239739.
37. J.-S. Rachoin, P. Olsen, J. Gaughan, E. Cerceo. Racial differences in outcomes and utilization after cardiac arrest in the USA: a longitudinal study comparing different geographical regions in the USA from 2006–2018. *Resuscitation* 2021; **169**: 115–23.
38. D. Epstein, M. Reibel, J.B. Unger, et al. The effect of neighborhood and individual characteristics on pediatric critical illness. *J Community Health* 2014; **39**: 753–9.
39. K.N. Kershaw, J.W. Magnani, A.V. Diez Roux, et al. Neighborhoods and cardiovascular health: a scientific statement from the American Heart Association. *Circ Cardiovasc Qual Outcomes* 2024; **17**: e000124.
40. K. Fullin, S. Keen, K. Harris, J.W. Magnani. Impact of neighborhood on cardiovascular health: a contemporary narrative review. *Curr Cardiol Rep* 2023; **25**: 1015–27.
41. A. Garg, A.A. Sochet, R. Hernandez, D. C. Stockwell. Association of the Child Opportunity Index and Inpatient Illness Severity in the United States, 2018–2019. *Acad Pediatr* 2024; **24**(7): 1101–9.
42. M.C. McCrory, M. Akande, K.N. Slain, et al. Child opportunity index and pediatric intensive care outcomes: a multicenter retrospective study in the United States. *Pediatr Crit Care Med* 2024; **25**: 323–34.
43. S.E. Erickson, E.E. Vasilevskis, M. W. Kuzniewicz, et al. The effect of race and ethnicity on outcomes among patients in the intensive care unit: a comprehensive study involving socioeconomic status and resuscitation preferences. *Crit Care Med* 2011; **39**: 429–35.
44. A.V. Diez Roux, C. Mair. Neighborhoods and health. *Ann N Y Acad Sci* 2010; **1186**: 125–45.

45. N. Kravitz-Wirtz, S. Teixeira, A. Hajat, et al. Early-life air pollution exposure, neighborhood poverty, and childhood asthma in the United States, 1990–2014. *Int J Environ Res Public Health* 2018; **15**: 1114.

46. S.E. Chambliss, E.C. Matsui, R.A. Zárate, C.M. Zigler. The role of neighborhood air pollution in disparate racial and ethnic asthma acute care use. *Am J Respir Crit Care Med* 2024; **210**: 178–85.

47. P.J. Ohtake, A.C. Lee, J.C. Scott, et al. Physical impairments associated with post-intensive care syndrome: systematic review based on the World Health Organization's international classification of functioning, disability and health framework. *Phys Ther* 2018; **98**: 631–45.

48. J. McPeake, L. Boehm, E. Hibbert, et al. Modification of social determinants of health by critical illness and consequences of that modification for recovery: an international qualitative study. *BMJ Open* 2022; **12**: e060454.

49. M.D. Low, B.J. Low, E.R. Baumler, P. T. Huynh. Can education policy be health policy? Implications of research on the social determinants of health. *J Health Polit Policy Law* 2005; **30**: 1131–62.

50. R.C. Palmer, D. Ismond, E.J. Rodriquez, J. S. Kaufman. Social determinants of health: future directions for health disparities research. *American Public Health Association*; 2019: S70–S1.

51. I. Dankwa-Mullan, E.J. Perez-Stable, K. Gardner, et al. *The science of health disparities research*. Hoboken, NJ: Wiley-Blackwell; 2021.

52. J.N. Hall, N. Mitchel, S.N. Halpin, G. A. Kilanko. Using focus groups for empowerment purposes in qualitative health research and evaluation. *Int J Soc Res Methodol* 2023; **26**: 409–23.

53. L.R. Cutler, M. Hayter, T. Ryan. A critical review and synthesis of qualitative research on patient experiences of critical illness. *Intensive Crit Care Nurs* 2013; **29**: 147–57.

54. J. King, B. O'Neill, P. Ramsay, et al. Identifying patients' support needs following critical illness: a scoping review of the qualitative literature. *Crit Care* 2019; **23**: 187.

55. C.L. Auriemma, M.O. Harhay, K.J. Haines, et al. What matters to patients and their families during and after critical illness: a qualitative study. *Am J Crit Care* 2021; **30**: 11–20.

56. M. Exworthy. Policy to tackle the social determinants of health: using conceptual models to understand the policy process. *Health Policy Plan* 2008; **23**: 318–27.

57. F. Osei Baah, B.M. Brawner, A.M. Teitelman, et al. A mixed-methods study of social determinants and self-care in adults with heart failure. *J Cardiovasc Nurs* 2023; **38**: E59–e71.

58. M.J. Holosko. *Social Work Case Management: Case Studies From the Frontlines*. 1st ed. Los Angeles: SAGE; 2018.

59. S. Pathak, D.M. Low, L. Franzini, J. M. Swint. A review of Canadian policy on social determinants of health. *Rev Eur Stud* 2012; **4**: 15.

60. S. Kostelanetz, M. Pettapiece-Phillips, J. Weems, et al. Health care professionals' perspectives on universal screening of social determinants of health: a mixed-methods study. *Popul Health Manag* 2022; **25**: 367–74.

61. M.E. Kondrat. Actor-centered social work re-visioning "person-in-environment" through a critical theory lens. *Soc Work* 2002; **47**: 435–48.

62. S. Prenovitz. What happens when you wait? Effects of Social Security Disability Insurance wait time on health and financial well-being. *Health Econ* 2021; **30**: 491–504.

63. M G. Embrett, G.E. Randall. Social determinants of health and health equity policy research: exploring the use, misuse, and nonuse of policy analysis theory. *Soc Sci Med* 2014; **108**: 147–55.

64. S.L. Craig, R. Bejan, B. Muskat. Making the invisible visible: are health social workers addressing the social determinants of health? *Soc Work Health Care* 2013; **52**: 311–31.

65. L. Petruzzi, N. Milano, Q. Chen, et al. Social workers are key to addressing social

determinants of health in integrated care settings. *Soc Work Health Care* 2024; **63**: 89–101.

66. S.L. Rizvi, M.M. Linehan. Dialectical behavior therapy for personality disorders. *Curr Psychiatry Rep* 2001; **3**: 64–9.

67. S.E. Schellinger, E.W. Anderson, M.S. Frazer, C.L. Cain. Patient self-defined goals: essentials of person-centered care for serious illness. *Am J Hosp Palliat Care* 2018; **35**: 159–65.

68. C.G. Bäckman, M. Ahlberg, C. Jones, G.H. Frisman. Group meetings after critical illness: giving and receiving strength. *Intensive Crit Care Nurs* 2018; **46**: 86–91.

69. J. McPeake, T.J. Iwashyna, L.M. Boehm, et al. Benefit of peer support for intensive care unit survivors: sharing experiences, care debriefing, and altruism. *Am J Crit Care* 2021; **30**(2): 145–9.

70. U. o. W. P. H. Institute. County Health Rankings & Roadmaps 2024. 2024. www.countyhealthrankings.org/.

Chapter 26
What Matters Most to Patients and Families

Sarah K. Andersen and Kirsten Fiest

Introduction

Critical illness is often a life-altering experience for both patients and families. Survivors of critical illness face many challenges – physical, cognitive, psychological, social, and existential – that are collectively known as post-intensive care syndrome (PICS) [1,2]. Families, meanwhile, frequently step into the role of informal caregiver and face their own struggles with the trauma of critical illness, including the physical, mental, social, and financial burdens of caregiving [3,4,5,6,7]. Increasingly, clinicians and researchers are engaging in dialogue with patients and families to better understand their lived experiences and what matters most to them in their recovery journey. Although every patient and family is unique, common themes may provide guidance for clinicians, researchers, and health systems looking to support critical illness recovery. In this chapter, we explore guiding principles for patient- and family-centered recovery, categories of shared and distinct patient and family needs, and areas for future research and engagement.

Guiding Principles for Patient- and Family-Centered Recovery

Although the support needs of patients and families are multifaceted and dynamic, certain principles may be useful to guide care across all phases of critical illness recovery (see Table 26.1).

Proactive, Structured, and Coordinated Care

First, patients and families want care that is proactive, structured, and coordinated across the entire critical illness recovery continuum. This requires hospital-based and community providers to share knowledge and resources with patients and their loved ones and to communicate effectively across care transitions [8]. In qualitative studies, patients and families describe a sense of loneliness and isolation following critical illness, amplified by poor communication, lack of preparation for the challenges of recovery, and limited knowledge of PICS among community health providers [9,10]. Survivors of critical illness and their families have consistently advocated for more information and community resources, particularly physical therapy and psychosocial support, to promote recovery [11]. Importantly, patients and families desire information that is tailored to the recovery stage and support that is individualized based on the unique needs and goals of each patient [9,10,11,12]. Early and frequent follow-up after hospital discharge, whether by phone call, virtual, or in-person visits, may provide much needed reassurance, particularly to family caregivers [12,13]. Interventions that are designed to be convenient for debilitated patients

Table 26.1 Guiding principles for patient and family-centered recovery

Principles of Care	Practical Examples
Proactive, structured, and coordinated	• Frequent communication between hospital and community clinicians • Introduction of critical illness recovery during ward-based ICU outreach and follow-up • Early phone check-in after discharge • Virtual follow-up appointments • Multidisciplinary clinics
Holistic, not reductionist	• Address disease management, symptom relief, and social/financial support at each clinic visit • Validate progress and address existential distress • Offer participation in peer support programs • Adopt holistic measures of quality of life in research and clinical practice
Prioritize recovery and resolution	• Deliver active interventions focused on regaining abilities • Conduct functional reconciliations at key time points to identify deficits and personalize a recovery plan • Explore functional goals and quality of life considerations at clinic visits
Dynamic and individualized	• Adopt *Timing-it-Right* framework to structure follow-up programs • Recognize distinct phases of recovery • Revisit patient and family needs and goals periodically

and strained caregivers, such as multidisciplinary joint appointments and telehealth visits, are also well-received [12].

Broadly speaking, patients and families express a desire to have intensive care unit (ICU) clinicians oversee care transitions and coordinate follow-up care [14]. ICU clinicians are viewed as experts on PICS who can best help manage expectations for recovery. Moreover, interactions with ICU teams on the ward and in ICU follow-up clinics, as well as opportunities to return to the ICU where they received care, may help patients and families process their critical illness experience [14,15]. In one study, survivors of critical illness voiced a desire for ongoing contact with the ICU team even one to two years after their ICU stay, highlighting both the longitudinal nature of recovery and the life-altering nature of critical illness [13]. These longitudinal relationships may, in turn, improve clinicians' understanding of PICS and enhance their ability to counsel future patients and families during their ICU stay [8].

Holistic, Not Reductionist

Second, patients and families desire care that is holistic rather than reductionist. PICS is often conceptualized by clinicians and researchers as deficits in distinct physical, cognitive, and psychological domains; patients and families, however, experience critical illness as a cataclysmic event that disrupts all aspects of life, including personal and social identity [16,17]. In a qualitative study of survivors of acute respiratory distress syndrome and their informal caregivers, Cox and colleagues describe how critical illness impacts survivors' sense of self, leads to relationship strain, and provokes difficult and intrusive memories of ICU care [17]. Established family, professional, and social roles may be disrupted and reconfigured by critical illness, causing existential distress to both patients and family members. In a study examining patient and family priorities for ICU recovery programs, patients expressed a desire to achieve a "holistic reintegration of multiple areas of life" impacted by critical illness [14]. This holistic approach runs counter to prevailing reductionist approaches to care, where the focus is on discrete symptoms or diseases (see Chapter 23 for additional information). A holistic approach requires clinicians and recovery programs to integrate disease management, symptom relief, and support for social and financial needs [14]. McPeake and colleagues found that, from the perspective of patients, successful ICU follow-up clinics not only provided continuity of care and symptom management, but also normalized the recovery process, addressed feelings of guilt and helplessness, and provided internal and external validation of progress [14]. Clinic- or community-based peer support programs may also help patients and families process their illness experience in a more holistic way (see Chapter 49 for additional information) [18].

Focus on Recovery and Resolution

Lastly, patients and families want care that is centered on recovery and resolution, rather than adjusting to a "new normal" of reduced function and quality of life. To the extent possible, ICU follow-up programs should deliver active interventions focused on regaining important abilities, instead of simply screening for deficits [11]. Patients, in particular, view symptom and disease management as a means to regain their former lives, rather than ends in themselves [19]. Although survival is an important first step, survival with severe functional impairment, continued dependence on machines, or intractable pain may be worse than death. Physical and cognitive function, as well as quality of life, are heavily valued by patients and families [20,21]. To ensure that patients receive effective, targeted interventions, functional status should be assessed and documented across the critical illness continuum and ideally include baseline function prior to hospitalization. In the same way that pharmacists reconcile medications across transitions of care, Elliot and colleagues have proposed that clinicians conduct "functional reconciliations" at key time points to identify important deficits and enhance rehabilitation supports [10].

Timing It Right

It is important for clinicians and health systems to understand that patient and family needs evolve over time. For many patients and families, recovery from critical illness is a journey that takes months to years. A dynamic approach to care following critical illness is therefore key [11]. The "timing it right" model, which was originally developed to guide post-stroke care [22], is a useful framework to map the dynamic nature of patient and family needs and experiences across critical illness recovery (see Table 26.1) [11,13,23].

Timing it right conceptualizes critical illness recovery in five phases. Phase 1 consists of the *acute critical illness event*, where the focus is on survival and stabilization. There is often a high degree of uncertainty and little thought of the future. In this phase, patients and families require emotional support and clear, comprehensible information [20]. Patients desire comforting words and touch, family presence, and personal care and hygiene, while families desire specific information about the illness and associated acute complications, such as delirium.

Phase 2 is a period of *stabilization*, where the focus shifts to recovery in hospital and determining the extent of disability. In this phase, patients and families both desire more detailed illness information, including realistic expectations for recovery, and ongoing emotional support. This phase often signals a transition from the ICU to ward. Non-abandonment, fostering realistic hope, and structured continuity of care (e.g., from critical care outreach teams) are particularly important during this transition. Many families start to learn caregiving skills in this phase and take on a more active role in their loved one's care.

Phase 3 involves *preparation* for discharge home to the community. Patients and families often experience apprehension and fear related to the upcoming transition home. Emotional support and reassurance, along with more detailed information on recovery-focused treatments, are important aspects of care in this phase. Family caregivers may worry about their readiness for unsupervised caregiving and desire additional training and supervised practice, as well as information on signs of potential new and serious health events and available community supports.

Phase 4 signals *implementation* of the post-hospital phase of care and recovery. Patients must cope with the loss of their former pre-critical illness self and adapt to new functional impairments and the home environment. Families must adjust to the role of primary caregiver and work to coordinate community-based services and healthcare follow-up. In this phase, patients and families may start to process their critical illness experience more fully and want to make sense of their illness story. Counseling, peer support, and reconnecting with ICU staff may be helpful to validate and normalize their emotional journey. Patients and families in this phase also desire early cognitive and physical rehabilitation and tangible resources to support recovery.

Lastly, phase 5 involves ongoing *adaptation* to life following critical illness. Patients continue to adjust to their new sense of self and may begin to rebuild their social networks, form new life goals, and strive for increased independence. In this phase, family members must recalibrate their caregiving role based on patient recovery and may start to return to preexisting social and workplace roles. Family caregivers in this phase may also start to think more about their own future and seek out peer support to process their lived experiences of critical illness.

Categories of Patient and Family Needs

Patients and families travel parallel paths through recovery from a critical illness, and they have both shared and distinct needs. Understanding where patient and family needs overlap and where they differ is important for clinicians looking to support critical illness recovery (see Figure 26.1).

Shared Needs (Patients and Families)

We report shared patient and family needs across the recovery trajectory into categories initially proposed by House [24] and expanded by King and colleagues [23] to focus on critical illness: informational, emotional, appraisal, instrumental, and spiritual. We further propose social/relational support needs as an additional category shared by ICU patients and their family members.

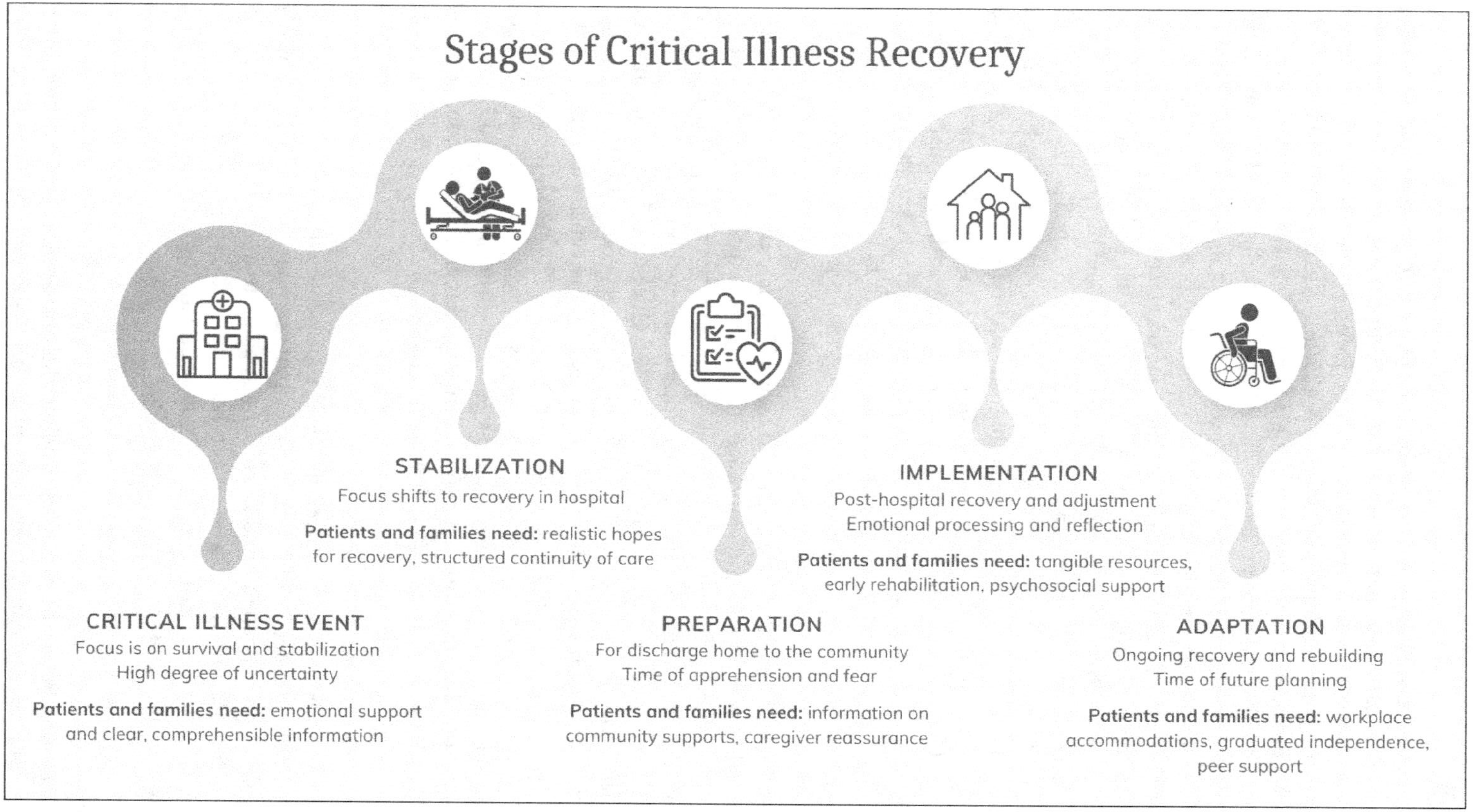

Stages of Critical Illness Recovery

CRITICAL ILLNESS EVENT
Focus is on survival and stabilization
High degree of uncertainty

Patients and families need: emotional support and clear, comprehensible information

STABILIZATION
Focus shifts to recovery in hospital

Patients and families need: realistic hopes for recovery, structured continuity of care

PREPARATION
For discharge home to the community
Time of apprehension and fear

Patients and families need: information on community supports, caregiver reassurance

IMPLEMENTATION
Post-hospital recovery and adjustment
Emotional processing and reflection

Patients and families need: tangible resources, early rehabilitation, psychosocial support

ADAPTATION
Ongoing recovery and rebuilding
Time of future planning

Patients and families need: workplace accommodations, graduated independence, peer support

Figure 26.1 Critical illness recovery across five stages for patients and families.

Informational

Informational needs are supported by providing information to patients and families to address problems [23], and these needs vary across the "timing it right" recovery trajectory. During the acute illness event, informational needs focus on details about the illness, treatments, potential complications, and prognosis [25,26]. At this stage, information is more likely to be provided to families, given the severity of illness of many critically ill patients; because of this, information about what happened during an ICU stay is often provided to patients *after* the acute illness has resolved [13]. Given the stressful and uncertain nature of the acute illness, information needs to be repeated to patients and families in clear and understandable terms [25,26]. During the stabilization and recovery stages, informational needs should focus on providing realistic expectations for recovery and treatments that focus on recovery. The transfer from ICU to ward must be accompanied by clear communication from clinician to clinician and from clinicians to patients and families [27]. During the discharge process, clinicians should review treatments and medications that will support ongoing recovery, including information regarding the long-term effects of critical illness [25]. Once in the community (during the adaptation phase), shared informational needs include a continued focus on long-term symptoms and recovery, with particular emphasis on supports that are available in the community. Patients and families desire information to be provided in written form so that it can be referred to in perpetuity [25].

Emotional

Emotional needs include empathy, love, trust, and caring [23]. The emotions of ICU patients and families change over time, and thus emotional supports must also evolve to support these changing needs [28]. During the acute critical illness event, emotional supports should focus on the terror, dread, anxiety, and the unknown of critical illness for both patients and families; comfort in words and touch is particularly helpful [29,30]. Once on the ward, the transition from the familiar environment of the ICU is difficult for some, coupled with the changing intensity of care, including the nurse to patient ratio [31,32]. For others, leaving the ICU is seen as part of the care process and a sign that progress is happening [32], however slowly [31]. During the implementation and adaptation stages of recovery, emotional supports should focus on reintegrating with a new role, as either a survivor of critical illness or as caregiver of a survivor. Since this time is marked by anxiety, fear, and isolation, supports need to be tailored to provide confidence and independence [33,34].

Appraisal

Appraisal needs include feedback, affirmation, and social comparison [23]. These needs often manifest upon transfer to the ward, where patients may be less well-known by clinicians [35]. Once home, patients and families must adapt to a new state and appreciate affirmation that focuses on strengths (e.g., survival and recovery progress) rather than deficits [36]. Setting recovery goals may be helpful as patients and families return to life outside the hospital and adjust to a new sense of self.

Instrumental

Instrumental needs can be met by providing tangible aids and services [23]. Throughout the entire recovery journey, structured continuity of care is essential; this means providing sufficient support for all needs at different times, such as meetings focused on medication needs before discharge and provision of a critical care outreach service following hospital discharge [28,33]. On the ward, support to undertake basic care needs once provided by nurses is often filled by family [35]. Physical and cognitive disability may be pronounced across all stages but becomes particularly apparent once patients are home. Supports needed at this time include assistance with personal care and household activities [37]. When such support is provided by the family, patients may feel as if they are a burden, given their reduced ability to work or to afford the cost of hospital bills [13,38].

Spiritual
Spiritual needs do not always mean religious needs and mainly focus on believing in a higher power and having near-death experiences while in the ICU (see Chapter 15 for additional information) [23]. Spiritual healing may be as important to some patients as physical healing [39]. Positive spiritual experiences can lead to a sense of acceptance and hope and open the door to recovery [40,41].

Social/Relational
While in the ICU, support for social needs can include extending or opening visiting hours to allow for the maintenance of important social connections [42]. Navigating changed and new relationships and positions in society is an important social/relational need during and after critical illness for both patients and families. This includes integrating into changed social networks and navigating new roles as "survivor" and "caregiver."

Patient-Specific Needs
While patients and families often have shared and overlapping needs during and after critical illness, they also experience critical illness as individuals, and thus their needs also differ in important ways.

Throughout the acute critical illness, transfer to the ward, and return to the community, patients' physical, cognitive, and psychological needs are constantly changing. High severity of illness necessitating intensive care is coupled with invasive therapies and their side effects, including sedation and mechanical ventilation, which can lead to delirium, memory loss, and post-traumatic stress disorder [13,26,29,30]. Longer ICU stays result in more pronounced physical impairment, and deficits begin to develop early in an ICU admission. These effects are not limited to the ICU stay itself and often persist long after discharge from the ICU [43], making the provision of support for these new impairments essential [17,37]. Support must focus on adapting and adjusting to new physical states, such as loss of limbs, loss of strength, and reduced endurance and stamina [13,17,29]. Patients should be made aware of the spectrum of possible deficits to mobility, cognition, and psychological health, all of which will require support following ICU discharge. Early visits to ICU follow-up clinics and prompt initiation of rehabilitation are desired by many [34]. For some survivors of critical illness, returning to the ICU may help them process their illness and prepare for recovery; others, however, may not want to return to the site of their trauma, making personalization of recovery supports essential [44]. While many survivors of critical illness are unable to return to work and are often dependent on others to provide basic care [25,38], others sustain less disability and can reintegrate more quickly. Regardless, a focus on graduated independence is important to support realistic recovery goals. Validation by others who have survived critical illness (e.g., via peer support groups) is important to patients, as they may gain comfort from hearing that their experiences are normal and valid [45]. Patients often worry about the toll that their critical illness has on family members and want to ensure the well-being of their families throughout the critical illness journey.

Family-Specific Needs

Family members and loved ones of survivors of critical illness experience unique challenges related to caregiving that often go underappreciated (see Chapter 48 for additional information). In the ICU, inadequate communication and a failure to convey realistic expectations for critical illness recovery can be emotionally distressing [9,46]. At home, caregiver burden, financial strain, and social isolation may contribute to symptoms of anxiety, depression, and post-traumatic stress disorder [4,6,47,48,49]. In general, supports tailored to family caregivers are lacking; instead, many families rely on personal resourcefulness and resilience to cope [9,50]. It is important for clinicians to have an appreciation for the distinct needs of families, who largely shoulder the burden of caregiving following critical illness alone.

Families have several distinct needs. First, they have a need to be included and involved throughout the recovery journey. As patients regain the ability to participate in their own care, family members often receive less information and are less included in decision-making. Even as patients gain independence, it is important to family caregivers that they continue to receive information and be included in the circle of care [13]. In a study of patient and caregiver opinions of a telehealth ICU program, family caregivers appreciated the ability to participate in appointments and were important facilitators of patient attendance by installing video conferencing software and encouraging patients to attend scheduled visits [12].

Family members also have unique informational, logistical, and emotional support needs that differ from those of patients. Families want specific information on caregiving so that they may be sufficiently prepared for the role. They desire anticipatory guidance from ICU clinicians to develop realistic expectations for their loved one's recovery and to prepare for important transitions in care, including potential challenges and timeframes. Advice should be concrete and practical and should facilitate future planning. Logistical support needs include assistance obtaining workplace modifications, accessing disability insurance, and connecting with community programs [15]. Social workers may be best positioned to provide this type of support (see Chapter 25 for additional information).

Emotional and social support for family members is often overlooked but crucially important to address caregiver fatigue and burnout. Caregivers often feel the need to hold everything together by acting as a bridge between their loved one and the healthcare system, ensuring financial stability, and maintaining prior home and family routines in the face of disruptions from critical illness [51]. Caregivers may struggle with feelings of guilt related to the belief that they should have encouraged loved ones to seek medical attention earlier or the wish that their loved one would die so that they could be released from the burden of caregiving [15]. They may also struggle to balance the need to protect and supervise loved ones with the need for their own self-care. Family caregivers may come to feel like their caregiving role is overshadowing their identity and wish to be seen as individuals with distinct needs and concerns. By taking an active interest in the well-being of family members, healthcare teams can provide much-needed validation and recognition. Family-oriented support groups may also be beneficial; in one study, family members found that providing support to others in similar situations helped them find meaning and purpose from their experience [15].

Lastly, family members have a deep, abiding need to trust in healthcare professionals across all phases of their loved one's critical illness journey. In a systematic review of family support needs, Millward and colleagues found that the need for trust impacted how families perceived information, their emotional state, and their ability to tend to their own self-care needs [51]. Families who trusted their healthcare teams were more optimistic, more secure, and better able to cope with the challenges of critical illness recovery. Healthcare teams can build trust through timely, consistent, and clear communication with families. Compassion, approachability, and competence are other traits that families identified as being important for them to have trust in their loved one's clinicians.

Knowledge Gaps and Future Directions

Measuring Outcomes That Matter to Patients and Families

Selecting research outcomes that represent patient and family priorities is necessary to promote patient- and family-centered, evidence-based care. Although measures of survival are often used to evaluate new ICU interventions, patients and families may care more about long-term function and quality of life [20]. Importantly, established measures of health-related quality of life, such as the EQ-5D [52] and the 36 Item Short Form Health Survey (SF-36) [53], which are widely used in research and clinical practice, do not include social or spiritual domains and may fail to capture the whole picture of a patient and family's critical illness experience [19,21]. Across multiple studies, patients and families have described the importance of drawing on inner strengths, social connection, and spirituality to help them maintain optimism and hope during the recovery journey [9,17,23]. Critical illness may provoke self-reflection, causing people to revisit the purpose of their lives and seek new experiences, along with deepening their sense of gratitude and faith in a higher power [16,17,19]. Researchers should prioritize the development of more holistic measures of quality of life following critical illness that reflect this experiential complexity. In the meantime, studies should consider adopting more holistic measures such as the World Health Organization Quality-of-Life Scale (WHOQOL-BREF) [54] to better capture recovery from the perspective of patients and families [21].

Whose Voices Have Not Been Heard?

The generalizability of ICU research is limited by the patients and families included in ICU trials and observational studies. When the demographics of included participants are provided, studies tend to measure age and sex (binary); few studies measure race or ethnicity, housing, employment, income, education, disability, or sexual orientation [55]. When reported [56], included participants do not represent societal demographics, with studies more likely to include white men [55]. ICU research must represent the population served, and greater efforts should be made to justify inclusion and exclusion criteria and diversify recruitment so that study data are applicable to the patients seen in ICUs day-to-day [57].

Partnering with Patients and Families

To ensure ICU research is responsive and addresses the needs of patients and families, they must be engaged at each stage of the research process. This includes idea generation, grant writing, data collection and interpretation, and knowledge translation [58]. Patients and families want to be involved in research beyond the role of participant, but for this to be a successful partnership, they must be provided with training and support (including financially) to succeed [58,59]. Tokenism should be avoided in favor of building meaningful connections and opportunities for patients and families to contribute [58]. Patient engagement does not have to be restricted to clinical ICU research, and there is also a movement toward engaging them in preclinical laboratory research [60,61]. The lived experience of patients and families should also be incorporated into priority setting initiatives [62] and guideline development [63].

Key Points

1. Patient and family priorities are dynamic and evolve over distinct phases of critical illness recovery.
2. Patients and family support needs can be organized into distinct categories, including informational, emotional, appraisal, instrumental, social, and spiritual.
3. Patients and families desire recovery-oriented care that is proactive, coordinated, and holistic.
4. Future research efforts should include diverse patient and family perspectives and prioritize holistic and functional outcomes.

References

1. D.M. Needham, J. Davidson, H. Cohen, et al. Improving long-term outcomes after discharge from intensive care unit: report from a stakeholders' conference. *Crit Care Med* 2012; **40**(2): 502–9.
2. T.J. Iwashyna, E.W. Ely, D.M. Smith, K.M. Langa. Long-term cognitive impairment and functional disability among survivors of severe sepsis. *JAMA* 2010; **304**(16): 1787–94.
3. E. Azoulay, F. Pochard, N. Kentish-Barnes, et al. Risk of post-traumatic stress symptoms in family members of intensive care unit patients. *Am J Respir Crit Care Med* 2005; **171**(9): 987–94.
4. J.I. Cameron, L.M. Chu, A. Matte, et al. One-year outcomes in caregivers of critically ill patients. *NEJM* 2016; **374**(19): 1831–41.
5. C.C. Johnson, M.R. Suchyta, E.S. Darowski, et al. Psychological sequelae in family caregivers of critically ill intensive care unit patients: a systematic review. *Ann Am Thorac Soc* 2019; **16**(7): 894–909.
6. J. McPeake, H. Devine, P. MacTavish, et al. Caregiver strain following critical care discharge: an exploratory evaluation. *J Crit Care* 2016; **35**: 180–4.
7. I. van Beusekom, F. Bakhshi-Raiez, N.F. de Keizer, et al. Reported burden on informal caregivers of ICU survivors: a literature review. *Crit Care* 2016; **20**: 16.
8. N. Leggett, K. Emery, T.C. Rollinson, et al. Clinician and patient identified solutions to reduce the fragmentation of post-icu care in Australia. *Chest* 2024; **166**(1): 95–106.
9. K.J. Haines, E. Hibbert, N. Leggett, et al. Transitions of care after critical illness-challenges to recovery and adaptive problem solving. *Crit Care Med* 2021; **49**(11): 1923–31.

10. D. Elliott, J.E. Davidson, M.A. Harvey, et al. Exploring the scope of post-intensive care syndrome therapy and care: engagement of non-critical care providers and survivors in a second stakeholders meeting. *Crit Care Med* 2014; **42**(12): 2518–26.

11. K.J. Haines, N. Leggett, E. Hibbert, et al. Patient and caregiver-derived health service improvements for better critical care recovery. *Crit Care Med* 2022; **50**(12): 1778–87.

12. M.A. Kovaleva, A.C. Jones, C.C. Kimpel, et al. Patient and caregiver experiences with a telemedicine intensive care unit recovery clinic. *Heart Lung* 2023; **58**: 47–53.

13. A.I. Czerwonka, M.S. Herridge, L. Chan, et al. Changing support needs of survivors of complex critical illness and their family caregivers across the care continuum: a qualitative pilot study of towards recover. *J Crit Care* 2015; **30**(2): 242–9.

14. J. McPeake, L.M. Boehm, E. Hibbert, et al. Key components of icu recovery programs: what did patients report provided benefit? *Crit Care Explor* 2020; **2**(4): e0088.

15. S. Watland, L. Solberg Nes, E. Hanson, et al. The caregiver pathway, a model for the systematic and individualized follow-up of family caregivers at intensive care units: development study. *JMIR Form Res* 2023; **7**: e46299.

16. L.P. Scheunemann, J.S. White, S. Prinjha, et al. Post-intensive care unit care: a qualitative analysis of patient priorities and implications for redesign. *Ann Am Thorac Soc* 2020; **17**(2): 221–8.

17. C.E. Cox, S.L. Docherty, D.H. Brandon, et al. Surviving critical illness: acute respiratory distress syndrome as experienced by patients and their caregivers. *Crit Care Med* 2009; **37**(10): 2702–8.

18. J. McPeake, E.L. Hirshberg, L.M. Christie, et al. Models of peer support to remediate post-intensive care syndrome: a report developed by the society of critical care medicine thrive international peer support collaborative. *Crit Care Med* 2019; **47**(1): e21–e7.

19. M.D. Hashem, A. Nallagangula, S. Nalamalapu, et al. Patient outcomes after critical illness: a systematic review of qualitative studies following hospital discharge. *Crit Care* 2016; **20**(1): 345.

20. C.L. Auriemma, M.O. Harhay, K.J. Haines, et al. What matters to patients and their families during and after critical illness: a qualitative study. *Am J Crit Care* 2021; **30**(1): 11–20.

21. C. Konig, B. Matt, A. Kortgen, et al. What matters most to sepsis survivors: a qualitative analysis to identify specific health-related quality of life domains. *Qual Life Res* 2019; **28**(3): 637–47.

22. J.I. Cameron, M.A. Gignac. "Timing it right": a conceptual framework for addressing the support needs of family caregivers to stroke survivors from the hospital to the home. *Patient Educ Couns* 2008; **70**(3): 305–14.

23. J. King, B. O'Neill, P. Ramsay, et al. Identifying patients' support needs following critical illness: a scoping review of the qualitative literature. *Crit Care* 2019; **23**(1): 187.

24. J. House. *Work Stress and Social Support.* Reading, MA: Addison-Wesley Pub. Co; 1981.

25. C.M. Lee, M.S. Herridge, A. Matte, J.I. Cameron. Education and support needs during recovery in acute respiratory distress syndrome survivors. *Crit Care* 2009; **13**(5): R153.

26. S.L. Williams. Recovering from the psychological impact of intensive care: how constructing a story helps. *Nurs Crit Care* 2009; **14**(6): 281–8.

27. E.H. Strahan, R.J. Brown. A qualitative study of the experiences of patients following transfer from intensive care. *Intensive Crit Care Nurs* 2005; **21**(3): 160–71.

28. B. O'Neill, N. Green, B. Blackwood, et al. Recovery following discharge from intensive care: what do patients think is helpful and what services are missing? *PLoS One* 2024; **19**(3): e0297012.

29. H. Adamson, M. Murgo, M. Boyle, et al. Memories of intensive care and experiences of survivors of a critical illness: an interview study. *Intensive Crit Care Nurs* 2004; **20**(5): 257–63.

30. J.E. Hupcey. Feeling safe: the psychosocial needs of ICU patients. *J Nurs Scholarsh* 2000; **32**(4): 361–7.

31. A.A. McKinney, P. Deeny. Leaving the intensive care unit: a phenomenological study of the patients' experience. *Intensive Crit Care Nurs* 2002; **18**(6): 320–31.

32. M. Odell. The patient's thoughts and feelings about their transfer from intensive care to the general ward. *J Adv Nurs* 2000; **31**(2): 322–9.

33. V.C. Chiang. Surviving a critical illness through mutually being there with each other: a grounded theory study. *Intensive Crit Care Nurs* 2011; **27**(6): 317–30.

34. S. Prinjha, K. Field, K. Rowan. What patients think about ICU follow-up services: a qualitative study. *Crit Care* 2009; **13**(2): R46.

35. K. Field, S. Prinjha, K. Rowan. "One patient amongst many": a qualitative analysis of intensive care unit patients' experiences of transferring to the general ward. *Crit Care* 2008; **12**(1): R21.

36. M. Maddox, S.V. Dunn, L.E. Pretty. Psychosocial recovery following ICU: experiences and influences upon discharge to the community. *Intensive Crit Care Nurs* 2001; **17**(1): 6–15.

37. A.S. Agard, I. Egerod, E. Tonnesen, K. Lomborg. Struggling for independence: a grounded theory study on convalescence of ICU survivors 12 months post ICU discharge. *Intensive Crit Care Nurs* 2012; **28**(2): 105–13.

38. C. Palesjo, L. Nordgren, M. Asp. Being in a critical illness-recovery process: a phenomenological hermeneutical study. *J Clin Nurs* 2015; **24**(23–24): 3494–502.

39. S. Willemse, W. Smeets, E. van Leeuwen, et al. Spiritual care in the intensive care unit: an integrative literature research. *J Crit Care* 2020; **57**: 55–78.

40. J.M. Magarey, H.H. McCutcheon. "Fishing with the dead": recall of memories from the icu. *Intensive Crit Care Nurs* 2005; **21**(6): 344–54.

41. T.Y. Bulut, Y. Cekic, B. Altay. The effects of spiritual care intervention on spiritual well-being, loneliness, hope and life satisfaction of intensive care unit patients. *Intensive Crit Care Nurs* 2023; **77**: 103438.

42. E.L. Leong, C.C. Chew, J.Y. Ang, et al. The needs and experiences of critically ill patients and family members in intensive care unit of a tertiary hospital in Malaysia: a qualitative study. *BMC Health Serv Res* 2023; **23**(1): 627.

43. P.P. Pandharipande, T.D. Girard, J.C. Jackson, et al. Long-term cognitive impairment after critical illness. *N Engl J Med* 2013; **369**(14): 1306–16.

44. L. Haraldsson, L. Christensson, L. Conlon, M. Henricson. The experiences of ICU patients during follow-up sessions: a qualitative study. *Intensive Crit Care Nurs* 2015; **31**(4): 223–31.

45. K.S. Deacon. Re-building life after ICU: a qualitative study of the patients' perspective. *Intensive Crit Care Nurs* 2012; **28**(2): 114–22.

46. E. Iverson, A. Celious, C.R. Kennedy, et al. Factors affecting stress experienced by surrogate decision makers for critically ill patients: implications for nursing practice. *Intensive Crit Care Nurs* 2014; **30**(2): 77–85.

47. D.S. Davydow, C.L. Hough, K.M. Langa, T.J. Iwashyna. Depressive symptoms in spouses of older patients with severe sepsis. *Crit Care Med* 2012; **40**(8): 2335–41.

48. A.C. Blok, T.S. Valley, L.E. Weston, et al. Factors affecting psychological distress in family caregivers of critically ill patients: a qualitative study. *Am J Crit Care* 2023; **32**(1): 21–30.

49. S.A. van den Born-van Zanten, D.A. Dongelmans, D. Dettling-Ihnenfeldt, et al. Caregiver strain and posttraumatic stress symptoms of informal caregivers of intensive care unit survivors. *Rehabil Psychol* 2016; **61**(2): 173–8.

50. E.L. Zale, T.J. Heinhuis, T. Tehan, et al. Resiliency is independently associated with greater quality of life among informal caregivers to neuroscience intensive care unit patients. *Gen Hosp Psychiatry* 2018; **52**: 27–33.

51. K. Millward, C. McGraw, L.M. Aitken. The expressed support needs of families of adults who have survived critical illness: a thematic synthesis. *Int J Nurs Stud* 2021; **122**: 104048.

52. R. Rabin, F. de Charro. Eq-5d: a measure of health status from the euroqol group. *Ann Med* 2001; **33**(5): 337–43.

53. P.S. Chrispin, H. Scotton, J. Rogers, et al. Short form 36 in the intensive care unit: assessment of acceptability, reliability and validity of the questionnaire. *Anaesthesia* 1997; **52**(1): 15–23.

54. S. Vahedi. World health organization quality-of-life scale (WHOQOL-BREF): analyses of their item response theory properties based on the graded responses model. *Iran J Psychiatry* 2010; **5**(4): 140–53.

55. S. Mehta, A. Ahluwalia, A. Ahluwalia, et al. The diversity of research participants in randomized controlled trials and observational studies conducted by the Canadian critical care trials group. *Ann Am Thorac Soc* 2024; **21**(9): 1309–15.

56. K.D. Krewulak, F. Sheikh, A. Heirali, et al. Core sociodemographic data variables in ICU trials (code-it): a protocol for generating core data variables using a Delphi consensus process. *BMJ Open* 2024; **14**(7): e082912.

57. Y. Li, K. Fiest, K.E.A. Burns, et al. Addressing health care inequities in Canadian critical care through inclusive science: a pilot tool for standardized data collection. *Can J Anaesth* 2023; **70**(6): 963–7.

58. K.M. Fiest, B.G. Sept, H.T. Stelfox. Patients as researchers in adult critical care medicine: fantasy or reality? *Ann Am Thorac Soc* 2020; **17**(9): 1047–51.

59. K.E.A. Burns, E. McDonald, S. Debigare, et al. Patient and family engagement in patient care and research in Canadian intensive care units: a national survey. *Can J Anaesth* 2022; **69**(12): 1527–36.

60. G. Fox, D.A. Fergusson, Z. Daham, et al. Patient engagement in preclinical laboratory research: a scoping review. *EBioMedicine* 2021; **70**: 103484.

61. M.M. Lalu, D. Richards, M. Foster, et al. Protocol for co-producing a framework and integrated resource platform for engaging patients in laboratory-based research. *Res Involv Engagem* 2024; **10**(1): 25.

62. E. McKenzie, M.L. Potestio, J.M. Boyd, et al. Reconciling patient and provider priorities for improving the care of critically ill patients: a consensus method and qualitative analysis of decision making. *Health Expect* 2017; **20**(6): 1367–74.

63. J.W. Devlin, Y. Skrobik, C. Gelinas, et al. Clinical practice guidelines for the prevention and management of pain, agitation/sedation, delirium, immobility, and sleep disruption in adult patients in the ICU. *Crit Care Med* 2018; **46**(9): e825–e73.

Chapter 27

A Brief History of ICU Follow-Up Clinics

John C. Madara and Michael Baram

Introduction

Intensive care unit (ICU) follow-up clinics have gained traction as a solution to the complex needs assessments and ongoing care required by survivors of critical illness. For the past 30 years, clinics worldwide have been describing their experiences and outcomes, and the number of clinics has grown as the post-intensive care syndrome (PICS) has become increasingly recognized as a condition that merits attention by the medical community.

In the late 1980s, a multidisciplinary group in the United Kingdom (UK) convened to review the state of ICU literature at the time. The panel met often in 1988 to address the paucity of data and the lack of a standardized approach to the care of critically ill patients across the UK. It was clear that while survival of patients with life-threatening conditions was increasing, comparatively little attention was being paid to quality of life and long-term outcomes in this growing population of critical illness survivors. The collaborative group concluded that literature was needed to address these concerns and recommended that every ICU should identify a system to collect data on individual patient outcomes [1].

The First ICU Follow-Up Clinics

In 1993, the first ICU follow-up clinic was established in Reading, UK (see Figure 27.1). Termed "Intensive After Care After Intensive Care," this predecessor of modern ICU follow-up clinics was staffed by nurses and an ICU consultant and saw patients twice monthly. Since this initial model, ICU follow-up clinics have significantly expanded in the UK, with data suggesting that the number of ICUs with dedicated follow-up clinics has increased from 27% in 2013 to 74% in 2020 [2].

The early 2000s saw continued interest and growth in the field of long-term outcomes after critical illness with the development of ICU follow-up clinics in several European countries. Kvale and Flatten established an ICU follow-up clinic in Bergen, Norway from 1999 to 2001, where patients were seen in a 60-minute consultation with an ICU physician approximately 7–8 months after hospital discharge. They noted that 76% of patients who were offered follow-up consultation in their clinic accepted the invitation, demonstrating that such a service was both wanted and needed by patients to address the impact of critical illness on their lives [3]. Flatten editorialized that ICU physicians were best suited to provide ICU follow-up care, recognizing well before PICS was defined that intensivists needed to lead the charge to care for this patient population and their unique pathologies.

Literature addressing long-term outcomes in survivors of critical illness began to grow from single site experiences to international collaborative efforts. The 2002 "Surviving Intensive Care" conference held in Brussels and sponsored by the European Society of

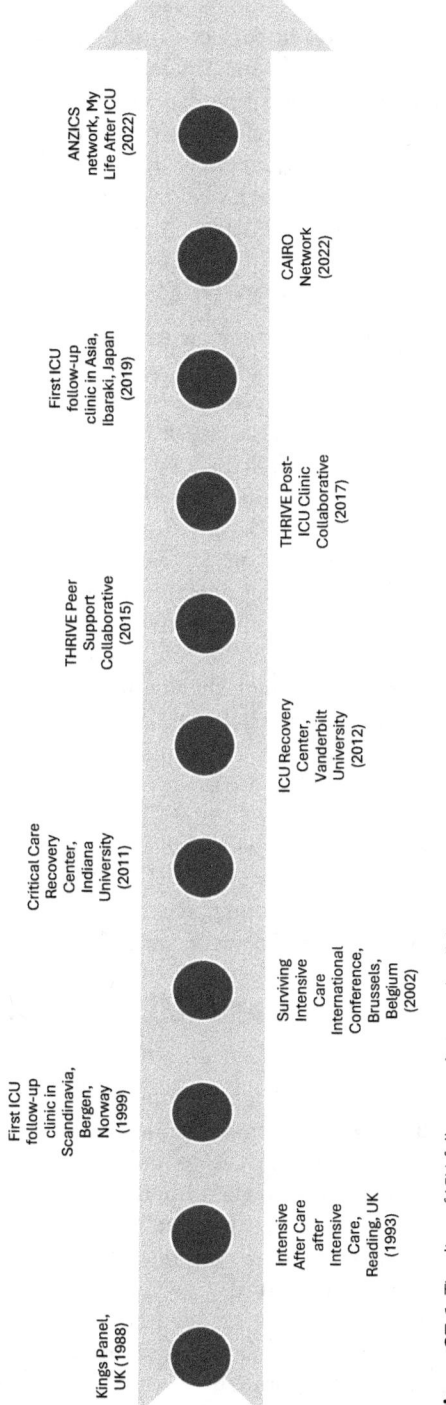

Figure 27.1 Timeline of ICU follow-up clinics and collaboratives.

Intensive Care Medicine (ESICM), the American Thoracic Society (ATS), and the Society of Critical Care Medicine (SCCM) brought together leaders in critical care medicine to discuss long-term outcomes of survivors of critical illness. This conference highlighted the importance and necessity of focusing on the impact of critical illness on patient- and family-centered outcomes, and a call was made to encourage future observational, interventional, and methodological research to include outcomes like quality of life and functional status in their methodologies. In addition, new alternatives to the traditional model of ICU care, which included roles for critical care providers in both ward and outpatient follow-up care, were introduced. This group helped to raise global awareness that care of the ICU patient should not be limited to time spent in the ICU [4].

Continued Growth of ICU Follow-Up Clinics

With no evidence-based recommendations for how to best care for this patient population, nascent ICU follow-up clinics empirically adopted an interprofessional, multidisciplinary approach to address the numerous and complex issues faced by critical illness survivors. The first ICU follow-up clinic in the United States began in 2011, with the opening of Indiana University's Critical Care Recovery Center (CCRC). Patients requiring more than 48 hours of mechanical ventilation or experiencing more than 48 hours of delirium were invited to participate in weekly clinics staffed by a collaborative team, including a critical care physician, nurse, and social worker, with additional support from physical therapy, psychology, and psychiatry, utilizing the Healthy Aging Brain Care (HABC) Monitor tool. Guided by the goal to maximize recovery after critical illness by improving the quality of transitional care, reducing hospital readmission, and enhancing patient and caregiver satisfaction, data from the CCRC suggested that patients seen longitudinally in follow-up had enhanced recovery from persistent cognitive, physical, and psychological disabilities [5].

In 2012, the ICU Recovery Center at Vanderbilt University opened, utilizing a multidisciplinary approach modeled after the interprofessional team of the ICU, including ICU physicians and nurse practitioners, an ICU pharmacist, case managers, and a neuropsychologist (see Table 27.1). Individualized assessments by team members are combined to formulate a comprehensive, multimodal treatment plan for patients with the goals of improving patient outcomes, educating patients and their caregivers about PICS, and gaining further insight into the recovery process to guide future research [6].

Development of Peer Support and ICU Follow-Up Clinic Collaboratives

As a complement to ICU follow-up clinics, peer support groups, first proposed by Mark Mikkelsen and others, are another mechanism to both aid in the recovery of survivors of critical illness and their loved ones and to enlighten ICU providers about this recovery process [7]. There are many formats for how peer support may be delivered (see Chapter 49 for additional information), but regardless of the model, creating a community of shared experiences for survivors and their loved ones may augment the recovery process of others facing similar challenges. In 2015, SCCM created the THRIVE Peer Support Collaborative with six inaugural members who met monthly to exchange ideas in providing peer support for their respective patient panels and to discuss strategies to enhance the development of additional peer support groups. Two

Table 27.1 Roles and responsibilities of the multidisciplinary team at the ICU Recovery Center at Vanderbilt University. From: E.L. Huggins, S.L. Bloom, J.L. Stollings, et al. A Clinic Model: Post-intensive Care Syndrome and Post-Intensive Care Syndrome-Family. *AACN Adv Crit Care* 2016; **27(2)**: 204–11. Reproduced with permissions from the American Association of Critical Care Nurses.

Role	Responsibility
Medical Intensive Care Unit Nurse Practitioner	• Discusses work status and supports persons involved in care • Ensures that services arranged for at hospital discharge have been received; for example, access to medications and/or home health services (notifies case manager as indicated) • Educates patient and patient's family regarding health promotion, tracheostomy/wound care, nutritional assessment • Reviews level of independence for activities of daily living with patient and patient's family
Clinical Pharmacist	• Medication reconciliation • Vaccine review/recommendation (e.g., influenza and pneumococcal)
Neurocognitive Psychologist	• Screens for presence of anxiety, depression, and/or posttraumatic stress disorder • Therapeutic dialogue, referrals for ongoing therapy
Pulmonary Critical Care Physician	• Reviews and interprets 6-minute walk and spirometry results with patient and patient's family
Case Manager	• Accesses medications and durable medical equipment as indicated • Follows up with home health services if needed

years later, in 2017, SCCM created the THRIVE Post-ICU Clinic Collaborative to foster new ICU follow-up clinics, to improve quality of life and other long-term outcomes following critical illness, and to act as a vehicle for data collection and quality improvement. These collaboratives were the catalyst for much of the PICS-related research that has been published since their inception.

The SCCM THRIVE Peer Support and Post-ICU Clinic Collaboratives ended in 2020 but served as the model for the Critical and Acute Illness Recovery Organization (CAIRO) network, which began in 2020 and continues to add new members on a yearly basis. Much like THRIVE, CAIRO has both ICU follow-up clinic and peer support divisions, which meet on a monthly basis to exchange ideas regarding models of patient care, to enhance the visibility of PICS as an increasingly important public health challenge, and to develop a research agenda to address lingering unanswered questions in the field of ICU survivorship. As of the time of this writing, the CAIRO network consisted of 29 programs from 6 countries unified in the goal of promoting innovations in critical illness recovery through outreach and research.

Development in Australasia

Coincident with the increased recognition and credibility that PICS has garnered in both the medical and lay communities has been the continued international growth in ICU follow-up clinics. In 2019, the first ICU follow-up clinic in Asia was started in Ibaraki, Japan using a multidisciplinary model including ICU physicians, ICU nurses, and physical therapists. In a 2021 survey performed by the Japanese Society of Intensive Care Medicine, however, only 4% of institutions in Japan that responded to the survey offered an ICU follow-up clinic [8]. Similarly, in a 2020 survey, only 2% of responding institutions in Australia operated an ICU follow-up clinic [9]. Recognizing the need for more resources for providers and their families, the Australia and New Zealand Intensive Care Society (ANZICS) network launched a campaign called "My Life After ICU" in 2022 as an online resource for patients and families who have survived a critical illness.

Impact of the COVID-19 Pandemic

In 2019, the outbreak of the SARS-CoV-2 pandemic posed significant challenges to healthcare systems worldwide. As the pandemic progressed, long-term effects in survivors of SARS-CoV-2 infection, irrespective of its severity, were recognized and termed post-acute sequelae of COVID-19, or the long-COVID syndrome (see Chapter 53 for additional information). Though some unique complications in this patient population exist, several of the persistent physical and cognitive difficulties experienced after SARS-CoV-2 infection are similar to those seen in patients with PICS. Many models of support were created for these patients, including multidisciplinary follow-up clinics and peer support groups, based upon ICU follow-up clinics and collaboratives, which pioneered multidisciplinary and interprofessional models of care for patients in the decades leading up to the pandemic. Accompanying the increased recognition of the long-term sequalae of COVID was the rapid development of over 150 long-COVID clinics in the United States alone over a two-year period, a growth rate in stark contrast to the much slower establishment of ICU follow-up clinics, despite the similarity in the syndromes.

Current Models and Outcomes

In the decade since the first ICU follow-up clinic opened in the US, it is currently estimated that there are fewer than 30 medical centers that offer an ICU follow-up clinic. A survey performed by Danesh and colleagues during the pandemic demonstrates the changing landscape of resource utilization and support in critical illness recovery: in the months leading up to the surge of ICU patients related to COVID-19, multiple ICU follow-up clinics opened, but since the middle of 2020, all new recovery clinics that had opened by the time of the survey were specifically dedicated to COVID recovery rather than to critical illness recovery at large (see Figure 27.2).

Due to variability in health care systems and resources and the diversity of ICU survivors, many models of ICU follow-up clinics exist, but most are based on a series of central tenets. One such tenet is the idea that care of survivors of critical illness and their families requires an interprofessional, multidisciplinary team, and accordingly, more than half of the centers surveyed in one study included pharmacists, physical therapists, and care coordinators. A second tenet is that to maximize delivery of care, follow-up services cannot be restricted to visits at large, urban centers. As such, 80% of ICU follow-up clinics offer telehealth services to provide care to those who may not otherwise be able to receive it (see Chapter 29 for more information). Third, most centers rely on volunteerism to staff their clinics, and only one-third of ICU follow-up clinics are supported by institutional funding. Danesh and colleagues argue that as demand for ICU follow-up clinics increases,

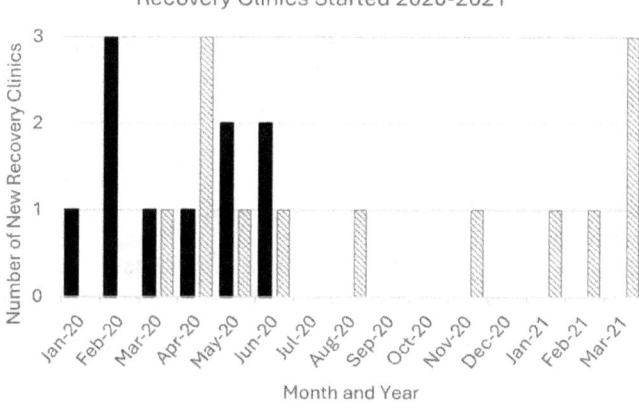

Figure 27.2 The number of ICU-recovery clinics and COVID-recovery clinics opened between 2020 and 2021. From: V. Danesh, L. Boehm, T. Eaton, et al. Characteristics of post-ICU and post-Covid recovery clinics in 29 U.S. health systems. *Crit Care Explor* 2022; 9; **4**(3): e0658. Reproduced with permission from Wolters Kluwer Health, Inc.

volunteerism and lack of institutional funding will be insufficient to meet the needs of the healthcare system. The variability in clinic structures, screening tools used, and outcome metrics measured demonstrates that although there has been considerable growth in the science of ICU survivorship, much is still unknown about the processes and structures that provide the best outcomes in this patient population [10].

The establishment of ICU follow-up clinics and collaboratives across the world has promoted much research regarding long-term outcomes in survivors of critical illness and has provided educational resources for physicians, patients, and caregivers. As studies continue to investigate the benefits of outpatient follow-up to survivors of critical illness, it is becoming clearer that there may be improvements seen in certain outcome measures. For example, in one study, when compared to the standard of care, patients who participated in a combined inpatient and outpatient PICS program received more care interventions then those who did not, and of patients requiring hospital readmission, time to readmission was longer in patients receiving the intervention [11]. In a second study, patients who participated in an ICU survivor program demonstrated both reduced mortality and healthcare cost expenditures when compared to those receiving the standard of care [12].

Conclusion

From the 1980s to the present, there has been a gradual evolution from the recognition of the need for long-term outcomes research to the establishment of individual ICU follow-up clinics to the development of international collaboratives to enhance patient care, promote education, and drive the future research agenda. The growth of ICU follow-up clinics continues. Due to a number of factors, ICU follow-up clinics across the world have different structures, but despite their differences, they are united by a focus on patient and family needs and ultimately an improvement in the quality of life for survivors of critical illness.

Like with many health care initiatives, change can be slow. Clinicians have long recognized the need for continued care of survivors of critical illness, and the development and refinement of ICU follow-up clinics and peer support programs is helping to achieve that goal. Collaboratives are currently leading a robust research agenda to help further improve the care that our patients and their families deserve.

Key Points

1. In the late 1980s, it was recognized that there was no standard approach to the care of survivors of critical illness and data on long-term outcomes following critical illness were limited.
2. Initial ICU follow-up clinics were single center programs that started in the UK before spreading across Europe and subsequently around the world.
3. International critical care organizations such as SCCM created collaboratives focused on peer support groups and ICU follow-up clinics to provide important care to survivors of critical illness and to help drive education and research in the field.
4. Many current models and systems exist to provide care to survivors of critical illness.

References

1. Intensive care in the United Kingdom: report from the King's Fund panel. *Anaesthesia* 1989; **44**: 428–31.
2. Life after critical illness: a guide for developing and delivering aftercare services for critically ill patients. The Faculty of Intensive Care Medicine; 2021. www.ficm.ac.uk/criticalfutures/life-after-critical-illness. Accessed June 2025.
3. R. Kvale, A. Ulvik, H. Flaatten. Follow up after intensive care: a single center study. *Intensive Care Med* 2003; **29**; 2149–56.
4. D. Angus, J. Carlet. Surviving intensive care; a report from the 2002 Brussels Roundtable. *Intensive Care Med* 2003; **29**: 368–77.
5. B. Khan, S. Lasiter, M. Boustani. The critical care recovery center: an innovative collaborative care model for ICU survivors. *Am J Nurs* 2015; **115**: 24–31.
6. E. Huggins, S. Bloom, J.L. Stollings, et al. A clinic model: post-intensive care unit syndrome and post-intensive care syndrome-family. *AACN Adv Crit Care* 2016; **27**: 204–11.
7. M. Mikkelson, J. Jackson, R.O. Hopkins, et al. Peer support as a novel strategy to mitigate post-intensive care unit syndrome. *AACN Adv Crit Care* 2016; **27**: 221–9.
8. Japanese Society of Intensive Care Medicine. A questionnaire survey regarding follow-up after ICU discharge in Japan. *J Jpn Soc Intensive Care Med* 2022; **29**:165–76.
9. K. Cook, R. Bartholdy, M. Raven, et al. A national survey of intensive care follow-up clinics in Australia. *Aust Crit Care* 2020; **33**: 533–7.
10. V. Danesh, L. Boehm, T. Eaton, et. al. Characteristics of post-ICU and post-Covid recovery clinics in 29 U.S. Health Systems. *Crit Care Explor* 2022; 4 (3): e0658.
11. S. Bloom, J. Stollings, O. Kirkpatrick, et al. Randomized clinical trial of an ICU recovery pilot program for survivors of critical illness. *Crit Care Med* 2019; **47**: 1337–45.
12. K. Snell, C. Beiter, E.L. Hall, et al. A novel approach to ICU survivor care: a population health quality improvement project. *Crit Care Med* 2020; **48**: 1164–70.

Chapter 28
Fundamentals of ICU Follow-Up Clinics

Brad W. Butcher

Introduction

The need to design and implement effective interventions to ameliorate the constellation of physical, cognitive, psychological, and social impairments characteristic of critical illness survivorship is a priority [1]. Such durable impairments following critical illness place a burden on public health and society by increasing healthcare cost and resource utilization (see Chapter 33 for additional information), creating new disability (see Chapter 24 for additional information), and impacting financial health and the ability to resume employment and driving (see Chapter 44 for additional information) [2]. A stakeholders meeting held by the Society of Critical Care Medicine (SCCM) in 2012 concluded that systematic recognition of the various impairments associated with post-intensive care syndrome (PICS) is required during transitions of care across the continuum of critical illness and recovery [3].

Intensive care unit (ICU) follow-up clinics, particularly when combined with peer support groups, are the most comprehensive approach to improve long-term outcomes and quality of life in survivors of critical illness and their loved ones. Despite their existence since 1993, the number of ICU follow-up clinics remains insufficient, both in the United States and worldwide [2], particularly in light of the millions of people who survive critical illness annually. The reasons for this are several and include: a relative paucity of data that demonstrate clear and consistent clinical benefits or financial solvency (see Chapter 30 for additional information) and a significant amount of institutional inertia that must be overcome to initiate a complex, multi-component clinic that often spans multiple departments.

This chapter examines the evidence for ICU follow-up clinics; discusses the current landscape of ICU follow-up clinics and their operational characteristics; reviews key components necessary to implement ICU follow-up clinics; explores screening strategies, both to identify patients who may benefit from clinic participation and to identify impairments during appointments; offers potential interventions that clinics can provide; highlights enablers and barriers to clinic development; and describes benefits of ICU follow-up programs that extend beyond patients and families.

Evidence for ICU Follow-Up Clinics

The earliest randomized trials of interventions for survivors of critical illness failed to show benefit, yet these studies were limited in meaningful ways, including prolonged time to follow-up and interventions inconsistent with the modern concept of an ICU follow-up clinic. Rather, in these trials, the interventions tested included informative pamphlets and facilitated discussions with trained nurses, primarily via telephone [4]; a self-directed home physical rehabilitation program complemented by two nurse visits for psychiatric assessment [5]; and intensive case management and decision support for primary care physicians (PCPs) [6].

Two more recent randomized controlled trials, however, demonstrated modest clinical benefit from participation in an ICU follow-up program. In a trial by Bloom and colleagues, patients requiring critical care for at least 48 hours and with a predicted 30-day readmission risk of at least 15% were randomized to either usual care as determined by their treating clinicians or to a structured 10-part ICU recovery program that included both inpatient and outpatient components. Even though patients randomized to the ICU recovery program received a median of only two of the ten components and only 8.1% of them attended an ICU follow-up clinic visit, those patients were less likely to either die or be readmitted within 30 days of hospital discharge compared with those who received usual care (18% versus 30%, respectively) [7].

A subsequent study by Snell and colleagues compared clinical outcomes in 48 patients who participated in an ICU follow-up clinic with 118 patients who either did not meet criteria for clinic participation or who were offered a clinic visit but declined [8]. Patients who participated in the ICU follow-up clinic had significantly lower mortality, lower unadjusted readmission rates at both 30 and 60 days, and shorter average length of stay in those who required readmission when compared to patients who did not participate in the ICU follow-up clinic. Moreover, this study suggested a positive financial impact of ICU follow-up clinics by demonstrating a lower average cost per readmission for patients who received care in the ICU follow-up clinic; although this cost benefit did not carry over to emergency department visits or post-acute facility costs, the estimated total annual cost savings to the health plan, after accounting for the clinic's operating costs, was over $400,000 when using 90-day readmission data. The main driver of savings was the reduction in the readmission rate, which, although not statistically significant between the two groups in adjusted analyses, was indeed financially significant [8].

Although important, single-center studies alone are likely insufficient to definitively answer the question of how impactful ICU follow-up clinics are. Unfortunately, given the heterogeneity among current clinics with respect to patient population, timing and duration of follow-up, screening tests performed, and interventions administered, multicenter studies have proven to be challenging. International collaboratives, such as the former SCCM THRIVE initiative and the current Critical and Acute Illness Recovery Organization (CAIRO), have sought and continue to seek means to overcome these logistical hurdles.

Despite the paucity of data regarding their efficacy, there are several reasons why ICU follow-up clinics are an important resource for survivors of critical illness. Such clinics provide continuity of care; providers who are knowledgeable of the diagnoses and interventions common in the ICU can competently review the patient's ICU course and help patients reconstruct memories of their ICU experience, supplement their illness narrative, and review an ICU diary if present (see Chapter 18 for additional information). Over the course of an appointment that frequently lasts more than two hours [2], clinicians familiar with PICS can spend more time therapeutically listening to patients and their families, normalizing their experience, and setting realistic expectations for the depth and breadth of their recovery, while comprehensively evaluating them for PICS and constructing a patient-centered, goal-directed rehabilitation plan. PICS is neither a uniform syndrome nor a static set of problems but rather an individualized chronic illness that changes over time; serial assessments and flexible interventions are required to care for patients with PICS, and this need is integral to the design of most ICU follow-up clinics.

Operational Characteristics

A study by Danesh and colleagues gives insight into the similarities and differences in operational characteristics of 26 ICU follow-up clinics representing 133 hospitals in 26 health systems that participate in the CAIRO ICU follow-up clinic collaborative [2]. Over two-thirds of clinics in the survey operated in large, metropolitan areas, and 80% of them offered telemedicine services, extending their geographical reach to more rural and resource-limited areas. Approximately three-quarters of clinics served health systems that included both large academic medical centers and smaller community hospitals.

The median number of clinic days per month was four, and 80% of clinics operated between four and eight hours during a clinic day. Over half of the clinics reported seeing patients for at least one hour, and nearly one-quarter of clinics had patient visits consistently lasting more than two hours. ICU follow-up clinic services varied considerably and were largely dependent on the composition of the multidisciplinary team staffing the clinic [2]. Alongside ICU follow-up clinics, the COVID-19 pandemic resulted in the rapid development of COVID-19 recovery clinics, which, given the similarities between PICS and the post-COVID condition (see Chapter 53 for additional information), were largely modeled on the interprofessional care paradigm of ICU follow-up clinics [2,9].

Key Components for ICU Follow-Up Clinics

Developing an ICU follow-up clinic is a challenging endeavor, and interested parties must take the following factors into consideration to design and implement a clinic that is compatible with locally available resources.

Finding an Appropriate Space

Finding sufficient space in which to hold an ICU follow-up clinic can be difficult. Unused clinic and office space is often unavailable, and developers of ICU follow-up clinics may need to negotiate with hospital leadership to find a space that can meet their needs [10]. As resources dictate, clinic space may need to be shared with other specialty clinics that are occurring contemporaneously. Importantly, the size of the clinic space and the number of available clinic rooms may determine how many patients and providers can be accommodated at a given time. Ensuring that there is sufficient space for providers to work and document in the electronic medical record (EMR) is important, and this may also impact the size of the multidisciplinary team and determine whether learners can be present. The layout of the clinic space may be as important as its size; having a communal area for providers to gather and develop a collaborative, patient-centered plan of care is important. Although many assessments performed during a clinic visit can occur inside a conventional room, a more robust physical assessment, such as a six-minute walk test, may require a neighboring space or hallway to perform the test consistently and accurately [10]. The majority of telemedicine-based clinic models require only a sufficiently confidential workspace with adequate information technology support, whether in an outpatient clinic or a clinician's office. Depending on the telemedicine platform being utilized, multidisciplinary team members can securely join the visit from disparate locations [10]. In some telemedicine-based operations, a visiting nurse or home health aide is present in the patient's home during the visit to examine the patient and administer screening tests under a physician's real-time supervision.

On a larger scale, hospital-based clinics seeking to expand services to accommodate patients throughout a larger healthcare system must decide whether one centralized clinic providing services to the entire system or several satellite clinics serving various regions of the system is the preferred strategy. This will need to be decided alongside healthcare system executives, administrators, and financial personnel [10].

Assembling the Multidisciplinary Team

Comprehensive ICU follow-up relies on coordinated care that is provided by a multidisciplinary team with expertise in the various domains of recovery and rehabilitation following critical illness (see Chapters 23 and 31 for additional information) [10]. In many clinic models, the multidisciplinary team of the ICU is effectively transplanted into the outpatient setting, thereby allowing sophisticated evaluation of every component of the patient's health: physical, cognitive, emotional, and social. Not every institution can recruit a full complement of providers, as personnel resources may be limited by staff availability, interest, and lack of financial compensation [10]. Securing dedicated financial support for providers, even if partial, is often the most significant challenge. In some models, ICU follow-up clinic responsibilities are built into larger roles; for example, ICU-based pharmacists, respiratory therapists, and dietitians may have ICU follow-up clinic time folded into their job descriptions and compensation schemes [10]. Over half of ICU follow-up clinics rely partially on volunteerism to staff the clinic; although not a sustainable model, volunteerism may allow sufficient time to establish the benefit of the clinic to the healthcare system and its patients [2].

In the aforementioned survey of ICU follow-up clinics, the composition of the multidisciplinary teams staffing the clinics varied considerably [2]. Most clinic physicians and advanced practice providers were trained in critical care medicine or the combination of pulmonology and critical care medicine, and fewer clinics were staffed by providers trained in internal medicine or physical medicine and rehabilitation. Pharmacists, social workers, and physical therapists were present in the majority of clinics, and other providers participating in ICU follow-up clinics to varying degrees included: nurses, respiratory therapists, speech-language pathologists, occupational therapists, dietitians, psychiatrists, psychologists, geriatricians, palliative care providers, spiritual care providers, and trainees of various disciplines [2]. If the ICU follow-up clinic will support a research agenda alongside its clinical mission, it is important to partner with researchers who may be not be directly involved in patient care but who are skilled in crafting a research program [10].

Equipment, Supplies, and Other Costs

Depending on the disciplines staffing the clinic and the patient evaluations that will be performed, there are certain pieces of equipment that may need to be purchased unless resources can be shared with or donated by other clinics at the institution [10]. If a spirometric evaluation will be performed and pulmonary function testing is not readily available, a spirometer, plastic mouthpieces (flow tubes), nose clips, and a dedicated printer may need to be purchased. Swallowing evaluations require food and drink of varying consistencies, which need to be restocked as they approach their expiration dates.

Physical assessments may require mobile pulse oximetry and sphygmomanometers, a stopwatch, activity cones, handgrip strength dynamometers, and various assistive devices, including canes, walkers, and rollators [10].

Print Materials

ICU follow-up clinics benefit from advertisement and the provision of patient and family education. Such materials, which may need to be created and printed, include brochures to advertise the clinic, literature about PICS, ICU journals (see Chapter 18 for additional information), and handbooks of patient resources. Access to graphic design services and the hospital's marketing department is often beneficial and may be required if materials are branded with the hospital or health system's logo [10].

Technology

The EMR is an important component to the success of an ICU follow-up clinic, and establishing a relationship with the hospital's information technology team is important to ensure that data is captured in a manner that is beneficial to both clinical and research goals. Given the significant amount of clinical data collected during visits, note templates should be designed to organize the data in the most logical manner, such that notes are easily interpretable by clinicians in disparate specialties [10]. Certain outpatient EMRs have built-in flowsheets to facilitate data entry for commonly used screening instruments, such as the Montreal Cognitive Assessment (MoCA) tool or the Hospital Anxiety and Depression Scale (HADS), which can be incorporated into the note template. If a research program is being considered, it is important to determine how data placed in the EMR can subsequently be extracted into a database for organization and analysis [10].

Financial Resources

Financial support is essential for implementing and sustaining an ICU follow-up clinic. ICU follow-up clinics are not inherently revenue-generating enterprises, and the positive financial impact realized is typically one of value-based care and cost savings (see Chapter 30 for additional information) [8,10]. Preventing hospital readmissions [7,8], discovering near misses (e.g., an inferior vena cava filter that is not removed in a timely fashion or potentially adverse medication interactions), providing preventative services (e.g., vaccine administration), and readdressing goals of care to ensure that future care is concordant with patient goals, values, and preferences are all arguments for ICU follow-up clinics to be fiscally sound investments.

In addition to seeking funding from the hospital system, it is worth exploring whether health plans or insurers are willing to provide financial support. If the hospital system has a close relationship with an insurer, they may be interested in sharing resources, such as a case manager or transitions coordinator, to specifically follow clinic patients who are also members of the health plan [10]. Internal or external grant funding for research or quality improvement projects, health system endowments, diagnosis-specific advocacy groups, philanthropic donations, and volunteerism are all possible funding sources. Providing data regarding the value of the ICU follow-up clinic, such as decreased readmission rates or improvements in patient-perceived value of care, may enhance the possibility of receiving ongoing funding from the health system. Using personal stories of the impact of PICS on patients and families may also sway recalcitrant hospital administrators; nearly everyone will know someone whose life fundamentally changed as a consequence of critical illness and who might have benefited from such a resource had it been available to them [10,11].

Screening

Inpatient Screening for Clinic Candidates

Existing tools and clinical judgment are insufficient to reliably predict PICS-related problems in all survivors of critical illness, but certain patient- and illness-related risk factors can reasonably identify those at highest risk [12]. Patients at risk for physical impairment following critical illness include those with pre-existing frailty, functional disability, and cognitive impairment and those whose critical illness was complicated by prolonged bed rest and ICU-acquired weakness [13,14]. Patients at risk for cognitive impairments following critical illness include those with pre-existing cognitive dysfunction and those whose critical illness was characterized by delirium, receipt of sedation (particularly with benzodiazepines), sepsis, shock, hypoxemic respiratory failure, and receipt of life support, including mechanical ventilation [13]. Patients at risk for psychological impairments following critical illness include those with preexisting depression, anxiety, and post-traumatic stress disorder and those whose illness was complicated by memories of frightening experiences [13]. A contemporaneous systematic review and meta-analysis of PICS risk factors also identified, in addition to the above, advanced age, female gender, and disease severity as additional predisposing factors [15].

As part of their initial evaluation in the ICU, patients should have an assessment of their pre-morbid functional capabilities (e.g., independence or dependence with activities of daily living and instrumental activities of daily living) to serve as a reference point for future clinicians engaged in their care. At the time of hospital discharge, brief, standardized assessments should be performed and compared with the patient's pre-morbid function, a process known as "functional reconciliation," which may help identify the patient's care needs and determine their discharge destination [13].

As there is currently no consensus regarding screening for post-ICU impairments, each clinic may tailor screening to their specific needs, complement of providers, and patient populations. Recruitment criteria for ICU follow-up clinics are highly variable and are largely based on the aforementioned risk factors and institutional resources (i.e., how many patients can be accommodated on a given clinic day; see Chapter 22 for additional information). Such criteria may be based on lengths of stay, diagnoses (e.g., hypoxemic respiratory failure, acute respiratory distress syndrome, sepsis, shock requiring vasopressor or inotropic support, or ICU-acquired weakness), receipt of specific interventions (e.g., emergency surgery, mechanical ventilation, tracheotomy, or extracorporeal membrane oxygenation), or patient-specific factors (e.g., pre-existing frailty, cognitive impairment, or mental health problems). Exclusion criteria for ICU follow-up clinics are similarly variable and may include high risk of imminent death (i.e., over the next six months), pre-existing dependence in performing activities of daily living, persistent coma, prolonged dependence on mechanical ventilation, or severe dementia or psychiatric disorder. Screening and eligibility determinations are often performed by members of the ICU care team (e.g., pharmacists or nurse practitioners) or members of the ICU follow-up clinic care team (e.g., social workers); the EMR can also be harnessed to identify patients who meet certain clinical criteria and to order referrals to the ICU follow-up clinic.

In-Clinic Evaluation

Despite the lack of robust data supporting ICU follow-up clinics, the United Kingdom National Institute for Health and Care Excellence guidelines recommend that adults who required critical care for more than four days have a clinical evaluation within three months of hospital discharge [16]. Similarly, the SCCM International Consensus Conference on prediction and identification of long-term impairments after critical illness recommends serial and dynamic assessments of patients at heightened risk for PICS beginning within two to four weeks of hospital discharge and following important health and life changes, both anticipated and unanticipated [13]. Serial assessments establish a longitudinal framework to more effectively prepare survivors to reengage with employment and society, mitigate the sense of isolation and abandonment that often accompany survivorship, address patient needs in a timely manner, and prevent complications through a deliberate, coordinated, longitudinal approach to care [13]. In some clinics, serial assessments occur at specified time points (e.g., at 3 months, 6 months, and 12 months after discharge), and in others, assessments are variable and based on patients' rehabilitation needs or following setbacks, such as hospital readmission.

Of the numerous screening tools that can be administered in a clinic setting (see Chapter 29, Table 29.1 and Chapter 48, Table 48.2), the aforementioned SCCM International Consensus Conference recommends the following based on degree of consensus from the expert participants: the MoCA for assessment of cognitive impairment (strong consensus), the HADS for assessment of both anxiety and depression (strong consensus), the Impact of Events Scale-Revised (IES-R) or the abbreviated IES-6 for assessment of post-traumatic stress disorder (weak consensus), and the 6-minute walk test and/or the EuroQol-5D-5L for assessment of physical impairment (weak consensus) [13]. More detailed information regarding these and other screening tools commonly used in ICU follow-up clinics can be found in Chapters 15 (spiritual concerns), 34 (quality of life), 35 (pulmonary disorders), 37 (sleep disorders), 38 (swallowing disorders), 40 (nutritional disorders), 41 (physical impairments), 42 (functional impairments), 43 (cognitive impairments), 46 (psychiatric impairments), and 48 (assessments for PICS-Family). Irrespective of the screening tools used, the concept of functional reconciliation should be a guiding principle throughout the patient's recovery trajectory and included in every ICU follow-up clinic visit [13].

Clinic Interventions

As with the screening tools administered, the interventions that clinics can provide are dependent on the composition of the multidisciplinary team and the amount of time available to spend with the patient. In the aforementioned study of 26 ICU follow-up clinics, the most commonly offered services, in descending order of frequency, included physical assessment (100%), medication reconciliation (96%), global needs assessment (85%), behavioral health referral (85%), cognitive assessment (77%), debriefing of the ICU stay (77%), communication with primary care (77%), care coordination (73%), and referral to pulmonology and sleep medicine (73%). Other less frequently offered services included immunization review and administration, spirometry, education distribution, advanced care planning, caregiver assessment and support, and referral to various other specialties and disciplines [2]. Importantly, devoting a portion of the visit to having a thoughtful conversation about the patient's future goals, values, and preferences is an opportunity to both deliver future care that is concordant with patients' wishes and to reduce healthcare utilization costs by not providing expensive care that is inconsistent with patients' values.

Table 28.1 demonstrates a list of potential assessments and interventions that can be performed by various providers in an ICU follow-up clinic.

Table 28.1 Potential providers, assessments, and interventions in an ICU follow-up clinic

Provider	Potential Assessments	Potential Interventions
Intake nurse	Vitals and weight Frailty score EQ–5D quality of life questionnaire* Symptom burden questionnaire Sleep assessment questionnaire	Relay patient concerns to team
Pharmacist	Medication reconciliation Vaccine history review	Provide medication education Discontinue unnecessary medications started during hospitalization Resume medications held during hospitalization Identify adverse drug events or drug-drug interactions Assist in fee reduction for expensive medications Recommend and provide vaccinations Provide pill boxes
Respiratory therapist	Spirometric evaluation MRC Dyspnea score Tracheotomy evaluation Assess home oxygen/NIPPV needs Participate in/perform 6-minute walk test	Provide smoking cessation counseling Provide inhaler teaching Provide spacers for inhalers Perform tracheotomy care Recommend patients for pulmonary rehabilitation
Occupational therapist	Katz ADL screen Lawton IADL screen Handgrip strength dynamometry	Refer to home-based or outpatient occupational therapy Refer to vocational rehabilitation Refer to driving rehabilitation
Physical therapist	6-minute walk test* Gait speed Balance assessment 5 times sit to stand	Referral for home-based or outpatient physical therapy Recommend a home exercise program
Speech language pathologist	Swallowing evaluation Montreal Cognitive Assessment tool (MoCA)*	Refer to swallowing therapy Refer to speech therapy Refer to home-based or outpatient cognitive therapy
Dietitian	Nutrition assessment screen for malnutrition Weight trend Assessment of current diet and GI symptoms	Refer to outpatient dietitian or food programs (Meals on Wheels, local food pantries) Provide education and information regarding diets and meal planning

Table 28.1 (cont.)

Provider	Potential Assessments	Potential Interventions
		Provide supplement samples and coupons for supplements
Social worker	Social determinants of health screening Psychiatric screening tools (HADS*, IES–6*, IES-R*) Assess caregiver burden and depression, anxiety, and PTSD in caregiver	Provide short term psychotherapy Assist with resources for transportation, food, housing, and financial insecurity Refer to support groups for survivors and their loved ones
Psychologist or psychiatrist	Psychiatric screening tools (HADS*, IES–6*, IES-R*) Assess caregiver burden and depression, anxiety, and PTSD in caregiver	Provide short-term psychotherapy Refer to outpatient mental health provider Refer to support groups for survivors and their loved ones
Spiritual care provider	Spiritual assessment tools (e.g., FICA, HOPE)	Help patients and loved ones cope with stress and uncertainty Address spiritual or religious needs Pray with patients
Palliative care provider	Symptom management tool (e.g., PEACE Tool) Address code status and surrogate decision maker	Refer to primary palliative care or pain management Document changes in goals of care or surrogate decision makers Address caregiver burden and PICS-F
Intensivist/APP	Review hospitalization/ICU course Debrief about ICU experiences Review symptoms and concerns EQ–5D quality of life assessment* Sleep assessment questionnaire Review data learned about patient during appointment Address code status and surrogate decision maker Goal setting with patient Assess caregiver burden and depression, anxiety, and PTSD in caregiver	Document changes in goals of care or surrogate decision makers Refer to other subspecialists as appropriate Provide education about PICS and manage expectations about recovery Normalize the recovery process Address caregiver burden and PICS-F

Abbreviations: APP, advanced practice provider; EQ-5D, EuroQol 5 dimension; MRC, Medical Research Council; NIPPV, non-invasive positive pressure ventilation; ADL, activities of daily living; IADL, instrumental activities of daily living; HADS, Hospital Anxiety and Depression Scale; IES-6, Impact of Events Scale – 6 item; IES-R, Impact of Events Scale-Revised; PTSD, post-traumatic stress disorder; FICA, Faith, Importance/Influence, Community, Action/Address in care; HOPE, Hope, Organized religion, Personal spirituality, Effects on medical care and end-of-life issues; PEACE Tool, Physical, Emotive, Autonomy, Communication, Economic, and Transcendent domains; PICS-F, post-intensive care syndrome – family; * denotes recommended screening tools by the SCCM International Consensus Conference [13]

Clinic Attendance

Failing to attend clinic appointments or becoming lost to follow-up are common among survivors of critical illness. Patients must often overcome many deterrents to make appointments, and these obstacles frequently overlap with the primary manifestations of PICS. Patients may be too physically weak to come, may fail to remember the appointment, may be too depressed to leave their home, or may prefer to avoid the location of their recent trauma. To circumvent these challenges, clinicians staffing the clinic must be adept, persistent, and creative at problem solving. Social determinants of health (see Chapter 25 for additional information) may also play a significant role in a patient's inability to make an appointment, including lack of transportation, insufficient funds to pay for the visit, limited health literacy, or living too far from the clinic [17]. Social workers often play a significant role in navigating these barriers, which likely impact the patient's healthcare far beyond an ICU follow-up clinic appointment alone.

Enablers and Barriers to ICU Follow-Up Clinics

Qualitative analysis of interviews of international experts in ICU aftercare revealed several enablers and barriers to successful implementation of ICU follow-up clinics and peer support groups. Key ingredients to the success of both interventions included: using patient stories to create a human connection for other clinicians and hospital administrators to generate interest in the program, recruiting motivated clinician champions to lead an interprofessional team forward using creative problem solving, and building relationships with supportive administrators to help overcome bureaucratic "red tape" with defined operational processes [18]. Common barriers to the development of ICU follow-up clinics and peer support programs included limited access to and sustainability of funding, difficulty in recruiting skilled clinicians to staff these programs, a lack of consensus on identifying those survivors who might derive the greatest benefit from participation, and lack of mechanisms to support patient attendance [18].

Feedback to ICU Care

In a companion study, the same group of international experts in ICU survivorship identified mechanisms to improve care provided in the ICU informed by engagement in ICU follow-up programs [19]. Organizational improvements included: identifying targets for quality improvement or education programs, such as enriching discharge summaries with important information (e.g., stop dates for antibiotics or anticoagulation) or developing patient-facing information about expectations following discharge; creating a new role for survivors, harnessing their spirit of altruism to adopt advocacy roles in professional societies, volunteer in the ICU, or provide real-time support to families in the ICU waiting room; and inviting colleagues to ICU follow-up clinics to learn about recovery trajectories, which may inform goals of care discussions for patients in the ICU [19]. Improvements at the clinician level included: strengthening one's own understanding of the patient experience (i.e., becoming a better clinician by recognizing, anticipating, and pre-empting patient and family needs following ICU discharge) and improving morale and decreasing burnout and compassion fatigue by sharing with ICU staff positive outcomes in challenging cases [19]. Indeed, in a field fraught with death and burnout, seeing patients thrive following their illness can be therapeutic to a clinician's soul.

The Patient Perspective

In a qualitative study of participants' impressions of ICU follow-up programs, patients and their care providers identified five key processes that ICU follow-up programs provided: continuity of care, management of debilitating symptoms, management of expectations regarding recovery, internal and external validation of progress, and mitigation of feelings of guilt and helplessness [20]. Continuity of care was necessary to coordinate otherwise fragmented care, ensuring that ongoing physiological problems were addressed longitudinally. Symptom management was fundamental to improving functional trajectories, with an emphasis on care delivery that linked healthcare and social care, ensuring that physical, emotional, and social problems were being addressed contemporaneously. By providing guidance in setting, meeting, and resetting personal goals, ICU follow-up programs enhanced motivation for improvement and cultivated an increased sense of self-efficacy. Patients appreciated direct and honest anticipatory guidance about managing expectations during recovery and described value in both recognizing their own progress (internal validation) and having their progress recognized by their healthcare providers (external validation). Having a safe space to share their emotions regarding recovery, both positive and negative, and having those feelings validated were critical for maintaining optimism and self-esteem and assuaging feelings of guilt and helplessness [20].

Collaboration with Primary Care Physicians

ICU follow-up clinics are not intended to replace PCPs but instead complement them by focusing on the rehabilitative components of care that have heretofore largely been overlooked, providing psychological support for the patient and their family, and exploring the patient's nutritional, financial, environmental, and social resources, or lack thereof. Realistically, given the limited number of ICU follow-up clinics available and the millions of people who require their services annually, the vast majority of ICU aftercare will be provided by PCPs. Enhanced PICS advocacy is needed at the local and national levels to educate PCPs about the needs of survivors of critical illness (see Chapter 55 for additional information). Curricula in medical schools and graduate medical education programs need to incorporate both didactics and clinical experiences surrounding PICS to ensure exposure begins early in medical training and not just for those who intend to practice critical care (see Chapter 22 for additional information). Moreover, structural and organizational changes in the primary care setting may be required, given that conventional 15–30-minute appointments are largely inadequate to meet the needs of this patient population. Accordingly, PCP practice managers may need to redesign clinic scheduling patterns to provide adequate time to properly care for survivors of critical illness and harness additional resources that the clinic may have, such as a social worker, to provide more comprehensive care. Ultimately, intensivists and the critical care community at large must explore partnerships with internists and generalists to assist them in providing the most sophisticated care possible for patients who do not have access to ICU follow-up clinic services. Such engagement likely requires collaboration among various medical societies at the national and international levels.

Conclusion

Given the increasing number of survivors of critical illness, PICS is likely to become one of the leading public health challenges of the twenty-first century. Developing and sustaining ICU follow-up clinics to address PICS in survivors of critical illness and their loved ones pose significant challenges, and clinics need to be tailored to the physical, personnel, and financial resources available at a given institution. Although no standard recipe guarantees a successful ICU aftercare program, emerging clinics need to address a common set of hurdles, including securing an adequate space; assembling an invested, multidisciplinary staff; and procuring the necessary equipment, technological, and financial support to be successful [10]. Although certain risk factors for the development of PICS are defined, there remains no consensus on screening tools to determine which patients would derive most benefit, and recruitment strategies for clinic participants remain institution-dependent. Although there is modest expert consensus on some screening tools to detect durable impairments associated with PICS, significant additional investigation is needed to refine these recommendations. The benefits derived by patients and their families, feedback mechanisms to improve in-ICU care at the organizational and clinician level, and the general lack of awareness of PICS among the critical care, medical, and lay communities demand that motivated clinicians with a commitment to interprofessional teamwork, defined operational processes, and creative problem-solving skills continue their efforts to further encourage the promise of the ICU follow-up clinic.

Key Points

1. ICU follow-up clinics, particularly when combined with peer support groups, are the most comprehensive approach to improve long-term outcomes and quality of life in survivors of critical illness and their loved ones.
2. Although a robust evidence base does not exist, some single-center studies demonstrate clinical and financial benefits rendered by participation in ICU follow-up clinics.
3. Over the course of an appointment that frequently lasts more than two hours, clinicians familiar with PICS can spend more time therapeutically listening to patients and their families, normalizing their experience, and setting realistic expectations for the depth and breadth of their recovery, while comprehensively evaluating patients and their families for PICS and constructing a patient-centered, goal-directed rehabilitation plan.
4. Those interested in developing and growing an ICU follow-up clinic must consider finding appropriate space and staff, purchasing equipment and supplies, securing information technology and financial resources, and advertising the clinic.
5. Existing tools and clinical judgment are insufficient to reliably predict PICS-related problems in all survivors of critical illness, but certain patient- and illness-related risk factors can reasonably identify those at highest risk.
6. Patients at heightened risk should be screened for PICS beginning within two to four weeks of hospital discharge and following important health and life changes, both anticipated and unanticipated; screening tools vary by institution, but may include the MoCA, HADS, IES-6, 6-minute walk test, and EQ-5D.

References

1. C.M. Sevin, S.L. Bloom, J.C. Jackson, et al. Comprehensive care of ICU survivors: development and implementation of an ICU recovery center. *J Crit Care* 2018; **46**: 141–8.
2. V. Danesh, L.M. Boehm, T.L. Eaton, et al. Characteristics of post-ICU and post-COVID recovery clinics in 29 U.S. health systems. *Crit Care Explor* 2022; **4** (3): e0658.
3. D. Elliott, J.E. Davidson, M.A. Harvey, et al. Exploring the scope of post-intensive care syndrome therapy and care: engagement of non-critical care providers and survivors in a second stakeholders meeting. *Crit Care Med* 2014; **42**: 2518–26.
4. J.F. Jensen, I. Egerod, M.H. Bestle, et al. A recovery program to improve quality of life, sense of coherence and psychological health in ICU survivors: a multicenter randomized controlled trial, the RAPIT study. *Intensive Care Med* 2016; **42**(11): 1733–43.
5. B.H. Cuthbertson, J. Rattray, M. K. Campbell, et al. The PRaCTICaL study of nurse led, intensive care follow-up programmes for improving long term outcomes from critical illness: a pragmatic randomized controlled trial. *BMJ* 2009; **339**: b3723.
6. K.F. Schmidt, D. Schwarzkopf, L-M. Baldwin. Long-term courses of sepsis survivors: effects of a primary care management intervention. *Am J Med* 2020; **133**(3): 381–5.
7. S.L. Bloom, J.L. Stollings, O. Kirkpatrick, et al. Randomized clinical trial of an ICU recovery pilot program for survivors of critical illness. *Crit Care Med* 2019; **47**(10): 1337–45.
8. K.P. Snell, C.L. Beiter, E.L. Hall, et al. A novel approach to ICU survivor care: a population health quality improvement project. *Crit Care Med* 2020; **48**(12): e1164–e1170.
9. M.A. Martillo, N.S. Dangayach, L. Tabacof, et al. Postintensive care syndrome in survivors of critical illness related to Coronavirus disease 2019: cohort study from a New York City critical care recovery clinic. *Crit Care Med* 2021; **49**(9): 1427–38.
10. B.W. Butcher, T.L. Eaton, A. A. Montgomery-Yates, C.M. Sevin. Meeting the challenges of establishing intensive care unit follow-up clinics. *Am J Crit Care* 2022; **31**(4): 324–8.
11. J. McPeake, L.M. Boehm, E. Hibbert, et al. Key components of ICU recovery programs: what did patients report provided benefit? *Crit Care Explor* 2020; **2** (4): e0088.
12. K.J. Haines, E. Hibbert, J. McPeake, et al. Prediction models for physical, cognitive, and mental health impairments after critical illness: a systematic review and critical appraisal. *Crit Care Med* 2020; **48** (12): 1871–80.
13. M.E. Mikkelsen, M. Still, B.J. Anderson, et al. Society of Critical Care Medicine's International Consensus Conference on prediction and identification of long-term impairments after critical illness. *Crit Care Med* 2020; **48**(11): 1670–9.
14. E. Fan, D.W. Dowdy, E. Colantuoni, et al. Physical complications in acute lung injury survivors: a two-year longitudinal prospective study. *Crit Care Med* 2014; **42** (4): 849–59.
15. M. Lee, J. Kang, Y. J. Jeong. Risk factors for post–intensive care syndrome: a systematic review and meta-analysis. *Aust Crit Care* 2020; **33**: 287–94.
16. National Institute for Health and Care Excellence (NICE). 2018 surveillance of rehabilitation after critical illness in adults (NICE guideline CG83). www.nice.org.uk/guidance/cg83. Accessed: December 6, 2024.
17. K.P. Mayer, H. Boustany, E.P. Cassity, et al. ICU recovery clinic attendance, attrition, and patient outcomes: the impact of severity of illness, gender, and rurality. *Crit Care Explor* 2020; **2**: e0206.
18. K.J. Haines, J. McPeake, E. Hibbert, et al. Enablers and barriers to implementing ICU follow-up clinics and peer support groups following critical illness: the Thrive Collaboratives. *Crit Care Med* 2019; **47**(9): 1194–200.

19. K.J. Haines, C.M. Sevin, E. Hibbert, et al. Key mechanisms by which post-ICU activities can improve in-ICU care: results of the international THRIVE collaboratives. *Intensive Care Med* 2019; **45** (7): 939–47.

20. J. McPeake, L.M. Boehm, E. Hibbert, et al. Key components of ICU recovery programs: what did patients report provided benefit? *Crit Care Explor* 2020; 2(4): e0088.

Chapter 29: Telemedicine-Based ICU Follow-Up Clinics and Digital Health

Neha S. Dangayach and Jenna M. Tosto-Mancuso

Introduction

Care delivery for critically ill patients necessitates coordinated multidisciplinary models during both the acute care setting and long-term recovery [1]. Telemedicine has recently evolved to improve the quality of care provided in both the intensive care unit (ICU) and in outpatient settings. Telehealth is defined as "the use of telecommunications technologies to deliver health-related information that supports patient care, administrative activities, and health communications" [2]. While telemedicine solutions and their use in critical care have been in development over the past two decades, deployment of such innovations accelerated and became a cornerstone of care during the COVID-19 pandemic [3]. Telehealth can be leveraged to improve patient health status; optimize access to patient care; address healthcare system disparities; and overcome physical, logistical, and socioeconomic barriers to accessing care [2]. Moreover, development and implementation of remote technologies (e.g., video conferencing) and asynchronous data acquisition and transfer (e.g., from Bluetooth-enabled wearables and sensors) have been shown to improve outcomes in both the ICU and post-ICU settings [4,5,6,7,8,9,10].

Post-discharge follow-up and coordination of care is paramount to address the long-term morbidities for survivors of critical illness. The interdisciplinary care model of ICU follow-up clinics can be supported and complemented by the deployment of technology-enabled care to address the long-term side effects of post-intensive care syndrome (PICS) and reduce fragmentation of outpatient care [11,12]. Advances in digital technology, further accelerated by the COVID-19 pandemic, have allowed many ICU follow-up clinics to adopt either primary or hybrid telemedicine models. This chapter discusses the role of telemedicine in ICU follow-up clinics and the opportunity to leverage digital health and digital therapeutics to optimize patient care and long-term outcomes.

Tele-ICU and Improvements in Quality of Care

To better understand the role telemedicine plays across the continuum of care for critically ill patients, it is important to appreciate how telemedicine can be used in the ICU to reduce risk factors associated with PICS. "Tele-ICU" is a network of audiovisual communication devices and computer systems that provides the foundation for a collaborative, interprofessional care model focusing on critically ill patients. Tele-ICU services are not specifically designed to replace in-person care but to augment care through leveraging resources and standardization of processes [13]. Models for tele-ICU care include a centralized continuous monitoring model and a decentralized consultative model, the latter of which is designed to respond to a patient's evolving clinical status (e.g., trigger alerts, virtual consultations, and facilitation of patient rounds) [13].

A systematic review of 25 studies on the utility of tele-ICU identified four principal roles: improving the availability of critical care expertise, particularly in community or rural settings; delivering high-quality, evidence-based care, particularly in tertiary care settings; increasing compliance with interventions promoting patient safety; and facilitating transfer of critically ill patients to another institution [14]. A second systematic review of 20 studies concluded that enhanced decision-making capacity utilizing tele-ICU services was associated with decreased mortality and ICU length of stay compared with tele-expert consultation alone [15]. Tele-ICU has also been shown to improve the quality of care delivery in the ICU by increasing adherence to effective practices such as the Society of Critical Care Medicine's (SCCM) ABCDEF bundle (see Chapter 11 for additional information), the utilization of which could potentially decrease the development of PICS [16].

Telemedicine-Based ICU Follow-Up Clinics

The number of ICU follow-up clinics utilizing telemedicine exclusively or in a hybrid model consisting of both in-person and telemedicine options increased during the COVID-19 pandemic. In a single-center study during the first wave of the COVID-19 pandemic in New York City, a telehealth-based ICU follow-up clinic evaluated 45 COVID-19 survivors and diagnosed a high burden of PICS one month after hospital discharge [17]. In a study describing characteristics of ICU follow-up and COVID-19 recovery clinics, 18 of 26 ICU follow-up clinics employed a hybrid model and four provided telehealth services exclusively [18].

Types of Assessments

Survivors of critical illness need assessments for impairments associated with PICS and other morbidities throughout the continuum of care, but universal consensus on what assessments should be performed does not currently exist. The SCCM International Consensus Conference on Prediction and Identification of Long-Term Impairments After Critical Illness provides guidance on appropriate patient assessments based on expert opinion [19]. Patients' pre-hospitalization functional status should be assessed at the time of ICU admission to identify those at greatest risk of developing new or worsening deficits following hospital discharge. At the time of hospital discharge, providers should perform "functional reconciliation," a process in which a patient's current functional status, as assessed by brief, standardized surveys, is compared with their pre-morbid capabilities. This is then followed by serial assessments beginning at two to four weeks following hospital discharge for high-risk patients to enable more detailed assessments and prompt referral to appropriate services [19].

This section summarizes different assessment tools for each PICS domain that can be employed during telehealth visits, offering an opportunity to improve access to timely assessments for patients who are unable to access face-to-face clinical care because of distance from an ICU follow-up clinic, financial limitations, lack of transportation, impaired mobility, or active avoidance of returning to the site of a traumatic experience (see Table 29.1).

Physical Domain

Assessments of physical function aim to inform the physical and functional status of survivors of critical illness. Physical impairments following critical illness include but are not limited to:

Table 29.1 Details of primary domains of PICS and relevant and recommended outcomes assessments to appropriately screen for impairment in each domain. While many of these outcomes measures have been validated for remote administration, care should be taken when implementing outcomes measures with limited or no evidence. This is especially true of assessments in the physical domain requiring the use of wearables or sensors for accurate kinematic or spatiotemporal data.

PICS Domain	Outcome Measure
Physical	Glasgow Coma Scale (GCS)
	Katz Index of Independence in Activities of Daily Living (ADL)
	The Lawton Instrumental Activities of Daily Living (IADL) Scale
	Boston University Activity Measure for Post-Acute Care Short Form (AM–PAC)
	MRC Dyspnea Scale
	10 Meter Walk Test (10MWT)
	6 Minute Walk Test (6MWT)
	Eating Assessment Tool–10 (EAT–10)
	Nestle Nutrition Institute Mini Nutrition Assessment (MNA)
	Neuro–QOL Upper Extremity Function–Short Form
	PROMIS Fatigue Scale
Cognitive Impairment	Telephonic–Montreal Cognitive Assessment (T–MoCA)
	Repeatable Battery for the Assessment of Neuropsychological Status (RBANS)
	Patient Reported Outcome Measure Information System (PROMIS)
	Mini Mental State Exam (MMSE)
Mental Health	Patient Health Questionnaire–9 (PHQ–9)
	General Anxiety Disorder–7 (GAD–7)
	Beck Depression Inventory (BDI)
	PTSD Checklist (PCL–5)
	Impact of Event Scale–6 (IES–6)
	Insomnia Severity Scale (ISS)
	Hospital Anxiety and Depression Scale (HADS)
Quality of Life (QOL)	Neuro–QOL Stigma Short
	EuroQOL 5–level EQ–5D (EQ 5D–5L)
Spirituality and Religiosity	Duke University Religion Index (DUREL)
	Conor–Davidson Resilience Scale 10 (CD–RISC 10)
	FICA Spirituality Tool
Caregiver and PICS-F	Burden Scale for Family Caregivers–Short Version (BSFC-s)
	Zarit Caregiver Burden Interview

strength, endurance, exercise capacity, range of motion, upright tolerance, balance, gait and locomotion, and the ability to perform activities of daily living (ADLs) and instrumental activities of daily living (IADLs). Physical function is the most challenging PICS domain to assess in a telemedicine-based ICU follow-up clinic, as the ability to assess strength, endurance, balance, and gait largely rely on physical interaction with the patient or use of equipment that may not be readily available to patients or practitioners. Validated questionnaires to assess independence with ADLs and IADLs, such as the Katz Index of Independence in Activities of Daily Living and The Lawton Instrumental Activities of Daily Living Scale, respectively, can be performed via telemedicine with either the patient or their care provider, as can basic self-report mobility questionnaires such as the Boston University Activity Measure of Post-Acute Care (AM-PAC) mobility questionnaire. Evaluations of dysphagia and nutritional status can also be performed via telemedicine using questionnaires such as the Eating Assessment Tool-10 (EAT-10) and the Nestle Nutrition Institute Mini Nutrition Assessment (MNA), respectively.

The reliability of strength and functional mobility measures, including grip strength, endurance, and gait speed, continues to be evaluated in the literature. These functional measures have been largely correlated with prediction of secondary health conditions beyond their intended domain target in traditional assessments. Despite great promise for applications in telehealth, there exist a number of challenges in effectively and reliably administering these assessments via telehealth. In their standard administration, many of these evaluations require specific environmental setups and trained personnel to appropriately evaluate the patient and ensure validity.

The six-minute walk test (6MWT) is well-validated to evaluate functional capacity and cardiopulmonary function and is recommended for use in patients following critical illness [19,20]. Several approaches have been utilized to validate the 6MWT performed via telemedicine. While such patient-centered assessments have preliminary evidence to suggest they can be done by patients alone, the most well-validated studies suggest the use of sensors to accurately track the distance ambulated and spatiotemporal parameters of gait [21,22]. Additionally, mobile applications, including the Apple iPhone's Health Kit, may be implemented for valid measures of the 6MWT [23,24].

The 10-meter walk test (10MWT), which is used to evaluate gait speed, is highly correlative with numerous other health outcomes. While preliminary findings support the remote adoption of the 10MWT, emerging literature suggests that employing the 10MWT in telehealth should include gait sensors, such as chronometers and accelerometers, which measure spatiotemporal parameters [25]. Grip strength requires addition research to validate home-based testing, including the use of sensors and wearables, that can be performed via telemedicine [26].

Cognitive Domain

Several cognitive assessment tools have been validated to be performed via telemedicine. The Telephonic Montreal Cognitive Assessment tool (T-MoCA) is a telephonically adapted version of the Montreal Cognitive Assessment tool, which has been validated to evaluate cognitive impairment in several patient populations and demonstrates high sensitivity (72%) and moderate specificity (59%) compared to the standard in-person assessment [27]. Use of the Mini Mental State Examination (MMSE) via telemedicine is non-inferior to traditional in-person assessment with respect to scoring and accuracy [28,29]. The Repeatable Battery for the Assessment of Neuropsychological Status (RBANS), which is used to assess several domains of cognitive function, including immediate and delayed memory, visuospatial skills, language, and attention, has also been validated for completion via telemedicine [30]. Comprehensive batteries of patient-reported outcomes that include cognitive domains are the Patient-Reported Outcome Measurement Information System (PROMIS) and Neuro Quality of Life (Neuro-QOL) questionnaires, which have both been validated for remote administration with the advent of computerized adaptive testing [31,32,33,34,35].

A gold standard intervention for evaluating consciousness and wakefulness in patients with critical illness, the Glasgow Coma Scale (GCS), is traditionally evaluated at the bedside; however, recent work has aimed to evaluate validity and reliability of remote assessment of the GCS to expand clinical adoption and application [36]. Studies have shown that GCS scores obtained remotely and in-person are highly correlated, suggesting that the GCS can be leveraged for longitudinal monitoring in telemedicine-based ICU follow-up clinics, particularly in patients with profound disorders of consciousness.

This broad array of validated neurocognitive screening instruments offers multiple approaches for providers to screen survivors of critical illness for cognitive deficits when evaluated in a telemedicine-based ICU follow-up clinic appointment.

Mental Health Domain

Deploying validated outcomes assessments in telemedicine-based ICU follow-up clinic appointments may allow providers to thoroughly screen for symptoms of depression, anxiety, post-traumatic stress disorder (PTSD), and sleep disturbances. As these assessments are generally patient reported outcomes (PROs), telehealth administration has established validity and reliability more readily than other traditionally face-to-face assessments. The Patient Health Questionnaire-9 (PHQ-9) is a 9-item screening tool for depression validated for use across populations that can be administered remotely and via phone-based applications [37]. The Generalized Anxiety Disorder-7 (GAD-7), Post Traumatic Stress Disorder Checklist-5 (PCL-5), and Impact of Event Scale-6 (IES-6) are screening tools for anxiety and PTSD, respectively, that are adopted from the Diagnostic and Statistical Manual of Mental Disorders 5 (DSM-5) and easily administered remotely [38]. Although commonly used in ICU follow-up clinics to screen patients and their loved ones for depression and anxiety, use of the Hospital Anxiety and Depression Scale (HADS) has not been validated for use in telemedicine. To evaluate sleep disturbance in ICU survivors, the Insomnia Severity Index (ISI) has been validated for telemedicine administration [39].

Quality of Life

To evaluate quality of life (QOL), the EuroQol-5Dimension-5Level (EQ-5D-5L) is a highly validated metric that evaluates mobility, self-care activities, usual activities, pain, depression and anxiety, and a numerical assessment of global health that is commonly used both in person and via telemedicine [19,40].

Care Partner Evaluation and PICS-F

Limited evidence has evaluated the psychometric properties of both spirituality and caregiver-facing outcomes delivered remotely. Future work is needed to evaluate the validity of such metrics to ensure reliable administration and evaluation in ICU follow-up clinics.

Comprehensive outcomes assessments are pivotal to develop a thorough patient-centered plan of care and evaluate for changes in clinical status in survivors of critical illness. The number of validated outcomes assessments that can be deployed via telehealth further supports the evolution of ICU follow-up clinics' abilities to leverage telemedicine to maximize impact and access to care.

Digital Health and Wearables

Digital health uses technology to improve the quality of care in both medical settings and the community [41,42]. Digital health may leverage wearables, sensors, and healthcare data collection to maximize objective patient assessments and improve access to care [43,44]. For patients following critical illness, digital health technologies may serve to detect changes in medical or functional status and increase access to care when geographic location, cost, or mobility are barriers [8,9,45,46,47]. This increase in connectivity to the healthcare system may reduce the risk of developing sequelae following critical illness and reduce fragmentation of care [46]. ICU follow-up clinics that leverage such technologies serve to maximize patient support throughout the transition from hospital to home and to address primary domains often left unmanaged by general practitioners in patients with PICS, including physical, cognitive, mental health, and spiritual domains of recovery (see Figure 29.1) [1,46,47,48].

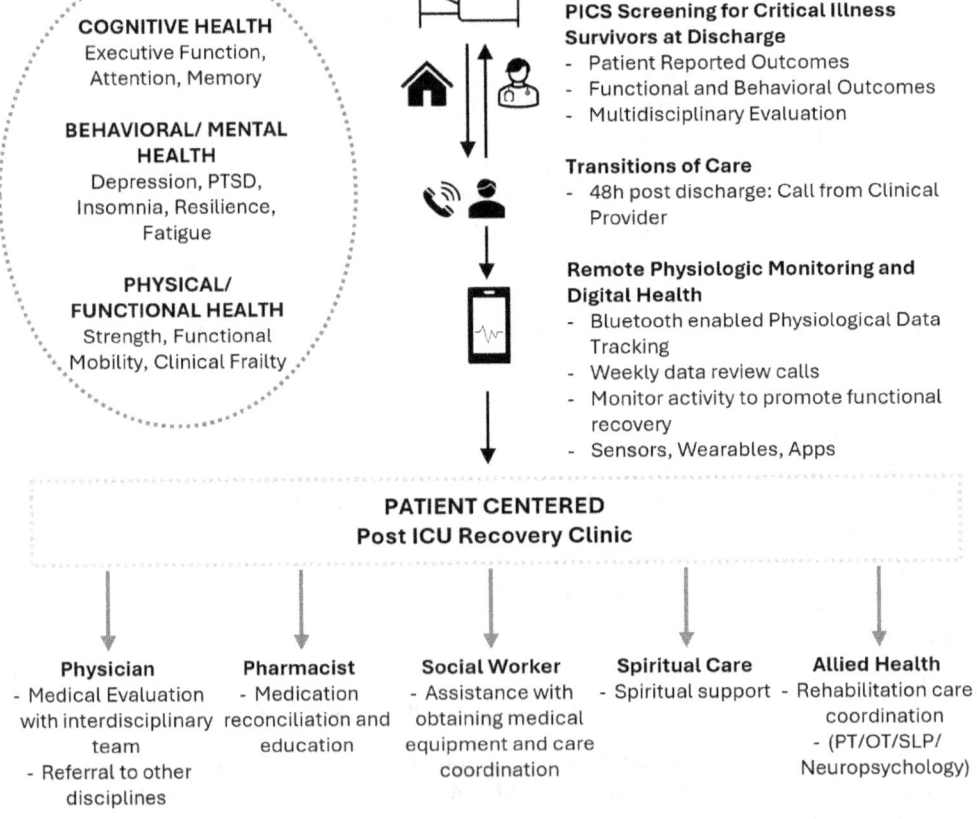

Figure 29.1 Interdisciplinary collaboration can leverage digital health solutions to improve patient care, including sensors, wearables, remote physiological monitoring, and remote therapeutic monitoring solutions. These technologies may improve the continuum of care in telemedicine-based ICU follow-up clinics.

Remote Patient Monitoring

Remote patient monitoring (RPM) is a home-based telehealth modality that has become increasingly prevalent in telemedicine practice over the last decade [49,50]. RPM allows for the automatic or "asynchronous" longitudinal collection of physiological data using sensors or Bluetooth-enabled devices [49,51]. Data may be continuously or intermittently transmitted to a healthcare team in real time for clinical evaluation and intervention as necessary, and some RPM platforms may flag abnormal or out-of-range data for rapid clinical evaluation [50]. Furthermore, modern RPM solutions may include bidirectional communication features that allow patients and providers to interact in real time, thus increasing access to healthcare.

RPM was initially developed to support care management in patients with chronic diseases, including cardiovascular disease and diabetes, and it has been shown to promote adherence to recovery programs following hospital discharge [7,49,52,53]. Since its original deployment, RPM applications have evolved to cater to the complexities of ICU survivorship, with a special interest in early detection of abnormal physiological parameters [54]. RPM may provide survivors of critical illness and their care partners a sense of agency over their healthcare: by providing patients and their caregivers access to physiological data, they may become empowered in the active monitoring and management of their health.

RPM provides an additional means of connection to the healthcare system for patients navigating recovery following critical illness, allowing for improved patient management, monitoring of physiological status, and reduced fragmentation of care. A recent systematic review identified the most common physiological data monitored remotely in patients following critical illness, including blood pressure (continuous and intermittent), electrocardiography, respiratory rate, pulse oximetry, skin temperature, posture, falls detection, and activity and step counts [54]. Such consistent and comprehensive data tracking may allow healthcare providers to asynchronously detect concerning changes that may herald the early development of complications in survivors of critical illness.

In survivors of stroke, for example, RPM has been significantly leveraged to monitor blood pressure and promote improved health management in the outpatient setting. In a study by Naqvi and colleagues, 50 patients discharged after acute stroke were randomized to either usual care or a novel Telehealth After Stroke Care (TASC) model that included remote physiological monitoring of blood pressure, infographics, and multidisciplinary telehealth visits [55]. Patients randomized to the TASC group demonstrated a significant decrease in systolic blood pressure when compared with those in the usual care group, and this effect was notably prominent in otherwise underserved Black and Hispanic patients [55].

Additional studies have demonstrated RPM's ability to facilitate triage in the setting of abnormal vital sign excursions. Tosto-Mancuso and colleagues utilized RPM of blood pressure in 12 stroke survivors, demonstrating frequent excursions of systolic and diastolic blood pressure above established parameters, which lead to 16 triage events for care escalation to either the referring neurologist or neurosurgeon, primary care physician, or emergency department [10]. Similarly, remote monitoring of pulse oximetry in patients following COVID-19 infection may expedite care escalation and mitigate further physiological worsening [6]. Altogether, RPM may provide an additional layer of security to vulnerable outpatient populations, including survivors of stroke and COVID-19, to detect physiological abnormalities early and expedite clinician evaluation to reduce the risk of further decompensation [5,6,56]. Accordingly, those caring for survivors of critical illness may consider incorporating RPM technology in ICU follow-up clinics to maximize comprehensive care across the recovery trajectory and improve patient outcomes and quality of life.

Wearables and Sensors

Wearables and sensors have become increasingly popular in both consumer and healthcare settings for their ability to accurately track vital signs and markers of activity, which can be asynchronously delivered to healthcare teams for interpretation. Such wearables may include activity trackers, step counters, accelerometers, heat rate monitors, and pulse oximeters. In an exploratory observational study, Kim and colleagues evaluated the use of a consumer-grade wearable to monitor frailty in survivors of critical illness. They found that frail survivors of critical illness demonstrated significantly lower daily step counts than those who were not frail based on the Clinical Frailty Scale (p=.02; d=1.81) [57], suggesting that data generated by a commercial-grade wearable may be used to contextualize a diagnosis of frailty in survivors of critical illness [57]. Wearables can also detect vital sign abnormalities in survivors of critical illness as demonstrated by Kroll and colleagues, who found that wearables had moderate sensitivity and high specificity for detecting tachycardia [45]. Furthermore, there is significant correlation between wearable-derived sleep data and results from the Richards-Campbell Sleep Questionnaire ($r = 0.33$, $p = 0.03$, 95% confidence interval [CI] 0.04–0.58) [45]. Digital health and wearables continue to evolve to better inform the recovery journey of patients following critical illness.

Technology and Regulatory Guidance

Regulatory requirements for audio-video visits, which were relaxed during the COVID-19 pandemic, vary by state in the United States. Licensure laws and practice acts should be consistently followed when delivering care in telemedicine-based ICU follow-up clinics. Furthermore, special regulatory and compliance considerations should be taken when deploying digital health solutions outside of the patient's electronic medical record to ensure succinct monitoring and capturing of both synchronous and asynchronous data. This includes digital health solutions using cloud-based data capture tools to store and transmit patient health information.

Novel Current Procedural Terminology (CPT) codes and billing strategies have emerged to support the development of telemedicine clinics. Transitions of care CPT codes facilitate discharge from hospital to home by ensuring that patients are contacted by a member of the clinical team within 48 hours of discharge. Chronic care management CPT codes support a financially sustainable path of developing chronic care management plans for survivors of critical illness, leveraging the evaluations and skillsets of the ICU follow-up clinic interdisciplinary team, even when performed via telemedicine. Remote physiological monitoring CPT codes provide reimbursement for collecting and interpreting physiological and activity data, while remote therapeutic (RTM) CPT codes allow for the prescription and monitoring of therapeutic exercise and physical rehabilitation. Behavioral Health Integration (BHI) allows for the provision of mental health services in the context of ICU follow-up clinics and can be supported by BHI CPT codes enacted in the Physician Fee Schedule in 2017. These novel reimbursement strategies propose a means of sustainability for emerging telemedicine practices at large and are particularly meaningful in providing comprehensive care for survivors of critical illness in ICU follow-up clinics.

Future Directions and Conclusion

For survivors of critical illness and their caregivers, quality clinical care and support are needed beyond discharge. To improve access and to reduce fragmentation of care, ICU follow-up clinics may leverage telemedicine and digital health technologies to overcome barriers to accessing traditional care and to enhance patient care by providing physiological, mobility, and other data to clinicians. With novel reimbursement pathways including the use of transitions of care, chronic care management, remote patient monitoring, and remote therapeutic monitoring CPT codes, telemedicine-based ICU follow-up clinics have become more financially sustainable and scalable. Telemedicine-based ICU follow-up clinics present a novel approach to reducing fragmentation and maximizing coordinated, patient-centered care for survivors of critical illness and their care partners.

Key Points

1. Critical illness survivors benefit from continuous follow-up beyond the acute phases of care to facilitate recovery and support survivorship.
2. Digital health and telemedicine-based ICU follow-up clinics may serve to support the dynamic needs of survivors of critical illness and their care partners.
3. A great number of objective assessments are validated for use in telemedicine and may better identify patients and care partners experiencing post intensive care syndrome (PICS) or post intensive care syndrome-family (PICS-F).
4. Wearables, sensors, and asynchronous monitoring of physiological data may further inform clinical decision-making in survivors of critical illness.
5. Regulatory bodies have supported the adoption of telemedicine practices with sustainable billing pathways for these care paradigms.

References

1. C.M. Sevin, S.L. Bloom, J.C. Jackson, et al. Comprehensive care of ICU survivors: development and implementation of an ICU recovery center. *J Crit Care* 2018; **46**: 141–8.
2. O.J. Mechanic, Y. Persaud, A.B. Kimball. Telehealth Systems 2024. www.ncbi.nlm.nih.gov/books/NBK459384/ (Accessed October 18, 2024.)
3. J. Shaver. The state of telehealth before and after the COVID-19 pandemic. *Prim Care* 2022; **49**(4): 517.
4. A.R. Watson, R. Wah, R. Thamman. The value of remote monitoring for the COVID-19 pandemic. *Telemed J E-Health Off J Am Telemed Assoc* 2020; **26**: 1110–12.
5. L. Tabacof, J. Wood, N. Mohammadi, et al. Remote patient monitoring identifies the need for triage in patients with acute COVID-19 infection. *Telemed E-Health* 2022; **28**(4): 495–500.
6. L. Tabacof, C. Kellner, E. Breyman, et al. Remote patient monitoring for home management of coronavirus disease 2019 in New York: a cross-sectional observational study. *Telemed E-Health* 2021; **27**: 641–8.
7. R. Benzo, J. Hoult, C. McEvoy, et al. Promoting chronic obstructive pulmonary disease wellness through remote monitoring

and health coaching: a clinical trial. *Ann Am Thorac Soc* 2022; **19**: 1808–17.

8. V.A.J. Block, E. Pitsch, P. Tahir, et al. Remote physical activity monitoring in neurological disease: a systematic review. *PLoS ONE* 2016; **11**: e0154335.

9. A. Davoudi, N.S. Lee, C. Chivers, et al. Patient interaction phenotypes with an automated remote hypertension monitoring program and their association with blood pressure control: observational study. *J Med Internet Res* 2020; **22**: e22493.

10. J.M. Tosto-Mancuso, D. Putrino, J. Wood, et al. Remote patient monitoring of blood pressure is feasible poststroke and can facilitate triage of care. *Telemed Rep* 2022; **3**: 149–55.

11. L.M. Boehm, V. Danesh, T.L. Eaton, et al. Multidisciplinary ICU recovery clinic visits: a qualitative analysis of patient-provider dialogues. *Chest*. 2023; **163**(4): 843–54.

12. M. Cadde, M. Nunn. The transition from ventilator to video call: the ICU recovery clinic. *Chest* 2023; **163**(4): 742–3.

13. T.M. Davis, C. Barden, S. Dean, et al. American Telemedicine Association Guidelines for TeleICU Operations. *Telemed E-Health* 2016; **22**: 971–80.

14. C. Guinemer, M. Boeker, D. Fürstenau, et al. Telemedicine in intensive care units: scoping review. *J Med Internet Res* 2021; **23**: e32264.

15. C. Kalvelage, S. Rademacher, S. Dohmen, et al. Decision-making authority during tele-ICU care reduces mortality and length of stay: a systematic review and meta-analysis. *Crit Care Med* 2021; **49**: 1169–81.

16. B. Weiss, N. Paul, F. Balzer, et al. Telemedicine in the intensive care unit: a vehicle to improve quality of care? *J Crit Care* 2021; **61**: 241–6.

17. M.A. Martillo, N.S. Dangayach, L. Tabacof et al. Postintensive care syndrome in survivors of critical illness related to coronavirus disease 2019: cohort study from a New York City critical care recovery clinic. *Crit Care Med* 2021; **49**: 1427–38.

18. V. Danesh, L.M. Boehm, T.L. Eaton, et al. Characteristics of post-ICU and post-COVID recovery clinics in 29 U.S. health systems. *Crit Care Explor* 2022; **4**: e0658.

19. M.E. Mikkelsen, M. Still, B.J. Anderson, et al. Society of critical care medicine's international consensus conference on prediction and identification of long-term impairments after critical illness. *Crit Care Med* 2020; **48**: 1670–9.

20. P.L. Enright. The six-minute walk test. *Respir Care* 2003; **48**: 783–5.

21. T. LaPatra, G.L. Baird, R. Goodman, et al. Remote 6-minute-walk testing in patients with pulmonary hypertension: a pilot study. *Am J Respir Crit Care Med* 2022; **205**: 851–4.

22. I.M. Pires, H.V. Denysyuk, M.V. Villasana, et al. Development technologies for the monitoring of six-minute walk test: a systematic review. *Sensors* 2022; **22**: 581.

23. J. Mak, N. Rens, D. Savage D, et al. Reliability and repeatability of a smartphone-based 6-min walk test as a patient-centred outcome measure. *Eur Heart J Digit Health* 2021; **2**: 77–87.

24. D. Salvi, E. Poffley, E. Orchard, et al. The mobile-based 6-minute walk test: usability study and algorithm development and validation. *JMIR MHealth UHealth* 2020; **8**: e13756.

25. C.L. Gabriel, I.M. Pire, P.J. Coelho, et al. Mobile and wearable technologies for the analysis of Ten Meter Walk Test: a concise systematic review. *Heliyon* 2023; **9**: e16599.

26. P.A. Heslop, C. Hurst, A.A. Sayer, et al. Remote collection of physical performance measures for older people: a systematic review. *Age Ageing* 2023; **52**: afac327.

27. M.J. Katz, C. Wang, C.O. Nester, et al. T-MoCA: a valid phone screen for cognitive impairment in diverse community samples. *Alzheimers Dement Diagn Assess Dis Monit* 2021; **13**: e12144.

28. E.L. Ciemins, B. Holloway, P.J. Coon, et al. Telemedicine and the mini-mental state examination: assessment from a distance.

Telemed J E-Health Off J Am Telemed Assoc 2009; **15**: 476–8.

29. W. McEachern, A. Kirk, D.G. Morgan, et al. Reliability of the MMSE administered in-person and by telehealth. *Can J Neurol Sci* 2008; **35**: 643–6.

30. J.M. Galusha-Glasscock, D.K. Horton, M.F. Weiner, et al. Video teleconference administration of the repeatable battery for the assessment of neuropsychological status. *Arch Clin Neuropsychol* 2016; **31**: 8–11.

31. M.S. Fidai, B.M. Saltzman, F. Meta et al. Patient-reported outcomes measurement information system and legacy patient-reported outcome measures in the field of orthopaedics: a systematic review. *Arthroscopy* 2018; **34**: 605–14.

32. M. Hung, M.W. Voss, J. Bounsanga, et al. Psychometrics of the patient-reported outcomes measurement information system physical function instrument administered by computerized adaptive testing and the disabilities of arm, shoulder and hand in the orthopedic elbow patient population. *J Shoulder Elbow Surg* 2018; **27**: 515–22.

33. P.A. Borowsky, O.M. Kadri, J.E. Meldau, et al. The remote completion rate of electronic patient-reported outcome forms before scheduled clinic visits: a proof-of-concept study using patient-reported outcome measurement information system computer adaptive test questionnaires. *JAAOS Glob Res Rev* 2019; **3**: e19.00038.

34. K.F. Cook, S.W. Choi, P.K. Crane, et al. Letting the CAT out of the bag: comparing computer adaptive tests and an eleven-item short form of the Roland-Morris disability questionnaire. *Spine* 2008; **33**: 1378–83.

35. D. Cella, R. Gershon, J.S. Lai, et al. The future of outcomes measurement: item banking, tailored short-forms, and computerized adaptive assessment. *Qual Life Res* 2007; **16** (Suppl 1): 133–41.

36. A.K. Adcock, H. Kosiorek, P. Parikh, et al. Reliability of robotic telemedicine for assessing critically ill patients with the full outline of unresponsiveness score and Glasgow coma scale. *Telemed J E Health* 2017; **23**: 555–60.

37. K. Kroenke, R.L. Spitzer, J.B. Williams. The PHQ-9: validity of a brief depression severity measure. *J Gen Intern Med* 2001; **16**: 606–13.

38. L.S. Taylor, S.G. Caloudas, L.C. Haney, et al. Asynchronous assessment with the PCL-5: practice considerations and recommendations. *Psychol Serv* 2023; **21**: 552–9.

39. F.P. Thorndike, L.M. Ritterband, D.K. Saylor, et al. Validation of the insomnia severity index as a web-based measure. *Behav Sleep Med* 2011; **9**: 216–23.

40. N. Nakanishi, K. Liu, A. Kawauchi, et al. Instruments to assess post-intensive care syndrome assessment: a scoping review and modified Delphi method study. *Crit Care Lond Engl* 2023; **27**: 430.

41. Health C for D and R. What is Digital Health? FDA 2020. www.fda.gov/medical-devices/digital-health-center-excellence/what-digital-health.

42. Y. Ronquillo, A. Meyers, S.J. Korvek. Digital Health. In: StatPearls [Internet]. StatPearls Publishing; 2024. www.ncbi.nlm.nih.gov/books/NBK470260/.

43. D.H. Solomon, R.S. Rudin. Digital health technologies: opportunities and challenges in rheumatology. *Nat Rev Rheumatol* 2020; **16**: 525–35.

44. E. Murray, E.B. Hekler, G. Andersson, et al. Evaluating digital health interventions: key questions and approaches. *Am J Prev Med* 2016; **51**: 843–51.

45. R.R. Kroll, E.D. McKenzie, J.G. Boyd, et al. Use of wearable devices for post-discharge monitoring of ICU patients: a feasibility study. *J Intensive Care* 2017; **5**: 64.

46. L. Rose, C.E.Cox. Digital solutions and the future of recovery after critical illness. *Curr Opin Crit Care* 2023; **29**: 519.

47. I. McElroy, S. Sareh, A. Zhu, et al. Use of digital health kits to reduce readmission after cardiac surgery. *J Surg Res* 2016; **204**: 1–7.

48. L. Jalilian, M. Cannesson, N. Kamdar. Post-ICU recovery clinics in the era of digital

health and telehealth. *Crit Care Med* 2019; **47**: e796–7.

49. F.A.C. de Farias, C.M. Dagostini, Y. Bicca, et al. Remote patient monitoring: a systematic review. *Telemed J E-Health* 2020; **26**: 576–83.

50. R. Wootton. Twenty years of telemedicine in chronic disease management: an evidence synthesis. *J Telemed Telecare* 2012; **18**: 211–20.

51. A. Vegesna, M. Tran, M. Angelaccio, et al. Remote patient monitoring via non-invasive digital technologies: a systematic review. *Telemed J E-Health* 2017; **23**: 3–17.

52. P.A. Lee, G. Greenfield, Y. Pappas. The impact of telehealth remote patient monitoring on glycemic control in type 2 diabetes: a systematic review and meta-analysis of systematic reviews of randomised controlled trials. *BMC Health Serv Res* 2018; **18**: 495.

53. M. Ando, Y.C. Kao, Y.C. Lee, et al. Remote cognitive behavioral therapy for older adults with anxiety symptoms: a systematic review and meta-analysis. *J Telemed Telecare* 2024; **30**: 1376–85.

54. D. Viderman, E. Seri, M. Aubakirova, et al. Remote monitoring of chronic critically ill patients after hospital discharge: a systematic review. *J Clin Med* 2022; **11**: 1010.

55. I.A. Naqvi, K. Strobino, Y. Kuen Cheung, et al. Telehealth after stroke care pilot randomized trial of home blood pressure telemonitoring in an underserved setting. *Stroke* 2022; **53**: 3538–47.

56. A. Alboksmaty, T. Beaney, S. Elkin, et al. Effectiveness and safety of pulse oximetry in remote patient monitoring of patients with COVID-19: a systematic review. *Lancet Digit Health* 2022; **4**: e279–89.

57. B. Kim, M. Hunt, J. Muscedere, et al. Using consumer-grade physical activity trackers to measure frailty transitions in older critical care survivors: exploratory observational study. *JMIR Aging* 2021; **4**: e19859.

Chapter 30

Financial Considerations for ICU Follow-Up Clinics

Karen A. Korzick, Ross H. Perfetti, and Janet F. Tomcavage

Introduction

Understanding the financial implications of intensive care unit (ICU) survivor care is critical to the success of ICU follow-up clinics. Patients who require intensive care during hospitalization experience higher rates of mortality, hospital readmission, hospital costs, and healthcare resource utilization in the years following their initial episode of critical illness (see Chapter 33 for additional information) [1,2,3,4,5]. This body of literature and our evolving understanding of post-intensive care syndrome (PICS) provide ample evidence that the goal of improving health after critical illness should be of interest to patients and their families as well as providers and payors of healthcare. Two core aspects of contemporary American healthcare must be understood when measuring the impact of ICU follow-up clinics and advocating for financial support from health system administrators and payors: value-based healthcare and population health management.

Value-Based Healthcare

We argue that value-based healthcare models, rather than fee-for-service models, must be used when considering the value of ICU follow-up clinics. Fee-for-service models have historically driven healthcare in the United States (US) until the early 2000s. The fee-for-service model determines the value of healthcare services in terms of the revenue generated for providers and their employers at the point of service, with inadequate consideration of the quality and cost of healthcare and other patient-centered concerns. If ICU follow-up clinics are evaluated using this framework, they are highly likely to be viewed as financially unsustainable. For instance, an intensivist providing outpatient care rather than inpatient care results in an opportunity cost to their employer, as the revenue generated by providing outpatient care cannot match that generated by providing inpatient care over the same period of time.

In contrast, value-based healthcare models entail a holistic valuation process attained from the combined perspectives of all stakeholders (e.g., patients, families, providers, payors, and society) relative to the costs, benefits accrued, burdens endured, and consumption of healthcare resources *over time* [6,7,8]. A general equation to calculate the value of patient-centered healthcare within the value-based health care model is:

$$\text{Value} = \frac{\text{quality}}{\text{cost}}$$

One of the challenges of value-based care models is identifying reliable methods for measurement of both quality (with consideration of the patient experience) and cost. The ratio of quality to cost depends on several factors, including who is paying the cost, who defines the "quality" of care, and the nature and timing of quality assessments. For example, a person with advanced malignancy refractory to treatment may value hospitalization and receipt of life-sustaining care to extend quantity of life, while providers and payors may argue that the cost of care for the length of life attained is financially unjustifiable. Suggested metrics and targets for assessing value are presented in Table 30.1.

Porter and Teisburg argue that a zero-sum competition model of healthcare results in competition to shift costs, increase bargaining power, capture patients, and restrict both patient choice and access to services in the name of cost reduction, despite the fact that none of these maneuvers increases *value* for patients [6]. Instead, they argue that the following principles should drive value-based competition in value-based healthcare design: (1) the focus should be on value for patients and not just on lowering costs; (2) there should be unrestricted competition based on results; (3) competition should center on medical conditions over the full cycle of care; (4) high quality care should be less costly; (5) value should be driven by provider experience, scale, and learning at the medical condition level; (6) competition should be regional and national, not just local; and (7) information on results and prices needed for value-based competition must be widely available.

There are multiple mechanisms to achieve value-based aims, including enhanced care coordination, establishment of accountable care organizations (ACOs), quality performance benchmarking, pay-for-performance schemes, and other necessary preconditions, such as multi-payer alignment and risk adjustment [9,10].

Population Health Management and Transitions of Care: An Opportunity to Increase Value

Through disciplined design of care processes, population health management addresses a range of social, economic, environmental, and behavioral factors that affect the health of specific patient populations, including survivors of critical illness [11]. ICU follow-up clinics attempt to bridge the known gaps in transitions of care and quality of care, as patients move from hospital to home, with the goal of improving long-term outcomes for survivors of critical illness. Patients and their families, healthcare providers, and payors would all prefer to see processes to enhance both financial sustainability and improvements in long-term metrics – as supported by data collection and analysis – incorporated in the design, implementation, and subsequent development of ICU follow-up clinics.

Patients report significant benefits from participating in ICU follow-up clinics [12], but to date, only one ICU follow-up clinic has reported statistically significant reductions in the one-year mortality rate and 30-, 60-, and 90-day readmission rates compared to usual care processes (see Table 30.2) [13,14]. Financial data analysis of the first 13 months of this ICU follow-up clinic demonstrated the following when compared with the control cohort of patients who received usual care: a significant cost savings to the payor (first stakeholder); an unclear cost impact on the hospital (second stakeholder), which funded the ICU follow-up clinic; and slightly higher out-of-pocket expenses to the clinic patients (third stakeholder) [13].

This study demonstrates two additional challenges to ICU follow-up clinic valuation. First, policy reform remains incomplete in the US, and the financial policies of health systems and payors are not uniform. Thus, the various stakeholders that are involved in providing and paying for ICU follow-up clinics may be distinct from the stakeholders to

Table 30.1 Suggested stakeholders, metrics, and targets for value-based care assessment of ICU follow up-clinics

Patient/Family	Providers and Healthcare systems	Payors (Private Health Care Insurance)	Society
Improve mortality rate	Improve mortality rate	Optimize costs of effective health care	Maximize opportunity for all citizens who are survivors of critical illness to attain optimal achievable recovery
Avoid unplanned hospital readmissions	Decrease unplanned readmission rates and length of readmission, when readmission occurs		
Decrease co-morbidities in physical, cognitive, and emotional health	Decrease co-morbidities in physical, cognitive, and emotional health	Avoid expenditure on health care that is ineffective	Maximize value of care delivered to cost-of-care ratio from socially funded payor sources
Decrease time to return to independent activities of daily living			
Decrease time to return to work	Decrease in unplanned utilization of post-discharge healthcare	Expenditure per patient	Maximize opportunity to avoid preventable disability insurance payouts from socially funded payor sources
Decrease time to return to ability to engage in role(s) within the household and/or family networks	Improve Medicare Star rating for the organization	Expenditure per readmission in recovery from index ICU admission	

Table 30.1 (cont.)

Patient/Family	Providers and Healthcare systems	Payors (Private Health Care Insurance)	Society
Minimize negative financial impact of ICU illness and recovery on family finances	Meet Pay-for-performance (P4) targets	Optimize value of care delivered to cost-of-care ratio	
	Cost of clinic space/tele-medicine infrastructure		
Minimize negative career impact of ICU illness on patient and family caregivers	Cost of staffing the clinic	**Payors (Private Disability Insurance)**	
	Reimbursement rates for ICU follow up clinic	Optimize recovery time from disability acquired in the ICU	
Control out-of-pocket costs for health insurance premiums, copays, co-insurance, and deductibles	Impact of ICU follow-up clinic on inpatient bed capacity/new inpatient admission opportunity	Maximize opportunity to avoid preventable disability insurance payouts from private disability payor sources	

Table 30.2 Geisinger ICU survivor clinic care versus usual care, three-year cohort outcomes, preliminary data

	ICU Survivor Clinic Full Participation (N=96)	Usual Care (N=177)	Chi-Square p value	95% Confidence Intervals	Hazard Ratio
1 Year Mortality	17 (17.7%)	74 (41.8%)	p<0.0001	0.193, 0.558	0.329
30-Day Readmission	11 (11.5%)	42 (23.7%)	p=0.0186	0.232, 0.876	0.451
60-Day Readmission	16 (16.7%)	56 (31.6%)	p=0.0081	0.273, 0.824	0.475
90-Day Readmission	20 (20.8%)	66 (37.3%)	p=0.0052	0.301, 0.810	0.494

whom the financial value attained accrues, which generates problems when evaluating value (e.g., one policy may bring cost savings to the payor while increasing expenses for the provider). This lack of alignment between the value attained and the costs borne by healthcare institutions supporting ICU follow-up clinics is a challenging proposition for many hospital administrators in the current US healthcare model. Second, while the benefit of mortality rate reduction was evident after the first 13 months, the benefit of readmission rate reduction was not apparent until a time point between 13 and 36 months of clinic operation [14]. This finding highlights the lack of alignment between the conventional benchmark of 30-day readmission rates set by payors and the time frame often required for sufficient recovery from PICS and therefore the beneficial impact of ICU follow-up clinics.

Challenges to Understanding the Financial Implications of ICU Follow-Up Clinics

In addition to the above challenges, several other factors must be considered when evaluating the financial implications of ICU follow-up clinics, including the inherent heterogeneity in the presentation of PICS, the current variability in ICU follow-up clinic models and the clinical outcomes measured, and the need to determine which costs borne by which stakeholders should be included in the value equation.

Sepsis and the acute respiratory distress syndrome (ARDS) are the diagnoses that have received the most significant attention with respect to long-term outcomes in survivors of critical illness, but they represent only two of the commonly encountered diagnoses in survivors of critical illness. In addition to the diversity in primary ICU diagnoses necessitating follow-up care, PICS is a similarly heterogeneous syndrome, with wide-ranging effects that differ greatly among patients, translating into considerable variability in the care needs of survivors of critical illness (see Chapter 2 for additional information). To date, there is no definitive consensus on the most effective screening process for the detection of PICS, nor has there been convincing evidence that any one ICU follow-up clinic design or care pathway for PICS is superior [15,16,17,18].

There is significant variability in the outcome measures reported in studies of ICU follow-up clinic care processes, with reported outcomes including: mortality and readmission rates, health-related quality of life and quality-adjusted life years, the ability to engage independently in activities of daily living and instrumental activities of daily living, objective measures of physical and cognitive impairment, and the ability to resume driving and employment, among others [13,15,16,17,18]. These outcome measures are not intrinsically comparable, as some have no standard associated cost assigned to them, and little to no financial data has been included in most published studies.

ICU follow-up clinic models vary by geographic location, health system design and ecology, and the composition of the multidisciplinary care team staffing them, making it particularly challenging to elucidate the drivers of variable direct costs among them [13,19,20,21,22]. In the US, multiple regional and local factors impact the cost to deliver care. Factors responsible for these regional variations include: the six Centers for Medicare and Medicaid Services (CMS) cost regions, social determinants of health, health resources available to patients, and staffing costs. Resource shortages, especially for mental healthcare, are more prevalent in rural health systems [23]. Telemedicine interventions for ICU follow-up care are just beginning to be studied by some organizations (see Chapter 29 for additional information) [24], and the use of artificial intelligence to improve healthcare outcomes at a financially sustainable cost is now being demonstrated [25].

Historically, only the direct costs to providers or payors of healthcare have been included in value calculations; however, patient-centered care demands that the direct and indirect costs incurred by the patient and their family be included in the value calculation of healthcare delivered and those assessing the financial benefit of ICU follow-up clinics. Table 30.3 provides examples of direct and indirect costs which may accrue to each stakeholder.

Rather than a need for care process or study standardization, this variability demands the need for critical reflection on multiple topics. The most pressing issues to address include: how metrics are chosen to represent "cost" and "quality," whose perspective is included in developing and choosing said metrics, how cost and quality are calculated and reported, how clinics are designed and optimally staffed to meet the needs of the local population, what time period is under study, and how financial siloes can be nullified.

Pragmatic Considerations: Making the Financial Case for an ICU Follow-Up Clinic

Using the principles of value-based health care and population health management and integrating the identified concerns above, the following are suggestions to design, implement, and increase the presence and accessibility of ICU follow-up clinics.

1. Recruit a financial champion to the ICU follow-up clinic leadership team. The constantly changing rules and regulations for population health management, coding, billing and payment, revenue sources, and variations in laws regarding the ability of non-physicians to bill, require a full-time financial specialist who can update clinicians on these concerns at the national, state, and local health system levels. Table 30.4 provides a list of possible billing codes that may be appropriate for an ICU follow-up clinic.
2. Recruit somebody with knowledge of the strategic priorities with respect to managing population health within the organization. They should identify items of value to the

Table 30.3 Direct and indirect costs by stakeholder to consider in the value-based healthcare value equation denominator: value = quality/cost

Stakeholder	Direct Cost(s)	Indirect Cost(s)
Patients	Out-of-pocket payments per insurance benefit contract (premium payments for insurance, deductibles, co-pays and co-insurance).	Reduction in employment income for patients because of hospitalization and recovery, or need to retrain for employment due to newly acquired temporary or permanent disability that prevents return to prior occupation.
Members of patient household	Out-of-pocket expenses for healthcare items needed to recover but not covered by insurance, (e.g., bandages, ointments, lotions).	Reduction in employment income for family or household members caring for patient.
Members of patient family	Cost of travel to acquire care	Loss of career advancement opportunities while not working or due to newly acquired temporary or permanent disability for patient.
		Loss of career advancement opportunities while not working for family/household members caring for patient.
		Loss of mentoring for patient or family/household members while not working.
		Cost associated with loss of home/homelessness or need to move to a different home due to newly acquired/permanent disability, medical expenses, and/or loss of income.
		Cost of modifying the current home to allow patient with newly acquired temporary or permanent disability to remain in the home.
		Bankruptcy caused by medical expenses.

Table 30.3 (cont.)

Stakeholder	Direct Cost(s)	Indirect Cost(s)
Providers – privately owned practices, group practices, health system-owned practices, health systems facilities, non-physician providers eligible to receive payments for care delivered.	Staff Pharmaceuticals Durable medical equipment Consumable medical supplies	Infrastructure costs Technology planning and acquisition costs
Payors of healthcare – private insurance companies, Medicare, Medicaid, advocacy groups who raise funds for patient care and/or medical research for various diagnoses or patient populations, philanthropic sources.	Payouts per contractual obligations with patients, ACOs, or providers.	Avoidable cost due to inefficient or ineffective healthcare processes.
Employers of patient/families/household members	Cost to replace employee temporarily (i.e., while out on disability) or permanently (i.e., if unable to return to work).	Cost of lost productivity of the company due to employee out on medical leave or due to ramp up time for new employee to be trained.
Payors of disability insurance benefits	Cost of payments to disabled patient as per contractual obligations.	Cost of avoidable prolonged payments to disabled survivor of critical illness due to inefficient or ineffective ICU follow-up care process which prolong recovery time.

Table 30.4 Current Procedural Technology (CPT)® codes that may be appropriate for ICU follow-up clinic billing. Consult your coding and billing manager for guidance on which codes are appropriate for your clinic and www.cms.gov/medicare/coding-billing/healthcare-common-procedure-system for further information on the Healthcare Common Procedure Coding System (HCPCS).

CPT Code	Care Delivered	Notes
99205	Evaluation/Management (E/M) new patient, level 5	-
99215	E/M established patient, level 5	-
G2212	Per each 15-minute block above established maximum time for above two codes	Prolonged code for Medicare, Medicaid, and Medicare Advantage plans
99417	Per each 15-minute block above established maximum time for above two codes	Prolonged code for all other insurance plans
99495	Transition of care (TOC) moderate visit within 14 days	-
99496	TOC advanced visit within 7 days	-
Modifier 93	Audio only telemedicine visit	-
Modifier 95	Audio-visual telemedicine visit	-
94010	Spirometry, when performed	-
99417	Prolonged goals of care discussion	-
99406	3–10 minutes tobacco counseling, if provided	-
99407	10+ minutes tobacco counseling, if provided	-
96160	Administration of health risk assessment	A range of assessments may qualify
Z23	Vaccine given during encounter	A secondary code to the code for the diagnosis which is the indication for the vaccine
Vaccine product billing code	Varies with vaccine product, needs to be included with Z23	-

organization and the major payors for the organization's services. They should also help craft a care process that optimizes concordance with the organization's strategic priorities, leverages the existing population health management infrastructure, and ensures that pre-existing transitions of care processes are integrated into the process designed.
3. Identify sources of funding to support the follow-up clinic. If highly trained (i.e., expensive to employ) providers are utilized, the cost of staffing the clinic may exceed the revenue generated by the clinic's billing and collections, while if less trained providers

are used, the clinic may lack the expertise required to deliver high-value healthcare. This reality underscores why a value-based approach is key in gaining the financial support for an ICU follow-up clinic and why metrics other than billing, revenue, and relative value units (RVUs) need to be integrated into the value assessment. Internal and external research funds, quality improvement funds, health system endowments, and diagnosis-specific advocacy group grants are all possible funding sources. Providing data regarding the value of the ICU follow-up clinic may enhance the possibility of negotiating with payors for contracts to deliver ICU follow-up care.

4. Develop a data collection and management system for the clinic. How will value and cost data be captured? What metrics are considered valuable by patients and their families, providers, the organization, and the payor mix? What data should be collected and analyzed to support the value metrics you intend to use? How will dollar values be assigned to items of value not traditionally associated with a specific dollar amount? For instance, consider the negative financial impact of a preventable readmission on revenue generation for the hospital, in which an occupied bed by a disallowed readmission generates no revenue to offset cost incurred to provide care and simultaneously prevents the bed from being occupied by a patient for whom revenue can be collected. How will information be collected on the cost of care incurred by the clinic versus the cost of current usual care delivered to survivors of critical illness by the organization? Think about creating a population health dashboard to compare care and costs for survivors of critical illness enrolled in the clinic versus those who are not.

5. Identify the financial siloes that exist within the organization and address them in a strategic plan for the clinic. If the billing will be bundled to the Critical Care Department to promote patient uptake of the clinic but providers from other departments are used to staff the clinic, how will those departments be made financially whole? Is there an opportunity, given local system priorities and goals, to argue for support for the clinic from the perspective of revenue loss management?

6. Consider if the clinic will occur in a discrete clinic location or if it will be a more diffuse care process not tied to a single physical space. While it might be intellectually appealing to have a discrete clinic space with all needed disciplines present simultaneously, it may not be pragmatic from staffing, space availability, patient throughput, or cost versus revenue perspectives.

7. Understand that the majority of ICU follow-up care is delivered by outpatient primary care providers (PCPs), which is likely to always be the case, both from cost of care and patient preference perspectives. How can those providers be captured to improve ICU follow-up care and what are the anticipated costs of attempting to make that capture?

8. Consider the use of telemedicine as a component of the clinic. What is the cost of the telemedicine infrastructure used to deliver care? Does it currently exist at the organization, and does it have the capacity to add on an ICU follow-up clinic? What reimbursement will be attained from telemedicine visits? Does the organization have a home-based program, and could early follow-up be provided via a home visit with a nurse or community health worker supervised by the clinic provider via telemedicine?

9. Identify the care elements that should be included in the clinic. What experts will the clinic employ and how will they be recruited if not currently available? What will be the impact on the home departments of any providers included in the clinic? What is the right balance between the skill of the provider, the cost of their time, and the

potential revenue generated by their activities? Will bills be bundled under one provider or will services rendered by each provider be billed separately?
10. Consider the socioeconomic limitations faced by survivors of critical illness. Is there value in attempting to mitigate the costs of local barriers, like transportation, as the design and cost of the clinic are considered?

Areas for Future Study and Advocacy

In some complex diseases, there is evidence that the level of expertise attained by providers improves with the volume of care, leading to better patient clinical outcomes and decreases in the cost of care [26,27]. Likewise, there is literature suggesting that PCPs are inadequately trained and lack sufficient support services to care properly for complexly ill outpatients [28,29]. Taken together, and congruent with the notion that value is driven by provider experience, scale, and learning at the medical condition level, these ideas reinforce that team expertise is essential in clinically and financially efficacious care delivery for complex syndromes like PICS. This area would benefit from further research.

To be truly patient-centered in assessing the value of any care process for recovery from critical illness, future research should identify and quantify the direct and indirect costs to patients, their households, and their family units. These costs should then be included in the denominator of the value equation. Hidden costs to employers and society are similarly consequential and should be included in future research to better understand the broader financial impact of ICU follow-up clinics. Moreover, the time frame for assessing value in the current system is driven by mortality and 30-day hospital readmission rates, but physiological recovery from PICS can take as long as two years or more, if it occurs at all [30,31]. Further research and policy changes are needed to align the time frames for recovery from PICS and for assessing the value of care delivery models.

Currently existing financial silos in US healthcare between the components of the healthcare delivery system that bear the immediate direct cost of delivering ICU follow-up care versus the components of the healthcare delivery system that may benefit financially from these clinics need to be addressed both within individual healthcare systems as well as at the national policy level. For instance, development of an International Classification of Diseases tenth edition (ICD-10) code for PICS, similar to calls for an ICD-10 code for sepsis survivor aftercare, is needed to ensure adequate reimbursement to ICU follow-up clinics [32]. The application of behavioral economics to patients with PICS is another area of future study that may impact the financial considerations of ICU follow-up clinics and encourage survivors of critical illness with PICS to attend these clinics [33].

To optimize outcomes in survivors of critical illness, PCPs must be educated about PICS, including the needs for patient and family education about deficits and therapies, expectation management about the timeline for recovery, and high intensity follow-up that may be needed for a prolonged time. PCP practice managers must also be educated about PICS, with corresponding re-design of PCP clinic scheduling patterns to align expertise and provide adequate time to properly care for survivors of critical illness [13].

Conclusion

It would be premature to conclude that ICU follow-up clinics lack value, as suggested by some interpretations of the scant literature on the financial aspects of these clinics [20,21]. Although an ICU follow-up clinic may be a cost center in the healthcare system budget, it contributes significant items of value, including improved Medicare Five Star and patient satisfaction scores, operational excellence, customer service, and product value by virtue of saving lives and reducing readmissions. If these aspects are combined with revenue generated from patient care billing and cost savings to insurers attained through decreased readmission rates, ICU follow-up clinics are a smart choice for health system leadership and ACOs to include in the services offered to this patient population.

Key Points

1. Value-based healthcare models should be used to develop and value ICU follow-up clinics.
2. Population health methodology should be incorporated into models of ICU survivor care.
3. Value *for patients* rather than to providers or payors should be the key driver of value.
4. Financial silos in US healthcare need to be neutralized.
5. All types of cost for all stakeholders in cost modeling and accounting need to be included in valuations of ICU follow-up clinics.

References

1. N.I. Lone, M.A. Gillies, C. Haddow, et al. Five-year mortality and hospital costs associated with surviving intensive care. *Am J Respir Crit Care Med* 2016; **194**(2): 109–208.
2. I. van Beusekom, F. Bakhshi-Raiez, N.F. de Keizer, et al. Health costs of ICU survivors are higher before and after ICU admission compared to a population-based control group: a descriptive study combining healthcare insurance data and data from a Dutch national quality registry. *J Crit Care* 2018; **44**: 345–51.
3. A.N. Chalupka and D. Talmor. The economics of sepsis. *Crit Care Clin* 2012; **28**: 57–76.
4. B. Tiru, E.K. DiNino, A. Orenstein, et al. The economic and humanistic burden of severe sepsis. *PharmacoEconomics* 2015: **33**: 925–37.
5. A.P. Ruhl, M. Huang, E. Colantuoni, et al. Healthcare utilization and costs in ARDS survivors: a 1-year longitudinal national US multicenter study. *Int Care Med* 2017; **43**: 980–91.
6. M.E. Porter and E.O. Teisburg. *Redefining Health Care: Creating Value-Based Competition on Results*. Boston: Harvard Business School Press; 2006.
7. M. Young and M.A. Smith. Standards and evaluation of healthcare quality, safety and person-centered care. [Updated 2022 Dec 13]. In: StatPearls [Internet]. Treasure Island (FL): StatPearls Publishing; 2024 Jan–. www.ncbi.nlm.nih.gov/books/NBK576432/# (Accessed November 4, 2024.)
8. K.H. Ken Lee, J.M. Austin, P.J. Pronovost. Developing a measure of value in health care. *Value Health* 2016; **19**(4): 323–5.
9. Centers for Medicare and Medicaid Services. What are the value-based programs? www.cms.gov/medicare/quality/value-based-programs (Accessed November 11, 2024.)
10. Centers for Medicare and Medicaid Services. Key Concepts. www.cms.gov/priorities/innovation/key-concepts (Accessed October 26, 2024.)
11. University of Minnesota Online. https://online.umn.edu/story/population-health-what-it-why-it-important (Accessed October 31, 2024.)

12. J. McPeake, L.M. Boehm, E. Hibbert, et al. Key components of ICU recovery programs: what did patients report provided benefit? *Crit Care Explor* 2020; **2**(4): e0088.
13. K.P. Snell, C.L. Beiter, E.L. Hall, et al. A novel approach to ICU survivor care: a population health quality improvement project. *Crit Care Med* 2020; **48**(12): e1164–e1170.
14. K.A. Korzick, unpublished data, manuscript in development. Geisinger ICU survivor clinic impact on mortality and readmission rates compared to usual care, a three-year cohort experience, 2024.
15. J.F. Jensen, T. Thomsen, D. Overgaard, et al. Impact of follow-up consultations for ICU survivors on post-ICU syndrome: a systematic review and meta-analysis. *Int Care Med* 2015; **41**: 763–75.
16. S. Lasiter, S.K. Oles, J. Mundell, et al. Critical care follow-up clinics, a scoping review of interventions and outcomes. *Clin Nurse Spec* 2016; **30**(4): 227–37.
17. A.E. Turnbull, A. Rabiee, W.E. Davis, et al. Outcome measurement in ICU survivorship research from 1970–2013: a scoping review of 425 publications. *Crit Care Med* 2016; **44**(7): 1267–77.
18. O.J. Schofield-Robinson, S.R. Lewis, J. McPeake, et al. Follow-up services for improving long-term outcomes in intensive care unit (ICU) survivors (review). *Cochrane Database Syst Rev* 2018; **11**: 1–69.
19. B.H. Cuthbertson, J. Rattray, M.K. Campbell, et al. The PRaCTICaL study of nurse led, intensive care follow-up programmes for improving long term outcomes from critical illness: a pragmatic randomized controlled trial. *BMJ* 2009; **339**: b3723.
20. R.A. Hernandez, D. Jenkinson, L. Vale, et al. Economic valuation of nurse-led intensive care follow-up programmes compared with standard care: the PRaCTICaL trial. *Eur J Health Econ* 2014; **15**: 243–52.
21. X. Willaert, B.K.T. Vijayaraghavan, B.H. Cutherbertson. Cost-effectiveness of Post-intensive Care Clinics. In: J. Preiser, M. Herridge, E. Azoulay, eds. *Post-Intensive Care Syndrome*. Springer e-book 2020, 367–77.
22. V. Danesh, L.M. Boehm, T.L. Eaton, et al. Characteristics of post-ICU and post-COVID recovery clinics in 29 U.S. health systems. *Crit Care Explor* 2022; **4**(3): e0658.
23. C. Andrilla, A. Holly, G. Davis, et al. Geographic variation in the supply of selected behavioral health providers. *Am J Prev Med* 2018; **54**(6, Supplement 3): S199–207.
24. M.A. Kovaleva, A.C. Jones, C.C. Kimpel, et al. Patient and caregiver experiences with a telemedicine intensive care unit recovery clinic. *Heart Lung* 2023; **58**: 47–53.
25. A. Kasyanau. Balancing the cost of AI in healthcare: future savings vs. current spending. Forbes. www.forbes.com/sites/cognizant/2024/10/16/the-ai-revolution-when-is-it-going-to-really-arrive/? (Accessed November 11, 2024.)
26. K. Slicker, W.G. Lane, O.O. Oyetayo, et al. Daily cardiac catheterization procedural volume and complications at an academic medical center. *Cardiovasc Diagn Ther* 2016; **6**(5): 446–52.
27. S.O. Cawich, D.A. Thomas, N.W. Pearce, et al. Whipple's pancreaticoduodenectomy at a resource-poor, low-volume center in Trinidad and Tobago. *World J Clin Oncol* 2022; **13**(9): 738–47.
28. T. Bodenheimer, E. Chen, H.D. Bennett. Confronting the growing burden of chronic disease: can the U.S. health care workforce do the job? *Health Affairs* 2009; **28**(1): 64–74.
29. D.F. Loeb, E.A. Bayliss, C. Candrian, et al. Primary care providers' experiences caring for complex patients in primary care: a qualitative study. *BMC Fam Prac* 2016; **17**:34.
30. A.M. Cheun, C.M. Tansey, G. Tomlinson, et al. Two-year outcomes, health care use, and costs of survivors of acute respiratory distress syndrome. *Am J Respir Crit Care Med* 2006; **174**: 538–44.

31. M.S. Herridge, C.M. Tansey, G. Tomlinson et al. Functional disability 5 years after acute respiratory distress syndrome. *N Engl J Med* 2011; **364**(14): 1293–304.

32. S. Oh, M.E. Mikkelson, M. O'Connor, et al. Why sepsis survivors need an ICD-10 code for "sepsis aftercare." *Chest* 2022; **162**(5): 979–81.

33. L.L. Chang, A.D. DeVore, B.B. Granger, et al. Leveraging behavioral economics to improve heart failure care and outcomes. *Circulation* 2017; **136**: 765–72.

Chapter 31

Best Practices for Interprofessional Teams

Aysar Al-Husseini, Deepali Dixit, and Sugeet Jagpal

What Is Currently Being Taught

Interprofessional teamwork is critical in healthcare to address complex patient needs and deliver safe, efficient, and patient-centered care [1,2]. As a result, developing and teaching teamwork skills among healthcare professionals have become increasingly essential in educational curricula and professional development programs [1,2].

Interprofessional education initiatives aim to equip healthcare professionals with skills necessary for collaborative practice, such as teamwork, communication, and mutual respect. Health professions curricula include various topics devoted to working in interprofessional teams, including understanding professional roles and responsibilities, effective communication strategies, conflict resolution techniques, shared decision-making, and collaborative problem-solving [3]. The curricular content also emphasizes the significance of cultural competence, ethical considerations, and patient-centered care in interprofessional teamwork [3]. Educators use various teaching methods to facilitate the learning of teamwork in interprofessional teams. These methods may include didactic lectures, case-based discussions, interactive scenarios, and experiential learning activities. In particular, interprofessional simulations provide opportunities for students to practice their teamwork skills in realistic clinical scenarios, which helps foster collaboration and communication among different healthcare disciplines [3,4].

Three well-known frameworks have been used in healthcare to improve training in teamwork: High-Reliability Organizations (HRO), the Sunnybrook Framework, and TeamSTEPPS (Team Strategies and Tools to Enhance Performance and Patient Safety). Enacting any of these frameworks can help create a safety culture, enhance communication and teamwork dynamics, and ultimately improve the quality of patient care [5].

The concept of the HRO, which emphasizes managing complex systems with a high potential for catastrophic failures, originated from the aviation and nuclear power industries. In healthcare, HRO principles focus on developing a culture of safety, mindfulness, and continuous learning to prevent errors and adverse events. The HRO principles that apply to interprofessional teamwork include preoccupation with failure, reluctance to simplify interpretations, sensitivity to operations, commitment to resilience, and deference to expertise. By adopting these principles, healthcare organizations can promote a proactive approach to risk management, encourage open communication, and improve situational awareness among team members [6,7,8].

The Sunnybrook Framework is a model developed by the Sunnybrook Health Sciences Centre in Toronto, Canada, to guide the integration of interprofessional collaboration into clinical practice by providing a structured approach to enhance teamwork dynamics and foster a culture of collaboration among healthcare professionals [9]. This model focuses on four core elements: patient and family engagement, team effectiveness, communication, and interprofessional education. The aim of this framework is to promote patient-centered care and shared decision-making through interdisciplinary teamwork, ultimately enhancing the quality and safety of healthcare delivery.

TeamSTEPPS is an evidence-based teamwork system developed by the Agency for Healthcare Research and Quality (AHRQ) with the aim of improving communication and teamwork skills among healthcare professionals [5]. It offers a comprehensive set of tools, strategies, and training modules designed to enhance team effectiveness, facilitate collaboration, foster mutual respect, and optimize patient outcomes.

Integrating HRO, the Sunnybrook Framework, or TeamSTEPPS into interprofessional teamwork within healthcare settings can yield numerous benefits. First, these shared models foster a culture of safety and continuous improvement, encouraging healthcare professionals to anticipate and mitigate potential risks. Second, by emphasizing effective communication, mutual support, and situational awareness, these frameworks enhance teamwork processes and reduce the likelihood of errors. Additionally, the patient-centered approach advocated by the Sunnybrook Framework promotes collaborative decision-making and enhances patient satisfaction [9].

Training healthcare workers and students to work effectively in interprofessional teams is crucial for promoting collaborative practice within healthcare organizations. The HRO, Sunnybrook Framework, and TeamSTEPPS are three highly effective platforms that offer valuable insights and strategies for enhancing interprofessional teamwork. By integrating these models into organizational policies, training programs, and clinical practice, healthcare organizations can foster a culture of safety, improve communication and coordination among healthcare professionals, and ultimately enhance patient outcomes.

What Is Currently Being Researched

Research on healthcare teams is important because the quality of teamwork is directly associated with the quality and safety of care [10]. Although the frameworks for interdisciplinary care presented above (HRO, Sunnybrook, and TeamSTEPPS) are well known in healthcare, social scientists and anthropologists look at healthcare teamwork through a different lens. Their insights are important, as they could impact future training frameworks. As stated above, various techniques to educate teams (including simulation) are being used based on the currently accepted frameworks; if our understanding of healthcare team function changes over time, the current curricula may need to be modified.

Some research demonstrates that teamwork and communication challenges in healthcare are indicative of coordination neglect in organizational systems. Coordination neglect is defined by cognitive scientists as an individual's incomplete understanding of organizational structure, leading to a lack of integration of that individual's goals and actions into the organization as a whole [11]. To address coordination neglect, organizations must solve two challenges: motivate individuals so that their goals are aligned (the agency problem), and organize individuals so that their actions are aligned (the coordination problem). Accordingly, training healthcare team members outside of the context of their current organization is unlikely to be successful; even if the team members' goals are naturally aligned at a high level (e.g., providing high-quality patient care), they can be unsuccessful in the organization if their actions are not aligned with the organization's endeavors at a granular level.

Serendipitously, this interest in teams as focal units for research coincided with rising interest in multilevel theory (MLT) [12]. MLT focuses on connecting the levels (often defined by disciplinary boundaries) that separate the science of organizations into micro- (individual), meso- (group or team), and macro- (organizational) levels of analysis. Because teams are at the micro-macro juncture, research has focused on the antecedents of team-work (i.e., team inputs), team member interactions (i.e., team processes), and effectiveness facets (i.e., team outputs) [13]. MLT offers a broader lens through which coordination neglect can be understood, and it also draws attention to the unique challenges faced by multiteam systems, such as in healthcare. Multiteam systems need to coordinate within the team (meso), between teams, and at organizational levels (macro) [14]. To add to the complexity, there are administrative and research teams in healthcare that clinical teams may not appreciate [14]. This has led to additional focus on "teams of teams" and how they function; as the science of teams evolves, healthcare stands to benefit from any break-throughs [14].

Another area of research in teams is leader and follower relations. It has been established that leader-follower relations allow for safe and effective patient care [15], and it has become increasingly common to have dyad or dual leadership structures in healthcare teams [14]. These leadership models unite a clinician co-leader and a leader from a complementary background (nonclinical) to lead a division or service line, enhancing coordination with the organization as a whole [14]. As the paradigm shifts from individual leaders to shared leadership, additional opportunities for future development of frameworks for training become available.

Researchers also suggest that having adaptive capacity, defined as the ability to coordinate activities under routine and novel conditions responding to situational change, needs to be further studied in healthcare teams [16]. This would first require observation in the natural environment and then integration of contextual influences into study designs [16]. Exploratory research designs could prove helpful with further data in this field.

How Can We Use the Above in the ICU and Post-ICU Settings?

The majority of teams research in healthcare focuses on co-located, hospital-based action teams (e.g., surgery teams, intensive care unit (ICU) teams, and emergency medicine teams), and although many of the research findings may generalize to outpatient teams, it is likely that outpatient teams need unique investigation [16]. The ICU is a clinical area that consistently has high acuity patients, variability in resource availability, and frequent and rapid changes in clinical team composition, particularly at academic medical centers. ICU teams have little temporal stability, with individual team members changing very frequently (e.g., nurses, respiratory therapists, and physician trainees), and unlike other teams with little temporal stability (e.g., code teams), the tasks assigned to the ICU team have a duration longer than the shift of any individual team member [17]. The persons fulfilling each position are expected to bring shared knowledge about caring for critically ill patients and shared expectations about their specific roles in the ICU [18], but the literature does not suggest unconditional mutual support and shared mental models [19].

Work on team function in the ICU indicates that the level of collaboration or conflict amongst the team fluctuates on the basis of six key catalysts: authority, education, patient needs, knowledge, resources, and time [20]. Research states that, in order to foster optimal team function, we need to understand the relationship and interactions between professionals, including between specialists such as the ICU team and external consultants [19]. Team collaboration is rooted in ownership and exchange of information and skills (i.e., commodities). Ownership is categorized as either individual or collective, and exchange of commodities can vary based on what is being exchanged (i.e., the pharmacist knows the optimal dose of a medication, while the nurse knows the optimal set up of the IV pump). These factors suggest that our understanding of teamwork must move beyond the rhetoric of cooperation towards a more authentic depiction of ownership and commodity exchange, while simultaneously acknowledging the often-competitive nature of teams. A salient example of this competitive nature is that collective ownership of a patient's clinical outcome is accepted by the ICU team as opposed to delegated to external consultant teams. Individual ownership is thought of as ownership by an individual or specific profession, such as the nursing role in sedation management, and it is not unusual for professions to strongly advocate for their ownership.

ICU follow-up clinics are largely multidisciplinary endeavors in which the interprofessional team from the ICU is "transplanted" to the outpatient setting, with preservation of the goal to provide the highest quality of care possible. It is reasonable to surmise that outpatient multidisciplinary teams would function similarly to inpatient teams but at a different pace. Being cognizant of perceptions of ownership of distinct components of clinical care and the rules for interacting with others from different professions will allow outpatient teams to deliver effective care. The aforementioned Sunnybrook Framework of interprofessional collaboration highlights core competencies that aid in team function: communication, interprofessional conflict resolution, shared decision-making, reflection, role clarification, and interprofessional values and ethics [21]. We suggest that role clarification is similar to the ownership concept proposed by Lingard and colleagues [20] and that shared decision-making occurs most beneficially when all professions take ownership over their areas of expertise.

All models for teamwork emphasize behavior-based competencies, as they are actionable, applicable, and can be embedded into evaluations [21]. Importantly, the Sunnybrook Framework is distinct in that it considers patients and families as part of both the team and the organizational culture [21]. This is an important consideration for outpatient work as well, and incorporation of patient and family feedback is critical to team reflection.

Key Points

1. There are various models currently being taught for health professions teamwork. The HRO, Sunnybrook Framework, and TeamSTEPPS are three highly effective platforms that offer valuable insights and strategies for enhancing interprofessional teamwork.
2. Social scientists and anthropologists look at healthcare teamwork through a different lens, and several current lines of research may change the models through which teamwork is taught in the future.

3. ICU follow-up clinics are largely multidisciplinary endeavors in which the interprofessional team from the ICU is "transplanted" to the outpatient setting, with preservation of the goal to provide the highest quality of care possible. Therefore, understanding the current landscape of teamwork research is useful for leaders of ICU follow-up clinics.

References

1. S. Reeves, L. Perrier, J. Goldman, D. Freeth, M. Zwarenstein. Interprofessional education: effects on professional practice and healthcare outcomes (update). *Cochrane Database Syst Rev* 2013; **2013**: CD002213.

2. J. Thistlethwaite. Interprofessional education: a review of context, learning and the research agenda. *Med Educ* 2012; **46**: 58–70.

3. H. Barr. Interprofessional education: the fourth focus. *J Interprof Care* 2007; **21** (Suppl 2): 40–50.

4. S. Reeves, M. Zwarenstein, J. Goldman, et al. The effectiveness of interprofessional education: key findings from a new systematic review. *J Interprof Care* 2010; **24**: 230–41.

5. H.B. King, J. Battles, D.P. Baker, et al. TeamSTEPPS(): Team Strategies and Tools to Enhance Performance and Patient Safety. In: K. Henriksen, J. B. Battles, M.A. Keyes, M.L. Grady (eds.), *Advances in Patient Safety: New Directions and Alternative Approaches* (Vol 3: Performance and Tools). Rockville, MD: Agency for Healthcare Research and Quality (US); 2008.

6. L. Melby, P.J. Toussaint. Coping with the unforeseen in surgical work. *Int J Med Inform* 2011; **80**: e39–47.

7. D.P. Baker, R. Day, E. Salas. Teamwork as an essential component of high-reliability organizations. *Health Serv Res* 2006; **41**: 1576–98.

8. D.P. Baker, S. Gustafson, J.M. Beaubien, et al. Medical team training programs in health care. In: K. Henriksen, J.B. Battles, E. S. Marks, D.I. Lewin (eds.), *Advances in Patient Safety: From Research to Implementation* (Volume 4: Programs, Tools, and Products). Rockville, MD: Agency for Healthcare Research and Quality (US); 2005.

9. E. McLaney, S. Morassaei, L. Hughes, et al. A framework for interprofessional team collaboration in a hospital setting: advancing team competencies and behaviours. *Healthc Manage Forum* 2022; **35**: 112–17.

10. L. Rosengarten. Teamwork in nursing: essential elements for practice. *Nurs Manag (Harrow)* 2019; **26**: 36–43.

11. C. Heath, N. Staudenmayer. Coordination neglect: how lay theories of organizing complicate coordination in organizations. *Research in Organizational Behavior* 2000; **22**: 153–91.

12. K.J. Klein. S.W.J. Kozlowski. *Multilevel theory, research, and methods in organizations: foundations, extensions, and new directions.* Hoboken, NJ: Pfeiffer; 2013.

13. S.W.J. Kozlowski. Enhancing the effectiveness of work groups and teams: a reflection. *Perspect Psychol Sci* 2018; **13**: 205–12.

14. D.J. Ingels, S.A. Zajac, M.P. Kilcullen, et al. Interprofessional teamwork in healthcare: observations and the road ahead. *J Interprof Care* 2023; **37**: 338–45.

15. M. Murphy, A. McCloughen, K. Curtis. The impact of simulated multidisciplinary trauma team training on team performance: a qualitative study. *Australas Emerg Care* 2019; **22**: 1–7.

16. J.E. Anderson, M. Lavelle, G. Reedy. Understanding adaptive teamwork in health care: progress and future directions. *J Health Serv Res Policy* 2021; **26**: 208–14.

17. J.N. Ervin, J.M. Kahn, T.R. Cohen, L. R. Weingart. Teamwork in the intensive care unit. *Am Psychol* 2018; **73**: 468–77.
18. J.A. Alexanian, S. Kitto, K.J. Rak, S. Reeves. Beyond the team: understanding interprofessional work in two north American ICUs. *Crit Care Med* 2015; **43**: 1880–6.
19. L. Lingard, S. Espin, C. Evans, L. Hawryluck. The rules of the game: interprofessional collaboration on the intensive care unit team. *Crit Care* 2004; **8**: R403–8.
20. L.A. Hawryluck, S.L. Espin, K.C. Garwood, et al. Pulling together and pushing apart: tides of tension in the ICU team. *Acad Med* 2002; **77**: S73–6.
21. M.D. Jensen, D.H. Ryan, C.M. Apovian, et al. 2013 AHA/ACC/TOS guideline for the management of overweight and obesity in adults: a report of the American College of Cardiology/American Heart Association Task Force on Practice Guidelines and The Obesity Society. *Circulation* 2014; **129**: S102–38.

Section 5   Diagnosis and Management of PICS

Chapter 32: Medication Management across the Continuum of Care

Joanna L. Stollings and Taylor J. Miller

Introduction

Critically ill patients require focused attention on medications both during and after their hospitalization to minimize medication-related problems, such as adverse drug effects, drug-drug interactions, and continuation of unnecessary therapies. Pharmacists are optimally positioned to provide comprehensive medication services to facilitate transitions of care from the intensive care unit (ICU) to the post-hospital setting [1].

Medication Management Strategies in the ICU

Certain medications used in the ICU are risk factors for the development of delirium, ICU-acquired weakness, and other untoward effects, and they may ultimately contribute to long-term physical and cognitive impairments in survivors of critical illness. Although a comprehensive review of the deleterious side effects of medication classes used in the ICU is beyond the scope of this chapter, we briefly highlight the potential impact of analgesic and sedating medications, neuromuscular blockers, corticosteroids, insulin, antipsychotics, and antimicrobials on outcomes in survivors of critical illness.

Analgesics, Sedating Medications, and Neuromuscular Blockade

The 2018 Clinical Practice Guidelines for the Prevention and Management of Pain, Agitation/Sedation, Delirium, Immobility, and Sleep Disruption in Adult Patients in the ICU (PADIS guidelines) published by the Society of Critical Care Medicine (SCCM) provide evidence-based recommendations for the prescription of analgesic and sedating medications. In patients requiring mechanical ventilation, analgesic medications should be administered prior to sedating medications (analgesia-first sedation or analgesia-based sedation), and for both categories of medication, bolus administration should precede initiation of continuous infusions [2]. The thoughtful use of medication to address pain and agitation dovetails with the remaining elements of the SCCM ABCDEF bundle (see Chapter 11 for additional information), increasing the likelihood of earlier extubation, minimizing the incidence of delirium, enhancing early mobilization, and promoting interaction with loved ones.

Opioids are associated with numerous adverse effects, including respiratory depression, constipation, and dependence, and they have been linked with both an increased and decreased risk of delirium [3,4,5,6]. Utilization of a protocol-based pain assessment and management program is important to minimize exposure to opioids and their attendant negative effects. This includes routine assessment of pain with validated tools, such as numeric pain scales in verbal patients and the Critical Care Pain Observation Tool or the

Behavioral Pain Scale in nonverbal patients, and thoughtful prescribing using multimodal therapy (i.e., incorporating acetaminophen, non-steroidal anti-inflammatory drugs, neuropathic pain medications, lidocaine, and ketamine into pain regimens) and non-pharmacological strategies to ensure the least amount of medication needed to adequately treat pain [7].

In mechanically ventilated patients, the PADIS guidelines recommend light sedation over deep sedation and the preferred use of either propofol or dexmedetomidine over benzodiazepines [2], which have been shown in numerous studies to increase delirium risk [3,8,9,10,11,12]. To decrease the likelihood of myopathy and ICU-acquired weakness, prolonged use of neuromuscular blockers in patients with severe acute respiratory failure should be minimized [13,14].

Corticosteroids and Insulin

Use of corticosteroids has been associated with the development of both delirium and ICU-acquired weakness, which increase the risk for long-term cognitive and physical impairments, respectively. In two separate studies of patients undergoing mechanical ventilation, use of systemic corticosteroids was found to be an independent risk factor for the development of delirium and to increase the risk of developing ICU-acquired weakness by a factor of 15 [14,15]. Furthermore, the absence of steroids during hospitalization was associated with better functional status at one year among patients with the acute respiratory distress syndrome (ARDS) [16]. Given their broad indications, corticosteroids need not be completely avoided, but limiting the dose and duration of therapy can help minimize the risk of developing long-term impairments.

Both intensive and relaxed glucose control have been linked with adverse cognitive and physical outcomes. A retrospective study of patients with ARDS found that a blood glucose value of 153.5 mg/dL or higher resulted in a nearly threefold greater chance of long-term cognitive impairment [17], while in another study, ICU patients who experienced at least one episode of hypoglycemia demonstrated higher cognitive impairment ($p<0.01$) [18]. In studies of surgical and medical ICU patients, intensive insulin therapy to maintain glucose < 110 mg/dL significantly decreased the incidence of critical illness polyneuropathy (CIP) and critical illness myopathy (CIM) [19,20]. SCCM guidelines suggest titrating insulin infusions to a blood glucose target range of 140–200 mg/dL to reduce the risk of hypoglycemia and its attendant consequences [21].

Antipsychotics and Antibiotics

Although antipsychotic medications are commonly prescribed in the ICU, the 2018 PADIS guidelines suggest against routinely using haloperidol or atypical antipsychotics to treat delirium [2]. A study comparing haloperidol, ziprasidone, and placebo for treating delirium in patients with acute respiratory failure or shock found no difference in the incidence of delirium, duration of mechanical ventilation, ICU or hospital lengths of stay, or mortality between the three groups [22]. While the risk of arrhythmia, extrapyramidal symptoms, and neuroleptic malignant syndrome is low, nearly one-fourth of ICU survivors in one evaluation were continued on an antipsychotic after hospitalization, increasing the possibility of long-term side effects [23]. These studies argue against using antipsychotics except in cases of severe agitation and highlight the importance of discontinuing these medications as soon as the indication has resolved.

The use of antimicrobials has also been associated with the development of delirium. In a cohort study of non-neurological critically ill adults, use of first- to third-generation cephalosporins was associated with transition to delirium, whereas penicillins, carbapenems, fluroquinolones, macrolides, or the fourth-generation cephalosporin cefepime were not associated with delirium [24]. In contrast, a prospective trial comparing cefepime and piperacillin-tazobactam suggested a lower rate of days alive and free of delirium and coma in patients treated with cefepime [25].

Medication Reconciliation at Transitions of Care

Medication reconciliation is the process of comparing a patient's current medication orders to a list of medications that the patient has been taking to evaluate for medication errors, including omissions, duplications, inappropriate continuation of medications no longer indicated, failure to resume chronic maintenance medications (e.g., to avoid withdrawal syndromes), dosing errors, or drug-drug interactions [26]. Medication reconciliation should be performed at all transitions of care, including hospital/ICU admission, discharge from the ICU, readmission to the ICU (if required), discharge from the hospital, and arrival at the post-acute care facility or home; lower rates of errors are found when pharmacists perform the reconciliation [27,28,29,30,31]. When performing medication reconciliation, pharmacists must additionally gauge patient (and family) understanding of the medications, ensure adherence, and determine any barriers to medication management. Given the frequency of delirium in hospitalized patients, involvement of the family in medication reconciliation at all transitions of care is key in obtaining the most accurate report [32].

Transitions of care are recognized as a frequent source of adverse drug events (ADEs) [33,34], which have been associated with increased hospital length of stay, healthcare expenditures, and mortality [35,36]. In response to the growing amount of data demonstrating medication errors at transitions of care, The Joint Commission on Accreditation of Healthcare Organizations has consistently emphasized the importance of maintaining and communicating accurate medication information as a part of their National Patient Safety Goals.

Failure to Discontinue Medications Started in the ICU at Discharge

Continuation of medications initiated in the ICU at the time of ICU or hospital discharge, even though they may no longer be indicated or appropriate, has been frequently described. In a single-center study of elderly survivors of critical illness, potentially inappropriate medications (PIMs), as defined by Beers criteria, were frequently identified, with 36% deemed to be actually inappropriate medications by an interprofessional team. At hospital discharge, the medication categories with the highest positive predictive values for being actually inappropriate medications were anticholinergics (55%), non-benzodiazepine hypnotics (67%), benzodiazepines (67%), atypical antipsychotics (71%), and muscle relaxants (100%), and nearly two-thirds of these medications were started in the ICU [37].

Failure to stop medications once no longer indicated can increase the potential for ADEs and drug-drug interactions. For example, in one study, prescriptions for new sedative agents at hospital discharge were identified in one in 15 sedative-naïve older adults following ICU admission, with more than half filling prescriptions serially [38], a factor linked with more than a twofold increase in risk of falls and healthcare resource utilization [39]. Many studies have documented the inappropriate continuation of acid suppressive therapy at hospital discharge [40,41,42,43]; numerous acute and chronic complications have been associated with persistent acid suppressive therapy, including *Clostridium difficile* infection, pneumonia, hip fracture, and dementia [44,45,46,47,48].

Failure to Initiate Home Medications During Admission

Along with the inappropriate continuation of medications without indication at hospital discharge, practitioners often fail to continue maintenance medications for chronic conditions when patients are admitted to the hospital. A Canadian cohort study of 396,380 elderly patients evaluated inpatient and outpatient records for medications prescribed from at least one of the five following groups: statins, antiplatelet or anticoagulant agents, levothyroxine, respiratory inhalers, and gastric acid-suppressing drugs [49]. Compared to patients who were hospitalized without an ICU stay, there was a higher risk of medications not being restarted in all medication groups except for respiratory inhalers in patients hospitalized with an ICU admission. The composite risk of death, hospitalization, and emergency department visits up to one year after hospital discharge was found to be significantly higher in patients in which a statin, antiplatelet, or anticoagulant was unintentionally discontinued. Attention to chronic medications and continuation of necessary maintenance therapy as soon as it is safe to do so is an important responsibility for physicians and pharmacists.

Polypharmacy and Deprescribing

Polypharmacy is typically defined as the use of five or more medications, and although sometimes required in medically complex patients, polypharmacy increases the risk of adverse health outcomes, particularly in older adults. Elderly patients with cognitive impairment or low health literacy [50] or patients with polypharmacy are at high risk for ADEs during transitions of care [33], and ADEs related to polypharmacy are often implicated in sustaining traumas and hospital readmissions. The number of medications a patient is taking has been shown to be a risk factor for drug-drug interactions [51], delirium [52], and increased mortality in the elderly [53].

"Deprescribing" is defined as tapering or discontinuing medications to reduce polypharmacy and theoretically improve patient outcomes; it should be performed in consultation with a pharmacist at transitions of care, including the transitions from ICU to ward and from hospital to home. The following five-step protocol for deprescribing has been recommended:

(1) Determine that each medication has an appropriate indication
(2) When determining the number of medications that should be discontinued, the overall potential harm of the medications should be considered
(3) Determine if each individual drug should be discontinued
(4) Prioritize which medications should be discontinued first
(5) Start and monitor a drug discontinuation plan.

Deprescribing at the time of ICU discharge should focus on medications initiated in the ICU that may no longer be indicated and that have the highest risk of adverse events, including benzodiazepines, anticholinergics, and antipsychotics. If newly prescribed medications are still required, a clear plan for discontinuation should ideally be discussed with the provider assuming care, the patient, and the family. When inpatient providers consider deprescribing chronic medications, collaboration with primary care providers can be helpful in understanding the reason the medication was initiated, determining whether it has an ongoing indication, and building consensus on a safe strategy for deprescribing.

Discharge Counseling

Following hospital discharge, up to 20% of patients experience an adverse event, with approximately 60% being related to a medication and deemed to be preventable [54,55,56]. These adverse events have been linked to emergency department visits, hospital admissions, and increased healthcare utilization and expenditures [57,58,59,60]. Given the number of medication changes that occur during hospitalization, particularly hospitalizations that require critical care, many patients and their families may not fully understand what medications the patient should be taking at home, highlighting the critical role of medication counseling at the time of hospital discharge. In one evaluation of patients' medication knowledge, less than 60% of patients understood the indications for their new medications at the time of hospital discharge, and only 12% knew possible side effects [61].

Discharge counseling on medications is an important patient safety initiative, and given their expertise, pharmacists are best positioned to provide discharge counseling. A study found that all pharmacists surveyed considered medication counseling at the time of discharge helpful in improving patient knowledge of their medication regimen [32]. Discharge medication reconciliation performed by pharmacists is cost effective [62], improves patient satisfaction, and increases medication adherence [63], but its impact on hospital readmission rates has not been consistently demonstrated [57,64,65,66,67].

Discharge medication counseling should include the following: a plan for filling medications, troubleshooting anticipated barriers to adherence, utilization of adherence aids such as a pill box, and a teach-back approach to verify understanding. Family presence during discharge counseling is imperative and has been reported to be helpful by pharmacists [32]. A study seeking to identify predictors of medication nonadherence in patients who had received discharge medication counseling by a pharmacist found that patients who lived alone, who were discharged on more than 10 medications, or who had lower incomes were more likely to be nonadherent [68].

Pharmacists in ICU Follow-Up Clinics

Pharmacists are an important member of the multidisciplinary team caring for patients with post-intensive care syndrome (PICS) in ICU follow-up clinics. While individual responsibilities may vary depending on specific population needs, pharmacists are well-positioned to provide comprehensive medication reconciliation and immunization reviews as well as screening for PIMs, drug-drug interactions, ADEs, nonadherence, and untreated or undertreated conditions (see Tables 32.1 and 32.2). Additionally, pharmacists can utilize interactions in ICU follow-up clinics to provide focused medication education and counseling to patients and their loved ones, which may be difficult to provide in the inpatient setting. Pharmacists can also have an impact in connecting patients to available resources to assist with medication access and affordability (see Box 32.1). A suggested template for pharmacist workflow can be found in Box 32.2.

Medication-related problems detected by pharmacists in ICU follow-up clinics are common and often considered severe (see Table 32.1). In a single-center evaluation of 47 patients cared for in an ICU follow-up clinic, 81% of patients were found to have

Table 32.1 Summary of pharmacists' interventions in ICU recovery centers

Citation	Population	Outcomes
Stollings et al. [70]	56 patients seen in a PICS Clinic	• Median of 4 medication interventions per patient • Medication discontinuation in 39% of patients and initiation in 32% of patients • ADE in 16% of patients • 18 ADE preventative measures were implemented • Influenza vaccine administration in 23% of patients and pneumococcal vaccine administration in 4% of patients
MacTavish et al. [74]	47 patients seen in a PICS Clinic [Intensive Care Syndrome: Promoting Independence and Return to Employment (InS:PIRE)] 5-week rehabilitation program for ICU survivors assessing medication related problems (single-center)	• 69 MRP identified in 81% of patients • Drug omissions identified in 29% of patients • Dose adjustments made in 19% of patients • Treatment duration clarification in 17% of patients • 64% of MRP were deemed severe • 55% were not aware of any medication changes at discharge • 60% of patients vocalized concerns to the PharmD regarding their medications • Drug classes requiring the most intervention included CV (26%), analgesics (22%), and respiratory (10%)
MacTavish et al. [75]	183 patients seen in InS:PIRE (Multicenter)	• 62.8% of patients requiring ≥ 1 intervention • Treatment duration clarification occurred 44 times • Counseling occurred 33 times • Drug omissions were identified 27 times • 171 clinically significant PharmD interventions were made • 27.4% increase in regular analgesia when comparing before ICU to PICS clinic visit • 16.3% increase in opioid use when comparing before ICU to PICS clinic visit
Bottom-Tanzer et al. [76]	82 surgical and trauma ICU survivors in PICS Clinic	• PharmD performed medication reconciliations on 96.5% of visits with 94.6% having 1 or more actionable change • 116 interventions were performed by the PharmD, with 19 dose adjustments, 23 medication initiations, 27 medication discontinuations, and 47 counseling sessions

MacTavish et al. [69]	78 COVID–19 survivors in PICS Clinic	• Full medication review in 78 patients • 29.5% of patients had previous medications discontinued which were never restarted after discharge • 32 CV medications were new or increased doses (50% anticoagulants, 16% antiarrhythmics, 25% statins/antihypertensives) • 37 CNS medications were new or increased doses (84% analgesics and 16% mental health/insomnia agents) • 23 (29.5%) patients required analgesics prior to hospitalization, which increased to 39 (50%) after discharge
Mohammad et al. [73]	52 control vs 52 intervention patients with sepsis, septic shock, and/or respiratory failure survivors in PICS Clinic	• 84 MRP in control vs 110 MRP identified in intervention group • Reduction in interventions and MRP from initial visit compared to follow up in intervention arm: 3.5 vs 2.4 • Most common drugs with MRP were neurologic and CV
Stollings et al. [71]	472 patients that received a full medication review in 12 ICU-RCs	• Pharmacy interventions made in 84% of patients • Median of 2 pharmacy interventions per patient • Medications were stopped in 26% of patients • Medications were started in 19% of patients • A dose was decreased in 11% of patients • A dose was increased in 9% of patients • There was no difference in the total number of medications that the patient was prescribed at the start and end of the patient visit • ADE preventive measures were implemented in 24% of patients • ADE events were identified in 15% of patients • Medication interactions were identified in 6% of patients

Abbreviations: ADE=Adverse drug event; CMM=Comprehensive medication management; CNS=Central nervous system; CV=Cardiovascular; ICU=Intensive care unit; MICU=Medical intensive care unit; MRP=Medication related problem; PharmD=Doctor of pharmacy; QI=Quality improvement; SAT=Spontaneous awakening trial; SBT=Spontaneous breathing trial

Table 32.2 Vaccine assessment recommendations for adults in an ICU recovery clinic

Vaccine	Criteria for Use
COVID–19	Unvaccinated: - 1 dose of updated Moderna or Pfizer-BioNTech vaccine - 2-dose series of updated Novovax at 0, 3–8 weeks Previously vaccinated with 1 or more doses of any COVID–19 vaccine: - 1 dose of any updated COVID–19 vaccine at least 8 weeks after the most recent COVID–19 vaccine dose
Influenza	Age 19+: 1 dose annually Age 65+: 1 dose annually of quadrivalent high-dose, recombinant, or quadrivalent adjuvanted influenza vaccines
Pneumococcal	Age 65+ or Age 19–64 with select underlying medical conditions or risk factors*: Not previously received a dose of PCV13, PCV15, or PCV20, or with unknown vaccination history: 1 dose PCV15 or PCV20 - If PCV15 used, administer 1 dose of PPSV23 at least 1 year after the PCV15 dose
RSV	Routine: Pregnant at 32–36 weeks from September through January Age 60+: based on shared decision-making, 1 dose RSV for persons at increased risk for severe RSV
Tdap or Td	1 dose Tdap then Td or Tdap booster every 10 years
Zoster	Age 50+: 2-dose recombinant zoster vaccine, 2–6 months apart

Source: CDC.gov/vaccines/schedules/index.html

Abbreviations: PCV=pneumococcal conjugate vaccine; PPSV=pneumococcal polysaccharide vaccine; RSV=Respiratory syncytial virus; Tdap=Tetanus, diphtheria, and pertussis; Td=Tetanus and diphtheria

*Underlying medical conditions or risk factors include alcoholism, chronic heart/liver/lung disease, chronic renal failure, cigarette smoking, cochlear implant, congenital or acquired asplenia, CSF leak, diabetes mellitus, generalized malignancy, HIV infection, Hodgkin disease, immunodeficiencies, iatrogenic immunosuppression, leukemia, lymphoma, multiple myeloma, nephrotic syndrome, solid organ transplant, or sickle cell disease or other hemoglobinopathies

Box 32.1 Case vignette

A 58-year-old man named Joe presents to the ICU follow-up clinic for his first visit after admission to the hospital for management of a traumatic subarachnoid hemorrhage. The initial 16-day hospital stay included nine days in the ICU and was complicated by hyperactive delirium as well as seizures. After hospital discharge, he spent 20 days in an inpatient rehabilitation hospital prior to his discharge to home.

The patient's medical history includes coronary artery disease, heart failure, hypertension, and atrial fibrillation. He reports adherence to his medication list as noted below and uses a pill box to assist with medication adherence. He is up-to-date on his scheduled vaccinations.

Medication List

Amiodarone 200 mg daily

Apixaban 5 mg twice daily

Atorvastatin 20 mg daily

Carvedilol 3.125 mg twice daily

Cholecalciferol 1000 units daily

Digoxin 250 mcg daily

Furosemide 40 mg daily

Melatonin 10 mg at bedtime

Omeprazole 20 mg daily

Sacubitril/Valsartan 24–26 mg twice daily

Phenytoin 100 mg twice daily

He reports that his medication list has been unchanged since discharge, but he expresses concern about being able to afford his apixaban and asks if the pharmacist has access to drug samples to get through the last month of the year. Additionally, he has questions about his new medications – omeprazole, melatonin, and phenytoin – that were started during his time in the ICU.

The pharmacist reviews his prescription coverage with the clinic social worker and determines that he would be eligible for a manufacturer assistance program that would reduce his monthly co-pay for apixaban to $10. The pharmacist provides the enrollment paperwork to the social worker for review and helps to get the patient enrolled in the assistance program to lower his monthly out-of-pocket expenses.

During the interview, the patient reports that he has never had a history of gastroesophageal reflux disease or related symptoms and has never experienced gastrointestinal bleeding. He was started on omeprazole to "protect his stomach" while in the hospital. He has never had difficulty sleeping, and he reports that since his hospitalization he often feels excessive drowsiness. A review of the medical records from hospitalization reveals that phenytoin was started for seizures.

The pharmacist recommends discontinuing omeprazole as it was only used for stress ulcer prophylaxis and is no longer indicated. Melatonin is suggested to be reduced to 3 mg and changed from scheduled use to as-needed only. Lastly, the pharmacist notes that a drug-drug interaction between the new phenytoin prescription and apixaban could result in increased metabolism of apixaban. A recommendation is made to discontinue the phenytoin and transition therapy to levetiracetam 500 mg twice daily.

> **Box 32.2** Pharmacist workflow example in an ICU recovery clinic
>
> 1. Review/reconcile medication list, comparing with patient/facility supplied medication list and hospital discharge summary.
> 2. Review each medication with the patient: drug, dose, frequency, indication.
> 3. Does the patient take any additional over-the-counter (OTC) medications/herbal supplements? If so, which?
> 4. How frequently does the patient take as needed (PRN) doses of medications?
> 5. Is the patient experiencing any side effects from medications?
> 6. Is the patient adherent to the prescribed medication regimen?
> 7. Does the patient use a pill box? If not, was one provided to the patient?
> 8. Is medication cost or any other barrier prohibiting obtaining medications?
> 9. Does the patient use one pharmacy?
> 10. Do any medications need to be discontinued?
> 11. Do any medications need to be started?
> 12. Do any medications need to be modified?
> 13. Does the patient need an influenza vaccination today?
>   ☐Yes ☐Already received ☐Not indicated ☐Declined
> 14. Does the patient need a pneumonia vaccination today?
>   ☐Yes ☐Already received ☐Not indicated ☐Declined
> 15. Does the patient need a shingles vaccination today?
>   ☐Yes ☐Already received ☐Not indicated ☐Declined
> 16. Does the patient need a COVID-19 vaccination today?
>   ☐Yes ☐Already received ☐Not indicated ☐Declined
> 17. Does the patient need a tetanus vaccination today?
>   ☐Yes ☐Already received ☐Not indicated ☐Declined

a medication-related problem, 64% of which were graded as severe [69]. A multisite study of more than 500 patients evaluated in ICU follow-up clinics demonstrated that over 80% of patients undergoing a comprehensive medication review required at least one intervention by a pharmacist, with 26% of patients having an inappropriate therapy discontinued [70]. Additionally, 19% of patients had new therapy initiated based on pharmacist recommendation, with commonly initiated therapies including anti-depressants, bronchodilators, and neuropathic pain agents [71]. Another study occurring over a three-year period demonstrated that 100% of patients receiving counseling from a pharmacist in an ICU follow-up clinic had at least one medication intervention, with the median number of interventions per patient being four [70]; interventions in addition to medication review and reconciliation included stopping inappropriate medication(s), starting new medication(s), identification of ADEs, and initiation of measures to prevent ADEs. Comprehensive medication review by pharmacists in an ICU follow-up clinic can help to minimize medication-related problems as well as limit the use of PIMs and other nonindicated therapies. In addition to identifying and addressing medication-related problems, pharmacists in an ICU follow-up clinic can also play an important role in the assessment of lingering impacts from the ICU stay, including pain, insomnia, and post-traumatic stress disorder [72,73].

Conclusion

As ICU survivorship continues to improve, diagnosis and treatment of PICS must also continue to improve, with proper medication management of patients with PICS a critical component of their care. Pharmacists are essential to ensure that in the ICU, during transitions of care, and following hospital discharge, medications are managed properly to prevent and treat PICS.

Key Points

1. Critically ill patients require focused attention on medications both during and after their hospitalization to minimize medication-related problems.
2. Medication reconciliation should be performed at all transitions of care, including hospital/ICU admission, discharge from the ICU, readmission to the ICU (if required), discharge from the hospital, and arrival at the post-acute care facility or home.
3. Deprescribing at the time of ICU discharge should focus on medications initiated in the ICU that may no longer be indicated and which have the highest risk of adverse events.
4. Medication-related problems detected by pharmacists in ICU follow-up clinics are common and often noted to be severe.

References

1. D.M. Needham, J. Davidson, H. Cohen, et al. Improving long-term outcomes after discharge from intensive care unit: report from a stakeholders' conference. *Crit Care Med* 2012; **40**(2): 502–9.
2. J.W. Devlin, Y. Skrobik, C. Gelinas, et al. Clinical practice guidelines for the prevention and management of pain, agitation/sedation, delirium, immobility, and sleep disruption in adult patients in the ICU. *Crit Care Med* 2018; **46**(9): 825–73.
3. P. Pandharipande, B.A. Cotton, A Shintani et al. Prevalence and risk factors for development of delirium in surgical and trauma intensive care unit patients. *J Trauma* 2008; **65**(1): 34–41.
4. M.J. Dubois, N. Bergeron, M. Dumont, et al. Delirium in an intensive care unit: a study of risk factors. *Intensive Care Med* 2001; **27**(8): 1297–304.
5. S. Ouimet, B.P. Kavanagh, S.B. Gottfried, et al. Incidence, risk factors and consequences of ICU delirium. *Intensive Care Med* 2007; **33**(1): 66–73.
6. B. Van Rompaey, M.M. Elseviers, M. J. Schuurmans, et al. Risk factors for delirium in intensive care patients: a prospective cohort study. *Crit Care* 2009; **13**(3): R77.
7. M.A. Pisani, T.E. Murphy, K.L. Araujo KL, et al. Benzodiazepine and opioid use and the duration of intensive care unit delirium in an older population. *Critical care medicine* 2009; **37**(1): 177–83.
8. V. Agarwal, P.J. O'Neill, B.A. Cotton, et al. Prevalence and risk factors for development of delirium in burn intensive care unit patients. *J Burn Care Res* 2010; **31**(5): 706–15.
9. P. Pandharipande, A. Shintani, J. Peterson, et al. Lorazepam is an independent risk factor for transitioning to delirium in intensive care unit patients. *Anesthesiology* 2006; **104**(1): 21–6.
10. B.B. Kamdar, T. Niessen, E. Colantuoni, et al. Delirium transitions in the medical ICU: exploring the role of sleep quality and other factors. *Crit Care Med* 2015; **43**(1): 135–41.

11. C.W. Seymour, J.M. Kahn, C.R. Cooke, et al. Prediction of critical illness during out-of-hospital emergency care. *JAMA* 2010, **304**(7): 747–54.

12. R.B. Serafim, M.F. Dutra, F. Saddy, et al. Delirium in postoperative nonventilated intensive care patients: risk factors and outcomes. *Ann Intensive Care* 2012; **2**: 51.

13. J.W. Leatherman, W.L. Fluegel, W. S. David, et al. Muscle weakness in mechanically ventilated patients with severe asthma. *Am J Respir Crit Care Med* 1996; **153**(5): 1686–90.

14. I.A. MacFarlane, F.D. Rosenthal. Severe myopathy after status asthmaticus. *Lancet* 1977; **2**(8038): 615.

15. B. De Jonghe, T. Sharshar, J.P. Lefaucheur, et al. Paresis acquired in the intensive care unit: a prospective multicenter study. *JAMA* 2002; **288**(22): 2859–67.

16. M.S. Herridge, A.M. Cheung, C.M. Tansey, et al. One-year outcomes in survivors of the acute respiratory distress syndrome. *N Engl J Med* 2003; **348**(8): 683–93.

17. R.O. Hopkins, M.R. Suchyta, G.L. Snow, et al. Blood glucose dysregulation and cognitive outcome in ARDS survivors. *Brain Inj* 2010; **24**(12): 1478–84.

18. T. Duning, I. van den Heuvel, A. Dickmann, et al. Hypoglycemia aggravates critical illness-induced neurocognitive dysfunction. *Diabetes Care* 2010; **33**(3): 639–44.

19. G. Van den Berghe, K. Schoonheydt, P. Becx, et al. Insulin therapy protects the central and peripheral nervous system of intensive care patients. *Neurology* 2005; **64**(8): 1348–53.

20. G. Hermans, A. Wilmer, W. Meersseman, et al. Impact of intensive insulin therapy on neuromuscular complications and ventilator dependency in the medical intensive care unit. *Am J Respir Crit Care Med* 2007; **175**(5): 480–9.

21. K. Honarmand, M. Sirimaturos, E. L. Hirshberg EL, et al. Society of Critical Care Medicine guidelines on glycemic control for critically ill children and adults 2024. *Crit Care Med* 2024; **52**(4): e161–e181.

22. T.D. Girard, M.C. Exline, S.S. Carson, et al. Haloperidol and ziprasidone for treatment of delirium in critical illness. *N Engl J Med* 2018; **379**(26): 2506–16.

23. J.E. Tomichek, J.L. Stollings, P. P. Pandharipande, et al. Antipsychotic prescribing patterns during and after critical illness: a prospective cohort study. *Crit Care* 2016; **20**(1): 378.

24. J.J. Grahl, J.L. Stollings, S. Rakhit, et. al. Antimicrobial exposure and the risk of delirium in critically ill patients. *Crit Care* 2018; **22**(1): 337.

25. E.T. Qian, J.D. Casey, A. Wright, et al. Cefepime vs piperacillin-tazobactam in adults hospitalized with acute infection: the ACORN randomized clinical trial. *JAMA* 2023; **330**(16): 1557–67.

26. Joint Commission on Accreditation of Healthcare Organizations, USA. Using medication reconciliation to prevent errors. *Sentinel Event Alert* 2006; **35**: 1–4.

27. T.A. Reeder, A. Mutnick. Pharmacist-versus physician-obtained medication histories. *Am J Health Syst Pharm* 2008; **65**(9): 857–60.

28. J.R. Pippins, T.K. Gandhi, C. Hamann, et al. Classifying and predicting errors of inpatient medication reconciliation. *J Gen Intern Med* 2008; **23**(9): 1414–22.

29. E. Patel, J.M. Pevnick, K.A. Kennelty. Pharmacists and medication reconciliation: a review of recent literature. *Integr Pharm Res Pract* 2019; **8**: 39–45.

30. E. Bajeux, L. Alix, L. Cornee, et al. Pharmacist-led medication reconciliation at patient discharge: a tool to reduce healthcare utilization? An observational study in patients 65 years or older. *BMC Geriatr* 2022; **22**(1): 576.

31. H. Studer, T.L. Imfeld-Isenegger, P. E. Beeler, et al. The impact of pharmacist-led medication reconciliation and interprofessional ward rounds on drug-related problems at hospital discharge. *Int J Clin Pharm* 2023; **45**(1): 117–25.

32. K.T. Haynes, A. Oberne, C. Cawthon, et al. Pharmacists' recommendations to improve

care transitions. *Ann Pharmacother* 2012; 46(9): 1152–9.

33. A.L. Hume, J. Kirwin, H.L. Bieber, et al. Improving care transitions: current practice and future opportunities for pharmacists. *Pharmacotherapy* 2012; 32 (11): e326–337.

34. A.J. Leendertse, A.C. Egberts, L.J. Stoker, et al. Frequency of and risk factors for preventable medication-related hospital admissions in the Netherlands. *Arch Intern Med* 2008; 168(17): 1890–6.

35. D.W. Bates, N. Spell, D.J. Cullen, et al. The costs of adverse drug events in hospitalized patients: adverse drug events prevention study group. *JAMA* 1997; 277(4): 307–11.

36. B.L. Hug, C. Keohane, D.L. Seger, et al. The costs of adverse drug events in community hospitals. *Jt Comm J Qual Patient Saf* 2012; 38(3): 120–6.

37. A. Morandi, E.E. Vasilevskis, P. P. Pandharipand, et al. Inappropriate medication prescriptions in elderly adults surviving an intensive care unit hospitalization. *J Am Geriatr Soc* 2013; 61: 1128–34.

38. L.D. Burry, C.M. Bell, A. Hill, et al. New and persistent sedative prescriptions among older adults following a critical illness: a population-based cohort study. *Chest* 2023; 163(6): 1425–36.

39. D.T. Amari, T Juday, F.H. Frech, et al. Falls, healthcare resources and costs in older adults with insomnia treated with zolpidem, trazodone, or benzodiazepines. *BMC Geriatr* 2022; 22: 1–12.

40. C.L. Tasaka, C. Burg, S.J. VanOsdol, et. al. An interprofessional approach to reducing the overutilization of stress ulcer prophylaxis in adult medical and surgical intensive care units. *Ann Pharmacother* 2014; 48(4): 462–9.

41. C.E. Murphy, A.M. Stevens, N. Ferrentino, et al. Frequency of inappropriate continuation of acid suppressive therapy after discharge in patients who began therapy in the surgical intensive care unit. *Pharmacotherapy* 2008; 28(8): 968–76.

42. A. Pavlov, R. Muravyev, Y. Amoateng-Adjepong, et al. Inappropriate discharge on bronchodilators and acid-blocking medications after ICU admission: importance of medication reconciliation. *Respir Care* 2014; 59(10): 1524–9.

43. S. Shin. Evaluation of costs accrued through inadvertent continuation of hospital-initiated proton pump inhibitor therapy for stress ulcer prophylaxis beyond hospital discharge: a retrospective chart review. *Ther Clin Risk Manag* 2015; 11: 649–57.

44. W. Gomm, K. von Holt, F. Thome, et al. Association of proton pump inhibitors with risk of dementia: a pharmacoepidemiological claims data analysis. *JAMA Neurol* 2016; 73(4): 410–16.

45. B. Lazarus, Y. Chen, F.P. Wilson, et al. Proton pump inhibitor use and the risk of chronic kidney disease. *JAMA Intern Med* 2016; 176(2): 238–46.

46. T.A. Miano, M.G. Reichert, T.T. Houle, et al. Nosocomial pneumonia risk and stress ulcer prophylaxis: a comparison of pantoprazole vs ranitidine in cardiothoracic surgery patients. *Chest* 2009; 136(2): 440–7.

47. H. Khalili, E.S. Huang, B.C. Jacobson, et al. Use of proton pump inhibitors and risk of hip fracture in relation to dietary and lifestyle factors: a prospective cohort study. *BMJ* 2012; 344: e372.

48. J.F. Barletta, D.A. Sclar. Proton pump inhibitors increase the risk for hospital-acquired Clostridium difficile infection in critically ill patients. *Crit Care* 2014; 18(6): 714.

49. C.M. Bell, S.S. Brener, N. Gunraj, et al. Association of ICU or hospital admission with unintentional discontinuation of medications for chronic diseases. *JAMA* 2011; 306(8): 840–7.

50. T.C. Davis, M.S. Wolf, P.F. Bass, et al. Literacy and misunderstanding prescription drug labels. *Ann Intern Med* 2006; 145(12): 887–94.

51. D.M. Qato, G.C. Alexander, R.M. Conti, et al. Use of prescription and over-the-counter medications and dietary

supplements among older adults in the United States. *JAMA* 2008; **300**(24): 2867–78.

52. S.K. Inouye, P.A. Charpentier. Precipitating factors for delirium in hospitalized elderly persons: predictive model and interrelationship with baseline vulnerability. *JAMA* 1996; **275**(11): 852–7.

53. J. Jyrkka, H. Enlund, M.J. Korhonen, et al. Polypharmacy status as an indicator of mortality in an elderly population. *Drugs Aging* 2009; **26**(12): 1039–48.

54. A.J. Forster, H.D. Clark, A. Menard, et al. Adverse events among medical patients after discharge from hospital. *Can Med Assoc J* 2004; **170**(3): 345–9.

55. A.J. Forster, H.J. Murff, J.F. Peterson, et al. The incidence and severity of adverse events affecting patients after discharge from the hospital. *Ann Int Med* 2003; **138**(3): 161–7.

56. M. Pirmohamed, S. James, S. Meakin, et al. Adverse drug reactions as cause of admission to hospital: admissions to ear, nose, and throat departments were not mentioned: reply. *Brit Med J* 2004; **329**(7463): 460.

57. B.W. Jack, V.K. Chetty, D. Anthony, et al. A reengineered hospital discharge program to decrease rehospitalization: a randomized trial. *Ann Intern Med* 2009; **150**(3): 178–87.

58. S.F. Jencks, M.V. Williams, E.A. Coleman. Rehospitalizations among patients in the Medicare Fee-for-Service Program. *N Engl J Med* 2009; **360**(14): 1418-22

59. B. Friedman, J. Basu. The rate and cost of hospital readmissions for preventable conditions. *Med Care Res Rev* 2004; **61**(2): 225–40.

60. R. Raschetti, M. Morgutti, F. Menniti-Ippolito, et al. Suspected adverse drug events requiring emergency department visits or hospital admissions. *Eur J Clin Pharmacol* 1999; **54**(12): 959–63.

61. H. Kerzman, O. Baron-Epel, O. Toren. What do discharged patients know about their medication? *Patient Educ Couns* 2005; **56**(3): 276–82.

62. C. Chinthammit, E.P. Armstrong, T. L. Warholak. A cost-effectiveness evaluation of hospital discharge counseling by pharmacists. *J Pharm Pract* 2012; **25**(2): 201–8.

63. P. Sarangarm, M.S. London, S.S. Snowden, et al. Impact of pharmacist discharge medication therapy counseling and disease state education: Pharmacist Assisting at Routine Medical Discharge (project PhARMD). *Am J Med Qual* 2013; **28**(4): 292–300.

64. S.A. Al-Rashed, D.J. Wright, N. Roebuck, et al. The value of inpatient pharmaceutical counselling to elderly patients prior to discharge. *Brit J Clin Pharmacol* 2002; **54**(6): 657–64.

65. M. Kilcup, D. Schultz, J.Carlson, et al. Postdischarge pharmacist medication reconciliation: impact on readmission rates and financial savings. *J Am Pharm Assoc* 2013; **53**(1): 78–84.

66. P.C. Walker, S.J. Bernstein, J.N. Jones, et al. Impact of a pharmacist-facilitated hospital discharge program: a quasi-experimental study. *Arch Intern Med* 2009; **169**(21): 2003–10.

67. R. Holland, J. Desborough, L. Goodyer, et al. Does pharmacist-led medication review help to reduce hospital admissions and deaths in older people? A systematic review and meta-analysis. *Brit J Clin Pharmacol* 2008; **65**(3): 303–16.

68. K. Wooldridge, J.L. Schnipper, K. Goggins, et al. Refractory primary medication nonadherence: Prevalence and predictors after pharmacist counseling at hospital discharge. *J Hosp Med* 2016; **11**(1): 48–51.

69. P. MacTavish, J. McPeake, A. Breslin, et al. Evaluation of medication changes following severe COVID-19 infection: a multicentre evaluation. *BMJ Open Respir Res* 2021; **8**(1): 001037.

70. J.L. Stollings, S.L. Bloom, L. Wang, et al. Critical care pharmacists and medication management in an ICU recovery center. *Ann Pharmacother* 2018; **52**(8): 713–23.

71. J.L. Stollings, J.O. Poyant, C.M. Groth, et al. An international, multicenter evaluation of comprehensive medication management

72. J.L. Stollings, M.M. Caylor. Postintensive care syndrome and the role of a follow-up clinic. *Am J Health-Syst Pharm* 2015; **72**: 1315–23.

73. R.A. Mohammad, C. Eze, V.D. Marshall, et al. The impact of a clinical pharmacist in an interprofessional intensive care unit recovery clinic providing care to intensive care unit survivors. *J Am Coll Clin Pharm* 2022; 5(10): 1027–38.

74. P. MacTavish, T. Quasim, M. Shaw, et al. Impact of a pharmacist intervention at an intensive care rehabilitation clinic. *BMJ Open Qual* 2019; 8(3): e000580.

75. P. MacTavish, T. Quasim, C. Purdie, et al. Medication-related problems in intensive care unit survivors: learning from a multicenter program. *Ann Am Thorac Soc* 2020; **17**(10): 1326–9.

76. S.F. Bottom-Tanzer, J.O. Poyant, M.T. Louzada, et al. High occurrence of postintensive care syndrome identified in surgical ICU survivors after implementation of a multidisciplinary clinic. *J Trauma Acute Care Surg* 2021; **91**(2): 406–12.

by pharmacists in ICU recovery centers. *J Intensive Care Med* 2023; **38**(10): 957–65.

Chapter 33

Mortality, Chronic Disease, and Healthcare Utilization in Survivors of Critical Illness

Hiam Naiditch, Florian B. Mayr, and Brad W. Butcher

Introduction

More than 5.7 million patients in the United States are admitted to the intensive care unit (ICU) annually [1], and roughly 85% of them will survive at least one year after hospital discharge [2,3,4]. Because of improvements in technology and the provision of critical care, the mortality rate among patients with sepsis, for example, has decreased globally from approximately 30% in 1990 to 20% in 2017, and the mortality rate among patients with acute respiratory distress syndrome (ARDS) has experienced a similar decline [5,6]. Consequently, there is a growing population of survivors of critical illness that is at risk for significant morbidity and future mortality.

Recovery trajectories in survivors of critical illness can vary significantly (see Figure 33.1). While some patients are able to return to their pre-morbid baseline, others experience a subsequent, gradual decline in their overall health; across patients, the slope of this decline is variable and can be influenced by a number of factors, including their baseline health status and recurrent episodes of critical illness. Iwashyna classified recovery trajectories following critical illness into three basic patterns: the "big hit," the "slow burn," and "relapsing recurrences." In some, a "big hit" is associated with an acute loss of function from which the patient may gradually recover, while others experience either a "slow burn," associated with a more accelerated decline in functional status than might have been expected, or a course of "relapsing recurrences," characterized by disease exacerbations interspersed with periods of partial recovery [7]. Although this is a helpful classification scheme, patients may not neatly fit into one of these three trajectories, which are influenced by the burden of preexisting comorbidities and shaped by the development of chronic disease following critical illness.

Regardless of trajectory, survivors of critical illness exhibit a prolonged vulnerability that challenges the idea that critical illness ends at the doors of the ICU. For many, the need for critical care is not a transient phenomenon but instead the beginning of a significant burden of illness that far exceeds the time spent in the ICU, and in many respects, mimics the course of a chronic disease. In addition to the development of the post-intensive care syndrome (PICS) [8], these patients are at increased risk of death, worsening of preexisting chronic conditions or the development of new ones, hospital readmission, and healthcare resource utilization [9]. Healthcare providers caring for survivors of critical illness are uniquely positioned to recognize these complications and risks, and appreciating them can help providers contextualize healthcare burden for survivors on both the individual and healthcare system levels.

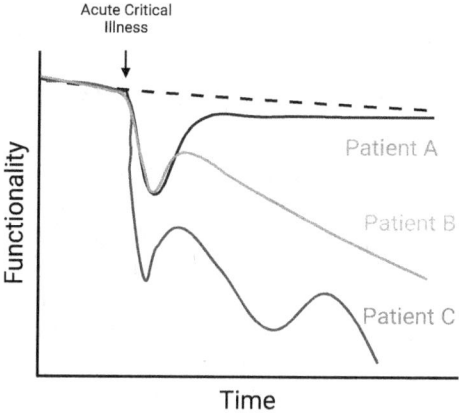

Figure 33.1 Three recovery trajectories in survivors of critical illness. Patient A demonstrates the "Big Hit" trajectory, in which an acute illness results in a brisk decline in functionality that ultimately recovers to their previous baseline over time. Patient B demonstrates the "Slow Burn" trajectory, in which an acute illness results in an incomplete recovery to baseline functionality and initiates a more accelerated decline than would have been expected in the absence of an acute illness. Patient C demonstrates the "Relapsing Recurrences" trajectory, in which an acute illness results in an incomplete recovery to baseline functionality and additional episodes of illness punctuate the recovery period, leading to further decline. Adapted from T. J. Iwashyna. *Am J Respir Crit Care Med* 2012; **186(4)**: 302–4. Adapted with permission of the American Thoracic Society. Copyright © 2024 American Thoracic Society. All rights reserved. The American Journal of Respiratory and Critical Care Medicine is an official journal of the American Thoracic Society. Readers are encouraged to read the entire article for the correct context at www.atsjournals.org/doi/10.1164/rccm.201206-1138ED. The authors, editors, and The American Thoracic Society are not responsible for errors or omissions in adaptations.

Mortality Among Survivors of Critical Illness

Until recently, population-level estimates of the excess mortality risk attributed to surviving critical care were poorly defined, with varying findings likely related to clinical and demographic differences [10]. It is now clear that survivors of critical illness carry a significantly increased risk of mortality for years following their initial illness. In a matched, retrospective cohort study using a sample of Medicare beneficiaries from 2002 to 2006, Wunsch and colleagues demonstrated that the excess mortality risk among those who received critical care extended well beyond the first year after hospital discharge. At 3 years, mortality for survivors of critical illness was 40% compared to 34.5% for hospital controls not requiring critical care and 15% for the general population; the need for mechanical ventilation significantly increased the risk of death by 3 years [11].

Ou and colleagues showed that survivors of sepsis have higher all-cause mortality (hazard ratio [HR] 2.18, 95% confidence interval [CI] 2.14–2.22) and risks of sudden cardiac death or ventricular arrhythmias (HR 1.65; 95% CI 1.57–1.74) compared with propensity-matched control patients, which persisted up to 5 years following discharge [12]. Similarly, a study by Prescott and colleagues demonstrated that a hospitalization for sepsis was associated with a 22.1% (95% CI 17.5%-26.7%) and a 16.2% (95% CI 10.2%-22.2%) absolute mortality risk increase relative to nonhospitalized adults and to those hospitalized with non-septic/sterile inflammatory conditions, respectively, suggesting that sepsis may have a more significant impact on mortality than others illnesses [13]. This was complemented by another study in which patients with severe sepsis exhibited significantly higher 1-year mortality than patients hospitalized for non-sepsis conditions (44.2% [95% CI 41.3–47.2%] vs. 31.4% [95% CI 28.6–34.2%]) [14].

The Relationship Between Chronic Disease and ICU Outcomes

Chronic disease has a bidirectional relationship with critical illness and its outcomes: those with preexisting chronic disease are more likely to develop critical illness, and critical illness may accelerate underlying co-morbid conditions or result in the development of new ones. In an analysis of over 56,000 patients requiring critical care and 75,000 control patients, van Beusekom and colleagues found that patients with no preexisting conditions who required critical care were nearly fivefold more likely to develop new chronic conditions than control patients who did not require critical care. The increase in risk for chronic disease was demonstrated across multiple organ systems and increased with age. Hyperlipidemia, heart disease, chronic obstructive pulmonary disease (COPD), depression, diabetes, and epilepsy were the most prevalent newly developed chronic conditions in survivors of critical illness in the year following discharge [15]. The development of new chronic conditions or worsening of preexisting chronic disease has important implications for survivors of critical illness, impacting their quality of life as well as their ability to resume employment and reintegrate into previous social roles.

Cardiovascular Disease

Risk of cardiovascular events is particularly increased in survivors of sepsis relative to matched controls, suggesting that sepsis may contribute directly to the development of or progression of cardiovascular disease. A systematic review and meta-analysis of 27 studies demonstrated that sepsis was associated with a higher long-term risk of myocardial infarction, stroke, and congestive heart failure compared to non-sepsis controls. In an observational study, the incidence of new cardiovascular events aside from myocardial infarction, including stroke, sudden cardiac death, and ventricular arrhythmias, was increased almost two-fold relative to population controls [16]. Survivors of sepsis have a higher risk of major cardiovascular events (HR 1.37, 95% CI 1.34–1.41), myocardial infarction (HR 1.22, 95% CI 1.14–1.30), and heart failure (HR 1.48, 95% CI 1.43–1.53) [12], and they are 1.9 times more likely to be hospitalized for cardiovascular events within one year compared with matched controls [17].

Respiratory Disease

The odds of a new diagnosis of COPD is higher among survivors of critical illness than matched controls (odds ratio [OR] 4.32, 95% CI 3.33–5.590 for males, OR 6.01, 95% CI 4.49–8.05) for females), and this is also true for a new diagnosis of asthma (OR 1.67, 95% CI 1.29–2.17); OR 2.41, 95% CI 1.85–3.13). [15]. Respiratory viruses including SARS-CoV-2 have been found to be associated with incident respiratory disease such as asthma [18,19]. Survivors of ARDS may experience reductions in the diffusing capacity of the lungs for carbon monoxide (DLCO) and a decreased distance covered during a 6-minute walk test 12 months following discharge when compared with age- and sex-matched controls [20]; exertional hypoxemia may also be present [21]. In some patients, persistent pulmonary effects can be radiographically present in the form of reticular changes on chest radiography and fibrosis or bronchiectasis on computed tomography (see Chapter 35 for additional information) [21]. Changes in the understanding of optimal mechanical ventilation parameters, such as the benefit of low-tidal volume ventilation, may have impacted pulmonary outcomes among patients who received mechanical ventilation [22].

Neurological and Muscular Disease

The risk of developing a new diagnosis of epilepsy is markedly higher among survivors of critical illness than matched controls (OR 24.35, 95% CI 14.00–42.34 for males, OR 20.91, 95% CI 11.77–37.15 for females) [15]. Additionally, survivors of sepsis have higher rates of ischemic stroke (HR 1.27, 95% CI 1.23–1.32) and hemorrhagic stroke (HR 1.36, 95% CI 1.26–1.46) than propensity-matched controls [12]. Approximately 86% of survivors of ARDS experience new onset muscle weakness and fatigue, which can persist for months to years following discharge and is often attributable to critical illness myopathy and neuropathy (see Chapters 4 and 41 for additional information) [23,24,25]. Other patient-reported neurological outcomes include sensory changes, such as visual impairment and hearing loss (see Chapter 36 for additional information) [26].

Renal Disease

Critical illness is often complicated by the development of acute kidney injury (AKI), with one study suggesting that over half of all patients experience AKI during an ICU admission [27]. Nearly one-fifth of patients who develop AKI in the setting of sepsis may develop chronic kidney disease (CKD) by one year [28]. Indeed, patients who develop AKI are approximately 13 times as likely to ultimately develop end-stage renal disease (ESRD) than those who do not, a risk magnified nearly threefold in patients who develop AKI superimposed on preexisting CKD, which is itself a risk factor for the development of AKI in the ICU [29,30]. Even patients with no or mild AKI (Kidney Disease Improving Global Outcomes [KDIGO] stage 1) while in the ICU exhibit a 10% decrease in estimated glomerular filtration rate (eGFR) in the first 6 months following discharge, while those with moderate to severe AKI (KDIGO AKI stages 2 and 3, respectively) were estimated to have a 20% increased risk for mortality or need for dialysis within 7 years [31]. Given how common AKI is in the ICU, the astute provider should seek to recognize early signs of CKD using standard laboratory testing, such as serum creatinine, cystatin-C, and urine albumin to creatinine ratio, to identify patients in need of referral to nephrology.

Hospital Readmission and Healthcare Resource Utilization

An important measure of vulnerability in survivors of critical illness is the frequent need for hospital readmission and increased healthcare resource utilization. In a cohort study of nearly 500,000 patients with a hospitalization requiring critical care between 2008 and 2010, 16% of patients discharged after an ICU stay were readmitted within 30 days, and 35% were readmitted within 6 months, over one-quarter of whom required intensive care once again. Readmission was more likely in patients with older age, more comorbidities, a longer index hospitalization, need for tracheostomy or dialysis, a diagnosis of severe sepsis, and in those discharged to a skilled nursing facility. Only 17% of patients had the same admission diagnoses for both hospitalizations, and the five most common reasons for early readmission were congestive heart failure, sepsis, complications from a procedure, dysrhythmia, and pneumonia [32]. Similarly, among a large cohort of patients hospitalized for both critical and non-critical illness in the US Nationwide Readmissions Database (NRD), the most common reasons for unplanned 30-day hospital readmission were exacerbations of congestive heart failure, exacerbations of COPD, and sepsis [33].

Readmission rates are particularly high in survivors of sepsis, occurring in roughly 40% of survivors within 90 days of hospital discharge, accounting for 12.2% of all hospital readmissions and 14.5% of readmission costs in the United States. Sepsis accounts for more readmissions and higher cost per readmission than congestive heart failure, pneumonia, myocardial infarction, and exacerbations of COPD, the four core conditions for which the Centers for Medicare and Medicaid Services track 30-day readmission rates to measure quality of care and guide pay-for-performance. The most common reason for readmission in survivors of sepsis is recurrent infection, including pneumonia and urinary tract infections, as well as exacerbations of underlying heart failure and COPD, similar to general populations of survivors of critical illness; such admissions are considered potentially preventable [34,34,35].

In addition to hospital readmissions, survivors of critical illness also visit emergency departments and outpatient clinics more frequently. In a study of inpatient admissions, emergency department visits, and outpatient visits in the year prior to and following ICU admission in a cohort of over 4,000 survivors of critical illness, readmission rates at 30 days, 90 days, and 1 year were 15%, 26%, and 43%, respectively; 24% of readmissions were classified as preventable. Compared with the pre-ICU period, hospital admissions increased by 60% in the post-ICU period, whereas emergency department and outpatient visits increased by 8% and 33%, respectively. Perhaps surprisingly, only 8% of all survivors in this study received support from physical therapy, occupational therapy, cognitive therapy, or mental health services in the year following ICU discharge [36].

A Korean study comparing readmission rates and medical expenditures between ICU and non-ICU survivors demonstrated that, compared with survivors who did not require critical care, survivors who did require critical care were much more likely to be readmitted within the first 6 months following discharge (40% versus 9%) and incurred consistently higher medical expenses [37]. Lone and colleagues showed that, over five years of follow-up, when compared with control subjects, survivors of critical illness were more likely to have one or more hospital admissions (81.6% versus 73.3%), to use more hospital resources (4.8 admissions per person per 5 years versus 3.3 admissions per person per 5 years), to spend more days in the hospital (mean 32.6 days versus 21.5 days), and to have higher mean costs of hospital admissions ($133.5 million vs $88.2 million). Factors present before the ICU admission (e.g., the presence of co-morbidities and history of prior hospitalization) were stronger predictors of hospital resource utilization than factors associated with the acute illness [38].

Among diagnoses that commonly require intensive care, sepsis and ARDS are particularly associated with increased healthcare costs and resource utilization. In a longitudinal follow-up study of patients from the multicenter ARDSNet trials from 2006 to 2013, 40% of ARDS survivors required at least one hospital readmission within one year, with a median estimated hospital cost of $18,760 USD (interquartile range [IQR] $7,852–46,174) [39]. Moreover, in a prospective cohort study of 126 adults requiring prolonged mechanical ventilation, there were 457 transitions in care location during follow-up, with a median of 4 transitions per patient, and nearly 75% of days were spent in hospitals, post-acute care facilities, or receiving paid home care. Consistent with earlier studies, there were 150 readmissions in 68 of the 103 hospital survivors, most of which occurred within the first 3 months and half of which were related to sepsis. The mean total 1 year cost for cohort members was $306,000, and costs incurred by the total cohort exceeded $38.5 million [40]. This increase in healthcare utilization by survivors of critical illness also highlights a remarkably altered day-to-day life, often spent away from home. Patients spend a higher proportion of days alive in hospitals, long-term acute care hospitals, and skilled nursing facilities following discharge for severe sepsis than in the year prior (median 9.6%, IQR 1.4–33.8% versus 1.9%, IQR 0.0–7.9%; p < 0.001) [14].

Limitations

Among some of the studies presented, health insurance claims databases were employed, implying the use of diagnostic codes. The presence of a new diagnostic code does not necessarily imply new-onset disease but instead provides a rough estimate for disease using available data.

Conclusion

The care of survivors of critical illness requires a comprehensive approach that takes into account a patient's preexisting risk of mortality and of multiorgan morbidity. It is likewise important to recognize new-onset chronic diseases and exacerbations of preexisting diseases to direct resources appropriately. In addition to increased mortality and morbidity risk, healthcare resource utilization is likely to increase for patients who survive critical illness, with the potential for increased costs to the patient and increased care complexity overall. Future studies should examine how post-ICU interventions, including ICU follow-up clinics, may help to reduce the burden of chronic disease and resource utilization for survivors of critical illness.

Key Points

1. Survivors of critical illness have higher rates of mortality that extend to at least three to five years following initial hospital discharge.
2. Chronic disease has a bidirectional relationship with critical illness and its outcomes: those with preexisting chronic disease are more likely to develop critical illness, and critical illness may accelerate underlying co-morbid conditions or result in the development of new ones.
3. Healthcare utilization, including hospital readmissions, emergency department visits, and outpatient clinic visits, is higher among survivors of critical illness, leading to significantly increased cost of care.

References

1. E.M. Viglianti, T.J. Iwashyna. Toward the ideal ratio of patients to intensivists: finding a reasonable balance. *JAMA Intern Med* 2017; **177**: 396–8.
2. E. Gayat, A. Cariou, N. Deye, et al. Determinants of long-term outcome in ICU survivors: results from the FROG-ICU study. *Crit Care* 2018; **22**: 8.
3. K. Rockwood, T.W. Noseworthy, R. T. Gibney, et al. One-year outcome of elderly and young patients admitted to intensive care units. *Crit Care Med* 1993; **21**: 687–91.

4. M. Niskanen, A. Kari, P. Halonen. Five-year survival after intensive care–comparison of 12,180 patients with the general population: Finnish ICU study group. *Crit Care Med* 1996; **24**: 1962–7.

5. K.E. Rudd, S.C. Johnson, K.M. Agesa, et al. Global, regional, and national sepsis incidence and mortality, 1990–2017: analysis for the Global Burden of Disease Study. *Lancet* 2020; **395**: 200–11.

6. Z. Zhang, K.M. Ho, H. Gu, et al. Defining persistent critical illness based on growth trajectories in patients with sepsis. *Crit Care* 2020; **24**: 57.

7. T.J. Iwashyna. Trajectories of recovery and dysfunction after acute illness, with implications for clinical trial design. *Am J Respir Crit Care Med* 2012; **186**: 302–4.

8. M.S. Herridge, E. Azoulay. Outcomes after critical illness. *N Engl J Med* 2023; **388**: 913–24.

9. A.D. Hill, R.A. Fowler, R. Pinto, et al. Long-term outcomes and healthcare utilization following critical illness: a population-based study. *Crit Care* 2016; **20**: 76.

10. J. Máca, O. Jor, M. Holub, et al. Past and present ARDS mortality rates: a systematic review. *Respir Care* 2017; **62**: 113–22.

11. H. Wunsch, C. Guerra, A.E. Barnato, et al. Three-year outcomes for Medicare beneficiaries who survive intensive care. *JAMA* 2010; **303**: 849–56.

12. S.M. Ou, H. Chu, P.W. Chao, et al. Long-term mortality and major adverse cardiovascular events in sepsis survivors: a nationwide population-based study. *Am J Respir Crit Care Med* 2016; **194**: 209–17.

13. H.C. Prescott, J.J. Osterholzer, K.M. Langa, et al. Late mortality after sepsis: propensity matched cohort study. *BMJ* 2016; **353**: i2375.

14. H.C. Prescott, K.M. Langa, V. Liu, et al. Increased 1-year healthcare use in survivors of severe sepsis. *Am J Respir Crit Care Med* 2014; **190**: 62–9.

15. I. van Beusekom, F. Bakhshi-Raiez, M. van der Schaaf, et al. ICU Survivors have a substantial higher risk of developing new chronic conditions compared to a population-based control group. *Crit Care Med* 2019; **47**: 324–30.

16. L.B. Kosyakovsky, F. Angriman, E. Katz, et al. Association between sepsis survivorship and long-term cardiovascular outcomes in adults: a systematic review and meta-analysis. *Intensive Care Med.* 2021; **47**: 931–42.

17. S. Yende, W. Linde-Zwirble, F. Mayr, et al. Risk of cardiovascular events in survivors of severe sepsis. *Am J Respir Crit Care Med* 2014; **189**: 1065–74.

18. N.G. Hansbro, J.C. Horvat, P.A. Wark, et al. Understanding the mechanisms of viral induced asthma: new therapeutic directions. *Pharmacol Ther* 2008; **117**: 313–53.

19. H. Lee, B.G. Kim, S.J. Chung, et al. New-onset asthma following COVID-19 in adults. *J Allergy Clin Immunol Pract* 2023; **11**: 2228–31.

20. M.S. Herridge, A.M. Cheung, C.M. Tansey, et al. One-year outcomes in survivors of the acute respiratory distress syndrome. *N Engl J Med* 2003; **348**: 683–93.

21. M.F. Mart, L.B. Ware. The long-lasting effects of the acute respiratory distress syndrome. *Expert Rev Respir Med* 2020; **14**: 577–86.

22. J.A. Palakshappa, J.T.W. Krall, L.T. Belfield, et al. Long-term outcomes in acute respiratory distress syndrome: epidemiology, mechanisms, and patient evaluation. *Crit Care Clin* 2021; **37**: 895–911.

23. M.S. Herridge, C.M. Tansey, A. Matté, et al. Functional disability 5 years after acute respiratory distress syndrome. *N Engl J Med* 2011; **364**: 1293–304.

24. S. Koch, T. Wollersheim, J. Bierbrauer, et al. Long-term recovery in critical illness myopathy is complete, contrary to polyneuropathy. *Muscle Nerve* 2014; **50**: 431–6.

25. K. Cheung, A. Rathbone, M. Melanson, et al. Pathophysiology and management of critical illness polyneuropathy and myopathy. *J Appl Physiol* 2021; **130**: 1479–89.

26. M.N. Eakin, Y. Patel, P. Mendez-Tellez, et al. Patients' outcomes after acute respiratory failure: a qualitative study with the PROMIS framework. *Am J Crit Care* 2017; **26**: 456–65.

27. S. Mo, T.W. Bjelland, T.I.L. Nilsen, et al. Acute kidney injury in intensive care patients: incidence, time course, and risk factors. *Acta Anaesthesiol Scand* 2022; **66**: 961–8.

28. A. Arshad, A. Ayaz, S. Rehman, et al. Progression of acute kidney injury to chronic kidney disease in sepsis survivors: 1-year follow-up study. *J Intensive Care Med* 2021; **36**: 1366–70.

29. T.J. Loftus, A.C. Filiberto, T. Ozrazgat-Baslanti, et al. Cardiovascular and renal disease in chronic critical illness. *J Clin Med* 2021; **10(8)**: 1601.

30. P. Fidalgo, S.M. Bagshaw. Chronic kidney disease in the intensive care unit. *Management of Chronic Kidney Disease*. 2014; 417–38.

31. R.W. Haines, J. Powell-Tuck, H. Leonard, et al. Long-term kidney function of patients discharged from hospital after an intensive care admission: observational cohort study. *Sci Rep* 2021; **11**: 9928.

32. M. Hua, M.N. Gong, J. Brady, et al. Early and late unplanned rehospitalizations for survivors of critical illness. *Crit Care Med* 2015; **43**: 430–8.

33. F.B. Mayr, V. Balakumar, V. Talisa, et al. 1336: Understanding the burden of unplanned sepsis readmissions. *Crit Care Med* 2016; **44**(12): 409.

34. F.B. Mayr, V. B. Talisa, V. Balakumar, et al. Proportion and cost of unplanned 30-day readmissions after sepsis compared with other medical conditions. *JAMA* 2017; **317** (5): 530–1.

35. H.C. Prescott, K.M. Langa, and T. J. Iwashyna. Readmission diagnoses after hospitalization for severe sepsis and other acute medical conditions. *JAMA* 2015; **313** (10): 1055–7.

36. E.L. Hirshberg, E.L. Wilson, V. Stanfield, et al. Impact of critical illness on resource utilization: a comparison of use in the year before and after ICU admission. *Crit Care Med* 2019; **47**: 1497–504.

37. J. Kang, K.M. Lee. Three-year mortality, readmission, and medical expenses in critical care survivors: a population-based cohort study. *Aust Crit Care* 2024; **37**: 251–7.

38. N.I. Lone, M.A. Gillies, C. Haddow, et al. Five-year mortality and hospital costs associated with surviving intensive care. *Am J Respir Crit Care Med*. 2016; **194** (2):198–208.

39. A.P. Ruhl, M. Huang, E. Colantuoni, et al. Healthcare utilization and costs in ARDS survivors: a 1-year longitudinal national US multicenter study. *Intensive Care Med* 2017; **43**: 980–91.

40. M. Unroe, J.M. Kahn, S.S. Carson, et al. One-year trajectories of care and resource utilization for recipients of prolonged mechanical ventilation: a cohort study. *Ann Intern Med* 2010; **153**: 167–75.

Chapter 34

Quality of Life in Survivors of Critical Illness

Rita Bakhru and Howard Saft

History of Quality of Life and Quality of Life in Critical Illness

The term "quality of life" (QOL) first appeared in the academic literature in the late 1950s in the context of population planning in health economics and public health research [1,2,3]. As interest in clinical research increased, clinicians and researchers opted to use the term to evaluate the impact of interventions on both quantity and quality of life.

Interest in measuring health-related quality of life (HRQOL) across populations grew with the creation of Medicare and Medicaid, the Health Care Finance Administration, and private health insurance programs [4]. Administrators and researchers who had an interest in evaluating the impact of healthcare delivery needed a population-based measure for HRQOL that was more nuanced than mortality alone. Early QOL measures included the Sickness Impact Profile [5,6] among others [7], which were first used to measure outcomes in survivors of acute respiratory distress syndrome (ARDS). At the same time, to facilitate a population-level view of the healthcare system, policymakers sought to develop a comprehensive and rigorous HRQOL measurement tool that could be applied to everyone rather than to those with a specific disease or to those who received a specific intervention. In the United States, the RAND Medical Outcomes Study was used to create the Short Form 36 item health survey (SF-36) [8], which quantified QOL based on a combination of physical and mental health components, including limitations in physical activities, social activities, and usual roles; bodily pain; general mental health; limitations due to emotional problems; vitality (energy level); and general health perceptions [8]. Contemporaneously, from 1987 to 1991, a European collaborative, EuroQol, developed a more compact QOL measurement named the EQ-5D [9], whose dimensions include: mobility, self-care, usual activities, pain/discomfort, anxiety/depression, and a numerical score of overall health [10].

The use of these general HRQOL measures, such as the SF-36 and the EQ-5D, expanded in both population-level research and clinical domains. Health economists, public health officials, and healthcare administrators incorporated these measures to evaluate the costs and effectiveness of specific interventions to promote discussions of judicious resource use. From the clinical perspective, results of QOL assessments increase the granularity of outcomes beyond mortality; they promote patient-centered decision-making and help clinicians think more deeply about how patients' QOL can be optimized beyond simply surviving. Additionally, when clinicians and clinical researchers use more granular information derived from these measures, they can identify specific QOL dimensions that may be adversely affected, which promotes the development of specific interventions to target the impacted dimensions.

While a comprehensive clinical assessment may identify QOL concerns, screening tools like the SF-36 and EQ-5D enabled clinical researchers and clinicians to quantify and communicate about the global health of patients who survived ARDS. Studies by Davidson [11] and Angus [12] in the late 1990s and early 2000s demonstrated significant decrements in QOL in survivors of ARDS and highlighted that worsening QOL was not attributed to respiratory issues alone. Herridge and colleagues confirmed that impaired QOL in ARDS survivors, as measured by the SF-36, was impacted in multiple domains, including general health, vitality, physical functioning, physical role, emotional role, pain, and social functioning [13,14].

Multiple systematic reviews and meta-analyses of QOL following critical illness using the SF-36 or the EQ-5D have furthered our understanding of the deleterious impact of a critical illness on patients' perceptions of their general health and its trajectory over time. For example, in a systematic review of 21 studies including 7320 patients, Dowdy and colleagues found that survivors of critical illness had significantly lower QOL scores in each domain of the SF-36 than healthy controls; over time, most patients' scores improved except in the mental health and general health domains (see Figure 34.1) [15].

In this chapter, we focus on the use of the SF-36 and EQ-5D due to their inclusion in core outcomes data sets and their common use by clinicians, policymakers, and administrators.

Practical Utility in ICU Follow-Up Clinics

Measuring QOL in an ICU follow-up clinic has several benefits, including identifying and prioritizing areas of concern, facilitating communication and shared decision-making, screening for hidden or undivulged problems, and longitudinal monitoring of responses to treatment [16]. As above, QOL can be measured with a variety of tools, most commonly the SF-36, a more compact version known as the SF-12 [17], and the EQ-5D; other, less commonly used tools include the Sickness Impact Profile [5], Nottingham Health profile [18], Assessment of Quality of Life Multi-Attribute Utility Instrument (AQoL-8D) [19], and various qualitative methods using focus groups and interviews [20].

The SF-36 and EQ-5D have significant thematic overlap (see Figure 34.2), but given that the SF-36 asks more questions, the data derived is more granular and divided into more domains. The SF-36 consists of 36 questions (see Table 34.1) and requires approximately 9 minutes to administer, while the EQ-5D consists of 6 questions and requires approximately 2 minutes to administer [9]. The SF-36 has some questions with five levels of responses and some with three levels of responses, while the EQ-5D has two versions – the 5L and the 3L; the 5L has five levels of responses, while the 3L has three levels of responses. Both instruments have been used extensively in the critical care literature, with over 50 publications utilizing each instrument. Panels of experts on survival after acute respiratory failure and general critical illness recommended the EQ-5D as the preferred QOL measurement [21,22]; the SF-36 is considered an acceptable alternative [21]. One benefit of using the EQ-5D is that it can be used to calculate Quality-Adjusted Life Years (QALYs), a metric used by clinicians, researchers, and health economists to understand the cost-effectiveness of particular interventions or treatments. Policy makers may use a cost-per-QALY calculation to approve certain therapeutic interventions; a cost-per-QALY cutoff is often decided by healthcare system administrators and policy makers within their country or location.

Source	N[a]	Follow-up time[b]	Physical QOL domains[c]				Mental QOL domains[c]			
			Physical function	Role physical	Bodily pain	General health	Vitality	Social function	Role emotional	Mental health
Studies of QOL prior to ICU admission[d]										
Wehler [26]	318	—	↓*	↓*	↓*	↓*	→	↓*	↓*	↓*
Graf [27]	153	—	↓*	↓*	↓*	↓*	→	↓*	↓*	↓*
Ridley [32][e]	75	—	→	↓*	↓*	→	→	→	→	→
Studies of QOL after ICU stay										
Wehler [26]	171	6 months	↓*	↓*	↓*	↓*	→	↓*	↓*	↓*
Ridley [32][e]	75	6 months	↓*	↓*	→*	↓*	→	→	→	→
Vedio [31][f]										
Elective	66	6 months	—	↓*	↑	—	—	—	—	—
Emergency	49	6 months	↓*	↓*	→	↓*	↓*	↓*	↓*	↓*
Graf [27]	153	9 months	↓*	↓*	—	→	↓*	→	↓*	→
Pettila [23]	298	12 months	↓*	↓*	→	↓*	—	—	—	—
Kaarlola [24][g]	169	6 years	↓*	↓*	—	↓*	—	↓*	—	↓*
Flaatten [33]	51	13–14 years	↓*	↓*	→	↓*	→	↓*	↓*	↓*

[a] Sample size at the time of follow-up
[b] Length of time from ICU or hospital discharge until quality of life measurement
[c] ↓*/↑* clinically meaningful (i.e., >5-point) decrement/improvement in quality of life; ↓*↑* clinically meaningful and statistically significant ($p<0.05$) decrement in quality of life; – non-clinically meaningful (i.e., ≤5-point) change in quality of life
[d] QOL prior to ICU admission was measured retrospectively from patient or proxy.
[e] Includes only patients <65 years old
[f] Separately analyzed patients with emergency and elective diagnoses on ICU admission
[g] The study population in [24] is a subset of that in [23]. No measure of significance was reported in [24].

Figure 34.1 Quality of life measurements in adult survivors of critical illness versus age- and gender-matched controls in the general population (ICU, Intensive Care Unit; QOL, Quality of Life). From: D.W. Dowdy, M.P. Eid, A. Sedrakyan, et al. Quality of life in adult survivors of critical illness: a systematic review of the literature. *Intensive Care Med* 2005; **31**: 611–20. Reproduced with permission from Springer Nature.

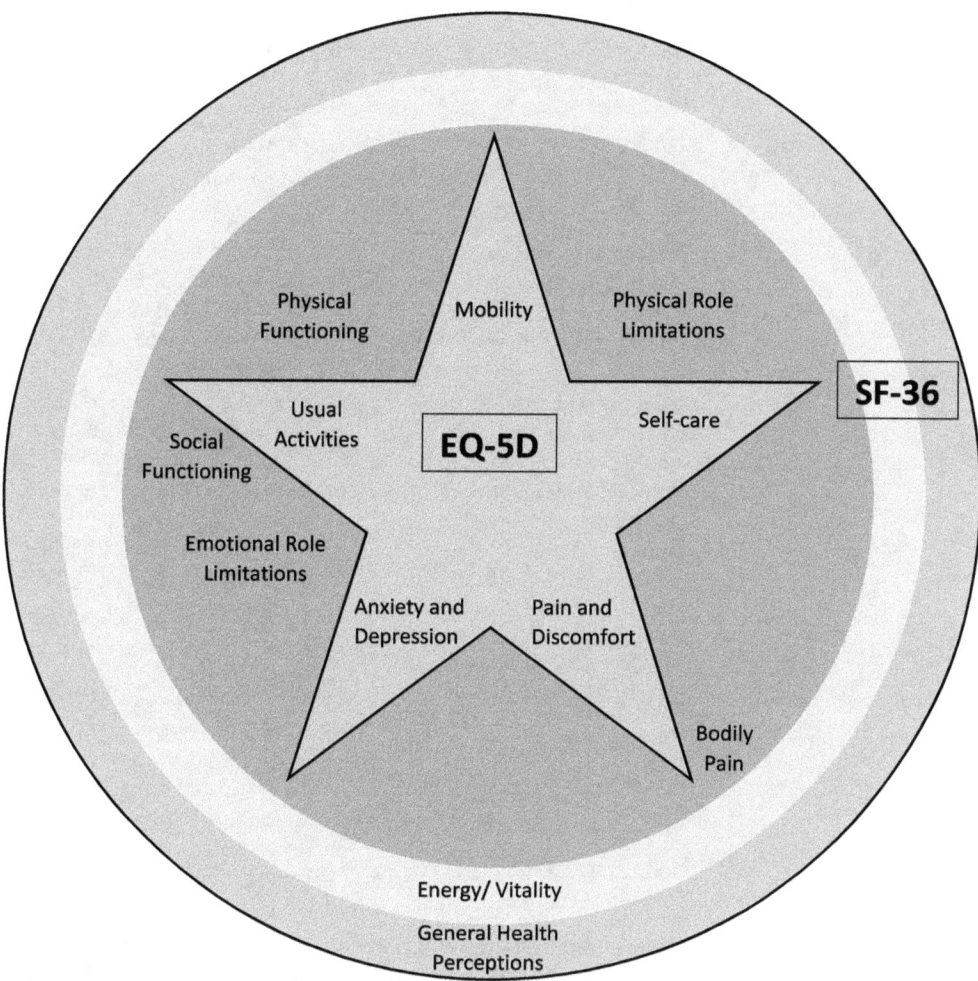

Figure 34.2 Domains of the EQ-5D and the SF-36 quality of life measures

Assessing QOL in ICU follow-up clinics, particularly with the EQ-5D, is common and can help direct the visit to address concerns that are of primary importance to the patient, particularly if time is limited. Mobility problems as identified by the EQ-5D, for example, may lead to a more detailed assessment of physical function and physical therapy referral, while concerns regarding self-care may prompt occupational therapy referral. Difficulties with usual activities may elicit further discussion about the ability to resume driving and employment or engage in social roles, which may result in cognitive therapy referral. Concerns regarding pain may lead to examination of the involved area and possible initiation of pharmacological or non-pharmacological treatment, while the presence of anxiety and depression may lead to a more thorough assessment with screening tools, such as the Hospital Anxiety and Depression Scale, and referrals to psychiatry, psychology, and peer support groups. Additionally, QOL screening tools may prompt patients and their families to raise issues that they may not have thought about without being prompted.

Table 34.1 A comparison of the SF-36 and EQ-5D

QOL Measure	SF–36	EQ–5D
Total Questions	36	6
Estimated Time to Complete	9 minutes	2 minutes
Recall Period	4 weeks	Today
Scoring Information	Two-step process: 1) Each question scored according to scoring key to obtain a score between 0 and 100. 2) Questions in each scale averaged together to get 8 subscale scores, including physical functioning, social functioning, role limitations caused by physical problems, role limitations caused by emotional problems, general mental health, energy and fatigue, bodily pain, and general health. 3) Can also create the Mental Health Component Scale and the Physical Component Scale	5L version: 5 levels of severity – 1: No problems, 2: Slight problems, 3: Moderate problems, 4: Severe problems, 5: Extreme problems. 3L version: 3 levels of severity – 1: No problems, 2: Some problems, 3: Extreme problems The visual analog scale is scored 0 to 100, with higher scores reflecting better health-related QOL.
Mode of Administration	Mail, in-person, phone	Mail, in-person, phone

Despite their utility, there are limitations to QOL screening tools. For example, although these measures are static, they are highly subjective, person-specific (i.e., two patients with similar impairments may rate their importance differently), may change in their meaning to a patient over time, and may be modified by the patient's experience [23]. This "response shift" may be due to recalibration, reprioritization, and reconceptualization, making the true assessment of QOL after critical illness more difficult [24]. Additionally, translating scores between different measures of QOL is not accurate [25], suggesting that different instruments may measure different aspects of QOL. While broad QOL measures are often helpful in research applications, they may be inadequate for testing interventions that target specific domains of health.

The Human Perspective

Understanding and improving patients' QOL following critical illness is the ultimate goal of any intervention. Importantly, there is no universal definition of QOL, and so assessing it is patient-specific and based on several factors, including their pre-morbid function, familial and societal roles, vocation and avocations, and their general belief system and worldview. One helpful model to consider is displayed in Figure 34.3 [27]. When assessing QOL in survivors of critical

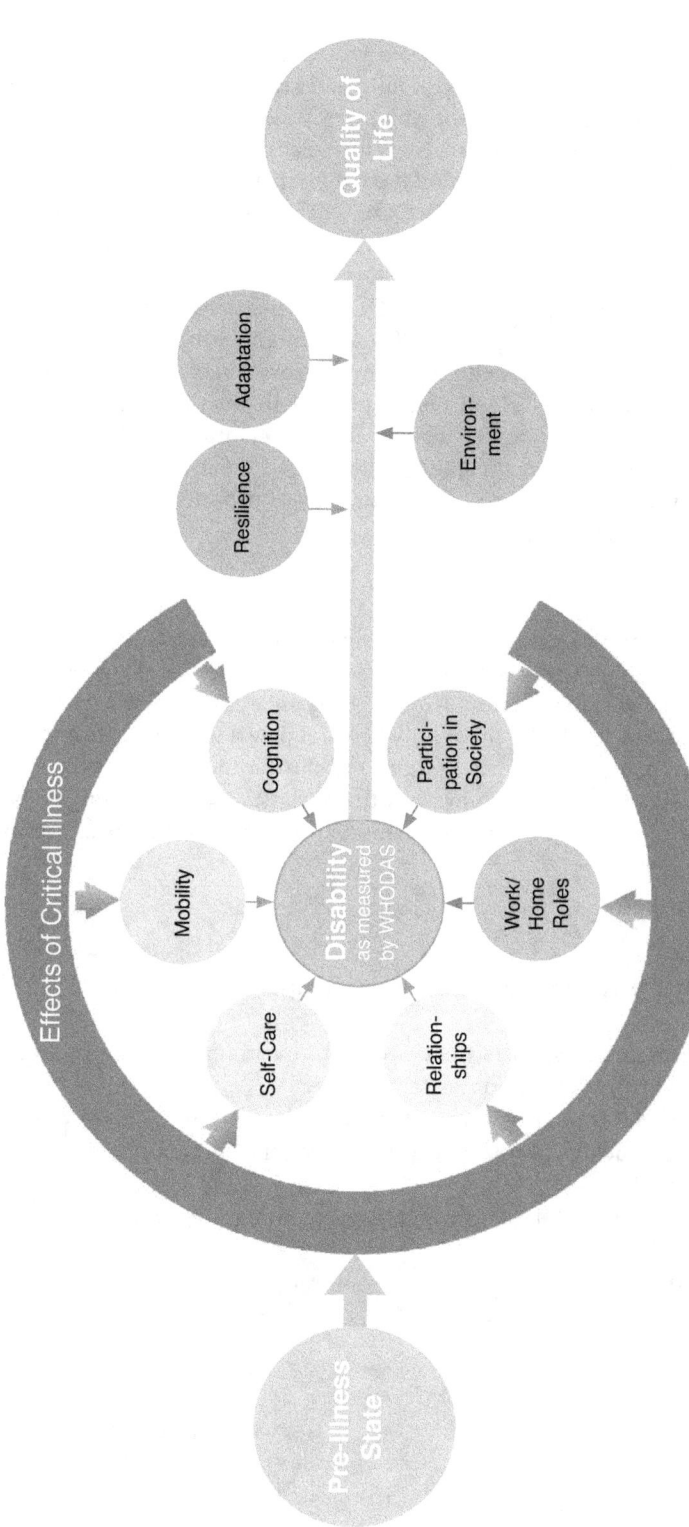

Figure 34.3 Conceptual model of the factors that are included in the World Health Organisation's International Classification of Functioning after critical illness. [27] From: C.L. Hodgson, A.A. Udy, M. Bailey, et al. The impact of disability in survivors of critical illness. *Intensive Care Med* 2017; **43**: 992-1001. Reproduced with permission from Springer Nature.

illness, it is essential to determine their pre-morbid function to better appreciate the impact of critical illness on their self-care, mobility, cognition, and relationships, as well as their work, home, and social roles. For example, a patient with preexisting paraplegia may not interpret an additional loss in mobility as meaningful, whereas for an athlete, any loss of mobility may be catastrophic to their QOL. A deeper understanding of the patient's environment, resilience, and adaptation leads to a fuller view of the patient's QOL. This detailed understanding of QOL can help the patient and their family, clinicians, and researchers better appreciate the impact of post-intensive care syndrome (PICS) on people's lives.

Understanding one patient's perspective on QOL compared with another patient or to the population as a whole may be important. These differences provide an opportunity to look more closely at how we can help patients improve their QOL. Some may have particular symptoms that may not be identified in general medical assessments, while others may have specific goals that they want to achieve in order to attain a perceived minimally acceptable QOL. Clinicians can use their understanding of a patient's goals and values to design a patient-specific rehabilitation plan and to counsel patients and families regarding goals of care in the setting of a future illness.

Conclusion

Understanding QOL and its measurement is important to care for patients with PICS. The SF-36 and EQ-5D, two instruments commonly used to measure QOL in this patient population, complement a clinical assessment and identify problem areas that require intervention. Discussing QOL data from studies of survivors of critical illness with patients and families in ICU follow-up clinics can help manage expectations and illustrate potential recovery trajectories. QOL measures can also be used to communicate with nonclinicians, such administrators, public health officials, and economists, who play an increasingly important role in healthcare delivery.

Key Points

1. The term HRQOL was first introduced by economists and policy makers in the late 1950s.
2. HRQOL measures are helpful to assess a patient's overall health status and to measure health outcomes beyond mortality.
3. HRQOL questionnaires are useful in ICU follow-up clinics to measure different domains of health, such as physical health, functional health, mental health, and other related domains.
4. Despite their utility, HRQOL questionnaires have limitations and vary in areas of focus.
5. Overall, HRQOL measures complement a comprehensive history and physical examination and help clinicians communicate with policy makers.

References

1. J.K. Galbraith. Economics and the Quality of Life. *Science* 1964; **145**: 117–23.
2. J. Huxley. Population planning and quality of life. *Eugen Rev* 1959; **51**: 149–54.

3. F.S. Jaffe. Health policy and population policy: a relationship redefined. *AJPH* 1973; **63**: 401–4.
4. Key milestones in Medicare and Medicaid history, selected years: 1965–2003. *Health Care Financ Rev* 2005; **27**: 1–3.
5. B.S. Gilson, J.S. Gilson, M. Bergner, et al. The sickness impact profile: development of an outcome measure of health care. *Am J Public Health* 1975; **65**: 1304–10.
6. L.G. McHugh, J.A. Milberg, M. E. Whitcomb, et al. Recovery of function in survivors of the acute respiratory distress syndrome. *Am J Resp Crit Care Med* 1994; **150**: 90–4.
7. C. Jones, R. Hussey, R.D. Griffiths. A tool to measure the change in health status of selected adult patients before and after intensive care. *Clin Intensive Care* 1993; **4**: 160–5.
8. J.E. Ware, Jr., C.D. Sherbourne. The MOS 36-item short-form health survey (SF-36). I. Conceptual framework and item selection. *Med Care* 1992; **30**: 473–83.
9. N. Devlin, D. Parkin, B. Janssen. *An Introduction to EQ-5D Instruments and Their Applications*. New York: Springer International Publishing; 2020.
10. R. Rabin, F. de Charro. EQ-5D: a measure of health status from the EuroQol Group. *Ann Med* 2001; **33**: 337–43.
11. T.A. Davidson, E.S. Caldwell, J.R. Curtis, et al. Reduced quality of life in survivors of acute respiratory distress syndrome compared with critically ill control patients. *JAMA* 1999; **281**: 354–60.
12. D.C. Angus, A.A. Musthafa, G. Clermont, et al. Quality-adjusted survival in the first year after the acute respiratory distress syndrome. *Am J Resp Crit Care Med* 2001; **163**: 1389–94.
13. M.S. Herridge, M. Moss, C.L. Hough, et al. Recovery and outcomes after the acute respiratory distress syndrome (ARDS) in patients and their family caregivers. *Intensive Care Med* 2016; **42**: 725–38.
14. M.S. Herridge, C.M. Tansey, A. Matte, et al. Functional disability 5 years after acute respiratory distress syndrome. *N Engl J Med* 2011; **364**: 1293–304.
15. D.W. Dowdy, M.P. Eid, A. Sedrakyan, et al. Quality of life in adult survivors of critical illness: a systematic review of the literature. *Intensive Care Med* 2005; **31**: 611–20.
16. I.J. Higginson, A.J. Carr. Using quality of life measures in the clinical setting. *BMJ (Clinical research ed)* 2001; **322**: 1297–300.
17. J. Ware, Jr., M. Kosinski, S.D. Keller. A 12-Item Short-Form Health Survey: construction of scales and preliminary tests of reliability and validity. *Med Care* 1996; **34**: 220–33.
18. S.M. Hunt, J. McEwen, S.P. McKenna. Measuring health status: a new tool for clinicians and epidemiologists. *Br J Gen Pract* 1985; **35**: 185–8.
19. J. Richardson, A. Iezzi, M.A. Khan, A. Maxwell. Validity and reliability of the Assessment of Quality of Life (AQoL)-8D multi-attribute utility instrument. *Patient* 2013; **7**: 85–96.
20. C.R. Weinert, C.R. Gross, J.R. Kangas, et al. Health-related quality of life after acute lung injury. *Am J Resp Crit Care Med* 1997; **156**: 1120–8.
21. D.M. Needham, K.A. Sepulveda, V. D. Dinglas, et al. Core outcome measures for clinical research in acute respiratory failure survivors. an international modified delphi consensus study. *Am J Resp Crit Care Med* 2017; **196**: 1122–30.
22. M.E. Mikkelsen, M. Still, B.J. Anderson, et al. Society of Critical Care Medicine's international consensus conference on prediction and identification of long-term impairments after critical illness. *Crit Care Med* 2020; **48**: 1670–9.
23. A.J. Carr, B. Gibson, P.G. Robinson. Is quality of life determined by expectations or experience? *BMJ (Clinical Research ed)* 2001; **322**: 1240–3.
24. A.E. Turnbull, M.S. Hurley, I. M. Oppenheim, et al. Curb your enthusiasm: definitions, adaptation, and expectations for quality of life in icu survivorship. *AnnalsATS* 2020; **17**: 406–11.

25. D. Rowen, J. Brazier, J. Roberts. Mapping SF-36 onto the EQ-5D index: how reliable is the relationship? *Health Qual Life Outcomes* 2009; 7: 27.
26. I. Buchholz, M.F. Janssen, T. Kohlmann, Y.-S. Feng. A systematic review of studies comparing the measurement properties of the three-level and five-level versions of the EQ-5D. *PharmacoEconomics* 2018; **36**: 645–61.
27. C.L. Hodgson, A.A. Udy, M. Bailey, et al. The impact of disability in survivors of critical illness. *Intensive Care Med* 2017; **43**: 992–1001.

Chapter 35
Pulmonary and Diaphragmatic Complications in Survivors of Critical Illness

Megan Trieu, Le T. Ho, and Amy Bellinghausen

Introduction

One of the most commonly reported physical symptoms in survivors of critical illness is dyspnea, which is often multifactorial and can be caused by numerous pulmonary and diaphragmatic complications as well as extra-pulmonary problems [1,2]. Several measurements are used to characterize pulmonary function, including spirometry, plethysmography, diffusing capacity of the lung for carbon monoxide (DLCO), blood gas analysis, maximal oxygen consumption (VO_2 max), and the six-minute walk test (6MWT) [3]. It is imperative that these measures be evaluated and interpreted in the context of patient-centered outcomes, such as health-related quality of life (HRQL). An approach to the care of patients with post-intensive care syndrome (PICS) should encompass the timely identification of pulmonary impairments and support for their acute respiratory needs. In this chapter, we review the most common pulmonary and diaphragmatic complications following critical illness, discuss the different outcome measures used to assess pulmonary function, and suggest a framework for pulmonary follow-up of patients in intensive care unit (ICU) follow-up clinics.

Pulmonary and Diaphragmatic Complications after Critical Illness

Pulmonary Complications

Various pulmonary complications following critical illness may benefit from early detection and targeted interventions. In cases of acute lung injury, radiographic manifestations exist on a spectrum, including organizing pneumonia, acute fibrinous and organizing pneumonia, and diffuse alveolar damage [4]. Depending on the degree of initial lung injury and other contributing patient-related factors, the acute inflammation may evolve into pulmonary fibrosis. Longitudinal studies have found that residual fibrotic changes on computed tomographic (CT) imaging occurred more frequently in survivors of COVID-related acute respiratory distress syndrome (ARDS) compared to ARDS due to other etiologies and in patients with older age, lower body mass index (BMI), lower mean Richmond Agitation Sedation Scale (RASS) scores, longer total duration of supplemental oxygen, and longer ICU length of stay [5]. CT imaging most commonly revealed nonspecific interstitial pneumonia (NSIP) or usual interstitial pneumonia (UIP) patterns of fibrosis, with combined ground-glass opacities and reticulations, architectural distortion, and bronchial dilatation [4,6].

Tracheal stenosis is another notable complication, often associated with prolonged intubation or tracheostomy (see Chapter 39 for additional information). Web-like stenosis may develop due to tracheal injury at the site of the endotracheal tube cuff or around the tracheal stoma [7,8]. Additionally, a malpositioned endotracheal tube cuff or a high tracheostomy site may result in subglottic stenosis [8]. The presenting symptoms of tracheal stenosis include dyspnea, wheezing or stridor, and cough. It occasionally mimics other obstructive lung diseases, but can be differentiated on pulmonary function testing, chest imaging, and bronchoscopy if a high index of suspicion is maintained [9]. Patient characteristics and comorbidities that may increase the risk of developing tracheal stenosis include autoimmune disease, gastroesophageal reflux disease, radiation injury, infection, obesity, and smoking [7,9]. Management strategies typically involve bronchoscopic interventions, such as laser or mechanical dilatation, electrosurgery, or stenting. Pharmacologic treatment with mitomycin C and intralesional or systemic steroids has also been described [7,10]. Definitive management with surgical tracheal resection may be considered for restenosis after multiple interventional bronchoscopy treatments but is often precluded by comorbidities or length and location of the stricture [9].

Critical illness, especially in the context of prolonged immobility, can predispose individuals to venous thromboembolism (VTE). Following an ICU hospitalization, patients may be at increased risk for VTE, including acute pulmonary embolism (PE), for up to six weeks [11]. Appropriate follow-up for patients diagnosed with VTE/PE during hospitalization should include an assessment of timely discontinuation of anticoagulation. Further testing with echocardiography and a pulmonary ventilation-perfusion (VQ) scan may be considered in persistently symptomatic patients to evaluate for post-PE complications, such as chronic thromboembolic disease (CTED) or chronic thromboembolic pulmonary hypertension (CTEPH).

Chronic chest pain is a complex and debilitating complication that can arise after critical illness. Many ICU patients experience acute pain related to their underlying illness, injury, or invasive procedures. Identifying and managing pain in the ICU is a fundamental component of supportive critical care; however, the transition from acute pain to chronic pain and the role of chronic opioid use in the development of persistent pain remain poorly understood [12]. Literature on chronic chest pain and long-term respiratory disability is currently limited primarily to patients with blunt trauma to the chest, where over 60% of patients reported persistent pain at three months post-injury [13]. Anecdotal experiences in ICU follow-up clinics, however, suggest chronic chest pain is more prevalent than described in the literature and is present in patients with many diagnoses. Chronic chest pain is likely under-recognized in post-ICU settings; however, its association with poorer health-related quality of life (HRQL) emphasizes the need for improved recognition and treatment [14].

Diaphragmatic Complications

Many critically ill patients with respiratory failure require mechanical ventilation. While clinicians are often vigilant about monitoring for complications of mechanical ventilation, including infection, ventilator-induced lung injury, and hemodynamic instability, they may be less attentive to diaphragmatic complications. Recently, a growing body of evidence suggests that mechanically ventilated patients may develop diaphragmatic dysfunction due to respiratory muscle inactivity and unloading as well as consequences of systemic inflammation and medications, such as sedatives, analgesics, or neuromuscular blocking agents [15,16]. Sometimes referred to as ventilator-induced diaphragmatic dysfunction (VIDD) or critical illness-associated diaphragmatic weakness, this complication occurs in a majority of patients in the ICU. Studies report that clinically significant diaphragmatic dysfunction may develop in 60 to 80% of patients requiring mechanical ventilation and occurs twice as often as ICU-acquired limb weakness [16]. While the extent of diaphragmatic dysfunction is correlated with duration of ventilator support, significant diaphragmatic atrophy and weakness may occur even after relatively short periods (> 18 hours) of mechanical ventilation [17,18].

Various mechanisms may contribute to the development of VIDD. Animal studies and, more recently, human studies performed on brain-dead organ donors suggest that muscle fiber atrophy and injury occurs following prolonged mechanical ventilation and complete diaphragmatic inactivity [15,17,18]. The subsequent reduction in force-generating capacity of the diaphragm seen with VIDD can be assessed by measuring the transdiaphragmatic twitch pressure (PdiTw) in response to bilateral anterior magnetic phrenic nerve stimulation. Compared to an average PdiTw of 30 cm H_2O observed in normal healthy adults, studies have shown that mechanically ventilated patients generate a mean PdiTw of 8 cm H_2O [16].

Recognition of VIDD is critical, as it is associated with poor short- and long-term outcomes [19]. While it is a diagnosis of exclusion, it nonetheless should be considered in any patient requiring mechanical ventilation. Some findings that may be suggestive of VIDD include difficulty weaning from mechanical ventilation despite treatment of the underlying pulmonary disorder, recurrent unexplained respiratory failure, presence of paradoxical abdominal movement, or unexpectedly high rapid shallow breathing index (RSBI) despite improved respiratory mechanics [16]. In addition to extubation failure, VIDD may be associated with increased ICU mortality and hospital readmission [16,20]. The effects of diaphragmatic dysfunction additionally extends to the post-ICU setting. Low maximal inspiratory pressure (MIP) is independently associated with decreased one-year mortality [21]. Further research is necessary to determine the impact of diaphragmatic dysfunction on long-term survival, HRQL, and physical function.

Pulmonary Function Outcome Measures After Critical Illness

There is substantial heterogeneity in the pulmonary disorders and diaphragmatic dysfunction that patients may encounter following critical illness. The diverse nature of these conditions makes it challenging to establish universal instruments to effectively evaluate pulmonary function in the post-ICU setting. Identifying a set of core outcome measures would not only guide clinicians assessing and screening for pulmonary disorders in survivors of critical illness but also facilitate clinical research on long-term pulmonary outcomes after critical illness; however, achieving consensus on such measures remains elusive. An international modified Delphi study, conducted to identify core outcome measures for clinical research in acute respiratory failure patients, did not reach consensus on any measure considered for pulmonary function [22]. The Society of Critical Care Medicine's international consensus conference on PICS prediction and assessment suggests the use of the 6MWT for evaluating both physical and pulmonary function in post-ICU patients [23].

Despite the absence of precise outcome measures for pulmonary function, most studies investigating long-term outcomes in patients with ARDS utilize spirometry, plethysmography, and carbon monoxide diffusion capacity assessments. These studies have shown that mild abnormalities in static and dynamic lung volumes are common but gradually improve over several months [1,24,25]. Similarly, based on studies that employed the 6MWT, patients frequently show improvement over 12 months, though distances tend to remain below predicted values [1]. Beyond these measures, other assessments used to assess pulmonary function in the clinical setting include blood gas analysis, maximal respiratory pressures (MIP and maximal expiratory pressure [MEP]), and maximal oxygen capacity as determined via cardiopulmonary exercise testing (CPET). CPET is a noninvasive evaluation of the integrated physiological response to symptom-limited incremental exercise that can identify cardiac, respiratory, musculoskeletal, and metabolic impairments. As such, CPET is commonly used to evaluate unexplained dyspnea or exercise intolerance and to assess functional capacity, such as with pre-operative or pre-transplant risk assessment. Studies evaluating the application of CPET as an outcome measure after critical illness are limited. While survivors of critical illness frequently have abnormalities in pulmonary function, these studies suggest that the etiology of exercise intolerance is often multifactorial, largely driven by musculoskeletal and metabolic limitations [26,27,28,29]. Further studies are needed to confirm the role of CPET in distinguishing pulmonary and extra-pulmonary complications in this patient population.

Pulmonary Follow-Up Aims in ICU Follow-Up Clinics

In ICU follow-up clinics, clinicians care for a diverse group of patients, each with unique needs and challenges. Therefore, the focus of this section will be to provide a practical, multidisciplinary, patient-centered approach to the follow-up of survivors of critical illness focusing on early identification of pulmonary and diaphragmatic complications and management of acute and chronic respiratory needs.

The routine use of cross-sectional chest imaging to monitor for pulmonary complications of critical illness should be approached judiciously and in the context of the individual patient. Prior studies have shown that while a majority of patients will have abnormal radiologic findings, there may be limited correlation between these findings and patient symptoms, pulmonary function testing, 6MWT, or HRQL [30]. This suggests that functional limitations experienced by survivors of critical illness may be multifactorial or partially attributable to extrapulmonary causes, such as ICU-acquired weakness. In populations with a risk of underlying malignancy (e.g., tobacco use or advanced age), however, a repeat CT scan to ensure resolution of areas of dense consolidation and rule out a hidden mass may be warranted. Pulmonary function testing may have more consistent correlation with patient-centered outcomes, such as HRQL, and can provide valuable information when used as a diagnostic or monitoring tool within a comprehensive assessment [25,31,32].

Assessing and addressing the acute and chronic respiratory needs of survivors of critical illness is paramount to their recovery and quality of life. Various measures are used to characterize the severity of dyspnea, which is helpful in determining the impact on functional disability and monitoring for progression or improvement over time. Tools utilized to evaluate activity limitation due to dyspnea include the Modified Medical Research Council (mMRC) Dyspnea Scale, Baseline Dyspnea Index (BDI)/Transition Dyspnea

Table 35.1 Various measures used to evaluate activity limitation due to dyspnea

Measure	Description
Modified Medical Research Council (mMRC) Dyspnea Scale	Self-rating scale used to stratify the severity of breathlessness in individuals, particularly those with chronic respiratory conditions. It ranges from Grade 0 to Grade 4, with higher grades indicating greater perceived disability due to dyspnea.
Baseline Dyspnea Index (BDI)/ Transition Dyspnea Index (TDI)	Interviewer-administered tool used to assess the severity of dyspnea at baseline (BDI) and at subsequent visits (TDI). The interviewer selects grades based on an individual's responses to open-ended questions regarding 3 components (functional impairment, magnitude of task, and magnitude of effort) that provoke breathlessness during activities of daily living. Scores range from 0 to 12, with lower scores indicating greater severity of dyspnea.
Oxygen Cost Diagram (OCD)	Visual representation used to estimate the oxygen expenditure of various activities. Individuals are asked to select the level of activity at which they are limited by dyspnea.
Borg Rating of Perceived Exertion (RPE)	Self-rating scale used to measure an individual's perceived level of exertion during physical activity. It ranges from 6 (no exertion) to 20 (maximum exertion).

Index (TDI), Oxygen Cost Diagram (OCD), and Borg Rating of Perceived Exertion (RPE) (see Table 35.1). Blood gas analysis, ambulatory oxygen saturation, and 6MWT can additionally be employed to further assess respiratory status. Once identified, acute respiratory needs can be addressed through: managing symptoms such as dyspnea and cough with pharmacological and non-pharmacological interventions; prescribing supplemental oxygen when indicated based on ambulatory oxygen saturation or blood gas measurements; treating pre-existing pulmonary conditions, such as asthma and chronic obstructive pulmonary disease (COPD), that are diagnosed or exacerbated in the post-ICU setting; collaborating with various sub-specialists for comorbid conditions, such as anxiety and post-traumatic stress disorder (PTSD); and facilitating referrals to pulmonary rehabilitation programs. In contrast to conventional physical therapy, pulmonary rehabilitation is a structured program designed for individuals experiencing persistent symptoms of chronic respiratory conditions despite optimal medical management. The goal is to reduce dyspnea, improve exercise tolerance, and enhance quality of life through a comprehensive schedule of supervised exercise training, education sessions, and behavioral interventions.

ICU follow-up clinics frequently operate as a collaborative effort involving various healthcare professionals, including respiratory therapists (RTs), physical therapists, pharmacists, dietitians, social workers, and case managers, with each contributing expertise to optimize patient experience and outcomes. RTs can play a pivotal role within this multidisciplinary team [33]. Similar to physicians who work both in the ICU and in the clinic, respiratory therapists can provide a bridge from inpatient to outpatient care. In an ICU follow-up clinic, RTs can screen for symptoms of dyspnea; provide education on underlying respiratory diseases, such as COPD; and assess respiratory function using pulmonary function testing, blood gas analysis, and the 6MWT. Additionally, RTs are integral in educating patients on how to use inhalers and secretion clearance equipment correctly; evaluating challenges related to home oxygen, continuous positive airway pressure (CPAP) devices, or bilevel positive airway pressure (BiPAP) devices; performing routine tracheostomy care; and providing smoking cessation counseling.

Clinical Vignette 1

A 58-year-old previously healthy woman presented to the emergency department with progressive dyspnea. She reported associated fevers, chills, cough, and myalgias for the past week. Her temperature was 38.5°C, heart rate 118 beats per minute, blood pressure 134/62 mmHg, respiratory rate 24 breaths per minute, and oxygen saturation 82% breathing ambient air. Her chest radiograph showed bilateral patchy opacities in a predominantly peripheral and mid-to-lower lung zone distribution. A nasopharyngeal reverse transcription-polymerase chain reaction assay detected the presence of SARS-CoV-2 RNA, and the patient was diagnosed with COVID-19 pneumonia.

She was initially admitted to the intermediate care unit and was treated with remdesivir, dexamethasone, and supplemental oxygen via high-flow nasal cannula. However, on hospital day two, she was transferred to the ICU for worsening hypoxia and intubated. A chest CT scan demonstrated diffuse bilateral ground-glass opacities with a posterior predominance and subpleural sparing. Arterial blood gas analysis revealed a PaO_2 of 120 mmHg on an FiO_2 of 1.0 and a PEEP of 10 cm H_2O. She was placed in the prone position for 16 hours per day and completed the course of remdesivir and dexamethasone. Her oxygenation improved and she was eventually extubated. On hospital day 15, she was discharged to an acute rehabilitation facility with follow up in the ICU follow-up clinic.

Three months later, she is evaluated in the ICU follow-up clinic after returning home from acute rehabilitation. Although she can now perform her activities of daily living (ADL) independently, she reports ongoing dyspnea with exertion and associated non-productive cough. Her oxygen saturation is 93% breathing ambient air. A pulmonary function test (PFT) is notable for mild restriction and moderate reduction in DLCO. Chest CT shows mild residual lower lobe reticulation and architectural distortion. She is able to walk 284 meters during her 6MWT.

Clinical Vignette 2

A 79-year-old man with congestive heart failure (New York Heart Association [NYHA] functional class III) was admitted to the ICU with mixed hypoxemic hypercapnic respiratory failure due to acute decompensated heart failure. He was placed on noninvasive positive pressure ventilation and given intravenous diuretics but developed progressively worsening encephalopathy. Arterial blood gas analysis revealed a pH of 7.16, $PaCO_2$ of 72 mmHg, and PaO_2 of 109 mmHg. He was intubated and continued on intravenous diuretics. Over the course of the next several days, his volume status was optimized, and his respiratory mechanics on the mechanical ventilator improved. However, ongoing delirium prohibited extubation until hospital day nine, when he was successfully extubated to non-invasive positive pressure ventilation. He was discharged five days later to a skilled nursing facility.

Two months later, he presents to the ICU follow-up clinic. He describes breathlessness with minimal exertion, equivalent to grade 4 on the mMRC dyspnea scale. Using a front-wheel walker, he requires two rests to ambulate from the clinic waiting room to the examination room. His oxygen saturation is 92% on 2 liters per minute of supplemental oxygen via nasal cannula. His spirometry in clinic is suggestive of mild restriction. His scores on a 36-item short form survey (SF-36) reveal decreased HRQL.

Key Points

1. Dyspnea, a common symptom among survivors of critical illness, is often multifactorial. It can be caused by various pulmonary and diaphragmatic complications as well as extra-pulmonary problems.
2. Pulmonary complications, such as pulmonary fibrosis, tracheal stenosis, and pulmonary embolism, occur frequently after critical illness. Early detection and targeted interventions are crucial for managing these complications effectively.
3. Ventilator-induced diaphragmatic dysfunction is prevalent among survivors of critical illness and can have detrimental effects on short- and long-term outcomes.
4. Due to substantial heterogeneity in the pulmonary disorders and diaphragmatic dysfunction that occurs following critical illness, establishing universal instruments to evaluate pulmonary function in the post-ICU setting is challenging. Spirometry, plethysmography, DLCO, and 6MWT are commonly used measures.
5. ICU follow-up clinics can facilitate early identification of pulmonary and diaphragmatic complications and management of acute and chronic respiratory needs through a multidisciplinary approach. RTs play a pivotal role by evaluating respiratory complaints, assessing pulmonary function, managing equipment and treatments, and providing education.

References

1. M.S. Herridge, A.M. Cheung, C.M. Tansey, et al. One-year outcomes in survivors of the acute respiratory distress syndrome. *N Engl J Med* 2003; **348**: 683–93.
2. K. Nanwani-Nanwani, L. López-Pérez, C. Giménez-Esparza, et al. Prevalence of post-intensive care syndrome in mechanically ventilated patients with COVID-19. *Sci Rep* 2022; **12**: 7977.
3. D. Chiumello, S. Coppola, S. Froio, et al. What's next after ARDS: long-term outcomes. *Respir Care* 2016; **61**: 689–99.
4. S. Kligerman. Pathogenesis, imaging, and evolution of acute lung injury. *Radiol Clin North Am* 2022; **60**: 925–39.
5. J.L. Sturgill, K.P. Mayer, A.G. Kalema, et al. Post-intensive care syndrome and pulmonary fibrosis in patients surviving ARDS-pneumonia of COVID-19 and non-COVID-19 etiologies. *Sci Rep* 2023; **13**: 6554.
6. M. Balbi, C. Conti, G. Imeri, et al. Post-discharge chest CT findings and pulmonary function tests in severe COVID-19 patients. *Eur J Radiol* 2021; **138**: 109676.
7. N. Zias, A. Chroneou, M.K. Tabba, et al. Post tracheostomy and post intubation tracheal stenosis: report of 31 cases and review of the literature. *BMC Pulm Med* 2008; **8**: 18.
8. J.D. Cooper. Tracheal injuries complicating prolonged intubation and tracheostomy. *Thorac Surg Clin* 2018; **28**: 139–44.

9. N. Ravikumar, E. Ho, A. Wagh, et al. The role of bronchoscopy in the multidisciplinary approach to benign tracheal stenosis. *J Thorac Dis* 2023; **15**: 3998–4015.

10. M.B. Shadmehr, A. Abbasidezfouli, R. Farzanegan, et al. The role of systemic steroids in postintubation tracheal stenosis: a randomized clinical trial. *Ann Thorac Surg* 2017; **103**: 246–53.

11. K. MacDougall and A.C. Spyropoulos. New paradigms of extended thromboprophylaxis in medically ill patients. *J Clin Med* 2020; **9**: 1002.

12. K.A. Puntillo and R. Naidu. Chronic pain disorders after critical illness and ICU-acquired opioid dependence: two clinical conundra. *Curr Opin Crit Care* 2016; **22**: 506–12.

13. C. Carrie, Y. Guemmar, V. Cottenceau. Long-term disability after blunt chest trauma: don't miss chronic neuropathic pain! *Injury* 2019; **50**: 113–18.

14. M. Boyle, M. Murgo, H. Adamson. The effect of chronic pain on health related quality of life amongst intensive care survivors. *Aust Crit Care* 2004; **17**: 104–106, 108–113.

15. T. Vassilakopoulos, B.J. Petrof. Ventilator-induced diaphragmatic dysfunction. *Am J Resp Crit Care Med* 2004; **169**: 336–41.

16. G.S. Supinski, P.E. Morris, S. Dhar, et al. Diaphragm dysfunction in critical illness. *Chest* 2018; **153**: 1040–51.

17. S. Jaber, B.J. Petrof, B. Jung, et al. Rapidly progressive diaphragmatic weakness and injury during mechanical ventilation in humans. *Am J Resp Crit Care Med* 2011; **183**: 364–71.

18. S. Levine, T. Nguyen, N. Taylor, et al. Rapid disuse atrophy of diaphragm fibers in mechanically ventilated humans. *N Engl J Med* 2008; **358**: 1327–35.

19. M. Dres, E.C. Goligher, L.M.A. Heunks, et al. Critical illness-associated diaphragm weakness. *Intensive Care Med* 2017; **43**: 1441–52.

20. D. Adler, E. Dupuis-Lozeron, J.-C. Richard, et al. Does inspiratory muscle dysfunction predict readmission after intensive care unit discharge? *Am J Resp Crit Care Med* 2014; **190**: 347–50.

21. C. Medrinal, G. Prieur, É. Frenoy, et al. Respiratory weakness after mechanical ventilation is associated with one-year mortality: a prospective study. *Crit Care* 2016; **20**: 231.

22. D.M. Needham, K.A. Sepulveda, V.D. Dinglas, et al. Core outcome measures for clinical research in acute respiratory failure survivors. an international modified Delphi consensus study. *Am J Resp Crit Care Med* 2017; **196**: 1122–30.

23. M.E. Mikkelsen, M. Still, B.J. Anderson, et al. Society of Critical Care Medicine's international consensus conference on prediction and identification of long-term impairments after critical illness. *Crit Care Med* 2020; **48**: 1670–9.

24. T.A. Neff, R. Stocker, H.-R. Frey, et al. Long-term assessment of lung function in survivors of severe ARDS. *Chest* 2003; **123**: 845–53.

25. G. Schelling, C. Stoll, C. Vogelmeier, et al. Pulmonary function and health-related quality of life in a sample of long-term survivors of the acute respiratory distress syndrome. *Intensive Care Med* 2000; **26**: 1304–11.

26. M. Joris, P. Minguet, C. Colson, et al. Cardiopulmonary exercise testing in critically ill coronavirus disease 2019 survivors: evidence of a sustained exercise intolerance and hypermetabolism. *Crit Care Explor* 2021; **3**: e0491.

27. S. Benington, D. McWilliams, J. Eddleston, et al. Exercise testing in survivors of intensive care: is there a role for cardiopulmonary exercise testing? *J Crit Care* 2012; **27**: 89–94.

28. N. Van Aerde, P. Meersseman, Y. Debaveye, et al. Aerobic exercise capacity in long-term survivors of critical illness: secondary analysis of the post-EPaNIC follow-up study. *Intensive Care Med* 2021; **47**: 1462–71.

29. K.-C. Ong. Pulmonary function and exercise capacity in survivors of severe

acute respiratory syndrome. *Eur Respir J* 2004; **24**: 436–42.

30. M.E. Wilcox, D. Patsios, G. Murphy, et al. Radiologic outcomes at 5 years after severe ARDS. *Chest* 2013; **143**: 920–6.

31. J. Orme, J.S. Romney, R.O. Hopkins, et al. Pulmonary function and health-related quality of life in survivors of acute respiratory distress syndrome. *Am J Resp Crit Care Med* 2003; **167**: 690–4.

32. D.K. Heyland, D. Groll, M. Caeser. Survivors of acute respiratory distress syndrome: relationship between pulmonary dysfunction and long-term health-related quality of life. *Crit Care Med* 2005; **33**: 1549–56.

33. A.L. Bellinghausen, B.W. Butcher, L.T. Ho, et al. Respiratory therapists in an ICU recovery clinic: two institutional experiences and review of the literature. *Respir Care* 2021; **66**: 1885–91.

Chapter 36
Common Somatic Concerns in Survivors of Critical Illness

Hiam Naiditch and Brad W. Butcher

Introduction

Although the physical challenges of post-intensive care syndrome (PICS) are typically thought of in terms of impaired endurance, strength, and balance, survivors of critical illness often report additional debilitating physical symptoms that can have a significant impact on their quality of life (see Figure 36.1). While some of these conditions may be minimized by patients or potentially embarrassing for them to share, the identification of these symptoms by astute providers through a thoughtful review of systems can facilitate referral to specialty care providers, improve functional outcomes among survivors of critical illness, and alleviate some of the suffering with which they must contend.

Fatigue

About one-half to two-thirds of all survivors of critical illness experience fatigue, making it the most commonly reported symptom, and female patients are more than twice as likely as males to experience fatigue (odds ratio [OR] for males 0.47, 95% interval [CI] 0.30–0.74) [1,2,3]. Fatigue can persist for at least five years following hospital discharge [3], and it can have a substantial impact on one's ability to return to normal routines, including performing activities of daily living and instrumental activities of daily living, resuming employment, and reengaging in previously held social, avocational, and community roles. Fatigue is a heterogenous symptom that eludes a clear and consistent definition in the literature [4], and in many conditions, including PICS, its cause is often multifactorial. Homeostatic mechanisms mediate fatigue through altered autonomic nervous system regulation based on inflammatory and energetic feedback, while psychological mechanisms, based largely in the frontal lobe, may mediate fatigue through depression and chronic fatigue syndrome [4]. Fatigue can also be a manifestation of intensive care unit-acquired weakness (ICUAW), a heterogeneous entity composed of critical illness polyneuropathy (CIN), critical illness myopathy (CIM), or a combination thereof that can be associated with prolonged weaning from mechanical ventilation and may contribute to persistent weakness and fatigue for years following hospital discharge (see Chapter 4 for additional information) [5,6,7,8,9].

While there is no gold standard, several tools are available for measuring fatigue, which are typically administered in the form of questionnaires answered by the patient. These include the Chalder Fatigue Scale (CFS), the Fatigue Impact Scale (FIS) [10], and the Functional Assessment of Chronic Illness Therapy – Fatigue (FACIT-F) [2]. FACIT-F has been shown to be reproducible and correlative with other fatigue measures in at least one rheumatologic condition [11] and has also been used in survivors of critical illness [2]. While more data is needed to determine the most valid fatigue screening tool in this patient

Common Somatic Concerns in Survivors of Critical Illness

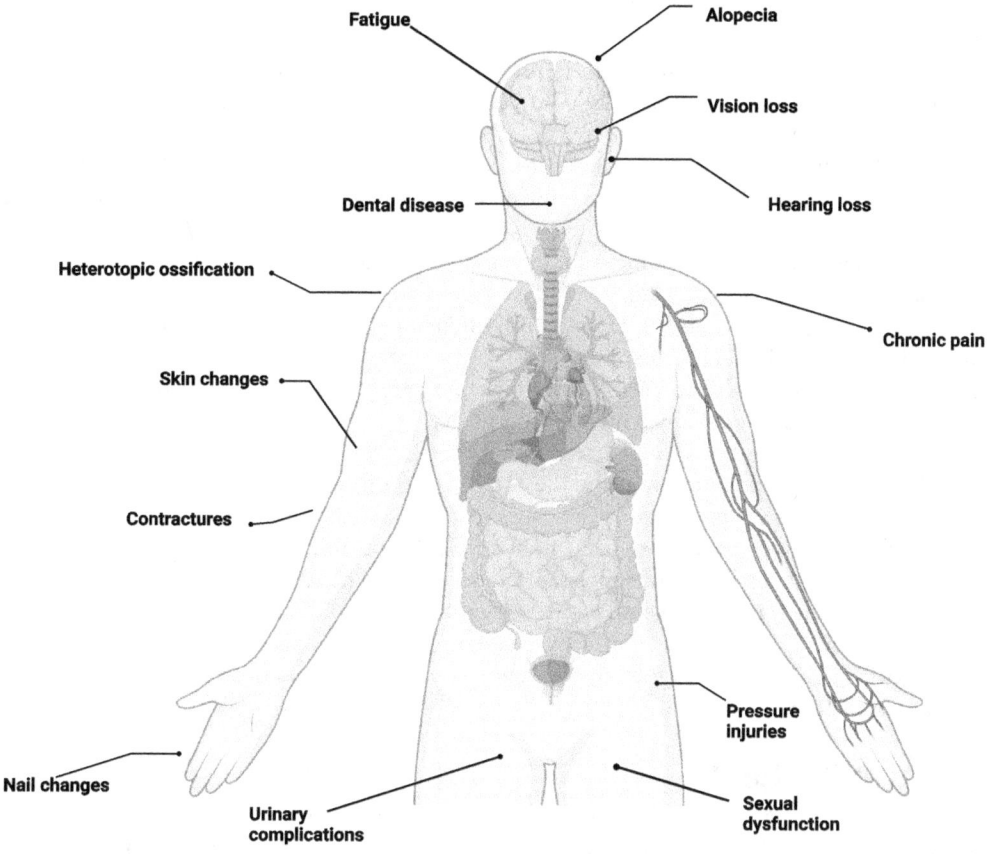

Figure 36.1 Common somatic concerns in survivors of critical illness. Common somatic concerns encountered in ICU survivors can include fatigue, chronic pain, hearing and vision loss, contractures, and pressure injuries. *Image generated using Biorender.com.*

population, clinicians would likely benefit from choosing a standard tool with which to measure baseline fatigue and follow patients longitudinally.

Interventions aimed to address fatigue are numerous and include regular fatigue assessments; use of notebooks, handbooks, and electronic resources; goal setting with tracking of progress; and counseling [12]. Structured exercise routines, which vary in content and duration based on the patient's condition and needs, are likely to be of benefit in managing fatigue and may also have a beneficial impact on cognition and mood [13,14,15]. When recommending graduated exercise programs and other rehabilitation therapies for survivors of critical illness, it is important to consider barriers to care, including financial and transportation difficulties [13]. Identifying and addressing comorbid conditions that overlap with fatigue, such as sleepiness, obstructive sleep apnea, depression, or apathy, may also be helpful in improving patients' symptoms and quality of life [4].

Chronic Pain

In a comprehensive review, the prevalence of chronic pain in survivors of critical illness ranged from 14% to 77%, while the incidence of new-onset chronic pain following critical illness is 22–33% [16]. One study identified a 23% increase in pain among patients previously hospitalized in a surgical intensive care unit (ICU) as compared to the general population, a number that is likely to be impacted by preexisting disease [17,18]. Interestingly, the most commonly reported site of chronic post-ICU pain was the shoulder, a finding that may be explained at least in part by the higher incidence of brachial plexus injuries in patients who require mechanical ventilation in the prone position for severe respiratory failure [16,19].

Several pain scales exist to measure chronic pain, and other tools incorporate pain as a component of an overall health-related quality of life (HRQoL) assessment, such as the Short Form 36 (SF-36) and the EuroQol-5Dimensions (EQ-5D; see Chapter 34 for additional information) [19]. Similar to the scales used for fatigue, these are subjective questionnaires that are useful in establishing baseline symptoms and measuring progress in survivors of critical illness receiving follow-up care.

Among the interventions studied, reasonable approaches involve a biopsychosocial appreciation for the nature of chronic pain and the employment of a multimodal treatment plan. Such treatment plans may include integrative treatments, such as massage and acupuncture; pharmacotherapy, including acetaminophen, non-steroidal anti-inflammatory drugs (NSAIDs), antiepileptic agents, analgesic antidepressants, localized anesthetics (e.g., lidocaine or capsaicin), or opioid analgesics; transcutaneous electrical nerve stimulation (TENS); and invasive procedures, such as image-guided injections (see Chapter 45 for additional information) [16]. Future studies are needed to identify the most effective interventions to address chronic pain in this patient population.

Joint Contractures

A joint contracture is a pathologic decrease in the size of periarticular connective tissue and muscle, leading to limitation in passive motion of a joint [20]. Prolonged bed rest and immobility can predispose patients to joint contractures, and one-third of patients with an ICU length of stay of greater than two weeks are likely to experience a functionally significant contracture of a major joint [20]. Elbows and ankles are the most frequently affected joints, but contractures of the knees, hips, shoulders, and even fingers are also relatively common [20,21]. Although data are limited, occupational therapy consultation for consideration of dynamic splinting, stretching exercises, and surgery, where appropriate, can be considered for management [22]. Botulinum toxin A injections may also help reduce contractures and may have a role early in the course of ICU recovery (see Chapter 45 for additional information) [23].

Heterotopic Ossification

Heterotopic ossification (HO) is the abnormal development of bone in soft tissues, particularly near large joints, resulting in pain, enlargement of the joint, and functional limitation [24]. HO may be identified as a palpable tender mass, and radiographs or computed tomography scans may identify a mass outlined by peripheral calcification [24]. Prolonged immobility is an important risk factor, including among critically ill patients with acute respiratory distress syndrome [21]. Its presence in patients with central nervous system injury is considered a distinct entity known as neurologic heterotopic ossification [25]. Functional limitations in the distance covered during a six-minute walk test have been at least partially attributable to HO [21]. Potential treatment options include NSAIDs, bisphosphonates, radiation therapy, and surgical excision, all of which have variable outcomes [25].

Pressure Injuries

Approximately 14–27% of critically ill patients develop pressure injuries or ulcers during hospitalization, two-thirds of which are acquired in the ICU; the sacrum and the heel are the most commonly affected sites [26,27]. Pressure ulcers are a frequent consequence of prolonged immobilization and inadequate turning, and receipt of corticosteroids may predispose patients to an increased risk for their development [28,29]. Pressure ulcers are associated with increased mortality: the presence of stage III pressure injuries increases the risk of in-hospital mortality two- to three-fold. Best practices to prevent pressure injury development include ensuring adequate nutritional supplementation and offloading pressure through repositioning and appropriate mattress use [30,31,32,33]. Specific nutritional supplements that may be of benefit are arginine, vitamin C, zinc, and enhanced protein delivery, although evidence for these interventions is limited [34,35]. Vitamin A may be useful for wound healing in patients receiving corticosteroids [36,37]. Among mattresses, reactive air surfaces or alternating pressure air surfaces may reduce pressure ulcer risk or, in the case of reactive air surfaces, may foster ulcer healing as compared to foam surfaces [38]. Consultation with a wound care specialist can streamline optimal care of pressure injuries in this patient population.

Skin, Hair, and Nail Changes

In addition to pressure injuries, changes to the skin that occur during critical illness may be disease-related or iatrogenic [39]. Although rare, vasopressor use can be associated with peripheral gangrene, which may be related to duration of intensive care and dose of vasopressor administered [40,41]. Intravenous and intra-arterial catheters can be associated with scars or keloid formation [42]. Tracheotomy tube insertion sites may also develop scars that patients may consider cosmetically unacceptable, and these may be amenable to surgical revision for cosmesis [21]. Dry skin has been reported in survivors of critical illness and may be a function of systemic disease, the duration of the ICU stay, or the comparatively arid environments of the ICU and hospital [43].

Alopecia has been reported in one-sixth to one-third of survivors of critical illness and can present as localized hair loss to diffuse hair-thinning [4]. Sepsis and septic shock have been identified as a risk factors for alopecia, and the duration of hair loss may extend from three weeks to seven months [43,44]. Although hair loss may be temporary, treatment for prolonged hair loss guided by a dermatologist might be warranted and conventionally mirrors that used for hair loss in the general population, including topical minoxidil, finasteride, or spironolactone, depending on the etiology and gender of the patient [45,46].

Brittle nails are also common and may be related to ICU-related trauma, repeated wetting and drying during ICU care, and the relatively dry ICU environment [47,48]. Application of moisturizers can aid in the management of dry skin and brittle nails [47].

Dental Disease

Oral health is often negatively impacted during hospitalization as manifested by increased plaque accumulation and gingival inflammation [49,50]. An increase in the number of bacteria on dental plaque and colonization by hospital-acquired pathogenic bacteria likely contribute to poor dental health [51]. Several oral health assessments have been proposed for use in the ICU and include evaluation of the lips, tongue, mucosa, gingiva, teeth, and saliva, as well as assessment for the presence of plaque, debris, bleeding, redness, ulceration, or halitosis [52]. An oral evaluation by the patient's primary care physician or post-ICU provider focusing on these elements can help identify the need for a dedicated dental evaluation.

Hearing Loss

Preexisting hearing loss is a risk factor for poor functional recovery in survivors of critical illness aged 70 years and older [53]. Roughly one-sixth of patients experience hearing loss following an ICU stay, as defined as a >10dB increase in the pure tone average (PTA) threshold [54]. Possible mechanisms include altered perfusion to key audiological structures, hypercoagulability, and the use of ototoxic agents, including aminoglycoside and macrolide antibiotics, salicylates, loop diuretics, and NSAIDs [54]. Given the association of hearing loss with cognitive decline, providers caring for survivors of critical illness should seek to identify and address hearing loss [55,56]. Methods of screening include examination maneuvers such as finger rub and whispered voice as well as in-office audiometry [54]. Abnormal results should prompt referral to an audiologist for further evaluation and management.

Ophthalmologic Sequelae

Ocular surface disease is a relatively common phenomenon among critically ill patients, affecting one-fifth to one-third of all patients [57,58]. Patients who are sedated and mechanically ventilated may experience conjunctival swelling (chemosis) and complications resulting from inadequate eye closure (lagophthalmos), including corneal abrasions, exposure keratopathy, and infectious keratitis [57,59,60,61]. Prone positioning may also be a risk factor for ocular complications, including optic neuropathy and potentially blindness [59,61]. The use of agents with α-adrenergic activity can decrease perfusion to key ocular structures and may also increase intra-ocular pressure, thereby exacerbating glaucoma [62]. Vascular occlusions, including central retinal artery occlusion, central retinal vein occlusion, and ischemic optic neuropathy, may occur due to presenting conditions such as vasculitis and systemic hypertension and can be associated with long-term vision loss [63,64]. A patient's self-reported symptoms, ideally accompanied by screening tests such as a Snellen eye chart evaluation, may prompt early referral to ophthalmology for identification and management of these ophthalmologic sequelae of critical illness.

Sexual Dysfunction

The incidence of sexual dysfunction among survivors of critical illness is likely underappreciated. Sexual health may not be discussed with survivors during clinic appointments, and some patients may be embarrassed to raise concerns with their healthcare providers. When surveyed, however, 43.6% of survivors of critical illness reported symptoms of sexual dysfunction [65]. Among survivors of severe physical trauma, approximately one-third have persistent symptoms, which may be influenced by the development of post-traumatic stress disorder in some of these patients [65,66]. While the prevalence may be similar to that in the general population, recognizing and addressing sexual dysfunction in survivors of critical illness is likely to positively impact quality of life [67,68]. Assessment should include the identification of potentially contributing comorbidities, including hypertension, diabetes, and tobacco use, and a review of medication side effects, including selective serotonin reuptake inhibitors, antihypertensives, and α-adrenergic blockers [69,70,71,72]. Referral to the appropriate specialist, including gynecology or urology, can help provide directed evaluation and treatment for sexual dysfunction.

Urinary Complications

The use of indwelling urinary catheters is common (and often overused) among ICU patients [73]. Prolonged use of indwelling urinary catheters, prolonged immobility, and use of midazolam, opioid analgesics, and propofol are all associated with acute urinary retention [74]. In addition to catheter-associated urinary tract infections, long-term complications of urethral catheterization can include urethral strictures, urethral fracture, and rarely, iatrogenic hypospadias [75]. It is unclear whether suprapubic or urethral catheters are preferable for patients with neurogenic bladder; among patients with spinal cord injuries, rates of urinary tract infection, nephrolithiasis, bladder calculi, and urothelial cancer were found to be similar with both types of catheters [76].

Conclusion

Caring for survivors of critical illness requires a holistic and detailed approach that evaluates all organ systems. A thorough review of systems, use of validated questionnaires, and targeted questions about common problems following critical illness are essential to elucidating challenges that patients may minimize or feel uncomfortable sharing with a provider. Recognizing the various somatic complications that survivors of critical illness may suffer, normalizing how common such complications are following critical illness, educating about treatments and management strategies, and supporting and reassuring patients are required to facilitate recovery.

Key Points

1. Post-ICU sequelae span multiple organ systems that can be identified through a thorough, knowledge-based review of systems and targeted questionnaires.
2. Fatigue and chronic pain are among the most common symptoms in survivors of critical illness and may benefit from regular assessments using validated questionnaires and comprehensive multimodal treatment strategies.
3. Identification of varying symptoms among survivors of critical illness may warrant referral to subspecialty providers, including dermatology, ophthalmology, and urology.

References

1. G-B. Wintermann, J. Rosendahl, K. Weidner, et al. Self-reported fatigue following intensive care of chronically critically ill patients: a prospective cohort study. *J Intensive Care* 2018; **6**: 27.
2. K.J. Neufeld, J.S. Leoutsakos, H. Yan, et al. Fatigue symptoms during the first year following ARDS. *Chest* 2020; **158**: 999–1007.
3. J. Morel, P. Infantino, L. Gergelé, et al. Prevalence of self-reported fatigue in intensive care unit survivors 6 months–5 years after discharge. *Sci Rep* 2022; **12**: 5631.
4. B.M. Kluger, L.B. Krupp, R.M. Enoka. Fatigue and fatigability in neurologic illnesses: proposal for a unified taxonomy. *Neurology* 2013; **80**: 409–16.
5. I. Vanhorebeek, N. Latronico, G. Van den Berghe. ICU-acquired weakness. *Intensive Care Med* 2020; **46**: 637–53.
6. C.F. Bolton, J.J. Gilbert, A.F. Hahn, et al. Polyneuropathy in critically ill patients. *J Neurol Neurosurg Psychiatr* 1984; **47**: 1223–31.
7. L. Gutmann, L. Gutmann. Critical illness neuropathy and myopathy. *Arch Neurol* 1999; **56**: 527–8.
8. S. Shepherd, A. Batra, D.P. Lerner. Review of critical illness myopathy and neuropathy. *Neurohospitalist* 2017; **7**: 41–8.
9. W. Zink, R. Kollmar, S. Schwab. Critical illness polyneuropathy and myopathy in the intensive care unit. *Nat Rev Neurol* 2009; **5**: 372–9.
10. R. Billones, J.K. Liwang, K. Butler, et al. Dissecting the fatigue experience: a scoping review of fatigue definitions, dimensions, and measures in non-oncologic medical conditions. *Brain Behav Immun Health* 2021; **15**: 100266.
11. M.O. Machado, N.C. Kang, F. Tai, et al. Measuring fatigue: a meta-review. *Int J Dermatol* 2021; **60**: 1053–69.
12. S.E. Brown, A. Shah, W. Czuber-Dochan, et al. Non-pharmacological interventions for self-management of fatigue in adults: an umbrella review of potential interventions to support patients recovering from critical illness. *J Crit Care*. 2023; **75**: 154279.
13. K. Liu, O. Tronstad, D. Flaws, et al. From bedside to recovery: exercise therapy for prevention of post-intensive care syndrome. *J Intensive Care* 2024; **12**: 11.
14. C.L.A. Wender, M. Manninen, P. J. O'Connor. The effect of chronic exercise on energy and fatigue states: a systematic review and meta-analysis of randomized trials. *Front Psychol* 2022; **13**: 907637.
15. P. Zalewski, S. Kujawski, M. Tudorowska, et al. The impact of a structured exercise programme upon cognitive function in chronic fatigue syndrome patients. *Brain Sci* 2019; **10**(1): 4.
16. H.I. Kemp, H. Laycock, A. Costello, et al. Chronic pain in critical care survivors: a narrative review. *Br J Anaesth* 2019; **123**: e372–84.
17. T.K. Timmers, M.H. Verhofstad, K. G. Moons, et al. Long-term quality of life after surgical intensive care admission. *Arch Surg* 2011; **146**: 412–18.
18. L. Orwelius, A. Nordlund, U. Edéll-Gustafsson, et al. Role of preexisting disease in patients' perceptions of health-related quality of life after intensive care. *Crit Care Med* 2005; **33**: 1557–64.
19. J. King-Robson, E. Bates, E. Sokolov, et al. Prone position plexopathy: an avoidable complication of prone positioning for COVID-19 pneumonitis? *BMJ Case Rep* 2022; **15**(1): e243798.
20. H. Clavet, P.C. Hébert, D. Fergusson, et al. Joint contracture following prolonged stay in the intensive care unit. *CMAJ* 2008; **178**: 691–7.
21. M.S. Herridge, A.M. Cheung, C. Tansey, et al. One-year outcomes in survivors of the acute respiratory distress syndrome. *N Engl J Med* 2003; **348**: 683–93.
22. L.A. Harvey, O.M. Katalinic, R.D. Herbert, et al. Stretch for the treatment and prevention of contracture: an abridged republication of a Cochrane Systematic Review. *J Physiother* 2017; **63**(2): 67–75.

23. C. Lindsay, S. Ispoglou, B. Helliwell, et al. Can the early use of botulinum toxin in post stroke spasticity reduce contracture development? A randomised controlled trial. *Clin Rehabil* 2021; **35**: 399–409.

24. C. Meyers, J. Lisiecki, S. Miller, et al. Heterotopic ossification: a comprehensive review. *JBMR PLUS* 2019; **3**: e10172.

25. K.R. Wong, R. Mychasiuk, T.J. O'Brien, et al. Neurological heterotopic ossification: novel mechanisms, prognostic biomarkers and prophylactic therapies. *Bone Res* 2020; **8**: 42.

26. J. Cox, L.E. Edsberg, K. Koloms, et al. Pressure injuries in critical care patients in US hospitals: results of the international pressure ulcer prevalence survey. *J Wound Ostomy Continence Nurs* 2022; **49**: 21–8.

27. S.O. Labeau, E. Afonso, J. Benbenishty, et al. Prevalence, associated factors and outcomes of pressure injuries in adult intensive care unit patients: the DecubICUs study. *Intensive Care Med* 2021; **47**: 160–9.

28. A. de O. Ramalho, L.M. Santiago, L. Meira, et al. Pressure injury prevention in adult critically ill patients: best practice implementation project. *JBI Evid Implement* 2023; **21**: 218–28.

29. H-L Chen, W-Q. Shen, Y-H. Xu, et al. Perioperative corticosteroids administration as a risk factor for pressure ulcers in cardiovascular surgical patients: a retrospective study. *Int Wound J* 2015; **12**: 581–5.

30. J. Rivera, E. Donohoe, M. Deady-Rooney, et al. Implementing a pressure injury prevention bundle to decrease hospital-acquired pressure injuries in an adult critical care unit: an evidence-based, pilot initiative. *Wound Manag Prev* 2020; **66**: 20–8.

31. W.V. Padula, J.M. Black. The Standardized Pressure Injury Prevention Protocol for improving nursing compliance with best practice guidelines. *J Clin Nurs* 2019; **28**: 367–71.

32. J. Kottner, J. Cuddigan, K. Carville, et al. Prevention and treatment of pressure ulcers/injuries: the protocol for the second update of the international Clinical Practice Guideline 2019. *J Tissue Viability* 2019; **28**: 51–8.

33. K.J. Desneves, B.E. Todorovic, A. Cassar, et al. Treatment with supplementary arginine, vitamin C and zinc in patients with pressure ulcers: a randomised controlled trial. *Clin Nutr* 2005; **24**: 979–87.

34. G. Langer, C.S. Wan, A. Fink, et al. Nutritional interventions for preventing and treating pressure ulcers. *Cochrane Database Syst Rev* 2024; **2**: CD003216.

35. J.D. Phillips, C.S. Kim, E.W. Fonkalsrud, et al. Effects of chronic corticosteroids and vitamin A on the healing of intestinal anastomoses. *Am J Surg* 1992; **163**: 71–7.

36. D.U. Talas, A. Nayci, S. Atis, et al. The effects of corticosteroids and vitamin A on the healing of tracheal anastomoses. *Int J Pediatr Otorhinolaryngol* 2003; **67**: 109–16.

37. C. Shi, J.C. Dumville, N. Cullum, et al. Beds, overlays and mattresses for preventing and treating pressure ulcers: an overview of Cochrane Reviews and network meta-analysis. *Cochrane Database Syst Rev* 2021; **8**: CD013761.

38. M. Badia, J.M. Casanova, L. Serviá, et al. Dermatological manifestations in the intensive care unit: a practical approach. *Crit Care Res Pract* 2020; **2020**: 9729814.

39. M. Bromley, S. Marsh, A. Layton. Dermatological complications of critical care. *BJA Educ* 2021; **21**: 408–13.

40. J.W. Kwon, M.K. Hong, B.Y. Park. Risk factors of vasopressor-induced symmetrical peripheral gangrene. *Ann Plast Surg* 2018; **80**: 622–7.

41. S. Munjal, J. Kumar, P. Kumar, et al. Keloid formation on neck after jugular central venous catheter placement: an unsightly unusual complication in a young female. *Indian J Anaesth* 2018; **62**: 82–4.

42. M.J. Lee, J.Y. Chang, C.S. Shin, et al. Analysis of increased xerosis in intensive care unit patients. *Ann Dermatol* 2006; **18** (1): 1–4.

43. C.E. Battle, C. Lynch, C. Thorpe, et al. Incidence and risk factors for alopecia in

survivors of critical illness: a multi-centre observational study. *J Crit Care* 2019; **50**: 31–5.

44. C.E. Battle, K. James, and P. Temblett. Alopecia in survivors of critical illness. *J Intensive Care Soc* 2016; **17**: 270.

45. A.L. Mounsey, S.W. Reed. Diagnosing and treating hair loss. *Am Fam Physician* 2009; **80**: 356–62.

46. T. Scott, M. Davies, C. Dutton, et al. Intensive care follow-up in UK military casualties: a one-year pilot. *J Intensive Care Soc* 2014; **15**(2): 113–16.

47. M.A. Chessa, M. Iorizzo, B. Richert, et al. Pathogenesis, clinical signs and treatment recommendations in brittle nails: a review. *Dermatol Ther (Heidelb)* 2020; **10**: 15–27.

48. S. Saran, M. Gurjar, A. Baronia, et al. Heating, ventilation and air conditioning (HVAC) in intensive care unit. *Crit Care* 2020; **24**: 194.

49. E. Terezakis, I. Needleman, N. Kumar, et al. The impact of hospitalization on oral health: a systematic review. *J Clin Periodontol* 2011; **38**: 628–36.

50. M-K. Jun, J.K. Ku, I.H. Kim, et al. Hospital dentistry for intensive care unit patients: a comprehensive review. *J Clin Med* 2021; **10**(16): 3681.

51. M. Sachdev, D. Ready, D. Brealey, et al. Changes in dental plaque following hospitalisation in a critical care unit: an observational study. *Crit Care* 2013; **17**: R189.

52. L. Winning, F.T. Lundy, B. Blackwood, et al. Oral health care for the critically ill: a narrative review. *Crit Care* 2021; **25**: 353.

53. L.E. Ferrante, M.A. Pisani, T.E. Murphy, et al. Factors associated with functional recovery among older intensive care unit survivors. *Am J Respir Crit Care Med* 2016; **194**: 299–307.

54. J.J. Walker, L.M. Cleveland, J.L. Davis, et al. Audiometry screening and interpretation. *Am Fam Physician* 2013; **87**: 41–7.

55. T. Fujiwara, M. Sato, S.I. Sato, et al. Sensorineural hearing dysfunction after discharge from critical care in adults:

a retrospective observational study. *J Otol* 2021; **16**: 144–9.

56. F.R. Lin, K. Yaffe, J. Xia, et al. Hearing loss and cognitive decline in older adults. *JAMA Intern Med* 2013; **173**: 293–9.

57. L. Płaszewska-Żywko, A. Sega, A. Bukowa, et al. Risk factors of eye complications in patients treated in the intensive care unit. *Int J Environ Res Public Health* 2021; **18** (21): 11178.

58. B.J. Hearne, E.G. Hearne, H. Montgomery, et al. Eye care in the intensive care unit. *J Intensive Care Soc* 2018; **19**: 345–50.

59. P. Sanghi, M. Malik, I.T. Hossain, et al. Ocular complications in the prone position in the critical care setting: the COVID-19 pandemic. *J Intensive Care Med* 2021; **36**: 361–72.

60. T.B. Saritas, B. Bozkurt, B. Simsek, et al. Ocular surface disorders in intensive care unit patients. *Scientific World Journal* 2013; **2013**: 182038.

61. F. Mayr, N. Asher, K. Scanlan, et al. 1953: Bilateral blindness after prone positioning for acute respiratory distress syndrome. *Crit Care Med* 2016; **44**(12): 563.

62. F. Mercieca, P. Suresh, A. Morton, et al. Ocular surface disease in intensive care unit patients. *Eye* 1999; **13**(Pt 2): 231–6.

63. P.H. Parekh, C.S. Boente, R.D. Boente, et al. Ophthalmology in critical care. *Ann Am Thorac Soc* 2019; **16**: 957–66.

64. H.M.J. Blegen, D.S. Reed, G.B. Giles, et al. Long-term outcomes after central retinal artery occlusion treated acutely with hyperbaric oxygen therapy: a case series. *J Vitreoretin Dis* 2021; **5**: 142–6.

65. J. Griffiths, M. Gager, N. Alder, et al. A self-report-based study of the incidence and associations of sexual dysfunction in survivors of intensive care treatment. *Intensive Care Med* 2006; **32**: 445–51.

66. A. Ulvik, R. Kvåle, T. Wentzel-Larsen, et al. Sexual function in ICU survivors more than 3 years after major trauma. *Intensive Care Med.* 2008; **34**: 447–53.

67. R.C. Rosen. Prevalence and risk factors of sexual dysfunction in men and women. *Curr Psychiatry Rep* 2000; **2**: 189–95.

68. K.E. Flynn, L. Lin, D.W. Bruner, et al. Sexual satisfaction and the importance of sexual health to quality of life throughout the life course of U.S. adults. *J Sex Med* 2016; **13**: 1642–50.

69. A.R. Polland, M. Davis, A. Zeymo, et al. Association between comorbidities and female sexual dysfunction: findings from the third National Survey of Sexual Attitudes and Lifestyles (Natsal-3). *Int Urogynecol J* 2019; **30**: 377–83.

70. J. Das, S. Yadav. Comorbidities of male patients with sexual dysfunction in a psychiatry clinic: a study on industrial employees. *Ind Psychiatry J* 2022; **31**: 81–8.

71. C. Valeiro, C. Matos, J. Scholl, et al. Drug-induced sexual dysfunction: an analysis of reports to a national pharmacovigilance database. *Drug Saf* 2022; **45**: 639–50.

72. B. Volk and F. Grassi. Treatment of the post-ICU patient in an outpatient setting. *Am Fam Physician* 2009; **79**: 459–64.

73. S. Saint, R.H. Savel, M.A. Matthay. Enhancing the safety of critically ill patients by reducing urinary and central venous catheter-related infections. *Am J Respir Crit Care Med* 2002; **165**: 1475–9.

74. D.A. Schettini, F.G. Freitas, D.Y. Tomotani, et al. Incidence and risk factors for urinary retention in critically ill patients. *Nurs Crit Care* 2019; **24**: 355–61.

75. G. Garg, V. Baghele, N. Chawla, et al. Unusual complication of prolonged indwelling urinary catheter: iatrogenic hypospadias. *J Family Med Prim Care* 2016; **5**: 493–4.

76. H.K. Katsumi, J.F. Kalisvaart, L.D. Ronningen, et al. Urethral versus suprapubic catheter: choosing the best bladder management for male spinal cord injury patients with indwelling catheters. *Spinal Cord* 2010; **48**: 325–9.

Chapter 37

Sleep Impairments in Survivors of Critical Illness

Janna R. Raphelson and Robert L. Owens

Introduction

Sleep problems often predate a hospital admission with critical illness, as they are common in the general population and even more so in those with chronic medical conditions. Critical illness can lead to or exacerbate preexisting sleep problems that can persist well into recovery. Impaired sleep can impact other symptoms in all three post-intensive care syndrome (PICS) domains (physical, cognitive, and psychological). Addressing sleep concerns, which are often overlooked, can provide significant relief to patients who may find these symptoms distressing. This chapter provides an approach to the outpatient evaluation of a survivor of critical illness with poor sleep (see Figure 37.1).

Sleep after the ICU

While knowledge about sleep in the recovery period after critical illness remains limited, recent studies highlight concerning trends. A systematic review of 22 studies characterizing sleep disturbances following an intensive care unit (ICU) admission found a high prevalence of abnormal sleep at all timepoints examined, with a general trend toward improvement over time: 50–66% of patients had a sleep disturbance at one month following hospital discharge, 34–64% at 1–3 months, 22–57% at 3–6 months, and 10–61% at more than 6 months [1]. Patients recovering from critical illness reported greater difficulty falling asleep, worse sleep quality, and greater sleep deficit compared to patients who were hospitalized but not critically ill [2]. A qualitative study of patient experiences following an episode of critical illness performed by an ICU follow-up clinic in Northern Ireland noted that the most frequently reported physical complaint was "difficulty getting to sleep," while another qualitative study of survivors of critical illness identified major themes of "longing for normal sleep" and "being tormented by nightmares" [3]. The underlying causes of impaired sleep after critical illness are not clear; however, by assessing sleep symptoms, screening for underlying pathology, and offering treatments and coping strategies, providers can comprehensively address this patient-centered concern.

Approach to Patients with Sleep Problems

First, it is important to define the specific sleep disturbance(s) and determine its impact on the patient's daytime functioning. Typical complaints include insomnia, defined as difficulty falling asleep or staying asleep despite an adequate opportunity to do so, and excessive daytime sleepiness. Sleepiness is the propensity to fall asleep, and when it interferes with normal functioning, it is referred to as excessive daytime sleepiness. It can be difficult to distinguish excessive daytime sleepiness from fatigue, which is a lack of energy with or

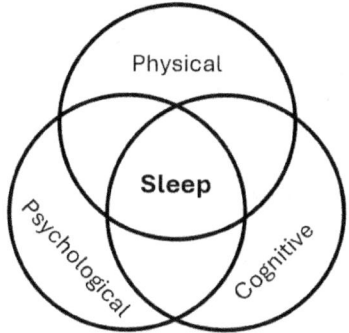

Figure 37.1 Sleep can impact symptoms in all three post-intensive care syndrome domains: physical, cognitive, and psychological.

without a tendency to fall asleep easily. Patients often use these terms interchangeably. Both complaints are common after critical illness and often improve along the recovery trajectory. Sleep quality can be more objectively evaluated by using tools such as the Pittsburgh Sleep Quality Index or the Functional Outcomes of Sleep Questionnaire.

After assessing the patient's satisfaction with their sleep quality and addressing any specific sleep concerns they have, the patient's medications should be reviewed, with particular attention paid to sedating or stimulating side effect profiles. Insomnia in the hospital is often addressed with sedative-hypnotic agents, but the continuation of these medications in the outpatient setting may impair sleep recovery [4]. Culprit medications often include benzodiazepines, atypical antipsychotics, and sedating antidepressants, such as trazodone and mirtazapine, which are often used for insomnia or agitation in the hospital, but many other medication classes can also cause daytime drowsiness (e.g., beta blockers) [5]. Selective serotonin reuptake inhibitors (SSRIs) can exacerbate symptoms of restless leg syndrome (RLS), which can also contribute to poor sleep [6,7]. In cases where an offending medication is deemed essential, educating the patient on its potential impact on sleep can manage expectations in patients struggling with fatigue.

Common Sleep Disturbances

Following assessment of general sleep quality and examination of the role medications might be playing in sleep disturbances, the patient should be screened for common sleep disorders (insomnia, nightmares, obstructive sleep apnea [OSA], and RLS), excessive daytime sleepiness, and evidence of inadequate nocturnal oxygenation or ventilation.

Insomnia

Chronic insomnia is a subjective disturbance in sleep initiation, duration, consolidation, or quality despite adequate opportunity for sleep that results in daytime impairment [8]. It is common, debilitating, and frequently associated with many conditions, including other sleep disorders. Predisposing factors can include poor sleep hygiene (see Box 37.1); medications, including glucocorticoids, stimulants, opioid analgesics, and diuretics causing nocturia; and psychological stressors, which are particularly common in patients with PICS. Insomnia symptom severity can be evaluated with the Insomnia Severity Index. The American Association of Sleep Medicine recommends multicomponent cognitive behavioral therapy for insomnia (CBT-i) as first-line treatment [9]; components of CBT-i

> **Box 37.1** Sleep hygiene recommendations [10]
>
> 1. Reduce blue light exposure: stop all electronic use 30 minutes before bed.
> 2. Limit time in bed: use bed only for sleep, sex, and sickness.
> 3. Sleep routine: keep a set bedtime and waketime.
> 4. Limit caffeine: avoid four to six hours before bed.
> 5. Improve environment: reduce noise and light in sleeping area.

> **Box 37.2** Dedicated Worry Time technique
>
> - Useful for patients struggling with insomnia who endorse "mind racing" at night.
> - Involves accepting that worry is a natural and normal process that helps keep us safe.
> - Patients select a specific 15–20-minute time period during the day to actively spend worrying.
> - Practice deferring worries that arise at bedtime and throughout the day to the dedicated worry time.
> - Can be helpful to write the worries down to refer to during the worry time.
> - With practice, the technique can allow the brain to do the important function of worrying and protect sleep.
> - Read more at www.copingwithcoronavirus.co.uk/ [12].

include sleep restriction therapy (i.e., limiting time in bed while awake), relation therapy, and stimuli control techniques (e.g., avoid clock watching). Improving sleep hygiene, defined as a combination of sleeping conditions, environmental factors, and lifestyle habits intended to promote consistent, uninterrupted sleep, is important; however, improving sleep hygiene alone may be insufficient to effectively treat insomnia [9]. Patients with PICS may struggle to improve sleep hygiene because of physical impairments that preclude daytime activity to promote nighttime tiredness; a delayed return to work, school, or other activities, which makes establishing a routine difficult; and an inability to control their environment, especially if discharged to a location other than home. Patients who endorse feeling overwhelmed by worries when they lie down to sleep can be offered instruction on the Dedicated Worry Time technique (see Box 37.2), which can easily be provided in clinic without dedicated sleep staff or expertise.

Some patients with PICS may have experienced acute situational insomnia during hospitalization, and these patterns can continue following discharge. For patients who were discharged with sedative-hypnotic medications initiated during hospitalization, it may be reasonable to provide a limited prescription for use in times of severe sleep symptoms to provide symptom relief, improve daytime functioning, and prevent the development of an antagonistic relationship with sleep. Long-term use of sedative-hypnotic agents is not recommended due to an association with decreased long-term cognitive function (specifically with Z-hypnotics, e.g., zolpidem) [11]. Once sleep is stabilized, the goal is to help patients return to normal sleep patterns and wean off sedative medications. Despite this, some patients may nevertheless require long-term sedative-hypnotics to manage their insomnia; if weaning off these medications is challenging, consultation with a sleep specialist for further evaluation should be considered. Addressing other health concerns that may be contributing to impaired sleep and providing complementary non-pharmacological therapies may be helpful in this transition.

Nightmares

Nightmares are a commonly reported sleep disturbance during and after critical illness, and in one qualitative study of patient experiences, 47% reported having nightmares after hospital discharge [13]. This finding is particularly worrisome, as the ability to recall nightmares following critical illness has been identified as a predictor of post-traumatic stress disorder (PTSD) in this patient population [14]. In one study, in-depth, face-to-face interviews with patients after ICU admission identified major themes of "longing for normal sleep" and "being tormented by nightmares" [3]. Nightmares may contribute to ongoing psychosocial distress resulting from hospitalization, especially in patients who experienced significant delirium, and they are a common manifestation of PTSD (see Chapter 46 for additional information). Occasionally, they may signify another sleep disorder (e.g., OSA); although sleep disordered breathing rarely presents with nightmares, its high prevalence makes it important to consider, particularly in patients who describe dreams involving choking, drowning, or suffocating. The American Academy of Sleep Medicine now recommends imagery rehearsal therapy as the first-line treatment for patients with PTSD-related nightmares rather than pharmacotherapy with prazosin [15,16,17]. Imagery rehearsal therapy is a technique in which patients experiencing nightmares with recurring themes take time when awake to rewrite these dreams, either literally or by active reflection, with positive alternative endings; with practice, many begin to dream their conceived alternative ending instead. There are few therapists trained to provide this technique, so evaluation in an ICU follow-up clinic may be the only opportunity for a patient to benefit from this methodology.

Obstructive Sleep Apnea

Estimated to affect one billion people worldwide, OSA is characterized by recurrent upper airway obstruction during sleep [18,19]. Apnea is defined as a total cessation of respiratory flow for at least 10 seconds, and hypopnea is defined as a reduction of ventilation with an associated desaturation [20]. Although data are still emerging, OSA has been identified as a risk factor for the development of Post-Acute Sequelae of SARS-CoV-2 infection (PASC; see Chapter 53 for additional information) [21]. Screening questionnaires for OSA, such as the STOP-BANG questionnaire, can be easily woven into other evaluations during a comprehensive PICS assessment [22]; other questionnaires that evaluate OSA include the Berlin Questionnaire, OSA50, and the Calgary Sleep Apnea Quality of Life Index.

OSA is common globally, but patients with PICS may be at especially high risk, as many sequelae of critical illness may predispose to upper airway collapse. These include muscular weakness of the upper airway, narrowing of the upper airway secondary to edema, and hyperarousal [8,23]. If it is difficult for a patient to breathe during the day due to ICU acquired weakness, pulmonary fibrosis, or another preexisting lung pathology, it may be even more difficult to maintain normal breathing patterns at night. During REM sleep, all skeletal muscles, with the exception of the diaphragm, are paralyzed to avoid dream enactment [24], and this can exacerbate breathing issues in patients with a baseline dependence on accessory respiratory muscles for adequate ventilation. Patients with an "overlap" between chronic lung disease and OSA may experience increased hypopneas and greater desaturations with airflow cessations [25], making even mild sleep apnea that predated the hospital admission more severe. Screening for and addressing OSA in ICU follow-up clinics may improve quality of life, reduce risk of motor vehicle accidents, and even help normalize blood pressure in vulnerable patients [26]. Of note, treatment of OSA is one of the few reversible causes of fatigue.

Central sleep apnea (CSA) is much less common than OSA; however, predisposing factors include opioid analgesic use and medical disorders, such as congestive heart failure or stroke, which may be prevalent in patients with PICS. CSA is characterized by cessation in airflow due to an abnormal respiratory pattern rather than obstruction of the upper airway. It can cause symptoms of fragmented sleep and daytime tiredness similar to OSA.

Restless Leg Syndrome

RLS is a sleep and sensorimotor disorder marked by the intense and uncomfortable urge to move one's legs that generally abates with leg movement. It is fairly common, occurring in 2.7% of the general population [6]. Iron deficiency has been noted to be associated with this disease entity, and guidelines recommend therapy with iron supplementation for patients with serum ferritin ≤75 μg/L. Patients are particularly at risk for iron depletion after an ICU stay given phlebotomy, malnutrition, and other overlapping anemias; this may result in de novo RLS presentations or worsening of preexisting disease [27]. RLS can be highly distressing for patients, but it is infrequently asked about by providers despite its high prevalence and treatability, and the unusual nature of the symptoms may prevent patients from volunteering the relevant information needed to make the diagnosis.

Nocturnal Hypoventilation

Critical illness myopathy affecting the muscles of ventilation during sleep, specifically the diaphragm, is a poorly studied but worrisome complication of critical illness. Patients with generalized muscle weakness from critical illness often maintain adequate ventilation while awake. In the upright position, gravity aids respiratory mechanics and helps to offload the work of the diaphragm; when asleep and supine, this benefit may disappear. Even marked symmetric diaphragmatic weakness may be missed on sniff fluoroscopy, as this common test for diaphragmatic dysfunction is insensitive in the absence of unilateral diaphragmatic paralysis. A rising serum bicarbonate, which signifies renal compensation for a persistently elevated partial pressure of carbon dioxide, may be a clinical clue. The consequences of severe nocturnal hypoxemia and hypoventilation in the absence of clear sleep disordered breathing are still being researched. Other similar conditions, such as stable persistent hypercapnic chronic obstructive pulmonary disease, have clear guidelines to suggest treatment with positive pressure (PAP) therapy. In other cases of suspected nocturnal hypoventilation or severe nocturnal hypoxemia, clinicians may consider a trial of supplemental oxygen delivered via nasal cannula or nocturnal PAP to see if there is a symptomatic benefit, but until there are further data to recommend a specific approach, treatment should be tailored to patient preference.

Conclusion

Sleep concerns are common, often debilitating, and frequently persist for 6–12 months following hospital discharge. Despite this, sleep disorders are treatable, and normal sleep patterns can ultimately be restored. An ICU follow-up clinic is an ideal place for an evaluation of sleep impairments, which can easily be integrated into the patient's comprehensive PICS assessment. Practitioners in ICU follow-up clinics can offer reassurance to patients suffering from these symptoms, screen for common sleep disorders, and refer to specialty care when necessary. Sleep affects all three PICS domains, and if left unaddressed, can hinder recovery and even endanger patients with undiagnosed sleep disorders.

Key Points

1. Sleep problems are common and may be exacerbated by critical illness.
2. Critical illness may foster sleep concerns that extend beyond the acute care setting.
3. Sleep affects all three PICS domains.
4. Sleep concerns may be underdiagnosed in the PICS population due to lack of screening.

References

1. M.T. Altman, M.P. Knauert, M.A. Pisani. Sleep disturbance after hospitalization and critical illness: a systematic review. *Ann Am Thorac Soc* 2017; **14**: 1457–68.
2. L. Orwelius, A. Nordlund, P. Nordlund, et al. Prevalence of sleep disturbances and long-term reduced health-related quality of life after critical care: a prospective multicenter cohort study. *Crit Care* 2008; **12**: R97.
3. A.C. Tembo, V. Parker, I. Higgins. The experience of sleep deprivation in intensive care patients: findings from a larger hermeneutic phenomenological study. *Intensive Crit Care Nurs* 2013; **29**: 310–16.
4. C.M. Gillis, J.O. Poyant, J.R. Degrado, et al. Inpatient pharmacological sleep aid utilization is common at a tertiary medical center. *J Hosp Med* 2014; **9**: 652–7.
5. F.A.J.L. Scheer, C.J. Morris, J.I. Garcia, et al. Repeated melatonin supplementation improves sleep in hypertensive patients treated with beta-blockers: a randomized controlled trial. *Sleep* 2012; **35**: 1395–402.
6. S.G. Matar, Z.S. El-Nahas, H. Aladwan, et al. Restless leg syndrome in hemodialysis patients: a narrative review. *Neurologist* 2022; **27**: 194–202.
7. H.K. Walia, G. Shalhoub, V. Ramsammy, et al. Symptoms of restless legs syndrome in a palliative care population: frequency and impact. *J Palliat Care* 2013; **29**: 210–16.
8. S. Schutte-Rodin, L. Broch, D. Buysse, et al. Clinical guideline for the evaluation and management of chronic insomnia in adults. *J Clin Sleep Med* 2008; **4**: 487–504.
9. J.D. Edinger, J.T. Arnedt, S.M. Bertisch, et al. Behavioral and psychological treatments for chronic insomnia disorder in adults: an American Academy of Sleep Medicine clinical practice guideline. *J Clin Sleep Med* 2021; **17**: 255–62.
10. https://sleep.hms.harvard.edu/education-training/public-education/sleep-and-health-education-program/sleep-health-education-68. Accessed June 5, 2025.
11. H.I. Shih, C.C. Lin, Y.F. Tu, et al. An increased risk of reversible dementia may occur after zolpidem derivative use in the elderly population: a population-based case-control study. *Medicine* 2015; **94**: e809.
12. Coping With Coronavirus [Internet]. Self-Help Guides. https://copingwithcoronavirus.co.uk/self-help-guides. Accessed February 27, 2024.
13. E. Strahan, J. Mccormick, E. Uprichard, et al. Immediate follow-up after ICU discharge: establishment of a service and initial experiences. *Nurs Crit Care* 2003; **8**: 49–55.

14. D.S. Davydow, J.M. Gifford, S.V. Desai, et al. Posttraumatic stress disorder in general intensive care unit survivors: a systematic review. *Gen Hosp Psychiatry* 2008; **30**: 421–34.

15. M. Albanese, M. Liotti, L. Cornacchia, F. Mancini. Nightmare rescripting: using imagery techniques to treat sleep disturbances in post-traumatic stress disorder. *Front Psychiatry* 2022; **13**: 866144.

16. D.E. Yücel, A.A.P. van Emmerik, C. Souama, J. Lancee. Comparative efficacy of imagery rehearsal therapy and prazosin in the treatment of trauma-related nightmares in adults: a meta-analysis of randomized controlled trials. *Sleep Med Rev* 2020; **50**: 101248.

17. T.I. Morgenthaler, S. Auerbach, K.R. Casey, et al. Position paper for the treatment of nightmare disorder in adults: an American academy of sleep medicine position paper. *J Clin Sleep Med* 2018; **14**: 1041–55.

18. A.V. Benjafield, N.T. Ayas, P.R. Eastwood, et al. Estimation of the global prevalence and burden of obstructive sleep apnoea: a literature-based analysis. *Lancet Respir Med* 2019; **7**: 687–98.

19. D.J. Eckert, A. Malhotra. Pathophysiology of adult obstructive sleep apnea. *Proc Am Thorac Soc* 2008; **5**: 144–53.

20. G. Mbata, J. Chukwuka. Obstructive sleep apnea hypopnea syndrome. *Ann Med Health Sci Res* 2012; **2**:74–7.

21. S.F. Quan, M.D. Weaver, M.E. Czeisler, et al. Association of obstructive sleep apnea with post-acute sequelae of SARS-CoV-2 infection. *Am J Med* 2024; Available from: http://dx.doi.org/10.1016/j.amjmed.2024.02.023.

22. B. Oktay Arslan, Z.Z. Uçar Hoşgör, M.N. Orman. Which screening questionnaire is best for predicting obstructive sleep apnea in the sleep clinic population considering age, gender, and comorbidities? *Turk Thorac J*. 2020; **21**: 383–9.

23. J.A. Verbraecken, W.A. De Backer. Upper airway mechanics. *Respiration* 2009; **78**: 121–33.

24. J.J. Fraigne, Z.A. Torontali, M.B. Snow, J.H. Peever. REM sleep at its core: circuits, neurotransmitters, and pathophysiology. *Front Neurol* 2015; **6**: 123.

25. R.L. Owens, M.M. Macrea, M. Teodorescu. The overlaps of asthma or COPD with OSA: a focused review. *Respirology* 2017; **22**: 1073–83.

26. S.P. Patil, I.A. Ayappa, S.M. Caples, et al. Treatment of adult obstructive sleep apnea with positive airway pressure: an American academy of sleep medicine systematic review, meta-analysis, and grade assessment. *J Clin Sleep Med* 2019; **15**: 301–34.

27. M.M. Ohayon, R. O'Hara, M.V. Vitiello. Epidemiology of restless legs syndrome: a synthesis of the literature. *Sleep Med Rev* 2012; **16**: 283–95.

Chapter 38

Persistent Dysphagia in Survivors of Critical Illness

Lauren Costa, Kirra Mediate, Lauren Tusar Van Fleet, and Veronica Tyszkiewicz

Background and Prevalence of Dysphagia in PICS

Dysphagia is common in critically ill patients, particularly among those who require intubation and mechanical ventilation (see Chapter 6 for additional information). Of patients requiring mechanical ventilation, dysphagia is present in 80% of patients immediately following extubation [1], remains present in up to 60% of patients at hospital discharge [1], and persists in 25% of patients 6 months thereafter [2]. Dysphagia in common in survivors of the acute respiratory distress syndrome (ARDS), although the exact prevalence is not known given the variability of dysphagia screening protocols across hospitals [2]. In studies of critically ill patients with SARS-CoV-2 infection, 83% of whom required intubation and mechanical ventilation, there was a 29% prevalence of dysphagia at hospital discharge [3]. Patient outcomes related to ongoing dysphagia are influenced by increasing age, worsening severity of illness, and duration of intubation and mechanical ventilation [4].

Swallowing impairments following a prolonged stay in the intensive care unit (ICU) may be influenced by medical conditions that directly impact the patient's anatomy and physiology and by treatments required during critical illness, including endotracheal intubation and the provision of sedating medications, which may impact neurological function and increase the risk of delirium. Generally, dysphagia may result from direct traumatic injury to the head and neck region, brain injury, weakness (either pre-existing or ICU-acquired), impaired sensation, and impaired coordination of breathing and swallowing [1].

Dysphagia following hospital discharge results from persistent impairment in neuromuscular function, which is critical to ensure the timely initiation and coordination of swallowing [1]. The ability to swallow safely may therefore be impacted by both the physical and cognitive disabilities that are commonly associated with post-intensive care syndrome (PICS), and rehabilitation efforts targeting both domains are often necessary to improve swallowing function and safety [5]. For patients with PICS, outpatient therapy with a speech language pathologist (SLP) targeting dysphagia rehabilitation is recommended to help them return to their prior or highest level of functioning. The implementation of dysphagia rehabilitation, compensatory strategies, and diet modifications has been shown to be effective in reducing the risk of aspiration-related complications and hospital readmission [2]. Patient and family training are also critical to the success of therapy services [6].

Characteristics of Dysphagia

The act of swallowing is composed of three phases: the oral, pharyngeal, and esophageal phases, and signs of dysphagia may be associated with each phase (see Table 38.1 and Figure 38.1). Signs of oral dysphagia include poor secretion management (i.e., drooling),

Table 38.1 The three phases of swallowing

Phase	Description
Oral Phase	• Voluntary movement • Food enters the oral cavity • Mastication and bolus formation • Tongue elevates against soft palate and propels bolus to the pharynx
Pharyngeal Phase	• Involuntary movement • Soft palate elevates to seal the nasopharynx • Larynx and hyoid bone move anteriorly and upwards • True and false vocal cords adduct • Epiglottis retroflexion occurs (respiration is inhibited) • Pharyngeal stripping wave • Upper esophageal sphincter relaxes and opens
Esophageal Phase	• Involuntary movement • Bolus passes through the esophagus • Esophagus contracts • Lower esophageal sphincter relaxes

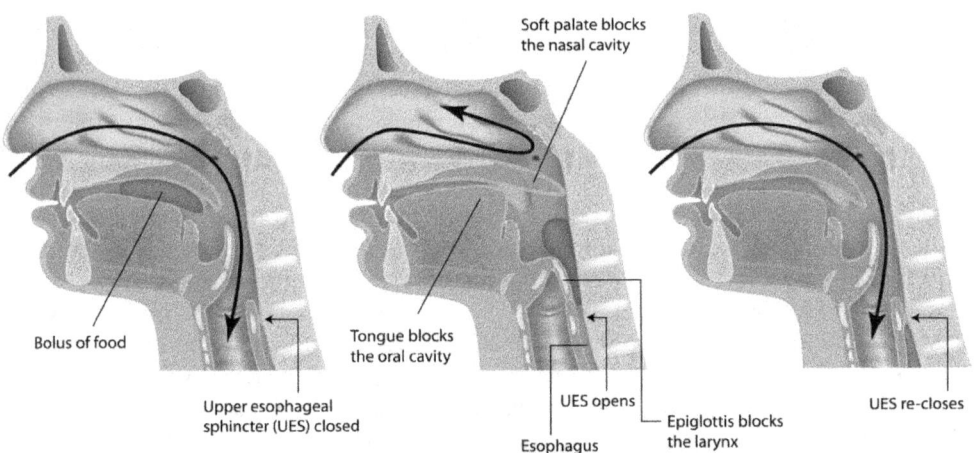

Figure 38.1 Anatomical representation of the three phases of swallowing: the oral phase, the pharyngeal phase, and the esophageal phase. From: Y. Fujiso, N. Perrin, J. van der Giessen, et al. Swall-E: A robotic in-vitro simulation of human swallowing. *PLOS ONE* 2018; **13**(12): e0208193. Reproduced with permission from PLOS ONE via CC BY (Creative Commons Attribution) https://journals.plos.org/plosone/article/figure?id=10.1371/journal.pone.0208193.g00.1

anterior loss of a bolus (i.e., food escaping from the mouth unintentionally during mastication), impairment with mastication, and difficulty with bolus propulsion. Pharyngeal and esophageal deficits require instrumental imaging to be observed. A delayed swallow initiation, reduced hyolaryngeal excursion, and incomplete closure of the airway are indicators of pharyngeal impairments. Esophageal dysphagia may include esophageal motility issues, incomplete or delayed opening of the upper esophageal sphincter (UES), or backflow of the bolus to the pharynx [7]. Additional clinical signs of dysphagia, most likely indicative of pharyngeal swallow phase impairments, include post prandial coughing, throat clearing, and a wet vocal quality. Symptomatically, patients may complain of food being stuck in their throat, referred to as a globus sensation. The presence of any of these signs and symptoms of dysphagia warrants a comprehensive assessment.

Outpatient Evaluation Process

Patients experiencing dysphagia following hospital discharge are often referred to an SLP for outpatient dysphagia rehabilitation. The evaluation process begins with obtaining the patient's case history through review of the medical record and patient interview. A chart review involves gathering information such as the patient's medical diagnoses, comorbidities, past treatments, nutritional status, respiratory status, cognitive status, imaging results, and medications. A patient interview assists with understanding the patient's current diet and their overall nutritional status, their symptoms, the timeline of dysphagia, patterns or changes observed since hospital discharge, and information regarding coexisting conditions. An interview can also shed light on the patient's pleasure with eating and drinking, which can impact their performance and willingness to participate in therapy.

The evaluation process includes an oral mechanism examination to assess oral motor and sensory function. Patients are asked to complete a series of lingual, labial, and buccal movements to assess symmetry, strength, speed, and range of motion. Results may demonstrate cranial nerve impairments that can impact swallowing function (see Chapter 6 for additional information). A bedside clinical swallowing evaluation (CSE) is administered to assess for signs and symptoms of dysphagia. During this evaluation, patients are administered foods and liquids of various consistencies, including thin and/or thickened liquids, pureed solids, and regular solids, to assess bolus consumption. Patients are monitored for signs of aspiration, including post-prandial coughing, throat clearing, wet vocal quality, and decreases in oxygen saturation as measured by pulse oximetry. The SLP palpates hyolaryngeal excursion to manually assess swallowing movements [7]. The patient is asked to report symptoms, such as globus sensation or odynophagia. If signs and symptoms of aspiration are present, compensatory strategies may be trialed, including postural techniques and swallowing maneuvers. The Yale Swallow Protocol (YSP) may also be incorporated into the CSE to assess swallowing abilities. The YSP is a quick, pass/fail standardized screen to predict aspiration risk. Patients are asked to drink three ounces of water in sequential swallows; the patient fails if they stop drinking, cough, or have changes in their vocal quality [8].

In addition to a CSE, instrumental imaging studies, which are the gold standard for diagnosing dysphagia severity, may be warranted. These include a flexible endoscopic evaluation of swallowing (FEES) or modified barium swallow study (MBSS) [9]. Completion of a FEES allows direct visualization of the horizontal plane for swallowing and is therefore ideal for assessing laryngeal and pharyngeal symmetry, laryngeal function, and potential laryngeal injury or abnormalities. Completion of an MBSS allows for lateral or anterior-posterior views of a swallow, provides visualization of the oral phase of swallowing, and enables clinicians to assess synchrony and coordination between oral, pharyngeal, and esophageal phases. FEES is generally superior for identifying laryngeal abnormalities, as it provides direct visualization of these structures in real time, while the MBSS may not capture detailed laryngeal views. MBSS is generally a better option for evaluating the entire swallowing process, as it observes all phases of the swallow. Both assessments may be used to complement each other, but the clinical question or abnormality being specifically investigated may help the clinician choose between FEES or MBSS initially (see Chapter 6 for additional information). The results of both MBSS and FEES examinations inform diet texture and viscosity recommendations and compensatory strategy recommendations for safe eating. SLPs follow the International Dysphagia Diet Standardisation Initiative (IDDSI) Framework to make appropriate liquid and solid recommendations (see Figure 38.2).

Various outcome measures are used in the outpatient setting along with the CSE, including, but not limited to, the Dysphagia Outcome and Severity Scale (DOSS), Functional Oral Intake Scale (FOIS), and Eating Assessment Tool (EAT-10). Measures can be readministered throughout the recovery trajectory to assess progress and changes with swallowing function. The DOSS is a seven-point scale used to rate the functional severity of dysphagia and considers a patient's level of independence, nutrition, and diet level or modifications. Ratings are based on objective assessment, such as an MBSS [10]. The FOIS characterizes the functional oral intake of patients with dysphagia using a scale from 1 to 7, with lower

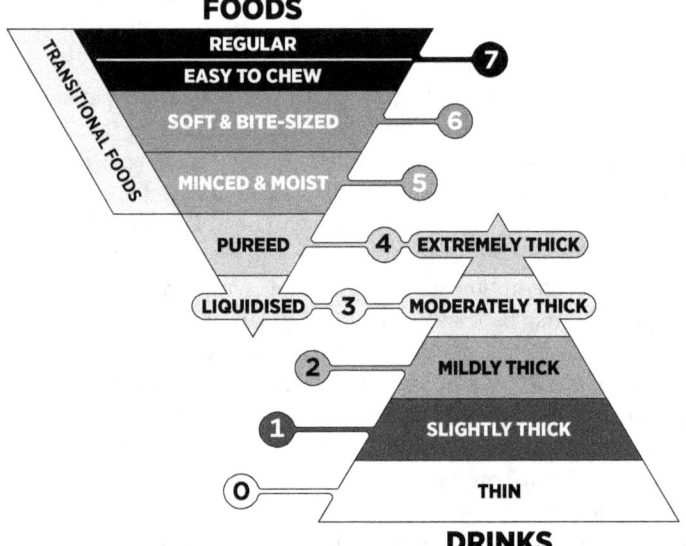

Figure 38.2 The IDDSI Framework. © The International Dysphagia Diet Standardisation Initiative 2019 @ https://iddsi.org/framework. Licensed under the CreativeCommons Attribution Sharealike 4.0 License https://creativecommons.org/licenses/by-sa/4.0/legalcode. Derivative works extending beyond language translation are NOT PERMITTED. This is NOT an official IDDSI resource, educational material, or education program and it is NOT meant to replace materials and resources on www.IDDSI.org. Please refer to the IDDSI website for the most current information and resources.

scores reflecting dependency on enteral nutrition and higher scores reflecting increasing independence with an oral diet [11]. The EAT-10 is a self-administered 10-item questionnaire to identify dysphagia risk by asking patients to rate various characteristics of or potential difficulties with swallowing on a severity scale from 0 to 4; total scores of 3 or more are concerning for dysphagia [12].

Referrals

Given the anatomical and physiological complexity of swallowing, the management of dysphagia may require multiple specialists working as part of an interprofessional team [13]. An otolaryngologist may play an important role in dysphagia care if vocal cord dysfunction is involved, as vocal cord weakness or hypomobility may further increase risk of aspiration (see Chapter 39 for additional information). Patients with esophageal symptoms or other comorbidities such as gastroesophageal reflux disease (GERD) may benefit from referral to a gastroenterologist. When diet texture modifications are needed to reduce the risk of aspiration, a dietitian can help manage nutrition and caloric intake. Other notable referrals may be to neurology and psychology if the patient has significant neurological deficits or if their swallowing deficits negatively impact their mood, respectively.

The development of ICU-acquired weakness (see Chapter 4 for additional information) may contribute to the incidence and persistence of dysphagia, and patients may also benefit from receiving physical therapy due to general deconditioning alongside targeted swallowing therapy. Some individuals, particularly those with underlying neurological or pulmonary disease or those who are immunocompromised, may not be able to tolerate any amount of aspiration and its attendant risk of aspiration-related infection. Additionally, patients with PICS may demonstrate cognitive deficits, which can also impact the risk for dysphagia and aspiration, as patients may not recall dysphagia exercises or precautionary measures; cognitive rehabilitation may help improve a patient's management of their dysphagia. In general, SLPs act as a coordinator between team members to facilitate communication regarding dysphagia [13].

Dysphagia Treatment

Outpatient dysphagia therapy is generally tailored to the individual based on the etiology of their dysphagia, instrumental assessment results, and CSE. Dysphagia therapy includes diet modifications, swallowing exercises, and compensatory strategies to improve the safety of oral intake. The SLP will set goals with the patient to improve strength, coordination, timing, and swallow efficiency and develop strategies to optimize swallow biomechanics and reduce aspiration risk. Most goals are achieved in 6 to 12 weeks, with sessions 1 to 2 times per week, each lasting 30 to 45 minutes. Patients are given a home exercise program (HEP) to complete in between therapy sessions.

Dysphagia Exercises

The dysphagia exercises and maneuvers performed during therapy and included in the HEP are chosen based primarily on the impairments noted on instrumental imaging (see Table 38.2). These exercises and maneuvers contribute to the rehabilitation of impaired swallow function across all swallow phases, as many muscles work together to impact the efficiency of swallowing. While there is significant research backing the effectiveness of

Table 38.2 Swallowing exercises and their intended effect

Exercise/Maneuver	Target of exercise
Tongue Tethered Exercise (known as Masako Maneuver)	Increases pharyngeal constriction and improves tongue base retraction during the swallow
Tongue Range of Motion Exercises (including tongue propulsion, lateralization, and elevation exercises)	Improves tongue strength and range of motion
Effortful swallow	Improves pharyngeal constrictor strength and base of tongue strength; helps with improved bolus clearance and strengthening of the swallow muscles
Shaker Maneuver	Strengthens the muscles that open the UES, improves hyolaryngeal movements, and reduces pharyngeal residue
Mendelsohn Maneuver	Maintains longer UES opening by holding larynx in a raised position for reduced aspiration risk
Supraglottic Swallow	Improves ability to close the airway before swallow; clears any food or liquid remaining in the pharynx
Chin Tuck Against Resistance	Promotes anterior movement of the hyoid bone and larynx; also improves airway entrance closure, facilitation of bolus propulsion, and improved swallow strength and efficiency

exercises and strategies as key components of dysphagia rehabilitation, there is little research available regarding specific methods for patients with PICS; however, all exercises and strategies can be applied to patients with dysphagia irrespective of the etiology.

The act of swallowing itself is the best therapy for dysphagia, and high intensity repetitions of dysphagia exercises along with trials of various food textures and liquid viscosities is generally the foundation of treatment. Commonly used dysphagia exercises include the effortful swallow, the supraglottic swallow, chin tuck against resistance (CTAR), the Mendelsohn maneuver, and the Shaker exercise. The effortful swallow exercise helps to increase oral and pharyngeal pressures to propel a bolus with extra force through the oropharynx [14]. The supraglottic swallow exercise targets improved airway closure to prevent aspiration by closing off the airway prior to the swallow. The patient is cued to hold their breath, swallow, cough, and then complete a dry swallow to reduce pharyngeal residuals after the initial swallow. This exercise can be challenging for patients to coordinate, and a visual cue can improve patient performance. The CTAR helps improve coordination and strength of swallowing muscles. During the exercise, the patient commonly places a rolled towel under their chin and is instructed to tuck their chin towards their chest by applying gentle pressure against the towel. This resistance helps to engage and strengthen the muscles involved in swallowing, and the exercise can be completed in an isometric hold or in several repetitions.

Other exercises involve strengthening the UES, including the Mendelsohn maneuver and the Shaker exercise. During the Mendelsohn maneuver, which can be challenging for patients to learn, the patient is asked to keep the UES open longer by holding the larynx in a raised position, which reduces the risk of aspiration and improves efficiency of swallowing. The Shaker exercise aims to strengthen the muscles that open the UES. During this exercise, the patient is asked to lay down flat on a bed and lift their head, tucking their chin to their chest to look at their toes. As with other exercises, this exercise can be completed in an isometric hold or in several repetitions.

There are several lingual and lip strengthening exercises that promote an improved oral phase, such as lingual protrusion exercises against resistance and the tongue tethered exercise, also known as the Masako maneuver. During this exercise, the patient is asked to place their tongue between their teeth and gently bite down to hold their tongue in place. They then swallow their saliva to promote base of tongue retraction and improved bolus transfer.

Compensatory Strategies

Compensatory strategies are another key component of dysphagia rehabilitation. These may include postural adjustments and positional techniques such as a chin tuck, lateral head turn, or lateral flexion of the head and neck to reduce aspiration risk. Aspiration precautions describe a bundle of behaviors and strategies that can improve the safety of eating, such as pacing, taking small bites and drinking small sips, performing a cough after every swallow, and completing multiple swallows for each bolus to reduce pharyngeal residue. Some techniques may be used for both compensatory and rehabilitative purposes. For example, the supraglottic swallow is an exercise that increases airway closure and may also serve as a compensation to protect the airway [15]. If a patient has cognitive impairments, family members may play an important role in implementing strategies at mealtimes to improve safety.

The Role of Technology

Technology has been shown to be useful in dysphagia rehabilitation. The Iowa Oral Performance Instrument (IOPI) objectively measures the strength and endurance of the lips and tongue against normative data, allowing therapists to track progress with rehabilitation over time. The IOPI improves anterior and posterior tongue strength, specifically enhancing the efficiency of bolus transfer and the ability to manage oral food residue [16]. The Expiratory Muscle Strength Trainer-150 (EMST-150) increases the strength and activation of weakened respiratory muscles that may contribute to difficulty swallowing [17]. This is often incorporated into dysphagia rehabilitation for patients with concomitant respiratory compromise, which is commonly found in patients with PICS.

Discharge Considerations

The overall goal for discharge from dysphagia rehabilitation is for the patient to safely tolerate the least restrictive diet. The SLP takes a holistic approach to determine a plan that maximizes each patient's quality of life. Repeat instrumental imaging may be recommended to assess readiness for diet advancement and discharge. A patient's achievement of goals and independence with their HEP are also factors for discharge consideration.

Decision making regarding discharge can be challenging due to multiple factors. A model for ethical decision making proposed by Jonsen and colleagues is a helpful framework for clinicians to consider, which includes medical indications, patient preferences, quality of life, and implications for caregiver burden [18]. The patient and family may decide to accept or reject recommendations with which they are uncomfortable, such as choosing not to utilize thickened liquids; indeed, eating a patient-preferred diet and accepting the risk of aspiration is something that patients with dysphagia may choose to improve their quality of life [19]. Family training, education, and communication is essential for the success of patients adopting this risk [19]. It is the clinician's responsibility to provide education regarding possible health outcomes and provide family training. Overall, embracing aspiration precautions and other lifestyle behaviors, such as maintaining an active lifestyle and keeping the lungs clear, are strategies to reduce occurrence of aspiration-related infection.

Case Study: Dysphagia After Severe Burns

A 39-year-old male was admitted to the ICU for management of a severe burn after a house fire. His 36-day hospitalization included 34 days in the ICU, and he required 7 days of mechanical ventilation, which included paralysis and prone positioning for severe respiratory failure thought to be secondary to ARDS and aspiration pneumonitis. During hospitalization, he was found to have significant dysphagia, requiring the provision of enteral nutrition via a naso-duodenal tube as well as total parenteral nutrition. Following discharge from acute care to inpatient rehabilitation, he had several instrumental studies that allowed him to progressively advance to an oral diet. His diet first required texture modifications and thickened liquids, but he was ultimately discharged home on a regular diet with thin liquids with no straws. In concert with a comprehensive rehabilitation plan developed an at outpatient ICU follow-up clinic appointment, he participated in outpatient dysphagia rehabilitation once weekly for 8 weeks, with a treatment plan focused on initiation of EMST-150, compensatory strategies, and swallowing exercises, including the Masako and Mendelsohn maneuvers. He was independent with his HEP and compliant with compensatory strategies.

In his ICU follow-up clinic appointments, the SLP collaborated with a dietician to align his nutrition and dysphagia goals. The SLP provided pertinent education to the family, such as reviewing recent MBSS results and aspiration precautions. He was able to be discharged from dysphagia rehabilitation, tolerating a regular diet with thin liquids, remaining independent with his HEP and compensatory strategies, and showing no evidence of aspiration-related complications or infections.

Case Study 2: Dysphagia Following COVID-19

A 78-year-old male required an extended ICU stay due to SARS-CoV-2 infection. His hospitalization was complicated by aspiration pneumonia and the placement of a feeding tube due to the severity of his dysphagia. During hospitalization, the patient was followed by SLPs and participated in multiple instrumental studies. He was discharged home from the hospital on a full-liquid diet and referred to outpatient dysphagia therapy.

The initial evaluation included a CSE and oral motor exam to determine the deficits and treatment goals. His oral motor assessment was significant for decreased lingual strength, particularly lingual protrusion and retraction; no deficits in labial strength or oral motor asymmetry were observed. At the initial assessment, a comprehensive plan of care was developed, including recommendations to participate in dysphagia therapy twice weekly, targeting lingual strength, base of tongue retraction, hyolaryngeal elevation, pharyngeal

Table 38.3 Case study #2 summarized regarding pre-and post-dysphagia treatment

	Pre-Dysphagia Therapy	Post-Dysphagia Therapy
Diet (solid oral intake)	NPO	Regular consistency
Diet (liquid oral intake)	NPO	Thin liquids
Aspiration	Noted with thin and nectar thick liquids	None
Vallecular Residue	Compensatory strategies were ineffective in clearance	Liquid wash and cough-re-swallow were effective in clearance

strength, and glottic closure. A HEP consisted of the Masako maneuver, effortful swallow, the Mendelsohn maneuver, and CTAR.

At the culmination of outpatient dysphagia therapy, the patient received an MBSS, which resulted in the recommendation for a regular diet with thin liquids. He was also taught strategies to perform during mealtimes, such as a liquid wash and a cough re-swallow strategy (see Table 38.3).

Key Points

1. Dysphagia is common in critically ill patients and may persist following ICU discharge, where it may be identified in ICU follow-up clinic evaluations in patients with PICS.
2. Outpatient dysphagia therapy includes restorative exercises, compensatory strategies, and diet modifications.
3. An outpatient dysphagia evaluation includes the following: review of medical records, instrumental assessment, oral mechanism exam, outcome measures, and bedside swallowing evaluation.
4. The act of swallowing itself is the best rehabilitative exercise for dysphagia therapy.
5. The goal of dysphagia rehabilitation is for the patient to tolerate the least restrictive diet.

References

1. P. Zuercher, C.S. Moret, R. Dziewas, J. C. Schefold. Dysphagia in the intensive care unit: epidemiology, mechanisms, and clinical management. *Crit Care* 2019; **23**(1): 103.
2. J.M. Kruser, H.C. Prescott. Dysphagia after acute respiratory distress syndrome. another lasting legacy of critical illness. *Ann Am Thorac Soc* 2017; **14**(3): 307–8.
3. N.A. Clayton, A. Freeman-Sanderson, E. Walker. Dysphagia prevalence and outcomes associated with the evolution of covid-19 and its variants in critically ill patients. *Dysphagia* 2023; **39**(1): 109–18.
4. F.C. Sassi, A.P. Ritto, M.S. de Lima, et al. Characteristics of postintubation dysphagia in ICU patients in the context of the COVID-19 outbreak: a report of 920 cases from a Brazilian reference center. *PLOS ONE* 2022; **17**(6): e0270107.

5. C. Renner, M.M. Jeitziner, A. Tran, et al. Guideline on multimodal rehabilitation for patients with post-intensive care syndrome. *Crit Care* 2023; **27**(1): 301.

6. N. Nakanishi, K. Liu, J. Hatakeyama, et al. Post-intensive care syndrome follow-up system after hospital discharge: a narrative review. *J Intensive Care* 2024; **12**(1): 2.

7. C. Roseberry-McKibbin, M.N. Hegde, G. Trellis. *An advanced review of speech-language pathology: preparation for the SLP praxis and comprehensive examination*. 5th ed. Austin, Texas: PRO-ED, Inc; 2019.

8. D.M. Suiter, J. Sloggy, S.B. Leder. Validation of the Yale swallow protocol: a prospective double-blinded videofluoroscopic study. *Dysphagia* 2013; **29**(2): 199–203.

9. S. Brady, J. Donzelli. The modified barium swallow and the functional endoscopic evaluation of swallowing. *Otolaryngolog Clin North Am* 2013; **46**(6): 1009–22.

10. K.H. O'Neil, M. Purdy, J. Falk, L. Gallo. The dysphagia outcome and severity scale. *Dysphagia* 1999; **14**(3): 139–45.

11. M.A. Crary, G.D.C. Mann, M.E. Groher. Initial psychometric assessment of a functional oral intake scale for dysphagia in stroke patients. *Arch Phys Med Rehabil* 2005; **86**(8): 1516–20.

12. P.C. Belafsky, D.A. Mouadeb, C.J. Rees, et al. Validity and reliability of the Eating Assessment Tool (EAT-10). *Ann Otol Rhinol Laryngol* 2008; **117**(12): 919–24.

13. ASHA. Adult Dysphagia: Overview. Asha.org. 2019 (accessed March 22, 2024). Available from: www.asha.org/Practice-Portal/Clinical-Topics/Adult-Dysphagia/.

14. H. Park, D. Oh, T. Yoon, J. Park. Effect of effortful swallowing training on tongue strength and oropharyngeal swallowing function in stroke patients with dysphagia: a double-blind, randomized controlled trial. *Int J Lang Commun Disord* 2019; **54**(3): 479–84.

15. J. Ashford, D. McCabe, K. Wheeler-Hegland, et al. Evidence-based systematic review: oropharyngeal dysphagia behavioral treatments. Part IV: impact of dysphagia treatment on individuals' postcancer treatments. *J Rehabil Res Dev* 2009; **46**(2): 195–204.

16. J.S. Park, H.J. Kim, D.H. Oh. Effect of tongue strength training using the Iowa Oral Performance Instrument in stroke patients with dysphagia. *J Phys Ther Sci* 2015; **27**(12): 3631–4.

17. Aspire Respiratory Products. EMST150 for Difficulty Swallowing (Dysphagia) • Aspire [Internet]. Aspire. 2021 (accessed April 8, 2024). Available from: https://emst150.com/health-challenges/difficulty-swallowing/#:~:text=The%20EMST150%20is%20the%20most%20clinically%20validated%20expiratory%20muscle%20trainer.

18. A.R. Jonsen, M. Siegler, W.J. Winslade. *Clinical ethics: a practical approach to ethical decisions in clinical medicine*. New York: McGraw-Hill, Health Professions Division; 1992.

19. N. Soar, J. Birns, P. Sommerville, et al. Approaches to eating and drinking with acknowledged risk: a systematic review. *Dysphagia*.2020; **36**(1): 54–66.

20. Y. Fujiso, N. Perrin, J. van der Giessen, et al. Swall-E: a robotic in-vitro simulation of human swallowing. *PLOS ONE* 2018; **13**(12): e0208193.

Chapter 39
Laryngeal Disorders in Survivors of Critical Illness

Libby J. Smith and Laura Habich

Introduction and Anatomy

The larynx sits at the intersection of breathing, swallowing, and voice production. In the critically ill patient who requires intubation, the endotracheal tube traverses the glottis, defined as the area between the vocal folds. This can result in several anatomic and behavioral alterations that can have variable impact on the patient's ability to breathe, swallow, and speak following extubation. The larynx is composed of the supraglottis, glottis, and subglottis. The supraglottis contains the epiglottis, false vocal folds, and arytenoids; the true vocal folds comprise the glottis; the subglottis starts below the vocal folds and ends at the cricoid cartilage; and the trachea extends caudally from the cricoid cartilage (see Figure 39.1).

Endotracheal Tube Size and Cuff Pressure

Endotracheal intubation requires passage of an endotracheal tube through the vocal folds to control the airway during mechanical ventilation. Endotracheal tube size should be chosen based upon patient height, as the subcricoid diameter and patient height are directly correlated (see Figure 39.2) [1]. Inappropriately large endotracheal tubes may result in difficulty with intubation; laryngeal injury, either during intubation or as a sequela of having an oversized tube spanning the glottis; or subglottic/tracheal injury secondary to cuff over-inflation. There is a misconception that smaller endotracheal tubes (that still allow for flexible bronchoscopy) are inappropriate in the critically ill patient. In a study by Esianor and colleagues, hospital length of stay was similar regardless of the appropriateness of endotracheal tube size, and patients with inappropriately large endotracheal tubes based on height were intubated for longer periods of time [2]. Women are more often intubated with inappropriately large endotracheal tubes due to their shorter average height [3].

There is a correlation between intubation, especially with inappropriately large endotracheal tubes, and laryngeal injury. Acute laryngeal injury, defined as the development of mucosal ulceration or granulation tissue of the larynx, is seen in over half of mechanically ventilated patients after 12 hours of intubation. The risk of acute laryngeal injury is increased by comorbid diabetes, larger body habitus, and use of an endotracheal tube size greater than 7.0. Patients who sustain laryngeal injury may have progressively worsening dyspnea and voicing, but this is often unappreciated during the remainder of their hospitalization, and symptomatic dyspnea or dysphonia may only become evident to the patient and their clinical care team four to eight weeks after extubation. By that time, patients are typically no longer hospitalized, and their

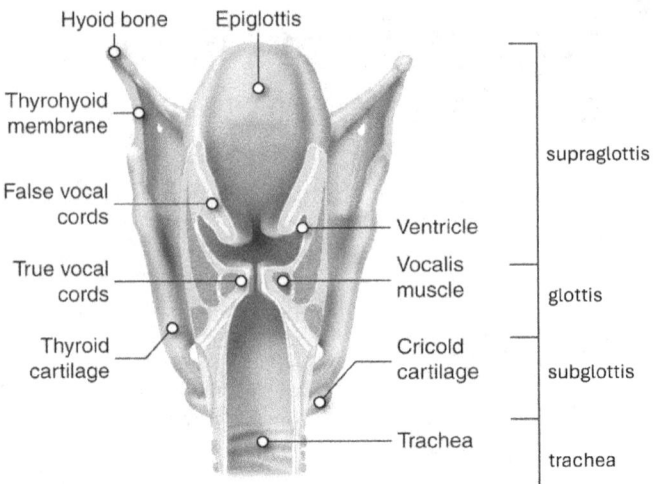

Figure 39.1 Anatomy of the larynx. The airway areas contained by the laryngeal structures are categorized as the supraglottis, glottis, and subglottis. Supraglottis and glottis configuration changes because of false vocal fold constriction and true vocal fold motion, respectively. The subglottis is fixed since the cricoid cartilage is a complete cartilage ring. Supraglottic structures include the epiglottis, aryepiglottic folds, arytenoids, false vocal folds, and ventricle. Glottic structures include the true vocal folds. Subglottic structures include the cricoid cartilage. The trachea begins at the end of the subglottis. Anatomy tool larynx and vocal cords English © Cenveo (https://anatomytool.org/content/cenveo-drawing-larynx-and-vocal-cords-english-labels). CC BY 4.0.

"new complaints" of dyspnea and dysphonia are usually managed by an otolaryngologist in the outpatient setting. A high index of suspicion for laryngeal injury, signified by hoarseness, dyspnea, or stridor, could result in earlier engagement with the otolaryngology team, with whom prompt intervention can help reduce long-term sequelae for the patient, as discussed later in this chapter.

Appropriate endotracheal tube cuff pressure is an important consideration. When endotracheal tube cuff pressures exceed that of the capillary perfusion pressure (>25 cmH$_2$O or >18.5 mmHg), delivery of mucosal nutrients is compromised and often inadequate, resulting in mucosal ischemia and subsequent stenosis or tracheomalacia. Stenosis results from collagen deposition at the site of injury, while tracheomalacia is defined as loss of structure and stability of the tracheal wall without the presence of scarring. Clinically symptomatic stenosis is often amenable to surgical dilation, while tracheomalacia requires resection, stenting, or T-tube placement. Vigilant monitoring of endotracheal tube cuff pressure, which is recommended at least every 8 hours, reduces the incidence of long-term tracheal injury. Use of a cuff pressure manometer is recommended, as tactile and visual feedback of the pilot balloon provides an inaccurate measure of cuff pressure [4].

To minimize the risk of both acute and chronic laryngeal injury, critically ill patients in the intensive care unit (ICU) require meticulous, coordinated multidisciplinary care. Specialty-specific skills of critical care physicians and nurses, otolaryngologists, thoracic surgeons, respiratory therapists, and speech language pathologists (SLP) help navigate laryngeal and tracheal issues, such as difficulties and aberrations with airway patency, swallowing, and voicing.

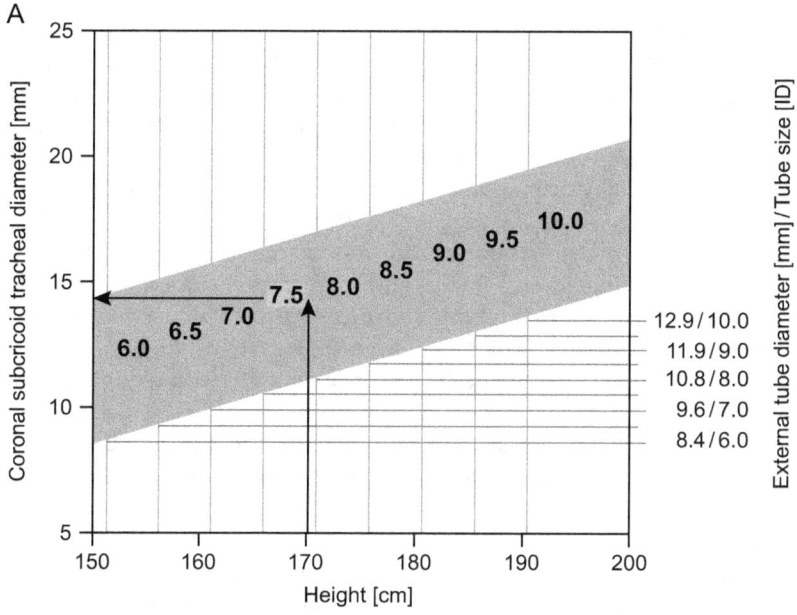

Figure 39.2 Nomograms for tube size selection based on height. Nomograms for tube size selection were developed based on simple confidence intervals (gray bars) of regression analyses. Calculations were performed using Rüsch tubes as a model. (A) Tube size selection: for any given patient height (x-axis), the appropriate tube size can be determined according to the vertical lines, which represent the limits for the selection of different tube sizes. Vertical lines were drawn to illustrate the intersection point of the lower confidence interval limit for the regression analysis tracheal diameter and the external tube diameter for every tube size (dotted lines). For example, patients with a height of 170 cm and a mean tracheal diameter of 14.5 mm require a maximum tube size of 7.5, which has an external tube diameter of 10.2 mm. **Note: Different brands of endotracheal tubes can have different internal and external diameters. Please check your institution's endotracheal tubes to determine which tubes are most appropriate for your patients.** From: R.O Seidl, B. Estel, A. Ernst, et al. Selection and placement of oral ventilation tubes based on tracheal morphometry. *Laryngoscope* 2011; **121(6)**: 1225–30. Reprinted by permission of John Wiley and Sons.

Vocal Cord Dysfunction

Since the larynx is at the intersection of breathing, swallowing, and voice production, behavioral alterations in the patient that may occur as a response to being intubated, critically infirm, or highly stressed can impact any of these three processes. A particularly concerning entity is paradoxical vocal fold motion disorder (PVFMD), also known as vocal cord dysfunction (VCD) or inducible laryngeal obstruction (ILO). Typical symptoms of PVFMD include difficulty with inspiration, throat tightness, and stridor, which can be very loud and distressing to the patient and the clinical team [5]. With severe attacks, patients may describe a sense of impending doom; despite this, oxygen saturations usually remain normal, although tachycardia and hypertension may be present. PVFMD is not responsive to bronchodilators, distinguishing it from asthma, which is typically bronchodilator-responsive and characterized by wheezing, chest tightness, and difficulty with exhalation. Notably, patients can have concurrent PVFMD and asthma, which makes accurate diagnosis challenging, as symptoms often overlap [6]. Flexible laryngoscopy is performed to ensure airway patency and evaluate for other laryngeal abnormalities, such as stenosis or vocal fold paralysis, that may account for a patient's abnormal breathing patterns. During a PVFMD attack, aberrant vocal fold closure during respiration (usually during inhalation and less often during exhalation) is seen. Spirometry and pulmonary function testing are often performed in patients with PVFMD to rule out asthma or other significant pulmonary disease. For patients with PVFMD, spirometry might reveal a blunted inspiratory loop, indicating a variable extra-thoracic obstruction [7].

While PVFMD is usually diagnosed and treated in the outpatient setting, occurrence in the ICU is possible. There are many triggers for PVFMD attacks, including stress, anxiety, environmental irritants (such as cleaning products), exercise, gastroesophageal reflux, post-nasal drip, talking/laughing, strong smells, and temperature changes. Proper diagnosis is crucial to prevent inappropriate intubation of these patients, as once intubated, it can be difficult to successfully extubate, which may necessitate tracheotomy [8]. When accurately identified, PVFMD is managed medically and behaviorally with anxiolytic medications, antacid medications if reflux is suspected, and bronchodilators, if coexistent asthma is suspected. Recalcitrant laryngospasms despite medical and behavioral interventions are rare but are treated with laryngeal botulinum toxin, chronic anxiolytic medications, and rarely, tracheotomy.

Behavioral management is the gold standard treatment for PVFMD and includes working with an SLP and often a mental health professional if stress, anxiety, and depression are playing a significant role. Behavioral therapy administered by the SLP involves education about the diagnosis, review of diet and lifestyle modifications that can reduce known irritants (e.g., gastroesophageal reflux disease, allergens, etc.), identification of breathing "attack" triggers, provision of relaxation techniques, and most importantly, education regarding breathing techniques (including lower abdominal breathing) to prevent or reduce the severity of the breathing "attack" episodes [9,10].

The treating SLP may teach a variety of breathing techniques, all of which aim to reduce the severity, length, and frequency of the breathing episodes. These breathing techniques often involve semi-occlusion of the vocal tract, which changes the inspiratory laryngeal configuration to optimize opening at the levels of the glottis and supraglottis [11]. One common example of this is teaching patients to breathe in through their nose and out through tightly pursed lips. Often this is synced with a breathing "rhythm" that aligns with the patient's needs. For example, "Breathe in through your nose on one, and breathe out through tightly pursed lips on two, three, and four," or "Breathe in through your nose on one and two and breathe out with a 'shhhh' on three, four, five, and six." The specific posturing of the upper airway (e.g., nasal breathing, "shhhh" breathing, and pursed lip breathing) and rate of breathing (e.g., 1:3; 2:4, as above) are tailored to the patient. Most patients will require several rounds of these breathing techniques to prevent an episode or to stop one that is occurring. Close collaboration with the hospital or outpatient SLP team is critical to start appropriate treatment for these patients, thus mitigating the risk of unneeded and morbid treatments, such as inappropriate intubation.

Anatomic Sequelae of Laryngeal Injury

The endotracheal tube lays in the posterior glottis, contacting the vocal folds, medial face of both arytenoids, and the posterior glottic mucosa. The incidence of vocal fold edema is unknown but is likely common. More serious mucosal injury occurs in approximately 50% of patients and can result in ulceration or granulation tissue formation on the vocal folds (see

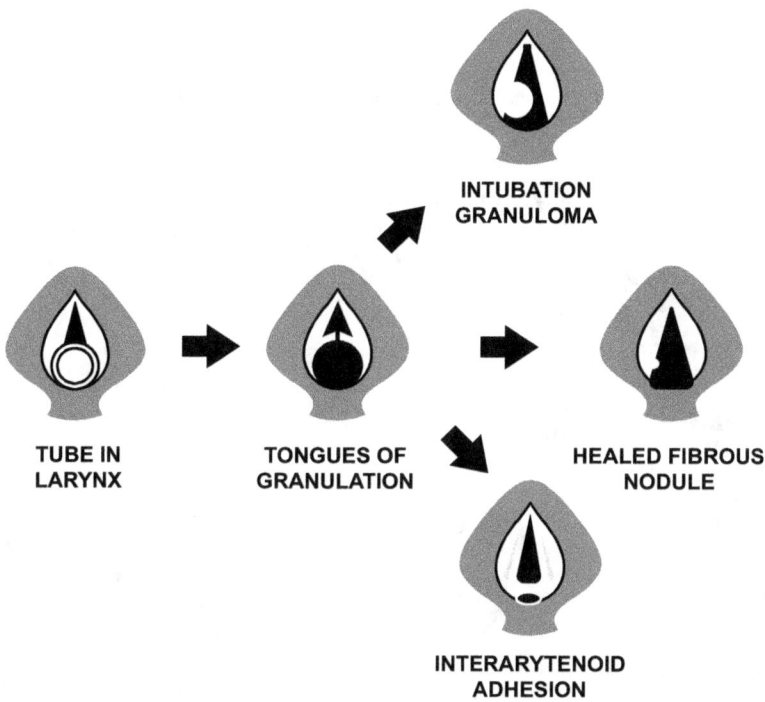

Figure 39.3 Flow chart showing consequences of granulation tissue formation during prolonged intubation and three distinct chronic changes that can occur: intubation granuloma, healed fibrous nodule, and interarytenoid adhesion. From: B. Benjamin. Prolonged intubation injuries of the larynx: endoscopic diagnosis, classification, and treatment. *Ann Otol Rhinol Laryngol* 2018; **127(8)**: 492–507. ©2018 Sage Publications. Reprinted by permission of Sage Publications.

Figures 39.3 and 39.4) [12]. While it is common to convert intubation to tracheotomy within 7–10 days of mechanical ventilation, the time to injury can be shorter in patients with diabetes, small vessel disease, or critical illness. Conversion of endotracheal intubation to tracheotomy in a timely manner can mitigate the risk of lifelong sequelae from laryngeal injury. Additionally, early identification of acute laryngeal injury by the otolaryngology service can reduce or eliminate the possibility of lifelong dyspnea, tracheotomy, and decreased quality of life [13].

Dysphonia

Hoarseness is common after intubation and results from vocal fold edema caused by endotracheal tube irritation. This edema changes how the vocal folds vibrate, resulting in a raspy voice. In addition, ICU-acquired weakness (see Chapter 4 for additional information) can result in reduced strength of the muscles of respiration, which is key to "power" the voice with an adequate and appropriately forceful flow of air through semi-closed vocal folds. Even though this condition is benign and typically improves as the vocal fold edema resolves, it is important to examine the larynx to confirm the etiology of the hoarseness. More nefarious etiologies may be present and will be discussed next.

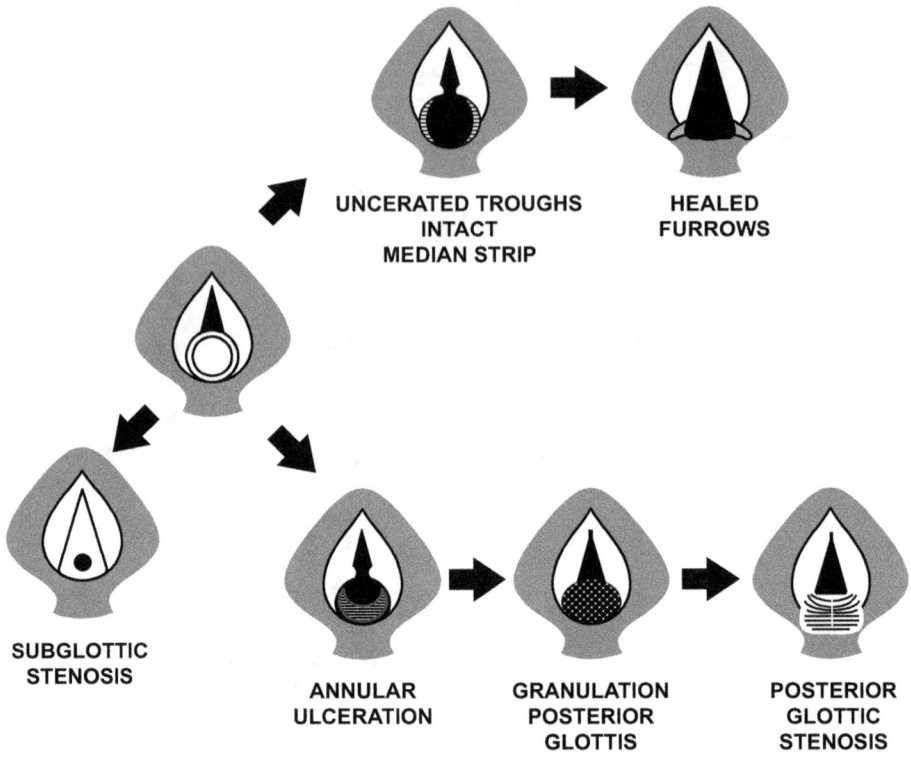

Figure 39.4 Flow chart showing consequences of ulceration following prolonged intubation: healed furrows, posterior glottic stenosis, and subglottic stenosis. From: B. Benjamin. Prolonged intubation injuries of the larynx: endoscopic diagnosis, classification, and treatment. *Ann Otol Rhinol Laryngol* 2018; **127(8)**: 492–507. ©2018 Sage Publications. Reprinted by permission of Sage Publications.

Vocal Process Granuloma

Vocal process granulomas are the result of impaired healing of a mucosal injury and are most commonly located at the vocal process of the arytenoid cartilage. "Tongues" of granulation tissue usually resolve in time after extubation but may cause ipsilateral throat soreness, globus sensation, and occasionally dysphonia if they persist in the form of a vocal process granuloma. Inhaled corticosteroids, aggressive antacid management, endoscopic corticosteroid injection, laser treatment, or ipsilateral vocal fold botulinum toxin injection are graduated treatment options.

Interarytenoid Adhesion

When the tongues of granulation tissue coalesce anterior to the endotracheal tube, they form an adhesion. When the endotracheal tube is removed, this interarytenoid adhesion will restrict vocal fold abduction (opening), which can result in dyspnea. Treatment involves lysis of the interarytenoid adhesion with either "cold" incision or laser, often accompanied by corticosteroid injection of the base, which often restores at least some vocal fold motion. Persistent restriction in vocal fold motion is usually the result of posterior glottic stenosis.

Posterior Glottic Stenosis

Posterior glottic stenosis (PGS) is a dreaded outcome of acute laryngeal injury because it can have a significantly negative impact on the patient's quality of life and is difficult to improve with surgical intervention, particularly when diagnosed late. Mucosal ulceration of contact points between the endotracheal tube and the medial face of both arytenoid cartilages and the posterior glottic mucosa can result in fibrosis. This "circumferential" scar contracts as it matures, which can "pull" both arytenoid cartilages to the midline. It takes approximately two months for this contracture to result in subjective dyspnea, at a time when the voice quality is often improving.

Early detection of PGS is possible with serial flexible laryngoscopy examinations by the otolaryngology team after extubation, particularly in patients with prolonged intubation, traumatic intubation, inhalational burn injuries, or comorbid diabetes; a high index of suspicion is required. Visualization of the larynx shows bilateral vocal fold immobility, often with a critically small glottic opening. PGS severity is variable, and the severity impacts expectations of surgical treatment. When detected early, treatment involves glottal dilation, corticosteroid injection, and often tracheotomy if identified within one to two months after extubation [14]. Surgical success is thought to be related to how quickly surgery is performed after the injury, with better success after early surgery due to the natural history of scar maturation. If early intervention is unsuccessful or diagnosis is delayed, there is a greater negative impact on the patient's quality of life.

When PGS is identified late, treatments are limited to glottal opening surgeries or lifelong tracheotomy. Endoscopic glottal opening surgeries include transverse cordotomy, medial arytenoidectomy, and arytenoidectomy, which create a permanent glottal opening to breathe through at the expense of vocal quality and possible dysphagia. Transverse cordotomy, the most common surgery performed for PGS, uses a CO_2 laser to make an incision across the thyroarytenoid muscle from medial to lateral, starting just anterior to the vocal process, and then extending laterally to the extent of the inner table of the cricoid. Contraction and scarring of the vocal fold results in a small defect through which the patient will pass more air. Medial arytenoidectomy is only possible if there is no scar intervening between the medial face of both arytenoid cartilages. CO_2 laser ablation of a medial portion of the arytenoid cartilage results in a small defect through which to pass more air. Endoscopic arytenoidectomy similarly uses the CO_2 laser to remove more of the arytenoid cartilage, often in conjunction with a transverse cordotomy, creating a much larger defect through which the patient can breathe.

Tracheotomy bypasses the glottic obstruction entirely. Although most patients prefer to avoid tracheotomy, depending upon the medical circumstances, tracheotomy may be the best treatment for some and is often needed in order to safely secure the airway for glottic-opening surgery, in which case it is hopefully a temporary treatment. Permanent hoarseness and dysphagia can occur with any of these procedures. Preoperative swallowing evaluations are needed to assess if it is safe to proceed with surgery, since the patient's baseline swallowing function can permanently worsen due to the lack of glottic closure to protect the airway from aspiration and the "weaker" swallow that results in the setting of glottic incompetence. Importantly, these surgeries are irreversible, and patients must understand the trade-off between breathing and voice/swallowing and that, despite surgery, decannulation may not ultimately be possible.

Posterior Glottic Diastasis

Ulceration of the posterolateral glottic mucosa can result in a deficiency along the medial face of the arytenoid, which results in dysphonia by causing posterior glottic incompetence during vocal fold adduction while voicing. Posterior glottic diastasis can be difficult to identify on laryngeal examination without high-quality endoscopic equipment but should be considered in cases of dysphonia in the setting of previous intubation and grossly normal vocal fold motion. Posterior glottic diastasis is difficult to surgically correct with mucosal flaps, and these patients often have permanent dysphonia, which can be detrimental to their professional livelihood and quality of life.

Subglottic/Tracheal Stenosis and Tracheomalacia

Mucosal ulceration at the subglottis results from intubation with an inappropriately large endotracheal tube or the prolonged presence of endotracheal tube cuff pressures that exceed capillary perfusion pressure at the cricoid cartilage, which can lead to subglottic or tracheal stenosis or tracheomalacia. Malacia of the cricoid cartilage can occur but is fortunately uncommon; as the only complete cartilaginous ring of the airway, cricoid malacia results in the need for permanent tracheotomy. Reconstruction of the cricoid is highly successful in the pediatric population, but it is more challenging and less successful in older, more infirm patients.

Tracheal stenosis is often managed with surgical tracheal dilation, while tracheomalacia is more challenging to treat and not amenable to dilation. Tracheomalacia results in a collapse of the airway in the area of injury, resulting in dyspnea. Controlled breathing techniques may reduce the inhalation pressures that cause airway collapse, resulting in a more patent airway during inhalation. Surgically, tracheal stents can be deployed, but they must be closely monitored for formation of granulation tissue, which may ultimately cause airway obstruction. Future treatments may include resorbable stents that create a more stable tracheal wall after the stent has resorbed.

Management of Issues Related to Tracheotomy

Early tracheotomy should be performed when appropriate, as it reduces risk of laryngeal injury and is correlated with less sedation, fewer days of mechanical ventilation, shorter ICU lengths of stay, and reduced long-term mortality [15]. Tracheotomy is a surgical airway created via dissection from the anterior neck through the anterior wall of the trachea. Ideal tracheotomy placement is between the second and third tracheal rings; higher tracheotomy placement abutting the cricoid can cause cricoid chondritis, ultimately resulting in subglottic stenosis or cricoid malacia. Tracheotomy can be performed via an "open" or "percutaneous" approach. Open tracheotomy involves a skin incision followed by dissection of tissue between the skin and anterior tracheal wall, often including mobilization or lysis of the thyroid isthmus, and subsequent placement of the tracheotomy tube under direct visualization into the trachea. Occasionally, "stay sutures" are placed around the tracheal ring above and below the entry into the trachea; these are used to facilitate the first tracheotomy tube change and are then removed. Open tracheotomy is recommended for patients with difficult neck anatomy, previous tracheotomy, coagulopathy, or high-riding innominate artery. Percutaneous tracheotomy, in contrast, requires that the patient already be intubated. A small incision is made on the anterior neck with minimal to no dissection of the soft tissue overlying the trachea, and progressive dilation of the tract allows for tracheotomy tube placement via the modified Seldinger technique. Flexible bronchoscopy through the existing endotracheal tube helps verify proper trocar placement, which is then followed by the tracheotomy tube. Candidates for percutaneous tracheotomy must have favorable anatomy and no previous surgery in the surgical field, thyroid disease, or coagulopathy. After either procedure, the tracheotomy tube is secured with a neck collar (twill, Velcro) and sutures through the tube faceplate.

While both open and percutaneous tracheotomy can be performed in the ICU, safety concerns may necessitate completing open tracheotomy in the operating room. Complication rates are comparable between the two approaches when performed by experienced surgeons in appropriately chosen patients.

Considerations for Tracheotomy Tube Decannulation

Once tracheotomized patients no longer require mechanical ventilation, decannulation should be considered. Most institutions have "decannulation protocols," which vary among hospitals. Despite the variability, the intent is consistent: appropriate decannulation without the need for urgent replacement of the tracheotomy tube or endotracheal intubation. There is often strong pressure for decannulation when patients are transitioned to long-term care facilities, as many will not care for tracheotomized patients. If returning home to the care of loved ones, tracheotomy tube care requires manual dexterity, intellectual aptitude, and many durable supplies, which may present challenges for some patients and caregivers. In general, for a patient to be considered for decannulation, the following must be verified:

1. The indication for tracheotomy has resolved or improved such that the patient no longer requires mechanical ventilation.
2. There is no upcoming planned procedure that requires general anesthesia; if so, consider decannulation after planned episodes of general anesthesia.
3. The patient has an appropriate level of consciousness to protect the airway from aspiration and possesses the ability to effectively expectorate aspirated material. Importantly, tracheotomy does *not* prevent aspiration, which is defined as passage of liquid, food, or saliva past the level of the vocal folds. Since tracheotomy tubes are usually placed between the second and third tracheal rings, material has already been aspirated when it reaches the tracheotomy tube. Tracheotomy tubes do, however, allow for more effective retrieval of aspirated material via suctioning.
4. The patient should be able to adequately handle secretions and require suctioning less than four to six times per day.
5. The patient should have a patent airway. If airway obstruction was a factor for intubation initially, then flexible nasolaryngoscopy should be performed to assess upper airway patency. If a patient does not respond well to tracheotomy tube capping or speaking valve placement, then visualization of the larynx while the patient is awake is valuable to identify reasons for the patient's poor response.
6. The patient should be able to tolerate a tracheotomy tube capping trial with an appropriately sized, uncuffed tracheotomy tube, with no resultant respiratory distress or stridor. Patients are often sequentially moved from tracheotomy to decannulation after successfully passing through both a speaking valve trial and capping trial. A speaking

valve allows the patient to produce "hands-free" speech. On exhalation, inhaled air from the tracheotomy tube passes around the shaft of the tube and through the volitionally semi-closed vocal folds, which produces sound. This requires sufficient space between the outer diameter of the tracheotomy tube and the tracheal wall; if this space is too small, the patient will feel resistance and not tolerate the speaking valve. It is safest to place speaking valves on *uncuffed* tracheotomy tubes, as inadvertent cuff inflation in cuffed tracheotomy tubes results in the inability to exhale, which will lead to death if not rectified. Speaking valve placement requires the expertise of a respiratory therapist to assess patient appropriateness and their response to placement. If the patient does not tolerate placement of a speaking valve, flexible laryngoscopy and tracheoscopy by an otolaryngologist is valuable to identify the reasons for intolerance. After a successful speaking valve trial, a capping trial is performed, which prevents air from passing through the tracheotomy tube. All air passage is restricted to the space between the tracheotomy tube and tracheal wall; if the tracheotomy tube is too large, then this space will be too small, and downsizing the tracheotomy tube may be required. Women more often require downsizing, as they are more likely to have an inappropriately large tracheotomy tube placed. As with endotracheal tubes, tracheotomy tube size should be chosen based on height. Capping trials usually last for 24–48 hours, depending upon the clinical team's concern for successful decannulation. Under special circumstances, speaking valve and capping trials can be avoided when airway patency is confirmed with endoscopy.
7. The patient should demonstrate effective coughing, which correlates with adequate pulmonary drive. This is sometimes used instead of laryngoscopy when otolaryngology services are not available. An audibly "crisp" cough is suggestive of adequate vocal fold closure, which may protect against aspiration. Peak expiratory flow rates should be greater than 160 L/min.

Sequalae of Decannulation

After successful decannulation, the tracheostoma is taped in a more closed configuration, and a dressing is placed over the stoma. Patients are asked to press on the dressing when speaking to reduce air passage through the stoma, which increases the chances of tracheostoma closure. If there is a persistent tracheocutaneous fistula, surgical closure is needed.

Granulation tissue associated with tracheotomy tube placement is common. If suprastomal granulation tissue (above the tracheotomy tube as it enters the tracheal lumen) obstructs the airway after decannulation, it must be treated to improve air passage. Granulation tissue usually resolves without treatment after the tracheotomy tube is removed, so not all granulation tissue requires treatment. Granulation tissue at the distal tip of the tracheotomy tube would have already been assessed and treated when the tracheotomy tube was in place.

Unique to tracheotomy, anterior tracheal wall malacia, termed "A-frame deformity," can occur. The anterior tracheal wall sustains injury with tracheotomy, regardless of the method of placement. The tube itself is larger than the tracheal ring interspace and thus exerts pressure on the tracheal ring above and below the tracheotomy tube shaft. This pressure not unexpectedly can result in loss of nutrient exposure to the adjacent cartilaginous rings, resulting in malacia. Since the tracheal rings are "C-shaped" with a membranous portion posteriorly, loss of the anterior component of the ring results in two lateral cartilaginous segments that collapse medially in the shape of an "A-frame," analogous to removing the keystone from an arch. Clinically significant tracheomalacia requires treatment, including tracheal stent placement, T-tube placement, or tracheal resection.

Key Points

1. Endotracheal intubation required in the care of the critically ill places the larynx at risk of injury. The larynx is the critical intersection of airway, swallowing, and voice production.
2. Interdisciplinary care of tracheal disorders requires the specialized skill sets of otolaryngologists, speech-language pathologists, respiratory therapists, thoracic surgeons, and critical care physicians and nurses.
3. Appropriately sized endotracheal tubes and early tracheotomy mitigate the risk of lifelong laryngeal injury, including need for permanent tracheotomy. Appropriate endotracheal tube and tracheotomy tube cuff pressure requires manometric monitoring to reduce the risk of tracheal injury.
4. Nonstatic laryngeal obstruction (e.g., paradoxical vocal fold motion disorder) should be considered when patients exhibit respiratory distress despite maintaining excellent oxygen saturation. Flexible laryngoscopy will confirm or refute the diagnosis. Treatment in the acute setting involves anxiolytic medications and behavioral breathing techniques.
5. Anatomic sequelae of laryngeal injury include dysphonia, vocal process granuloma, interarytenoid adhesion, posterior glottic stenosis, posterior glottic diastasis, and subglottic/tracheal stenosis and tracheomalacia, which are all managed differently.
6. Attempts at tracheotomy tube decannulation should be made, provided that the patient meets appropriate criteria and can tolerate speaking valve and capping trials with uncuffed tracheotomy tubes.

References

1. A. Coordes, G. Rademacher, S. Knopke, et al. Selection and placement of oral ventilation tubes based on tracheal morphometry. *Laryngoscope* 2011; **121**(6): 1225–30.
2. B.I. Esianor, B.R. Campbell, J.D. Casey, et al. Endotracheal tube size in critically ill patients. *JAMA Otolaryngol Head Neck Surg* 2022; **148**(9): 849–53.
3. A.C. Cao, S. Rereddy, N. Mirza. Current practices in endotracheal tube size selection for adults. *Laryngoscope* 2021: **131**; 1967–71.
4. L.G. Morris, R.A. Zoumalan, J. D. Roccaforte, et al. Monitoring tracheal tube cuff pressures in the intensive care unit: a comparison of digital palpation and manometry. *Ann Otol Rhinol Laryngol* 2007; **116**(9): 639–42.
5. J.A. Koufman, C. Block. Differential diagnosis of paradoxical vocal fold movement. *Am J Speech Lang Pathol* 2008; **17**: 327–34.
6. E.O. Shay, E. Sayad, and C.F. Milstein. Exercise-induced laryngeal obstruction (EILO) in children and young adults: from referral to diagnosis. *Laryngoscope* 2020; **130**: 400–6.
7. A. Fretzayas, M. Moustaki, I. Loukou, et al. Differentiating vocal cord dysfunction from asthma. *J Asthma Allergy* 2017; **10**: 277–83.
8. N. Denipah, C.M. Dominguez, E.P. Kraai, et al. Acute management of paradoxical

9. B.A. Mathers-Schmidt. Paradoxical vocal fold motion: a tutorial on a complex disorder and the speech-language pathologist's role. *Am J Speech Lang Pathol* 2001; **10**: 111–25.

10. R.R. Patel, R. Venediktov, T. Schooling, et al. Evidence-based systematic review: effects of speech-language pathology treatment for individuals with paradoxical vocal fold motion. *Am J Speech Lang Pathol* 2015; **24**: 566–84.

11. M. Shaffer, J.K. Litts, E. Nauman, et al. Speech-language pathology as a primary treatment for exercise-induced laryngeal obstruction. *Immunol Allergy Clin North Am* 2018; **38**: 293–302.

vocal fold motion (vocal cord dysfunction). *Ann Emerg Med* 2017; **69**: 18–23.

12. B. Benjamin. Prolonged intubation injuries of the larynx: endoscopic diagnosis, classification, and treatment. *Ann Otol Rhinol Laryngol* 1993; **160**: 1–15.

13. A.S. Lowery, J.A. Malenke, A.J. Bolduan, et al. Early intervention for the treatment of acute laryngeal injury after intubation. *JAMA Otolaryngol Head Neck Surg* 2021; **147**(3): 232–7.

14. C.A. Rosen, H. Wang, D.J. Cates, et al. The glottis is not round: teardrop-shaped glottic dilation for early posterior glottic stenosis. *Laryngoscope* 2019; **129**: 1428–32.

15. K. Hosokawa, M. Nishimura, M. Egi, et al. Timing of tracheotomy in ICU patients: a systematic review of randomized controlled trials. *Crit Care* 2015; **19**: 424.

Nutrition Impairments in Survivors of Critical Illness

Kathlene E. Hendon, Melissa A. Jacobs, and Matthew D. Smith

Introduction

An intensive care unit (ICU) admission is frequently characterized by the delivery of inadequate nutrition, and patients who were well-nourished prior to hospitalization often develop malnutrition during critical illness. Nutrition rehabilitation is an essential component of regaining muscle mass, strength, and independence following critical illness and should begin as soon as possible. The constellation of disabilities associated with post-intensive care syndrome (PICS) can significantly impact the nutritional status of survivors of critical illness.

The physical, functional, cognitive, and psychosocial impairments present in patients with PICS are potential barriers to optimal nutrition [1,2]. Well-intentioned practitioners, patients, and families often mistakenly assume that once nutrition support is discontinued, a patient's appetite, weight, and nutritional status will return to premorbid levels with minimal ongoing intervention. The inability to appreciate the numerous obstacles to obtaining adequate nutrition in the outpatient setting can lead to failed nutrition rehabilitation. Recognizing the presence of malnutrition, barriers to achieving adequate nutrition, and strategies to guide the patient, their family, and their medical team in nutrition rehabilitation is essential for the best outcomes.

This chapter examines the outpatient nutrition needs of survivors of critical illness. The convalescent phase following critical illness requires the skill of a registered dietitian (RD), in concert with the patient's multidisciplinary care team, to manage continuity of nutrition care. The dietitian's understanding of the clinical course of critical illness, nutrition diagnosis at discharge, and barriers to nutrition associated with PICS are essential to develop individualized care plans for successful nutrition rehabilitation.

Nutrition Challenges After Discharge

The prevalence of malnutrition in patients requiring intensive care ranges from 38% to 78% due to a variety of confounding factors [3]. Malnutrition is described as a state of subacute or chronic under-nutrition or over-nutrition, often accompanied by systemic inflammation, that leads to changes in body composition and diminished physical and mental function [4]. Nutrition is compromised by suboptimal nutrient delivery during hospitalization along with the development of impairments associated with PICS, new or existing comorbidities, and/or advancing age of the survivor of critical illness. In some studies, more than 80% of survivors of critical illness develop PICS, symptoms of which can persist for years after their index illness [5]. Following discharge, patients may develop appetite changes, fatigue, weight loss, dysgeusia, dysosmia, dysphagia, cognitive impairment, and socioeconomic challenges, all either precipitated or worsened by their critical illness. Specific nutrient deficiencies may develop related to critical care treatments, such as continuous renal replacement therapy, certain medications, and gastrointestinal surgery, which may impact digestion and nutrient absorption. Commonly prescribed medications that can contribute to nutrient depletion include anticonvulsants, corticosteroids, proton pump inhibitors, loop and thiazide diuretics, estrogen, bile acid sequestrants, and H_2 receptor antagonists (see Table 40.1) [6,7,8]. Comorbidities, including preexisting

Table 40.1 Medications associated with vitamin and mineral deficiencies

Vitamin/Mineral	Medication
Vitamin A [6,7]	Bile sequestrants Proton pump inhibitors (PPIs)
Vitamin B–1 (Thiamine) [6,7]	Loop and thiazide diuretics
Vitamin B–6 (Pyridoxine) [7, 8]	Isoniazid Estrogens/progesterone
Vitamin B–9 (Folic acid) [6, 7]	Anticonvulsants Estrogens Pancreatic enzymes Calcium channel blockers
Vitamin B–12 (Cobalamin) [6,7]	Metformin Histamine 2 receptor antagonists (H_2RAs) PPIs
Vitamin C [7] (Ascorbic acid)	Aspirin PPIs
Vitamin D [6,7]	Anticonvulsants Bile acid sequestrants H_2RAs Selective serotonin reuptake inhibitors (SSRIs) Bronchodilators (inhaled) Hypoglycemics Statins
Vitamin E [7]	Estrogen/progesterone Statins
Vitamin K [6]	Bile acid sequestrants

Table 40.1 (cont.)

Vitamin/Mineral	Medication
Co-Q10 [6,7]	Hydralazine
	Statins
Calcium [6,7]	Anticonvulsants
	Corticosteroids
	H_2RAs
	SSRIs
	Estrogen/progesterone
	Loop diuretics
	Bronchodilators (inhaled)
	Hypoglycemics
	PPIs
Iron [7]	Aspirin
Magnesium [6,7]	Estrogens
	H_2RAs
	Thiazide diuretics
	PPIs
Potassium [6,7]	Corticosteroids
	Loop and thiazide diuretics
Sodium [6,7]	Loop and thiazide diuretics
Zinc [6,7]	Loop and thiazide diuretics
	H_2RAs
	ACE-inhibitors, specifically captopril
	Antihypertensives

Note: Vitamin and mineral supplementation should be individualized while receiving long-term medication administration.

malnutrition or obesity, cancer, endocrinopathies, specific organ dysfunctions, and wounds, may require targeted nutrition therapies outside of the provision of adequate calories and protein. Furthermore, as survivors of critical illness are living well beyond their index hospitalization, the physiological challenges more commonly associated with elderly critical illness survivors must be considered, including the anorexia of aging, senescence, chewing difficulties, dysphagia, underhydration, and changes in sensory perception.

Malnutrition has not been universally defined, although the Global Leadership Initiative on Malnutrition (GLIM) and International Classification of Diseases (ICD) are developing a comprehensive approach to its identification. GLIM recommends using a validated

Table 40.2 Nutrition screening tools

Screening Tool	Number of Questions	Low Risk Score	Moderate Risk Score	High Risk Score	Population	Setting
Mini Nutrition Assessment Short Form (MNA-SF) [11]	4–5	12–14	8–11	0–7	Older Adults	Inpatient Outpatient
Malnutrition Universal Screening Tool (MUST) [12]	5	0	1–2	≥2	Adults	Inpatient Outpatient
Malnutrition Screening Tool (MST) [13]	2–3	0–1	No moderate scoring	≥ 2 at risk	Adults	All

Note: MNA-SF parallels deficits common to PICS patients. Validation studies are warranted in PICS patients.

nutrition screening tool administered by a trained individual to identify the risk of malnutrition (see Table 40.2) [9]. If risk of malnutrition is identified with the screening tool, a thorough nutrition assessment should be conducted by an RD to definitively diagnose the presence of malnutrition. The nutrition assessment should include a medical history, nutrition history, social history, medication review, nutrition-focused physical examination (NFPE), anthropometrics, biochemical data, and diagnostic information. These two steps are required to gather information for the GLIM model, which includes five diagnostic criteria: three phenotypic criteria (weight loss, underweight, and reduced muscle mass) and two etiologic criteria (reduced food/nutrition intake and inflammation/high disease burden). At least one criterion from each phenotypic and etiologic category is required to determine a malnutrition diagnosis. Malnutrition is graded as moderate or severe based on the degree of deviation from normal [9,10].

Discharge to Post-Acute Facilities

Compared with ongoing medical issues, the patient's nutritional status is often undervalued as they approach hospital discharge. Given the complexity of this patient population, the discharge planning process should be multidisciplinary and include the patient, family, support persons, and resources to address any anticipated nutritional barriers. At the time of care transitions, a comprehensive nutrition discharge summary, including anthropometrics, NFPE findings, nutrition diagnosis, and the nutrition prescription, should be made available to the RD.

Post-acute facility food service limitations and high patient-to-staff ratios can negatively impact nutritional rehabilitation. While protected mealtimes aim to limit disruptions, patients with PICS often have early satiety, taste changes, and loss of appetite, which limit their ability to consume adequate calories and protein at mealtime. Food quality and the use of texture-modified foods are contributory factors to poor intake [14]. Meals are often served at the bedside rather than in a communal space, which can inadvertently worsen delirium or contribute to feelings of social isolation and depression [15,16]. Furthermore, nursing and RD staffing ratios may not be conducive to providing one-to-one feeding assistance and close monitoring of oral intake. Adopting family-style dining with family visitation can foster a community environment and allow for social interaction. Volunteers can provide feeding assistance and help ensure patients have the best opportunity to reach their energy and protein needs. The family should be encouraged to supply the patient's favorite foods to help improve intake.

Appetite and Weight Loss

Although there is little dedicated research on nutrition rehabilitation in survivors of critical illness, appetite changes, early satiety, and weight loss are commonly observed in this patient population, and disruption in the natural desire to eat is a significant barrier to adequate nutrition. Medications; changes in the microbiome, gut hormones, and sensory perception; persistent inflammation and disease burden; and depression and anxiety can all worsen the appetite and precipitate weight loss. Medications that cause loss of appetite include antibiotics, amphetamines, chemotherapeutic agents, digoxin, fluoxetine, hydralazine, and opioid analgesics [17]. Survivors of critical illness have been found to have reduced appetite and oral intake for at least three months after discharge [18,19]. Microbiome alterations in critical illness have undesirable effects on the appetite by impacting hormone regulation and hedonic feelings [20]. It remains possible that altered gut microbiota may negatively influence host appetite through modifying the secretion of appetite-related hormones [20], including peptide YY, which inhibits the appetite, and ghrelin, which stimulates the appetite. The appetite tends to improve in the fourth week following critical illness [21].

Weight loss is commonly present following critical illness, with average weight loss of 3.3 kg three months following hospital discharge [19]. This may be driven, in part, by a prolonged inflammatory response, which can suppress appetite during recovery. Pro-inflammatory biomarkers, including the cytokines interleukin (IL)-1β, tumor necrosis factor (TNF)-α, and IL-6, are implicated in anorexia. Although the mechanisms by which this occurs are not fully understood, pro-inflammatory cytokines activate neuropathways in the hypothalamus that repress the desire for food and activate autonomic nervous system signaling, which modulates gastric motility and emptying. Furthermore, cytokines stimulate the release of leptin and insulin, which both suppress food intake [22]. Should appetite, early satiety, and weight loss persist, oral supplements are a useful tool in the nutrition prescription; enteral or parenteral nutrition support should also be considered if appetite does not sufficiently improve to correct malnutrition.

Taste and Smell Changes

Altered taste and smell after critical illness are common complaints contributing to decreased appetite and a diminished desire to eat. Disorders of taste are classified as ageusia (total loss of taste sensation), hypogeusia (diminished taste sensation), and dysgeusia (persistent, unpleasant taste sensation). Conditions commonly associated with taste changes are numerous and include respiratory illness, COVID-19, infections, organ failures, malnutrition, nutrient deficiencies, slowed turnover of taste receptors, cancer, medications, chemotherapy, radiation, inflammation, head/neck trauma, surgeries, and changes in the microbiome [23]. Specific nutrient deficiencies associated with taste alterations include zinc, vitamin A, vitamin C, vitamin D, vitamin E, vitamin B-3 (niacin), vitamin B-9 (folate), and vitamin B-12 (cobalamin) [24,25,26].

Patients presenting with taste alterations may have multiple etiologies affecting their sensory perception. After reviewing the critical illness history, the RD may determine that the taste alteration is related to a nutrient deficiency. It is feasible to counsel the individual to improve diet quality to ensure essential nutrients are consumed. The RD may recommend empirical supplementation if a deficiency is suspected to be related to a poor diet, nutrient losses that occurred during hospitalization, or malabsorption. In some instances, obtaining laboratory values may be required to determine appropriate supplementation to correct a deficiency; of note, persistent inflammation and the volume status of the patient can impact the laboratory values and lead to an inaccurate reflection of nutrient levels.

Olfaction disorders (OD) can be described as anosmia (total loss of smell), hyposmia (reduced ability to smell), and phantosmia (perception of an odor despite the absence of an identifiable stimulus) [27]. Conditions commonly associated with OD include depression, malnutrition, cognitive impairment, head injury, neurological disorders, advanced age, and COVID-19 [28]. With respect to COVID-19, there is a high rate of olfaction recovery between one month and one year, but approximately 5% of individuals with long-COVID syndrome have persistent OD [27]. Distortions or loss of sensory perception reduce enjoyment and hedonic feelings associated with eating, which may lead to decreased appetite, suboptimal oral intake, reduced quality of life, and malnutrition. Options for treatment are limited, but research is exploring new therapies and lifestyle modifications that may improve disorders of sensory perception.

Physical and Functional Impairments

Physical deficits resulting from atrophy of skeletal and respiratory muscles among patients with PICS are characterized by the term ICU-acquired weakness (ICU-AW; see Chapter 4 for additional information) [29,30,31]. The pathophysiology of ICU-AW involves complex structural and functional changes within the myofibers and neurons, which can result in an increased likelihood of poor long-term outcomes and need for long-term care characterized by an inability to perform activities of daily living (ADLs) and instrumental activities of daily living (IADLs) [32]. Previously simple tasks such as feeding oneself (including chewing and swallowing), grocery shopping, and meal preparation, all of which are impacted by weakness and impaired endurance, become significant barriers to optimal nutrition status. Close collaboration with the patient, caregivers, and a comprehensive rehabilitation team composed of speech-language pathologists (SLP), occupational therapists (OT), physical therapists (PT), and an RD is critical to ensure that the patient meets their nutritional needs. As the patient progresses through recovery and regains muscle mass, strength, and function, their energy and protein needs change accordingly.

Dysphagia

Patients with PICS may present with dysphagia because of prolonged mechanical ventilation, ICU-AW, damage to the central nervous system, or the presence of naso-enteric or tracheotomy tubes [33]. Additionally, poor dentition and advanced age may contribute to dysphagia. While some patients may transiently experience swallowing difficulty following extubation, others may require further assessment and treatment with SLPs (see Chapter 38 for additional information). The International Dysphagia Diet Standardization Initiative (IDDSI) is a guide for practitioners designed to characterize the consistency of texturally modified diets and should be employed to provide the most appropriate diet consistency (see Figure 38.2) [34].

Patients experiencing the combination of dysphagia and poor appetite have increased difficulty achieving and maintaining their nutrient and hydration needs. Mechanically altered food and liquids may not be as visually appealing or nutrient dense as foods with conventional consistency, and acceptance of texturally modified foods and liquids may be limited, making treatment of malnutrition even more challenging. Under such circumstances, use of oral nutrition supplements and micronutrient supplementation may be warranted. The RD should also provide education to the patient, family, and caregivers regarding strategies to optimize oral intake. These include small, frequent meals; assistance with feeding; limiting external distractions at mealtimes; and use of adaptive equipment if necessary. Close collaboration with SLP to provide the most effective nutrition care is warranted. Should patients be unable to meet nutrition needs orally, supplementation with enteral nutrition following the placement of a naso-enteric tube or gastrostomy tube may be required.

Mental Health Disorders

Nutritional psychiatry is a nascent field addressing the role of nutrition on mental illness [35]. Though studies are lacking in patients recovering from critical illness, balanced nutrition should be integrated into the management of psychiatric disorders that develop after critical illness. There is growing evidence that the gut microbiome influences the neurotransmitter serotonin and its connection to mood, appetite, sleep, and pain. Short-chained fatty acids (SCFAs) are produced by healthy bacteria in the presence of fermentable fiber in the colon and provide the main source of energy for cells lining the colon. The SCFA butyrate has been found to regulate the gut production of serotonin and gut peptides, which affect the gut-brain hormones [36]. Several gut bacterial species have been found to have serotonin-producing properties through tryptophan synthetase mediation [37]. Ghrelin, peptide YY, glucagon-like peptide 1 (GLP-1), glucose dependent insulinotropic polypeptide (GIP), and cholecystokinin (CCK) are gut hormones thought to be key to gut-brain crosstalk in humans. These gut hormones are known to have a role in depression and anxiety disorders [38].

The population of beneficial organisms in the human gut microbiome dramatically decreases in critical illness [39]. A quality diet, such as the Mediterranean diet, may be beneficial in recovery to repopulate healthy gut species during the nutrition rehabilitation period. The Mediterranean meal pattern consists primarily of fish, chicken, whole grains, legumes, nuts, vegetables, fruits, and moderate consumption of full-fat dairy, red meat, and olive oil. The known benefits of adopting this diet include reduction of inflammation, oxidative stress, and free radicals and the provision of probiotics to the gut microbiome [40]. In contrast, processed foods and refined carbohydrates have been observed to have a detrimental effect on mood [40].

Avoidance of alcohol is recommended, as alcohol consumption can intensify symptoms of anxiety and depression due to its effect on serotonin levels [41]. Limiting caffeine is also recommended, as caffeine consumption can cause anxiety in healthy individuals and exacerbate symptoms in those with preexisting anxiety disorders [42].

Cognitive Disorders

The complex relationship between gut and brain function reveals the influence of nutrition on cognition [43], and the detrimental results of critical illness on the gut microbiome and its effect on cognition should be considered during recovery. The PREDIMED substudy assessed cognitive performance at baseline and after four years in subjects eating a Mediterranean diet compared with those on a control diet; participants eating a Mediterranean diet were found to have improved cognitive function, while those eating the control diet exhibited a decline in cognitive function [44]. Based on these results, the Mediterranean diet may be encouraged as a potential strategy to improve the health of the microbiome and potentially slow the development of cognitive decline.

Executive function deficits affect the patient's ability to perform the complex activities of meal planning, shopping, kitchen organization, and meal preparation. Survivors of critical illness may find that the once simple tasks of meal planning and preparation have become daunting, time-consuming, and overly complex. Safety awareness in the kitchen may be altered, leading to accidents and injury. Preparing a grocery list, navigating the grocery store, organizing groceries in a pantry, and preparing meals may require support from friends, family, or support services during recovery. Educating the patient and their support persons, along with enrollment in occupational and cognitive therapies, is essential to navigate these challenges until patients can once again assume these responsibilities.

Socioeconomic Barriers

Unemployment can lead to loss of savings or the inability to save, loss of health insurance, and the inability to afford food (or food that is high quality and nutritionally replete). Financial insecurity experienced by many survivors of critical illness could impact the ability to secure adequate nutrition in recovery. Food insecurity can play a significant role in the overall health and recovery of a patient and can be measured with the Food and Agricultural Organization's (FAO) Food Insecurity Experience Scale (FIES; see Table 40.3) [45]. In patients who remain dependent on enteral or parenteral nutrition following hospital discharge, loss of insurance coupled with financial insecurity may disrupt nutrition support, leading to inappropriate substitutes or foregoing the nutrition care plan entirely. Identifying financial constraints regarding access to quality nutrition is important to direct the patient to the appropriate support services.

Survivors of critical illness without a strong social network often struggle to maintain adequate nutrition. Social isolation can contribute to diminished appetite or lack of desire to eat [46]. Given that eating is often a communal experience, socialization and eating have a symbiotic relationship benefiting the recovering patient. In an elder care facility, those

Table 40.3 Food and Agricultural Organization (FAO) food insecurity experience scale (FIES) [45]

Scale	Description
Mild Food Insecurity	Concerns about food with worry about the ability to obtain foods
Moderate Food Insecurity	Associated with the inability to regularly eat a healthy, nutritious diet; an important indicator of poor dietary quality/variety; risk of micronutrient deficiencies
Severe Food Insecurity	Inadequate quantity of food and risk of hunger

who share meals with others consume 36% more than those who eat alone [47]. Qualitative studies have found an association between social isolation or loneliness and one or more food/eating behaviors that would negatively affect health (e.g., lower fruit and vegetable intake, higher intake of energy-dense-nutrient-poor foods, and lower overall diet quality) [46]. Recognizing social isolation and encouraging strategies to share meals with others will benefit those in nutrition rehabilitation.

The ICU Follow-Up Clinic Experience

An RD is an essential member in an ICU follow-up clinic multidisciplinary team directing nutrition rehabilitation. Prior to the scheduled clinic appointment, the RD should review the patient's critical illness course, nutrition diagnosis, and recommendations made at hospital discharge.

At an ICU follow-up clinic visit, a nutrition screen should be completed and scored by trained office personnel or by the RD. The nutrition screening tool should be selected for ease of administration and putative validity in identifying nutrition risk in survivors of critical illness. The Mini Nutrition Assessment-Short Form (MNA-SF) from the Nestle Nutrition Institute, for example, is a screening tool validated for use in geriatric patients, which reasonably parallels nutrition barriers in patients with PICS, including appetite loss, weight loss, impaired mobility, and psychological and cognitive problems. For patients at risk of or with malnutrition, the RD should then complete an in-depth nutrition assessment by obtaining a nutritional history, performing an NFPE, developing a nutrition care plan, and providing education to the patient and their loved ones. If a patient continues to attend the clinic, the score obtained on the nutrition screening tool can be used to objectively track nutrition progress in recovery.

In instances where ICU follow-up clinics are unavailable, or if an ICU follow-up clinic does not have an RD as a multidisciplinary team member, the patient should be referred to a general ambulatory clinic for continued nutrition care. A nutrition screen should be administered by qualified personnel or, in some cases, filled out by the patient or caregiver, and a nutrition care plan should be developed if the screen is concerning for malnutrition risk. If an RD is unavailable, professionally developed materials should be used to guide the patient, such as ICUsteps [48]. Scheduled follow-up appointments with an RD should be made if malnutrition fails to improve. Communication with patients, their loved ones, and their primary care provider, including shared decision-making regarding nutrition goals, is paramount to successful recovery.

The Nutrition Care Plan

The nutrition care plan should include a personalized summary of short-term goals, strategies, and resources to facilitate success. The plan should specify patient-specific needs for energy, macronutrients, and micronutrients; hydration; a meal schedule; simple menu ideas; recommended oral nutritional supplements; and contact information for meal delivery services, grocery delivery services, and other community resources. These recommendations are provided to optimize nutritional status, gain strength and independence, and improve the quality of life (see Box 40.1). A summary of the nutrition care plan can be used as a cover letter for educational materials given to the patient and caregivers. If a patient has a language, literacy, cognitive, visual, or hearing impairment, the nutrition care plan method should be adapted to their preferred method of communication. Coordination with other multidisciplinary team members is critical for effective nutrition rehabilitation.

Box 40.1 Strategies to optimize nutrition

General

- Obtain a written nutrition care plan with individualized specific goals and strategies
- Consume four to six balanced, regularly scheduled meals
- Eat the least restrictive diet possible
- Encourage the Mediterranean Diet
- Determine supplementation needs based on nutrition status
- Consume an oral nutrition supplement if eating < 50% of balanced meals
- Encourage adequate hydration
- Share mealtime with others daily
- Maintain a food journal

Appetite Loss

- Consider an appetite stimulant if indicated
- Avoid intense aromas that may decrease appetite
- Refer to pharmacy to optimize medication schedules

Taste/Smell Changes

- Identify cause of taste or smell disorder when possible
- Check zinc, vitamin A, vitamin B-12, niacin, folate, and vitamin D levels or supplement empirically
- Rinse mouth before eating and maintain oral hygiene
- Drink seltzer water or ginger ale with meals
- Smell foods to help elicit the memory of flavors
- Ageusia: Add citrus ingredients to recipes/foods; tart and sour flavors may boost taste
- Dysgeusia: Use marinades, strong seasonings, and lemon, vinegar, or other ingredients to mask off flavors; drink tea, carbonated beverages, or ginger ale to mask off flavors; chew sugar-free mint chewing gum or mints before meals; consider simple meals with few ingredients; serve cold foods rather than hot
- Hypogeusia: Add salt and herbs for enhanced flavor; use marinades and citrus or vinegar ingredients; try sour or tart flavors
- Consider OD exposure therapy of floral, resinous, fruity, and spicy scents in morning and evening for six to nine months.

Nausea/Vomiting

- Consume four to six dry meals at regular times; do not skip meals
- Avoid fatty or fried foods
- Drink fluids between meals
- Ginger and peppermint may be helpful
- Keep salty dry snacks handy
- Use oral rehydration solution if needed
- Consider antinausea/antiemetic medications

Diarrhea

- Avoid sorbitol-containing medications
- Avoid foods and beverages with refined carbohydrates
- Encourage adequate hydration
- Rule out an infectious origin
- Monitor electrolyte losses
- Consider antidiarrheal medication

Dysphagia

- Consider SLP consultation
- Keep thickened liquids cold for best enjoyment
- Present a textured modified diet in an attractive manner
- Thickening methods, premade thickened products for convenience, recipe resources
- Nutrition support as required

Cognitive Deficit

- Consider meal services determined by level of independence, including ready-to-eat meal delivery, meal kit services, and grocery delivery
- Meal program delivery services provided by insurance or government assistance
- Volunteer agencies or faith-based community meal programs
- Senior meal programs

Depression/Anxiety

- Eat meals with family and friends in a social setting
- Eat a clean diet with minimal processed foods and carbohydrates
- Avoid caffeinated beverages
- Avoid alcoholic beverages

Clinical Vignette

A 59-year-old female was discharged home after a two-month hospital stay, including two weeks in the ICU, where she required mechanical ventilation for acute respiratory distress syndrome (ARDS) secondary to community-acquired pneumonia. While in the ICU, the patient was diagnosed with severe malnutrition related to weight loss, muscle wasting, and fat loss. At hospital admission, her weight and body mass index (BMI) were 75 kg and 32.2, respectively, while at hospital discharge, they were 67.5 kg and 28.9, respectively. An appointment for the ICU follow-up clinic was scheduled.

At the initial ICU follow-up clinic appointment, four weeks after hospital discharge, the MNA-SF [11] indicated that malnutrition was present. The weight was 63.5 kg, with a BMI of 27.3. The RD obtained a detailed diet history, indicating an oral intake of less than 50% of the minimum recommended calorie and protein requirements. The NFPE demonstrated that severe malnutrition worsened since discharge from the ICU. The patient demonstrated impairments related to PICS, including weakness, mild cognitive impairment, depression, decreased appetite, weight loss, hypogeusia, and social isolation. Her diet indicated that she was missing essential foods to provide a balanced diet.

Severe malnutrition in the setting of recent critical illness was diagnosed, as evidenced by consuming less than 50% of her estimated energy requirement (EER) and protein needs for more than one month; weight loss of 15% in 3 months; moderate triceps and buccal fat losses; and severe temporal, clavicular, and calf muscle losses. Education illustrating a balanced diet was provided, and the written nutrition care plan and rationale were presented in the following letter to the patient:

Dear Ms. M.,
Your suggested nutrition care plan is summarized below.

Estimated Nutrition Needs:
~1780–2030 kcal/d (28–32 kcal/kg)
~95–110 g protein/d (1.5–1.7 g/kg)

We suggest six small meals per day, each with 300–350 kcal/meal and 15–20 g protein/meal. These goals are guidelines to prevent further weight loss and to regain muscle mass already lost. Oral nutrition supplements with 220–350 calories and 10–20 g protein should be worked into your schedule if you are eating less than 50% of your meals. Eat whether you are feeling hungry or not and avoid skipping meals. Share mealtimes with loved ones daily. The meal setting should be attractive, with minimal distractions, to focus on meal enjoyment.

Use seltzer water or an oral rinse before meals to cleanse the palate. Season food with salt (if permitted), pepper, citrus, herbs, and marinades to help intensify the flavor. Recall aromas and taste memories of foods to help stimulate the senses.

Resources provided: ICUsteps.org [48], ready-to-eat meal programs, grocery delivery services, PICS clinic support group schedule, Mediterranean diet materials, a menu of small balanced meals to meet nutrition goals, sample oral nutrition supplements, and coupons for purchasing oral nutrition supplements.

Best regards,
K. Smith RD, CNSC
Advanced Practice Dietitian

The RD communicated the visit's findings to the clinic physician, recommending zinc and vitamin A supplementation. The visit was documented in a brief note in the patient's chart. Social isolation and depression were discussed with the social worker. Involvement in a community meal program and participation in the PICS peer support group were recommended. Nutrition follow-up was recommended in two to three weeks.

Conclusion

Nutrition is fundamental to recovery following critical illness and improving quality of life. The physical, functional, cognitive, and psychosocial impairments common in patients with PICS can present significant barriers to patients meeting their basic nutrition needs. Indeed, the relationship between PICS and nutrition health is reciprocal, as patients with malnutrition are less likely to see and sustain improvements in their recovery. RDs are the practitioners best equipped to recognize and manage the complex course of nutrition rehabilitation after critical illness, but unfortunately, they are infrequently consulted or included as part of the multidisciplinary team caring for patients with PICS. Further research regarding the role of nutrition rehabilitation in critical illness recovery is warranted.

Key Points

1. Nutrition rehabilitation and the continuity of nutrition care in patients with PICS requires the expertise of a RD on the multidisciplinary care team.
2. Nutrition rehabilitation addresses the physical, functional, cognitive, and psychosocial impairments present in patients with PICS that are potential barriers to optimal nutrition.
3. Identification of malnutrition risk through a validated screening tool in the outpatient setting is imperative to determine if an in-depth nutrition assessment by an RD is required.
4. If a malnutrition diagnosis is assigned, a nutrition care plan should be developed to identify specific strategies to address and potentially resolve malnutrition to enhance quality of life and independence.

References

1. D.M. Needham, J. Davidson, H. Cohen, et al. Improving long-term outcomes after discharge from intensive care unit. *Crit Care Med* 2012; **40**: 502–9.
2. C. Renner, M.M. Jeitziner, A. Tran, et al. Guideline on multimodal rehabilitation for patients with post-intensive care syndrome. *Crit Care* 2023; **27**: 301.
3. K. Sharma, K.M. Mogensen, M.K. Robinson. Pathophysiology of critical illness and role of nutrition. *Nutr Clin Pract* 2019; **34**: 12–22.
4. P.B. Soeters, A.M. Schols. Advances in understanding and assessing malnutrition. *Curr Opin Clin Nutr Metab Care* 2009; **12**: 487–94.
5. E. Schwitzer, K. Schwab, L. Brinkman, et al. Survival ≠ Recovery. *ChestCC* 2023; **1**: 100003.
6. C.M. Mospan. Drug-induced nutrient depletions: what pharmacists need to know. *U.S. Pharm* 2019; **44**: 18–24.
7. E.S. Mohn, H.J. Kern, E. Saltzman, et al. Evidence of drug-nutrient interactions with chronic use of commonly prescribed medications: an update. *Pharmaceutics* 2018; **10**: 36.
8. D.E. Snider. Pyridoxine supplementation during isoniazid therapy. *Tubercle* 1980; **61**: 191–6.
9. T. Cederholm, G.L. Jensen, M.I.T.D. Correia, et al. GLIM criteria for the diagnosis of malnutrition: a consensus report from the global clinical nutrition community. *J Cachexia Sarcopenia Muscle* 2019; **10**: 207–17.
10. A. Malone, K.M. Mogensen. Key approaches to diagnosing malnutrition in adults. *Nutr in Clin Pract* 2021; **37**: 23–34.
11. M.J. Kaiser, J.M. Bauer, C. Ramsch, et al. Validation of the Mini Nutritional Assessment short-form (MNA®-SF): a practical tool for identification of nutritional status. *J Nutr Health Aging* 2009; **13**: 782–8.
12. BAPEN. "MUST" Calculator [Internet]. BAPEN. 2023. www.bapen.org.uk/must-and-self-screening/must-calculator/ (Accessed October 22, 2024.)
13. M. Ferguson, S. Capra, J. Bauer, et al. Development of a valid and reliable malnutrition screening tool for adult acute hospital patients. *Nutrition* 1999; **15**: 458–64.
14. L.L. Moisey, J.L. Merriweather, J. W. Drover. The role of nutrition rehabilitation in the recovery of survivors of critical illness: underrecognized and underappreciated. *Crit Care* 2022; **26**: 270.
15. J.L. Merriweather, P. Smith, T. Walsh. Nutritional rehabilitation after ICU – does it happen: a qualitative interview and observational study. *J Clin Nurs* 2014; **23**: 654–62.
16. J.L. Merriweather, L.G. Salisbury, T. S. Walsh, et al. Nutritional care after

critical illness: a qualitative study of patients' experiences. *J Hum Nutr Diet* 2014; **29**: 127–36.

17. J. Gotfried. Loss of Appetite – Digestive Disorders – Merck Manual Consumer Version. 2023. www.merckmanuals.com/home/digestive-disorders/symptoms-of-digestive-disorders/loss-of-appetite (Accessed October 22, 2024)

18. M. Fadeur, J.C. Preiser, A.M. Verbrugge, et al. Oral nutrition during and after critical illness: SPICES for quality of care. *Nutrients* 2020; **12**: 3509.

19. L.S. Chapple, L.M. Weinel, Y. A. Abdelhamid, et al. Observed appetite and nutrient intake three months after ICU discharge. *Clin Nutri* 2019; **38**: 1215–20.

20. H. Han, B. Yi, R. Zhong, et al. From gut microbiota to host appetite: gut microbiota-derived metabolites as key regulators. *Microbiome* 2021; **9**: 162.

21. M. Nematy, J.E. O'Flynn, L. Wandrag, et al. Changes in appetite related gut hormones in intensive care unit patients: a pilot cohort study. *Crit Care* 2005; **10**: R10.

22. J.L. Merriweather, D.M. Griffith, T. S. Walsh. Appetite during the recovery phase of critical illness: a cohort study. *Eur J of Clin Nutr* 2018; **72**: 986–92.

23. R. Leung, M. Covasa. Do gut microbes taste? *Nutrients* 2021; **13**: 2581.

24. S. Younes. The impact of micronutrients on the sense of taste. *Hum Nutri Met* 2024; **35**: 200231.

25. S. Redzic, M.F. Hashmi, V. Gupta. Niacin Deficiency [Internet]. PubMed. Treasure Island (FL): StatPearls Publishing; 2023.

26. R.A. Bernard, B.P. Halpern. Taste changes in vitamin A deficiency. *J Gen Physiol* 1968; **52**: 444–64.

27. A.L. Pendolino, G. Ottaviano, A. V. Navaratnam, et al. Clinical factors influencing olfactory performance in patients with persistent COVID-19 smell loss longer than 1 year. *Laryngoscope Investig Otolaryngol* 2023; **8**: 1449–58.

28. M.M. Speth, U.S. Speth, A.R. Sedaghat, et al. Smell and taste disorders. *ENT* 2022; **70**: 157–66.

29. Y.F.N. Boelens, M. Melchers, A.R.H. van Zanten. Poor physical recovery after critical illness: incidence, features, risk factors, pathophysiology, and evidence-based therapies. *Curr Opin Crit Care* 2022; **28**: 409–16.

30. A.F. Rousseau, H.C. Prescott, S.J. Brett, et al. Long-term outcomes after critical illness: recent insights. *Crit Care* 2021; **25** (1): 108.

31. M.S. Herridge, E. Azoulay. Outcomes after critical illness. *N Engl J of Med* 2023; **388**: 913–24.

32. A.A. Hssain, N. Farigon, H. Merdji, et al. Body composition and muscle strength at the end of ICU stay are associated with 1-year mortality, a prospective multicenter observational study. *Clin Nutr* 2023; **42**: 2070–9.

33. P. Zuercher, C.S. Moret, R. Dziewas, et al. Dysphagia in the intensive care unit: epidemiology, mechanisms, and clinical management. *Crit Care* 2019; **23**: 103.

34. J. Cichero, P. Lam, C.M. Steele, et al. Development of international terminology and definitions for texture-modified foods and thickened fluids used in dysphagia management: The IDDSI framework. *Dysphagia* 2016; **32**: 293–314.

35. R. Adan, E.M. van der Beek, J.K. Buitelaar, et al. Nutritional psychiatry: towards improving mental health by what you eat. *Eur Neuropsychopharmacol* 2019; **29**: 1321–32.

36. J. Appleton. The gut-brain axis: influence of microbiota on mood and mental health. *Integra Med* 2018; **17**: 28–32.

37. A. Mhanna, N. Martini, G. Hmaydoosh, et al. The correlation between gut microbiota and both neurotransmitters and mental disorders: a narrative review. *Medicine* 2024; **103**: e37114–4.

38. L.J. Sun, J.N. Li, Y.Z. Nie. Gut hormones in microbiota-gut-brain crosstalk. *Chin Med J (Engl)* 2020; **133**: 826–33.

39. J. Sung, S.S. Rajendraprasad, K. L. Philbrick, et al. The human gut microbiome in critical illness: disruptions,

consequences, and therapeutic frontiers. *J Crit Care* 2023; **79**: 154436.

40. A. Ventriglio, F. Sancassiani, M.P. Contu, et al. Mediterranean diet and its benefits on health and mental health: a literature review. *Clin Pract Epidemiol in Ment Health* 2020; **16**: 156–64.

41. National Institute on Alcohol Abuse and Alcoholism. Alcohol and the Brain: An Overview | National Institute on Alcohol Abuse and Alcoholism (NIAAA). www.niaaa.nih.gov/publications/alcohol-and-brain-overview (Accessed October 22, 2024).

42. C. Liu, L. Wang, C. Zhang, et al. Caffeine intake and anxiety: a meta-analysis. *Frontiers Psych* 2024; **15**: 1270246.

43. L. Gutierrez, A. Folch, M. Rojas, et al. Effects of nutrition on cognitive function in adults with or without cognitive impairment: a systematic review of randomized controlled clinical trials. *Nutrients* 2021; **13**: 3728.

44. D. Kargin, L. Tomaino, L. Serra-Majem. Experimental outcomes of the mediterranean diet: lessons learned from the Predimed randomized controlled trial. *Nutrients* 2019; **11**: E2991.

45. H. Ritchie. How is food insecurity measured? Our World in Data 2023. Available from: https://ourworldindata.org/food-insecurity (Accessed October 23, 2024)

46. K. Hanna, J. Cross, A. Nicholls, et al. The association between loneliness or social isolation and food and eating behaviours: a scoping review. *Appetite* 2023; **191**: 107051.

47. L. Wright, M. Hickson, G. Frost. Eating together is important: using a dining room in an acute elderly medical ward increases energy intake. *J Hum Nutr Diet* 2006; **19**: 23–6.

48. ICUsteps [Internet]. https://icusteps.org/ (Accessed October 23, 2024).

Chapter 41: Physical Impairments in Survivors of Critical Illness

Sara U. Dorn, Felipe González-Seguel, Kirby Mayer, Selina Parry, and Hallie Zeleznik

Introduction

More than half of survivors of critical illness experience new or worsening physical impairments after hospital discharge [1]. Physical symptoms and impairments related to post-intensive care syndrome (PICS) may occur in isolation but frequently affect multiple body structures and domains. Thus, the assessment and treatment of physical disability following hospital discharge requires engagement and coordination with the interprofessional healthcare team. This chapter reviews the literature highlighting the frequency and severity of physical impairment and disability related to PICS and describes physical therapy approaches for screening, assessment, and interventions.

Physical disability is defined as a physical limitation or condition that limits, inhibits, or prevents the performance of physical function or basic physical activities in daily life [2]. The World Health Organization (WHO) International Classification of Functioning, Disability, and Health (ICF) [3] classifies health and disability into three domains: impairments, activity limitations, and participation restrictions. In this chapter, we use the term physical disability to be inclusive of the physical symptoms, impairments, and limitations in physical function in survivors of critical illness.

Incidence and Prevalence of Physical Disability in Survivors of Critical Illness

The **incidence** of new physical disability in survivors of critical illness is difficult to examine due to several confounding factors both before and hospital discharge. Frequently, long-term outcome studies are unable to quantify patients' baseline functional status before hospitalization and rarely capture the entire at-risk population, limiting analysis of the true incidence of physical disability associated with PICS. Geense and colleagues found that, when controlling for pre-hospital status, 58% of 2,345 survivors of critical illness reported a new physical disability one year after discharge, demonstrating that self-report disability is common in a diverse group of survivors of critical illness [1].

More frequently reported in the literature is the **occurrence** or **prevalence** of physical disability related to PICS. The prevalence of physical disability is estimated to be as low as 20% [4] and as high as 99% [5] in survivors of critical illness. This variance in prevalence may be explained by several study-related factors, including study design and timepoints of assessment; severity of illness factors; and patient-related factors, such as age, sex, and pre-existing health conditions. Quantification of prevalence of physical disability is also influenced by whether the outcome measure utilized is self-reported or performance-based. Often, physical disability is ascertained using a self-reported measure of health-related quality of life that has components of physical functioning (e.g., physical functioning on the 36-item Short Form Survey [SF-36] or mobility impairment on the EuroQol-5D-5L [EQ-5D-5L]). Furthermore, variance may be explained by the definition of physical disability employed by the study: study definitions of physical disability range from mild mobility deficits to full dependence, potentially biasing the prevalence to higher or lower rates, respectively. These challenges prevent definitive conclusion on the prevalence of physical disability after critical illness, with the best estimates ranging from 50% to 80%.

Physical disability has been measured with diverse approaches in survivors of critical illness. Studies examining physical disability related to PICS range from a focus on one impairment in a body structure (e.g., muscle weakness) to multi-domain restrictions in societal participation (e.g., return to work). It is important to recognize that physical impairments rarely occur in isolation [5,6,7]. A cluster analysis of 430 acute respiratory distress syndrome (ARDS) survivors assessed with a battery of physical, cognitive, and emotional health screening tools identified four distinct subtypes of disability: (1) mildly impaired physical and mental health in 22%, (2) moderately impaired physical and mental health in 39%, (3) severely impaired physical health and moderately impaired mental health in 15%, and (4) severely impaired physical and mental health in 24% [6]. In another large secondary analysis of the ALTOS project, a high prevalence of fatigue (70% of 711 intensive care unit [ICU] survivors at 6 months) was strongly associated with co-occurrence of physical, cognitive, and mental health impairments [7]. Clinicians who evaluate and manage physical disability associated with PICS must also consider the impact of impairments in cognitive and emotional health on the patient's plan of care.

Trajectory of Physical Disability in Survivors of Critical Illness

Despite surviving critical illness, limitations in physical function can be present for months to years following hospital discharge [8,9,10,11,12,13]. Landmark studies by Herridge and colleagues in 2003 and 2011 demonstrated persistent impairments in exercise capacity and physical function as measured by the six-minute walk test (6MWT) at 1 year and 5 years after hospital discharge. These findings were confirmed by large systematic reviews demonstrating significant reductions in the 6MWT at 3 and 12 months after discharge [12,14]. Performance on the 6MWT generally improved between 3 months and 12 months, however, indicating the potential for recovery of physical functioning within the first year [12].

Trajectory analyses enhance understanding of recovery after critical illness by improving the ability to prognosticate which patients are at risk of poor recovery. Physical function testing in 260 acute respiratory failure survivors demonstrates four different trajectory phenotypes from hospital discharge to 6 months of follow-up: (1) poor physical functioning at baseline that does not improve, (2) poor physical functioning at baseline that minimally improves, (3) poor physical functioning at baseline that improves to intermediate functional status, and (4) intermediate physical functioning at baseline that improves rapidly to high functional status (at 2 months) and is sustained at the 6-month timepoint [15]. Neumeier and colleagues found that the rate of functional recovery from 3 to 6 months after hospitalization, as measured by the Continuous Scale Physical Functional Performance short form (CS-PFP -10), was largely influenced by age, with older age being associated with slower recovery [16]. Finally, in a study of 291 older adult survivors of critical illness with a mean age of 84 years, over half (53%) of patients suffered functional decline or early death after ICU admission regardless of their functional trajectory and level of disability as described by self-report [17].

In summary, patients surviving critical illness are at high risk of physical disability. Clinicians and scientists should focus efforts to refine the prevalence, severity, and trajectories of physical disability in survivors of critical illness. Research is necessary to examine how patient- and illness-related factors influence physical disability and to develop interventional strategies to improve outcomes.

Screening and Evaluation of Physical Disability in Survivors of Critical Illness

The physical therapy evaluation of patients surviving critical illness is derived from the aforementioned WHO ICF domains of physical disability, with assessments of impairments in body structure, limitations in activity (i.e., physical function), and societal participation restrictions. For this section, we primarily focus on the subjective and objective assessments of physical impairments in body structure and physical function; participation restrictions, such as the inability to resume employment and driving, are covered in Chapter 44. When available, dedicated physiotherapists in ICU follow-up clinics perform individualized assessments to address physical disability that align with patient values [18], but unfortunately, in most healthcare institutions worldwide, such specialization is not an option. Accordingly, we review common measures that may be performed in any community physical therapy setting that may evaluate and treat survivors of critical illness.

Timing

It is becoming widely accepted that there is benefit in screening survivors of critical illness for multidisciplinary needs within the first two to four weeks after hospital discharge [19], with additional assessments occurring at scheduled intervals thereafter based on the patient's individual recovery trajectory, acuity of needs, and access to services. Screening for physical disability related to PICS may also begin at hospital discharge.

Early assessment of physical disability in survivors of critical illness may be particularly important for patient-centered outcomes, such as the need for hospital readmission. Recent Australian and Korean studies demonstrate 1-year unplanned readmissions for survivors of critical illness to be as high as 40% (see Chapter 33 for additional information) [20,21]. In a multisite study in North America, sepsis survivors with poor functional status had a 22% risk of readmission in the first 30 days and a higher rate of 30-day mortality (7%) when compared to the overall average (3.5%). Of clinical significance, the findings of this study suggest that nearly half of the 30-day readmissions in this group were "potentially avoidable" [22] and could have been addressed or prevented with appropriate outpatient care. Collectively, these findings strongly support early assessment in ambulatory settings after discharge.

With respect to the appropriate interval between physical assessments, survivors of ARDS experience the greatest improvement in physical function within the first three months after hospital discharge, often with a plateau beginning around six months [23]. For this reason, assessment of physical function should occur at routine intervals to identify patients at risk for persistent physical disability, which may prompt referral for new or additional rehabilitation treatment. General timelines for assessment have been proposed, including at: 1 week, 1 month, 3 months, 6 months, and 12 months following discharge [24], although such frequent assessments may not be feasible in resource-constrained environments. Most importantly, physiotherapists should perform an assessment of physical disability as early as possible, with subsequent follow-up evaluations individualized to the patient's needs (i.e., more frequent follow-up in at-risk patients or those with significant disability on the initial evaluation). The frequency of physical assessments can be reduced as physical function is restored to pre-ICU levels, a process consistent with the concept of functional reconciliation [19].

Standardized Assessments

The assessment of physical disability associated with PICS should be performed using standardized measures with strong psychometric properties. Outcome measures in physical therapy practice typically occur in two domains:

1. Subjective or self-reported outcome measures, typically in the form of questionnaires, selected by the physiotherapist. Subjective measures quantify the patient's *perceived* physical disability.
2. Performance-based measures, which examine or observe the patient's participation in or performance of an activity, providing objective data on the *actual* physical disability.

In survivors of critical illness, self-report and performance measures are not always commensurate; for example, in one study, objective, performance-based muscle strength testing identified ICU-acquired weakness (ICU-AW) in only 12% of the cohort, yet 75% of patients subjectively reported suffering from ICU-AW [25].

Physical therapists should consider the purpose (i.e., the construct) of each assessment when selecting a measure to administer. Given the importance of the recovery trajectory, it is critical that measures have the ability to detect change over time and to assess the effectiveness of rehabilitation interventions. For example, the Medical Research Council-Sum Score (MRC-SS) is the clinical standard for diagnosing ICU-AW at ICU discharge and is frequently used in the recovery phase [26], but the MRC-SS is at high risk of ceiling effects (i.e., subjects achieving the maximal score), thereby reducing the sensitivity to capture responsiveness at 12 and 24 months after discharge [8].

In 2024, physical function was identified by a multifaceted initiative including patients, clinicians, and researchers as a critically important outcome for ICU rehabilitation trials, reaching the highest agreement (100%, n = 300 participants) [27]. A previous modified Delphi consensus process composed of internationally recognized experts in recovery following critical illness recommended physical function as a core domain for assessment of ICU survivors of acute respiratory failure [28] and SARS-CoV-2 infection (COVID) [29]; however, consensus on the specific measures to assess physical function was not reached [30]. Of those proposed, the 6MWT received the most agreement from experts to be used as an assessment of physical functioning.

The 6MWT is a valid and reliable performance-based outcome measure assessing functional capacity and exercise tolerance. The test measures the distance an individual can walk in a 6-minute period, performing laps on a walking track 100 feet (30 meters) in length. Physical therapists should follow the American Thoracic Society (ATS) guidelines when performing the test to ensure standardization among multiple evaluations. Data from a systematic review and meta-analysis in survivors of critical illness demonstrate the pooled mean 6MWT distance was 361 meters (95% confidence interval [CI]: 321–401 m) and 436 meters (95% CI: 391–481 m) at 3 and 12 months after hospital discharge, respectively [12], significantly lower than normative data (age 40–80 years: 571 ± 90 m) [31].

A modified Delphi consensus process composed of experts from the Japanese Society of Intensive Care Medicine identified the 6MWT, the MRC-SS, and handgrip strength dynamometry as instruments to assess the physical domain of PICS [32]. Likewise, a modified Delphi consensus process composed of experts primarily from Germany initially recommended handgrip strength dynamometry and the Timed-up and Go Test (TUG) as instruments to screen the physical domain of PICS; they subsequently augmented the screen with the 2-Minute Walk Test (2MWT) and the Short Physical Performance Battery (SPPB) for a more robust evaluation [33]. The EQ-5D-5L, although not specific to physical disability, is recommended by expert consensus for acute respiratory failure survivors [30] and ECMO survivors [34].

Expert recommendations from Delphi methodologies help narrow the selection of outcome measures to assess patients surviving critical illness; however, these methodologies are based exclusively on expert opinion and recommendations and may not capture each component of physical disability in survivors of critical illness. Furthermore, Delphi panels are at risk of variance in their processes and have the potential to undervalue the psychometric properties necessary for outcome measures. A summary of additional outcome measures to assess physical disability in individuals surviving critical illness is provided in Table 41.1. The table provides general measures that evaluate the diverse spectrum of constructs examining physical disability, but it should not be considered comprehensive. In addition, the table does not represent the conventional, comprehensive physical therapy examination, which includes vital sign and pain assessments, a review of systems, and sensory testing. Physical therapists must consider patient safety during testing, including providing clear instructions, guarding for falls, and monitoring the response to testing with vital sign measurement and assessing for the development of clinical signs or symptoms. Figure 41.1 demonstrates a representative flow diagram describing the physical therapist approach for screening, examination, and development of a plan of care for survivors of critical illness.

Management and Treatment

PICS is not a clinical diagnosis but rather a syndrome representing a diverse range of symptoms and impairments. Physical disability related to PICS may present as a single deficit or as complex, multidomain challenges impacting multiple body structures, functions, and activities. Therefore, physical therapy management and treatment require individualized and targeted interventions. There is, however, little evidence on the effectiveness of physical rehabilitation interventions to improve physical functioning outcomes after hospital discharge. This section discusses physical therapy management and treatment in the community during the recovery period of critical illness; see Chapter 12 for physical rehabilitation treatment in the ICU and hospital.

Only a few high-quality randomized controlled trials (RCTs) examining physical rehabilitation treatment after hospital discharge have been conducted. In this section, we review these trials and discuss current treatment approaches based on clinical expertise. We address models of care delivery that physical therapists routinely practice and review specific exercise and rehabilitation treatment approaches aimed at improving physical functioning outcomes.

To enhance the comprehension of this section, it is important to understand that physical therapists receive general practice education, attaining the knowledge and skills to manage physical function across the lifespan, regardless of health condition; they may also pursue

Table 41.1 Outcome measures to assess physical disability in survivors of critical illness

ICF Category	Construct	Outcome Measures	Description
Body Structures and Function	Skeletal muscle strength	Handheld dynamometry, Handgrip dynamometry	• Performance-based assessment involves equipment to measure maximal isometric contraction (i.e., force production) • Quantified in pounds, kilograms, or Newton • Assessor should utilize standardized positions based on the muscle being tested [69]
		Manual Muscle Testing (MRC-SS)	• Performance-based measure to test muscle strength using an ordinal scale (6-point: 0 = no muscle contraction to 5 = muscle activation against resistance) • Subjectivity and ceiling effects in survivors of critical illness may reduce the clinical utility and psychometric value
	Pain	EQ–5D–5L (Pain Question), Numeric Pain Rating Scale	• Self-reported assessment of pain
	Pulmonary Function	Pulmonary function tests	• Performance-based measure of lung volumes, flows, and gas exchange
		Modified MRC dyspnea Scale, ATS dyspnea scale	• Self-reported measure of dyspnea
Physical Function (Activity Limitation)	Gait or walking speed	4-meter gait speed*	• Objective measurement of the habitual or self-selecting walking speed over 4-meter track • Reliable, valid, and responsive in ARDS survivors [70] • Gait speed in meters per second can be compared to normative values [71] • Cutoff scores exist to prognosticate or predict falling and morbidity [72]

Table 41.1 (cont.)

ICF Category	Construct	Outcome Measures	Description
	Sit to stand performance	5-times sit to stand test (STS)	• Time to achieve 5-repetitions of sit-to-stand from standard height chair (17 in.) without using arms • Measures constructs of muscle strength, power, and transfer capability
		30-second sit to stand test (STS)	• Number of repetitions achieved in 30 seconds from standard height chair (17 in.) without using arms • Measures constructs of muscle strength and endurance • Strong psychometric properties in survivors of critical illness [73]
		60-second sit to stand test (STS)	• Number of repetitions achieved in 60 seconds from standard height chair (17 in.) without using arms • Measures construct of muscle strength and endurance
	Functional Capacity	6-minute walk test	• Performance-based outcome of functional exercise capacity • Measures the distance an individual can walk in a 6-minute period, performing laps on a 100-foot (30 meter) walking track.
		2-minute walk test	• Performance-based outcome of functional exercise capacity • Measures the distance an individual can walk in a 2-minute period; alternative to 6MWT
	Balance	Berg Balance Scale, Mini-BESTest, Functional Gait Assessment, Tinetti Falls Efficacy Scale, Activities Specific Balance Confidence Scale	• Measures of static and dynamic balance that have been examined or validated in diverse populations • Objective balance assessment may require equipment • Measures can help identity patients at risk of falling, those with fear of falling, and those with balance deficits

Multi-component physical function	Short Physical Performance Battery (SPPB)	• Performance-based outcome measure assessing lower body functioning • Three components: sit-to-stand performance, standing balance, and 4-meter gait speed • Has been used in latent class analyses to demonstrate that survivors of critical illness experience multiple patterns of recovery [15]
	Timed-up and go test (TUG)	• Performance-based outcome measure assessing mobility and balance • Records the time required for an individual to stand up from a chair, walk 3-meters, and return to the chair. • The TUG-cognitive adds a cognitive task, such as serial subtraction by three while performing the physical task, thereby providing an opportunity to assess dual-task performance [64]
	36-item short form survey (SF–36)	• Self-reported measure with 36 items, including 2 domains for physical functioning and role performance
	EQ–5D–5L	• Self-reported measure with 6 questions • Questions address components of physical disability, including mobility, self-care, usual activities, and pain/discomfort. • The questionnaire has strong psychometric value [74,75] and is easy to administer.

* Gait speed may be measured with several protocols, including different lengths of track and different testing parameters (e.g., rolling versus static start). The 4-meter gait speed test is provided as a representative test given its psychometric properties [70].

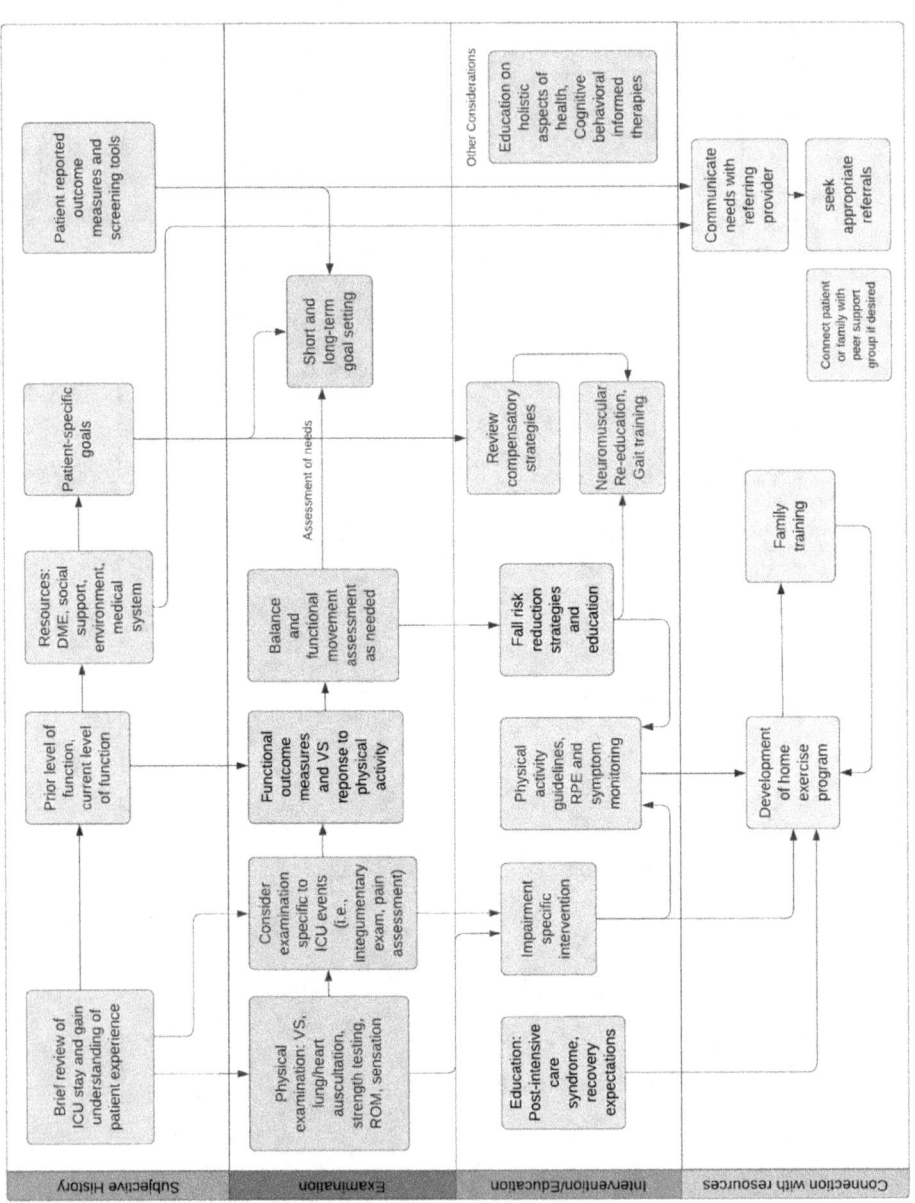

Figure 41.1 Representative flow diagram describing the physical therapist approach for screening, examination, and development of a plan of care for survivors of critical illness. DME: durable medical equipment; ICU: intensive care unit; RPE: rating of perceived exertion; ROM: range of motion; VS: vital signs.

advanced training, including sub-specialization certification, in areas including neurologic conditions and geriatric physical therapy. Although we will focus on physical functioning, it should be noted that physical therapists serve in diverse capacities to improve outcomes across multiple domains. Depending on the healthcare setting and the country of practice, physical therapists may address and treat emotional and cognitive challenges, especially when deficits occur in multiple domains; for example, a survivor of critical illness with depression may require motivational- and behavioral-based treatment before engaging in therapeutic exercise. Physical therapists working in the community must screen and refer for sinister pathologies and deficits outside of their scope of training.

Models of Delivery

Several models of rehabilitation care exist after hospital discharge. Models of care depend on location (i.e., country and regional practices), local resources, and patient-related factors, such as socioeconomic status. Patients may access community-based physical therapy treatment via referral from the discharging acute care facility, a primary care provider, a specialty clinic, an ICU-follow up clinic, or through direct access. There are three principal settings where physical therapy treatment is commonly delivered to survivors of critical illness:

Home-Based Physical Therapy Care

In general, home-based treatment is designed for individuals with significant impairments who are unable to participate in community ambulation or mobility. Physical therapists who provide treatment in the patient's home may be the sole clinician engaged in the plan of care or may be working as part of an interprofessional team. Theoretically, there is no limit to delivery of interventions in the home if modifications can be made to address the lack of exercise and medical equipment. In the United States, patients eligible to participate in home-based rehabilitation must be "homebound and require skilled care" per guidelines from the Centers for Medicare and Medicaid Services. Eligibility for home therapy in other regions, such as Australia, are less restrictive, focusing more on the patient's goals and preferences.

Outpatient (Ambulatory) Physical Therapy Care

"Brick and mortar" based rehabilitation clinics are common in several countries, particularly the United States and United Kingdom. Patients may access these clinics via referral or by seeking care directly. There are numerous models of outpatient clinics, including stand-alone physical therapy clinics, interprofessional clinics, specialty cardiac and pulmonary rehabilitation clinics, and aquatic centers.

Telerehabilitation Care

The advent of telecommunications in medicine coupled by the need for isolation during the COVID-19 pandemic increased the utilization of telerehabilitation. Like home-based therapy, interventions delivered via telecommunications may require modifications to address patient safety and potential lack of equipment. Data suggest that telerehabilitation may not be inferior to in-person treatment in survivors of critical illness [35], but high-level RCTs are needed. A pilot RCT of multi-component cognitive and physical rehabilitation using a mixed-methods approach with both in-person and telerehabilitation for physical training was effective at improving cognitive function and self-reported functional status compared to controls [36].

Although there are several avenues for referral and participation in physical therapy, data demonstrate that approximately 33% of Medicare beneficiaries in the United States will never receive physical therapy treatment following critical illness, and on average, patients receiving services only get one home-based visit per week in the first two months after discharge [37]. In the United Kingdom, post-hospital physical rehabilitation programs are present in only 31 of 176 hospital sites that offer adult critical care services [38]. Lack of referrals and limited participation in rehabilitation is multi-factorial; there is an urgent need for awareness, education, and high-quality evidence to demonstrate the benefits of physical rehabilitation for patients with impairments related to PICS [39,40].

Education and Disease Management

At the core of the physical therapy profession is education. Education regarding health, wellness, and physical activity is paramount for improving health-related outcomes and physical functioning. Physical therapists may provide education on a variety of topics inherent to improving physical functioning, which are highlighted below.

Physical Activity

A prospective study demonstrated that survivors of critical illness only achieve 1278 steps per day in their first week returning home [15]. Physical activity levels at home are significantly lower than the recommended 7,200–8,000 steps per day [41]. Physical activity includes any activity or bodily movement that leads to energy expenditure [42]; increased physical activity can improve physical fitness and address modifiable risk factors associated with metabolic diseases and cardiovascular morbidity. Several modifiable barriers limit physical activity in the hospital and community, including limited knowledge of clinicians and patients, access to equipment, and motivation [43]. Physical activity education should focus on gradually and safely increasing physical activity, such as increasing the number of steps walked per day, and monitoring the physiological response to exercise, including heart rate and perceived exertion, to achieve targeted zones. Patient education must include the importance of monitoring perceived rate of exertion, dyspnea, and other symptoms during physical activity; abnormal responses warrant contacting a qualified healthcare provider.

Fatigue

Fatigue, defined as a lack of energy negatively impacting performance of normal activities, is a complex physiological and emotional symptom that may include multiple body systems (see Chapter 36 for additional information). Fatigue education requires understanding of the underlying etiology (i.e., respiratory, neuromuscular, emotional, or a combination thereof) along with a comprehensive assessment to provide targeted strategies. For example, patients with fatigue primarily due to respiratory dysfunction may benefit from slowly progressive aerobic activity with close monitoring of pulse oximetry and rating of perceived exertion. Education may address breathing mechanics with diaphragmatic and deep breathing to enhance gas exchange in the lungs. Fatigue education may also incorporate education on pacing and identifying abnormal responses, such as post-exertional malaise, which may have an increased occurrence after viral infection (e.g., with influenza and SARS-CoV-2) [7,44]. Fatigue resulting from skeletal muscle deficits, in contrast, may benefit from an exercise prescription targeting muscular endurance adaptations. The complexity of fatigue and its potential for multi-domain involvement should be given thoughtful attention by rehabilitation clinicians and other members of the medical team. Occupational therapists also play an integral role in providing education on energy conservation techniques and modifications to daily activities to save energy for other tasks (see Chapter 42 for additional information).

Nutrition

Healthy eating supports numerous bodily functions, including muscle repair and growth following development of atrophy associated with ICU-AW. Nutrition is paramount for optimizing physical activity and functioning, and physical therapists should advocate for healthy eating choices that promote recovery. Optimizing nutrition with individualized prescriptions should be performed by a dietitian (see Chapter 40 for additional information). Physical therapists and dietitians should work in concert with the patient to understand the energy demands of daily physical activity and structured exercise.

Medication

Eighty percent of survivors of critical illness experience medication-related problems after hospital discharge (see Chapter 32 for additional information). While it is the role of physicians and pharmacists to perform medication reconciliation, physical therapists must understand, evaluate, and educate patients on how medications interact with physical activity and exercise. For example, patients requiring beta-blockers or anti-arrhythmic medications may have a blunted heart rate response to exercise [45], and responses to exercise should therefore be monitored using other methods as described above. Additionally, polypharmacy is a risk factor for falls in older adults with and without chronic illnesses and therefore a likely problem for survivors of critical illness [46].

Fall Prevention

Survivors of critical illness are at high risk of falling, with nearly 70% having one fall and almost 50% classified as a recurrent faller [47]. Reducing the risk of falling includes education regarding environmental factors, such as inadequate lighting and trip hazards, and education regarding symptoms and impairments, such as when fatigue or weakness may heighten the risk of falling. Although falling is highly prevalent, it may indicate that patients are trying to engage in high-level activities that promote recovery. Thus, modifiable factors should be addressed, and advocacy of physical activity should be promoted to ultimately reduce falling.

In addition to these areas, physical therapists may provide education for survivors of critical illness and their families on acute and chronic pain management, caregiver support (e.g., education on safe transfers with a dependent patient), skin integrity and wound healing, emotional health, and cognitive function.

Physical Therapy Interventions

Interprofessional expert consensus strongly supports physical rehabilitation treatment to improve physical functioning in survivors of critical illness, and clinical practice guidelines recommend rehabilitative implementation after hospital discharge [48,49,50]. Qualitative data from patients who participated in structured exercise following hospital discharge emphasize the need for tailored exercise to enhance recovery [51]. Patients report that exercise training is motivating, provides social interaction, improves confidence, and increases energy levels [52,53].

Survivors of critical illness and their caregivers report that recovery of physical functioning and restoration of societal roles is the primary focus of their recovery [54]. However, a systematic review comprising six studies of rehabilitation interventions provided after discharge for survivors of critical illness demonstrated little to no difference in functional exercise capacity and self-reported physical function [55]. A study conducted by Denehy and colleagues provided individualized exercise that began in the ICU and was followed by eight weeks of outpatient physical therapy after discharge [56]. When comparing the intervention group to standard care, there were no significant differences in functional outcomes up to 12 months after discharge. The REVIVE study demonstrated significant improvement in the incremental shuttle walk test in a 6-week structured exercise program compared to the control group that received no exercise; however, self-reported physical function on the SF-36 was not different between groups, and the walk test differences were not sustained at a 6-month follow-up evaluation [57]. Thus, the current literature on the efficacy of rehabilitation after hospital discharge for survivors of critical illness is equivocal and warrants additional high-quality RCTs.

Patient Safety

Patients surviving critical illness may be at heightened risk of altered or abnormal responses to rehabilitation and exercise interventions. Reasons for abnormal responses to exercise include a persistent inflammatory state associated with the underlying illness, medications that alter the physiologic response to physical activity, and anxiety disorders that alter the resting heart rate. It is imperative that physical therapists understand how patient-related and illness-related factors impact exercise response. Physical therapists should monitor vital signs (heart rate, blood pressure, respiratory rate, and pulse oximetry) and utilize a perceived exertion scale throughout treatment delivery. Due to the heterogeneity of patient populations, timing of recovery, and numerous non-modifiable characteristics, it is challenging to provide specific normative and targeted values for vital signs before, during, and after exercise for survivors of critical illness. In clinical practice, physical therapists should individualize interventions and prioritize patient safety.

Physical therapists provide a diverse range of interventions that promote improved physical functioning. Here, we explore several key areas, but this is not intended to be a comprehensive review.

Therapeutic Exercise

Therapeutic exercise is defined as "the systematic performance or execution of planned physical movements or activities intended to enable the patient to remediate or prevent impairments in body functions or structures, enhance activities and participation, reduce risk, and optimize overall health" [58]. In survivors of critical illness, therapeutic exercise is an umbrella term for structured and individualized exercise aimed at mitigating physical impairments and restoring physical functioning. There are multiple domains of therapeutic exercise:

- **Muscle strength training,** also known as resistance training, is performed to improve muscle strength. Strength training exercises are performed against resistance (e.g., resistance bands, weights, or bodyweight). Strength training exercises should target weak muscle groups, incorporate resistance to achieve physiological adaptations, and progressively increase the load or repetitions to sustain or optimize training effect [59]. The physical therapist should select a program that optimizes patient outcomes while maintaining safety. General recommendations suggest 2–3 resistance training sessions per week, each lasting 30–45 minutes. A sub-domain of strength training is **muscle power training**, in which the concentric phase of an exercise is performed as fast as possible. The emphasis on velocity of movement against lighter loads is different from traditional strength training. In literature on the aging population, muscle power training may be equivalent or slightly superior to traditional strength training for improving physical functioning [60]. Data suggest that older individuals lose muscle power earlier and more rapidly than muscle strength [61,62]. Survivors of critical illness may also be at risk for rapid deterioration of muscle power and thus may benefit from targeted muscle power training.

- **Aerobic training,** also known as endurance training, is performed to improve cardiorespiratory function or physical fitness. Aerobic training is typically performed to improve maximal oxygen uptake (VO_2max), which accounts for cardiovascular and pulmonary systems (central factors) and muscle oxygen utilization (peripheral factors). Aerobic training is typically performed at low-to-moderate target heart rate zones (40–60% of maximum heart rate; 4–6 on modified Borg Rating of Perceived Exertion). Target heart rates may be calculated with the Karvonen Formula or the Heart-Rate Reserve Method. In an RCT of 60 survivors of critical illness, moderate-intensity aerobic training with cycle ergometers had a small but unsustained benefit in cardiorespiratory fitness [63].
- **Neuromotor exercise** is an umbrella term that encompasses balance, coordination, and functional mobility (agility/gait). The American College of Sports Medicine (ACSM) recommends performing these exercises at least 2–3 days per week and preferably 20–30 minutes per session. Patients with neuropathy, altered sensation and proprioception, frailty, and high risk of falling may benefit from these types of exercises. Static and dynamic balance training focused on enhancing one's ability to maintain positioning in space may be particularly important to patient-centered outcomes.

Functional Task Training

The overarching focus of functional task training is reintegration into activities of daily living (ADLs), societal roles, and civic life. Training may focus on ADL capacity, such as improving bed mobility and toileting, by practicing sit-to-stand training from a low surface mimicking a standard height toilet. Functional training may include environments and tasks that simulate returning to driving, caregiving roles, and work duties. Functional task training frequently incorporates dual-task performance (i.e., performing motor and cognitive tasks simultaneously), which more closely simulates everyday tasks in the community and at work. Data demonstrate that survivors of severe SARS-CoV-2 infection have significant impairments in dual-task ability [64], but more research is needed to understand the best approach to improve multi-tasking.

Multicomponent or Circuit Training

To date, most RCTs examining rehabilitation for survivors of critical illness have incorporated multidomain or multicomponent training [36,55,65,66,67,68]. Multicomponent exercise typically includes strength training, aerobic training, and occasionally other components, such as chest physiotherapy. A small, single-site pilot RCT demonstrated improved anxiety levels and balance for individuals participating in a 6-week supervised program of cardiopulmonary, balance, and strengthening exercises [65], but no difference in the primary outcome of 6MWT distance was found. An RCT of multicomponent physiotherapy interventions paired with amino acid supplementation demonstrated improved physical recovery and reduced anxiety and depression in the intervention group compared to the control group [66]. The largest post-hospital rehabilitation RCT of 195 patients surviving critical illness comparing 8 weeks of multicomponent exercise to no exercise demonstrated no difference between the groups in physical functioning. The authors suggested that future studies adjusting the exercise dose from the original protocol by increasing intensity and frequency could potentially show a difference between the two groups [67].

Prescription and Dosing

The dosage of interventions is important, as patients respond differently based on personal-, environmental-, and illness-related factors. For general adults, the ACSM and Centers for Disease Control and Prevention (CDC) recommend 150 minutes of moderate-intensity aerobic exercise every week and two or more days of muscle-strengthening exercises that work all major muscle groups [2]. Moreover, the ACSM emphasizes that "exercise is medicine," providing general exercise prescriptions for a diverse range of conditions and diseases. Currently, there is limited guidance for dosing in survivors of critical illness, but data can be extrapolated from patients with cancer cachexia and chronic obstructive pulmonary disease; such recommendations are beyond the scope of this textbook, but they can be researched and considered judiciously. Physical rehabilitation for survivors of critical illness should be individualized and tailored to the patient's identified deficits. The dosage of interventions depends on the patient's response, with increases in intensity and frequency as the patient improves.

Conclusion

While the model of care for physical therapy services in the community may vary depending on country, regional practice, and patient accessibility, the commencement of physical rehabilitation shortly after hospital discharge may be influential in optimizing the safety and functional recovery of survivors of critical illness. Physical impairments in survivors of critical illness involve multiple body systems and are multifactorial in etiology; therefore, rehabilitation interventions should be individualized, multimodal, and progressive in nature. Collaborative and patient-centered goals should be established early, as should patient education covering a broad range of topics. It is essential that the physical therapist work collaboratively with the larger medical team to advocate for patient safety, health, and wellness.

Future research should focus on expanding the body of knowledge regarding the effectiveness and optimal dosage of specific physical therapy interventions. Due to the heterogeneity of patient characteristics and recovery trajectories after critical illness, implementation of a core outcomes measure set of patient-centered measures that can be tested longitudinally will facilitate consistency of reporting and allow meaningful comparisons.

Key Points

1. Survivors of critical illness are at risk of physical disability, with an estimated prevalence of 50–80%.
2. Physical disability for survivors of critical illness may present as an impairment in a single body function or as multidomain symptoms and deficits.
3. Physical therapists should utilize performance-based and self-report outcome measures to assess physical disability in individuals surviving critical illness; assessment should occur earlier during recovery and be repeated based on individual needs.
4. Physical therapy interventions after ICU admission should be individualized to the patient's needs and goals.
5. Data supporting physical therapy strategies after hospital discharge are limited, but expert consensus strongly support delivery of interventions for survivors. High-quality RCTs are necessary to understand the efficacy of rehabilitation to improve outcomes.

References

1. W.W. Geense, M. Zegers, M.A.A. Peters, et al. New physical, mental, and cognitive problems 1 year after icu admission: a prospective multicenter study. *Am J Respir Crit Care Med* 2021; **203**: 1512–21.
2. Centers for Disease Control and Prevention. Disability and Health Overview 2024 [updated April 3, 2024]. Available from: www.cdc.gov/ncbddd/disabilityandhealth/disability.html.
3. World Health Organization. International Classification of Functioning, Disability and Health (ICF) 2024. Available from: www.who.int/classifications/international-classification-of-functioning-disability-and-health.
4. M.C. Duggan, L. Wang, J.E. Wilson, et al. The relationship between executive dysfunction, depression, and mental health-related quality of life in survivors of critical illness: Results from the BRAIN-ICU investigation. *J Crit Care* 2017; **37**: 72–9.
5. A. Marra, P.P. Pandharipande, T.D. Girard, et al. Co-occurrence of post-intensive care syndrome problems among 406 survivors of critical illness. *Crit Care Med* 2018; **46**: 1393–401.
6. S.M. Brown, E.L. Wilson, A.P. Presson, et al. Understanding patient outcomes after acute respiratory distress syndrome: identifying subtypes of physical, cognitive and mental health outcomes. *Thorax* 2017; **72**: 1094–103.
7. K.J. Neufeld, J.S. Leoutsakos, H. Yan, et al. Fatigue symptoms during the first year following ARDS. *Chest* 2020; **158**: 999–1007.
8. E. Fan, D.W. Dowdy, E. Colantuoni, et al. Physical complications in acute lung injury survivors: a two-year longitudinal prospective study. *Crit Care Med* 2014; **42**: 849–59.
9. M.S. Herridge, A.M. Cheung, C.M. Tansey, et al. One-year outcomes in survivors of the acute respiratory distress syndrome. *N Engl J Med* 2003; **348**: 683–93.
10. M.S. Herridge, C.M. Tansey, A. Matté, et al. Functional disability 5 years after acute respiratory distress syndrome. *N Engl J Med* 2011; **364**: 1293–304.
11. D.M. Needham, A.W. Wozniak, C. L. Hough, et al. Risk factors for physical impairment after acute lung injury in a national, multicenter study. *Am J Respir Crit Care Med* 2014; **189**: 1214–24.

12. S.M. Parry, S.R. Nalamalapu, K. Nunna, et al. Six-minute walk distance after critical illness: a systematic review and meta-analysis. *J Intensive Care Med* 2021; **36**: 343–51.

13. E.R. Pfoh, A.W. Wozniak, E. Colantuoni, et al. Physical declines occurring after hospital discharge in ARDS survivors: a 5-year longitudinal study. *Intensive Care Med* 2016; **42**: 1557–66.

14. P.J. Ohtake, A.C. Lee, J.C. Scott, et al. Physical impairments associated with post-intensive care syndrome: systematic review based on the World Health Organization's international classification of functioning, disability and health framework. *Phys Ther* 2018; **98**: 631–45.

15. S. Gandotra, J. Lovato, D. Case, et al. Physical function trajectories in survivors of acute respiratory failure. *Ann Am Thorac Soc* 2019; **16**: 471–7.

16. A. Neumeier, A. Nordon-Craft, D. Malone, et al. Prolonged acute care and post-acute care admission and recovery of physical function in survivors of acute respiratory failure: a secondary analysis of a randomized controlled trial. *Crit Care* 2017; **21**: 190.

17. L.E. Ferrante, M.A. Pisani, T.E. Murphy, et al. Functional trajectories among older persons before and after critical illness. *JAMA Intern Med* 2015; **175**: 523–9.

18. K.J. Haines, N. Leggett, E. Hibbert, et al. Patient and caregiver-derived health service improvements for better critical care recovery. *Crit Care Med* 2022; **50**: 1778–87.

19. M.E. Mikkelsen, M. Still, B.J. Anderson, et al. Society of Critical Care Medicine's international consensus conference on prediction and identification of long-term impairments after critical illness. *Crit Care Med* 2020; **48**: 1670–9.

20. J.K. Pilowsky, A. von Huben, R. Elliott, M.A. Roche. Development and validation of a risk score to predict unplanned hospital readmissions in ICU survivors: a data linkage study. *Aust Crit Care* 2024; **37**: 383–90.

21. J. Kang, K.M. Lee. Three-year mortality, readmission, and medical expenses in critical care survivors: a population-based cohort study. *Aust Crit Care* 2024; **37**: 251–7.

22. S.P. Taylor, B.C. Bray, S.H. Chou, et al. Clinical subtypes of sepsis survivors predict readmission and mortality after hospital discharge. *Ann Am Thorac Soc* 2022; **19**: 1355–63.

23. M.S. Herridge, M. Moss, C.L. Hough, et al. Recovery and outcomes after the acute respiratory distress syndrome (ARDS) in patients and their family caregivers. *Intensive Care Med* 2016; **42**: 725–38.

24. K.P. Mayer, H. Boustany, E.P. Cassity, et al. ICU recovery clinic attendance, attrition, and patient outcomes: the impact of severity of illness, gender, and rurality. *Crit Care Explor* 2020; **2**: e0206.

25. C.H. Meyer-Frießem, N.M. Malewicz, S. Rath, et al. Incidence, time course and influence on quality of life of intensive care unit-acquired weakness symptoms in long-term intensive care survivors. *J Intensive Care Med* 2021; **36**: 1313–22.

26. O.D. Gustafson, M.A. Williams, S. McKechnie, et al. Musculoskeletal complications following critical illness: a scoping review. *J Crit Care* 2021; **66**: 60–6.

27. B.A. Connolly, M. Barclay, C. Davies, et al. PRACTICE: development of a core outcome set for trials of physical rehabilitation in critical illness. *Ann Am Thorac Soc* 2024; **21**(12): 1742-50.

28. A.E. Turnbull, K.A. Sepulveda, V.D. Dinglas, et al. Core domains for clinical research in acute respiratory failure survivors: an international modified delphi consensus study. *Crit Care Med* 2017; **45**: 1001–10.

29. M.A. Spruit, A.E. Holland, S.J. Singh, et al. COVID-19: interim guidance on rehabilitation in the hospital and post-hospital phase from a European respiratory society and American thoracic society-coordinated international task force. *Eur Respir J* 2020; **56**(6): 2002197.

30. D.M. Needham, K.A. Sepulveda, V.D. Dinglas, et al. Core outcome measures

for clinical research in acute respiratory failure survivors. an international modified Delphi consensus study. *Am J Respir Crit Care Med* 2017; **196**: 1122–30.

31. C. Casanova, B.R. Celli, P. Barria, et al. The 6-min walk distance in healthy subjects: reference standards from seven countries. *Eur Respir J* 2011; **37**: 150–6.

32. N. Nakanishi, K. Liu, A. Kawauchi, et al. Instruments to assess post-intensive care syndrome assessment: a scoping review and modified Delphi method study. *Crit Care* 2023; **27**: 430.

33. C.D. Spies, H. Krampe, N. Paul, et al. Instruments to measure outcomes of post-intensive care syndrome in outpatient care settings: results of an expert consensus and feasibility field test. *J Intensive Care Soc* 2021; **22**: 159–74.

34. C.L. Hodgson, B. Fulcher, F. P. Mariajoseph, et al. A core outcome set for research in patients on extracorporeal membrane oxygenation. *Crit Care Med* 2021; **49**: e1252–e4.

35. K.P. Mayer, S.M. Parry, A.G. Kalema, et al. Safety and feasibility of an interdisciplinary treatment approach to optimize recovery from critical coronavirus disease 2019. *Crit Care Explor* 2021; **3**: e0516.

36. J.C. Jackson, E.W. Ely, M.C. Morey, et al. Cognitive and physical rehabilitation of intensive care unit survivors: results of the RETURN randomized controlled pilot investigation. *Crit Care Med* 2012; **40**: 1088–97.

37. J.R. Falvey, T.E. Murphy, T.M. Gill, et al. Home health rehabilitation utilization among medicare beneficiaries following critical illness. *J Am Geriatr Soc* 2020; **68**: 1512–19.

38. B. Connolly, R. Milton-Cole, C. Adams, et al. Recovery, rehabilitation and follow-up services following critical illness: an updated UK national cross-sectional survey and progress report. *BMJ Open* 2021; **11**: e052214.

39. J.H. Vlake, E.J. Wils, J. van Bommel, et al. Familiarity with the post-intensive care syndrome among general practitioners and opportunities to improve their involvement in ICU follow-up care. *Intensive Care Med* 2022; **48**: 1090–2.

40. K.E. Hauschildt, R.K. Hechtman, H. C. Prescott, T.J. Iwashyna. Hospital discharge summaries are insufficient following icu stays: a qualitative study. *Crit Care Explor* 2022; **4**: e0715.

41. N.A. Stens, E.A. Bakker, A. Mañas, et al. Relationship of daily step counts to all-cause mortality and cardiovascular events. *J Am Coll Cardiol* 2023; **82**: 1483–94.

42. C.J. Caspersen, K.E. Powell, G. M. Christenson. Physical activity, exercise, and physical fitness: definitions and distinctions for health-related research. *Public Health Rep* 1985; **100**: 126–31.

43. S.M. Parry, L.D. Knight, B. Connolly, et al. Factors influencing physical activity and rehabilitation in survivors of critical illness: a systematic review of quantitative and qualitative studies. *Intensive Care Med* 2017; **43**: 531–42.

44. R. Gloeckl, R. H. Zwick, U. Fürlinger, et al. Practical recommendations for exercise training in patients with long COVID with or without post-exertional malaise: a best practice proposal. *Sports Med Open* 2024; **10**: 47.

45. E. Priel, M. Wahab, T. Mondal, et al. The impact of beta blockade on the cardio-respiratory system and symptoms during exercise. *Curr Res Physiol* 2021; **4**: 235–42.

46. Y. Ming, A. Zecevic. Medications & polypharmacy influence on recurrent fallers in community: a systematic review. *Can Geriatr J* 2018; **21**: 14–25.

47. S. Parry, L. Denehy, C. Granger, et al. The fear and risk of community falls in patients following an intensive care admission: an exploratory cohort study. *Aust Crit Care* 2020; **33**: 144–50.

48. M.E. Major, R. Kwakman, M.E. Kho, et al. Surviving critical illness: what is next? An expert consensus statement on physical rehabilitation after hospital discharge. *Crit Care* 2016; **20**: 354.

49. C. Renner, M.M. Jeitziner, M. Albert, et al. Guideline on multimodal rehabilitation for patients with post-intensive care syndrome. *Crit Care* 2023; **27**: 301.

50. R.C.H. Kwakman, M.E. Major, D.S. Dettling-Ihnenfeldt, et al. Physiotherapy treatment approaches for survivors of critical illness: a proposal from a Delphi study. *Physiother Theory Pract* 2020; **36**: 1421–31.

51. K. Ferguson, J.M. Bradley, D.F. McAuley, et al. Patients' perceptions of an exercise program delivered following discharge from hospital after critical illness (the revive trial). *J Intensive Care Med* 2019; **34**: 978–84.

52. W. Walker, J. Wright, G. Danjoux, et al. Project Post Intensive Care eXercise (PIX): a qualitative exploration of intensive care unit survivors' perceptions of quality of life post-discharge and experience of exercise rehabilitation. *J Intensive Care Soc* 2015; **16**: 37–44.

53. S. Goddard, H. Gunn, B. Kent, R. Dennett. The experience of physical recovery and physical rehabilitation following hospital discharge for intensive care survivors: a qualitative systematic review. *Nurs Rep* 2024; **14**: 148–63.

54. A.S. Agård, I. Egerod, E. Tønnesen, K. Lomborg. Struggling for independence: a grounded theory study on convalescence of ICU survivors 12 months post ICU discharge. *Intensive Crit Care Nurs* 2012; **28**: 105–13.

55. B. Connolly, L. Salisbury, B. O'Neill, et al. Exercise rehabilitation following intensive care unit discharge for recovery from critical illness. *Cochrane Database Syst Rev* 2015; **2015**: Cd008632.

56. L. Denehy, E.H. Skinner, L. Edbrooke, et al. Exercise rehabilitation for patients with critical illness: a randomized controlled trial with 12 months of follow-up. *Crit Care* 2013; **17**: R156.

57. K. McDowell, B. O'Neill, B. Blackwood, et al. Effectiveness of an exercise programme on physical function in patients discharged from hospital following critical illness: a randomised controlled trial (the REVIVE trial). *Thorax* 2017; **72**: 594–5.

58. American Physical Therapy Association. APTA Guide to Physical Therapist Practice 4.0; 2024 [Available from: https://guide.apta.org/].

59. G. Liguori. American College of Sports Medicine. ACSM's Guidelines for Exercise Testing and Prescription. Wilkins L.W., (ed.); 2020.

60. A.T. Balachandran, J. Steele, D. Angielczyk, et al. Comparison of power training vs traditional strength training on physical function in older adults: a systematic review and meta-analysis. *JAMA Network Open* 2022; **5**: e2211623-e.

61. J. Alcazar, A. Guadalupe-Grau, F.J. Garcia-Garcia, et al. Skeletal muscle power measurement in older people: a systematic review of testing protocols and adverse events. *J Gerontol A Biol Sci Med Sci* 2018; **17(7)**: 914-24.

62. J.F. Bean, S.G. Leveille, D.K. Kiely, et al. A comparison of leg power and leg strength within the InCHIANTI study: which influences mobility more? *J Gerontol A Biol Sci Med Sci* 2003; **58**: 728–33.

63. A.M. Batterham, S. Bonner, J. Wright, et al. Effect of supervised aerobic exercise rehabilitation on physical fitness and quality-of-life in survivors of critical illness: an exploratory minimized controlled trial (PIX study). *Br J Anaesth* 2014; **113**: 130–7.

64. N. Morelli, S.M. Parry, A. Steele, et al. Patients surviving critical COVID-19 have impairments in dual-task performance related to post-intensive care syndrome. *J Intensive Care Med* 2022; **37**: 890–8.

65. C. Battle, K. James, P. Temblett, H. Hutchings. Supervised exercise rehabilitation in survivors of critical illness: a randomised controlled trial. *J Intensive Care Soc* 2019; **20**: 18–26.

66. C. Jones, J. Eddleston, A. McCairn, et al. Improving rehabilitation after critical illness through outpatient physiotherapy classes and essential amino acid supplement: a randomized controlled trial. *J Crit Care* 2015; **30**: 901–7.

67. D. Elliott, S. McKinley, J. Alison, et al. Health-related quality of life and physical recovery after a critical illness: a multi-centre randomised controlled trial of a home-based physical rehabilitation program. *Crit Care* 2011; **15**: R142.

68. D.J. McWilliams, S. Benington, D. Atkinson. Outpatient-based physical rehabilitation for survivors of prolonged critical illness: a randomized controlled trial. *Physiother Theory Pract* 2016; **32**: 179–90.

69. A.F. Rousseau, N. Dardenne, I. Kellens, et al. Quadriceps handheld dynamometry during the post-ICU trajectory: using strictly the same body position is mandatory for repeated measures. *Intensive Care Med Exp* 2023; **11**: 39.

70. K.S. Chan, L. Aronson Friedman, V.D. Dinglas, et al. Evaluating physical outcomes in acute respiratory distress syndrome survivors: validity, responsiveness, and minimal important difference of 4-meter gait speed test. *Crit Care Med* 2016; **44**: 859–68.

71. R.W. Bohannon, Y.C. Wang. Four-meter gait speed: normative values and reliability determined for adults participating in the nih toolbox study. *Arch Phys Med Rehabil* 2019; **100**: 509–13.

72. A. Middleton, S.L. Fritz, M. Lusardi. Walking speed: the functional vital sign. *J Aging Phys Act* 2015; **23**: 314–22.

73. H.K. O'Grady, L. Edbrooke, C. Farley, et al. The sit-to-stand test as a patient-centered functional outcome for critical care research: a pooled analysis of five international rehabilitation studies. *Crit Care* 2022; **26**: 175.

74. N. Paul, J. Cittadino, B. Weiss, et al. Subjective ratings of mental and physical health correlate with EQ-5D-5L index values in survivors of critical illness: a construct validity study. *Crit Care Med* 2023; **51**: 365–75.

75. L.L. Porter, K.S. Simons, S. Corsten, et al. Changes in quality of life 1 year after intensive care: a multicenter prospective cohort of ICU survivors. *Crit Care* 2024; **28**: 255.

Chapter 42
Functional Impairments in Survivors of Critical Illness

Samantha Green, Meg Williamson, Maria Shoemaker, and Avital S. Isenberg

Introduction

Physical and cognitive impairments often lead to participation restrictions, including the inability to perform certain activities of daily living (ADLs) and instrumental activities of daily living (IADLS), which can compromise the ability to live independently. ADLs are defined as "activities oriented toward taking care of one's own body and completed on a routine basis," and IADLs are defined as "activities to support daily life within the home and community" (see Table 42.1) [1]. ADLs require physical strength, coordination, and cognitive skills including attention and sequencing, while IADLs require more sophisticated physical capabilities and cognitive processing skills.

Survivors of critical illness often experience new and enduring functional limitations that impact their abilities to perform ADLs and IADLs. Iwashyna and colleagues, for example, sought to determine changes in physical functioning, as measured by a composite score of ADLs and IADLs, among patients who survived sepsis by analyzing a nationally representative cohort study of older Americans. Participants were divided into three groups based on their pre-sepsis function: those with no limitations, those with mild to moderate limitations, and those with severe limitations, defined as requiring assistance with four or more ADLs or IADLs. Survivors of severe sepsis were at greater risk of developing functional limitations, particularly those with better baseline physical functioning. Severe sepsis was associated with the development of 1.6 new limitations among patients who had no prior limitations, 1.5 new limitations among patients who had mild to moderate limitations, and no significant new limitations in patients with severe pre-existing disability. This was the first demonstration that a hospitalization for severe sepsis is independently associated with enduring functional limitations with lasting implications for patients' independence [2]. Ehlenbach and colleagues found that nearly three quarters of older survivors of severe sepsis discharged to a skilled nursing facility (SNF) had hierarchal scales consistent with maximal or total dependence in ADLs. Additionally, the need for mechanical ventilation during hospitalization was associated with total dependence in ADLs and had a stronger relationship with ADL dependence than advanced age, prior SNF residence, or diagnosis of dementia [3].

Furthermore, a systematic review performed by Ohtake and colleagues noted that 35% of survivors of critical illness reported partial dependence in at least one ADL at 3 months following hospital discharge, which persisted in 33% of patients at 12 months after discharge [4]. Persistent impairments in IADL function are also observed, with only 30–38% of survivors of critical illness who were employed prior to their ICU stay capable of returning to work within 3 months of discharge and only 42–56% resuming employment 12 months following discharge (see Chapter 44 for additional information) [4].

Table 42.1 Common ADLs and IADLs [1]

ADLs	IADLs
Bathing/showering	Providing care for others
Toileting and toilet hygiene/continence	Pet/animal care
Dressing	Child rearing
Feeding	Communication management
Functional mobility/transferring	Community mobility and driving
Grooming/personal hygiene	Religious and spiritual practices/expression
Sexual activity	Shopping
	Health and medication management
	Education
	Work
	Food preparation
	Laundry
	Housekeeping
	Managing finances

The long-term sequalae of increased dependence in ADLs and IADLs is significant on both the individual level, impacting patient and caregiver safety and quality of life, and on the societal level, impacting healthcare utilization, cost of care, and need for institutionalization.

Role of Occupational Therapy

Occupational therapists (OTs) are trained to provide holistic, person-centered care to remediate impairments and teach compensatory approaches to improve a person's participation and independence in their daily activities [1]. OTs are skilled in the evaluation and treatment of the physical, cognitive, and mental health deficits that impact the daily functioning of survivors of critical illness. As experts in activity and performance analysis, OTs are equipped to provide interventions focused on maximizing patient independence despite existing impairments. Additionally, the profession's historical roots in mental health allow OTs to use assessments of both capacity and functional abilities to identify opportunities for patients to increase meaningful participation [5].

While evidence-based practice is regarded as the gold standard for the delivery of effective healthcare services [6], research specific to rehabilitation interventions for patients with post-intensive care syndrome (PICS) is limited. Accordingly, practitioners in this field have largely taken an evidence-informed practice approach, which combines the contributions of evidence-based practice with practice-based research and reflective practice, allowing practitioners to be flexible, adaptable, and pave the way for future providers and research [6]. The evaluation tools and interventions described in this chapter were derived by utilizing relevant empirical evidence in combination with clinical expertise for the delivery of occupational therapy in this unique patient population.

In addition to OTs who care for survivors of critical illness, there are several specialty practice areas which can be a beneficial resource for patients with PICS and specific additional needs. OT clinicians with Certified Driving Rehabilitation Specialist (CDRS) credentials complete in-depth assessments of driving skills and identify driving rehabilitation needs or adaptations for driving (see Chapter 44 for additional information). OT clinicians with Certified Low Vision Therapist (CLVT) credentials complete comprehensive functional visual assessments and train patients in adaptive visual strategies and technologies. Additionally, OTs with specializations in chronic pain, hand therapy, and neurological conditions can be consulted to provide specialized interventions based on patient needs.

Physical Impairments

OTs evaluate and treat physical impairments in strength, gross and fine motor coordination, and cardiorespiratory and muscular endurance by combining traditional cardiovascular exercise prescriptions with education regarding pacing strategies. This provides patients with various techniques to facilitate ADL participation and independence while utilizing remediation and compensatory techniques to improve endurance [7].

Evaluation of Physical Impairments

Strength, motor control, and endurance are typically evaluated through standardized performance assessments, details of which are listed in Table 42.2 and more comprehensively addressed in Chapter 41 [4,8,9,10].

Evaluation of ADL/IADL Impairments

The ability to perform ADLs and IADLs is an essential component of occupational therapy assessment and intervention in survivors of critical illness [8]. Each evaluation tool is briefly described below, and additional information regarding scoring and score interpretation is included in Table 42.3 [11,12,13,14,15].

The **Katz ADL** screening tool assesses six self-care areas in hierarchical order from most to least demanding, including bathing, dressing, toileting, transferring, continence, and feeding [11]. The **Barthel Index** assesses ten ADL self-care and mobility items, adding toilet hygiene, transferring to bed, walking, and climbing stairs to the items included in the Katz ADL screening tool [12,13]. The **Lawton IADL** screening tool assesses eight IADLs, including use of a telephone, shopping, housekeeping, food preparation, laundry, transportation management, financial management, and medication management [14]. **The Functional Activities Questionnaire (FAQ)** assesses the ability to perform tasks in 10 areas, including writing checks, paying bills, and balancing a check book; assembling tax records, business affairs, or papers; shopping alone for clothes, household necessities, or groceries; playing a game of skill or working on a hobby; heating water, making a cup of coffee, and turning off the stove after use; preparing a balanced meal; keeping track of current events; paying attention to, understanding, and discussing a television program, book, or magazine; remembering appointments, family occasions, holidays, and medications; and traveling out of the neighborhood, driving, or arranging public transportation [15].

Medical fitness to drive is an additional IADL that OTs are trained to assess, as the ability to drive is often limited following critical illness (see Chapter 44 for additional information) [16]. The **Rapid Pace Walk Test** (RPW), which requires patients to walk 10 feet, turn

Table 42.2 Physical impairment evaluation tools

Tool	Area of Measurement	Materials/Procedure	Scoring	Relation to function
Handgrip dynamometry [4,8]	Grip strength	• Patient holds the dynamometer, first in their dominant hand with their forearm supported on the chair armrest. • 3 measurements are taken for each hand and averaged	• Kilograms of force • Age/gender norms available	• Correlated with gross limb strength • Can be reduced for more than 24 months post discharge
Nine-hole peg test [9]	Fine motor coordination	Materials: • Rectangular board with well on one end and 9 holes on the other • 9 pegs Procedure: • Patient moves pegs from well into holes one by one, then immediately removes them one by one • Dominant or unaffected hand is tested first	• Time is recorded in seconds • Age/gender norms available	• Impacts tasks such as fastening clothing
Box and blocks test [10]	Gross manual dexterity	Materials: • Test box with lengthwise partition in the middle • 150 blocks placed on one side of the test box Procedure: • Transfer as many blocks as possible one by one across the partition • 60 seconds for each hand • Dominant or unaffected hand is tested first	• Number of blocks transferred • Age/gender norms available	• Ability to reach and grasp objects

Table 42.3 ADL, IADL, and functional cognition evaluation tools

Tool	Area of Measurement	Type	How Test is Scored	Maximum Score	Score Interpretation	Domain Assessed
Katz Activities of Daily Living Scale [11]	ADL independence	Performance-based or self-report ***	The clinician observes the patient completing tasks and rates each task. **Task Scoring:** 1: Independent 0: Requires assistance	6	6: Independent 3–5: Partially dependent 2 or less: dependent	ADLs
Barthel Index [12,13]	ADL independence	Performance based or self/caregiver report ***	The clinician observes the patient completing tasks and assigns scores based on the performance. **Task Scoring:** 0: Unable 5: Independent or partially independent (varies per item) 10: Independent or with minor help (varies per item) 15: Independent	100	0–20: "Total" dependency 21–60: "Severe" dependency 61–90: "Moderate" dependency 91–99: "Slight" dependency	ADLs
Lawton Instrumental Activities of Daily Living Scale [14]	IADL independence	Self-report or caregiver report	**Task Scoring:** 1: Completes portion of IADL independently 0: Cannot complete task without assistance, does not complete task	8	0: Low function/dependent 8: High function/independent	IADLs
Functional Activities Questionnaire (FAQ) [15]	IADL independence	Self-report or caregiver report	**Task Scoring:** 3: Dependent 2: Requires assistance	30	9: Dependent in 3 or more activities; indicative of impaired function and possible	IADLs

Assessment	Construct	Type	Scoring	Score Range	Interpretation	Category
PASS [30]	ADLs, IADLs, and functional mobility	Performance-based, standardized	Subtasks are rated for independence, safety and adequacy 1: Independent with difficulty or never did but would have difficulty now 0: Independent with no difficulty or never did but could do now	3	Higher scores indicative of more cognitive impairment; Higher scores indicative of more dependence	Functional Cognition
Kettle Test [31]	IADL independence	Performance-based	Therapist scores observed performance: 0: Intact performance 1: Questionable performance but completes independently 2: Receives general cues 3: Receives specific cueing or incomplete/deficit performance 4: Receives physical demonstration or assistance	52	52: Maximal assistance 0: Independent without difficulty Higher scores indicate greater independence, safety, and adequacy.	Functional Cognition
Pillbox Test [32]	Executive function	Performance-based	Clinician observation of types of errors (commission, omission, misplacement) Clinician identifies areas of executive function impairment: Purposive action/self-regulation Planning/attention Volition/inhibition	Varies	Pass: Completed in less than 5 minutes with fewer than 3 errors Fail: Completed in more than 5 minutes and/or	Functional Cognition

Table 42.3 (cont.)

Tool	Area of Measurement	Type	How Test is Scored	Maximum Score	Score Interpretation	Domain Assessed
			Effective performance/self-monitoring		more than 3 errors; Type of errors are recorded in addition to more detailed description of specific observations regarding areas of executive function impairments	
Multiple Errands Test [33]	Executive function	Performance-based	Time taken to complete the tasks (4–12 tasks) is recorded along with the types of errors made. Types of errors: Inefficiencies (use of poor strategies) Rule breaks (violation of rules) Interpretation failure (misunderstanding what is being asked) Task failure (incomplete performance)	30	Higher scores indicative of more errors and poorer performance	Functional Cognition

*** If the clinician is unable to observe the patient complete the task, self-and/or caregiver report can be utilized. The ideal application of these tests is to observe current patient performance.

around, and return to the starting point as quickly as possible, is one such screening tool used to assess driving skills [17]; requiring more than nine seconds to ambulate 20 feet is indicative of increased risk of an at-fault vehicle collision. The RPW is one component of the Assessment of Driving-Related Skills (ADReS), which includes a battery of tests addressing vision, cognition, motor function, and somatosensory function, all of which are necessary for safe driving [18]. If concerns arise during a clinical driving screen, OTs may make referrals to CDRS-specialized clinicians or recommend on-the-road evaluations.

Interventions for Physical Impairments

OTs use materials within the clinic or patient's home to build quality interventions to maximize function. Gross motor interventions such as weight training, activity circuits, floor transfers, and simulated ADLs can increase brain-derived neurotrophic factor (BDNF), leading to improved motor control for daily activities [19]. Additional examples of physical impairment interventions are listed in Table 42.4 [20].

Interventions for ADL Impairments

OTs provide multimodal interventions to improve ADL impairments. The performance and efficiency of ADLs can be improved through combining strength training, ADL training, and education during weekly, goal-directed sessions over 8 to 12 weeks [8,21,22]. Exercise prescriptions simulating the metabolic equivalent (MET) level of the impaired ADL can improve endurance needed to complete the functional task independently. Tasks are broken down into smaller components, allowing the patient to practice each part separately until they are competent with the entire task. If a patient is having difficulty standing at the sink to wash dishes, for example, task analysis is used to dissect the task into its key components, and interventions are then devised to engage a patient in those necessary components. A clinic activity may include standing while participating in a bimanual task, such as placing clips on a target outside of the patient's base of support; timing the activity can provide a baseline standing tolerance duration. This task can then be upgraded by manipulating height, horizontal location, and weight of items and targets [21,22,23]. OTs employ the "just right challenge" to create tasks that the patient can complete successfully without failure. The chosen intervention should challenge the patient, while not being too difficult or too easy. The ideology behind this approach is to have the patient meet the challenge while also seeing the purpose behind the chosen task [24]. Practice and repetition of the impaired ADL in the clinic setting with real-time feedback can enhance patient confidence to complete the task at home [25]. OTs address endurance impairments through energy conservation education and training (see Figure 42.1) [26].

Adaptive equipment prescription and training can increase patient independence in ADL completion despite decreased endurance. Shower chairs, tub transfer benches, bedside commodes, and rolling walkers all reduce metabolic demand for tasks, allowing patients to be more independent [21,27]. Additional examples of ADL interventions are listed in Table 42.4.

Functional Cognitive Impairments

Cognitive impairments can cause disruptions in ADL and IADL independence, limiting one's ability to return to pre-morbid roles, increasing morbidity rates, and often creating financial strain for survivors of critical illness and their caregivers [2]. Functional cognition

Table 42.4 Common OT interventions

Area Addressed	Activity Example(s)	Domain Addressed
Cardiovascular and muscular endurance [20]	Structured strength training and cardiovascular exercise twice weekly for 8 weeks Intensity can be personalized based on goal MET levels required for preferred activities	Physical Impairments
Fine motor coordination	Picking up coins, translating into and out of palm for in-hand manipulation Shoe tying Stringing beads	Physical Impairments
Gross motor coordination	Reach and grasp to place items on targets	Physical Impairments
Strategy-based training using guided facilitation and supervision [36]	**Returning to cooking:** OT will provide various levels of cueing, slowly reducing cueing to improve independence. External cues: Recipe, timer, verbal cues Internal cues: Evaluating own performance	Cognitive Impairments
Goal management training (GMT): facilitates goal management and overall executive function [37,38]	**Organizing weekly calendar:** OT will cue the patient to pause during the task and encourage the patient to identify the overall task goals and evaluate their performance.	Cognitive Impairments
Cognitive behavioral therapy [45]	Using problem-focused interventions to help patients identify and change maladaptive thought patterns	Mental Health Impairments
Behavioral activation [46]	Encourage patient to schedule a meaningful activity and a subsequent reward after completing the activity	Mental Health Impairments
Value based goal setting [47]	Help patients identify their intrinsic and extrinsic motivators Once values are identified, activity scheduling can increase patient participation	Mental Health Impairments

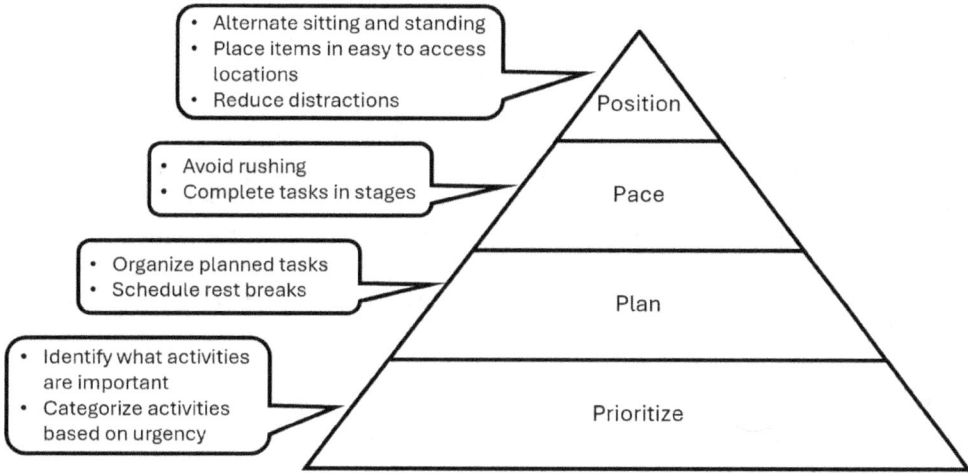

Figure 42.1 Energy conservation strategies [26].

is defined as the ability to use and integrate cognitive skills to perform complex everyday tasks [28]. Executive function refers to the collection of skills needed to plan, prioritize, organize, and focus to successfully manage tasks [29]. These skills can be assessed to provide valuable information for intervention planning (see Chapter 43 for additional information) [25].

Evaluation of Functional Cognitive Impairments

The use of functional cognitive assessment tools allows OTs to determine the impact of the identified impairment on the patient's daily life. Each evaluation tool is briefly described below, and additional information regarding scoring and score interpretation is included in Table 42.3 [30,31,32,33].

The PASS is a performance observation, criterion-based, standardized assessment tool that measures independence, safety, and task adequacy in 26 subtest areas of ADLs, IADLs, and functional mobility. Tasks can be completed as stand-alone assessments that take five to ten minutes to administer [30]. **The Kettle Test** is a performance-based IADL assessment where cognitive functional performance is assessed by having the patient follow specific instructions to prepare two different hot beverages [31]. **The Pillbox Test** is a performance-based assessment of executive function that evaluates medication management skills by having the patient read the instructions on pill bottles to organize one week's worth of five medications into a standardized pillbox [32]. The patient is successful if they complete the task with two or fewer errors within the allotted five-minute time frame. **The Multiple Errands Test** evaluates executive function by having the patient participate in 4 to 12 real-life activities, either in the hospital or community setting, such as purchasing specific items or arriving at a specific location [33]. The patient must complete the test within the constraints of the rules provided to them, and the therapist observes how efficiently the task is completed and records errors and failures where indicated.

Interventions for Functional Cognitive Impairments

Cognitive interventions aim to improve the patient's capacity to perform essential tasks within their ability. OTs create scenarios that simulate the cognitive demands that the patient will encounter while completing the task independently [34,35]. An OT may work on improving problem solving, safety, and executive functioning by asking the patient to follow a recipe for preparing a complex meal. To address planning, sequencing, and judgment, an OT may ask the patient to set up a load of laundry by sorting the clothes, reading the clothing labels, and setting the machine. Additional examples of cognitive interventions are listed in Table 42.4 [36,37,38].

Mental Health Impairments

New functional impairments combined with negative memories of their intensive care unit (ICU) experience can significantly impact the mental health of survivors of critical illness (see Chapter 46 for additional information). Given occupational therapy's roots in mental health, OTs possess skills to address the functional implications associated with mental health impairments [39].

Evaluation of Mental Health Impairments

OTs can evaluate and treat mental health deficits that interfere with the ability to complete daily activities. The Occupational Self-Assessment (OSA) and the Canadian Occupational Performance Measure (COPM) are self-report measures of occupational performance. The OSA is a self-report measure of the patient's perceptions on the importance of specific daily activities based on the Model of Human Occupation (MOHO) [40]. The MOHO is an occupation-based model categorized into components of volition, habituation, environment, and performance skills that has been used as a framework to guide OT practice [41]. The OSA is designed to encourage patient involvement in goal setting and to capture self-perceptions of how illness and disability affect occupational competence. COPM is a semi-structured interview that identifies patient-centered problem areas in daily function [42]. The patient rates tasks most important to them, their perceived performance, and how satisfied they are with their performance. The COPM addresses areas of self-care, productivity, and leisure to guide intervention and to assist patients in identifying and prioritizing concerns that restrict them from participating in daily activities.

Interventions for Mental Health Impairments

Occupational therapy mental health interventions are designed to empower patients to be active participants in the creation and completion of personalized goals with facilitated guidance from the OT. Collaborative goal setting, problem solving, self-monitoring, and active discussion are examples of ways that OTs can provide mental health interventions for this population [43,44]. Specific treatment techniques are listed in Table 42.4 [45,46,47].

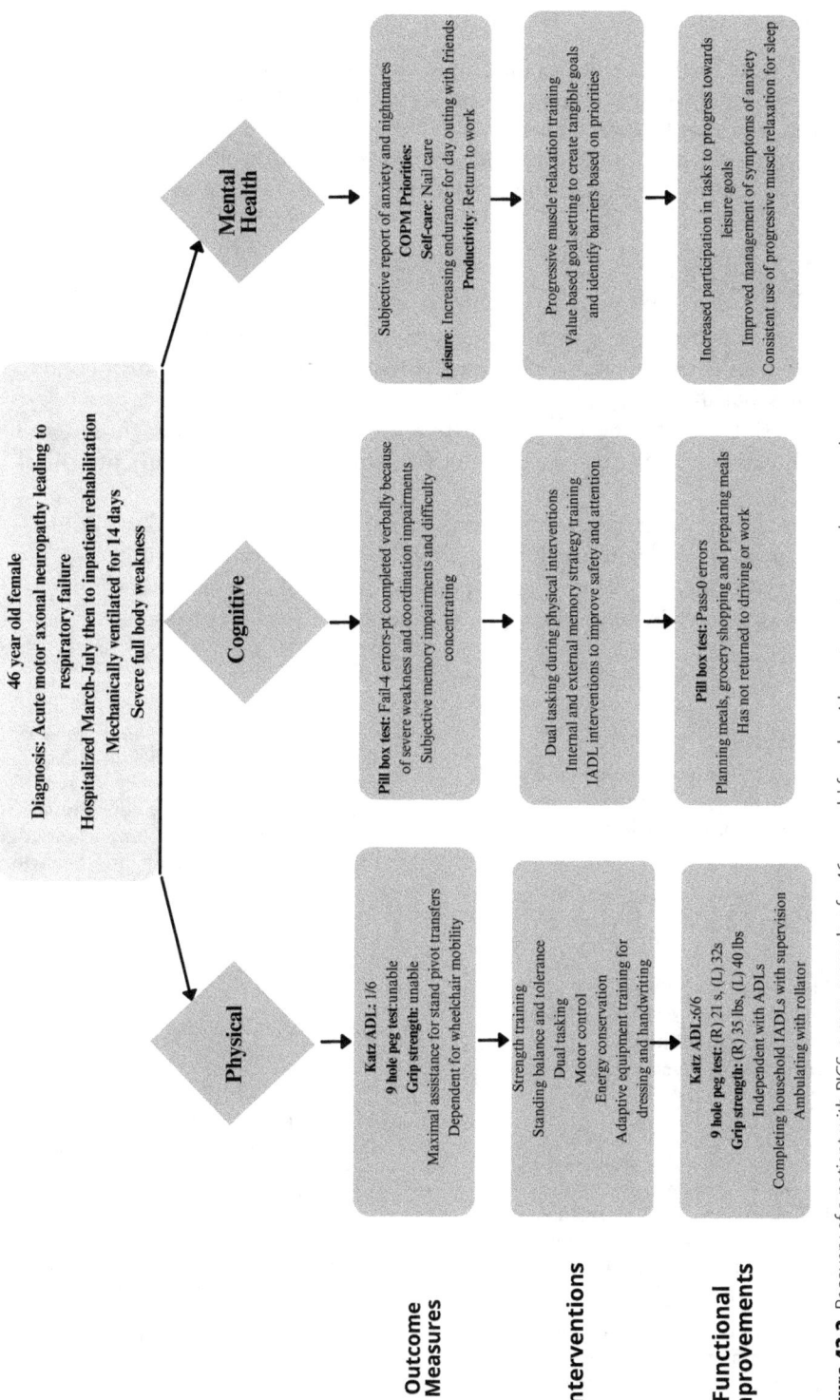

Figure 42.2 Recovery of a patient with PICS: a case example of a 46-year-old female with acute motor axonal neuropathy.

Conclusion

After an ICU stay, patient priorities have been shown to include restoring psychological health, connecting with others, feeling safe, participating in self-care, resuming normal roles and routines, and asserting personhood [48]. Through individualized treatment sessions and caregiver involvement, OTs can guide survivors of critical illness towards a life of fulfillment and healthy participation in meaningful activities (as seen in Figure 42.2).

Key Points

1. Survivors of critical illness are often impacted by residual functional impairments that can restrict participation in daily activities and cause significant disruption to their previous life roles.
2. OTs are skilled in the evaluation and treatment of the physical, cognitive, and mental health deficits that impact the daily functioning of survivors of critical illness.
3. A combination of standardized assessments, performance-based, and self-report evaluation tools should be used to adequately assess functional impairments.
4. OT interventions should focus on optimizing functional independence while addressing underlying physical, cognitive, and mental health impairments.

References

1. Occupational Therapy Practice Framework: Domain and Process – fourth edition. *Am J of Occup Ther* 2020; **74**(Supplement 2): 1–87.
2. T.J. Iwashyna, E.W. Ely, D.M. Smith, K.M. Langa. Long-term cognitive impairment and functional disability among survivors of severe sepsis. *JAMA* 2010; **304**(16): 1787.
3. W.J. Ehlenbach, A.G. Bykovskyi, M.D. Repplinger, et al. Sepsis survivors admitted to skilled nursing facilities: cognitive impairment, ADL dependence, and survival. *Crit Care Med* 2018; **46**(1): 37-44.
4. P.J. Ohtake, A.C. Lee, J.C. Scott, et al. Physical impairments associated with post-intensive care syndrome: systematic review based on the World Health Organization's International Classification of Functioning, Disability and Health framework. *Phys Ther* 2018; **98**(8): 631–45.
5. J.C. Rogers, M.B. Holm. Functional assessment in mental health: lessons from occupational therapy. *Dialogues Clin Neurosci* 2016 Jun 30; **18**(2): 145–54.
6. E.A. Kumah, R. McSherry, J. Bettany-Saltikov, et al. PROTOCOL: evidence-informed practice versus evidence-based practice educational interventions for improving knowledge, attitudes, understanding, and behavior toward the application of evidence into practice: a comprehensive systematic review of undergraduate students. *Campbell Syst Rev* 2019; **15**(1–2): e1015.
7. B. Fields, S. Smallfield. Occupational therapy practice guidelines for adults with chronic conditions. *Am J Occup Ther* 2022; **76**(2).
8. M.E. Major, R. Kwakman, M.E. Kho, et al. Surviving critical illness: what is next? An expert consensus statement on physical rehabilitation after hospital discharge. *Crit Care* 2016; **20**(1): 354.
9. V. Mathiowetz, K. Weber, N. Kashman, G. Volland. Adult norms for the nine hole peg test of finger dexterity. *OTJR (Thorofare N J)* 1985; **5**: 24–33.
10. V. Mathiowetz, G. Volland, N. Kashman, K. Weber. Adult norms for the Box and

Block Test of manual dexterity. *Am J Occup Ther* 1985; 39(6): 386–91.
11. S. Katz, A.B. Ford, R.W. Moskowitz, et al. Studies of illness in the aged: the index of ADL: a standardized measure of biological and psychosocial Function. *JAMA* 1963; **185**(12): 914–19.
12. N. Nakanishi, K. Liu, A. Kawauchi, et al. Instruments to assess post-intensive care syndrome assessment: a scoping review and modified Delphi method study. *Crit Care* 2023; 27(1): 430.
13. F.L. Mahoney, D.W. Barthel. Functional evaluation: Barthel Index. *Md State Med Jl* 1965; **14**: 61–5.
14. M.P. Lawton, E.M. Brody. Assessment of older people: self-maintaining and instrumental activities of daily living. *Gerontologist* 1969; **9**:179–86.
15. R.I. Pfeffer, T.T. Kurosaki, C.H. Harrah Jr, et al. Measurement of functional activities in older adults in the community. *J Gerontol* 1982; 37(3): 323–9.
16. J. Munn, S.M. Willatts, M.A. Tooley. Health and activity after intensive care. *Anaesthesia* 1995; **50**: 1017–21.
17. T.J. Mielenz, L.L. Durbin, J.A. Cisewski, et al. Select physical performance measures and driving outcomes in older adults. *Inj Epidemiol* 2017; 4(1): 14.
18. D.P. McCarthy, W.C. Mann. Process and outcomes evaluation of older driver screening programs: the assessment of driving-related skills (ADReS) older-driver screening tool. National Highway Traffic Safety Administration, United States National Highway Traffic Safety Administration & National Older Driver Research and Training Center (U.S.); 2009.
19. C.A. Grégoire, N. Berryman, F. St-Onge, et al. Gross motor skills training leads to increased brain-derived neurotrophic factor levels in healthy older adults: a pilot study. *Front in Physiol* 2019; **10**: 410.
20. A.P. Pillatt, J. Neilsson, R.H. Schneider. Efeitos Do Exercício Físico Em Idosos Fragilizados: Uma Revisão Sistemática. *Fisioter Pesqui* 2019; **18**: 225–32.
21. L. Finch, D. Frankel, B. Gallant, et al. Occupational therapy in pulmonary rehabilitation programs: A scoping review. *Respir Med* 2022; **199**: 106881.
22. K. Bendstrup, J. Jenson, S. Holm, B. Bengtsson. Outpatient rehabilitation improves activities of daily living, quality of life and exercise tolerance in chronic obstructive pulmonary disease. *Eur Respir J* 1997; **10**: 2801–6.
23. N. Martinez-Velilla, M. Saez de Asteasu, R. Ramirez-Velez, et al. Recovery of the decline in activities of daily living after hospitalization through an individualized exercise program: secondary analysis of a randomized clinical trial. *J of Gerontol* 2021; **76**(8): 1519–23.
24. H. Kuhaneck, S. Spitzer. The importance of conceptual origins: the case of the just right challenge. *Am J Occup Ther* 2024; **78**(4): 7804185110.
25. E.G. Hunter, P.J. Kearney. Occupational therapy interventions to improve performance of instrumental activities of daily living for community-dwelling older adults: a systematic review. *Am J Occup Ther* 2018; **72**(4):7204190050p1–9.
26. A. Weise, E. Ott, R. Hersche. Energy management education in persons with long covid-related fatigue: insights from focus group results on occupational therapy approach. *Healthc* 2024; **12**(2): 150.
27. A. Wingardh, C. Goransson, S. Larsson, et al. Effectiveness of energy conservation techniques in patients with COPD. *Respiration* 2020; **99**(5): 409–16.
28. G.M. Giles, D.F. Edwards, M.T. Morrison, et al. Health policy perspectives: screening for functional cognition in postacute care and the Improving Medicare Post-Acute Care Transformation (IMPACT) Act of 2014. *Am J Occup Ther* 2017; **71**: 7105090010.
29. Executive Function – The OT Toolbox. (2022, May 4). The OT Toolbox.
30. J.C. Rogers, M.B. Holm, (1989). Performance Assessment of Self Care Skills (PASS Home). Unpublished test, University of Pittsburgh, PA.

31. A. Hartman-Maeir, H. Harel, N. Katz. Kettle test: a brief measure of cognitive functional performance: reliability and validity in stroke rehabilitation. *Am J Occupl Ther* 2009; **63**(5): 592–9.
32. A.L. Zartman, R.C. Hilsabeck, C.A. Guarnaccia, A. Houtz. The Pillbox Test: an ecological measure of executive functioning and estimate of medication management abilities. *Arch Clin Neuropsychol* 2013; **28**(4): 307–19.
33. A. Poulin, A. McDermott. Multiple Errands Test (METS): Assessments In: Stroke Engine Intervention. Montreal. https://strokengine.ca/en/assessments/multiple-errands-test-met/. Accessed February 24, 2024.
34. G. Giles, D. Edwards, C. Baum, et al. Making functional cognition a professional priority. *Am J Occup Ther* 2020; **74**(1): 7401090010.
35. L. Chang, P. Chen, J. Wang, et al. High-ecological cognitive intervention to improve cognitive skills and cognitive-functional performance for older adults with mild cognitive impairment. *Am J Occup Ther* 2021; **75**(5): 7505205050.
36. L. Mowszowski, A. Lampit, C. Walton, S. Naismith. Strategy-based cognitive training for improving executive functions in older adults: a systematic review. *Neuropsychol Rev* 2016; **26**: 252–70.
37. B. Hagen, B. Lau, J. Joormann, et al. Goal management training as a cognitive remediation intervention in depression: a randomized controlled trial. *J Affect Disord* 2020; **275**: 268–77.
38. G.A. Colbenson, A. Johnson, M.E. Wilson. Post-intensive care syndrome: impact, prevention, and management. *Breathe (Sheff)* 2019; **15**(2): 98–101.
39. American Occupational Therapy Association. Specialized knowledge and skills in mental health. *Am J Occup Ther* 2010; **64**: S30–43.
40. K. Baron, G. Kielhofner, A. Iyenger, et al. The Occupational Self Assessment (OSA) Version 2.2. Chicago: University of Illinois of Chicago; 2006.
41. G. Kielhofner. *A model of human occupation: theory and application* (3rd ed.). Lippincott Philadelphia: Williams and Wilkins; 2002.
42. M. Law, S. Baptiste, M. McColl, et al. The Canadian occupational performance measure: an outcome measure for occupational therapy. *Can J Occup Ther* 1990; **57**(2): 82–7.
43. D.S. Davydow, C.L. Hough, D. Zatzick, W.J. Katon. Psychiatric symptoms and acute care service utilization over the course of the year following medical-surgical ICU admission: a longitudinal investigation. *Crit Care Med* 2014; **42**(12): 2473–81.
44. N. Alizadeh, T. Packer, Y-T. Chen, Y. Alnasery. What we know about fatigue self-management programs for people living with chronic conditions: a scoping review. *Patient Educ and Couns* 2023; **114**: 107866.
45. A. Carson, L. Mcwhirter. Cognitive behavioral therapy: principles, science, and patient selection in neurology. *Semin Neurol* 2022; **42**: 114–22.
46. A. Stein, E. Carl, P. Cuipers, et al. Looking beyond depression: a meta-analysis of the effect of behavioral activation on depression, anxiety, and activation. *Psychol Med* 2021; **51**: 1491–504.
47. D.R. Sullivan, X. Liu, D.S. Corwin, et al. Learned helplessness among families and surrogate decision-makers of patients admitted to medical, surgical, and trauma ICUs. *Chest* 2012; **142**(6): 1440–6.
48. L. Scheunemann, J. White, S. Prinjha, et al. Post-intensive care unit care: a qualitative analysis of patient priorities and implications for redesign. *Ann Am Thorac Soc* 2020; **17**(2): 221–8.

Chapter 43
Cognitive Impairments in Survivors of Critical Illness

Patsy Bryant, James C. Jackson, and Ramona O. Hopkins

Introduction

Many individuals experience new or worsening cognitive impairment as a component of post-intensive care syndrome (PICS), which is thought to occur from the effects of critical illness and treatments provided in the intensive care unit (ICU) [1,2,3,4]. Cognitive impairment is a broad term that refers to a wide array of neuropsychological deficits [5]. While cognitive impairment may develop in patients with chronic medical conditions, including diabetes, heart disease, lupus, multiple sclerosis, and Parkinson's disease, it is particularly common in survivors of critical illness. In general, between one-quarter and one-third of all survivors of critical illness appear to have significant neuropsychological challenges at remote timepoints after discharge [3].

These cognitive deficits span a variety of cognitive domains, including attention, executive functioning, language, memory (immediate, delayed, and working), processing speed, and visuospatial abilities, and the severity of impairment may be more pronounced in some cognitive domains than others [6]. Indeed, studies have consistently shown that problems in attention and executive functioning are quite common, while amnestic memory deficits and language difficulties are less common. Some individuals are impaired in multiple cognitive domains, while in others, deficits may be limited to a single cognitive ability [7]. The severity of cognitive deficits following critical illness may vary in degree over time but are generally stable, which differs from the progressively worsening cognitive impairments observed in patients with Alzheimer's disease.

Relatively few studies have sought to characterize the severity of cognitive impairment in survivors of critical illness, but two large studies provide insight on its prevalence and duration in this patient population. In a multicenter, prospective cohort study, Pandharipande and colleagues enrolled 821 patients with respiratory failure or septic shock, routinely evaluated them for delirium during hospitalization, and assessed global cognition with a battery of neuropsychological tests at 3 and 12 months after discharge. Three months after discharge, 40% of the patients had global cognition scores similar to patients with moderate traumatic brain injury, and 26% had scores similar to patients with mild Alzheimer's disease. These deficits persisted, such that at 12 months, 34% had cognitive scores similar to persons with moderate traumatic brain injury, and 24% had scores similar to persons with mild Alzheimer's disease. In this study, a longer duration of delirium was independently associated with worse global cognition and executive function at both 3 and 12 months. Moreover, little difference in cognitive functioning was found between younger and older patients, challenging a still popular misconception that only elderly patients are at risk for neurologic decline after severe illness [8].

In a second geographically diverse cohort of survivors of the acute respiratory distress syndrome, cognitive impairment, as measured by a validated test battery that included assessment of executive function, language, verbal reasoning, and immediate and delayed memory, occurred in 36% of patients at 6 months and 25% at 12 months [9], similar to findings in smaller single center cohort studies [10]. Although measures of physical functioning improved in this cohort between 6 and 12 months following discharge, measures of cognitive and psychological functioning did not, and quality of life assessments up to one year after discharge were substantially worse than estimated quality of life prior to hospitalization [9].

Understanding the natural history and trajectories of neuropsychological functioning after critical illness is a key concern of both patients and researchers. In a study by Schulte and colleagues assessing the association between critical illness and cognitive trajectories in a population of older adults, older adults admitted to the ICU during their hospital stay experienced greater decline in visuospatial abilities, memory, attention, and executive function than older adults who did not require ICU admission [11]. A systematic review of 46 studies examining cognitive impairment in survivors of critical illness found that, at 3 months, 35–81% of all survivors of critical illness experience some degree of cognitive impairment, and these impairments persisted in 42% at 1 year and 46% at 2 years [12]. The prevalence of cognitive impairment varied based on the method used to assess cognitive function; tools based on self-report demonstrated the lowest prevalence of cognitive impairment, validated cognitive screening tools like the Mini-Mental State Examination (MMSE) captured more patients with cognitive impairment, and comprehensive neuropsychological test batteries were the most effective strategy. Research to further characterize the various trajectories of cognitive impairment and factors that influence cognitive impairment is essential to better understand cognitive decline, how it may be predicted, and how to develop effective interventions to both prevent and treat it [13].

Risk Factors and Protective Factors

A variety of risk factors for cognitive impairment in survivors of critical illness have been studied, including both modifiable risk factors, such as severity of illness, and nonmodifiable risk factors, including age, race, and education level [14]. Among potentially modifiable risk factors, delirium has been the most widely studied, with nearly all investigations showing a strong relationship between the duration of delirium (with longer episodes presumed to be more "severe") and worse cognitive impairment [15,16,17]. In addition to delirium, a 2019 Society of Critical Care Medicine consensus conference statement identified several other potentially modifiable markers of illness severity that increase the risk of long-term cognitive impairment after critical illness, including sedating medications, sepsis, shock, hypoxia, acute respiratory distress syndrome, and mechanical ventilation [18]. Among nonmodifiable risk factors, preexisting cognitive impairment [19], older age, and a lower level of education [20] are associated with increased risk of long-term cognitive impairment.

Although risk factors for cognitive impairment following critical illness have been widely studied, less attention has been paid to protective factors – variables that make cognitive impairment less likely to happen. One candidate variable that may play a role is "cognitive reserve," the concept that the collective impact of one's educational attainment, occupation, and lifestyle may be protective in the face of a neurological insult [21].

Individuals with greater cognitive reserve, for example, may be better able to withstand neurologically harmful events occurring in the context of critical illness than those with less cognitive reserve. While cognitive reserve typical develops during childhood and adolescence, it may be possible to strengthen it during adulthood. If so, medically vulnerable patients could work to develop greater cognitive reserve to improve potential future cognitive outcomes against brain insults such as critical illness.

Duration of Impairment

The permanence of cognitive impairment after critical illness is unknown, as few studies have evaluated the natural history of cognitive functioning for more than 12 months after hospital discharge. The available data suggest that most individuals with cognitive impairment have slight to moderate improvement in the first year following discharge, with little to no improvement in the following year, depending on the cognitive domains assessed [12]. Although it is difficult to objectively determine preexisting cognitive function in individuals admitted to the ICU [20], patient and family reports suggest that it is rare that survivors of critical illness ultimately return to their cognitive baseline [21]. In some individuals, particularly those with unrecognized early dementia, cognitive impairments may increase rather than improve over time, displaying the hallmarks of a progressive neurodegenerative syndrome. These patients are often later diagnosed with Alzheimer's disease, which likely progresses at a more accelerated rate than would have been the case absent a critical illness [22]. In contrast, many patients, including those with multiple risk factors for cognitive decline, maintain robust cognitive function long after critical illness. A key goal of future research should be to better understand what protects these individuals from neuropsychological and functional decline despite experiencing substantial neurologic insult.

Understanding Cognitive Disability

Relatively little attention has been paid to the real-world consequences of cognitive impairment in survivors of critical illness. The consequences of cognitive impairment, whether mild, moderate, or severe, are often profound, and they may have a dramatic impact on the ability of a patient to perform functional activities of daily living, crossing the line from impairment to disability. While the definition of disability as it relates to cognitive impairment varies depending on the descriptive framework used, it can be broadly considered as the acute and chronic impact of pathological conditions on one's daily functioning and quality of life [23]. In general, the interrelationships between preexisting illness and the acute stressors of critical illness on long-term daily functioning are complex [24]. As such, additional long-term outcomes research is needed to show the impact of disability resulting from PICS-related cognitive impairment and to identify potential treatments.

According to some studies, executive dysfunction is the most common and potentially the most disabling cognitive impairment in survivors of critical illness. Executive function enables individuals to take part in purposeful, goal-directed activities via the mechanisms of initiating, shifting, planning, sequencing, and inhibiting ideas and actions [25,26] Although these functions may be partially retained when cognitive impairment occurs, key elements are often overlooked or disregarded when subjects are faced with both simple and demanding tasks. Many influential theorists consider executive dysfunction to be a "goal neglect" syndrome, in which individuals are unable

> **Box 43.1** The impacts of cognitive impairment (Richard's story)
>
> Sometimes people with executive dysfunction develop idiosyncratic workarounds that can be both inefficient and fraught with risk. One of my patients created his own system for taking about 20 different medications a day, as he was overwhelmed by the idea of setting up and keeping to a pill schedule. Instead of taking them as prescribed, he put one of each pill in a bottle every morning and swallowed them all together with a glass of water. One day, he came home from the pharmacy with a prescription for warfarin, a potentially lethal blood thinner, and, distracted by an old episode of his favorite television show "Wheel of Fortune," he inadvertently swallowed the full bottle of 30 warfarin pills, thinking he was taking the bottle filled with his daily supply. He spent a week in the hospital undergoing observation due to concerns about a cerebral hemorrhage.

to structure their behaviors to develop successful plans of action and achieve desired results [27,28,29]. These individuals often experience deficits in domains in addition to executive functioning, including problem-solving, memory, and attention, which can precipitate problems with retaining, recalling, and articulating information [30]. This inability to maintain sustained focus on tasks combined with neglect of task requirements often leads to real-world challenges, such as difficulty managing finances or medications, cooking meals, and shopping for groceries (see Box 43.1).

Distinguishing Cognitive Impairment from Dementia

Although PICS-related cognitive impairment has historically been considered by some studies to be a form of dementia due to similarities in symptom presentation (see Table 43.1), it is clinically far more similar to an acquired brain injury (ABI) given its acute onset during critical illness and subsequent trajectory. Unlike dementia, which usually has an inexorably progressive course, ABIs tend to be static rather than degenerative over time; they occur abruptly, driven by a medical event, and while they may or may not improve, they rarely get substantially worse, unless influenced by other variables such as aging or the experience of new insults. While ABIs typically involve structural damage, they are also characterized by alterations in neurotransmitters, such as increased glutamate release, and neuro-inflammation, both of which are associated with the development of brain injury [31]. Cognitive impairments due to critical illness impact patients across the entire spectrum of age, unlike dementia, which predominantly impacts older individuals. People experiencing PICS-related long-term cognitive impairment, such as those with ABI, frequently experience increased difficulty with daily functioning. For example, they may have diminished ability to take part in hobbies, engage in functional socialization, or perform in academic or professional settings, though these difficulties are typically less profound than those seen in the most common dementia, Alzheimer's disease [3,32,33]. Hindered by deficits in retaining information, maintaining attention, organizing, and planning, these individuals widely report moderately severe challenges with instrumental activities of daily living (IADLs), driving, and employment [34]. Indeed, nearly half of patients who are employed prior to critical illness are unable to return to work one year following hospital discharge (see Chapter 44 for additional information) [35].

Table 43.1 Acquired brain injury versus degenerative dementia

	Brain Injury	Dementia
Onset	Abrupt/Immediate	Gradual
Domains Effected	Multiple Domains	Predominately Single Domain
Trajectory	May Improve/Treatable	Degenerative
Risk Factors	ICU Hospitalization	Old Age/Genetics

Cognitive Screening

The importance of detecting cognitive impairment early is widely agreed upon by psychiatrists, neuropsychologists, neurologists, and other professionals caring for this patient population. Failure to identify cognitive impairment though cognitive screening or assessment may lead to diminished functional ability and increased caregiver burden when resources are not provided to support the patient and their family members. Delayed detection of cognitive impairment in the outpatient setting further postpones cognitive rehabilitation referral, which has been shown to improve cognitive functioning [36,37]. When one thinks about selection of cognitive screening tests, key considerations include ease and timing of administration in addition to their sensitivity and specificity for detecting cognitive impairment. Ideally, the tests used should be short enough to be tolerated by patients yet sensitive and specific enough to reliably identify cognitive impairments.

Delirium Screening Tools

Screening patients in the ICU for cognitive disorders is challenging as patients may be mechanically ventilated, sedated, delirious, fatigued, or have other difficulties communicating (see Chapters 8 and 13 for additional information). The Intensive Care Delirium Screening Checklist (ICDSC) [38,39] and the Confusion Assessment Method for the Intensive Care Unit (CAM-ICU) [40,41] are the most commonly used screening tools in the ICU to detect delirium quickly and accurately. Importantly, these screening tools do not assess cognitive function per se, but delirium, which is a robust risk factor for long-term cognitive impairment. Following transfer to a ward or hospital discharge, other instruments, including more comprehensive and sophisticated neuropsychological assessments, are used to assess cognition. Self-report measures, such as the Cognitive Failures Questionnaire, may be limited by self-assessment bias, but they provide insight on the patient's or family member's perceived level of impairment [42].

Outpatient Screening Tools

The MMSE was long considered the gold standard cognitive screening test and includes 11 questions that assess orientation, attention, memory, and calculation [43]. Despite many attractive features, including its brevity (can be administered in under 10 minutes) [44], in one study, it failed to predict cognitive impairment at 6 months in a population of critical illness survivors and should therefore be interpreted with caution in this patient population [45]. Indeed, data from Honarmand and colleagues found that the prevalence of cognitive impairment was lower when using the MMSE compared with more comprehensive neuropsychological test batteries [12]. The Montreal Cognitive Assessment (MoCA) tool is a rapid screening questionnaire that covers several domains of cognitive function, including visuospatial and executive function, naming, memory, attention, language, abstraction, delayed recall, and orientation [46]. It is scored out of a maximum of 30 points, with an additional point given to patients with 12 or fewer years of formal education; scores less than 26 are consistent with cognitive impairment. Alternate versions of the MoCA exist to accommodate patients with visual impairment (MoCA-BLIND) and those being evaluated via telephone (t-MoCA). The MoCA had been used to screen individuals with mild cognitive impairment who often obtain normal scores on the MMSE; one study validating its use among sepsis survivors found that it had lower sensitivity but higher specificity at six months, and as such, its threshold for detecting abnormalities may be too high in this population [47]. The Society of Critical Care Medicine's International Consensus Conference on Prediction and Identification of Long-Term Impairments after Critical Illness recommends using the MoCA in ICU follow-up assessments to screen for cognitive impairments [20].

Assessing for Preexisting Cognitive Impairment

A key challenge in screening for cognitive impairment after critical illness is determining whether the cognitive problems identified are a reflection of preexisting deficits or whether they are a consequence of the critical illness [14]. In patients undergoing elective surgery, for example, objective neuropsychological baselines can be obtained prior to hospitalization, but the same is not true for patients presenting with unpredictable illnesses necessitating hospital admission. In these patients, the most widely employed method of estimating a person's cognitive baseline is to use surrogate measures that provide estimates of a person's cognitive ability at specific points in time, including the presence or absence of a pattern of cognitive decline [8,48]. The most widely used surrogate measure of cognition is the Informant Questionnaire of Cognitive Decline in the Elderly (IQCODE) [49]. The IQCODE evaluates the magnitude of change (on a five-point scale that goes from "much better" to "much worse") that is observed across diverse areas of functioning, such as memory, learning, intelligence, and decision-making [50]. Patients with a mean score of 3.3 or more are believed to have preexisting cognitive impairment.

Self-Report Tools

The selection of instruments and approaches used to screen for cognitive impairment requires a nuanced and multifactorial approach that can vary widely depending on an individual's cognitive function, primary language, or hospitalization status at the time of screening. While cognitive screening tools aid in identifying mild, moderate, or severe cognitive impairment, self-report tools shed light on the individual's or caregiver's perception of impairment and its impact on activities of daily living (ADLs) [51]. The results of a positive screening test during hospitalization or immediately following discharge should be carefully considered alongside self- and caregiver reports regarding the ability to complete ADLs, manage financial and personal affairs, and meaningfully socialize. Informant-based measures, such as the Functional Activities Questionnaire (FAQ) [52], should be used in conjunction with cognitive assessments to best understand the full scope of impairment that a patient may be experiencing, as these are designed to capture even subtle deficits that are often overlooked in survivors of critical illness.

Approaches to Cognitive Rehabilitation

Since the advent of research on cognitive outcomes after critical illness, cognitive rehabilitation has rarely been employed in the treatment of impaired patients. Reasons for this are unclear, but it may be that the impairments experienced by survivors of critical illness have seldom been viewed as a brain injury with recovery potential and more often viewed as a persistent dementia unamenable to rehabilitation. Such thinking is incorrect and potentially harmful to patients, whose cognitive functioning could plausibly be enhanced by a variety of interventions. By viewing PICS-related cognitive impairment as an ABI, various forms of cognitive rehabilitation can be used to improve overall cognitive functioning and improve quality of life. Cognitive rehabilitation, defined as a functionally oriented and systematic approach to assess and improve one's cognitive deficits [53], is widely regarded as an effective treatment in many neurological diseases and injuries and has been shown to restore function or compensate for deficits in multiple cognitive domains, including memory, attention, and overall executive functioning [54,55,56,57].

Compensatory and Restorative Strategies

The strategies and methodologies implemented for cognitive rehabilitation can be described as either *compensatory* or *restorative*. A *compensatory* approach focuses on developing and reinforcing adaptive behaviors to accommodate cognitive limitations, while a *restorative* approach takes advantage of neuroplasticity to improve cognitive function [53,57,58]. Box 43.2 provides an example of the compensatory approach being used in the treatment of cognitive impairment and demonstrates the positive impact these strategies can have on daily functioning [59]. Unlike a restorative approach, a compensatory method is not designed to repair neural pathways or make structural changes to the brain, and as such, its key aims are to increase the individual's awareness of their deficits and to formulate compensatory strategies to improve daily functioning [60]. Examples of compensatory cognitive rehabilitation strategies include the use of aids (e.g., calendars and notebooks)

Box 43.2 Cognitive rehabilitation vignette using a compensatory approach

A 69-year-old woman enrolled in a cognitive rehabilitation study following discharge from the emergency department. She expressed frustration over consistently misplacing her bank card. In the past, she has hidden her bank card and then been unable to find it, causing her significant distress. She adds that she has difficulty with her mobility, and some days, she is unable to walk to her front door, leaving the bank card on her bedside table instead. Other days, she will leave the card somewhere by her front door.

To compensate for her thinking and memory problems, study staff suggests that she find a single, designated spot where she will always put her bank card, regardless of mobility, and place a post-it note at this location that reads "BANK CARD." They discuss how this novel approach may help her keep track of it, and she agrees to try it. The following week, study staff returns for the next cognitive rehabilitation session. She informs staff that the bank card strategy they had set up the week prior was a success. She explains, "I did not realize making such a slight change would make such an enormous difference. By always leaving the card in the same place, I never have to worry about it getting lost, and I have saved myself a lot of anxiety."

Table 43.2 Pros and cons of cognitive rehabilitation

Pros	Cons
Improves cognitive functioning	Not covered by most health insurance
Has lasting benefits	Not widely available
Adaptable and able to personalize	Requires time/dedication
May increase autonomy/independence	Less effective for severe cognitive impairment
Can be administered by a variety of healthcare professionals	Requires trained personnel

and association and organizational techniques to compensate for memory deficits. Another type of compensatory approach to improve daily functioning is the *metacognitive* approach, which aims to strengthen higher-order skills such as evaluating, monitoring, and regulating oneself by using self-talk techniques and problem-solving strategies to rehabilitate executive dysfunction [57].

In contrast, *restorative* approaches to cognitive rehabilitation promote neural growth and rely on the concept of neuroplasticity to improve cognitive function. Neuroplasticity is defined as the ability of the brain to alter its structure, function, or activity in response to internal or external stimuli [61]. Changes in brain structure and neuroplasticity can lead to behavioral changes and are the basis of restorative cognitive rehabilitation [62]. Cognitive rehabilitation of memory may be achieved through awareness training corresponding to various attention levels (i.e., focused, sustained, and selective) to repair neural networks. In contrast to the compensatory approach to cognitive rehabilitation, a restorative approach requires no awareness of deficits to be effective [61,62,63,64]. Table 43.2 highlights the advantages and limitations of cognitive rehabilitation approaches.

Pharmacology

Although pharmacologic agents have not conventionally been used in the management of cognitive impairment following critical illness, questions exist about appropriating pharmacologic strategies used in patients with other cognitive challenges including attention deficit disorder (ADD) and attention deficit hyperactivity disorder (ADHD). Alongside compensatory and restorative approaches to the treatment of cognitive impairment, the potential benefits of pharmacology should be considered, particularly when patients display an attention-deficit-related clinical phenotype. In other conditions that are similar to PICS-related cognitive impairment, such as the "brain fog" (i.e., confusion, lack of focus, and cognitive slowness) described in Long Covid survivors [65] (see Chapter 53 for additional information), one drug that is increasingly used is guanfacine. Guanfacine, a noradrenergic α_{2A} agonist that is primarily used in the treatment of ADHD and hypertension, has been shown in recent studies to improve network connections within the prefrontal cortex, leading to improvement in behavioral, thought, and emotional regulation [66]. As such, the potential cognitive benefits of guanfacine and related medications may be considered when developing a treatment plan for PICS-related cognitive impairment.

Conclusion, Limitations, and Future Directions

Despite being a serious problem that adversely impacts daily functioning and quality of life in millions of patients worldwide, cognitive impairment in survivors of critical illness receives much less attention than it deserves, although awareness is beginning to increase. As data from dozens of papers now attest, as many as one in three survivors of critical illness have personally meaningful and clinically significant neuropsychological deficits in wide-ranging domains, such as attention, executive functioning, memory, processing speed, visuospatial abilities, and language [67,68]. These problems have various clinical expressions, reflecting mild to moderate ABIs [3,32,33]. Risk factors for new or worsening cognitive impairment after critical illness have been extensively evaluated, and while researchers have been effective in determining the contributions of certain variables to cognitive decline, including advanced age, delirium duration, and prior cognitive abnormalities, efforts to prevent cognitive impairment from emerging after critical illness remain in their infancy.

While we look forward to one day implementing preventative strategies, clinicians must now rely on therapeutic and restorative strategies that have a long history of success in transforming the lives and functioning of other populations with neuropsychological deficits. Cognitive rehabilitation appears to have significant potential for the improvement of daily functioning in survivors of critical illness, although it remains a highly under-employed strategy [57]. Future research must prioritize more fully understanding the nature of cognitive impairment after critical illness – as insights about mechanisms and origins will no doubt accelerate the integration of effective treatments – while developing programs, practices, and protocols that will routinely engage patients in rehabilitation-related treatments, with the goal that such treatments will become the norm, not the exception.

Key Points

1. Long-term cognitive impairment following critical illness often persists, resulting in deficits in memory, attention, and executive functioning.
2. Protective factors, such as education level and lifestyle factors, contribute to cognitive reserve and may decrease the likelihood of cognitive impairment following critical illness.
3. Compensatory and restorative cognitive rehabilitation strategies may improve cognitive function and quality of life.
4. Further research is needed to better understand the trajectories of post-ICU cognitive impairment, potential protective factors, and treatment and intervention strategies.

References

1. M.S. Herridge, C.M. Tansey, A. Matte, et al. Functional disability 5 years after acute respiratory distress syndrome. *N Engl J Med* 2011; 364(14): 1293–304.
2. J.C. Jackson, P.P. Pandharipande, T.D. Girard, et al. Depression, post-traumatic stress disorder, and functional disability in survivors of critical illness in the BRAIN-ICU study: a longitudinal cohort study. *Lancet Respir Med* 2014; 2(5): 369–79.

3. P.P. Pandharipande, T.D. Girard, E.W. Ely. Long-term cognitive impairment after critical illness. *N Engl J Med* 2014; **370**(2): 185–6.

4. D.M. Needham, J. Davidson, H. Cohen, et al. Improving long-term outcomes after discharge from intensive care unit: report from a stakeholders' conference. *Crit Care Med* 2012; **40**(2): 502–9.

5. L. McCollum, J. Karlawish. Cognitive impairment: evaluation and management. *Med Clin North Am* 2020; **104**(5): 807–25.

6. T.D. Girard, R.S. Dittus, E.W. Ely. Critical illness brain injury. *Annu Rev Med* 2016; **67**: 497–513.

7. J.C. Jackson, R.P. Hart, S.M. Gordon, et al. Six-month neuropsychological outcome of medical intensive care unit patients. *Crit Care Med* 2003; **31**(4): 1226–34.

8. P.P. Pandharipande, T.D. Girard, J.C. Jackson, et al. Long-term cognitive impairment after critical illness. *N Engl J Med* 2013; **369**(14): 1306–16.

9. M.D. Hashem, R.O. Hopkins, E. Colantuoni, et al. Six-month and 12-month patient outcomes based on inflammatory subphenotypes in sepsis-associated ARDS: secondary analysis of SAILS-ALTOS trial. *Thorax* 2022; **77**(1): 22–30.

10. D.M. Needham, V.D. Dinglas, P.E. Morris, et al. Physical and cognitive performance of patients with acute lung injury 1 year after initial trophic versus full enteral feeding: EDEN trial follow-up. *Am J Respir Crit Care Med* 2013; **188**(5): 567–76.

11. P.J. Schulte, D.O. Warner, D.P. Martin, et al. Association between critical care admissions and cognitive trajectories in older adults. *Crit Care Med* 2019; **47**(8): 1116–24.

12. K. Honarmand, R.S. Lalli, F. Priestap, et al. Natural history of cognitive impairment in critical illness survivors: a systematic review. *Am J Respir Crit Care Med* 2020; **202**(2): 193–201.

13. R.O. Hopkins. Understanding cognitive outcome trajectories after critical illness. *Crit Care Med* 2019; **47**(8): 1164–6.

14. R.O. Hopkins, J.C. Jackson. Long-term neurocognitive function after critical illness. *Chest* 2006; **130**(3): 869–78.

15. J.F. Peterson, D.E. Penner, P. Harrison, et al. Clinical outcomes after implementing a computer-based protocol for sustained use of sedation and analgesia in the ICU. *Am J Respir Crit Care Med* 2004; **169**: A45.

16. D.H. Davis, G. Muniz Terrera, et al. Delirium is a strong risk factor for dementia in the oldest-old: a population-based cohort study. *Brain* 2012; **135**(Pt 9): 2809–16.

17. A.M. MacLullich, A. Beaglehole, R.J. Hall, D.J. Meagher. Delirium and long-term cognitive impairment. *Int Rev Psychiatry* 2009; **21**(1): 30–42.

18. M.E. Mikkelsen, M. Still, B.J. Anderson, et al. Society of Critical Care Medicine's International Consensus Conference on prediction and identification of long-term impairments after critical illness. *Crit Care Med* 2020; **48**(2): S208–19.

19. Y. Stern, Y. Gazes, Q. Razlighi, et al. A task-invariant cognitive reserve network. *NeuroImage* 2018; **178**: 36–45.

20. R.O. Hopkins, S. Brett. Chronic neurocognitive effects of critical illness. *Curr Opin Crit Care* 2005; **11**(4): 369–75.

21. J.C. Jackson, R.O. Hopkins, R.R. Miller, et al. Acute respiratory distress syndrome, sepsis, and cognitive decline: a review and case study. *South Med J* 2009; **102**(11): 1150–7.

22. C. Guerra, W.T. Linde-Zwirble, H. Wunsch. Risk factors for dementia after critical illness in elderly medicare beneficiaries. *Crit Care* 2012; **16**(6): R233.

23. L.M. Verbrugge, A.M. Jette. The disablement process. *Soc Sci Med* 1994; **38**(1): 1–14.

24. T.M. Gill. Disentangling the disabling process: insights from the precipitating events project. *Gerontologist* 2014; **54**(4): 533–49.

25. P.W. Burgess. Theory and methodology in executive function research. In: Rabbitt P. (ed.), *Methodology of Frontal and Executive Function*. London: Oxford University Press; 1997, pp. 79–108.

26. J.K. Foster, S.E. Black, B.H. Buck, M. J. Bronskill. Methodology of frontal and executive function. In: Rabbit P. (ed.), *Methodology of Frontal and Executive Function*. Hove: Psychology Press; 1997, pp. 117–34.

27. J. Duncan, E.H. Williams, P. Johnson, C. Freer. Intelligence and the frontal lobe: the organisation of goal-directed behavior. *Cogn Psychol* 1996; **30**: 257–303.

28. J. Duncan, A. Parr, A. Woolgar, et al. Goal neglect and Spearman's g: competing parts of a complex task. *J Exp Psychol Gen* 2008; **137**(1): 131–48.

29. S. Nieuwenhuis, B.A. Nielen, R. de Jong. A goal activation approach to the study of executive function: an application to antisaccade tasks. *Brain Cogn* 2004; **56**: 198–214.

30. E.J. Overdorp, R.P.C. Kessels, J. A. Claassen, J.M. Oosterman. The combined effect of neuropsychological and neuropathological deficits on instrumental activities of daily living in older adults: a systematic review. *Neuropsychol Rev* 2016; **26**(1): 92–106.

31. M. Pekna, M. Pekny. The neurobiology of brain injury. *Cerebrum* 2012; **2012**: 9.

32. J.M. Uomoto. Older adults and neuropsychological rehabilitation following acquired brain injury. *NeuroRehabilitation*. 2008 23(5): 415–24.

33. L.E. Ferrante, M.A. Pisani, T.E. Murphy, et al. Functional trajectories among older persons before and after critical illness. *JAMA Intern Med* 2015; **175**(4): 523–9.

34. D.B. Cooper, A.E. Bunner, J.E. Kennedy, et al. Treatment of persistent post-concussive symptoms after mild traumatic brain injury: a systematic review of cognitive rehabilitation and behavioral health interventions in military service members and veterans. *Brain Imaging Behav* 2015; **9**(3): 403–20.

35. H. Myhren, O. Ekeberg, O. Stokland. Health-related quality of life and return to work after critical illness in general intensive care unit patients: a 1-year follow-up study. *Crit Care Med* 2010; **38**(7): 1554–61.

36. M.R. Ho, T.L. Bennett. Efficacy of neuropsychological rehabilitation for mild-moderate traumatic brain injury. *Arch Clin Neuropsychol* 1997; **12**(1): 1–11.

37. S.M. Gordon, J.C. Jackson, E.W. Ely, et al. Clinical identification of cognitive impairment in ICU survivors: insights for intensivists. *Intensive Care Med* 2004; **30** (11): 1997–2008.

38. N. Bergeron, M.J. Dubois, M. Dumont, et al. Intensive Care Delirium Screening Checklist: evaluation of a new screening tool. *Intensive Care Med* 2001; **27**(5): 859–64.

39. M.J. Dubois, N. Bergeron, M. Dumont, et al. Delirium in an intensive care unit: a study of risk factors. *Intensive Care Med* 2001; **27**(8): 1297–304.

40. E.W. Ely, S.K. Inouye, G.R. Bernard, et al. Delirium in mechanically ventilated patients: validity and reliability of the confusion assessment method for the intensive care unit (CAM-ICU). *JAMA*. 2001 **286**(21): 2703–10.

41. E.W. Ely, R. Margolin, J. Francis, et al. Evaluation of delirium in critically ill patients: validation of the Confusion Assessment Method for the Intensive Care Unit (CAM-ICU). *Crit Care Med* 2001; **29**(7): 1370–9.

42. D.E. Broadbent, P.F. Cooper, P. FitzGerald, K.R. Parkes. The Cognitive Failures Questionnaire (CFQ) and its correlates. *Br J Clin Psychol* 1982; **21**(1): 1–16.

43. M.F. Folstein, L.N. Robins, J.E. Helzer. The Mini-Mental State Examination. *Arch Gen Psychiatry* 1983; **40**(7): 812.

44. E.R. Pfoh, K.S. Chan, V.D. Dinglas, et al. Cognitive screening among acute respiratory failure survivors: a cross-sectional evaluation of the Mini-Mental State Examination. *Crit Care* 2015; **19**: 220.

45. F.L. Woon, C.B. Dunn, R.O. Hopkins. Predicting cognitive sequelae in survivors of critical illness with cognitive screening tests. *Am J Respir Crit Care Med* 2012; **186** (4): 333–40.

46. Z.S. Nasreddine, N.A. Phillips, V. Bedirian, et al. The Montreal Cognitive Assessment (MoCA): a brief screening tool for mild

cognitive impairment. *J Am Geriatr Soc* 2005; **53**(4): 695–9.

47. S.M. Brown, D.S. Collingridge, E.L. Wilson, et al. Preliminary validation of the Montreal Cognitive Assessment tool among sepsis survivors: a prospective pilot study. *Ann Am Thorac Soc* 2018; **15**(9): 1108–10.

48. B. Johnstone, C.D. Callahan, C.J. Kapila, D.E. Bouman. The comparability of the WRAT-R reading test and NAART as estimates of premorbid intelligence in neurologically impaired patients. *Arch Clin Neuropsychol* 1996; **11**(6): 513–19.

49. A.F. Jorm, P.A. Jacomb. The Informant Questionnaire on Cognitive Decline in the Elderly (IQCODE): socio-demographic correlates, reliability, validity, and some norms. *Psychol Med* 1989; **19**(4): 1015–22.

50. A.F. Jorm. The Informant Questionnaire on cognitive decline in the elderly (IQCODE): a review. *Int Psychogeriatr* 2004; **16**(3): 275–93.

51. W.J. Lorentz, J.M. Scanlan, S. Borson. Brief screening tests for dementia. *Can J Psychiatry* 2002; **47**(8): 723–33.

52. R.I. Pfeffer, T.T. Kurosaki, C.H. Harrah Jr, et al. Measurement of functional activities in older adults in the community. *J Gerontol* 1982; **37**(3): 323–9.

53. K.D. Cicerone, D.M. Langenbahn, C. Braden, et al. Evidence-based cognitive rehabilitation: updated review of the literature from 2003 through 2008. *Arch Phys Med Rehabil* 2011; **92**(4): 519–30.

54. M. Mulhern. Cognitive rehabilitation interventions for post-stroke populations. *Dela J Public Health* 2023; **9**(3): 70–4.

55. J. Rajan, S. Udupa, S. Bharat. Hypoxia: can neuropsychological rehabilitation attenuate neuropsychological dysfunction? *Indian J Psychol Med* 2010; **32**(1): 65–8.

56. F.R. Freire, F. Coelho, J.R. Lacerda, et al. Cognitive rehabilitation following traumatic brain injury. *Dement Neuropsychol* 2011; **5**(1): 17–25.

57. L.T. Kirsch-Darrow, J.W. Tsao. Cognitive rehabilitation. *Continuum (Minneap Minn)* 2021; **27**(6): 1670–81.

58. R. Parente, M. Stapleton. History and systems of cognitive rehabilitation. *NeuroRehabilitation* 1997; **8**(1): 3–11.

59. D. Dirette. The development of awareness and the use of compensatory strategies for cognitive deficits. *Brain Inj* 2002; **16**(10): 861–71.

60. D.K. Bertens, E. Fiorenzato, D. Boelen, L. Fasotti. Do old errors always lead to new truths? A randomized controlled trial of errorless goal management training in brain-injured patients. *J Int Neuropsychol Soc* 2015; **21**(8): 639–49.

61. V. Galetto, K. Sacco. Neuroplastic changes induced by cognitive rehabilitation in traumatic brain injury: a review. *Neurorehabil Neural Repair* 2017; **31**(9): 800–13.

62. I.H. Robertson, J.M. Murre. Rehabilitation of brain damage: brain plasticity and principles of guided recovery. *Psychol Bull* 1999; **125**(5): 544–75.

63. Z. Warraich, J.A. Kleim. Neural plasticity: the biological substrate for neurorehabilitation. *PM R* 2010; **2**(12 Suppl 2): S208-19.

64. M.M. Sohlberg, K.A. McLaughlin, A. Pavese, et al. Evaluation of attention process training and brain injury education in persons with acquired brain injury. *J Clin Exp Neuropsychol* 2000; **22**(5): 656–76.

65. L.M. Laura, H.S. Heather, I.H. Ingrid, et al. What is brain fog? *J Neurol Neurosurg Psychiatry* 2023; **94**(4): 321.

66. A.F. Arnsten, L.E. Jin. Guanfacine for the treatment of cognitive disorders: a century of discoveries at Yale. *Yale J Biol Med* 2012; **85**(1): 45–58.

67. R.O. Hopkins, L.K. Weaver, D. Pope, et al. Neuropsychological sequelae and impaired health status in survivors of severe ARDS. *Am J Respir Crit Care Med* 1999; **160**(1): 50–6.

68. H.B. Rothenhausler, S. Ehrentraut, C. Stoll, et al. The relationship between cognitive performance and employment and health status in long-term survivors of the acute respiratory distress syndrome: results of an exploratory study. *Gen Hosp Psychiatry* 2001; **23**(2): 88–94.

Resuming Employment and Driving

Dharmanand Ramnarain, Ricarda Pingel, Maria Twichell, and Sjaak Pouwels

Introduction

For many, ideal recovery after critical illness means resuming normal activities and achieving an acceptable quality of life, which often includes returning to work and being able to drive a vehicle safely. Resumption of employment and driving are considerable challenges for many survivors of critical illness, as the constellation of physical, cognitive, and psychological impairments from which they suffer frequently makes resuming employment and driving difficult [1,2,3]. Driving, in particular, represents independence for many people and is frequently necessary to resume employment, enjoy leisure activities, and reintegrate into society.

Return to Work

The first major study demonstrating the inability to return to work in survivors of critical illness was by Herridge and colleagues, who found that only 49% of 109 survivors of the acute respiratory distress syndrome were able to return to work one year following hospital discharge [4]. In a five-year follow-up of the same patient cohort, 77% of patients had returned to work, and of these, 94% had returned to their original job; the majority of patients who returned to work did so by two years. Patients who resumed employment often required a gradual transition to work, a modified work schedule, or job retraining [5,6]. A subsequent study of 316 previously employed survivors of critical illness by Mattioni and colleagues highlighted the prevalence of impairments in survivors of critical illness that make the resumption of employment challenging: at the time of ICU discharge, cognitive dysfunction was present in 66% of survivors, muscle weakness in 76%, anxiety in 60%, and depression in 79%. Three months after discharge, 79% of patients remained physically dependent and 51% had functional impairments not present prior to their critical illness; consequently, only 39% of patients had returned to work despite an overwhelming desire to do so in those who could not [7]. Complementary studies suggest that although physical impairments often improve, cognitive impairment, emotional impairment, and interpersonal impairment remain present in a significant percentage of survivors of critical illness for as many as twelve months or longer after discharge. Perhaps not surprisingly, the more severe the impairments, the less likely the patient is to return to work [8,9].

Risk Factors Associated with Failure to Return to Work

The ability to return to work following critical illness is complex, and there are multiple patient-related and demographic factors that have been associated with a delayed return to work. Age is a major factor that negatively impacts the ability to successfully return to work;

the likelihood of returning to work decreases by 4% with each year of increasing age [10]. The severity of illness, including the hospital length of stay and the need for and duration of mechanical ventilation and other organ-supporting therapies, also decreases the ability to resume work after critical illness [6,10,11,12]. For example, in studies by both Fleischmann-Struzek and colleagues [11] and Skei and colleagues [12], the severity of sepsis was negatively associated with the ability to return to work. Survivors who were able to resume employment after one year were less likely to have had sepsis-related organ dysfunction than those who did not return to work. Similarly, in a study by Riddersholm and colleagues, the percentage of patients who returned to work after requiring organ support therapy was 65%, irrespective of the number of organs requiring support, while 75% of patients who did not receive organ support therapy returned to work within two years [13]. In addition to age and illness severity, a low level of education is also associated with a failure to return to work [14].

Return to Work Over Time

Several studies have investigated the extent to which survivors of critical illness are able to return to work at different points in time. These studies show that only 23–39% of patients return to work within three months after discharge from the intensive care unit (ICU) [4,7,12], a number which increases to approximately 40–53% at six months and 55–77% at one year [6,7,8,9,10,11]. Data on return to work in the long-term is scarce; in a study by Skei and colleagues, 52% of survivors of critical illness had returned to work after two years [12], and in the aforementioned study by Herridge and colleagues, 77% had returned to work within five years [5]. These findings are substantiated by a meta-analysis by Kamdar and colleagues, which found that 36% to 68% of survivors of critical illness had returned to work in a follow-up period of 1 to 60 months [15].

Return to Work and Employment Outcomes

After a critical illness, many patients have to take a prolonged absence or accept early retirement [11]. Many of those who do return to work have to change jobs (e.g., taking a role with lesser responsibility), have reduced employment status (e.g., transition from full-time to part-time employment), or ultimately lose their job entirely [15]. Up to 29% of those who return to work retire within the first year [13]. Not being able to return to work is associated with significant financial burden given the lack of generated income accompanied by persistent healthcare costs [4,14]; such financial stress is frequently associated with a negative impact on mental health and quality of life.

Medical Clearance and Functional Capacity Evaluations

Returning to work is an important goal for many survivors of critical illness, as health-related quality of life and mental health are positively influenced by being able to resume employment [14]. Early identification of survivors with a high risk of delayed return to work is important in order to provide targeted prevention and rehabilitation measures as well as aftercare. Employers can support their employees' return to work after a serious illness by recognizing the psychosocial challenges they may face, understanding each individual's unique needs, and encouraging open communication throughout the return-to-work process. It is also crucial that employers are aware of the physical and cognitive impacts of critical illness and are prepared to adapt the workplace to meet the employee's specific needs. Effective communication, the involvement of healthcare professionals, and a targeted rehabilitation approach can contribute significantly to the employee's successful reintegration into the labor market [1,5,6,16].

Medical clearance prior to resuming employment is often required by employers, particularly in the United States. Determining medical clearance requires an understanding of the patient's medical condition, residual deficits, and requirements for the job setting. Such requirements may be found in the employer-provided job description, which lists the physical, cognitive, and social skills required to perform the job safely and the frequency with which the employee needs to use these skills (e.g., constantly, frequently, occasionally, or never). Additional information from the multidisciplinary team is helpful in determining if the patient can safely meet their job requirements, including information gleaned from outpatient therapy notes detailing the patient's strength, endurance, range of motion, and progress. Speech and language pathologists can provide an assessment of the patient's cognitive strengths and deficits, and collateral information obtained (with appropriate medical releases in place) from a patient's psychological care provider can provide information regarding the patient's emotional state.

A functional capacity evaluation (FCE) is a specialized inventory of tasks outlining a patient's current physical abilities required for return to work [17]. Physicians write the prescription for the FCE, which is then performed by a physical therapist or occupational therapist trained to administer the assessment. The FCE evaluates the patient's abilities to lift prescribed weight to various heights, carry, push/pull, and to maintain positions such as sitting, standing, walking, and crawling. It also assesses the use of hands for manipulation of objects, grasping, and finger movements. Imbedded measures of validity and effort are documented [18]. The results are compared to the Dictionary of Occupational Titles published by the United States Department of Labor to categorize current physical abilities. An FCE can also be used to develop a treatment program and evaluate the results after completion.

If a patient is deemed unready (physically, cognitively, or psychologically) to return to their prior work environment, modifications to hours or responsibilities can be outlined by the physician. In the United States, employers are not obligated to adhere to these modifications unless the employee was injured at work, but it is beneficial to the employer and the worker to return to work as soon as possible [17].

Vocational Rehabilitation

Vocational rehabilitation is another tool to facilitate returning to work after a prolonged absence. Vocational rehabilitation utilizes multiple disciplines, including physical therapists, occupational therapists, occupational medicine, psychologists, psychiatrists, work counselors, job coaches, and others, depending on the available resources of the country [19]. Some countries have simulated work environments where the patient can be observed completing tasks specific to their work. Job coaches can suggest modifications to complete tasks more easily and may also accompany workers to their place of employment to provide suggestions on how to complete work within the patient's restrictions. The financial return after the initial cost of vocational rehabilitation can be 2–10 times the investment, accounting for mitigation of lost productivity [20].

Work disability is the disparity between an individual's capabilities and the demands of the workplace environment, and it includes biologic, mental, personal, and social aspects of disability [21], as defined by the World Health Organization's (WHO) International Classification of Functioning, Disability, and Health (ICF) [22]. Short-term disability forms can be filled out by any physician treating the patient, but a specialist with specific training in certifying work disability per the ICF should evaluate patients who are pursuing long-term disability.

Return to Driving

For many patients, the ability to drive represents independence and is important to reintegrate into social roles, return to employment, and resume avocations and leisure activities; as such, it is often considered a priority in a person's rehabilitation after critical illness [23]. Despite this, counseling regarding the ability to drive is largely absent from patient instructions provided at the time of hospital discharge. Meyer and colleagues, for example, reported that driving eligibility was mentioned in only 3% of affected patients' ICU discharge summaries, suggesting a clear deficiency in driving-related post-hospitalization guidance [23].

Cognitive impairments, such as deficits in attention, memory, and executive function, can hinder a driver's ability to process information, make decisions, and respond appropriately to traffic stimuli. Physical limitations, including weakness, decreased coordination, fatigue, and balance impairments, can affect a driver's ability to operate vehicular controls and execute maneuvers safely. Psychological sequelae, such as anxiety, depression, and post-traumatic stress disorder, can further strain a driver's confidence and decision-making ability, potentially leading to an accident or avoidance of driving altogether. Understanding the complex interplay of these factors is essential for effectively addressing driving disability following critical illness and promoting rehabilitation and road safety. Literature on resuming driving mainly focuses on patients with stroke, epilepsy, traumatic brain injury, and neurodegenerative disorders, such as Parkinson's disease and dementia. Little is known about driving disabilities in survivors of critical illness, who commonly experience the aforementioned cognitive, physical, and psychological impairments, collectively known as post-intensive care syndrome (PICS).

What Does the Available Literature in Survivors of Critical Illness Tell Us?

There are few studies regarding driving ability after critical illness. A report by Munn and colleagues found that 61% of patients who were able to drive before ICU admission were driving three months following hospital discharge, and the likelihood of regaining the ability to drive was inversely proportional to the severity of illness as defined by admission Acute Physiologic Assessment and Chronic Health Evaluation (APACHE) score [24]. In a study by Potter and colleagues, only 16 of 196 patients evaluated one month after ICU discharge had resumed driving; those who had returned to driving were less frail, more independent, and had better cognition scores (as determined by the Montreal Cognitive Assessment tool [MoCA]) than those who had not resumed driving. Perhaps surprisingly, 8 of the 16 patients who had resumed driving were cognitively impaired, as defined by a MoCA score less than 26 [25]. Importantly, lower MoCA scores are correlated with worse fitness-to-drive test ratings, questioning the ability to drive safely with even mild cognitive impairment [26].

Meyer and colleagues analyzed questionnaires given to 45 survivors of critical illness about their driving habits and found that 68%, 77%, and 84% had resumed driving at 3, 6, and 12 months, respectively [23]. In this group, 17 patients did not receive advice or information about how to resume driving safely. Thematic content analysis of patient interviews highlighted cognitive, psychological, and physical concerns about driving and a lack of information about when and how to safely return to driving. Cognitive and psychological concerns included lack of confidence in the ability to drive, lack of motivation to drive, and emotional lability and anxiety affecting driving performance, while physical concerns centered on weakness and fatigue. To receive guidance on how to resume driving, patients accessed several sources of information, including asking for advice from general practitioners or other medical providers. Advice received frequently focused on physical attributes requisite for driving with comparatively little attention paid to cognitive abilities and emotional state.

Many respondents reported different time frames in which they returned to driving, ranging from 1 to 52 weeks after hospital discharge, and some reported feeling unprepared to drive long distances [23]. Many patients valued information and exercises regarding how to safely return to driving, including taking a driving test and spending time with a driving instructor to build confidence and reacquaint themselves with previously familiar routes. Others practiced driving short distances initially to test their skills and then gradually increased their driving frequency and the distance covered.

In a qualitative study by Danesh and colleagues, a total of 15 survivors of critical illness participated in semi-structured interviews 3 weeks and 12 weeks after hospital discharge, with 3 major themes emerging: driving status, driving safety, and self-imposed driving modifications [27]. After 12 weeks, 4 patients reported driving without any subjective problems; 8 patients stopped driving because of fear of causing collisions, slow reaction time, lack of concentration, and daytime sleepiness; and 4 patients were driving with modifications, such as driving shorter distances, driving only to medical appointments, having another person ride along, or driving on private property only. This study demonstrated that, quite often, the decision to return to driving after critical illness is a personal one made by patients and their families rather than in consultation with healthcare professionals. These patients could, however, benefit from already existing driving assessment tools that are commonly employed in patients with dementia and neurological injuries as described below.

Assessment Tools Predicting Driving Ability

Driving ability is defined as the cognitive, perceptual, and motoric capacity of an individual to operate a vehicle safely [28,29]. Assessing driving ability after critical illness is important for ensuring safety on the road and promoting independence. These tools encompass various domains, including cognitive function, visual perception, motor skills, and on-road driving performance. Several assessment tools are available to evaluate different aspects of driving performance (see Table 44.1). The on-road driving test is considered the gold standard but is time consuming and costly [28,29].

To date, there is no single accepted clinical test or set of neuropsychological tests that can accurately predict the ability to safely return to driving in individual patients. Reasons for this include the heterogeneity of demographic and clinical characteristics of patients included in prior studies and the wide variability of the recovery process in patients with PICS. Because cognitive and behavioral impairment are the main causes of driving disability, some authors

Table 44.1 Overview of the most commonly used neuropsychological, cognitive, and physical tests to assess driving ability

Test Name	Description	Purpose	Interpretation
Trail Making Test Part B [36]	Assesses cognitive flexibility and executive functioning	Predicts on-road driving performance	A time of less than 78 seconds is considered within normal limits
Frontal Assessment Battery [37]	Evaluates executive functioning	Used for driving assessment after stroke or traumatic brain injury	A score of 12 or higher out of 18 suggests adequate executive function for safe driving
Stroke Driver Screening Assessment [38]	A screening tool that measures cognitive abilities important for driving	May have utility in predicting driving performance	Specific cut-off scores are used to determine the likelihood of passing or failing an on-road driving assessment
Useful Field of View Test [39]	Assesses visual attention and processing speed	Indicative of driving performance	A reduction of 40% or more in the useful field of view is associated with increased crash risk
Rey-O Complex Figure Test [40]	Measures visuospatial constructional ability and visual memory	Potential predictor of driving ability	No specific cut-off score provided but lower performance may indicate potential difficulties with driving
Mini-Mental State Examination (MMSE) [41]	A brief, 30-point questionnaire that is used to screen for cognitive impairment	Significant predictor of resuming driving after stroke	Scores below 24 out of 30 are generally considered indicative of cognitive impairment
Montreal Cognitive Assessment (MoCA) [42]	A rapid screening instrument for cognitive dysfunction assessing several cognitive domains	The test's attention and executive function tasks may be relevant for driving ability assessment	A score of 26 or higher is considered normal; scores below this may indicate cognitive deficits relevant to driving safety
On-Road Driving Test [43]	An actual driving test in a controlled environment to evaluate driving skills and behaviors	Directly assesses practical driving ability	This is a qualitative assessment, and the individual's performance is rated by a driving instructor or occupational therapist

Test	Description	Purpose	Guidelines
Brake Reaction Time [44]	Measures the time taken to respond to a stimulus by pressing the brake pedal	Assesses the driver's response time, which is critical for safe driving	Typically, a reaction time of less than 1.5 seconds is considered safe for driving
Range of Motion and Strength Assessment [45]	Evaluates the physical ability to control the vehicle, including steering and pedal operation	Determines if there are physical limitations affecting driving capability	There are no specific cut-off values, but the assessment determines if there are physical limitations affecting driving capability
Clock Drawing Test [46]	Assesses visuospatial and praxis abilities and may determine the presence of both impaired attention and executive dysfunction	Often used in conjunction with other screening tests like the MMSE for a quick assessment of cognitive functions relevant to driving	A markedly abnormal clock drawing is an important indication that the individual may have a cognitive deficit
Complex Figure Test [47]	Measures visuospatial constructional ability and visual memory	Used to evaluate cognitive functions that are relevant to driving	No specific guidelines provided, but performance may correlate with driving ability
Judgment of Line Orientation Test [48]	Assesses visuospatial abilities by requiring the individual to match the orientation of lines	Evaluates spatial perception	No specific guidelines provided, but performance may correlate with driving ability
Hooper Visual Organization Test [49]	Measures the ability to organize and categorize visual information	Assesses visual processing and organization skills relevant to driving	No specific guidelines provided, but performance may correlate with driving ability
Motor-Free Visual Perception Test [50]	Assesses visual perception independent of motor ability	Used to screen those with stroke or brain injury for visual perception deficits that could affect driving	No specific guidelines provided, but performance may correlate with driving ability

have advised performing a clinical neuropsychological evaluation prior to the resumption of driving, which can predict the probability of failing a driving test [30,31,32]. In a study by Fuermaier and colleagues, a combination of interviews, neuropsychological assessments, and driving simulator rides in patients with mild cognitive impairment showed high predictive accuracy in identifying patients unfit to drive when compared to an on-road driving evaluation (area under the curve [AUC] 0.944, standard error [SE] 0.052, $p = 0.003$) [30]. In a systematic review of existing guidelines and recommendations for patients with mild cognitive impairment and dementia, Stamatelos and colleagues found that there is no widely accepted approach to assess driving ability in these patient populations [33].

Rehabilitation for Regaining Driving Ability

Rehabilitation programs play a crucial role in helping individuals regain their driving abilities after a critical illness. Driving rehabilitation programs often use driving simulators and on-road training to address specific deficits and improve driving skills [34,35]. There are also online tools available for self-assessment of driving abilities (see Table 44.2). Given the complexity of driving, a multimodality therapy program may be necessary to adequately rehabilitate patients. Such a program may include physical therapy, which can improve the strength, coordination, and flexibility essential to operate a vehicle; occupational therapy, which focuses on improving activities of daily living, including driving, through cognitive and physical exercises; cognitive therapy, which enhances attention, memory, and problem-solving; and cognitive behavioral therapy, which addresses psychological barriers, such as fear of driving, which can impede the ability to drive [17]. Since visual skills are critical for driving, therapies to improve visual tracking, depth perception, and field of

Table 44.2 Available online assessment tools to determine cognitive fitness for driving

Assessment Tool	Description	Website Reference
CogniFit Driving Test	Evaluates cognitive abilities involved in driving and predicts vehicle handling capacity	www.cognifit.com/driving-test
CogniFit Brain Training for Driving	Trains essential cognitive abilities for safe and efficient driving	www.cognifit.com/driving-brain-training
Driving Decisions Workbook	Assesses functional ability and correlates scores with on-road driving scores	www.michigan.gov/-/media/Project/Websites/agingdriver/MDOT_DrivingDecisionsWorkbook.pdf?rev=94e63422849549b786042e3b990003f2
SkillCheck Driver Assessment Tool	Online course and assessment tool for improving employee driving skills	https://roadsafetyatwork.ca/resource/guide/skillcheck-driver-assessment-guide-and-form/
AAA Evaluate Your Driving Ability	Offers a self-rating tool and professional assessment for driving skills	https://exchange.aaa.com/safety/senior-driver-safety-mobility/evaluate-your-driving-ability/

vision can also be helpful. Rehabilitation programs often include education on adaptive driving equipment and techniques to compensate for any physical or cognitive limitations. It is important for survivors of critical illness to stay in close contact with their healthcare providers to determine the best approach for their individual needs.

Family Support Initiatives to Help Return to Driving

Family members can play a crucial role in supporting survivors of critical illness through their driving rehabilitation. They can provide emotional support and encourage patients to maintain a positive outlook during the rehabilitation process. They can help with prescribed physical and cognitive exercises at home; can coach skills necessary for driving; and offer rides to therapy sessions, driving evaluations, and medical appointments, attendance of which is vital for progress. Families can assist in communication with healthcare providers, therapists, and driving rehabilitation specialists and can keep track of improvements and challenges to help adjust the rehabilitation plan as needed. By being actively involved and supportive, family members can significantly contribute to the successful rehabilitation and eventual return to driving for survivors of critical illness.

Conclusion

Quantitative studies regarding return to work and driving are limited in survivors of critical illness. Patients with PICS have physical, cognitive, and psychological impairments that contribute to the inability to return to work and driving. The ability to return to work and driving may require a multimodal rehabilitation plan addressing these specific deficits in physical, cognitive, and psychiatric domains. No firm recommendations exist on the appropriate tests required to determine fitness to return to work or driving. Numerous neuropsychological screening tests for fitness to drive are available and applicable to patients with PICS, although the decision to resume driving is often made by patients in consultation with their loved ones rather than with medical professionals. More research is needed to bridge the knowledge gap and to develop clear guidelines for assessing return to work and driving in patients with PICS.

Key Points

1. The physical, cognitive, and psychiatric impairments associated with PICS can make it difficult to resume both employment and driving following hospital discharge.
2. Returning to work is not possible for many survivors of critical illness, and for those who can return to work, changes in employment, such as assuming a job with fewer responsibilities, working fewer hours, or retiring early, is frequently necessary.
3. Returning to driving is also challenging for many survivors of critical illness, and the decision to return to driving is often made by the patient in consultation with family members rather than with medical professionals.
4. There are no guidelines or evidence-based screening tools that have been specifically developed for returning to work or driving in patients with PICS.
5. Rehabilitation interventions should adopt a holistic approach, integrating cognitive rehabilitation, physical and occupational therapy, and psychological support to help survivors with PICS resume employment and driving and reintegrate into society.

References

1. D. Ramnarain, S. Pouwels, S. Fernández-Gonzalo, et al. Delirium-related psychiatric and neurocognitive impairment and the association with post-intensive care syndrome: a narrative review. *Acta Psychiatr Scand* 2023; **147**: 460–74.

2. D. Ramnarain, E. Aupers, B. den Oudsten, et al. Post Intensive Care Syndrome (PICS): an overview of the definition, etiology, risk factors, and possible counseling and treatment strategies. *Expert Rev Neurother* 2021; **21**: 1159–77.

3. D. Ramnarain, B. Den Oudsten, A. Oldenbeuving, et al. Post-intensive care syndrome in patients suffering from acute subarachnoid hemorrhage: results from an outpatient post-ICU aftercare clinic. *Cureus* 2023; **15**: e36739.

4. M.S. Herridge, A.M. Cheung, C.M. Tansey, et al. One-year outcomes in survivors of the acute respiratory distress syndrome. *New Engl J Med* 2003; **348**: 683–93.

5. M.S. Herridge, C.M. Tansey, A. Matté, et al. Functional disability 5 years after acute respiratory distress syndrome. *New Engl J Med* 2011; **364**: 1293–304.

6. M.S. Herridge, D.C. Angus. Acute lung injury: affecting many lives. *New Engl J Med* 2005; **353**: 1736–8.

7. M.F. Mattioni, C. Dietrich, D. Sganzerla, et al. Return to work after discharge from the intensive care unit: a Brazilian multicenter cohort. *Rev Bras Tera Intensiva* 2022; **34**: 492–8.

8. H. Su, R.O. Hopkins, B.B. Kamdar, et al. Association of imbalance between job workload and functional ability with return to work in ARDS survivors. *Thorax* 2022; **77**: 123–8.

9. H. Su, H.J. Thompson, S. May, et al. Association of job characteristics and functional impairments on return to work after ARDS. *Chest* 2021; **160**: 509–18.

10. M. Austenå, T. Rustøen, M.C. Småstuen, et al. Return to work during first year after intensive care treatment and the impact of demographic, clinical and psychosocial factors. *Intensive Crit Care Nurs* 2023; **76**: 103384.

11. C. Fleischmann-Struzek, B. Ditscheid, N. Rose, et al. Return to work after sepsis: a German population-based health claims study. *Front Med* 2023; **10**: 1187809.

12. N.V. Skei, K. Moe, T.I.L. Nilsen, et al. Return to work after hospitalization for sepsis: a nationwide, registry-based cohort study. *Crit Care* 2023; **27**: 443.

13. S. Riddersholm, S. Christensen, K. Kragholm, et al. Organ support therapy in the intensive care unit and return to work: a nationwide, register-based cohort study. *Intensive Care Med* 2018; **44**: 418–27.

14. J. McPeake, M.E. Mikkelsen, T. Quasim, et al. Return to employment after critical illness and its association with psychosocial outcomes: a systematic review and meta-analysis. *Ann Am Thorac Soc* 2019; **16**: 1304–11.

15. B.B. Kamdar, R. Suri, M.R. Suchyta, et al. Return to work after critical illness: a systematic review and meta-analysis. *Thorax* 2020; **75**: 17–27.

16. H. Su, H.J. Thompson, K. Pike, et al. Interrelationships among workload, illness severity, and function on return to work following acute respiratory distress syndrome. *Aust Crit Care* 2023; **36**: 247–53.

17. E.R. Soo Hoo. Evaluating return-to-work ability using functional capacity evaluation. *Phys Med Rehabil Clin N Am* 2019; **30**: 541–59.

18. D.L. Hart, S.J. Isernhagen, L.N. Matheson. Guidelines for functional capacity evaluation of people with medical conditions. *J Orthop Sports Phys Ther* 1993; **18**: 682–6.

19. C. Gobelet, F. Luthi, A.T. Al-Khodairy, M.A. Chamberlain. Vocational rehabilitation: a multidisciplinary intervention. *Disabil Rehabil* 2007; **29**: 1405–10.

20. The British Society of Rehabilitation. *Vocational Rehabilitation: The Way Forward*. London: BSRM; 2003.

21. A.M. Jette, P. Ni, E. Rasch, et al. The Work Disability Functional Assessment Battery

(WD-FAB). *Phys Med Rehabil Clin N Am* 2019; 30: 561–72.

22. World Health Organization. *International Classification of Functioning, Disability and Health: ICF.* Geneva: World Health Organization; 2001.

23. J. Meyer, C. Waldmann. Driving (or not) after critical illness. *J Intensive Care Soc* 2015; **16**: 186–8.

24. J. Munn, S.M. Willatts, M.A. Tooley. Health and activity after intensive care. *Anaesthesia* 1995; **50**: 1017–21.

25. K.M. Potter, V. Danesh, B.W. Butcher, et al. Return to driving after critical illness. *JAMA Intern Med* 2023; **183**: 493–5.

26. D. Kandasamy, K. Williamson, D.B. Carr, et al. The utility of the Montreal Cognitive Assessment in predicting need for fitness to drive evaluations in older adults. *J. Transp Health* 2019; **13**: 19–25.

27. V. Danesh, A.D. McDonald, J. McPeake, et al. Driving decisions after critical illness: qualitative analysis of patient-provider reviews during ICU recovery clinic assessments. *Int J Nurs Stud* 2023; **146**: 104560.

28. G.K. Fox, S.C. Bowden, D.S. Smith. On-road assessment of driving competence after brain impairment: review of current practice and recommendations for a standardized examination. *Arch Phys Med Rehabil* 1998; **79**: 1288–96.

29. J. Liddle, R. Hayes, L. Gustafsson, et al. Managing driving issues after an acquired brain injury: strategies used by health professionals. *Aust Occup Ther J* 2014; **61**: 215–23.

30. A.B. Fuermaier, D. Piersma, D. de Waard, et al. Assessing fitness to drive: a validation study on patients with mild cognitive impairment. *Traffic Inj Prev* 2017; **18**: 145–9.

31. H. Devos, A.E. Akinwuntan, A. Nieuwboer, et al. Screening for fitness to drive after stroke: a systematic review and meta-analysis. *Neurology* 2011; **76**: 747–56.

32. A. McKay, C. Liew, M. Schönberger et al. Predictors of the on-road driving assessment after traumatic brain injury: comparing cognitive tests, injury factors, and demographics. *J Head Trauma Rehabil* 2016; **31**: e44–e52.

33. P. Stamatelos, A. Economou, L. Stefanis, et al. Driving and Alzheimer's dementia or mild cognitive impairment: a systematic review of the existing guidelines emphasizing on the neurologist's role. *Neurol Sci* 2021; **42**: 4953–63.

34. H. Devos, C.A. Hawley, A.M. Conn, et al. Driving after stroke. In: Platz T. (ed.), *Clinical Pathways in Stroke Rehabilitation: Evidence-based Clinical Practice Recommendations.* Cham: Springer; 2021, pp. 243–60.

35. S. Hwang, C.S. Song. Driving rehabilitation for stroke patients: a systematic review with meta-analysis. *Healthcare (Basel)* 2023; **11**: 1637.

36. Y. Guo. A selective review of the ability for variants of the Trail Making Test to assess cognitive impairment. *Appl Neuropsychol Adult* 2022; **29**: 1634–45.

37. M. Hurtado-Pomares, M. Carmen Terol-Cantero, A. Sánchez-Pérez, et al. The frontal assessment battery in clinical practice: a systematic review. *Int J Geriatr Psychiatry* 2018; **33**: 237–51.

38. K.A. Radford, N.B. Lincoln. Concurrent validity of the stroke drivers screening assessment. *Arch Phys Med Rehabil* 2004; **85**: 324–8.

39. J.M. Wood, C. Owsley. Useful field of view test. *Gerontology* 2014; **60**: 315–18.

40. B.G. Lee, J.A. Kent, B.A. Marcopulos, et al. Rey-Osterrieth complex figure normative data for the psychiatric population. *Clin Neuropsychol* 2022; **36**: 1653–78.

41. I. Arevalo-Rodriguez, N. Smailagic, M. Roqué-Figuls, et al. Mini-Mental State Examination (MMSE) for the early detection of dementia in people with mild cognitive impairment (MCI). *Cochrane Database Syst Rev* 2021; **7**: Cd010783.

42. Z.S. Nasreddine, N.A. Phillips, V. Bédirian, et al. The Montreal Cognitive Assessment, MoCA: a brief screening tool for mild cognitive impairment. *J Am Geriatr Soc* 2005; **53**: 695–9.

43. M.A. Hird, A. Vetivelu, G. Saposnik, et al. Cognitive, on-road, and simulator-based driving assessment after stroke. *J Stroke Cerebrovasc Dis* 2014; **23**: 2654–70.

44. A.E. Dickerson, T.A. Reistetter, S. Burhans, et al. Typical brake reaction times across the life span. *Occup Ther Health Care* 2016; **30**: 115–23.

45. S. Bahrampouri, H.R. Khankeh, S. A. Hosseini, et al. Introducing practical tools for fit to drive assessment of the elderly: a step toward improving the health of the elderly. *J Educ Health Promot* 2021; **10**: 463.

46. B. Spenciere, H. Alves, H. Charchat-Fichman. Scoring systems for the Clock Drawing Test: a historical review. *Dement Neuropsychol* 2017; **11**: 6–14.

47. X. Zhang, L. Lv, G. Min et al. Overview of the complex figure test and its clinical application in neuropsychiatric disorders, including copying and recall. *Front Neurol* 2021; **12**: 680474.

48. E. Calderón-Rubio, J. Oltra-Cucarella, B. Bonete-López, et al. Regression-based normative data for independent and cognitively active spanish older adults: free and cued selective reminding test, Rey-Osterrieth complex figure test and judgement of line orientation. *Int J Environ Res Public Health* 2021; **18**: 12977.

49. I. Campagna, A. Ferreira-Correia. Hooper visual organization test: psychometric properties and regression-based norms for the Venezuelan population. *Appl Neuropsychol Adult* 2022; **29**: 1394–402.

50. E.C. Chiu, J.W. Hung, M.Y. Yu, et al. Practice effect and reliability of the motor-free visual perception test-4 over multiple assessments in patients with stroke. *Disabil Rehabil* 2022; **44**: 2456–63.

Chapter 45: The Role of Physiatry Consultation in PICS

Maria Twichell and Jean-Luc Banks

What Is a Physiatrist?

Physical Medicine & Rehabilitation (known as physiatry or PM&R) is a field of medicine that prioritizes the function and quality of life of patients who have become debilitated or disabled because of disease or injury. Physiatrists treat conditions related to the brain, spinal cord, nerves, muscles, and bones that may impair a person's ability to ambulate, complete self-care tasks, participate in recreational activities, and work. Common conditions treated by physiatrists include traumatic brain injury, spinal cord injury, stroke, amputation, and a variety of musculoskeletal disorders and chronic pain conditions. Physiatrists provide nonsurgical pain management and work together as part of a multidisciplinary team with physical therapy, occupational therapy, speech and language pathology, and neuropsychology to address patients' medical, physical, social, emotional, and vocational needs in both inpatient and outpatient settings.

The Role of the Physiatrist in PICS

Patients with post-intensive care syndrome (PICS) may experience skeletal and respiratory muscle weakness, difficulty walking, and impairments in executive functioning and mental processing speed, all of which may limit their ability to care for themselves [1]. Physiatrists can help address these deficits along the continuum of care, providing consultative services in the intensive care unit (ICU) and general wards, directing care in inpatient rehabilitation (IPR), and addressing lingering effects of debility in outpatient clinics. The initial physiatric assessment of a patient with PICS begins with a thorough history and physical examination.

The Physiatric History

The physiatric history is similar to that of general medical practitioners with a specialized emphasis on function. The physiatric history of a patient with PICS should be holistic, addressing the domains of physical, cognitive, mental, and social health. Collateral information from family members and caregivers may also be beneficial in assessing the presence of physical, cognitive, and emotional disabilities.

In assessing physical function, physiatrists perform a "functional reconciliation" to compare the patient's current functional status with their functional status prior to critical illness. This reconciliation should include the patient's abilities to perform activities of daily living (ADLs) and instrumental activities of daily living (IADLs; see Table 45.1), to tolerate exercise, and to return to work [2].

Table 45.1 Examples of activities of daily living and instrumental activities of daily living

ADLs	IADLs
Bathing	Housekeeping
Toileting	Managing Money
Dressing	Preparing Food
Grooming	Shopping for Groceries
Eating	Managing Medications
Transferring	Using Transportation

Physical Examination

A comprehensive physical examination should be performed when evaluating a patient with PICS. The examination should start with an assessment of the patient's overall appearance, including posture and vital signs, as this may provide insight into their functional status and current medical conditions. A thorough neurologic examination should be performed, including assessments of cranial and peripheral nerves, strength of all major muscle groups, and monosynaptic reflexes, which may indicate the presence of a myopathy or neuropathy. A cognitive evaluation, using validated tools such as the Mini–Mental Status Examination (MMSE) or the Montreal Cognitive Assessment tool (MoCA), should also be performed to screen for cognitive deficits that may prompt referral for more comprehensive neurocognitive testing (see Chapter 43 for additional information).

Muscle Weakness

Many of the prolonged physical impairments associated with PICS arise from weakness acquired during the ICU stay (see Chapter 4 for additional information). Referred to generally as ICU-acquired weakness (ICUAW), this condition is defined as a diffuse symmetric decrease in skeletal muscle strength for which other causes have been excluded, and it may manifest clinically as impairments in speaking and swallowing or generalized muscle weakness. Generalized muscle weakness may be further classified into deconditioning, critical illness myopathy, or critical illness polyneuropathy [3]. Critical illness myopathy (CIM) is characterized by weakness and atrophy primarily affecting proximal muscles with sensory preservation, while critical illness polyneuropathy (CIP) presents with prominent distal muscle weakness and limited atrophy [4]. Often, these conditions (CIM and CIP) can overlap and may be difficult to differentiate without electromyography (EMG). Deconditioning, or global weakness attributed to skeletal muscle atrophy, results primarily from disuse after prolonged immobility; however, excess inflammation, electrolyte imbalances, endocrine dysfunction, and malnutrition may all contribute to the weakness that patients with PICS experience.

Strength Evaluations

The muscle strength assessment is integral to the physiatric examination, as it provides valuable information on the degree of weakness and potential neurologic deficits. Manual muscle testing (MMT) is used to evaluate the function and strength of individual muscle groups based on the movement of a joint through a full range of motion against both gravity and manual resistance [5].

In performing MMT, it is important to determine if there are any precautions or contraindications to testing that may impact the examination's objectivity, including pain, weight bearing restrictions from prior fractures or surgical procedures, amputation of limbs that make certain muscles untestable, or cognitive barriers to full participation in testing. Proper positioning of the patient is key, as it both ensures that the appropriate muscle is tested and prevents the influence of other muscles in assisting with that movement. The unaffected side should be assessed prior to the affected side (if present, as in a patient with a stroke, for example). Muscles should be moved by the examiner through a full passive range of motion to detect any anatomic or neurologic deficits that may impact the patient's strength. Patients should then be instructed to range the muscle on their own against gravity, which informs the next steps of the exam. If a patient is unable to activate the muscle against gravity, their position should be adjusted to minimize the effects of gravity, with a subsequent attempt in the horizontal plane. If a patient can activate the muscle against gravity, the muscle's action against resistance should be tested to determine the force the patient can produce. Resistance should be performed in the mid-range of motion in muscles that cross two joints (such as the rectus femoris, hamstrings, and gastrocnemius), as this position produces the maximum force. In muscles that cross one joint (such as the deltoid), resistance should be applied at the end of the range of motion [6]. The examiner should provide slow and gradual resistance in the opposite direction of the patient's range of motion. Documentation should include the muscle being tested, any symptoms that may impact strength (e.g., pain), any changes in positioning needed to complete the test, and the numerical grade assigned based on the Medical Research Council Scale (also known as the Oxford Scale; see Table 45.2).

Although MMT is commonly performed, the reproducibility of results can be impacted by both patient and examiner factors. More objective evaluation of muscle strength can be performed using a handheld dynamometer, although the time required for comprehensive examination may be impractical for some outpatient appointments. Examination of handgrip strength with handheld dynamometers is more efficient, and handgrip strength has been associated with total muscle strength in both healthy adults and those with disease, making this a high-yield test that can be followed objectively over time [7].

Table 45.2 The Medical Research Council (Oxford) scale on grading muscular strength

Grade	Description
0	No muscular contraction
1	Flicker of muscle contraction
2	Full range of motion with gravity minimized
3	Full range of motion against gravity
4	Full range of motion against gravity with minimal resistance of examiner
5	Full range of motion against gravity with maximal resistance of examiner

Electrodiagnosis

In patients with prolonged muscle weakness or sensory deficits that do not respond to traditional therapies, electrodiagnostics such as electromyography (EMG) and nerve conduction studies (NCS) may be used. EMG analyzes electrical activity within muscles at rest and during contraction to provide data regarding the function of muscle fibers themselves. NCS measures the speed at which an electrical impulse propagates along a peripheral nerve (latency) and the degree to which that nerve is stimulated (amplitude) to determine the type and extent of nerve damage. Combining EMG and NCS is useful to diagnose the location and severity of a neuronal lesion as well as the status and level of nerve regeneration [8]. It is also helpful in diagnosing inflammatory and noninflammatory neuronal myopathies and dystrophies.

Therapy Referrals

An important aspect of physiatric practice is collaboration with therapists to achieve the patient's strength and functional goals. Physiatrists are well-educated in therapeutic techniques and write specific prescriptions for physical, occupational, and speech therapy that may include the types of exercises to be performed, duration of therapy, and any precautions or contraindications to certain therapeutic modalities. The therapist will then use this prescription, in addition to their own evaluation and assessment of the patient, to develop a treatment plan. Physiatrists may check in with patients throughout their therapy course to evaluate the efficacy of the treatment plan, assess patient satisfaction, and provide recommendations for the remaining therapy sessions.

Management of Specific Conditions

Contracture

Prolonged immobility from periods of critical illness can result in joint contracture. Contracture is the loss of joint mobility caused by replacement of elastic tissue with fibrous tissue in muscles, ligaments, tendons, and fascia. Common sites of contracture, which are largely preventable, include the shoulder, elbow, hip, knee, and ankle [9]. Physiatrists consulted in the ICU can recommend interventions to slow or prevent contractures, including passive range of motion exercises and stretching, although the effectiveness of these interventions is debated [10]. Once a contracture has developed, the joint must be continuously stretched through dynamic bracing or serial casting. Physiatrists work closely with occupational therapists and orthotists to ensure patients receive the best bracing to reduce the contracture and to treat any spasticity that might interfere with contracture reduction. Contractures have a profound impact on one's quality of life, including limited ability to perform ADLs or permanent immobility of the joint. In patients with contractures that significantly limit function or who have failed conservative therapies, surgical release with fasciectomy and fasciotomy may be required [9]. After surgery, these patients should continue to see a physiatrist to ensure durable functionality of the joint and to prevent further scar formation.

Spasticity

Spasticity, one manifestation of the upper motor neuron syndrome, is common in patients with PICS, particularly in those initially admitted with neurologic injury, and is frequently managed by a physiatrist. Spasticity results from loss of upper motor neuron inhibition of lower motor neuron pathways (found in the spinal arc reflex) due to a lesion or damage of the upper motor neuron that regulates muscle control. Clinically, it is characterized by a velocity-dependent increase in tonic stretch reflexes (muscle tone) with exaggerated tendon jerks [11]. The loss of inhibition of lower motor neurons results in uncontrolled, involuntary, intermittent, or sustained muscle activation, which can interfere with a patient's movement, balance, and ability to perform ADLs.

Spasticity is a velocity-dependent increase in muscle tone: if a muscle is moved or stretched quickly, more resistance is produced than if the muscle is moved or stretched slowly. Rigidity, in contrast, is a separate condition of increased tone that is not velocity dependent. When performing a spasticity evaluation, the muscle being tested is first moved through its full range of motion to establish a baseline. Then, the muscle will be brought from its neutral position to its end range at a faster rate, looking for a "catch," indicating the degree of tonicity present in the muscle. Common locations that may be tested for spasticity include the elbow, wrist, and finger flexors in the upper limb and the hip adductors, knee flexors and extensors, and plantar and dorsiflexors in the lower limb. Muscle tone is traditionally assessed using the Modified Ashworth Scale (see Table 45.3).

Spasticity management must be carefully considered, as some patients rely on their tone to help them maintain posture, transfer from bed to wheelchair, or ambulate with less assistance. It is also important to understand and mitigate triggers of spasticity prior to planning interventions to reduce tone. Common triggers of spasticity include pressure ulcers, constipation, urinary retention, restrictive clothing or ill-fitting orthotics, stress, and the development of other medical conditions [12], such as a latent infection or ingrown toenail.

Spasticity management begins with physical and occupational therapy to stretch and strengthen muscles to relieve stiffness and improve their resting position. Therapists may also use additional modalities such as orthotics, splints, heat, ice, ultrasound, or electrical stimulation to lessen spasticity. These additional modalities are often performed during outpatient therapy sessions and may require follow-up with a physiatrist.

Table 45.3 Modified Ashworth Scale

Grade	Description
0	No increase in muscle tone
1	Slight increase in muscle tone, characterized by a "catch and release" at the end range of motion
1+	Slight increase in muscle tone, characterized by a "catch" followed by minimal resistance through the remaining range of motion
2	Increased resistance to range of motion throughout, but affected part easily moved
3	Increase in muscle tone making passive movement difficult
4	Affected part is rigid in flexion or extension

Some individuals may benefit from systemic medications or focal interventions to manage spasticity. Common systemic medications used to manage spasticity include baclofen, dantrolene, tizanidine, and benzodiazepines such as diazepam. Baclofen, a GABA-B agonist, causes inhibition of mono- and polysynaptic reflexes at the spinal cord, leading to membrane hyperpolarization and skeletal muscle relaxation. Dantrolene acts as an antagonist to the ryanodine-1 receptor in skeletal muscle, decreasing intracellular calcium concentration and the force of skeletal muscle contraction. Tizanidine inhibits motor neurons at $α_2$ receptors, preventing the release of excitatory neurotransmitters that cause muscle spasms. Benzodiazepines also act on the GABA receptor to increase the influx of chloride ions across the terminal membrane, increasing the amount of presynaptic inhibition [13]. Benzodiazepines are often used as the last line agent for spasticity due to their sedative effects and potential for dependency. Medications should be started at a low dose with monitoring for common side effects, including fatigue, sedation, or dizziness, which may limit a patient's ability to perform daily activities. The medication can then be titrated depending on symptomatic relief of spasticity and any side effects the patient might experience.

For localized management of spasticity that may impair a patient's ability to perform ADLs, injection of a neurotoxin (e.g., botulinum toxin) may be used. Botulinum toxin binds to the presynaptic cholinergic nerve terminals, preventing the release of acetylcholine and causing a neuromuscular blockade effect [14]. Currently, there are three types of botulinum toxin A and one type of botulinum toxin B approved for spasticity management in the United States. Botulinum toxin is injected directly into the spastic muscle or group of muscles impairing the patient's function. This is often done in the outpatient clinic using electromyography or ultrasound guidance to ensure that the correct muscles are being injected; those without access to these modalities use anatomic landmarks to ensure proper injection location. Improvement with neurotoxin injection is seen within one to two weeks after injection, with a peak effect at three to four weeks, and a gradual washout period of three to four months. Neurotoxin cannot be dosed more frequently than every three months. Importantly, botulinum toxin has a black box warning regarding potential spread from the injection site and development of systemic effects, including diplopia, ptosis, dysphagia, dysphonia, dysarthria, and breathing difficulties [15]. Patients should be adequately informed of these risks prior to injection of the toxin.

Chronic Pain

Chronic pain is a common concern in patients with PICS, often impairing function and diminishing quality of life. Invasive devices and interventions in the ICU such as endotracheal tube and gastric tube insertion, vascular access devices, physical restraints, and prolonged immobility increase the risk of patients developing neuroplastic hyperalgesia and allodynia [16]. Physiatrists can be consulted during the ICU admission to facilitate early mobilization and rehabilitation and can also follow patients in the outpatient setting for longitudinal pain management using a multimodal approach.

Pain is divided into nociceptive and neuropathic components. Nociceptive pain arises from physical damage to tissues, while neuropathic pain results from damage to peripheral sensory nerves. While patients with PICS may have both nociceptive and neuropathic components of their pain, neuropathic pain, in which patients often report symptoms of burning or tingling, is more common after a prolonged ICU stay [17]. Neuropathic pain can be exacerbated by anxiety, sleep disturbances, and deconditioning; therefore, a multidisciplinary approach involving pharmacological management and non-pharmacological therapies, including neuropsychology, physical therapy, and massage, should be utilized.

Pharmacotherapy is the basis of neuropathic pain treatment, and the most commonly used medications include gabapentanoids, serotonin norepinephrine reuptake inhibitors (SNRIs), and tricyclic antidepressants (TCAs). Gabapentanoids, such as gabapentin and pregabalin, are often the initial treatment of choice. Gabapentanoids depress the excitability of neurons through calcium channel blockade, thereby decreasing glutamate, calcitonin gene-related peptide (CGRP), and substance P release. Analgesic effects are achieved by facilitating noradrenergic and serotonergic inhibition in the limbic system, the same mechanism by which SNRIs and TCAs work [18]. Medications should be started at a low dose and titrated slowly to minimize the commonly experienced side effects of fatigue, somnolence, and dizziness. In patients with co-morbid psychiatric conditions or sleep disorders or those who fail first-line therapy, SNRIs, such as duloxetine and venlafaxine, or TCAs, such as nortriptyline and amitriptyline, may be considered in addition to, or instead of, gabapentanoids. TCAs should be used with caution in the elderly to avoid potential side effects, including cardiac arrhythmias, urinary retention, orthostasis, and dry mouth.

In patients who fail or are unable to tolerate first- and second-line medications, interventional techniques, including epidural steroid injection or radiofrequency ablation, may be performed. These are most often performed in patients with disc herniation or radiculopathy, although the beneficial effects may be short-lived, and repeat injections may be needed. Interventional therapies are performed by physiatrists or anesthesiologists with specialized training in interventional pain management.

In patients with nociceptive pain, a combined approach of physical therapy and pharmacotherapy is recommended. Over-the-counter medications, such as acetaminophen and ibuprofen, are first-line therapies in those without severe hepatic or renal impairment, respectively. Opioids may be used as an adjunctive pain therapy in patients with refractory or breakthrough pain; however, they should not be used as the primary strategy for chronic pain management and should be tapered and discontinued as quickly as possible.

Impaired Ambulation

Some patients with PICS are at increased risk of falls because of generalized muscle weakness and impaired mobility. Generalized muscle weakness may be treated using a personalized therapy program; however, poor mobility can have many etiologies and therefore may require different modes of intervention.

The six-minute walk test (6MWT) and the timed get up and go (TUG) are two tests used to evaluate fall risk in the elderly and in patients with prolonged periods of immobility. The 6MWT evaluates the functional capacity of the cardiopulmonary and neuromuscular systems and is used as a measure of endurance (see Chapter 41 for additional information). The TUG measures a patient's ability to rise from a seated position, walk three meters (at their own pace), and return to a seated position. This test is useful for assessing the ability of a patient to maintain their balance in daily life. Physiatrists will use these tests in addition to their knowledge of gait mechanics to determine if a patient can ambulate safely on their own or if they require an assistive device.

Assistive devices are designed to maintain or improve a person's ability to navigate their environment. Common assistive devices include canes, crutches, walkers, and several types of wheelchairs, both manual and motorized. In a patient with impaired mobility, physiatrists perform a complete strength, neurological, and gait assessment to prescribe the appropriate device. Physiatrists are familiar with the regulatory documentation and evaluation practices required by various insurance companies (in the United States) to approve coverage of an assistive device and work closely with physical therapists, occupational therapists, and durable medical equipment companies to ensure the patient receives the best device. After receipt of the assistive device, the physiatrist will continue to follow the patient should any modifications to the device be required or should the patient need a new or different device. This longitudinal care ensures that patients, particularly those with degenerative conditions, have access to the best device for them, which may change along with their functional level.

Return to Work and Vocational Rehabilitation

Return to work is a signifier of recovery in patients with prolonged illness and development of PICS. Manifestations of PICS, such as physical weakness, cognitive impairment, and psychological distress may delay return to work after hospital discharge (see Chapter 44 for additional information). Prior studies cite only 49% of those with PICS who were previously employed are employed one year after discharge, with proximal muscle weakness and fatigue as the major contributors to the inability to resume work [19]. Low educational level, need for mechanical ventilation during the ICU stay, and persistent requirements for physical assistance are also associated with the inability to resume work. For those who returned to work, adjustments, including reduced working hours and a change in responsibilities, are frequently required to accommodate their deficits [20].

Physiatrists often work as part of a multidisciplinary team to facilitate the return to work. This may include providing medical clearance prior to returning to work, as often required by employers; writing prescriptions for functional capacity evaluations; recommending modifications to hours or responsibilities for patients deemed unready to return to their previous work responsibilities; and referring patients to vocational rehabilitation and job coaches (see Chapter 44 for additional information).

Conclusion

Physiatrists possess specialized training in addressing multiple conditions associated with PICS. Although physiatrists are not currently commonly incorporated into ICU follow-up clinics, physiatric consultation in select patients can be beneficial to maximize their functional recovery.

Key Points

1. Physiatrists specialize in Physical Medicine and Rehabilitation (PMR), an area of medicine that emphasizes work with multidisciplinary teams to enhance restoration of function after an injury or illness.
2. Physiatrists have deep knowledge of the musculoskeletal and neurological systems, allowing them to evaluate and treat conditions common after PICS.
3. Physiatrists address muscle weakness with a thorough examination to assess strength, spasticity, and contracture.

4. Physiatrists use medications, bracing, injections, and assistive device evaluation to promote restoration of function.
5. Physiatrists provide prescriptions for specific therapy interventions, including physical therapy, occupational therapy, speech therapy, cognitive therapy, and vocational rehabilitation.

References

1. P.J. Ohtake, A.C. Lee, J.C. Scott, et al. Impairments associated with post-intensive care syndrome: systematic review based on the World Health Organization's international classification of functioning, disability and health framework. *Physical Therapy* 2018; **98**: 631–45.

2. T. Hudson. Functional medicine: a view from physical medicine and rehabilitation. *Phys Med Rehabil Clin N Am* 2020; **31**: 527–40.

3. H. Farhan, I. Moreno-Duarte, N. Latronico, et al. Acquired muscle weakness in the surgical intensive care unit: nosology, epidemiology, diagnosis, and prevention. *Anesthesiology* 2016; **124**: 207–34.

4. S. Shepherd, A. Batra, D.P. Lerner. Review of critical illness myopathy and neuropathy. *Neurohospitalist* 2017; **7**: 41–8.

5. H.M. Clarkson. *Musculoskeletal Assessment: Joint Range of Motion and Manual Muscle Strength*. Philadelphia, PA: Lippincott Williams & Wilkins, 2013.

6. U. Naqvi, A.L. Sherman. Muscle strength grading. InStatPearls [Internet] 2021. StatPearls Publishing

7. R.W. Bohannon. Grip strength: an indispensable biomarker for older adults. *Clin Interv Aging* 2019; **14**: 1681–91.

8. K.S. Chen, R. Chen. Principles of electrophysiological assessments for movement disorders. *J Mov Disord* 2020; **13**: 27–38.

9. H. Clavet, P.C. Hébert, D. Fergusson, S. Doucette, G. Trudel. Joint contracture following prolonged stay in the intensive care unit. *CMAJ* 2008; **178**: 691–7.

10. K.R. Stiller, S. Dafoe, C.S. Jesudason, et al. Passive movements do not appear to prevent or reduce joint stiffness in medium to long-stay ICU patients: a randomized, controlled, within-participant trial. *Crit Care Explor* 2023; **5**: 1–13.

11. J.W. Lance, R.G. Feldman, R.R. Young, W.P. Koella. *Spasticity: Disordered Motor Control*. Chicago: Year Book Medical Publishers; 1980.

12. A. Kheder, K.P.S. Nair. Spasticity: pathophysiology, evaluation and management. *Practical Neurology* 2012; **12**: 289–98.

13. R.A. Davidoff. Antispasticity drugs: mechanisms of action. *Ann Neurol* 1985; **17**: 107–16.

14. A. Lagueny, P. Barbaud. Mechanism of action, clinical indications and results of treatment of botulinum toxin. *Neurophysiol Clin* 1996; **26**: 216–26.

15. B.M. Kuehn. FDA requires black box warnings on labeling for botulinum toxin products. *JAMA* 2009; **301**: 2316.

16. J. Sandkuhler. Models and mechanisms of hyperalgesia and allodynia. *Physiol Rev* 2009; **89**: 707–58.

17. A. Bourdoil, V. Legros, F. Vardon-Bounes, et al. Prevalence and risk factors of significant persistent pain symptoms after critical care illness: a prospective multicentric study. *Crit Care* 2023; **27**: 1–10.

18. M. Chincholkar. Gabapentinoids: pharmacokinetics, pharmacodynamics and considerations for clinical practice. *Br J Pain* 2020; **14**: 104–14.

19. M.S. Herridge, A.M. Cheung, C.M. Tansey, et al. One-year outcomes in survivors of the acute respiratory distress syndrome. *N Engl J Med* 2003; **348**: 683–93.

20. M.F. Mattioni, C. Dietrich, D. Sganzerla, et al. Return to work after discharge from

the intensive care unit: a Brazilian multicenter cohort. *Rev Bras Ter Intensiva* 2022; **34**: 492–8.

21. E.R. Soo Hoo. Evaluating Return-to-work ability using functional capacity evaluation. *Phys Med Rehabil Clin N Am* 2019; **30**: 541–59.

22. D.L. Hart, S.J. Isernhagen, L.N. Matheson. Guidelines for functional capacity evaluation of people with medical conditions. *J Orthop Sports Phys Ther* 1993; **18**: 682–6.

23. C. Gobelet, F. Luthi, A.T. Al-Khodairy, M. A. Chamberlain. Vocational rehabilitation: a multidisciplinary intervention. *Disabil Rehabil* 2007; **29**: 1405–10.

24. British Society of Rehabilitation Medicine. *Vocational rehabilitation: the way forward.* London: BSRM; 2003.

25. A.M. Jette, N. Pengsheng, E. Rasch, et al. The Work Disability Functional Assessment Battery (WD-FAB). *Phys Med Rehabil Clin N Am* 2019; **30**: 561–72.

26. World Health Organization. *International classification of functioning, disability and health: ICF.* Geneva: World Health Organization; 2001.

Chapter 46

Psychological Outcomes in Survivors of Critical Illness

Jamie L. Tingey, Jessica M. Hampton, and Megan M. Hosey

Introduction

Survivors of critical illness are exposed to unique stressors both during their hospitalization and throughout their recovery. Fighting a life-threatening illness, undergoing invasive procedures and treatments in an unfamiliar environment, and experiencing adverse side effects of medications can significantly contribute to the psychological vulnerability of this patient population. Psychological experiences such as frightening hallucinations and delusions, agitation, anxiety, sleep disturbances, upsetting memories, and perceived loss of control and autonomy are common for patients in intensive care units (ICUs; see Chapter 10 for additional information). Critical care research is seeking to better understand the long-term psychological outcomes of critical illness and how these contribute to the broader cluster of symptoms often seen with post-intensive care syndrome (PICS).

Anxiety

Anxiety symptoms are the most commonly reported psychological sequelae in survivors of critical illness, with more than 30% of survivors reporting clinically significant symptoms [1,2]. Symptoms include nervousness, restlessness, excessive worry about their health or the future, panic, and avoidance of anxiety triggers. Up to 38% of survivors report clinically significant, prolonged anxiety associated with their critical illness at five years after hospital discharge [2]. Most epidemiologic studies in this population use measures that do not assess physiologic symptoms of anxiety (e.g., increased heart rate and rapid breathing), but these are common among survivors of critical illness and can make distinguishing anxiety from medically sinister symptoms challenging for patients and clinicians [3]. The development of anxiety in survivors is associated with failure to return to work and reengage in social roles, increased healthcare resource utilization, and financial instability [1,4].

Risk and Protective Factors

Risk factors for anxiety after critical illness include a history of psychiatric diagnosis; lower socioeconomic status; delirium or fear of death during the ICU stay; memories of delusional experiences; and worse physiological functioning after critical illness, including impaired abilities to perform activities of daily living and persistent pain, fatigue, and breathlessness [1,2]. Age, gender, the need for mechanical ventilation (MV), and ICU type (e.g., trauma, surgical, or medical ICU) are not consistent predictors of clinically meaningful anxiety symptoms [1]. Protective factors that reduce the likelihood of anxiety symptoms in survivors of critical illness are insufficiently studied. It is hypothesized that self-management, early care coordination, and rehabilitation therapy in the ICU may reduce psychological morbidity [5,6]; however, this work is limited by significant heterogeneity in dosing, implementation strategies, and theoretical underpinnings.

Depression

Depressive symptoms are often seen in PICS and can lead to worse health outcomes for survivors of critical illness. Symptoms include low mood, anhedonia, fatigue, difficulty concentrating, sleep disturbances, and feelings of guilt or worthlessness [7]. Approximately 33% of individuals report clinically significant depressive symptoms within the first 12 months of recovery, and 32% report persistent symptoms 5 years after hospitalization [2,7]. Prevalence of depression in general American and European populations is 8–11%, thus survivors of critical illness have a prevalence of depression that is approximately 3–4 times that of the general population. Depressive symptoms in survivors of critical illness are associated with a higher burden of physical symptoms, poorer functional outcomes, and reduced health-related quality of life [7]. Consequently, individuals are more likely to experience challenges reintegrating into daily activities and returning to work, in addition to experiencing prolonged recovery and increased risk of disability [8]. The relationship between depression and the physical sequelae of PICS is bidirectional, as the physical and functional disabilities of PICS likely contribute to the onset and maintenance of depressive symptoms. Critical illness survivorship is also associated with higher risks of suicide compared with the general population [9]. Those who die of suicide are younger, have fewer medical comorbidities, and have greater physical independence on discharge.

Risk and Protective Factors

The largest predictor for depression following critical illness is the presence of a psychiatric diagnosis prior to ICU admission [7,10]. Neuroinflammation and metabolic disturbances implicated in the pathophysiology of delirium have been linked to subsequent emergence of neuropsychiatric disturbances, including depression [11]. Individuals with lower levels of education and income are at a greater risk of experiencing depressive symptoms following critical illness, possibly due to perceived financial strain and loss of control [12]. Aside from considering the inverse of identified risk factors, limited research has examined protective factors of depression among survivors of critical illness. Several reviews have supported the benefits of ICU diaries in reducing the risks of depression for survivors of critical illness [13,14], though this has not consistently been shown to be a significant protective factor (see Chapter 18 for additional information) [15].

Post-Traumatic Stress

Survivors of critical illness are at heightened risk for experiencing post-traumatic stress disorder (PTSD) and symptoms compared with the general population. PTSD symptoms (PTSS) include re-experiencing traumatic events (e.g., nightmares), avoiding trauma-related stimuli, negative alterations in mood and cognition, and hyperarousal. Prevalence rates are six times greater in survivors of critical illness compared to the general population, with approximately 20% of survivors experiencing clinically meaningful PTSS in the first year following discharge, and 23% with persistent symptoms 5 years after hospitalization [2,16]. The timeline for symptom onset remains equivocal, as psychological screening in the ICU is uncommon

Table 46.1 ICU-specific examples in relation to PTSD symptom domains

Symptom domain	Examples
Re-experiencing	Sudden onset of fear/stress when encountering reminiscent scent from the ICU (e.g., rotten egg smell, evocative of albuterol treatment), vasovagal syncope (i.e., fainting) in the context of medical/health-related factors (e.g., getting a physical exam or hearing of someone else's hospitalization)
Avoidance of thoughts, feelings, and reminders of the experience	Skipping medical appointments, turning off TV shows that take place in medical settings, not visiting a loved one in the hospital, avoiding physical activities/hobbies that inherently alter breathing (e.g., scuba diving, vigorous exercise, or hiking at high altitudes)
Negative alterations of cognition and mood	Self-conscious of image following surgical scarring and hair loss, reduced self-efficacy in managing health due to chronic fatigue, distrust of medical providers in the context of negative ICU memories/perceived mistreatment during ICU stay, irritability toward loved ones and social supports, health anxiety relating to worry of being ill or becoming ill
Hyperarousal symptoms	Increased heart rate and blood pressure at medical appointments, insomnia due to heightened cognitive arousal when in bed, somatic hypervigilance or perceiving expected bodily sensations as harmful

and existing research on PTSD in survivors has occurred following discharge [16,17]. Treatment in the ICU can be inherently traumatic: patients endure physical and emotional stressors that are actually life-threatening or are perceived to be (e.g., breathlessness with MV, painful procedures, and hallucinations caused by ICU delirium) [17]. Several systematic reviews have demonstrated a strong relationship between PTSS and reduced quality of life among ICU survivors, underscoring the need to improve prevention and management among survivors [16]. It is important to note that many survivors do not meet diagnostic criteria for PTSD, though experience isolated PTSS (e.g., hypervigilance and avoidance), which can nevertheless be debilitating and prevent them from obtaining necessary healthcare services. Table 46.1 provides examples of PTSS specific to ICU experiences.

Risk and Protective Factors

Prior psychological difficulties (e.g., anxiety, depression, and substance abuse) are associated with the development of PTSS following an ICU admission [16], as are memories of frightening experiences while in the ICU (e.g., a delusional memory of a nurse trying to cause harm or recalling a painful procedure). Receipt of benzodiazepines while critically ill has been inconsistently shown to increase risk of PTSS [16,18].

An important consideration for the majority of risk factors of psychological distress among survivors of critical illness is that they are highly interrelated [19]. For example, individuals with premorbid anxiety and depression frequently require increased sedating medications during an ICU stay [20], thereby increasing the incidence of delirium and frightening perceptual disturbances and, in turn, the risk of developing PTSS [21]. Fewer studies have examined protective factors for PTSS, though there is strong evidence that social support reduces risk. ICU diaries

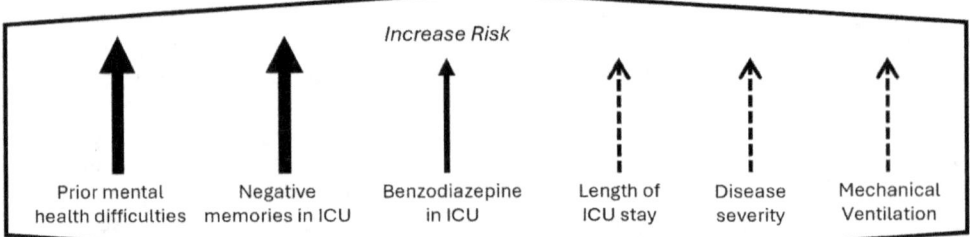

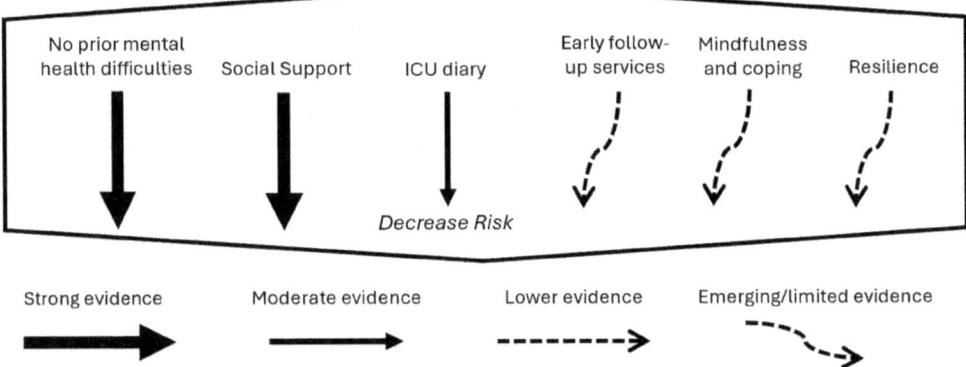

Figure 46.1 Strength of evidence on risk and protective factors of psychological distress in survivors of critical illness.

(see Chapter 18 for additional information) may reduce PTSS, but this is not a consistent finding [19,22]. Figure 46.1 illustrates the strength of evidence of risk and protective factors for the development of psychological distress following critical illness.

Physical Symptoms

Many physical symptoms experienced by survivors of critical illness with PICS are also manifestations of psychological distress, including anorexia, fatigue, and alopecia, which may complicate the assessment and treatment of somatic complaints related to psychiatric conditions (see Chapter 36 for additional information) [23]. Physical conditions pose further challenges to psychological recovery and coping. For example, more than half of survivors report having insomnia, nightmares, or reduced sleep quality following discharge (see Chapter 37 for additional information) [24], and approximately three-quarters report persistent pain [25]. In a study of survivors of critical illness one year after discharge, 66% reported clinically significant fatigue, which substantially overlapped with impaired physical function and clinically significant symptoms of anxiety or depression [26]. Fatigue, sleep dysregulation, and pain can precipitate and exacerbate psychological symptoms of distress; consequently, patient engagement and participation can be negatively impacted. Given the symptom overlap between psychiatric symptoms and physical manifestations of PICS, thorough assessments must carefully consider these relationships.

Post-Traumatic Growth and Resilience

Not all outcomes of critical illness are negative. Conceptualizing an adverse experience as an opportunity to grow in a way that positively impacts one's life is known as post-traumatic growth (PTG). Core facets of PTG involve a positive shift in personal, interpersonal, and existential domains [27]. Tedeschi and Calhoun, who first coined the term PTG, suggest that for growth to be possible, traumatic events must be impactful enough to force individuals to reassess their perspectives and beliefs [27]. While research regarding PTG in survivors of critical illness is limited, the expanding knowledge of psychological distress following critical illness suggests that PTG may be common among survivors. PTG has been associated with improved health-related quality of life, satisfaction with life, and happiness [28]. Resilience, one's ability to adapt to adverse experiences, also serves as an asset in the context of critical illness survivorship. While prevalence in survivors remains uncertain [29], sufficient resilience has been shown to mitigate adverse psychological symptoms associated with PICS and, consequently, to promote better outcomes for survivors. Understanding PTG and resilience in this patient population could inform treatment approaches and promote more desirable outcomes for survivors of critical illness.

Practical Application

Assessment

Appropriate assessment by trained professionals to detect symptoms of acute distress is an important first step to guide care in survivors of critical illness. Psychiatrists, psychologists, and social workers are trained in the assessment of psychiatric conditions and can provide valuable contributions to multidisciplinary teams in both the ICU and ICU follow-up clinics. Assessment and diagnosis of psychiatric morbidities should be undertaken systematically by trained mental health practitioners using standardized diagnostic classification of mental disorders (e.g., Diagnostic and Statistical Manual of Mental Disorders [DSM]) [30]. Semi-structured interviews are used to assist with the assessment and diagnosis of major DSM-5 diagnoses, such as mood, anxiety, or trauma and stressor-related disorders (e.g., The Structured Clinical Interview for DSM-5 [SCID-5]).

A Society of Critical Care Medicine (SCCM) taskforce recommends early screening for psychological symptoms after critical illness using a number of validated tools [31]. Several screening tools exist (see Table 46.2), and the most commonly used screening tools to assess for depression, anxiety, and PTSD in ICU follow-up studies are the Hospital Anxiety and Depression Scale (HADS) and the Impact of Events Scale – 6 (IES-6), respectively. The HADS has subscales for depression and anxiety, with scores of 11 or more suggesting severe symptoms, and scores between 8–10 suggesting mild symptoms. An item-average score of 1.6 or more on the IES-6 suggests clinically significant PTSS. Mental health practitioners can use these tools or others to quickly identify psychological symptoms of concern and inform treatment decision-making. Box 46.1 provides examples of other questions that can aid in eliciting information about survivors' experiences and help determine treatments.

Table 46.2 Brief self-report measures used in survivors of critical illness

Measure name	Constructs measured, items, and scaling
Patient Health Questionnaire 9 (PHQ–9) [33]	Symptoms of depression 9-items, 4-point scale
Generalized Anxiety Disorder–7 (GAD–7) [34]	Symptoms of anxiety 7-items, 4-point scale
*Hospital Anxiety and Depression Scale (HADS) [36]	Symptoms of anxiety and depression 14-items, 4-point scale
*Impact of Events Scale–6 (IES–6) [37]	Symptoms of PTSD 6-items, 5-point scale
Breathlessness Catastrophizing Scale (BCS) [32]	Catastrophic thinking related to breathlessness 13-items, 5-point scale
Montreal Cognitive Assessment (MoCA) [35]	Cognitive impairment 30-items, points vary by cognitive domain

*Included in the core outcomes measures for survivors of acute respiratory failure [38]

Box 46.1 Example questions for eliciting experiences and symptoms of survivors of critical illness

- Can you tell me about your experience in the ICU?
- Thinking back to your time in the ICU, what were the most challenging things about your experience?
- What have been the most difficult things you have faced since being in the ICU?
- How often do memories of your time in the ICU come to mind?
- How would you describe the nature of these memories (e.g., upsetting, fearful, anxiety-inducing, comforting, and/or peaceful)?
- How often do you have nightmares or flashbacks about your time in the ICU? What tends to trigger nightmares or flashbacks?
- What do you do when memories of your time in the ICU pop into your mind?
- How do these symptoms/problems impact
    - Your day-to-day life?
    - Your ability to work?
    - Your relationships?
    - Your view of yourself as a person?
    - How you manage your health now?
- In what ways have you grown since your time in the ICU (e.g., increased patience, more appreciation for life, closer to loved ones, and/or clarity of life goals/values)?

Interventions

A stepped care framework that provides the least intrusive and most effective intervention should be considered first when working with survivors with psychological distress. In the first step, psychological screening and offering education about the impact of medications, procedures, and critical illness can normalize changes in mental health. In the second step, education about self-monitoring symptoms can help individuals become more proactive in bolstering self-management skills and discern when additional specialized support is needed. Finally, survivors of critical illness who have ongoing distress after steps 1 and 2 may benefit from referral to specialized mental health professionals and peer support.

The United Kingdom's National Institute for Health and Care Excellence (NICE) guidelines recommend that patients discharged from the ICU receive psychological follow-up [39]. No specific guidelines for treating psychological symptoms of PICS exist, prompting providers to reference existing guidelines and evidence-based practices for conditions commonly experienced by survivors of critical illness. Cognitive behavioral therapy (CBT) is widely recognized as a frontline treatment for anxiety and depression, and trauma-focused CBT is used for treating PTSD symptoms [40]. Acceptance and commitment therapy (ACT), which has a strong evidence base in individuals with medical conditions, is also empirically supported for depression and anxiety [41]. CBT challenges unhelpful, negative thinking patterns and behaviors, while ACT invites a willingness to accept unwanted, challenging experiences. Accordingly, ACT is a particularly relevant treatment approach for survivors of critical illness coping with changes in physical and emotional health, as it emphasizes the pursuit of values (e.g., relationships, meaningful work, and health) in the face of challenging experiences. Irrespective of treatment interventions, psychotherapy is a valuable component of recovery from critical illness [42].

Strengths-based treatment approaches may also prove valuable in psychological follow-up. PTG literature underscores the importance of appreciating how distressing experiences, including psychological symptoms, can serve as catalysts for growth. Focusing only on challenging symptoms may slow progress and, importantly, mask opportunities for growth [43]. Survivors could benefit from leveraging personal strengths (e.g., altruism and resilience) and introducing positively valanced strategies (e.g., seeking social support, growth actions, and positive reappraisal) to aid in managing psychiatric manifestations of PICS [44].

Clinicians and researchers are integral in the continued development and implementation of interventions to advance psychological care for survivors of critical illness. Cox and colleagues developed a telephone-delivered intervention that taught survivors and caregivers coping strategies for managing psychological symptoms, which led to improved symptoms of anxiety, depression, and PTSD [45]. They also demonstrated that a coping skills intervention significantly improved symptoms of psychological distress and quality of life among patients with high levels of baseline distress when compared with an educational program intervention [45]. Cox has also developed mobile applications that provide coping skills and mindfulness training to address psychological distress in survivors, which have demonstrated effectiveness in reducing depressive symptoms [46].

Given the chronic and complex health outcomes of survivors of critical illness, innovative models of psychological care are needed for effective and equitable care. Danesh and colleagues developed a self-management program utilizing peer mentorship to address symptoms, treatments, and psychosocial outcomes in survivors of critical illness [47]. This program is exemplary for clinical innovation, as the intervention uniquely leverages protective factors that can reduce psychological distress (e.g., social support) by fostering connection among survivors; it also accommodates the insufficient infrastructure that many survivors experience when returning to their communities by using telephone and web-based technology to extend the reach of this support service.

Delivery modality is an important component of treatment for survivors of critical illness. Telemedicine can improve access to specialized care by reducing travel time, minimizing caregiver burden, and offering a delivery modality that accommodates common symptoms experienced by survivors, including fatigue, limited mobility, and anxiety induced by medical settings [48]. Care of survivors is likely to benefit from flexible modalities for treatment that consider individual-level differences, such as providing timely reminders to individuals with cognitive impairment, and systemic-level differences, such as offering telephone-delivered treatments to accommodate unreliable internet coverage.

Healthcare professionals should facilitate follow-up care that extends beyond the hospital. For example, psychologists can provide inpatient and outpatient consultation services that both directly support survivors and connect them to other important team members and treatment services [49,50,51]. Advanced nursing staff and social workers can also provide proactive care at individual and organizational levels through liaison and outreach services, which benefit patient outcomes and service utilization across the care continuum (see Chapter 25 for additional information) [52,53]. Primary care providers (PCPs) also play an important role in improving clinical care pathways for survivors, as follow-up with PCPs is routinely recommended after hospitalization and is, for the vast majority of survivors of critical illness, the only available resource for critical care follow-up. Table 46.3 provides select resources that survivors, families, friends, and providers can reference to obtain information that can further aid in promoting psychological adjustment after critical illness.

In addition to being cognizant of psychological manifestations of PICS, providers would benefit from having a general understanding of where survivors are in the psychological processing of events when considering treatment and appropriate points of intervention. Figure 46.2 illustrates a proposed process of psychological navigation, coping, and

Table 46.3 Selected resources for survivors of critical illness

Organization/Group	Website
Critical Illness, Brain Dysfunction, and Survivorship (CIBS) Center	www.icudelirium.org/patients-and-families/overview
Outcomes after Critical Illness and Surgery (OACIS) Group	www.hopkinsmedicine.org/pulmonary/research/outcomes_after_critical_illness_surgery/
Acute Respiratory Distress Syndrome (ARDS) Foundation	https://ardsglobal.org/other-resources/
Trauma Survivors Network (TSN)	www.traumasurvivorsnetwork.org/pages/home
Society for Critical Care Medicine (SCCM)	www.sccm.org/Education-Center/Clinical-Resources/Patient-and-Family
ICUsteps	https://icusteps.org/
ICU Diary Network	www.icu-diary.org/
My Life after ICU	www.mylifeaftericu.com/
American Thoracic Society	https://site.thoracic.org/advocacy-patients/patient-resources/acute-respiratory-distress-syndrome
ICU Unwrapped	https://icuunwrapped.co.uk/
The Conversation Project	https://theconversationproject.org/

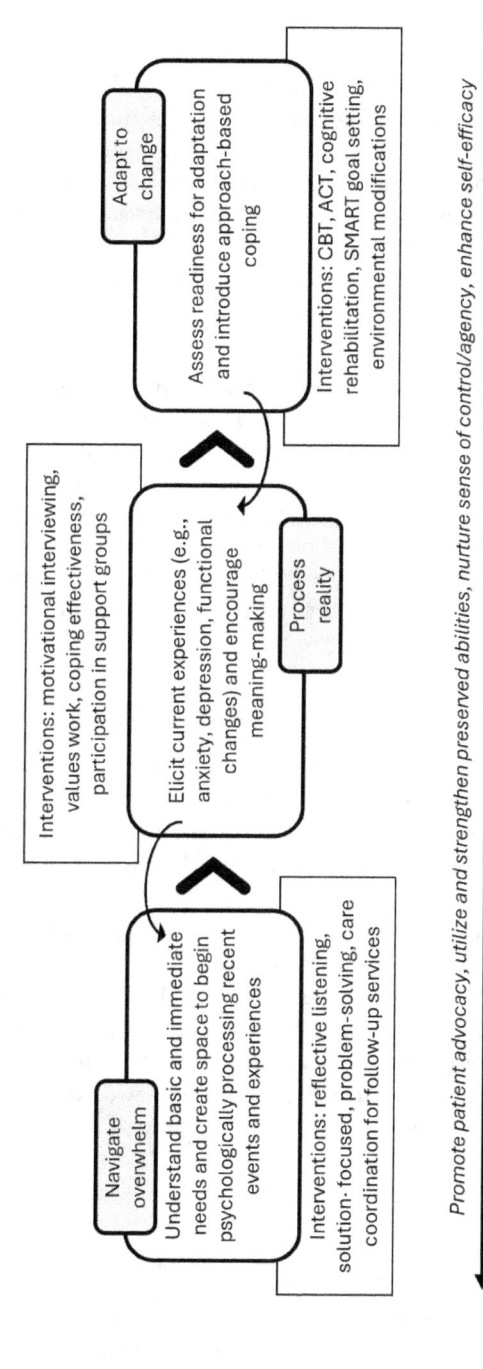

Figure 46.2 Proposed psychological process following ICU survivorship to aid providers in treatment planning.

adaptation following critical illness to help providers select appropriate interventions based on the patient's stage of processing. Understanding the impact of other physical conditions on psychological well-being could further improve patient-centered care. For example, providers who are aware of the high occurrence of sleep and pain disturbances could offer referrals to specialty sleep and pain clinics, respectively, for effective treatments to improve clinical outcomes (e.g., CBT for insomnia or chronic pain and image rehearsal therapy for nightmares; see Chapter 37 for additional information). Appreciating risk and protective factors for psychological symptoms among survivors is valuable for a systematic approach to treatment planning. Given that psychological assessment is not widely available in ICUs and variable treatment pathways exist following hospital discharge, advancing clinical care of survivors of critical illness requires providers of varied disciplines to screen for common psychological sequelae and assist patients in accessing specialized care.

Conclusion

Survivors of critical illness often experience significant psychological distress, including anxiety, depression, and PTSD. Risk factors, such as preexisting psychiatric conditions, traumatic ICU experiences, and episodes of delirium, frequently interact, compounding psychological burden of survivors. Protective factors, such as robust social support and timely psychological interventions, can mitigate these effects. Although further research is needed, early assessment to inform targeted interventions across the care continuum can aid in the early identification and treatment of PICS-related psychological symptoms, ultimately promoting more positive outcomes for survivors of critical illness.

Key Points

1. Psychological symptoms, including anxiety, depression, and post-traumatic stress, are common among survivors of critical illness.
2. The natural history of psychological symptoms among survivors of critical illness is poorly understood, and more research elucidating key intervention points to mitigate symptoms is needed.
3. Psychological symptoms have bidirectional effects with physical symptoms, such as pain, fatigue, sleep disturbances, and weakness.
4. Early evidence suggests that a continuum of psychological screening and interventions beginning during hospitalization and continuing throughout survivorship may mitigate psychological symptoms and improve quality of life.
5. In addition to distress, survivors of critical illness may also experience post-traumatic growth, framing the ICU experience as an opportunity to live life more fully.

References

1. S. Nikayin, A. Rabiee, M.D. Hashem, et al. Anxiety symptoms in survivors of critical illness: a systematic review and meta-analysis. *Gen Hosp Psychiatry* 2016; **43**: 23–9.
2. O.J. Bienvenu, L.A. Friedman, E. Colantuoni, et al. Psychiatric symptoms after acute respiratory distress syndrome: a 5-year longitudinal study. *Intensive Care Med* 2018; **44**: 38–47.

3. L.M. Boehm, C.M. Bird, A.M. Warren, et al. Understanding and managing anxiety sensitivity during critical illness and long-term recovery. *Am J Crit Care* 2023; **32**: 449–57.

4. I. Benjenk, J. Chen. Effective mental health interventions to reduce hospital readmission rates: a systematic review. *J Hosp Manag Health Policy* 2018; **2**: 45.

5. A. Parker, T. Sricharoenchai, D. M. Needham. Early rehabilitation in the intensive care unit: preventing physical and mental health impairments. *Curr Phys Med Rehabil Rep* 2013; **1**: 307–14.

6. M.M. Hosey, S.T. Wegener, C. Hinkle, D. M. Needham. A cognitive behavioral therapy-informed self-management program for acute respiratory failure survivors: a feasibility study. *J Clin Med* 2021; **10**: 1–8.

7. A. Rabiee, S. Nikayin, M.D. Hashem, et al. Depressive symptoms after critical illness: a systematic review and meta-analysis. *Crit Care Med* 2016; **44**: 1744–53.

8. C. Teixeira, R.G. Rosa, D. Sganzerla, et al. The burden of mental illness among survivors of critical care-risk factors and impact on quality of life: a multicenter prospective cohort study. *Chest* 2021; **160**: 157–64.

9. S.M. Fernando, D. Qureshi, M.M. Sood, et al. Suicide and self-harm in adult survivors of critical illness: population-based cohort study. *BMJ* 2021; **373**: n973.

10. D.S. Davydow, J.M. Gifford, S.V. Desai, et al. Depression in general intensive care unit survivors: a systematic review. *Intensive Care Med* 2009; **35**: 796–809.

11. R. Troubat, P. Barone, S. Leman, et al. Neuroinflammation and depression: a review. *Eur J Neurosci* 2021; **53**: 151–71.

12. N. Khandelwal, C.L. Hough, L. Downey, et al. Prevalence, risk factors, and outcomes of financial stress in survivors of critical illness. *Crit Care Med* 2018; **46**: e530–e9.

13. B.B. Barreto, M. Luz, M.N.O. Rios, et al. The impact of intensive care unit diaries on patients' and relatives' outcomes: a systematic review and meta-analysis. *Crit Care* 2019; **23**: 411.

14. P.A. McIlroy, R.S. King, M. Garrouste-Orgeas, et al. The effect of icu diaries on psychological outcomes and quality of life of survivors of critical illness and their relatives: a systematic review and meta-analysis. *Crit Care Med* 2019; **47**: 273–9.

15. A. Gazzato, T. Scquizzato, G. Imbriaco, et al. The effect of intensive care unit diaries on posttraumatic stress disorder, anxiety, and depression: a systematic review and meta-analysis of randomized controlled trials. *Dimens Crit Care Nurs* 2022; **41**: 256–63.

16. A.M. Parker, T. Sricharoenchai, S. Raparla, et al. Posttraumatic stress disorder in critical illness survivors: a metaanalysis. *Crit Care Med* 2015; **43**: 1121–9.

17. J.N. McGiffin, I.R. Galatzer-Levy, G. A. Bonanno. Is the intensive care unit traumatic? What we know and don't know about the intensive care unit and posttraumatic stress responses. *Rehabil Psychol* 2016; **61**: 120–31.

18. L. Kok, A.J. Slooter, M.H. Hillegers, et al. Benzodiazepine use and neuropsychiatric outcomes in the ICU: a systematic review. *Crit Care Med* 2018; **46**: 1673–80.

19. C. Jones, C. Backman, M. Capuzzo, et al. Intensive care diaries reduce new onset post traumatic stress disorder following critical illness: a randomised, controlled trial. *Crit Care* 2010; **14**: R168.

20. E. Prince, T.A. Gerstenblith, D. Davydow, O.J. Bienvenu. Psychiatric morbidity after critical illness. *Crit Care Clin* 2018; **34**: 599–608.

21. L. Kok, A.J. Slooter, M.H. Hillegers, et al. Benzodiazepine use and neuropsychiatric outcomes in the ICU: a systematic review. *Crit Care Med* 2018; **46**: 1673–80.

22. X. Sun, D. Huang, F. Zeng, et al. Effect of intensive care unit diary on incidence of posttraumatic stress disorder, anxiety, and depression of adult intensive care unit survivors: a systematic review and meta-analysis. *J Adv Nurs* 2021; **77**: 2929–41.

23. R. Thom, D.A. Silbersweig, R.J. Boland. Major depressive disorder in medical illness: a review of assessment, prevalence, and treatment options. *Psychosom Med* 2019; **81**: 246–55.

24. M.T. Altman, M.P. Knauert, M.A. Pisani. Sleep disturbance after hospitalization and critical illness: a systematic review. *Ann Am Thorac Soc* 2017; **14**: 1457–68.

25. C.J. Hayhurst, J.C. Jackson, K.R. Archer, et al. Pain and its long-term interference of daily life after critical illness. *Anesth Analg* 2018; **127**: 690–7.

26. K.J. Neufeld, J.S. Leoutsakos, H. Yan, et al. Fatigue symptoms during the first year Following ARDS. *Chest* 2020; **158**: 999–1007.

27. R.G. Tedeschi, L.G. Calhoun. *Trauma and transformation: growing in the aftermath of suffering.* Los Angeles: SAGE Publications; 1995.

28. T. Barskova, R. Oesterreich. Post-traumatic growth in people living with a serious medical condition and its relations to physical and mental health: a systematic review. *Disabil Rehabil* 2009; **31**: 1709–33.

29. D. Nehra, J.P. Herrera-Escobar, S.S. Al Rafai, et al. Resilience and long-term outcomes after trauma: an opportunity for early intervention? *J Trauma Acute Care Surg* 2019; **87**: 782–9.

30. American Psychiatric Association. *Diagnostic and statistical manual of mental disorders: DSM-5.* Washington, DC: American Psychiatric Association; 2013.

31. M.E. Mikkelsen, M. Still, B.J. Anderson, et al. Society of Critical Care Medicine's international consensus conference on prediction and identification of long-term impairments after critical illness. *Crit Care Med* 2020; **48**: 1670–9.

32. B.K. Solomon, K.G. Wilson, P.R. Henderson, et al. A Breathlessness Catastrophizing Scale for chronic obstructive pulmonary disease. *J Psychosom Res* 2015; **79**: 62–8.

33. K. Kroenke, R.L. Spitzer, J.B. Williams. The PHQ-9: validity of a brief depression severity measure. *J Gen Intern Med* 2001; **16**: 606–13.

34. R.L. Spitzer, K. Kroenke, J.B. Williams, B. Lowe. A brief measure for assessing generalized anxiety disorder: the GAD-7. *Arch Intern Med* 2006; **166**: 1092–7.

35. Z.S. Nasreddine, N.A. Phillips, V. Bedirian, et al. The Montreal Cognitive Assessment, MoCA: a brief screening tool for mild cognitive impairment. *J Am Geriatr Soc* 2005; **53**: 695–9.

36. A.S. Zigmond, R.P. Snaith. The hospital anxiety and depression scale. *Acta Psychiatr Scand* 1983; **67**: 361–70.

37. M.M. Hosey, J.S. Leoutsakos, X. Li, et al. Screening for posttraumatic stress disorder in ARDS survivors: validation of the Impact of Event Scale-6 (IES-6). *Crit Care* 2019; **23**: 276.

38. D.M. Needham, K.A. Sepulveda, V.D. Dinglas, et al. Core outcome measures for clinical research in acute respiratory failure survivors. an international modified Delphi consensus study. *Am J Respir Crit Care Med* 2017; **196**: 1122–30.

39. United Kingdom National Institute for Health and Care Excellence (NICE). Rehabilitation After Critical Illness 2009. www.nice.org.uk/guidance/cg83.

40. H. Murray, N. Grey, J. Wild, et al. Cognitive therapy for post-traumatic stress disorder following critical illness and intensive care unit admission. *Cogn Behav Therap* 2020; **13**: e13.

41. C.D. Graham, J. Gouick, C. Krahe, D. Gillanders. A systematic review of the use of Acceptance and Commitment Therapy (ACT) in chronic disease and long-term conditions. *Clin Psychol Rev* 2016; **46**: 46–58.

42. R. Clarke, V. Weare, H. Chow, et al. "It saved me": a thematic analysis of experiences of psychological therapy following critical illness and intensive care. *J Intensive Care Soc* 2024; **25**: 288–95.

43. L.J. Long, C.A. Phillips, N. Glover, et al. A meta-analytic review of the relationship between posttraumatic growth, anxiety, and depression. *J Happiness Stud* 2021; **22**: 3703–28.

44. C. Henson, D. Truchot, A. Canevello. What promotes post traumatic growth? A systematic review. *Eur J Trauma Dissoc* 2021; **5**: 100195.

45. C.E. Cox, C.L. Hough, S.S. Carson, et al. Effects of a telephone- and web-based coping skills training program compared with an education program for survivors of critical illness and their family members. a randomized clinical trial. *Am J Respir Crit Care Med* 2018; **197**: 66–78.

46. C.E. Cox, J.A. Gallis, M.K. Olsen, et al. Mobile mindfulness intervention for psychological distress among intensive care unit survivors: a randomized clinical trial. *JAMA Intern Med* 2024; **184**: 749–59.

47. V. Danesh, J. Hecht, R. Hao, et al. Peer Support for Post Intensive Care Syndrome Self-Management (PS-PICS): study protocol for peer mentor training. *J Adv Nurs* 2021; **77**: 2092–101.

48. M.A. Kovaleva, A.C. Jones, C.C. Kimpel, et al. Patient and caregiver experiences with a telemedicine intensive care unit recovery clinic. *Heart Lung* 2023; **58**: 47–53.

49. M. Beadman, M. Carraretto. Key elements of an evidence-based clinical psychology service within adult critical care. *J Intensive Care Soc* 2023; **24**: 215–21.

50. K. Stucky, J.E. Jutte, A.M. Warren, et al. A survey of psychology practice in critical-care settings. *Rehabil Psychol* 2016; **61**: 201–9.

51. Faculty of Intensive Care Medicine. Provision of Intensive Care Services: Faculty for Intensive Care Medicine; 2022. www.ficm.ac.uk/standards/guidelines-for-the-provision-of-intensive-care-services.

52. D.D. Carr. Building collaborative partnerships in critical care: the RN case manager/social work dyad in critical care. *Prof Case Manag* 2009; **14**: 121–32.

53. R. Endacott, S. Eliott, W. Chaboyer. An integrative review and meta-synthesis of the scope and impact of intensive care liaison and outreach services. *J Clin Nurs* 2009; **18**: 3225–36.

Chapter 47: Palliative Care Needs in Survivors of Critical Illness

Ross H. Perfetti, Jessica Lee, Taylor Lincoln, and Andrew L. Thurston

Introduction

Patients often face a variety of logistical challenges, overwhelming emotions, and debilitating physical symptoms after hospitalization requiring admission to an intensive care unit (ICU). Symptoms associated with post-intensive care syndrome (PICS) affect more than 50% of survivors of critical illness and may significantly impact quality of life, functional independence, and the abilities to drive, resume employment, and reestablish previous social roles [1,2,3]. Survivors of critical illness are often affected by their ICU experience in significant and unforeseeable ways, and they may emerge with new identities shaped by their critical illness journey. Exploring their ICU experience and how the emotional toll of critical illness overlaps with complicated symptoms following discharge is a key part of recovery, and studies have shown a range of patient priorities during the recovery period, including feeling safe, connecting with people, and seeking new life experiences (see Chapter 26 for additional information) [4,5]. The field of palliative care is uniquely equipped to evaluate this intersection of illness and identity, and it has particular relevance in survivors of critical illness, a population in which a high degree of unmet palliative care needs exists [6,7]. Integrating palliative care techniques into ICU follow-up clinics can help identify complicated challenges and symptoms during rehabilitation and allows clinicians to better coordinate recovery after critical illness [8,9].

In this chapter, we review the role of palliative care in survivors of critical illness, examine strategies for integration of palliative principles into ICU follow-up clinics, and explore specific communication techniques to facilitate expectation management and discussions of patient-centered goals in the recovery period.

Distinguishing Between PICS Challenges and Symptoms

To effectively integrate palliative care strategies into the evaluation and management of patients with PICS, it is important to distinguish challenges frequently encountered in patients with PICS and clinical symptoms commonly associated with PICS. While this may seem like a straightforward task, complicated clinical conditions, including fatigue, cognitive impairment, anxiety disorder, post-traumatic stress disorder (PTSD), and depression, are often interwoven with logistical challenges, such as access to transportation, paying hospital bills, and existential distress [10,11,12,13]. Key differences between PICS challenges and clinical symptoms are outlined in Table 47.1. Given the interconnected nature of PICS challenges and symptoms, the implementation of core palliative care principles may be helpful in identifying and isolating specific areas for focused management in survivors of critical illness [6,8].

Table 47.1 PICS challenges versus clinical symptoms

PICS Challenges	PICS Clinical Symptoms
Transportation	Physical
Food access	- Dyspnea
Insurance concerns/healthcare navigation	- Weakness
Identity crisis	- Pain
Existential or spiritual distress	- Impaired mobility
Caregiver burden	Cognitive
New or shifting family dynamics	- Memory difficulty
Financial burden/healthcare cost	- Impaired executive function
Job concerns and re-acclimation	- Impaired attention
Post-hospital appointments	- Impaired language/speech
Grief and feelings of loss	- Decreased processing speed
Medication questions	Psychological
	- Anxiety
	- Depression
	- PTSD

What Is Palliative Care?

Palliative care is an interdisciplinary specialty that addresses the needs of people with serious illness while focusing on improving quality of life for both patients and their families. These improvements can be achieved through relief of distressing symptoms; support of psychosocial, emotional, and spiritual concerns; and assistance with communication and decision-making. Research demonstrates that palliative care interventions improve quality of life, symptom management, and support for patients and families while lowering healthcare costs [14,15,16,17,18,19,20,21,22,23]. Palliative care is appropriate for any stage of serious illness and is provided either concurrently with curative treatment, such as organ transplantation or chemotherapy, or as the primary treatment focus [24,25]. Within this section, we provide a general overview of palliative care needs in survivors of critical illness, differentiate between primary and specialty palliative care, and review the various roles of specialty palliative care team members.

Palliative care addresses both symptomatic and nonsymptomatic needs [26,27]. As discussed in previous chapters, survivors of critical illness experience a myriad of distressing symptoms, both from the disease process itself and as a consequence of treatments delivered in the ICU [11]. Palliative care provides personalized and comprehensive options to address these symptoms with pharmacologic therapies, such as the use of opioids for dyspnea and antipsychotics for nausea, and non-pharmacologic interventions, such as guided imagery for anxiety. Additionally, patients and families experiencing serious illness have significant psychological, social, and spiritual needs that can be addressed using palliative care skills [8,9]. Communication and decision-making are often challenging for patients and their families, especially in situations with prognostic uncertainty or impaired decision-making capacity [28,29,30,31]. Utilizing specific palliative care skills, including empathetic response and active listening, may foster the growth of trusting relationships, clarify patient values and preferences, provide emotional support, and develop goal-concordant treatment plans moving forward [32,33].

Similar to other medical subspecialties, some components of palliative care can be implemented by healthcare professionals without specialized training [34]. These components, known broadly as primary palliative care, involve fundamental skills and competencies, including basic symptom management, delivering prognoses or bad news, and working with patients to develop an individualized plan of care [35]. In contrast, specialty palliative care is delivered by providers with extensive training in advanced therapeutic skills, such as managing refractory symptoms, navigating complex communication or decision-making dynamics, and exploring nuanced spiritual or psychosocial needs [36]. These palliative care specialists often work as part of an interdisciplinary team that includes clinicians, nurses, pharmacists, social workers, psychologists or counselors, therapists, and spiritual care professionals, who each contribute unique expertise and perspectives to the patient care plan [37]. While roles are collaborative and may overlap, clinicians generally oversee medical management, guide decision-making, and coordinate with other providers; nurses provide patient care, monitor symptoms, and offer support; social workers address psychosocial, emotional, and practical needs while connecting families to needed resources; and spiritual care providers address existential and spiritual support (see Chapter 15 for additional information) [38,39].

Individuals living with serious illness often carry a high risk of complications that may negatively impact their quality of life and excessively strain caregivers [40,41]. While specialty palliative care clinics are helpful in some of these situations, the application of primary palliative care principles in the management of patients with PICS can help identify complicated physical symptoms and potentially unrecognized needs in survivors, ultimately helping to promote post-traumatic growth after critical illness [42,43].

Application of Palliative Care Principles to Survivors of Critical Illness

Identifying Symptoms Across Critical Illness Survivorship

Given the impact of persistent clinical symptoms on survivors of critical illness, it is important to quickly identify and manage these symptoms before they further affect quality of life and recoverability. Current recommendations from an international consensus conference on the prediction and identification of long-term impairments following critical illness suggest serial assessments for symptoms associated with PICS beginning within two to four weeks of hospital discharge [44]. Clinical symptoms in PICS are classically divided into three categories: physical, cognitive, and psychological (see Table 47.1). As the management of these symptoms has been addressed in previous chapters, we focus instead on screening tools commonly used in the palliative care setting that may facilitate symptom identification in PICS. These screening tools are easily implemented without specialty palliative care training and are divided into two broad categories: psychosocial and physical.

Psychosocial screening tools, such as the Canadian Problem Checklist (CPC) and the Psychosocial Screen for Cancer (PSSCAN), are patient-reported tools validated in the cancer population for assessing patient distress, [45,46] and they may be similarly appropriate to screen for distress in survivors of critical illness. Distress is defined as "a multifactorial unpleasant emotional experience of a psychological (cognitive, behavioral, emotional), social, and/or spiritual nature that may interfere with the ability to cope effectively" with symptoms or treatment plans [47]. The CPC was developed by the Screening for Distress Toolkit Working Group to screen for the most common areas of distress experienced by patients and involves a self-reported list of problems in six key areas: practical, emotional, spiritual, social/family, information, and physical [48]. The PSSCAN more specifically assesses anxiety and depression, perceived social support, desired social support, and health-related quality-of-life, with scores greater than 11 showing high clinical correlation with depression and anxiety [49]. Cognitive screening tools frequently used in palliative care include the Montreal Cognitive Assessment (MoCA) tool and the Mini-Cog, both of which are easily implemented during the course of a clinic encounter and may be monitored for change over time [50,51,52,53]. While the MoCA is more comprehensive (see Chapter 43 for additional information), the Mini-Cog, which involves a three-word registration/recall separated by a clock drawing task for assessment of executive function, is faster and may be preferred if clinic time is limited [52,53]. Tools assessing mental health validated in survivors of critical illness include the Hospital Anxiety and Depression Scale (HADS) and the 9-Item Patient Health Questionnaire (PHQ-9; see Chapter 46 for additional information) [54,55].

Physical screening tools that target clinical symptoms and functional status include the Palliative Performance Scale (PPS) and the Edmonton Symptom Assessment System-Revised (ESAS-r) [56,57]. The PPS is frequently used in palliative care to guide discussions of prognosis based on functional parameters regardless of the primary diagnosis and may have an evolving role in survivors of critical illness [58,59]. The scale ranges from 0 (death) to 100 (fully functional with no limitations) and takes into account ambulation, activity level, evidence of disease, the ability to provide self-care, oral intake, and level of consciousness. A PPS of 30 (bed bound with extensive disease requiring total care) correlates with a prognostic range of 5–36 days [58]. The ESAS, first developed in 1991, has been validated in multiple patient populations and translated into over 20 languages. Originally covering 9 common symptoms using an 11-point numerical rating scale, the ESAS has since been modified into the ESAS-r based on patient feedback and clarification of terminology and symptom timeframe [60]. The ESAS-r is used for both initial symptom screening and longitudinal monitoring of symptom progression over time, can be completed by the patient typically in under one minute, and is free to use (see Figure 47.1) [61]. A third screening tool that may be considered in the post-ICU setting is the PEACE Tool (Physical, Emotive, Autonomy, Communication, Economic, and Transcendent domains), which similarly uses an 11-point numerical rating scale to assess physical symptoms, such pain, nausea, and weakness; cognitive and mental health symptoms, such as depression and anxiety; and psychosocial concerns, including the need for additional support and feeling abandoned by God. In contrast to the ESAS-r, which assesses how the patient is currently feeling, the PEACE Tool assesses symptom severity over the preceding week [62].

A potentially effective strategy that clinicians might consider in survivors of critical illness is the combination of the CPC with the ESAS-r. This practice has been implemented in the cancer population, is considered best practice by the Canadian Partnership Against Cancer [63], and may represent a quick and effective way to screen for distressing physical and psychosocial concerns in this patient population.

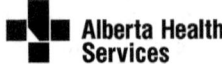

Alberta Health Services

Edmonton Symptom Assessment System Revised (ESAS-r)

Affix patient label within this box

Please circle the number that best describes how you feel NOW:

No Pain	0	1	2	3	4	5	6	7	8	9	10	Worst Possible Pain
No Tiredness *(Tiredness = lack of energy)*	0	1	2	3	4	5	6	7	8	9	10	Worst Possible Tiredness
No Drowsiness *(Drowsiness = feeling sleepy)*	0	1	2	3	4	5	6	7	8	9	10	Worst Possible Drowsiness
No Nausea	0	1	2	3	4	5	6	7	8	9	10	Worst Possible Nausea
No Lack of Appetite	0	1	2	3	4	5	6	7	8	9	10	Worst Possible Lack of Appetitie
No Shortness of Breath	0	1	2	3	4	5	6	7	8	9	10	Worst Possible Shortness of Breath
No Depression *(Depression = feeling sad)*	0	1	2	3	4	5	6	7	8	9	10	Worst Possible Depression
No Anxiety *(Anxiety = feeling nervous)*	0	1	2	3	4	5	6	7	8	9	10	Worst Possible Anxiety
Best Wellbeing *(Wellbeing = how you feel overall)*	0	1	2	3	4	5	6	7	8	9	10	Worst Possible Wellbeing
No _____ Other Problem *(For example constipation)*	0	1	2	3	4	5	6	7	8	9	10	Worst Possible _____

Patient Name _____

Date *(yyyy-Mon-dd)* _____

Time *(hh:mm)* _____

Completed by *(Check one)*
☐ Patient
☐ Family Caregiver
☐ Health Care Professional Caregiver
☐ Caregiver-assisted

Body Diagram on Reverse

Figure 47.1 The Edmonton Symptom Assessment System-Revised (ESAS-r). Reproduced with permission from Alberta Health Services.

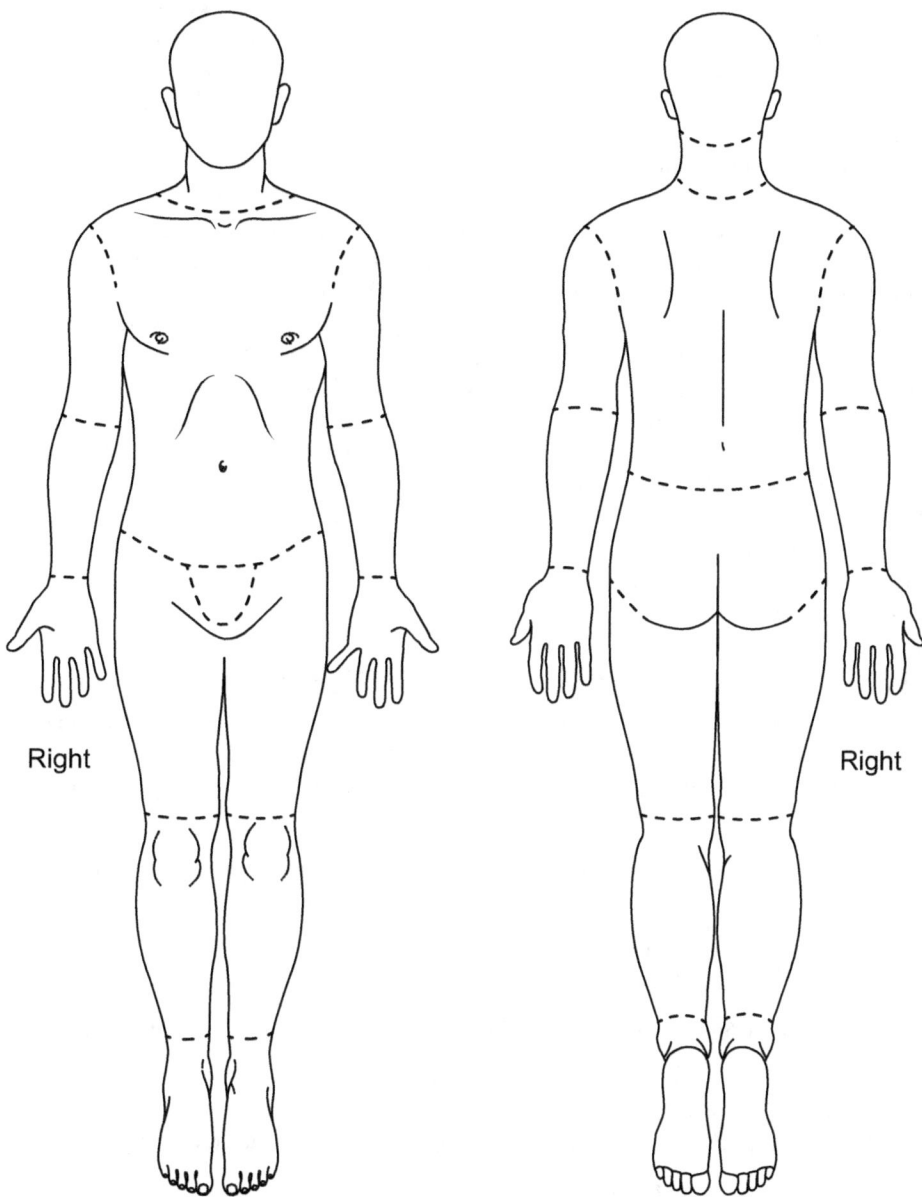

Figure 47.1 (cont.)

Facilitating Goal-Concordant Care

Facilitating discussions of patient-centered goals and managing expectations regarding the depth and breadth of recovery in survivors of critical illness can support rehabilitation that is both meaningful and aligned with patient wishes. Qualitative studies of patient priorities after hospital discharge for critical illness identify important, nonmedical components of recovery that may factor into patient goals. Survivors of critical illness participating in a peer support program articulated their goals for recovery in three broad categories: (1) physical, emotional, and psychosocial health (e.g., "improve balance" and "be able to deal with distressing memories of the ICU"), (2) management of health and setting expectations (e.g., "get back to work" and "increase confidence in caring for new stoma"), and (3) family and social engagement (e.g., "have some purpose . . . get back to hobbies" and "would like support for diabetes and would like to meet people in a similar position") [64]. In another study, patients reported a range of priorities, including feeling safe, asserting personhood, connecting with people, resuming previous roles and routines, and seeking new life experiences [5]. Attempts have been made to operationalize this array of recovery desires into the form of a validated "menu" of patient-centered goals that are set between the patient and care providers and then used to devise a rehabilitation plan to guide recovery [65].

Healthcare providers caring for patients in ICU follow-up clinics can use palliative communication principles to clarify patient goals and deliver clinical information [32,33]. Effective communication between patients and providers is linked to improvements in patients' quality of life and mood and results in increased adherence to recommended treatments [66,67,68]. Clinician recognition of family caregiver roles, exploring coping strategies, and demonstrating commitment to medical management are also key aspects of patient support [69].

Communication Techniques: Ask-Tell-Ask and NURSE Statements

There are several specific palliative communication techniques that aid in clarifying patient-centered goals and facilitating difficult conversations, and these can be implemented in an ICU follow-up clinic without requiring specialized training. One helpful technique is "Ask-Tell-Ask" [70].

1. **Ask** the patient/family to describe their current understanding (of their diagnosis, what happened in the hospital/ICU, bothersome symptoms, etc.)
   a. "What did the doctors tell you in the hospital?"
   b. "What are you hoping the next couple of months will look like?"

2. **Tell** the patient/family what you need to communicate in clear, straightforward language. Keep it short.
   a. "You almost died while you were in the ICU."
   b. "The symptoms you are feeling are related to your critical illness and ICU stay."

3. **Ask** the patient/family if they understood, giving them an opportunity to ask questions or restate their understanding in their own words.
   a. "What questions do you have about what we just discussed?"
   b. "If your family asks you later what we talked about, what will you say?"

Ask-Tell-Ask is a powerful inquiry technique that is used to explore patient insight, provide clinical information in a concise manner, and assess for any questions or concerns. As such, using this technique may trigger strong and potentially confusing emotions, especially after a difficult hospitalization.

Table 47.2 NURSE statements

Skill	Sample Statement
Name the emotion	"It sounds like the ICU experience was very scary."
Understand	"I can't imagine how hard it must be to feel so weak now that you're home."
Respect	"Thank you for sharing. I'm impressed by your fortitude."
Support	"Our PICS clinic team is here to help navigate these next steps with you."
Explore	"You mentioned feeling a loss of control. Tell me more … "

Pairing Ask-Tell-Ask with an emotional exploration framework is often helpful. The use of NURSE statements as an empathetic response to emotion can help patients and family members process these complex emotions and think more clearly about clinical goals and expectations (see Table 47.2) [71]. Utilizing techniques like "Naming" the emotion and "Exploring" statements (e.g., "Tell me more") may help facilitate discussions about feelings that are difficult to describe, while "Respect" and "Support" statements provide comfort in the form of reassurance and emotional validation. Navigating the emotional landscape with empathy is often a necessary step before any discussion of clinical planning may take place [72].

Discussing Future Healthcare Wishes and Advance Care Planning

Advanced care planning is important in the post-ICU period, especially given the increased risk of hospital readmission, development of new or worsening chronic diseases, and death among survivors of critical illness (see Chapter 33 for additional information) [73,74,75,76,77]. The months following critical illness represent an important window for patients to reflect on their illness experience and to make decisions regarding future care based on those reflections in a supportive environment distanced from the urgency of critical illness. This is especially true for older and frail survivors of critical illness, who face significant symptom burden and frequently poor prognoses, yet who often do not receive palliative care support during hospitalization [6,7]. ICU follow-up clinics provide an opportunity to revisit goals of care and conduct more formal advanced care planning, such as establishing code status, identifying surrogate decision-makers, and completing advance directives [8]. At one ICU follow-up clinic, four out of five patients had a documented goals of care conversation during their initial visit, and over 30% of patients who had such discussions requested future clinical de-escalation (e.g., a time-limited trial of critical care only, orders not to intubate, or orders not to return to the ICU during future hospitalizations) [78]. Navigating these conversations with both patients and their loved ones in an ICU follow-up clinic creates an opportunity to prevent future distress associated with medical decision-making among surrogates [79,80,81]. Empathetic exploration of the ICU experience using palliative principles in this setting can help patients and their families anticipate future decisions and draft documents that protect patient autonomy. Common documents discussed in the clinic setting include advance directives, healthcare powers of attorney, living wills, and physician orders for life-sustaining treatments (POLST) [82,83].

Spiritual Support

Critical illness is for many a life-altering experience [84], and as part of the healing process, patients may search for meaning within that experience [85]. Spirituality is one lens through which patients reflect on feelings of loss and changing relationships [9]. Among patients in a single-center study, 13% reported feeling "abandoned or punished by God or not supported by their church/faith" [86]. As spiritual and existential distress are frequently interwoven with psychosocial challenges and clinical symptoms, the evaluation of spiritual needs is a standard part of palliative practice (see Chapter 15 for additional information). Basic exploration is easily implemented using a NURSE "Explore" statement, as demonstrated in the following exchange [87,88]:

PATIENT: God granted me a miracle and helped me survive the ICU.
I hope He'll grant another miracle and help me recover.

PROVIDER: Tell me more. What would a miracle look like in the months ahead?

PATIENT: Well, I'd love to get stronger ... and maybe get back to fishing ...

PROVIDER: That sounds like a wonderful goal. Would it be helpful if we explored what the coming months might look like while focusing on your goal to get stronger?

Just as it is important to recognize the need for specialty palliative care referral, so, too, is it important to recognize the need for specialty spiritual care support. In such cases, if a spiritual care provider is not a member of the ICU follow-up clinic multidisciplinary team, then referral to a spiritual care provider may be appropriate [89].

Caregiver Support

Assisting caregivers in adapting to life after critical illness, finding adequate psychosocial supports, providing reassurance, and facilitating positive aspects of the caregiving experience are foundational components of supporting caregivers in the post-ICU period [90,91,92]. Critical illness may profoundly impact caregivers, with significant stress related to their loved one's illness and increased risk of anxiety, depression, and PTSD [93,94,95,96,97,98], commonly referred to as post-intensive care syndrome – family (PICS-F; see Chapter 48 for additional information). Providing support for caregivers' social, spiritual, and educational needs within one month of hospital discharge, as well as providing assistance with care management, are key to ensuring the success of follow-up care for patients [8]. In addition to curious and empathetic listening from clinicians, peer support groups for survivors of critical illness and their loved ones can be an important psychosocial resource for families (see Chapter 49 for additional information) [99].

Understanding the economic impact of critical illness on the patients' support network and working collaboratively with social workers to preemptively address financial problems are also important components of post-ICU care, as caregivers must often reduce working hours to assume the role of primary caregiver to their loved one [100]. Moreover, patients with multiple morbidities and compromised socioeconomic status experience disproportionate symptom burden, reinforcing the importance of addressing social determinants of health, including food insecurity and housing instability (see Chapter 25 for additional information) [101]. Using palliative communication principles as outlined above may facilitate the exploration of these psychosocial scenarios in an ICU follow-up clinic.

Expectation Management and Anticipatory Guidance

Patients want to understand their episode of critical illness and often have questions about what to expect next [102]. Many patients have difficulty remembering what happened to them during their time in the ICU and wonder if what they are experiencing is "normal" [103]. It is helpful to begin conversations regarding expectation management by reviewing the patient's diagnosis, course of illness, and treatments; this conversation can be complemented by a letter recapitulating this information in language that is easy to understand that patients can refer to in the future or bring to future physician appointments [103,104,105]. Using the Ask-Tell-Ask framework combined with NURSE statements may be helpful in exploring ICU memories and expectations for recovery. ICU diaries, which contain family and staff notes on a patient's ICU course, are another option for reviewing the ICU experience from a different perspective (see Chapter 18 for additional information) [106,107,108].

Patients hoping to understand the long-term ramifications of critical illness may benefit from individualized strategies for coping and stress management [105,109,110]. During preparation for return to community living, patients and their families may benefit from learning about their options for care and support at home, which can further alleviate anxiety related to this transition. Patients are often interested in how they can return to daily activities and prepare for resumption of employment [109], while families and caregivers struggle with anticipating how much care they will need to provide for their loved one [105]. As much as possible, clinicians should provide specific information to patients and their families about the expected length of recovery and the potential for functional independence, return to work, and reengagement in other social roles [90]. Such information may be overwhelming to many patients, and the exploration of such expectations and hopes using palliative techniques such as the "Some-Other" approach may be helpful [111].

> "Some people who have survived an ICU stay want a sense of what the months ahead might look like. Others want to focus on taking things one day at a time. What kind of person are you?"
> Or
> "It sounds like your critical illness experience was very overwhelming. Some people find it helpful to talk about their experience while it's fresh in their minds. Others aren't ready to talk about it, and that's ok. How do you feel about it?"

Using the "Some-Other" technique while exploring patient values may help clarify goals and simultaneously normalize differences in experiences, thereby minimizing the impact of emotional confounders like guilt and anger on decision-making.

Opportunities for Integration of Palliative Care into Critical Illness Survivorship

When to Refer to Specialty Palliative Care

Interdisciplinary ICU follow-up clinics offer unique opportunities to address interconnected symptoms and social challenges, with many clinicians viewing palliative care as essential to their practice [8,112]. ICU follow-up clinics could enhance patient care after critical illness by including palliative care practitioners in their treatment teams and by training staff in palliative care principles. Given challenges with patient attendance at in-person ICU follow-up clinic appointments, successful implementation of telehealth programs among many ICU follow-up

> **Box 47.1 Potential indications for specialty palliative care clinic referral [119]**
> - Severe physical symptoms
> - Severe emotional symptoms
> - Request for hastened death or alterations in advance care planning
> - Spiritual or existential distress
> - Delirium, cognitive change, or other symptoms impacting medical insight
> - Family conflict
> - New life-limiting diagnosis
> - Prognosis with median survival one year or less

clinics (see Chapter 29 for additional information), and the benefit of palliative care telehealth services to patients and providers alike, there may be a role for palliative care telehealth consultation in the post-ICU space as a means of increasing access to palliative care providers [113,114,115,116,117]. There are times, however, when referral to a specialty palliative care clinic is warranted. Although there are no palliative care referral guidelines specific to the post-ICU setting, ICU follow-up clinics could consider adapting current guidelines from the outpatient oncology setting (see Box 47.1) [118].

Barriers

Despite potential benefits, survivors of critical illness rarely receive palliative care consultation even though they have identified palliative care needs [6]. Clinicians caring for survivors of critical illness describe numerous challenges to the integration of palliative care in their practice, including limited primary palliative care skills among providers, patient prognostic uncertainty, worry about removing hope from patients, and the misconception that palliative care is solely for patients at the end of life. Additional barriers to the implementation of palliative care in the clinic setting include poor communication between healthcare providers, lack of after-hour palliative services, and lack of clarity around palliative roles and responsibilities [120,121]. Examples of integration of palliative care into clinical settings exist in other specialties, such as nephrology, with dedicated palliative care education for staff and the development of specific communication programs to facilitate training in primary palliative skills [122,123]. More research is needed to understand how barriers to the implementation of palliative care principles can be mitigated, how palliative care clinicians can best integrate into the workflow of ICU follow-up clinics, and how palliative services can establish continuity of care from the ICU.

Summary

Addressing psychosocial concerns, logistical limitations, overwhelming emotions, and physical symptoms in survivors of critical illness requires a multidisciplinary approach for optimal evaluation and management, and the field of palliative care is uniquely suited to explore these elements of PICS. Studies have identified numerous unmet palliative care needs in survivors of critical illness, along with a desires for patient-centered, goal-concordant medical management and clear provider communication. Utilization of primary palliative care communication techniques and principles in the exploration of patient needs is helpful in the post-ICU period. Referral to specialty palliative care services may be appropriate in some situations.

Key Points

1. Palliative care is an interdisciplinary specialty that addresses the complicated needs of people with serious illness while focusing on improving quality of life for both patients and their families.
2. Screening tools used in palliative care (e.g., ESAS-r and PPS) may be applicable in ICU follow-up clinics and implemented without prior palliative care training.
3. Palliative communication tools, such as NURSE statements, Ask-Tell-Ask, and the Some-Other technique, can be used by clinicians in ICU follow-up clinics to clarify goals and expectations in survivors of critical illness.
4. Referral to specialty palliative care clinics should be considered if there are additional unmet needs, including limited life expectancy, severe physical symptoms, or existential distress.

References

1. C. Yuan, F. Timmins, D.R. Thompson. Post-intensive care syndrome: a concept analysis. *Int J Nurs Stud* 2021; **114**: 103814.
2. J. McPeake, M.E. Mikkelsen, T. Quasim, et al. Return to employment after critical illness and its association with psychosocial outcomes: a systematic review and meta-analysis. *Ann Am Thorac Soc* 2019; **16**(10): 1304–11.
3. S.M. Brown, S. Bose, V. Banner-Goodspeed, et al. Approaches to addressing post–intensive care syndrome among intensive care unit survivors: a narrative review. *Ann Am Thorac Soc* 2019; **16**(8): 947–56.
4. L.M. Thurston, S.L. Milnes, C.L. Hodgson, et al. Defining patient-centered recovery after critical illness: a qualitative study. *J Crit Care* 2020; **57**: 84–90.
5. L.P. Scheunemann, J.S. White S. Prinjha, et al. Post–intensive care unit care: a qualitative analysis of patient priorities and implications for redesign. *Ann Am Thorac Soc* 2020; **17**(2): 221–8.
6. M.R. Baldwin, H. Wunsch, P.A. Reyfman, et al. High burden of palliative needs among older intensive care unit survivors transferred to post–acute care facilities: a single-center study. *Ann Am Thorac Soc* 2013; **10**(5): 458–65.
7. L.R. Pollack, N.E. Goldstein, W.C. Gonzalez, et al. The frailty phenotype and palliative care needs of older survivors of critical illness. *J Am Geriatr Soc* 2017; **65**(6): 1168–75.
8. T.L. Eaton, T.E. Lincoln, A. Lewis, et al. Palliative care in survivors of critical illness: a qualitative study of post-intensive care unit program clinicians. *J Palliat Med* 2023; **26**(12): 1644–53.
9. T.L. Eaton, A. Lewis, H.S. Donovan, et al. Examining the needs of survivors of critical illness through the lens of palliative care: a qualitative study of survivor experiences. *Intensive Crit Care Nurs* 2023; **75**: 103362.
10. A. Marra, P.P. Pandharipande, T.D. Girard, et al. Co-occurrence of post-intensive care syndrome problems among 406 survivors of critical illness. *Crit Care Med* 2018; **46**(9): 1393–401.
11. A.K. Langerud, T. Rustøen, M.C. Småstuen, et al. Intensive care survivor-reported symptoms: a longitudinal study of survivors' symptoms. *Nurs Crit Care* 2018; **23**(1): 48–54.
12. V.D. Dinglas, L.N. Faraone, D.M. Needham. Understanding patient-important outcomes after critical illness: a synthesis of recent qualitative, empirical, and consensus-related studies. *Curr Opin Crit Care* 2018; **24**(5): 401–9.

13. L.M. Cagino, K.S. Seagly, J.I. McSparron. Survivorship after critical illness and post-intensive care syndrome. *Clin Chest Med* 2022; **43**(3): 551–61.

14. D. Kavalieratos, J. Corbelli, D.I. Zhang, et al. Association between palliative care and patient and caregiver outcomes: a systematic review and meta-analysis. *JAMA* 2016; **316**(20): 2104–14.

15. P. Guo, M. Dzingina, A.M. Firth, et al. Development and validation of a casemix classification to predict costs of specialist palliative care provision across inpatient hospice, hospital and community settings in the UK: a study protocol. *BMJ Open* 2018; **8**(3): e020071.

16. M. Delgado-Guay, H.A. Parsons, Z. Li, et al. Symptom distress in advanced cancer patients with anxiety and depression in the palliative care setting. *Support Care Cancer* 2009; **17**(5): 573–9.

17. M.R. London, S. McSkimming, N. Drew, et al. Evaluation of a Comprehensive, Adaptable, Life-Affirming, Longitudinal (CALL) palliative care project. *J Palliat Med* 2005; **8**(6): 1214–25.

18. J.G. Rogers, C.B. Patel, R.J. Mentz, et al. Palliative care in heart failure. *J Am Coll Cardiol* 2017; **70**(3): 331–41.

19. J.S. Temel, J.A. Greer, A. Muzikansky, et al. Early palliative care for patients with metastatic non–small-cell lung cancer. *N Engl J Med* 2010; **363**(8): 733–42.

20. A.P. Abernethy, D.C. Currow, B.S. Fazekas, et al. Specialized palliative care services are associated with improved short- and long-term caregiver outcomes. *Support Care Cancer* 2008; **16**(6): 585–97.

21. H. Seow, K. Brazil, J. Sussman, et al. Impact of community based, specialist palliative care teams on hospitalisations and emergency department visits late in life and hospital deaths: a pooled analysis. *Br Med J* 2014; **348**: g3496.

22. S. Smith, A. Brick, S. O'Hara, C. Normand. Evidence on the cost and cost-effectiveness of palliative care: a literature review. *Palliat Med* 2014; **28**(2): 130–50.

23. R.S. Morrison, J. Dietrich, S. Ladwig, et al. Palliative care consultation teams cut hospital costs for Medicaid beneficiaries. *Health Aff* 2011; **30**(3): 454–63.

24. A. Berlin, T.J. Carleton. Concurrent palliative care for surgical patients. *Surg Clin North Am* 2019; **99**(5): 823–31.

25. E. Bruera, D. Hui. Integrating supportive and palliative care in the trajectory of cancer: establishing goals and models of care. *J Clin Oncol* 2010; **28**(25): 4013–17.

26. M. Swami, A.A. Case. Effective palliative care: what is involved? *Oncology* 2018; **32**(4): 180-4.

27. World Health Organization. *Why palliative care is an essential function of primary health care.* Geneva: World Health Organization; 2018.

28. R.F. Johnson Jr, J. Gustin. Acute lung injury and acute respiratory distress syndrome requiring tracheal intubation and mechanical ventilation in the intensive care unit: impact on managing uncertainty for patient-centered communication. *Am J Hosp Palliat Med* 2013; **30**(6): 569–75.

29. P. Butow, S. Dowsett, R. Hagerty, M. Tattersall. Communicating prognosis to patients with metastatic disease: what do they really want to know? *Support Care Cancer* 2002; **10**: 161–8.

30. A.B. Seckler, D.E. Meier, M. Mulvihill, et al. Substituted judgment: how accurate are proxy predictions? *Ann Intern Med* 1991; **115**(2): 92–8.

31. A. De Vleminck, K. Pardon, K. Beernaert, et al. Barriers to advance care planning in cancer, heart failure and dementia patients: a focus group study on general practitioners' views and experiences. *PLoS One* 2014; **9**(1): e84905.

32. O.A. Fawole, S.M. Dy, R.F. Wilson, et al. A systematic review of communication quality improvement interventions for patients with advanced and serious illness. *J Gen Intern Med* 2013; **28**: 570–7.

33. R.E. Bernacki, S.D. Block. Communication about serious illness care goals: a review and synthesis of best practices. *JAMA Intern Med* 2014; **174**(12): 1994–2003.

34. R.M. Thomson, C.R. Patel, R.B. Taylor. Palliative care principles primary care physicians should know. *Prim Care Rep* 2013; **19**(8).

35. T.E. Quill, A.P. Abernethy. Generalist plus specialist palliative care: creating a more sustainable model. *N Engl J Med* 2013; **368** (13): 1173–5.

36. National Consensus Project for Quality Palliative Care. Clinical Practice Guidelines for Quality Palliative Care, 4th ed. Richmond, VA: National Coalition for Hospice and Palliative Care; 2018. www.nationalcoalitionhpc.org/ncp.

37. J. Goldsmith, E. Wittenberg-Lyles, D. Rodriguez, S. Sanchez-Reilly. Interdisciplinary geriatric and palliative care team narratives: collaboration practices and barriers. *Qual Health Res* 2010; **20**(1): 93–104.

38. G. B. Crawford, S.D. Price. Team working: palliative care as a model of interdisciplinary practice. *Med J Aust* 2003; **179**(6): S32.

39. G. Gade, I. Venohr, D. Conner, et al. Impact of an inpatient palliative care team: a randomized controlled trial. *J Palliat Med* 2008; **11**(2): 180–90.

40. R. Schulz, S.R. Beach, E.M. Friedman, et al. Changing structures and processes to support family caregivers of seriously ill patients. *J Palliat Med* 2018; **21**(S2): S36-42.

41. A.S. Kelley, E. Bollens-Lund. Identifying the population with serious illness: the "denominator" challenge. *J Palliat Med* 2018; **21**(S2): S7–S16.

42. J.H. Maley, M.E. Mikkelsen. What happens to critically ill patients after they leave the ICU? In: Deutschman C.S., Neligan P.J. (eds), *Evidence-Based Practice of Critical Care*. New York: Elsevier; 2020, pp. 11–16.

43. H.H. Maley, I. Brewster, I. Mayoral, et al. Resilience in survivors of critical illness in the context of the survivor's experience and recovery. *Ann Am Thorac Soc* 2016; **13**(8): 1351–60.

44. M.E. Mikkelsen, M. Still, B.J. Anderson, et al. Society of Critical Care Medicine's international consensus conference on prediction and identification of long-term impairments after critical illness. *Crit Care Med* 2020; **48**(11): 1670–9.

45. W. Linden, D. Yi, M.C. Barroetavena, et al. Development and validation of a psychosocial screening instrument for cancer. *Health Qual Life Outcomes* 2005; **3**: 1–7.

46. W. Linden, A. Vodermaier, R. McKenzie, et al. The Psychosocial Screen for Cancer (PSSCAN): further validation and normative data. *Health Qual Life Outcomes* 2009; **7**: 1–8.

47. L.E. Carlson, M. Angen, J. Cullum, et al. High levels of untreated distress and fatigue in cancer patients. *Br J Cancer* 2004; **90**(12): 2297–304.

48. A. Srikanthan, B. Leung, A. Shokoohi, et al. Psychosocial distress scores and needs among newly diagnosed sarcoma patients: a provincial experience. *Sarcoma* 2019; **1**: 1–8.

49. W. Linden, A. Andrea Vodermaier, R. McKenzie, et al. The Psychosocial Screen for Cancer (PSSCAN): further validation and normative data. *Health Qual Life Outcomes* 2009; **7**: 1–8.

50. Z.S. Nasreddine, N.A. Phillips, V. Bédirian, et al. The Montreal Cognitive Assessment, MoCA: a brief screening tool for mild cognitive impairment. *J Am Geriatr Soc* 2005; **53**(4): 695–9.

51. P. Julayanont, Z.S. Nasreddine. Montreal Cognitive Assessment (MoCA): concept and clinical review. In: Larner A.J. (ed.), *Cognitive screening instruments: A practical approach*. Cham: Springer; 2017; 139–95.

52. A. Patel, R. Parikh, E.H. Howell, et al. Mini-cog performance: novel marker of post discharge risk among patients hospitalized for heart failure. *Circ Heart Fail* 2015; **8**(1): 8–16.

53. G. Eman, A. Marsh, M.N. Gong, A. A. Hope. Utility of screening for cognitive impairment at hospital discharge in adult survivors of critical illness. *Am J Crit Care* 2022; **31**(4): 306–14.

54. A. Milton, E. Brück, A. Schandl, et al. Early psychological screening of intensive care

55. A. Rhodes, C. Wilson, D. Zelenkov, et al. The psychiatric domain of post-intensive care syndrome: a review for the intensivist. *J Intensive Care Med* 2024; 08850666241275582.
56. E. Bruera, N. Kuehn, M.J. Miller, et al. The Edmonton Symptom Assessment System (ESAS): a simple method for the assessment of palliative care patients. *J Palliat Care* 1991; 7(2): 6–9.
57. F. Anderson, G.M. Downing, J. Hill, et al. Palliative performance scale (PPS): a new tool. *J Palliat Care* 1996; 12(1): 5–11.
58. D. Baik, D. Russell, L. Jordan, et al. Using the palliative performance scale to estimate survival for patients at the end of life: a systematic review of the literature. *J Palliat Med* 2018; **21**(11): 1651–61.
59. F. Lau, M. Downing, M. Lesperance, et al. Using the Palliative Performance Scale to provide meaningful survival estimates. *J Pain Symptom Manage* 2009; **38**(1): 134–44.
60. S.M. Watanabe, C. Nekolaichuk, C. Beaumont, et al. A multicenter study comparing two numerical versions of the Edmonton Symptom Assessment System in palliative care patients. *J Pain Symptom Manage* 2011; **41**(2): 456–68.
61. D. Hui, E. Bruera. The Edmonton Symptom Assessment System 25 years later: past, present, and future developments. *J Pain Symptom Manage* 2017; **53**(3): 630–43.
62. The PEACE Tool: Domains of Palliative Assessment. www.timeofcare.com/the-peace-tool-domains-of-palliative-assessment/ (Accessed January 24, 2025).
63. Canadian Partnership Against Cancer. Screening for distress, the 6th vital sign: a guide to implementing best practices in person-centred care. 2012. https://s22457.pcdn.co/wp-content/uploads/2018/12/Screening-Distress-6th-Vital-Sign-EN.pdf (Accessed January 24, 2025).
64. J.M. McPeake, M.O. Harhay, H. Devine, et al. Exploring patients' goals within the intensive care unit rehabilitation setting. *Am J Crit Care* 2019; **28**(5): 393–400.
65. C. Apps, K. Brooks, E. Terblanche, et al. Development of a menu of recovery goals to facilitate goal setting after critical illness. *Intensive Crit Care Nurs* 2023; **79**: 103482.
66. A. Dimoska, P.N. Butow, E. Dent, et al. An examination of the initial cancer consultation of medical and radiation oncologists using the Cancode interaction analysis system. *Br J Cancer* 2008; **98**(9): 1508–14.
67. K.E. Steinhauser, S.C. Alexander, I. R. Byock, et al. Do preparation and life completion discussions improve functioning and quality of life in seriously ill patients? Pilot randomized control trial. *J Palliat Med* 2008; **11**(9): 1234–40.
68. K.B. Zolnierek, M.R. DiMatteo. Physician communication and patient adherence to treatment: a meta-analysis. *Med Care* 2009; **47**(8): 826–34.
69. M. Engel, M.C. Kars, S.C.C. M. Teunissen, et al. Effective communication in palliative care from the perspectives of patients and relatives: a systematic review. *Palliat Support Care* 2023; **21**(5): 890–913.
70. A.L. Back, R.M. Arnold, W.F. Baile, et al. Approaching difficult communication tasks in oncology. *CA Cancer J Clin* 2005; **55**(3): 164–77.
71. A. Back, R. Arnold, J. Tulsky (eds.), *Mastering communication with seriously ill patients: balancing honesty with empathy and hope.* Cambridge: Cambridge University Press; 2009.
72. A.L. Back, R.M. Arnold. "Yes it's sad, but what should I do?": moving from empathy to action in discussing goals of care. *J Palliat Med* 2014; **17**(2): 141–4.
73. G. Hermans, H. Van Mechelen, B. Clerckx, et al. Acute outcomes and 1-year mortality of intensive care unit-acquired weakness: a cohort study and propensity-matched analysis. *Am J Respir Crit Care Med* 2014; **190**(4): 410–20.
74. V. Liu, X. Lei, H.C. Prescott, et al. Hospital readmission and healthcare utilization

following sepsis in community settings. *J Hosp Med* 2014; **9**(8): 502–7.

75. M. Hua, M.N. Gong, J. Brady, et al. Early and late unplanned rehospitalizations for survivors of critical illness. *Crit Care Med* 2015; **43**(2): 430–8.

76. T.K. Jones, B.D. Fuchs, D.S. Small, et al. Post-acute care use and hospital readmission after sepsis. *Ann Am Thorac Soc* 2015; **12**(6): 904–13.

77. N.I. Lone, M.A. Gillies, C. Haddow, et al. Five-year mortality and hospital costs associated with surviving intensive care. *Am J Respir Crit Care Med* 2016; **194**(2): 198–208.

78. T. Eaton, R. Castiglia, A. Qureshi, et al. 60: reexploring goals of care in patients surviving critical illness. *Crit Care Med* 2020; **48**(1): 30.

79. D. Wendler, A. Rid. Systematic review: the effect on surrogates of making treatment decisions for others. *Ann Intern Med* 2011; **154**(5): 336–46.

80. Y. Schenker, M. Crowley-Matoka, D. Dohan, et al. I don't want to be the one saying "we should just let him die": intrapersonal tensions experienced by surrogate decision makers in the ICU. *J Gen Intern Med* 2012; **27**(12): 1657–65.

81. J. Chiarchiaro, P. Buddadhumaruk, R. M. Arnold, et al. Prior advance care planning is associated with less decisional conflict among surrogates for critically ill patients. *Ann Am Thorac Soc* 2015; **12**(10): 1528–33.

82. R.L. Sudore, T.R. Fried. Redefining the "planning" in advance care planning: preparing for end-of-life decision making. *Ann Intern Med* 2010; **153**(4): 256–61.

83. E.K. Kross. Palliative care and end-of-life care planning after critical illness. In: Haines K.J., McPeake J., Sevin C.M. (eds), *Improving critical care survivorship: a guide to prevention, recovery, and reintegration.* Cham: Springer International Publishing; 2021; 185–96.

84. R. Collins, F. Vallières, G. McDermott. The experiences of post-ICU COVID-19 survivors: an existential perspective using interpretative phenomenological analysis. *Qual Health Res* 2023; **33**(7): 589–600.

85. S.L. Storli, R. Lind. The meaning of follow-up in intensive care: patients' perspective. *Scand J Caring Sci* 2009; **23**(1): 45–56.

86. T.L. Eaton, L.P. Scheunemann, B. W. Butcher, et al. The prevalence of spiritual and social support needs and their association with postintensive care syndrome symptoms among critical illness survivors seen in a post-ICU follow-up clinic. *Crit Care Explor* 2022; **4**(4): e0676.

87. C. Puchalski, G. Handzo, B. Ferrell. Religious conflicts: decision making when religious beliefs and medical realities conflict (P17). *J Pain Symptom Manage* 2016; **51**(2): 313–14.

88. R.S. Cooper, A. Ferguson, J.N. Bodurtha, et al. AMEN in challenging conversations: bridging the gaps between faith, hope, and medicine. *J Oncol Pract* 2014; **10**(4): e191–5.

89. L.F. Piotrowski. Advocating and educating for spiritual screening assessment and referrals to chaplains. *Omega J Death Dying* 2013; **67**(1–2): 185–92.

90. S. Prinjha, K. Field, K. Rowan. What patients think about ICU follow-up services: a qualitative study. *Crit Care* 2009; **13**(2): R46.

91. N. Pattison, G. O'Gara, J. Rattray. After critical care: patient support after critical care. A mixed method longitudinal study using email interviews and questionnaires. *Intensive Crit Care Nurs* 2015; **31**(4): 213–22.

92. J. Choi, Y.J. Son, J.A. Tate. Exploring positive aspects of caregiving in family caregivers of adult ICU survivors from ICU to four months post-ICU discharge. *Heart Lung* 2019; **48**(6): 553–9.

93. J.E. Davidson, C. Jones, O.J. Bienvenu. Family response to critical illness: postintensive care syndrome–family. *Crit Care Med* 2012; **40**(2): 618–24.

94. J. Torres, D. Carvalho, E. Molinos, et al. The impact of the patient post-intensive care syndrome components upon caregiver burden. *Med Intensiva* 2017; **41**(8): 454–60.

95. P. Henderson, T. Quasim, A. Asher, et al. Post-intensive care syndrome following cardiothoracic critical care: feasibility of a complex intervention. *J Rehabil Med* 2021; **53**(6): jrm00206.
96. A. Petrinec. Post-intensive care syndrome in family decision makers of long-term acute care hospital patients. *Am J Crit Care* 2017; **26**(5): 416–22.
97. P.L. Cairns, H.G. Buck, K.E. Kip, et al. Stress management intervention to prevent post-intensive care syndrome-family in patients' spouses. *Am J Crit Care* 2019; **28**(6): 471–6.
98. F. Gravante, F. Trotta, S. Latina, et al. Quality of life in ICU survivors and their relatives with post-intensive care syndrome: a systematic review. *Nurs Crit Care* 2024; **29**(4): 807–23.
99. J. McPeake, T.J. Iwashyna, L.M. Boehm, et al. Benefits of peer support for Intensive Care Unit survivors: sharing experiences, care debriefing, and altruism. *Am J Crit Care* 2021; **30**(2): 145–9.
100. A. Petrinec, B. Martin. Post-intensive care syndrome symptoms and health-related quality of life in family decision-makers of critically ill patients. *Pall Supp Care* 2018; **16**(6): 719–24.
101. S. Jain, L. Han, E.A. Gahbauer, et al. Changes in restricting symptoms after critical illness among community-living older adults. *Am J Respir Crit Care Med* 2023; **208**(11): 1206–15.
102. J. McPeake, L.M. Boehm, E. Hibbert, et al. Key components of ICU recovery programs: what did patients report provided benefit? *Crit Care Explor* 2020; **2**(4): e0088.
103. K.S. Deacon. Re-building life after ICU: A qualitative study of the patients' perspective. *Intensive Crit Care Nurs* 2012; **28**(2): 114–22.
104. S.L. Williams. Recovering from the psychological impact of intensive care: how constructing a story helps. *Nurs Crit Care* 2009; **14**(6): 281–8.
105. A.I. Czerwonka, M.S. Herridge, L. Chan, et al. Changing support needs of survivors of complex critical illness and their family caregivers across the care continuum: a qualitative pilot study of Towards RECOVER. *J Crit Care* 2015; **30**(2): 242–9.
106. C. Glimelius Petersson, M. Ringdal, G. Apelqvist, et al. Diaries and memories following an ICU stay: a 2-month follow-up study. *Nurs Crit Care* 2018; **23**(6): 299–307.
107. E. Åkerman, A. Langius-Eklöf. The impact of follow-up visits and diaries on patient outcome after discharge from intensive care: a descriptive and explorative study. *Intensive Crit Care Nurs* 2018; **49**: 14–20.
108. B. Brandao Barreto, M. Luz, S. Alves Valente do Amaral Lopes, et al. Exploring patients' perceptions on ICU diaries: a systematic review and qualitative data synthesis. *Crit Care Med* 2021; **49**(7): e707–18.
109. C. Lee, M. Herridge, A. Matte, et al. Education and support needs during recovery in acute respiratory distress syndrome survivors. *Crit Care* 2009; **13**(5): R153.
110. J. King, B. O'Neill, P. Ramsay, et al. Identifying patients' support needs following critical illness: a scoping review of the qualitative literature. *Crit Care* 2019; **23**(1): 187.
111. A. Thurston. The Some-Other Technique. 2025. https://momentsmattermd.com/2025/01/05/moments-matter-69-the-some-other-technique/ (Accessed January 24, 2005).
112. S.P. Taylor, C. Morley, M. Donaldson, et al. Characterizing program delivery for an effective multicomponent sepsis recovery intervention. *Ann Am Thorac Soc* 2024; **21**(4): 627–34.
113. K.J. Haines, J. McPeake, E. Hibbert, et al. Enablers and barriers to implementing ICU follow-up clinics and peer support groups following critical illness. *Crit Care Med* 2019; **47**(9): 1194–200.
114. R.N. Bakhru, J.F Davidson, R. E. Bookstaver, et al. Implementation of an ICU recovery clinic at a tertiary care

academic center. *Crit Care Explor* 2019; **1**(8): e0034.

115. V. Danesh, L.M. Boehm, T.L. Eaton, et al. Characteristics of post-ICU and post-COVID recovery clinics in 29 U.S. health systems. *Crit Care Explor* 2022; **4**(3): e0658.

116. T.L. Eaton, C.M. Sevin, A.A. Hope, et al. Evolution in care delivery within critical illness recovery programs during the COVID-19 pandemic: a qualitative study. *Ann Am Thorac Soc* 2022; **19**(11): 1900–6.

117. J.L. Bandini, A. Scherling, C. Farmer, et al. Experiences with telehealth for outpatient palliative care: findings from a mixed-methods study of patients and providers across the United States. *J Palliat Med* 2022; **25**(7): 1079–87.

118. D. Hui, Y. Heung, E. Bruera. Timely palliative care: personalizing the process of referral. *Cancers* 2022; **14**(4): 1047.

119. D. Hui, M. Mori, S.M. Watanabe, et al. Referral criteria for outpatient specialty palliative cancer care: an international consensus. *Lancet Oncol* 2016; **17**(12): e552–9.

120. M.L Carey, A.C. Zucca, M.A. Freund, et al. Systematic review of barriers and enablers to the delivery of palliative care by primary care practitioners. *Palliat Med* 2019; **33**(9): 1131–45.

121. N. Dudley, C.S. Ritchie, R.S. Rehm, et al. Facilitators and barriers to interdisciplinary communication between providers in primary care and palliative care. *J Palliat Med* 2019; **22**(3): 243–9.

122. P.M. Palevsky, S. Shreve, S.P. Wong. Implementation of kidney palliative care: lessons learned from the US Department of Veterans Affairs. *Ann Palliat Med* 2024; **13**(4): 85868.

123. J.O. Schell, R.A. Cohen, J.A. Green, et al. NephroTalk: evaluation of a palliative care communication curriculum for nephrology fellows. *J Pain Symptom Manage* 2018; **56**(5): 767–73.

Chapter 48

Post-Intensive Care Syndrome – Family

Ji Won Shin and Judith Tate

Introduction

Within the confines of the intensive care unit (ICU), families play a crucial role, offering emotional support, communication, and advocacy for their critically ill loved one [1]. The importance of family presence in the ICU cannot be overstated, as it significantly impacts patient outcomes, fosters enhanced communication with the medical team, and provides emotional solace to the patient during times of crisis [2,3]. Multiple terms are often used to refer to "family caregivers," including "informal caregivers," "family members," "loved ones," "relatives," or simply "families"; these terms are often used interchangeably but may be distinguished based on contextual definitions. Throughout this chapter, we use the term "family caregiver" to mean a person who is responsible for providing the patient's care, arranging additional treatments, and assisting in care decisions after hospital discharge without financial compensation. This person should have a significant relationship with the patient, but they need not be a blood relative [4].

The ICU experience is often stressful for families, as the hospitalization is usually unexpected and life-threatening for the patient, and outcomes are uncertain [5]. Long-term effects on families include adverse psychological, physical, and social impacts, collectively termed the post-intensive care syndrome – family (PICS-F) [5]. Family caregivers may experience PICS-F-related symptoms during the acute and rehabilitative phases of the patient's critical illness, and these symptoms may persist for months to years following the resolution of the critical illness.

Definition of PICS-F

Recently, a focus on the provision of family-centered care and family engagement in the ICU has received increased attention (see Chapter 17 for additional information). Psychological distress experienced by family caregivers during their loved one's ICU stay can be significant and persists long after hospital discharge. It was first recognized that family members of critically ill patients could experience clinically diagnosable psychological distress in the early 1990s [6], and more recently, researchers have sought to examine the significance of the problem and identify associated risk factors. PICS-F is defined as a cluster of common adverse outcomes that informal family caregivers of ICU patients may experience; psychological symptoms are the most frequently studied component of PICS-F, but physical, cognitive, and social difficulties may also be present. Although the symptom complex of PICS-F differs for each individual, it may directly impact family caregivers' involvement in patient care, their employment, and their quality of life. Figure 48.1 illustrates the burden of the psychological, physical, and social challenges experienced by family caregivers from ICU admission to the convalescent stage.

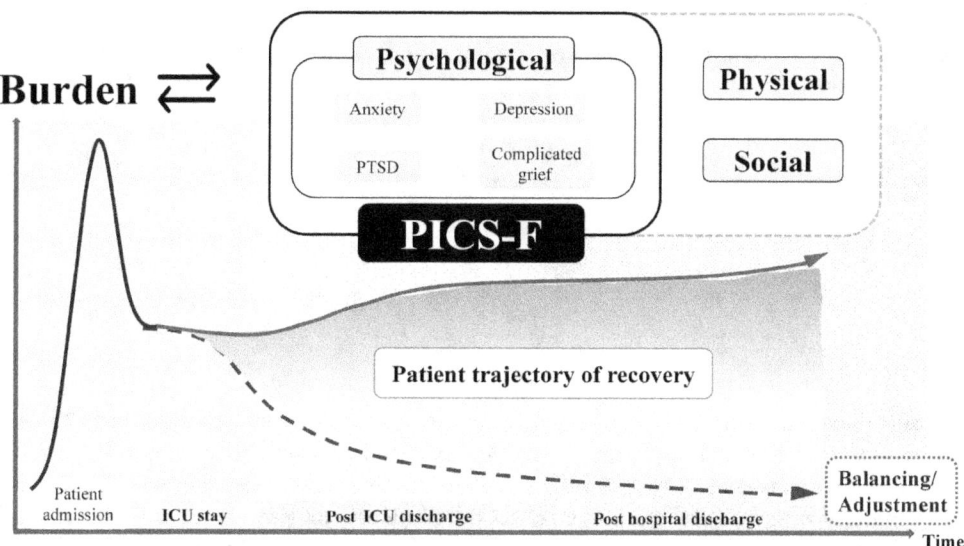

Figure 48.1 A conceptual diagram of PICS-F. From: K. Shirasaki, T. Hifumi, N. Nakanishi, et al. Postintensive care syndrome family: A comprehensive review. *Acute Med Surg* 2024; **11**: e939. Reproduced with permission from John Wiley & Sons.

Potential Etiologies

Critical illness is frequently characterized by instability of the patient's condition and uncertainty of the short-term and long-term outcomes. Due to the sudden nature of critical illness and its long-term sequelae, family caregivers of critically ill patients experience various challenges during and after hospitalization requiring intensive care. While the exact etiology of PICS-F remains unclear, its development is likely dependent on several factors. Possible etiologies for psychological distress in family caregivers of critically ill patients include fear of the potential loss of a loved one; the emotional burden associated with playing an integral, and occasionally unwanted, role in decision-making and patient care; uncertainty due to insufficient information and lack of effective communication with healthcare providers; personal and family conflict; sleep deprivation; and the social and economic impacts of hospitalization [7,8,9,10,11].

Problems, Prevalence, and Measurement Tools

Psychological Outcomes

Family caregivers of critically ill patients may endure high levels of psychological stress and develop psychological pathology as a consequence. PICS-F research is largely focused on these psychological challenges, including anxiety, depression, and stress-related disorders, such as post-traumatic stress disorder (PTSD), all of which are frequently experienced by families of critically ill patients (see Table 48.1). Other psychological manifestations that are significant but insufficient to merit a clinical diagnosis include generalized stress, feelings of fear and sadness, and learned helplessness. The prevalence of depressive symptoms in families of

Table 48.1 Summary of reported prevalence of common psychological symptoms among ICU family caregivers

Adverse psychological outcome	During ICU	3 months	6 months	1 year	2 years	General American population
Depression [12,13,14]	16–97%	12–26%	5–36%	23–43%	-	8.3%
Anxiety [12,13,14]	42–81%	24–63%	15–24%	-	-	19.1%
PTSD [12,13,14,15]	33–81%	30–52%	35–57%	32–80%	12–14%	6.8%

critically ill patients is considerable, ranging between 25 to 41% at two months and 23 to 43% at one year after hospital discharge [12,13,14]. Anxiety is particularly common during ICU admission, affecting 48 to 73% of family members, and the prevalence falls to approximately 15% 6 months after hospital discharge [12,13,14]. Similarly, the prevalence of PTSD in family members of critically ill patients is 30–52% at 3 months, 35–57% at 6 months, and 32–80% at 1 year following hospital discharge, which is considerably higher than the estimated lifetime prevalence of PTSD among adult Americans (6.8%) [12,13,14,15].

Physical and Functional Consequences

During a loved one's ICU admission, family caregivers may have difficulty paying attention to their own health. Impaired sleep affects between 53 and 64% of family caregivers due to high levels of psychological distress during their loved one's admission, nighttime interruptions for patient care needs, and intrusive thoughts and nightmares [16,17]. Among the sleep impairments, insomnia is common and can cause excessive daytime sleepiness and an impaired ability to perform daily activities [18]. Families also frequently experience clinically significant fatigue, which can persist for as long as four months after hospital discharge and is associated with worse caregiver strain [19,20].

Due to caregiving responsibilities for a seriously ill loved one, family caregivers may have difficulty paying attention to their own health, which can result in health-risk behaviors, defined as actions or habits that can potentially harm one's present or future physical or mental health. Although personal health decision-making in family members of critically ill patients has not been extensively examined, one study reported that family members' health-risk behaviors during the acute phase of their loved one's critical illness were worse than health-risk behaviors reported by family caregivers of community-dwelling older adults with disabilities [21,22]. In this study, 94% of family caregivers of critically ill patients reported one or more health-risk behaviors, including inadequate rest, inadequate exercise, and skipping meals. In addition, family caregivers often have difficulty managing their own chronic medical conditions and may fail to take medications as prescribed or attend their own physician appointments.

Caregiver Burden/Caregiver Strain

More than one in five Americans provide care for individuals with chronic health conditions or for those who are unable to function independently [23,24]. Caregiver roles vary widely based on family composition, the needs of the care recipient, the duration of the caregiving role, and transitions in care from the ICU to lower-intensity care settings (e.g., long-term acute care hospitals, inpatient rehabilitation facilities, skilled nursing facilities, or home) [25]. Common caregiving responsibilities include assistance with activities of daily living, management of complex medication regimens, and coordination of medical care.

Some family caregivers have described their experience as devastating and traumatic during the acute phase of the illness. During the patient's recovery phase, family caregivers must often accept additional responsibilities that require activation of internal and external support strategies to manage stress [26]. Of those patients who required care six months after hospital discharge, more than 25% required over 50 hours of care per week, with approximately 80% of care provided by family caregivers [27]. The need to perform care tasks during their loved one's convalescence may affect the caregiver's daily personal routines, financial health, societal roles, relationships with others, and their own physical and mental health.

Caregiver burden has been defined as "the extent to which caregivers perceive their emotional or physical health, social life, and financial status are suffering as a result of caring for their relative" [28]. Caregiver burden is experienced by individuals who care for persons with debilitating diseases, such as dementia, cancer, and chronic pulmonary disease, as well as for survivors of critical illness. While several studies have measured caregiver burden with standardized tools, including the Zarit Burden Inventory, others use psychological screening tools for anxiety, depression, and PTSD to elucidate the impact of caregiving responsibilities on the caregiver [29]. Recent studies suggest that 23 to 53% of caregivers of survivors of critical illness experience burden and strain [20,30]. Several studies correlate caregiver burden with the patient's clinical condition: caregiver burden is more common in patients whose recovery phase is complicated by adverse or worsening physical or psychological impairments [31]. A Portuguese study demonstrated that patient anxiety and depression in the three months following hospital discharge, but not continued physical limitations, also influenced the presence of caregiver burden [32]. Higher caregiver burden was associated with an increased risk of negative psychological outcomes, including anxiety, depression, and PTSD symptoms, and decreased mental health-related quality of life (HRQOL) for the caregiver [31].

Caregiving responsibilities can have a negative impact on recreation, lifestyle, and social activities, including visiting friends and engaging in hobbies [14,33,34]. While nearly 85% of caregivers prioritize the care of their loved one over social or recreational activities one month after hospital discharge, this falls to 46% of caregivers after one year, emphasizing the toll that being a caregiver takes over time.

Employment and Financial Strain

Many family members have to take time off from work due to caregiving demands, which may contribute to financial strain. During the patient's recovery period, family members may not be able to return to full employment, as caregiving responsibilities compete with the ability to resume work. In one study, 85% of family caregivers had returned to work one year following ICU discharge [35]; however, the return to work is often accompanied by changes in employment, including reduced work hours, which can lead to decreased wages; decreased responsibilities; or the need to assume a different job [36,37,38]. In a recent study, during a three-month follow-up period, caregivers reported using up to 90 days of sick leave as they assumed full caregiving responsibilities following hospital discharge [31].

Families also report financial burden during the ICU recovery period [36,37]. Direct impacts on family finances include loss of savings, delayed higher educational plans, or the need to change to more affordable housing [33]. Financial strain may directly impact psychological outcomes of family caregivers [37]. Families with lower levels of education, baseline financial health, emotional health, and quality of life are at greater risk for negative financial outcomes after the ICU [37].

Positive Aspects of Caregiving

While caregivers of survivors of critical illness experience many challenges that can have adverse effects on their health and well-being, many family members perceive the caregiving experience as positive. In a longitudinal study of family caregivers of survivors of critical illness, many described positive aspects of their caregiving experience, such as feeling needed, appreciating life more, and developing a more positive attitude toward life [39]. Participants reported that the experience of their loved one's critical illness often led to role reversal and presented new challenges, such as becoming the patient's advocate with the healthcare system and adjusting to changing family dynamics. Family caregivers of survivors of critical illness found satisfaction in their roles through fulfilling caregiving responsibilities; strengthening relationships; integrating caregiving into their identity; witnessing patient improvements; relying on social support, faith, and positivity to navigate challenges; and experiencing role changes [40]. The authors provided a conceptual diagram that illustrates the factors involved in positive appraisal of caregiving during the patient's recovery (see Figure 48.2).

Another potential area of research in PICS-F is the development of resilience and post-traumatic growth (PTG) in family caregivers during the recovery period. Resilience is defined as the capacity to withstand or recover from difficulties and to process traumatic events positively, allowing one to grow from the experience [41]. Studies of resilience in family caregivers of survivors of neurological critical illness found that higher resilience factors, such as mindfulness and coping skills, were associated with lower levels of depressive symptoms [42] and less severe PTSD symptoms [43]. Although some persons experiencing traumatic events ultimately develop PTSD, others recover from serious trauma with perceived beneficial changes and personal growth [44]; PTG refers to these positive psychological changes resulting from trauma [45]. Although PTG has been more frequently described in survivors of critical illness (see Chapter 46 for additional information), it may also occur in family caregivers of these patients as well [46,47,48].

Perceived positive aspects of caregiving, resilience, and PTG are examples of positive outcomes in family caregivers of survivors of critical illness that may yield potentially protective effects against psychological distress. These positive aspects of critical illness survivorship and their associations with psychological outcomes merit further examination.

Measures

Table 48.2 provides a comprehensive overview of measurement tools that have been used to examine PICS-F-related outcomes in family caregivers of critically ill patients. The majority of the measurement instruments are standardized self-report tools.

Psychological symptoms are the most frequently studied in this population, and there are many different measures used to assess anxiety, depression, and PTSD-related symptoms. For example, anxiety may be assessed with several tools, including the Hospital

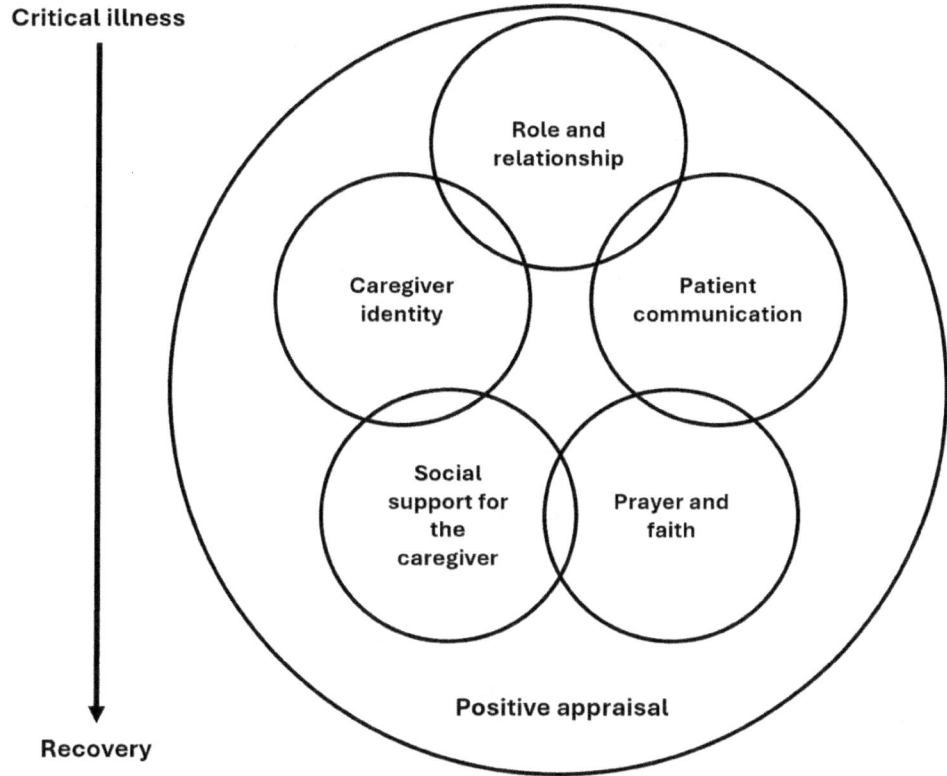

Figure 48.2 A conceptual model of positive appraisal of caregiving. From: J.A. Tate, J. Choi. Positive appraisal of caregiving for intensive care unit survivors: a qualitative secondary analysis. *Am J Crit Care* 2020; **29**: 340–9. Reproduced with permission from the American Association of Critical Care Nurses.

Anxiety and Depression Scale (HADS-A), the Generalized Anxiety Disorder-7 (GAD-7), and the Beck Anxiety Inventory (BAI). Depression may be assessed with the Hospital Anxiety and Depression Scale (HADS-D), the Beck Depression Inventory-II (BDI-II), and the Center for Epidemiologic Studies Depression Scale (CES-D). PTSD-related symptoms may be assessed with the Impact of Event Scale (IES), its revised version (IES-R), and the six-question version (IES-6); other PTSD screening tools include the Post-traumatic Symptom Scale (PTSS-10), the Posttraumatic Stress Diagnostic Scale (PDS), and the PTSD Checklist-5 (PCL-5; see Chapter 46 for additional information).

Physical and functional outcomes assessments include caregiver health-risk behavior, sleep disturbance, fatigue, caregiver burden, and quality of life questionnaires. Caregiver health-risk behavior is measured using the Caregiver Health Behavior Instrument, which includes 25 items that assess various health-risk behaviors, including physical activity, sleep patterns, substance use, and stress management. Sleep disturbance has also been assessed using several measures, including the General Sleep Disturbance Scale (GSDS), the Insomnia Severity Index (ISI), and the Pittsburgh Sleep Quality Index (PSQI; see Chapter 37 for additional information). Fatigue in family caregivers of critically ill patients has been measured using Lee's Fatigue Scale (LFS).

Table 48.2 PICS-F outcomes and measurement tools

Outcome	Measurement	Items/Scale	Score range
Psychological			
Anxiety	Hospital Anxiety and Depression Scale-Anxiety (HADS-A) [67]	7 items/4-point	0–21
	Depression Anxiety Stress Scales (DASS–12) [68]	12 items/4-point	0–36
	Generalized Anxiety Disorder – 7 (GAD–7) [69]	7 items/4-point	0–21
	Beck Anxiety Index (BAI) [70]	21 items/4-point	0–63
	State-Trait Anxiety Symptoms Questionnaire (STAI) [71]	40 items/4-point	20–80
Depression	Hospital Anxiety and Depression Scale-Depression (HADS-D) [67]	7 items/4-point	0–21
	Center for Epidemiologic Studies Depression Scale (CES-D) [72]	20 items/4-point	0–60
	Patient Health Questionnaire–9 (PHQ–9) [73]	9 items/4-point	0–27
	Patient Health Questionnaire–8 (PHQ–8) [74]	8 items/4-point	0–24
PTSD	Impact of Event Scale (IES) [75]	15 items/4-point	
	Impact of Event Scale-revised (IES-R) [76]	22 items/5-point	0–88
	Impact of Event Scale–6 (IES–6) [77]	6 items/4-point	0–24
	Posttraumatic Symptom Scale (PTSS–10) [78]	10 items/4-point	0–30
	Post-traumatic Stress Diagnostic Scale (PDS) [79]	24 items/5-point	
	PTSD Checklist–5 (PCL–5) [80]	20 items/5-point	0–80
	PTSD Checklist for Specific or Civilian Version (PCL-S or -C) [81]	17 items/5-point	17–85
Other trauma-related Symptoms	Peritraumatic Dissociative Experiences Questionnaire (PDEQ) [82]	10 items/5-point	10–50
	Trauma Screening Questionnaire (TSQ) [83]	10 items/yes-no	0–10
Prolonged grief	Inventory of Complicated Grief (ICG) [84]	19 items/5-point	0–76
Stress	Perceived Stress Scale [85]	10 items/5-point	0–40

Table 48.2 (cont.)

Outcome	Measurement	Items/Scale	Score range
Helplessness	Learned Helplessness Scale [86]	20 items/5-point	20–80
Physical/Functional			
Health risk behavior	Caregiver Health Behavior Instrument (CHBI) [87]	25 items/5-point	0–100
Sleep disturbance	General Sleep Disturbance Scale (GSDS) [88]	21 items/8-point	0–147
	Insomnia Severity Index (ISI) [89]	7 items/4-point Likert scale	0–28
	Pittsburgh Sleep Quality Index (PSQI) [90]	19 items/0–3 scale	0–21
Fatigue	Lee's Fatigue Scale (LFS) [91]	13 items/0–10 numeric rating scale	0–130
Caregiving burden	Caregiver Strain Index (CSI) [92]	13 items/yes-no	0–13
	Zarit Burden Interview [93,94]	22 items/5-point	0–88
	Zarit Burden Interview short version (Zarit–12) [95]	12 items/5-point	0–48
Quality of life	Short Form–36 (SF–36) [95]	36 items/scale varies across domains	0–100
	EuroQol-five dimensions (EQ–5D) [96]	5 items/visual analog scale	-
Social Endpoints			
Social support	Norbeck Social Support Questionnaire (NSSQ) [97]	9 items	score range varies
Family integrity/Role adaptation	Family Adaptability and Cohesion Evaluation Scale [98]	42 items / 5-point	

Several tools have been developed to measure caregiver burden. The Caregiver Strain Index (CSI) measures caregiver strain through the assessment of seven elements, including emotional adjustment, social issues, and physical and financial strain. The Zarit Burden Interview (ZBI) was developed specifically for caregivers of patients with dementia but has also been validated for other patient populations. Quality of life in family caregivers has been evaluated using tools including the Short Form-36 (SF-36), a comprehensive measure of overall quality of life, and the EuroQol-5 Dimensions (EQ-5D), which explores five dimensions of health: mobility, self-care, usual activities, pain/discomfort, and anxiety/depression, as well as an overall rating of health on a visual analog scale (see Chapter 34 for additional information).

Social endpoints of family caregivers of critically ill patients have also been measured in several different contexts. Social support has been measured using the Norbeck Social

Support Questionnaire (NSSQ), which is a self-administered tool designed to measure both the functional properties of social support (e.g., emotional and tangible support) and network properties (e.g., stability of relationships and frequency of contact). Family adaptation is assessed using the Family Adaptability and Cohesion Evaluation Scale (FACES), which measures family dynamics and adaptability.

Risk Factors

A systematic review and meta-analysis of 17 studies identified multiple potential risk factors for the development of PICS-F [49]. Risk factors were categorized into demographic factors, environmental and social factors, and experiential factors during the ICU admission. Of these, the most significant risk factor was a history of mental illness, which placed families at the greatest risk for adverse psychological outcomes, including the development of anxiety, depression, and PTSD. Demographic risk factors for increased psychological distress in family caregivers include the age of the patient [50], being a female caregiver [49,50], a low education level, and caring for a spouse as opposed to another relative [49]. Several personal traits in family caregivers are also associated with emotional distress, including decision-making preferences, understanding of the disease process, satisfaction with care, substance use habits, religiosity, and their own quality of life. Environmental and social factors may also play a role in the development of PICS-F, including distance from the hospital, social support, unemployment [51], and financial stability [37,50]. Other factors that influenced the risk of developing PICS-F were the severity of the patient's illness [49] and death of the patient [50], which significantly increased risk for anxiety and depression. Poor communication with ICU staff and perceived poor care [50] also affected families' risk for depression and anxiety, while higher levels of satisfaction were associated with lower levels of depression, anxiety, and PTSD in families three months following discharge [52].

Interventions for PICS-F

Given the profound impact that critical illness has on families, several interventions to prevent or overcome PICS-F have been evaluated. Interventions to *prevent* PICS-F include those that are delivered during the acute phase of the patient's illness. These include interventions designed to improve communication and information sharing, to express and document the experience of critical illness, to enable "making sense" of the ICU, and to increase family bedside presence. Interventions to *mitigate* the presence of PICS-F and improve the quality of life for family caregivers are delivered in the outpatient recovery period. These interventions include follow-up care directed at families, peer support, mental health services, and interventions directed at the patient-family dyad.

Interventions During the Acute Phase of Illness

Communication Facilitators

Communication facilitators are various strategies to help ensure effective and satisfactory communication between healthcare providers and family members, including important information regarding the patient's condition, prognosis, and care plan. Interventions to improve communication can consist of in-person, static, and technology-facilitated information sharing. Interventions that meet these criteria include regular family meetings, attendance during team rounds, information leaflets, and technology-based interventions, such as mobile applications and online platforms, which can provide caregivers with access to information, resources, and support. These resources can include educational materials, self-care tools, communication platforms, and remote monitoring systems [53].

ICU Diaries
By providing a sense of continuity, filling in memory gaps, and facilitating understanding and processing of the ICU experience, ICU diaries have been found to reduce PTSD symptoms in some patients and improve psychological well-being for some patients and families, but such improvements have not been seen across all studies (see Chapter 18 for additional information) [54,55].

Family-Centered Care/Family Presence
Involving and supporting family members in the care of ICU patients through open communication, shared decision-making, and collaboration has been shown to improve family satisfaction, reduce anxiety and stress, improve quality of life, and enhance the overall ICU experience for both patients and families (see Chapter 17 for additional information) [56].

Facilitated Sensemaking Model
The facilitated sensemaking model (FSM) is a middle range theory that provides a basis for the design of family-centered interventions in the ICU [57], the primary goal of which is to guide nursing interventions to prevent adverse psychological outcomes in family members of critically ill patients. After the disruption of an unplanned and serious illness in a loved one, family caregivers need a compensation period to overcome the challenges of the situation, to make sense of what has happened, and to accept their new roles as caregivers [57,58]. During this compensation period, family caregivers desire information, and nurses can facilitate the sensemaking process through directed interventions, including assisting the family with understanding the ICU environment, identifying and meeting their unmet needs, providing family support, and engaging them in bedside activities [57,59]. Nursing interventions derived from the FSM have been implemented and tested, and they have been shown to decrease families' anxiety [59,60,61], depression [61], and PTSD-related symptoms [61].

Post-ICU Interventions
Follow-up care for family caregivers of survivors of critical illness can be helpful in monitoring the family's well-being, addressing any ongoing concerns, and providing additional support [53]. It is recommended that a multidisciplinary team composed of critical care physicians, psychologists, social workers, and other specialists collaborate to provide comprehensive care for families caring for survivors of critical illness, but few formal programs have been tested to assist families in the recovery period.

Peer Support
Peer support programs, where caregivers connect with and receive support from others who have gone through similar experiences, have shown promise in reducing caregiver burden

and improving well-being. Peer support can provide emotional support, practical advice, and a sense of belonging and validation for caregivers (see Chapter 49 for additional information) [62,63].

Dyadic Intervention

Dyadic intervention focuses on addressing the construct of emotional distress by providing coping skills and support to the patient and informal caregiver together as a dyad. The Recovering Together intervention was found to be feasible and effective in reducing symptoms of depression, anxiety, and post-traumatic stress (PTS) among both survivors and caregivers, with improvements sustained through 12 weeks of follow-up [64].

Mental Health Interventions

A meta-analysis of 56 randomized controlled trials showed that mental health interventions that were implemented to improve psychological outcomes of informal family caregivers resulted in reduced anxiety and depression within 3 months following hospital discharge; however, there was no significant effect on PTSD or psychological distress. The interventions also increased humanity and transcendence and reduced caregiver burden. No significant effects of mental health interventions were observed after three months following discharge, however, leading the authors to conclude that clinicians should consider short-term prescriptions of mental health interventions for informal caregivers of critically ill patients [65]. A pilot study of cognitive behavioral therapy (CBT) delivered via smartphone to reduce the prevalence and severity of PICS-F symptoms in family members of survivors of critical illness demonstrated that anxiety and depression symptom severity decreased significantly over time in the intervention group but not in the control group [66].

Conclusion

Critical illness represents a significant source of psychological distress for family caregivers of critically ill patients. PICS-F is a complex phenomenon involving many related factors with etiologies that are not yet clearly understood. Given the significance of these problems and their durable impact on family caregivers' psychological, physical, and social outcomes, more attention to PICS-F is needed from healthcare providers and researchers. Early detection of PICS-F using standardized measurement tools from the ICU admission to the outpatient setting is helpful in identifying target family caregivers for interventions. Although recent studies have focused on developing and testing interventions to improve family caregivers' post-ICU outcomes using various strategies, larger studies with rigorous designs are still needed to generalize findings into practice. Recently, there has been growing interest in the positive aspects of critical illness, which may play a protective role in preventing or alleviating PICS-F.

Key Points

1. PICS-F is a complicated phenomenon involving psychological, physical, and social endpoints in family caregivers of critically ill patients.
2. Psychological outcomes, including anxiety, depression, and PTSD, are the most frequently studied and prevalent problems in family caregivers.

3. Early detection by assessing PICS-F outcomes throughout the continuum of care using standardized measures by providers is encouraged.
4. More attention is needed to develop and test interventions to prevent and alleviate PICS-F using rigorous research designs and larger samples to generalize findings into practice.

References

1. B.S. Cypress, K. Frederickson. Family presence in the intensive care unit and emergency department: a metasynthesis. *J Fam Theory Rev* 2017; **9**: 201–18.
2. S. Mohsen, S.J. Moss, F. Lucini, et al. Impact of family presence on delirium in critically ill patients: a retrospective cohort study. *Crit Care Med* 2022; **50**: 1628–37.
3. M.J. Goldfarb, L. Bibas, V. Bartlett, et al. Outcomes of patient-and family-centered care interventions in the ICU: a systematic review and meta-analysis. *Crit Care Med* 2017; **45**: 1751–61.
4. J.I. Cameron, L.M. Chu, A. Matte, et al. One-year outcomes in caregivers of critically ill patients. *N Engl J Med* 2016; **374**: 1831–41.
5. J.E. Davidson, C. Jones, O.J. Bienvenu. Family response to critical illness: postintensive care syndrome–family. *Crit Care Med* 2012; **40**: 618–24.
6. M.A. Pérez-San Gregorio, A. Blanco-Picabia, F. Murillo-Cabezas, et al. Psychological problems in the family members of gravely traumatised patients admitted into an intensive care unit. *Intensive Care Med* 1992; **18**: 278–81.
7. A.C. Long, E.K. Kross, J.R. Curtis. Family-centered outcomes during and after critical illness: current outcomes and opportunities for future investigation. *Curr Opin Crit Care* 2016; **22**: 613–20.
8. H. Myhren, O. Ekeberg, O. Stokland. Satisfaction with communication in ICU patients and relatives: comparisons with medical staffs' expectations and the relationship with psychological distress. *Patient Educ Couns* 2011; **85**: 237–44.
9. D. Wendler, A. Rid. Systematic review: the effect on surrogates of making treatment decisions for others. *Ann Intern Med* 2011; **154**: 336–46.
10. E. Azoulay, F. Pochard, N. Kentish-Barnes, et al. Risk of post-traumatic stress symptoms in family members of intensive care unit patients. *Am J Respir Crit Care Med* 2005; **171**: 987–94.
11. E. Azoulay, F. Pochard, N. Kentish-Barnes, et al. Risk of post-traumatic stress symptoms in family members of intensive care unit patients. *Am J Respir Crit Care Med* 2005; **171**: 987–94.
12. K.J. Haines, L. Denehy, E.H. Skinner, et al. Psychosocial outcomes in informal caregivers of the critically ill: a systematic review. *Crit Care Med* 2015; **43**: 1112–20.
13. C.C. Johnson, M.R. Suchyta, E. S. Darowski, et al. Psychological sequelae in family caregivers of critically-ill intensive care unit patients: a systematic review. *Ann Am Thorac Soc* 2019; **16(7)**: 894–909.
14. I. van Beusekom, F. Bakhshi-Raiez, N.F. de Keizer, et al. Reported burden on informal caregivers of ICU survivors: a literature review. *Crit Care* 2016; **20**: 16.
15. A.B. Petrinec, B.J. Daly. Post-traumatic stress symptoms in post-ICU family members: review and methodological challenges. *West J Nurs Res* 2016; **38**: 57–78.
16. A. Day, S. Haj-Bakri, S. Lubchansky, S. Mehta. Sleep, anxiety and fatigue in family members of patients admitted to the intensive care unit: a questionnaire study. *Crit Care* 2013; **17**: 1–7.
17. K. Dithole, G. Thupayagale-Tshweneagae, T. Mgutshini. Posttraumatic stress disorder among spouses of patients

discharged from the intensive care unit after six months. *Issues Ment Health Nurs* 2013; **34**: 30–5.

18. A.C. Verceles, D.S. Corwin, M. Afshar, et al. Half of the family members of critically ill patients experience excessive daytime sleepiness. *Intensive Care Med* 2014; **40**: 1124–31.

19. J. Choi, J.A. Tate, L.A. Hoffman, et al. Fatigue in family caregivers of adult intensive care unit survivors. *J Pain Symptom Manage* 2014; **48**: 353–63.

20. J. McPeake, H. Devine, P. MacTavish, et al. Caregiver strain following critical care discharge: an exploratory evaluation. *J Crit Care* 2016; **35**: 180–4.

21. J. Choi, L.A. Hoffman, R. Schulz, et al. Health risk behaviors in family caregivers during patients' stay in intensive care units: a pilot analysis. *Am J Crit Care* 2013; **22**: 41–5.

22. R. Schulz, S.R. Beach, B. Lind, et al. Involvement in caregiving and adjustment to death of a spouse: findings from the caregiver health effects study. *JAMA* 2001; **285**: 3123–9.

23. Centers for Disease Control and Prevention. Caregiving for family and friends – a public health issue 2019. www.cdc.gov/aging/agingdata/docs/caregiver-brief-508.pdf.

24. National Alliance for Caregiving, AARP Public Policy Institute. Caregiving in the U.S. 2020 [Internet]. Washington (DC): National Alliance for Caregiving and AARP; 2020 www.caregiving.org/research/caregiving-in-the-us/caregiving-in-the-us-2020/. Accessed May 26, 2025.

25. Committee on Family Caregiving for Older Adults, Board on Health Care Services, Health and Medicine Division, National Academies of Sciences, Engineering, and Medicine. Families caring for an aging America. Schulz R, Eden J, editors. Washington (DC): National Academies Press (US); 2016.

26. J. Kang. Being devastated by critical illness journey in the family: a grounded theory approach of post-intensive care syndrome-family. *Intensive Crit Care Nurs* 2023; **78**: 103448.

27. J. Griffiths, R.A. Hatch, J. Bishop, et al. An exploration of social and economic outcome and associated health-related quality of life after critical illness in general intensive care unit survivors: a 12-month follow-up study. *Crit Care* 2013; **17**: 1–12.

28. S. H. Zarit, P.A. Todd, J.M. Zarit. Subjective burden of husbands and wives as caregivers: a longitudinal study. *Gerontologist* 1986; **26**: 260–6.

29. I. van Beusekom, F. Bakhshi-Raiez, N.F. de Keizer, et al. Reported burden on informal caregivers of ICU survivors: a literature review. *Crit Care* 2015; **20**: 1–8.

30. A. Wolters, M. Bouw, J. Vogelaar, et al. The postintensive care syndrome of survivors of critical illness and their families. *J Clin Nurs* 2015; **24**: 876–9.

31. A. Milton, A. Schandl, I.M. Larsson, et al. Caregiver burden and emotional wellbeing in informal caregivers to ICU survivors: a prospective cohort study. *Acta Anaesthesiol Scand* 2022; **66**: 94–102.

32. J. Torres, D. Carvalho, E. Molinos, et al. The impact of the patient post-intensive care syndrome components upon caregiver burden. *Med Intensiva* 2017; **41**: 454–60.

33. S.M. Swoboda, P.A. Lipsett. Impact of a prolonged surgical critical illness on patients' families. *Am J Crit Care* 2002; **11**: 459–66.

34. J. Choi, M.P. Donahoe, T.G. Zullo, L. A. Hoffman. Caregivers of the chronically critically ill after discharge from the intensive care unit: six months' experience. *Am J Crit Care* 2011; **20**: 12–22.

35. A.S. Ågård, K. Lomborg, E. Tønnesen, I. Egerod. Rehabilitation activities, out-patient visits and employment in patients and partners the first year after ICU: a descriptive study. *Intensive Crit Care Nurs* 2014; **30**: 101–10.

36. J. McPeake, M.E. Mikkelsen, T. Quasim, et al. Return to employment after critical illness and its association with psychosocial

37. N. Khandelwal, C.L. Hough, L. Downey, et al. Prevalence, risk factors, and outcomes of financial stress in survivors of critical illness. *Crit Care Med* 2018; **46**: e530–e9.

38. J. Marti, P. Hall, P. Hamilton, et al. One-year resource utilisation, costs and quality of life in patients with acute respiratory distress syndrome (ARDS): secondary analysis of a randomised controlled trial. *J Intensive Care* 2016; **4**: 1–11.

39. J. Choi, Y.-J. Son, J.A. Tate. Exploring positive aspects of caregiving in family caregivers of adult ICU survivors from ICU to four months post-ICU discharge. *Heart Lung* 2019; **48**: 553–9.

40. J.A. Tate, J. Choi. Positive appraisal of caregiving for intensive care unit survivors: a qualitative secondary analysis. *Am J Crit Care* 2020; **29**: 340–9.

41. K.M. Connor, J.R. Davidson. Development of a new resilience scale: the Connor-Davidson resilience scale (CD-RISC). *Depress Anxiety* 2003; **18**: 76–82.

42. E. Meyers, A. Lin, E. Lester, et al. Baseline resilience and depression symptoms predict trajectory of depression in dyads of patients and their informal caregivers following discharge from the Neuro-ICU. *Gen Hosp Psychiatry* 2020; **62**: 87–92.

43. E.E. Meyers, K.M. Shaffer, M. Gates, et al. Baseline resilience and posttraumatic symptoms in dyads of neurocritical patients and their informal caregivers: a prospective dyadic analysis. *Psychosomatics* 2020; **61**: 135–44.

44. T. Barskova, R. Oesterreich. Post-traumatic growth in people living with a serious medical condition and its relations to physical and mental health: a systematic review. *Disabil Rehabil* 2009; **31**: 1709–33.

45. R.G. Tedeschi, L.G. Calhoun. The posttraumatic growth inventory: measuring the positive legacy of trauma. *J Trauma Stress* 1996; **9**: 455–71.

46. C. Cormio, F. Romito, G. Viscanti, et al. Psychological well-being and posttraumatic growth in caregivers of cancer patients. *Front Psychol* 2014; **5**.

47. K. Hefferon, M. Grealy, N. Mutrie. Post-traumatic growth and life threatening physical illness: a systematic review of the qualitative literature. *Br J Health Psychol* 2009; **14**: 343–78.

48. A. Sawyer, S. Ayers, A.P. Field. Posttraumatic growth and adjustment among individuals with cancer or HIV/AIDS: a meta-analysis. *Clin Psychol Rev* 2010; **30**: 436–47.

49. Y. Ito, M. Tsubaki, M. Kobayashi, et al. Effect size estimates of risk factors for post-intensive care syndrome-family: a systematic review and meta-analysis. *Heart Lung* 2023; **59**: 1–7.

50. Z. Putowski, N. Rachfalska, K. Majewska, et al. Risk factors for Post-Intensive Care Syndrome in Family Members (PICS-F) of adult patients: a systematic review. *Anaesthesiol Intensive Ther* 2023; **55(3)**: 168–78.

51. C.T. Lobato, J. Camões, D. Carvalho, et al. Risk factors associated with post-intensive care syndrome in family members (PICS-F): a prospective observational study. *J Intensive Care Soc* 2023; **24**: 247–57.

52. R. Naef, S. von Felten, J. Ernst. Factors influencing post-ICU psychological distress in family members of critically ill patients: a linear mixed-effects model. *Biopsychosoc Med* 2021; **15**: 1–9.

53. K. Shirasaki, T. Hifumi, N. Nakanishi, et al. Postintensive care syndrome family: a comprehensive review. *Acute Med Surg* 2024; **11**: e939.

54. J. Mellinghoff, M. Van Mol, N. Efstathiou. The caregiver. In H. Flatten, B. Guidet, H. Vallet (eds), *The very old critically ill patients*. Cham: Springer; 2022, pp.417–37.

55. R. Schofield, B. Dibb, R. Coles-Gale, C.J. Jones. The experience of relatives using intensive care diaries: a systematic review and qualitative synthesis. *Int J Nurs Stud* 2021; **119**: 103927.

56. G. Wang, R. Antel, M. Goldfarb. The impact of randomized family-centered interventions on family-centered outcomes in the adult Intensive Care Unit: a systematic review. *J Intensive Care Med* 2023; **38**: 690–701.

57. J.E. Davidson. Facilitated sensemaking: a strategy and new middle-range theory to support families of intensive care unit patients. *Crit Care Nurse* 2010; **30**: 28–39.

58. J.E. Davidson, B.J. Daly, D. Agan, et al. Facilitated sensemaking: a feasibility study for the provision of a family support program in the intensive care unit. *Crit Care Nurs Q* 2010; **33**: 177–89.

59. M. Skoog, K.A. Milner, J. Gatti-Petito, K. Dintyala. The impact of family engagement on anxiety levels in a cardiothoracic intensive care unit. *Crit Care Nurse* 2016; **36**: 84–9.

60. J.W. Shin, M.B. Happ, J.A. Tate. VidaTalk patient communication application "opened up" communication between nonvocal ICU patients and their family. *Intensive Crit Care Nurs* 2021; **66**: 103075.

61. H. Huang, H. Dong, X. Guan, et al. The facilitated sensemaking model as a framework for nursing intervention on family members of mechanically ventilated patients in the intensive care unit. *Worldviews Evid Based Nurs* 2022; **19**: 467–76.

62. L.M. Boehm, K. Drumright, R. Gervasio, et al. Implementation of a patient and family-centered ICU peer support program at a veterans affairs hospital. *Crit Care Nurs Clin North Am* 2020; **32**: 203.

63. M.B. Wasilewski, K.M. Kokorelias, M. Nonoyama, et al. The experience of family caregivers of ventilator-assisted individuals who participated in a pilot web-based peer support program: a qualitative study. *Digital Health* 2022; **8**: 20552076221134964.

64. A.-M. Vranceanu, E.C. Woodworth, M.R. Kanaya, et al. The Recovering Together study protocol: a single-blind RCT to prevent chronic emotional distress in patient-caregiver dyads in the Neuro-ICU. *Contemp Clin Trials* 2022; **123**: 106998.

65. S.J. Cherak, B.K. Rosgen, M. Amarbayan, et al. Mental health interventions to improve psychological outcomes in informal caregivers of critically ill patients: a systematic review and meta-analysis. *Crit Care Med* 2021; **49**: 1414–26.

66. A.B. Petrinec, C. Wilk, J.W. Hughes, et al. Self-care mental health app intervention for post–intensive care syndrome–family: a randomized pilot study. *Am J Crit Care* 2023; **32**: 440–8.

67. A.S. Zigmond, R.P. Snaith. The hospital anxiety and depression scale. *Acta Psychiatr Scand* 1983; **67**: 361–70.

68. M. Szabó. The short version of the Depression Anxiety Stress Scales (DASS-21): factor structure in a young adolescent sample. *J Adolesc* 2010; **33**: 1–8.

69. R.L. Spitzer, K. Kroenke, J.B. Williams, B. Löwe. A brief measure for assessing generalized anxiety disorder: the GAD-7. *Arch Intern Med* 2006; **166**: 1092–7.

70. A.T. Beck, N. Epstein, G. Brown, R.A. Steer. An inventory for measuring clinical anxiety: psychometric properties. *J Consult Clin Psychol* 1988; **56**: 893–7.

71. P. Skapinakis. Spielberger state-trait anxiety inventory. In: Michalos A.C. (ed.), *Encyclopedia of quality of life and well-being research*. Dordrecht: Springer Netherlands; 2014, pp. 6261–4.

72. L.S. Radloff. The CES-D Scale: a self-report depression scale for research in the general population. *Appl Psychol Meas* 1977; **1**: 385–401.

73. K. Kroenke, R.L. Spitzer, J.B. Williams. The PHQ-9: validity of a brief depression severity measure. *J Gen Intern Med* 2001; **16**: 606–13.

74. K. Kroenke, T.W. Strine, R.L. Spitzer, et al. The PHQ-8 as a measure of current depression in the general population. *J Affect Disord* 2009; **114**: 163–73.

75. M. Horowitz, N. Wilner, W. Alvarez. Impact of Event Scale: a measure of subjective stress. *Psychosom Med* 1979; **41**: 209–18.

76. D.S. Weiss, C.R. Marmar. *The Impact of Event Scale-Revised. Assessing psychological*

trauma and PTSD: a practitioner's handbook. New York: Guilford; 1995, pp. 399–411.

77. M.M. Hosey, J.S. Leoutsakos, X. Li, et al. Screening for posttraumatic stress disorder in ARDS survivors: validation of the Impact of Event Scale-6 (IES-6). *Crit Care* 2019; **23**: 276.

78. B. Raphael, T. Lundin, L. Weisaeth. A research method for the study of psychological and psychiatric aspects of disaster. *Acta Psychiatr Scand Suppl* 1989; **353**: 1–75.

79. E.B. Foa, L. Cashman, L. Jaycox, K. Perry. The validation of a self-report measure of posttraumatic stress disorder: the Posttraumatic Diagnostic Scale. *Psychol Assess* 1997; **9**: 445–51.

80. F.W. Weathers, B.T. Litz, et al. The PTSD Checklist for DSM-5 (PCL-5). National Center for PTSD; 2013. Available from: www.ptsd.va.gov.

81. F.W. Weathers, B.T. Litz, D.S. Herman, J.A. Huska, T.M. Keane (eds), *The PTSD Checklist (PCL): reliability, validity, and diagnostic utility. annual convention of the international society for traumatic stress studies.* San Antonio, TX; 1993.

82. C.R. Marmar, D.S. Weiss, T.J. Metzler. *The Peritraumatic Dissociative Experiences Questionnaire: assessing psychological trauma and PTSD.* New York: Guilford; 1997, pp. 412–28.

83. C.R. Brewin, S. Rose, B. Andrews, et al. Brief screening instrument for post-traumatic stress disorder. *Br J Psychiatry* 2002; **181**: 158–62.

84. H.G. Prigerson, P.K. Maciejewski, C.F. Reynolds, et al. Inventory of complicated grief: a scale to measure maladaptive symptoms of loss. *Psychiatry Res* 1995; **59**: 65–79.

85. S. Cohen, T. Kamarck, R. Mermelstein. A global measure of perceived stress. *J Health Soc Behav* 1983; **24**: 385–96.

86. F.W. Quinless, M.A. Nelson. Development of a measure of learned helplessness. *Nurs Res* 1988; **37**: 11–15.

87. R. Schulz, J. Newsom, M. Mittelmark, et al. Health effects of caregiving: the caregiver health effects study: an ancillary study of the Cardiovascular Health Study. *Ann Behav Med* 1997; **19**: 110–16.

88. K.A. Lee. Self-reported sleep disturbances in employed women. *Sleep* 1992; **15**: 493–8.

89. C.H. Bastien, A. Vallières, C.M. Morin. Validation of the Insomnia Severity Index as an outcome measure for insomnia research. *Sleep Med* 2001; **2**: 297–307.

90. D.J. Buysse, C.F. Reynolds, T.H. Monk, et al. The Pittsburgh Sleep Quality Index: a new instrument for psychiatric practice and research. *Psychiatry Res* 1989; **28**: 193–213.

91. K.A. Lee, G. Hicks, G. Nino-Murcia. Validity and reliability of a scale to assess fatigue. *Psychiatry Res* 1991; **36**: 291–8.

92. B.C. Robinson. Validation of a caregiver strain index. *J Gerontol* 1983; **38**: 344–8.

93. S.H. Zarit, K.E. Reever, J. Bach-Peterson. Relatives of the impaired elderly: correlates of feelings of burden. *Gerontologist* 1980; **20**: 649–55.

94. S.H. Zarit, N.K. Orr, J.M. Zarit. *The hidden victims of Alzheimer's disease: families under stress.* New York: New York University Press; 1985.

95. M. Bédard, D.W. Molloy, L. Squire, et al. The Zarit Burden Interview: a new short version and screening version. *Gerontologist* 2001; **41**: 652–7.

96. G. Balestroni, G. Bertolotti. [EuroQol-5D (EQ-5D): an instrument for measuring quality of life]. *Monaldi Arch Chest Dis* 2012; **78**: 155–9.

97. J.S. Norbeck. The Norbeck Social Support Questionnaire. *Birth Defects Orig Artic Ser* 1984; **20**: 45–57.

98. D.H. Olson, J. Portner, R.Q. Bell. *FACES II: Family Adaptability and Cohesion Evaluation Scales.* St. Paul (MN): University of Minnesota, Department of Family Social Science; 1982.

Chapter 49

Peer Support for Survivors of Critical Illness and Their Loved Ones

Heather Imperato-Shedden, Brad W. Butcher, and Annie B. Johnson

Introduction

To address the impact of post-intensive care syndrome (PICS), collaborative efforts to improve patient outcomes began organizing across the United States in 2015, while outside of the United States, organizations have implemented intensive care unit (ICU) recovery support group programs for over two decades. ICUsteps (icusteps.org), developed in 2005 in the United Kingdom, has been particularly instrumental in paving the way for the ongoing development of support resources globally. The specific focus on peer support in the ICUsteps program, where survivors of critical illness serve as group moderators, established a precedent for support groups in the ICU recovery space.

Collaboratives such as the Society of Critical Care Medicine's (SCCM) THRIVE program and the Critical and Acute Illness Recovery Organization (CAIRO; cairorecovery.com), both based in the United States but with international memberships, have advanced the development and science of ICU follow-up clinics and peer support groups [1,2]. Data from these efforts suggest that peer support groups for survivors of critical illness and their loved ones improve empowerment, self-advocacy, social support, shared coping, and key health outcomes, including depression [3,4].

Benefits of Peer Support

By allowing the development of social relationships that have a reciprocal influence on health and well-being, peer support programs exist for and have been studied in several chronic diseases, including cancer, diabetes, and stroke, and data suggest that peer support is effective in increasing psychological empowerment in these patient populations [4,5]. Given that PICS is in many respects a chronic disease that impacts reintegration into previous familial, social, and professional roles, peer support groups have been developed for survivors of critical illness and their loved ones as a tool to process the challenges of ICU survivorship and caregiver burden with others who have similar lived experiences. Survivors of critical illness have described three primary mechanisms by which peer support provides benefit: sharing experiences with others, care debriefing, and altruism [6]. Sharing experiences with one another results in decreased anxiety, increased hope and motivation, and, by speaking with patients further along the recovery trajectory, an appreciation that further improvement is possible. Care debriefing leads to a more sophisticated understanding of how to navigate complex healthcare systems, supports realistic goal setting, and manages expectations about the pace, depth, and breadth of recovery. Altruism derived from peer support yields a sense of purpose and allows survivors to give back to other patients, their caregivers, and often to the ICU staff who cared for them [6].

Peer support also contributes to increased social support for survivors of critical illness [3]. There is increasing evidence that social isolation and loneliness negatively impact both physical and mental health and are associated with all-cause mortality in several disease processes, highlighting the epidemic of loneliness as a public health concern. Effective interventions to mitigate loneliness include group modalities, such as peer support groups [7,8,9]. Peer support helps survivors of critical illness recast their traumatic experience as an opportunity to develop or refine new attributes, resulting in post-traumatic growth (PTG; see Chapters 46 and 48 for additional information) [10]. While more research is needed, there are opportunities for ICU clinicians and peers to educate survivors and their loved ones about PTG and for ICU follow-up clinics and peer support groups to help facilitate this experience [11]. A peer emulating the qualities of PTG by sharing their personal experiences can be a model to help others make positive meaning out of an otherwise challenging experience. Therefore, by giving patients a sense of purpose, mitigating social isolation and loneliness, and providing opportunities for PTG, peer support is a low-cost intervention that provides important psychosocial benefits and potentially even life-saving ones.

Despite these benefits, other data regarding the efficacy of peer support as an intervention to improve recovery in survivors of critical illness and their families are mixed. Haines and colleagues performed a systematic review of 8 studies, comprising 92 patients and 192 family members, in which the most common peer support model was an in-person, facilitated group for families that occurred during the hospitalization [3]. Two studies showed that peer support reduced anxiety and depression and improved social support and self-efficacy when using a peer-to-peer model that started in the hospital and extended beyond discharge, but similar findings were not found with facilitated group-based models. Only two of the eight studies assessed peer support for patients rather than family members, and nearly all of the peer support interventions occurred while patients were in the hospital, rather than in the months to years following critical illness, during the so-called adjustment and adaptation phases, when the reality of dealing with a new normal truly sets in. Despite the lack of robust evidence, there is little empirical reason to suspect that peer support would be ineffective with survivors of critical illness given its demonstrated effectiveness with other populations.

Models of Peer Support

Data from the organizational support group collaboratives cited above have demonstrated that multiple models of peer support groups for survivors of critical illness and their loved ones exist, each with its unique strengths and challenges. This structural variability helps promote the adaptation of support groups across a wide range of healthcare settings and ensures that the model chosen best accommodates the availability of local resources and individual participant needs. The SCCM THRIVE Peer Support Collaborative [12] has outlined the most commonly utilized models of peer support among collaborative sites, and the following is a brief description of each.

ICU-Based Groups

In this model, peer support groups are held within the hospital, either in the ICU or very near to it. This model is primarily aimed at loved ones and caregivers of patients who remain critically ill and is offered at various times during the patient's hospitalization [12]. As the patient's condition improves and loved ones feel more comfortable spending time away from the bedside, attendance at these groups is facilitated by physical proximity to the ICU.

Community-Based Groups

Community-based peer support groups typically meet in the community, but will occasionally meet on hospital grounds, usually in a location distant from the ICU. These groups often combine both survivors of critical illness and their families, and they can be led by survivors or by ICU recovery staff (e.g., physicians, advanced practice providers, social workers, and mental health professionals) who are trained to moderate such groups. Survivors and their loved ones are typically invited to participate in the peer support group in the months following hospital discharge, and participation is often open-ended, with participants determining when their support needs have been met [12].

Clinic-Based Groups

This model of peer support is integrated into ICU follow-up clinics and may occur at the same time and in the same space as the clinic, utilizing waiting rooms and other congregational spaces to allow for natural gathering of the participants. This model is largely unstructured and allows for participants at varied points of recovery to connect with one another [12].

Virtual Groups

Virtual peer support groups experienced a surge in popularity during the COVID-19 pandemic and have remained a popular model since. These groups operate similarly to in-person peer support groups but utilize virtual technology for facilitation, including video conferencing and teleconferencing technologies.

Online Groups

Online peer support models offer an asynchronous platform that enhances anonymity, convenience, and accessibility. Dedicated moderators are typically assigned to monitor these forums and provide a voice when needed, including introducing topics of conversation, replying to participants' concerns, providing additional resources to participants, and connecting participants with shared experiences. Participants engage per their comfort level and may use these sites for information gathering by reading others' submissions, active participation by sharing their own stories through written submissions and responses, or a combination thereof.

Peer Mentor Model

In this model, a survivor of critical illness or the family member of a survivor uses their lived experience as the vehicle to provide and foster peer support. The peer may have a leadership role facilitating a post-ICU peer support group, or they may volunteer their time to visit with patients and families in the ICU, hospital, or following discharge. When determining the scope of the role, the volunteer's interests and abilities should be aligned with the program's goals. Healthcare is an inherently hierarchal system with power differentials, which can be even more pronounced among interdisciplinary teams. A systematic review demonstrated that these factors negatively impact team effectiveness, as they reduce both effective communication and "speaking up" behaviors. To improve team effectiveness and collaboration, there must be an active awareness of power dynamics and purposeful efforts to mitigate them, such as shared leadership models and an open and supportive workplace culture [13].

The peer mentors leading the support group may still be under the care of providers with whom they are working alongside in this role. Clinicians need to be mindful of these power dynamics and work to mitigate them in order to prevent disempowering a peer volunteer. Peer mentors should be onboarded as a formal volunteer within the hospital's Volunteer Services department, and they should have access to a staff member, such as a social worker, psychologist, or other professional trained in supervising peer volunteers, to ensure they are receiving adequate supervision and support. Ideally, the peer volunteer will also have access to an existing or senior peer volunteer for mentorship and support.

Factors on the Post Traumatic Growth Inventory may help both interested peers and clinicians identify qualities that inform fit and readiness to serve and may help foster positive meaning in a volunteer experience [14]. The Substance Abuse and Mental Health Services Administration (SAMHSA) has developed core competencies for peer workers in behavioral health services and provides guidance on the potential use of these competencies to evaluate peer mentor performance and development. The SAMHSA core competencies include the knowledge, skills, and attitudes needed to successfully perform a role [15]; reviewing competencies provides a peer mentor with a standard for their development and growth in the role. In addition to developing competencies, SAMHSA's Bringing Recovery Supports to Scale Technical Assistance Center Strategy (BRSS TACS) has developed evidence-based resources to help programs successfully incorporate peers into behavioral health settings, including training for supervisors and methods of evaluating peer mentors' performance. SAMHSA's National Center for Trauma Informed Care has a series of trainings on delivering trauma-informed peer support that may benefit both peer volunteers and clinicians [15,16].

Social Gatherings

As social beings, we thrive on connection, belonging, and interaction with others [17]. Institutions that do not have the staff or resources to develop and sustain a peer support group or peer mentor volunteer role may consider hosting social gatherings instead. The attendees may eventually serve as the initial cohort for a future support group, or interested individuals may be recruited to provide one-on-one peer support. A social gathering can also be beneficial to institutions that have any component of post-ICU services, including ICU follow-up clinics, peer support groups, or volunteer services, by building awareness, engaging the community, and acting as a vehicle to connect survivors with one another. Furthermore, a gathering can reunite survivors and their families with the ICU staff who cared for them, potentially reducing ICU staff burnout [18,19]. Examples of social gatherings that have been successfully organized by member sites of the CAIRO Peer Support Collaborative are highlighted in Box 49.1.

> **Box 49.1** Examples of social gatherings
>
> A social work team hosted a pizza party at an outdoor plaza garden located on the hospital grounds. The location was close to restrooms and was accessible to individuals with different levels of mobility. Hosting the event outdoors enhanced inclusion for group members to safely gather in person during the COVID-19 pandemic. As this was a pilot event, a small number of staff were included, mainly the team members involved in the Post-ICU Program.
>
> The team worked with media services to arrange a speaker and microphone, and the program manager gave a welcome address to share the reasons for the gathering. Music was played throughout, and there were two optional activities. *Bracelets of Hope* provided guests the opportunity to create inspirational bracelets for themselves, other survivors, or staff, decorated with words that helped them during their experience. *Leaves of Gratitude* invited guests to share messages with those who helped them, including the staff who cared for them, fellow group members, or to their social support system. Messages were written on cut-out leaves and then displayed on branches; after the event, messages to staff were displayed on a bulletin board in the breakroom. The team provided hospital-branded tote bags with small blankets, as this event was held in the fall.
>
> With positive feedback from the pilot, the team utilized Critical Care Awareness and Recognition month in May to organize a larger social gathering. This event included current and former group members as well as former patients and families that were not yet engaged in post-ICU services. A large number of staff, including administrators, physicians, advanced practice providers, nurses, social workers, and spiritual care providers, attended. With assistance from Public Relations, photos were taken with the consent of attendees. In addition to the program manager's welcome address, a survivor was invited to speak and share their story.

Other event programming ideas include hosting and registering an event for the International Walk4PICS in September or renting a picnic pavilion at a local park. Given the role of expressive art in fostering PTG, hosting a workshop with an art therapist or writer may also be beneficial [20].

Guide to Developing Peer Support Programs

Understanding the facilitators and barriers that have been experienced by established peer support groups for survivors of critical illness and their loved ones provides a helpful foundation for those exploring starting their own group. In a qualitative study of established peer support groups in the THRIVE collaborative, Haines and colleagues describe the experiences of various professionals with developing and sustaining peer support groups in their respective organizations. Examples of key facilitators include finding skilled professional and peer moderators, clearly defining the operational aspects of the group, and collaborating with ICU follow-up clinics to recruit patients into the support group; barriers include lack of access to venues for patient recruitment, lack of skilled moderators, and bureaucratic organizational limitations [21].

Building upon this knowledge, the remainder of this section serves as a guide for those interested in developing a peer support group for patients recovering from critical illness and their loved ones. These steps were originally described in the qualitative work of Hope and colleagues and the CAIRO peer support collaborative [1].

Preparation

One of the most important aspects of preparing to develop a peer support group is to understand the needs of the participants and to choose a group platform that is most accommodating. In the post-COVID-19 pandemic era, a variety of platform options exist; however, the unofficial gold standard remains the in-person, face-to-face group meeting. Additional platforms that saw an increase in implementation during and after the COVID-19 pandemic include several virtual options, each of which has unique considerations. For example, video conferences work well for smaller, more intimate groups; phone calls are suited for areas where more advanced technology is either unavailable or undesired; and asynchronous internet-based forums cast a broad net and allow for participation when most convenient for participants.

Recruitment

Recruitment refers to finding participants to engage with the support group, and as previously noted, it can be one of the most difficult aspects of developing and growing peer support programs. Starting the recruitment process while patients remain hospitalized is one way that has been effective for some organizations, while others find success in collaborating with ICU follow-up clinics [1]. As virtual support groups become increasingly utilized, opportunities to share these resources among the broader critical care survivorship population grow, and accordingly, in areas where peer support groups are not available, referral to support groups that accept participants from outside of their organization is an attractive option. Similarly, online forums, such as Mayo Clinic Connect (connect.mayo-clinic.org), are another example of support available to the general public without specifically requiring one to be a patient of a particular organization, allowing highly resourced institutions to further their reach in helping improve the outcomes for survivors of critical illness and their loved ones.

Facilitation

Consideration must be paid to the anticipated needs of the group participants when choosing facilitators. Common choices for facilitators include social workers, psychologists or other mental health professionals, hospital chaplains, and trained survivors of critical illness. Effective facilitators are engaging, keep the conversation fluid and focused, and prioritize the safety and acceptance of all those participating [1]. It is common for groups to have more than one facilitator to help manage group dynamics and respond to individual participant needs as they arise [1].

Trauma-Informed Approach

Acknowledging that survivorship is associated with trauma is crucial when developing a peer support group. Centering the trauma helps inform several steps in group development, such as the location of the group setting (i.e., will it be near the ICU, in the hospital, or completely off-site), timing of group (i.e., will it be in the mornings, afternoon, or evenings, and what impact might that have on functioning at work or sleeping at night), and topics discussed during the group sessions. Choosing a facilitator with trauma-informed expertise, who can help guide the experience knowing that previous trauma can influence the dynamics and outcomes of the group, is critical [1].

Planning Logistics

Organizers will need a logistical plan for location, timing, frequency, size, and format of the developing group. In addition, a structured plan for collecting feedback from the participants can play an important role in improving the group to best meet participants' needs.

Planning for the In-Between

The "in-between" refers to the time period between group meetings or any time after the group has been completed. Participants may find group sessions triggering due to trauma associated with their critical care experience, highlighting the importance of having a plan for the in-between time. Having a compilation of readily available resources that participants can access if needed and ways to reach out if further help is required is one way to address this in-between time. Post-group debriefings by the facilitator team can also be a helpful exercise during this in-between time to reflect on what has worked well and what could be improved during group time [1].

Conclusion

Peer support has long been utilized by patients as: with chronic diseases to help meet their complex recovery needs, and despite a lack of definitive evidence, there is little reason to doubt that the same can be true for survivors of critical illness who participate in peer support groups. As awareness of the complex needs of survivors of critical illness grows within both the medical and lay communities, expectations will rise for the establishment of evidence-based resources to improve patient outcomes. Collaboratives composed of experts in critical care survivorship will continue to be vital in moving the science of critical illness recovery forward, including a focus on the crucial role that peer support can play.

Key Points

1. International collaboratives of experts in critical illness survivorship exist to promote development of evidence-based models to deliver peer support.
2. There is no "one-size-fits-all" approach to developing peer support groups for survivors of critical illness; variety promotes adaptation across a wide range of settings and helps meet individual participant needs.
3. Peer support can improve psychological empowerment, self-advocacy, social support, and shared coping.
4. Peer support has been shown to reduce feelings of loneliness and can improve key health outcomes, including depression.
5. To successfully integrate peers into volunteer roles, an on-boarding process that includes alignment of goals, supervision, and growth are important. Clinicians must

work to mitigate disempowerment by utilizing shared leadership models and creating an open and supportive culture.

References

1. A.A. Hope, A.A. Johnson, J. McPeake, et al. Establishing a peer support program for survivors of COVID-19: a report from the critical and acute illness recovery organization. *Am J Crit Care* 2021; **30**(2): 150–4.
2. M.E. Mikkelsen, J.C. Jackson, R. O. Hopkins, et al. Peer support as a novel strategy to mitigate post-intensive care syndrome. *AACN Adv Crit Care* 2016; **27**(2): 221–9.
3. K. J. Haines, S.J. Beesley, R.O. Hopkins, et al. Peer support in critical care: a systematic review. *Crit Care Med* 2018, **46**: 1522–31.
4. E. Ziegler, J. Hill, B. Lieske, et al. Empowerment in cancer patients: does peer support make a difference? A systematic review. *PsychoOncology* 2022; **31**(5): 683–704.
5. C. Bellamy, T. Schmutte, L. Davidson. An update on the growing evidence base for peer support. *Ment Health Soc Incl* 2017; **21**(3): 161–7.
6. J. McPeake, T.J. Iwashyna, L.M. Boehm, et al. Benefits of peer support for intensive care unit survivors: sharing experiences, care debriefing, and altruism. *Am J Crit Care* 2021; **30**(2): 145–9.
7. J. Holt-Lunstad. Our epidemic of loneliness and isolation: The U.S. surgeon general's advisory on the healing effects of social connection and community. Department of Health and Human Services 2023. www.hhs.gov/sites/default/files/surgeon-general-social-connection-advisory.pdf (Accessed May 5, 2024).
8. C.M. Masi, H-Y Chen, L.C. Hawkley, J. T. Cacioppo. A meta-analysis of interventions to reduce loneliness. *Pers Soc Psychol Rev* 2010; **15**(3): 219–66.
9. S.M. Fuller, A.A. Kotwal, S.H. Tha, et al. Key elements and mechanisms of a peer-support intervention to reduce loneliness and isolation among low-income older adults: a qualitative implementation science study. *J Appl Gerontol* 2022; **41**(12): 2574–82.
10. R.G. Tedeschi, L.G. Calhoun. Posttraumatic growth: conceptual foundations and empirical evidence. *Psychol Inq* 2004; **15**(1): 1–18.
11. A.C. Jones, R. Hilton, B. Ely, et al. Facilitating posttraumatic growth after critical illness. *Am J Crit Care* 2020; **29**(6): 108–15.
12. J. McPeake, E.L. Hirshberg, L.M. Christie, et al. Models of peer support to remediate post-intensive care syndrome: a report developed by the society of critical care medicine thrive international peer support collaborative. *Crit Care Med* 2019; **47**(1): 21–7.
13. E. Kearns, Z. Khurshid, S. Anjara, et al. P92 power dynamics in healthcare teams: a barrier to team effectiveness and patient safety: a systematic review. *BJS Open* 2021; 5(Suppl 1): zrab032.091.
14. R.G. Tedeschi, L.G. Calhoun. The posttraumatic growth inventory: measuring the positive legacy of trauma. *J Trauma Stress* 1996; **9**(3): 455–71.
15. Bringing Recovery Supports to Scale Technical Assistance Center Strategy. Substance Abuse and Mental Health Services Administration. www.samhsa.gov/brss-tacs (Accessed May 4, 2024).
16. National Association of State Mental Health Program Directors. Trauma Informed Peer Support. www.nasmhpd.org/content/webinar-series-trauma-informed-peer-support (Accessed May 5, 2024).
17. J. Holt-Lunstad. Social connection as a public health issue: the evidence and a systemic framework for prioritizing the "social" in social determinants of health.

Annu Rev Public Health 2022; **43**(1): 193–213.

18. L. Jarvie, C. Robinson, P. MacTavish, et al. Understanding the patient journey: a mechanism to reduce staff burnout? *Br J Nurs* 2019; **28**(6): 396–7.

19. T.L. Eaton, V. Danesh, C.M. Sevin, et al. Importance of reconnection with ICU survivors to ICU recovery program clinicians. *CHEST Critical Care* 2023; **1**(2): 1–4.

20. K. Perryman, P. Blisard, R. Moss. Using creative arts in trauma therapy: the neuroscience of healing. *J. Ment Health Couns* 2019; **41**(1): 80–94.

21. K.J. Haines, J. McPeake, E. Hibbert, et al. Enablers and barriers to implementing ICU follow-up clinics and peer support groups following critical illness: the thrive collaboratives. *Crit Care Med* 2019; **47**(9): 1194–200.

Section 6 PICS in Specific Populations

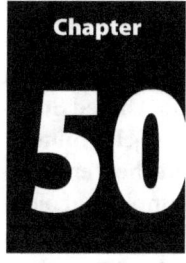

Chapter 50

PICS in Older Survivors of Critical Illness

Chisom A. Ikeji and Leslie P. Scheunemann

Introduction

The Age-Friendly Movement, an integrated model for intergenerational population health, comprises Age-Friendly Health Systems, Age-Friendly Communities, and Age-Friendly Public Health [1,2]. Age-Friendly Health systems include hospitals, clinics, and long-term care facilities that provide state-of-the art healthcare to older adults; Age-Friendly Communities promote healthy aging through community-based organizations, policy implementation, and advocacy; and Age-Friendly Public Health conceptually goes beyond Area Agencies on Aging to optimize functional health, facilitate social and civic engagement, and manage chronic conditions. The goals of caring for older adults with post-intensive care syndrome (PICS) align with the Age-Friendly Movement. Because millions of older adults survive critical illness each year, partnering with the Age-Friendly movement may be among the most efficient ways of delivering quality care to and improving outcomes for older adults with PICS.

Age-Friendly Health Systems are of most immediate relevance to clinicians caring for older adults with PICS. They provide evidence-based care delivery using five organizing principles known as the 5Ms of Age-Friendly Healthcare: Mobility, Mind, Medications, Multicomplexity, and What Matters Most. The 5Ms are interrelated and must be considered as a whole.

This chapter offers a novel application of the 5Ms to evidence-based care delivery for older adults with PICS; however, the 5Ms and core features of PICS overlap substantially. Thus, this chapter highlights issues particularly meaningful among older adults while also citing dedicated chapters on relevant topics (e.g., rehabilitation, frailty, etc.). The first section provides essential background on interpreting evidence about PICS through the lenses of ageism (bias related to age) and ableism (bias related to disability status). The next five sections explain the 5Ms construct and summarize related evidence in PICS. The final section offers a vision linking Age-Friendly Healthcare, Age-Friendly Communities, and Age-Friendly Public Health after critical illness.

Ageism and Ableism

For people over age 80, 3-year mortality is similar following ICU and non-ICU hospitalizations [3], suggesting that long-term mortality among survivors is not simply attributable to critical illness itself. Post-intensive care unit (ICU) disability is also not simply attributable to age [4], as disability is not an inevitable consequence of aging, and younger and older people experience post-ICU disability at similar rates [5,6,7,8]. The intersection of ageism and ableism contributes to ongoing knowledge and practice gaps by obscuring questions like: What factors in care delivery can make older adults more resilient to critical illness? What happens to younger adults with PICS?

Ageism is often structural, making it difficult to recognize [9]. For example, reliance on Medicare data to study the epidemiology of survivors of critical illness in the United States means that little is known about populations ineligible for Medicare, largely younger individuals whose insurance plans (e.g., through the Affordable Care Act or their employers) typically do not provide data for research. Further, nonrepresentative sampling of older adults in post-ICU research often goes unrecognized, especially when results confirm expectations of aging [9]. Finally, older adults often experience exclusion from care or suboptimal care quality, examples of which include policies that explicitly exclude them from ICUs [10,11], under-implementation of proven interventions that reduce their risk of disability (e.g., the ABCDEF bundle and Hospital Elder Life Program [HELP]) [12,13], and lack of adaptive resources to keep them at home instead of requiring long-term care. Addressing data and policy biases against age requires recognizing that multiple mechanisms – both biological and social – contribute to outcomes and that focusing on biomedical illness and disability generates radically different results than focusing on well-being and function [4].

These ways to address ageism invoke the social model of disability (see Chapter 24 for additional information), which emphasizes the importance of context, suggesting that social attitudes, inaccessible environments, and rigid organizations turn health impairments into disabilities [14,15]. It supports the idea that ableism is structural within many healthcare systems [16] and may be a problem among older adults after critical illness as well.

In contrast, the Age-Friendly model is designed for both age and disability. Rather than reacting to disability after it has predictably happened, it takes a preventative, systems-based approach. The Age-Friendly model creates systems that recognize that illness can coexist alongside well-being and that optimize well-being by ensuring access to basic human goods, including safety, belonging, and dignity; nutrition and hydration; hygiene, including bowel and bladder care; sensory support; sleep; mobility; relationships; and meaningful activities.

These goods are also key elements in healing trauma [17,18,19]. Optimizing critical care requires the integration of these elements with technological advances [20,21]. In fact, one of the most important themes in ICU research over the past two decades is that "less is more." The emerging principle is that we should minimize the use of life support and monitoring technology to that which is required to sustain life and promote function, while preserving, as much as possible, the habits and routines of healthy people, such as moving, thinking, and connecting. The following sections show how to apply that principle using the 5Ms. Notably, referral for comprehensive geriatric assessment can help with ongoing needs not addressed by the strategies discussed, although many communities lack geriatrics-trained providers.

Mobility

Mobility is foundational to the rhythms of loving, working, and playing, and it is part of all healthy habits and routines. Age-Friendly Health Systems are committed to the principle that everybody moves, and Age-Friendly Communities work towards enhanced community mobility for older adults. An additional principle is that preventing loss of function is much easier than regaining lost function. Finally, when function *is* lost, participation in meaningful activities can still be enabled by addressing patient barriers (e.g., strength and stamina), modifying tasks (e.g., energy conservation), or modifying environments (e.g., adaptive equipment and accessible transportation) [22,23].

Those principles should organize practice in several ways. First, clinicians should seize readily available opportunities to prevent mobility disability, which are under-implemented across the entire care trajectory. Functional and mobility decline often precede critical illness among older adults [24,25]. Whether early identification and intervention could prevent further decline and reduce incidence of critical illness is unknown. In the ICU, the ABCDEF bundle (see Chapter 11 for additional information) preserves the habits and routines of daily life to the greatest extent possible (see Table 50.1). The "E" is for exercise and early mobility (see Chapter 12 for additional information). While the specific impact of the ABCDEF bundle on older adults is unknown, overall implementation is poor, and older adults face increased barriers to implementation [26]. Clinicians should use published implementation strategies to scale up use of best practices [27,28]. Mobility may become even harder after transition from the ICU to general medical or surgical floors due to lower staffing ratios [29], a structural problem that contributes to permanent disability and institutionalization of older adults. Involving families in mobility is feasible, acceptable, and efficacious but underutilized both in the ICU and on the wards [30]. Training families in safe mobilization may free up staff while also optimizing discharge planning by making families more aware of what they will need to take the patient home safely (e.g., assistive devices, home modifications, and personal care assistance). Medicolegal concerns about falls can also impede mobilization efforts; however, it is unacceptable to permit large populations of older adults to quietly become permanently disabled in order to avoid any risk of falling. More work needs to be done to redefine what it means for hospitals to provide quality care that balances the basic need for mobility with the risk of falls.

Second, mobility disability after critical illness should prompt rehabilitation (see Chapters 41 and 42 for additional information); however, guidelines for screening and referral to rehabilitation services at the time of discharge are poorly implemented, even in countries with historically more integrated health systems than the United States [31,32,33,34,35]. Screening for fear of falling should also guide referral for physical therapy, since older adults who fear falling tend to self-restrict mobility, develop progressive disability, and experience high rates of injurious falls [36]. Home safety evaluations, often performed by occupational therapists, can identify environmental modifications that promote safe mobility. Patients whose Activity Measures for Post-Acute Care (AM-PAC) score worsens during hospitalization have three times the odds of discharge to a skilled nursing facility (SNF) rather than to home. Unfortunately, few older adults who survive severe sepsis respond to rehabilitation at SNFs: nearly three-quarters have high or total dependence in activities of daily living (ADLs), and most die within the year following discharge before achieving sufficient independence to return home [37,38].

Third, rehabilitation should shift from focusing on fixing deficits to enhancing strengths. The relative ineffectiveness of deficit-based approaches erodes support for them while preventing investment in the strategies offered by strengths-based solutions. For example, insurers in the United States frequently stop paying for rehabilitation when patients are not meeting their progress goals (e.g., improved gait speed, six-minute walk test distance, or ADL independence). These biomarkers are prognostically important but have less impact on well-being than positive measures of activity and participation, such as lifespace (the frequency and duration with which patients leave their primary living space), community participation indicators (a measure of participation in personally meaningful

Table 50.1 Mapping the 5Ms to the ABCDEF Bundle. These principles should be applied across the post-ICU trajectory, adapted to the context (i.e., the wards, post-acute care facilities, and community-based settings)

5Ms Construct	Related ABCDEF constructs	Mechanism
Mobility	Assess, treat, and manage pain Both SAT and SBT Delirium prevention and management Exercise and early mobilization Family support	• Pain & pain medications can impair mobility • Consciousness is necessary for mobility • Timely extubation facilitates mobility • Delirium impairs consciousness and gait, making mobility more difficult • Exercise is the intentional practice of mobility • Family can provide motivation, increased "dose" of mobility when staffing is thin, and enhance identification of new impairments that require support. Family involvement may include assistance with diaphragmatic breathing, strengthening exercises for upper and lower extremities, active transfers, and functional activity training.
Mind	Assess, treat, and manage pain Both SAT and SBT Choice of analgesia and sedation Delirium prevention and management Exercise and early mobilization	• Pain & pain medications can be deliriogenic • Timely extubation reduces ventilator-associated sleep disruption and exposure to deliriogenic tubes and drains • While no medications prevent delirium, use of least risky analgesia and sedation reduces its incidence • Delirium prevention and management is the intentional preservation of mind • Mobility itself reduces delirium risk
Medications	Assess, treat, and manage pain Both SAT and SBT Choice of analgesia and sedation Delirium prevention and management	• Optimal pain management involves choosing medications with the least side effects including delirium risk • SAT protocolizes rapid deprescribing of medications that impair mobility and mind • Optimal sedation includes choosing medications with least delirium risk that enable timely extubation

Multicomplexity	Both SAT and SBT Choice of analgesia and sedation Exercise and early mobilization	• Extubation timing must balance resolution of the underlying condition against functional impact of ongoing intubation • Comorbidities (e.g., hepatic, renal, and cardiac function) impact selection of analgesia and sedation • Preexisting functional impairment (e.g., frailty, neurodegenerative disease) can make patients more vulnerable to functional loss while increasing skill and resources required to mobilize them
What Matters Most	Assess, treat and manage pain Both SAT and SBT Choice of analgesia and sedation Delirium prevention and management Exercise and early mobilization Family support	Common values/health priorities among older adults include: • Managing health and symptoms (including pain) • Quality of life (including minimizing exposure to burdensome treatments) • Functioning (including optimizing cognitive and physical health to maintain dignity and independence) • Enjoying life (including optimizing cognitive and physical health to participate in personally meaningful activities, including hobbies, community service, and personal growth and development) • Connecting (including giving and receiving support, spending quality time, and promoting family well-being)

activities that is more equitable than many other functional measures), and measures of social participation and connection [39,40,41,42,43]. Optimizing such outcomes increases well-being and mobility, even if gait speed and ADL independence remain poor.

Mind

In Age-Friendly Health Systems, "Mind" comprises cognition (e.g., dementia, sensory impairment, and delirium) and mental health (e.g., depression and anxiety). The throughline is that neuroplasticity continues across the lifespan. While critical illness is undoubtedly neurotoxic, so are environments of care delivery, alternately providing sensory overstimulation (e.g., intubation, Foley catheters, bed alarms, pain, and sleep deprivation) and understimulation (e.g., immobility, social isolation, and boredom; see Chapter 12 for additional information). Person-environment interaction is key, and care provision must attend to both.

As in mobility, this should start with prevention. Community-based screening could assess sensory needs, cognition, and mood and intervene to promote daily routines that include physical activity, cognitive stimulation, and healthy sleep-wake cycles. Increased difficulty managing routine tasks could prompt assessment for an acute condition or progression of a chronic condition. Such upstream practices could reduce the incidence of both critical illness and PICS. In the hospital, including the ICU, prevention of cognitive and mood impairment focuses on optimal management of the acute condition and management of delirium risk factors (see Chapters 8 and 12 for additional information). Again, quality delivery is required because older adults generally have high rates of ICU delirium [44], and those with preexisting cognitive and mood disorders at are the highest risk [45,46]. Systems-based preventive strategies include the ABCDEF bundle in ICUs (see Chapter 11 for additional information) and HELP, an evidence-based intervention that promotes basic daily routines and reduces the incidence of delirium by approximately 50% in hospitalized older adults outside of ICUs.

Even more than with mobility, rehabilitation strategies for mind should focus on screening and providing supportive and adaptive resources for identified needs. While delirium is most often transient, at least 10% of older patients remain delirious at the time of hospital discharge, and up to 70% have long-term cognitive changes as a consequence [47]. While those with preexisting cognitive and mood disorders are at higher risk of developing PICS [48], the incidence among older adults is high enough to warrant screening in all-comers. Mood disorders cannot be assessed until delirium has resolved, but it is useful to identify apathy symptoms that may impair the motivation to participate, not just in rehabilitation, but in meaningful activities more generally. Approximately 10–20% of older adults have visual and hearing impairment before critical illness [24]; given increasing data showing associations between cognition, mood, and sensory impairments, visual and hearing needs, which are modifiable, should be identified and managed aggressively.

Successful discharge planning emphasizes communication, family involvement with hands-on training, early follow-up appointments, post-discharge cognitive testing (see Chapter 43 for additional information), and identification of community resources to help patients and families adapt to ongoing cognitive needs [49,50]. Most older adults with PICS require a structured care approach with emphasis on caregiver support. Family caregivers are essential in restoring mentation by establishing a point of familiarity, thereby helping to reorient patients and engage them in cognitively stimulating activity; however, they require additional resources and aid. Community resources, including geriatric psychiatrists and adult day centers that provide behavioral activation and caregiver support, are typically limited. Again, SNF discharge portends a poor prognosis, with over one-third of older adult sepsis survivors discharged to a SNF experiencing severe or very severe cognitive impairment accompanied by high short-term mortality. When efforts to avoid SNF discharges fail, those caring for these patients should provide appropriate anticipatory guidance and ensure that care aligns with values and goals [37].

Lastly, physical and cognitive impairments can impact patients' mental health. Loss of mobility and cognition for older adults who were previously independent can result in stigma, feelings of hopelessness, social isolation, and depression, particularly in those with preexisting depression and those without a solid support system (see Chapter 46 for additional information). As described in Chapter 24, these challenges need to be addressed via anti-ableist strategies emphasizing social support: friends, family, peer support groups, churches, and other community-based supports.

Medications

Older adults have higher rates of adverse drug events, drug-drug interactions, and polypharmacy compared to younger individuals (see Table 50.2). Several general principles should guide prescribing: new medications should have an evidence-based indication; when multiple options are available, the one with the least risky side effect profile should be selected; and providers along the care continuum should collaborate in developing a culture of deprescribing medications without an ongoing indication, especially those likely to affect function, cognition, and gait (see Chapter 32 for additional information). The American Geriatrics Society (AGS) BEERS criteria [51] and the Screening Tool of Older People's Prescriptions (STOPP) criteria [52] are evidence-based guides to reduce potentially inappropriate medications for older adults, and the Screening Tool to Alert to Right Treatment (START) criteria [52] can improve medication selection. Although numerous medications are potentially harmful to older adults, Table 50.2 is adapted from BEERS and STOPP criteria and focuses on common medications with significant impact.

Polypharmacy is typically defined as the use of more than five medications. While polypharmacy is sometimes required in medically complex patients, it raises the risk of adverse health outcomes in older adults, including adverse drug reactions, falls, reduced functional impairment, and increased hospital admission and mortality rates [53,54]. Adverse drug reactions related to polypharmacy often are causal factors in hospital admission, especially for trauma. Further, patients on three or more classes of medications are at increased risk of delirium, which in turn increases the risk for developing PICS.

In hospital follow-up, the same principles outlined above apply. Primary care providers should not defer to hospital-based providers and should seek to deprescribe new medications without a clear ongoing indication. Systems for communicating with pharmacists or checking with hospital-based teams about these choices would be valuable and are one goal of post-ICU transitional care programs and follow-up clinics.

Multicomplexity

In the 5Ms framework, multicomplexity encompasses both health and social needs. Medical needs are conceptualized as multiple chronic conditions, including geriatric syndromes.

Table 50.2 Proposed medications to discontinue or use with caution as adapted from BEERS criteria and STOPP criteria

Therapeutic category, Drug class, Drug(s) example	Rationale	Recommendations
Antihistamines (first generation) - Diphenhydramine - Hydroxyzine - Meclizine - Promethazine	Anticholinergic; reduced clearance with age; high risk for confusion, constipation, dry mouth; increased risk of falls	Avoid
Aspirin	Should not be used for primary prevention due lack of evidence supporting benefit and risk of major bleeding in older adults	Avoid initiating for primary prevention of cardiovascular disease. Consider deprescribing if the patient has no history of cardiovascular disease.
Atenolol	Should not be used as first-line agent to treat hypertension Increased risk of mortality Requires dose adjustment in renal impairment	Avoid Consider switching to alternative antihypertensive
Warfarin	High risk of major bleeding when compared with DOACs for treatment of nonvalvular atrial fibrillation and VTE	Avoid using warfarin as initial therapy for the treatment of nonvalvular atrial fibrillation or VTE. Consider switching to a DOAC medication unless contraindication or if patient has been on warfarin for a long period with well-controlled INR without adverse events.
Nonselective α1 blocker - Doxazosin - Prazosin - Terazosin	High risk of orthostatic hypotension	Avoid use in treatment for hypertension

Medication	Concerns	Recommendation
Clonidine	High risk for central nervous system effects, including hallucinations; risk for bradycardia, orthostatic hypotension, syncope	Avoid use in treatment for hypertension
Nifedipine	Hypotension, constipation, myocardial infarction	Avoid
Amiodarone	Multiple toxicities when used short-term and long-term	Avoid as first-line therapy for atrial fibrillation unless patient has heart failure or left ventricular hypertrophy. Consider switching to alternative rate/rhythm control medication once patient has left ICU.
Digoxin	Safer alternatives available, increased risk of toxicity with decreased renal clearance	Avoid as first-line treatment for atrial fibrillation or heart failure. Avoid dosages >0.125mg/day
Anticholinergics - Oxybutynin - Benztropine - Trihexyphenidyl - Prochlorperazine - Scopolamine - Atropine - Tricyclic antidepressants - Paroxetine - Olanzapine - Cyclobenzaprine (There are many other medications that have anticholinergic properties)	Increased risk for cognitive decline, delirium, dry mouth, blurry vison, constipation, urinary retention, falls, impaired psychomotor function	Avoid unless safer alternatives are unavailable. Use for the shortest duration possible

Table 50.2 (cont.)

Therapeutic category, Drug class, Drug(s) example	Rationale	Recommendations
Benzodiazepines - Alprazolam - Clonazepam - Diazepam - Lorazepam	Puts patients at risk for physical dependency, abuse, and misuse. Older adults have increased sensitivity and decreased metabolism Risk of cognitive impairment, delirium, falls, fractures, and motor vehicle collisions.	Avoid Consider taper to discontinuation May be appropriate for alcohol withdrawal, benzodiazepine withdrawal, and severe generalized anxiety disorder.
Non-benzodiazepine benzodiazepine receptor agonist hypnotics ("Z"-drugs) - Zolpidem - Zaleplon	Similar adverse events to benzodiazepines with minimal improvement in symptom control	Avoid
Antipsychotics (first and second generation) - Haloperidol - Quetiapine - Olanzapine - Risperidone	Increased risk of falls, delirium, parkinsonism, sedation, stroke. Greater risk of cognitive decline and mortality in people with dementia	Avoid use for behavior problems of dementia or delirium unless nonpharmacological interventions have been unsuccessful and/or the patient is deemed a threat to themselves or others. Deprescribing attempts should be made periodically or reduction to the lowest effective dose.
Sulfonylureas - Glipizide - Glimepiride	More hypoglycemia than alternative agents Increased risk of all-cause mortality and cardiovascular events	Avoid as first- and second-line therapy.
Proton Pump Inhibitors - Omeprazole - Pantoprazole	Increased risk of bone loss, fractures, *C. difficile*, and pneumonia	Avoid scheduled use for more than 8 weeks unless clinically indicted.

DOAC: direct-acting oral anticoagulants; VTE: venous thromboembolism; INR: international normalized ratio

Evidence increasingly shows that survivors of critical illness not only frequently develop functional impairments but also experience general loss of physiological reserve and heightened risk of developing new chronic conditions (see Chapter 33 for additional information). The American Geriatrics Society has published guidelines for care planning for patients with multiple chronic conditions that are relevant to post-ICU needs [55]. "What Matters Most" below applies their principles and action steps.

Geriatric syndromes are "clinical conditions in older persons that do not fit into disease categories but are highly prevalent in old age, multifactorial, associated with multiple co-morbidities and poor outcomes, and are only treatable when a multidimensional approach is used" [56]. The importance of geriatric syndromes in PICS is underscored by dedicated chapters on frailty (see Chapter 5 for additional information), dysphagia (see Chapter 38 for additional information), and delirium (see Chapter 8 for additional information), as well as the discussion of falls, depression, and dementia above.

Addressing social complexity starts with screening, including: functional history (especially ADLs, instrumental activities of daily living [IADLs], changes in driving status, use of assistive devices, cognitive changes, and lifespace); living environment (especially the number of steps to enter the home, the number of steps to the bathroom and laundry area, and bathroom modifications); social support (in-home or nearby care partner(s), hours of availability, frequency and types of other social contacts, and safety of social contacts); substance use (alcohol, tobacco, and cannabis, among others); and finances (employment status, Medicaid eligibility, and food, utility, or transportation insecurity). Given the extensive skilled assessments needed, care teams optimally include case managers or social workers through home health, insurance plans, or ICU follow-up clinics (see Chapter 25 for additional information).

Care planning should integrate the results of identified health and social needs. Care plans could be an even more powerful tool when three conditions are met: physicians consistently participate (e.g., as in hospice programs); care plans "belong" to patients and families, centering their engagement; and care plans are readily accessible and editable everywhere people receive healthcare. Doing so could reduce challenges of siloed care by providing an active and archived problem list, with details of evaluation, treatment, accountable care provider(s), and follow-up plans that could be updated as people transition across sites of care [57].

What Matters Most

What Matters Most should be the overarching driver of care delivery; clinicians who master the 5Ms use What Matters Most to organize care plans related to Mobility, Mind, Medications, and Multicomplexity.

Clinicians should determine patients' health priorities and take concrete steps to align care accordingly [55,58]. First, clarify the patient's top priority – whether it's a symptom, functional issue, healthcare task, or medication hindering their health goals [59]. Next, assess the conditions, symptoms, treatments, and life circumstances contributing to that issue. Then, evaluate which interventions and support services are most likely to help. Finally, clinicians can select two or three feasible interventions acceptable to the patient and their family. By focusing on culturally embedded priorities, clinicians provide care that respects patients' values, reduces self-stigma, and avoids imposing unnecessary interventions. Clinicians should use "need" carefully to avoid overshadowing patients' values and preferences with a focus on technical, life-sustaining therapy [60].

This holistic practice goes beyond the narrower notions of advance care planning or establishing goals of care. It requires curiosity and appreciation of the whole range of perspectives, experiences, and cultures encountered in practice. Clinicians often struggle to hear any but the most common values and to design care plans that do not readily align with standard payment models and referral mechanisms [61]. Patient-and-family centeredness requires a more expansive practice of listening for a wide range of values and tailoring treatments to those values in the context of available resources.

PatientPrioritiesCare.org offers training and tools to help identify patients' health priorities and align care with them [58,62,63,64]. These tools emphasize: identifying and communicating patients' health priorities and health trajectory; using them to weigh priorities, harms, burdens, and benefits of stopping, starting, or continuing care; and using them to align decisions and care among patients, caregivers, and other clinicians.

Given that adoption of advance care planning remains poor, and ICU clinicians have difficulty applying them even when available, Age-Friendly strategies may ultimately be more feasible, acceptable, and easier to disseminate widely into practice. Since no specific medical therapies are available for PICS, doing so may also help broaden clinicians' intervention strategies to include rehabilitative, palliative, and behavioral strategies that address function and the symptoms that have a large impact on well-being and quality of life. There is a need to innovate ways of rapidly communicating care plans organized around What Matters Most across transitions of care so that providers at each point along the trajectory do not need to reinvent the wheel.

Conclusion

Unless and until we have medications capable of regenerating damaged tissue, functional impairment will be a natural consequence of surviving previously fatal critical illnesses. That puts an onus on the healthcare system to reorganize to help people adapt to acquired functional impairment. Effective prevention and management of PICS in older adults involves implementation of the 5Ms principles of Age-Friendly Healthcare: Mobility, Mind, Medications, Multicomplexity, and What Matters Most.

Leaders at the American Thoracic Society and the Society of Critical Care Medicine have advanced an agenda for integrating principles of geriatric medicine into critical care [65]. This chapter attempted to show how 5Ms care aligns with the goals of both the ABCDEF bundle and ICU follow-up clinics [66]. It also showed opportunities for collaboration with interprofessional teams in the hospital and community to apply those principles across the entire critical illness continuum. Partnership with the Age-Friendly movement provides a vision for how to do that at scale.

Health services researchers focused on aging have a strong track record of innovating efficacious, cost-effective, scalable interventions addressing 5Ms needs (e.g., HELP, the Program for All-Inclusive Care for the Elderly, and the Transitional Care Model) [13,67,68]. Unfortunately, implementation of such programs remains limited. Under-implementation reflects the challenges of organizational change and aligning policy support with priorities. The post-ICU community could be excellent allies and advocates for this work. The post-ICU community can also support the development of Age-Friendly Communities, which provide infrastructure and resources capable of addressing physical, cognitive, psychological, and social needs that arise across the critical care continuum. Doing so could address the lived experiences of people who develop serious illness-related disability at all ages.

Key Points

1. The Age-Friendly Movement ties together Age-Friendly Health Systems, Age-Friendly Communities, and Age-Friendly Public Health to support intergenerational population health. Each of these focuses on different aspects of aging – from delivering quality care in hospitals and clinics to encouraging community engagement and optimizing public health approaches.
2. The 5Ms of Age-Friendly Healthcare (Mobility, Mind, Medications, Multicomplexity, and What Matters Most) are the guiding principles for providing evidence-based care to older adults. These elements are interconnected and must be applied together, particularly when managing post-intensive care syndrome (PICS).
3. The goals of the Age-Friendly Movement are directly in sync with the needs of older adults recovering from critical illness. The substantial overlap between the 5Ms and the core features of PICS makes this framework highly relevant and efficient for improving outcomes.
4. Interpreting evidence for older adults with PICS requires acknowledging the role of ageism and ableism. These biases, tied to age and disability, need to be addressed to ensure fair and effective care delivery.
5. Linking Age-Friendly Healthcare, Age-Friendly Communities, and Age-Friendly Public Health can create a comprehensive system that supports older adults after critical illness. This approach highlights the power and importance of working across systems to improve outcomes.

References

1. A. De Biasi, M. Wolfe, J. Carmody, et. al. Creating an age-friendly public health system. *Innov Aging* 2020; **4**(1): igz044.
2. D.V. Jeste, D.G. Blazer, K.C. Buckwalter, et al. Age-friendly communities initiative: public health approach to promoting successful aging. *Am J Geriatr Psychiatry* 2016; **24**: 1158–70.
3. A. Atramont, V. Lindecker-Cournil, J. Rudant, et al. Association of age with short-term and long-term mortality among patients discharged from intensive care units in France. *JAMA Netw Open* 2019; **2**: e1915529.
4. I. Mouchaers, H. Verbeek, G.I.J.M. Kempen, et al. The concept of disability and its causal mechanisms in older people over time from a theoretical perspective: a literature review. *Eur J Ageing* 2022; **19**: 397–411.
5. M. Herridge, A.M. Cheung, C.M. Tansey, et al. One-year outcomes in survivors of the acute respiratory distress syndrome. *N Engl J Med* 2011; **348**: 683–93.
6. M.S. Herridge, C.M. Tansey, A. Matte, et al. Functional disability 5 years after acute respiratory distress syndrome. *N Engl J Med* 2011; **364**: 1293–304.
7. P.P. Pandharipande, T.D. Girard, J.C. Jackson, et al. Long-term cognitive impairment after critical illness. *N Engl J Med* 2013; **369**: 1306–16.
8. J.C. Jackson, P.P. Pandharipande, T.D. Girard, et al. Depression, post-traumatic stress disorder, and functional disability in survivors of critical illness in the BRAIN-ICU study: a longitudinal cohort study. *Lancet Respir Med* 2014; **2**: 369–79.
9. L.P. Scheunemann, T.D. Girard, N.E. Leland. Epidemiological conceptual models and health justice for critically ill older adults. *Crit Care Med* 2021; **49**: 375–9.
10. C.L. Sprung, A. Artigas, J. Kesecioglu, et al. The Eldicus prospective, observational

study of triage decision making in European intensive care units. Part II: intensive care benefit for the elderly. *Intensive Care Med* 2012; **40**: 132–8.

11. T.W. Evans, S. Nava, G. Vazquez Mata, et al. Critical care rationing: international comparisons. *Chest* 2011; **140**: 1618–24.

12. L.P. Scheunemann, T.D. Girard, E.R. Skidmore, N.M. Resnick. The Hospital Elder Life Program: past and future. *Am J Geriatr Psychiatry* 2018; **26**: 1034–5.

13. J. Yue, P. Tabloski, S.L. Dowal, et al. The National Institute for Health and Clinical Excellence (NICE) to Hospital Elder Life Program (HELP): operationalizing NICE guidelines to improve clinical practice. *J Am Geriatr Soc* 2014; **62**: 754–61.

14. M. Oliver. The social model of disability: Thirty years on. *Disabil Soc* 2013; **28**: 1024–6.

15. J.M. Levitt. Exploring how the social model of disability can be re-invigorated: in response to Mike Oliver. *Disabil Soc* 2017; **32**: 589–94.

16. D.J. Lundberg, J.A. Chen. Structural ableism in public health and healthcare: a definition and conceptual framework. *Lancet Reg Health Am* 2023; **30**: 100650.

17. A.H. Maslow. A theory of human motivation. *Psychol Rev* 1943; **50**: 370–96.

18. S.B. Kaufman. *Transcend: the new science of self-actualization*. New York: Tarcher Perigree; 2020.

19. J. Herman. *Trauma and recovery: the aftermath of violence – from domestic abuse to political terror*. 4th ed. New York: Basic Books, Hachette Book Group; 2022.

20. J.C. Jackson, M.J. Santoro, T.M. Ely, et al. Improving patient care through the prism of psychology: application of Maslow's hierarchy to sedation, delirium, and early mobility in the intensive care unit. *J Crit Care* 2014; **29**: 438–44.

21. L.V. Karnatovskaia, O. Gajic, O.J. Bienvenu, et al. A holistic approach to the critically ill and Maslow's hierarchy. *J Crit Care* 2015; **30**: 210–11.

22. L. Scheunemann, J.S. White, S. Prinjha, et al. Barriers and facilitators to resuming meaningful daily activities among critical illness survivors in the UK: a qualitative content analysis. *BMJ Open* 2022; **12**: e057876.

23. M. Law, B. Cooper, S. Strong, et al. The Person-Environment-Occupation Model: a transactive approach to occupational performance. *Can J Occup Ther* 1996; **63**: 9–23.

24. T.J. Iwashyna, G. Netzer, K.M. Langa, C. Cigolle. Spurious inferences about long-term outcomes: the case of severe sepsis and geriatric conditions. *Am J Respir Crit Care Med* 2012; **185**: 835–41.

25. L.E. Ferrante, M.A. Pisani, T.E. Murphy, et al. Functional trajectories among older persons before and after critical illness. *JAMA Intern Med* 2015; **175**: 523–9.

26. L.B. Brunker, C.S. Boncyk, K.F. Rengel, C.G. Hughes. Elderly patients and management in intensive care units (ICU): clinical challenges. *Clin Interv Aging* 2023; **18**: 93–112.

27. M. Green, V. Marzano, I.A. Leditschke, et al. Mobilization of intensive care patients: a multidisciplinary practical guide for clinicians. *J Multidiscip Healthc* 2016; **9**: 247–56.

28. R. Dubb, P. Nydahl, C. Hermes, et al. Barriers and strategies for early mobilization of patients in intensive care units. *Ann Am Thorac Soc* 2016; **13**: 724–30.

29. M. Balas, R. Buckingham, T. Braley, et al. Extending the ABCDE bundle to the post-intensive care unit setting. *J Gerontol Nurs* 2013; **39**: 39–51.

30. J. Cussen, S. Mukpradab, G. Tobiano, et al. Early mobility and family partnerships in the intensive care unit: a scoping review of reviews. *Nurs Crit Care* 2024; **29**: 597–613.

31. M.E. Major, R. Kwakman, M.E. Kho, et al. Surviving critical illness: what is next? An expert consensus statement on physical rehabilitation after hospital discharge. *Crit Care* 2016; **20**: 354.

32. B. Connolly, A. Douiri, J. Steier, et al. A UK survey of rehabilitation following critical illness: implementation of NICE Clinical

Guidance 83 (CG83) following hospital discharge. *BMJ Open* 2014; 4: e004905.

33. National Institute for Health and Care Excellence. Rehabilitation after critical illness in adults: clinical guidelines. London, UK: National Institute for Health and Care Excellence. 2009. www.nice.org.uk/guidance/qs158. (Accessed September 12, 2024).

34. J.R. Falvey, T.E. Murphy, T.M. Gill, et al. Home health rehabilitation utilization among Medicare beneficiaries following critical illness. *J Am Geriatr Soc* 2020; 68: 1512–19.

35. B. Riegel, L. Huang, M.E. Mikkelsen, et al. Early post-intensive care syndrome among older adult sepsis survivors receiving home care. *J Am Geriatr Soc* 2019; 67: 520–6.

36. S. Parry, L. Denehy, C. Granger, et al. The fear and risk of community falls in patients following an intensive care admission: an exploratory cohort study. *Aust Crit Care* 2020; 33: 144–50.

37. W.J. Ehlenbach, A. Gilmore-Bykovskyi, M.D. Repplinger, et al. Sepsis survivors admitted to skilled nursing facilities: cognitive impairment, activities of daily living dependence, and survival. *Crit Care Med* 2018; 46: 37–44.

38. H.C. Prescott, K.M. Langa, V. Liu, et al. Increased 1-year healthcare use in survivors of severe sepsis. *Am J Respir Crit Care Med* 2014; 190: 62–9.

39. P.S. Baker, E.V. Bodner, R.M. Allman. Measuring life-space mobility in community-dwelling older adults. *J Am Geriatr Soc* 2003; 51: 1610–4.

40. C. König, B. Matt, A. Kortgen, et al. What matters most to sepsis survivors: a qualitative analysis to identify specific health-related quality of life domains. *Qual Life Res* 2018; 28: 637–47.

41. A.E. Turnbull, A. Rabiee, W.E. Davies, et al. Outcome measurement in ICU survivorship research from 1970–2013: a scoping review of 425 publications. *Crit Care Med* 2016; 44: 1267–77.

42. J. Kersey, L. Terhorst, J. Hammel, et al. Detecting change in community participation with the Enfranchisement scale of the community participation indicators. *Clin Rehabil* 2022; 36: 251–62.

43. E.A. Hahn, J.L. Beaumont, P.A. Pilkonis, et al. The PROMIS satisfaction with social participation measures demonstrated responsiveness in diverse clinical populations. *J Clin Epidemiol* 2016; 73: 135–41.

44. S.K. Inouye, R.G.J. Westendorp, J.S. Saczynski. Delirium in elderly people. *Lancet* 2014; 383: 911–22.

45. E.R. Marcantonio. Delirium in hospitalized older adults. *N Engl J Med* 2017; 377: 1456–66.

46. J.L. Stollings, K. Kotfis, G. Chanques, et al. Delirium in critical illness: clinical manifestations, outcomes, and management. *Intensive Care Med* 2021; 47: 1089–103.

47. M.G. Cole, A. Ciampi, E. Belzile, L. Zhong. Persistent delirium in older hospital patients: a systematic review of frequency and prognosis. *Age Ageing* 2009; 38: 19–26.

48. S.L. Hiser, A. Fatima, M. Ali, D.M. Needham. Post-intensive care syndrome (PICS): recent updates. *J Intensive Care* 2023; 11: 30.

49. G. Epstein-Lubow, A.T. Fulton, L.J. Marino, J. Teno. Hospice referral after inpatient psychiatric treatment of individuals with advanced dementia from a nursing home. *Am J Hosp Palliat Med* 2015; 32: 437–9.

50. S.M. Brown, S. Bose, V. Banner-Goodspeed, et al. Approaches to addressing post-intensive care syndrome among intensive care unit survivors: a narrative review. *Ann Am Thorac Soc* 2019; 16: 947–56.

51. American Geriatrics Society. 2023 updated AGS Beers Criteria® for potentially inappropriate medication use in older adults. *J Am Geriatr Soc* 2023; 71: 2052–81.

52. D. O'Mahony, D. O'Sullivan, S. Byrne, et al. STOPP/START criteria for potentially inappropriate prescribing in older people: version 2. *Age Ageing* 2015; 44: 213–8.

53. M. Gutiérrez-Valencia, M. Izquierdo, M. Cesari, et al. The relationship between frailty and polypharmacy in older people: a systematic review. *Br J Clin Pharmacol* 2018; **84**: 1432–44.
54. J.W. Wastesson, L. Morin, E.C.K. Tan, K. Johnell. An update on the clinical consequences of polypharmacy in older adults: a narrative review. *Expert Opin Drug Saf* 2018; **17**: 1185–96.
55. C. Boyd, C.D. Smith, F.A. Masoudi, et al. Decision making for older adults with multiple chronic conditions: executive summary for the American Geriatrics Society guiding principles on the care of older adults with multimorbidity. *J Am Geriatr Soc* 2019; **67**: 665–73.
56. A.J. Cruz-Jentoft, J.P. Baeyens, J.M. Bauer, et al. Sarcopenia: European consensus on definition and diagnosis. *Age Ageing* 2010; **39**: 412–23.
57. K.E. Hauschildt, R.K. Hechtman, H.C. Prescott, T.J. Iwashyna. Hospital discharge summaries are insufficient following ICU stays: a qualitative study. *Crit Care Explor* 2022; **4**: e0715.
58. M. Tinetti, A. Naik. Patient Priorities Care. 2018. https://patientprioritiescare.org/. (Accessed August 5, 2024).
59. A.D. Naik, L.N. Dindo, J.R. Van Liew, et al. Development of a clinically feasible process for identifying individual health priorities. *J Am Geriatr Soc* 2018; **66**: 1872–9.
60. J.M. Kruser, J.T. Clapp, R.M. Arnold. Reconsidering the language of serious illness. *JAMA* 2023; **330**: 587–8.
61. K.E. Hauschildt. Whose good death? Valuation and standardization as mechanisms of inequality in hospitals. *J Health Soc Behav* 2024; **65**: 221–36.
62. C.J. Gettel, A.K. Venkatesh, H. Dowd, et al. A qualitative study of "what matters" to older adults in the emergency department. *West J Emerg Med* 2022; **23**: 579–88.
63. M.E. Tinetti, D.M. Costello, A.D. Naik, et al. Outcome goals and health care preferences of older adults with multiple chronic conditions. *JAMA Netw Open* 2021; **4**(3): e211271.
64. M.E. Tinetti, A. Hashmi, H. Ng, et al. Patient priorities-aligned care for older adults with multiple conditions: a nonrandomized controlled trial. *JAMA Netw Open* 2024; **7**(1): e2352666.
65. N.E. Brummel, L.E. Ferrante. Integrating geriatric principles into critical care medicine: the time is now. *Ann Am Thorac Soc* 2018; **15**: 518–22.
66. B.T. Pun, M.C. Balas, M.A. Barnes-Daly, et al. Caring for critically ill patients with the ABCDEF bundle: results of the ICU Liberation Collaborative in over 15,000 adults. *Crit Care Med* 2019; **47**: 3–14.
67. M.D. Naylor, J.A. Sochalski. Scaling up: bringing the transitional care model into the mainstream. *Issue Brief (Commonw Fund)* 2010; **103**: 1–12.
68. V. Hirth, J. Baskins, M. Dever-Bumba. Program of All-Inclusive Care (PACE): past, present, and future. *J Am Med Dir Assoc* 2009; **10**: 155–60.

Chapter 51

PICS in Survivors of Cardiac Arrest

George E. Sayde and Sachin Agarwal

Introduction

In the United States, nearly 1,000 adults experience a sudden, out-of-hospital cardiac arrest (OHCA) each day, and an additional 500 patients suffer an in-hospital cardiac arrest (IHCA) due to various medical conditions [1,2]. Cardiac arrest (CA) is a life-threatening medical emergency that occurs when the heart suddenly stops beating, leading to the cessation of blood flow to the brain and other vital organs; causes include myocardial infarction, cardiac dysrhythmias, or other conditions affecting the heart's electrical system [3,4]. Over 10% of all OHCA patients (approximately 20,000 per year) and roughly 25% of all IHCA patients (approximately 50,000 per year) survive [5,6,7], largely due to effective public health campaigns for cardiopulmonary resuscitation [2,8], presence and use of defibrillators [9,10,11], and advances in bundled post-arrest intensive care [12,13,14,15,16,17] that are based on the American Heart Association's (AHA) original five links of the *Chain of Survival* [1,2]. Given the increasing number of survivors of CA, strategies must be identified to ensure that patients live longer, healthier, disability-free lives. National [5,18] and international [19] scientific bodies have issued scientific statements declaring that CA survivors have "unique and complex needs that are inadequately addressed by current treatment recommendations" [5], serving as a call to action for clinicians and researchers to address major knowledge gaps surrounding the critical "sixth link" of survivorship, the recovery phase after CA.

The Unique Experience of Cardiac Arrest Survivorship and Recovery

Unlike a myocardial infarction or cerebrovascular accident, CA results in near-instantaneous loss of consciousness, as blood flow to the brain ceases when the heart stops beating. Patients who regain consciousness typically awaken in an intensive care unit (ICU), are often receiving sedating medications, and have an average hospital length of stay of three weeks [20]. During this time, CA survivors who are no longer comatose must face the profound reality of having been "clinically dead" and subsequently revived [21].

Close family members often find themselves in the role of emergency responders, as 80% of all CA occur at home. Many family members witness the event, call 911, or provide initial cardiopulmonary resuscitation, and many must subsequently assume the roles of surrogate decision-maker during hospitalization and caregiver after hospital discharge [22]. These daunting responsibilities are thrust upon them with little to no preparation, making the experience both traumatic and life-altering [23,24]. Prognostic uncertainty extends beyond mere survival; it continues throughout the recovery process as survivors and their loved ones grapple with the fear of recurrent cardiac events and uncertainty regarding the degree of neurological recovery and the potential for significant impairments in functional status. This ambiguity can disrupt the survivor's sense of self-identity, lead to emotional instability, and strain familial relationships [25,26,27].

The recovery period following CA is marked by significant existential threat. Survivors and their families often experience feelings of insecurity and vulnerability, a need for support, and a reevaluation of life priorities. Themes of seeking explanations for why the event happened to them and a longing to regain a sense of normalcy frequently emerge within this population [28,29]. To address these challenges, there is a critical need for well-studied, interdisciplinary interventions aimed at improving outcomes and enhancing quality of life.

Studies Clarifying Long-Term Recovery Trajectories After Cardiac Arrest Are Needed

The extent and severity of impairments across multiple domains of health, including physical, cognitive, psychological, and social, that survivors of CA face and the risk factors [30] for their development remain unclear and are under active investigation [31]. Almost half of CA survivors have persistently poor functional outcomes [6,32,33,34,35,36], which result in impaired participation in social and leisure activities, an inability to return to work, and strained family relationships [35,37,38,39]. In a heterogeneous condition like CA, understanding why some patients experience a steady and meaningful recovery while others plateau or regress will inform future CA intervention trial designs, assist patients and families in planning transitions of care, and allow for personalized therapies and treatment plans. Currently, referrals to acute rehabilitation facilities after hospital discharge are not routine, in part because the clinical evidence regarding recovery trajectories of survivors of CA is insufficiently robust to determine the impact of intensive rehabilitation programs.

A larger evidence base exists regarding risk factors for survival, including demographics (e.g., age), CA-related characteristics (e.g., initial heart rhythm, duration of low-flow and no-flow time, and medications provided), and early interventions (e.g., targeted temperature management and cardiac revascularization) [13,40,41,42,43,44]. Less is understood regarding the range of long-term difficulties, including the physical, cognitive, psychological, interpersonal, and existential challenges, that patients encounter in the months to years following their CA. Interestingly, post-discharge factors, such as the presence of psychological distress and the degree of social support, along with other social determinants of health (SDOH; see Chapter 25 for additional information), may be more predictive of physical and mental health recovery than peri-arrest factors [34,45,46].

Prior research has identified sex and racial/ethnic disparities in the incidence of CA, receipt of guideline-concordant treatments [47], and rates of survival [47,48,49,50,51,52,53,54,55,56] but a significant knowledge gap remains regarding the impact of sex and racial/ethnic disparities in long-term outcomes after CA. The current literature suggests that females have worse functional, cognitive, and psychological status at the time of hospital discharge following CA [57] and may receive less rehabilitation compared with males [58]. Understanding which SDOH contribute to these discrepancies is critical for reducing disparities in outcomes. Limited data on other cardiac and general critical illnesses indicate that Black and Hispanic survivors are at higher risk of poor functional outcomes, including worse health-related quality of life (HRQoL) and impaired societal participation, compared with White patients

[59,60,61,62,63,64]. No national CA trials or registry data on SDOH exist at this time, so using this data for enhanced risk stratification and intervention work is challenging.

Understanding the Role of Psychological Distress Is a Crucial Step to Ensure Recovery

Nearly one-third of survivors of CA screen positive for post-traumatic stress disorder (PTSD) at both 1 month and 12 months after CA [20,65,66], a rate that is approximately 2.5–3 times greater than for other acute cardiovascular conditions (e.g., a PTSD prevalence of 11–15% in survivors of acute coronary syndrome or stroke) [67,68,69,70,71]. Similarly, depression and generalized anxiety disorders are common among survivors of CA, ranging from 14% to 45% [57,72,73,74,75,76,77]. This constellation of symptoms of PTSD and anxiety/stressor-related disorders, particularly hyperarousal [78], is associated with an increased risk of death and cardiovascular events during the first year of recovery [79]. Among general populations of survivors of critical illness, early symptoms of anxiety and depression experienced during critical illness increase the odds of future distress and poor perception of their functional recovery after discharge [80]. Irrespective of objectively measured physical and cognitive deficits, the presence of CA-induced psychological distress both at hospital discharge and at six months following discharge is a strong, independent risk factor for the survivor's perception of nonrecovery [81,82].

Given the lack of memory around CA events, it is unclear how certain hallmark reexperiencing symptoms of PTSD, such as flashbacks and intrusive memories, manifest in CA survivors. It may be that PTSD symptoms are not anchored on a discrete traumatic event per se, but rather manifest through daily somatic reminders of patients' near-death experiences and mortality. Common physiological sensations, such as increased heart rate, shortness of breath, and chest or shoulder pain during exercise, can trigger heightened awareness of bodily sensations, leading to a chronic, maladaptive fear of recurrence [7].

Cardiac anxiety, characterized by an ongoing fear of and heightened vigilance for cardiac-related sensations, emerges as a distinct form of distress among CA survivors. This anxiety frequently results in unnecessary visits to emergency departments, excessive medical interventions, and a reluctance to engage in physical activities [7,83,84]. As a unique and enduring psychological challenge for this population [76], cardiac anxiety represents a potential target for future transdiagnostic interventions that could enhance the recovery experience in survivors of CA.

The integrity of the family unit is critical to patients' recovery following CA. Post-intensive care syndrome-family (PICS-F; see Chapter 48 for additional information) after CA is inversely correlated with patients' physical and cognitive recovery after discharge [85]. The prevalence of clinically significant PTSD is higher for family caregivers (35–50%) than for survivors of CA (30%) at hospital discharge [85,86,87], and additional prospective data found that 61% of family members reported experiencing depressive symptoms, with 29% meeting criteria for major depressive disorder, one month after the CA [88]. Qualitative research identifies emotional disturbances as a significant challenge for family members of survivors of CA, often rooted in feelings of helplessness in restoring normalcy for both themselves and their loved ones [22,87].

Moreover, a family's perception of inadequate social support during the patient's hospitalization is correlated with more severe depressive symptoms at one month of follow-up. Compared with sleep quality prior to the event, a significant deterioration in sleep quality in loved ones was present one month after the CA, with concomitant psychological distress closely linked to this decline [89]. PTSD symptoms in survivors of CA, and not physical or cognitive impairments, notably correlated with the psychological distress experienced by their families [90]. These results highlight the pressing need for dyadic interventions aimed at improving psychosocial outcomes for both survivors of CA and their families.

Cognitive Impairment Is Highly Prevalent and Impacts Reintegration into Societal Roles

Up to 43% of survivors of CA, including those with seemingly promising early neurological recovery, experience long-term cognitive impairment, with deficits spanning the cognitive domains of memory, attention, language, and executive functioning [91]. Cognitive impairment (compared to mild Alzheimer's or moderate traumatic brain injury) occurs in 25–60% of CA survivors [32,35,57,92,93,94,95] and often persists for months to years after hospital discharge [6,96,97,98]. There is a high prevalence of cognitive impairment within the first year, with the most prominent impairments in attention, immediate memory, and delayed memory [99,100,101]. Survivors of CA with cognitive dysfunction generally have worse HRQoL and social functioning, a lower likelihood of returning to work, and more psychological distress than those without cognitive dysfunction [6,37,93,100,102]. When controlling for symptoms of depression and fatigue, both cognitive impairment and PTSD symptoms, including intrusive thoughts and avoidance, are major barriers to societal reintegration following CA [30,37]. Aside from cognitive impairment, in the largest population-based cohort study, survivors of CA had significantly increased rates of common neurological conditions, including stroke, epilepsy, Parkinson's disease, and dementia, particularly within the first year after discharge [103].

Cardiac Arrest Survivors with Disorders of Consciousness Are a Critical But Neglected Subgroup

Withdrawal of life-sustaining treatments for survivors of CA with disorders of consciousness (DoC), defined as persistent unresponsiveness and/or an inability to follow commands (typically resulting from anoxic brain injury following CA), within a few days of hospital admission is widespread [104,105], and it is estimated to be responsible for as many as 20,000 additional CA-related deaths per year [106]. This is due in part to limited data on long-term outcomes in patients with DoC and the common belief among clinicians that these patients are largely incapable of long-term improvement. Recent data has shown that up to 20% of patients discharged from the hospital after CA have a severe functional disability, and of those, 23% cannot follow commands at discharge [107]. Recovery of consciousness in up to 20% of survivors of CA discharged to inpatient acute rehabilitation facilities while still unconscious has been reported [107]. Nearly half (41%) of those who regained consciousness after discharge also experienced meaningful functional improvements that were not yet apparent at 3 months [108].

Targeted Interventions Along the Continuum of Cardiac Arrest-Related Critical Illness and Recovery Are Warranted

Fear- and cardiac anxiety-alleviating interventions aiming to reduce autonomic hyperactivity and to improve adherence to health behaviors, such as taking medications as prescribed, engaging in physical activity, and receiving adequate sleep, may lead to a reduced risk of cardiovascular disease. Cognitive behavioral therapy and interoceptive exposure interventions appear highly effective at improving the severity of cardiac anxiety [109]. Further, distress related to existential concerns and fear of future cardiac events also warrants unique treatment modalities, such as mindfulness, exposure-based interventions, and meaning-centered psychotherapy [110].

The identification of fear-based distress that reverberates between survivors of CA and their family members has led to novel treatments aimed at mitigating distress between dyads. Emerging research is actively investigating whether the treatment of distress in patients' family members, in turn, alleviates distress in the patients themselves [111]. The reduction of fear-based distress after CA may potentially improve the survivor's cardiovascular prognosis [20]; thus, building theory-based dyadic treatments that can be implemented to support family members of survivors of CA has the potential to be a powerful intervention.

In addition to interventions that target negative affect, therapies that bolster factors supportive of positive psychological well-being, such as optimism, positive affect, and purpose in life, should be studied in this patient population [112]. This may lead to the phenomenon of post-traumatic growth (see Chapter 46 for additional information), where psychological struggle following significant adversity leads to positive outcomes, such as the exploration of new possibilities, bolstering of personal strengths, and enhanced relationships [112]. Supporting positive psychological factors may negate some of the adverse effects of negative psychological factors and improve long-term recovery (e.g., reduced mortality and faster rate of return to normalcy) in non-cardiac arrest cohorts [7].

Most survivors feel ill-prepared for the multifaceted challenges of recovery, which is compounded by the lack of longitudinal, multidisciplinary follow-up services available to them. A recent systematic review found that survivors of CA improved over the course of an admission to an inpatient acute rehabilitation facility (medium-large effect size of 0.71) [113]. Following hospital discharge, cardiac rehabilitation programs are recommended for survivors of CA, along with patients enduring other types of cardiovascular disease (e.g., heart failure), due to their efficacy in improving both physical and psychological functioning [114,115]. In particular, the integration of psycho-education and addressing psychological distress into the traditional cardiac rehabilitation model appears to have promise in improving the quality of life of survivors of CA [66,116]. Incorporating this evidence into the development and structuring of ICU follow-up clinics is crucial. Table 51.1 and Table 51.2 highlight key existing studies and ongoing research, respectively, focused on understanding and improving survivorship outcomes for both CA survivors and their close family members.

Conclusion

The challenges faced by survivors of CA and their families following hospitalization are multifaceted, persistent, and under-recognized. Societal reintegration and healing from an existential threat are dynamic and nuanced processes. Certain psychological factors, such as cardiac-specific anxiety, are uniquely experienced by this population and mediate

Table 51.1 Completed studies to understand and enhance recovery in cardiac arrest survivors and their families

Authors	Purpose of Study	Study Design	Number of Subjects	Summary of Findings
Cowan et al. (2001) [117]	Assess the effect of psychosocial therapy on two-year cardiovascular mortality in OHCA survivors	Randomized controlled trial	129 survivors	Psychosocial intervention significantly reduced cardiovascular mortality in OHCA survivors over two years.
Moulaert et al. (2015) [118]	Evaluate the effectiveness of early neurologically focused follow-up in cardiac arrest survivors	Randomized controlled trial	185 survivors, 155 caregivers	Early neurologically focused follow-up in CA survivors improved their self-reported quality of life significantly over standard care.
Moulaert et al. (2016) [119]	Evaluate the cost-effectiveness of an early neurologically focused intervention for cardiac arrest survivors	Randomized controlled trial	136 survivors	Early neurologically focused intervention ("Stand still ... and move on") was cost-effective and improved long-term quality of life for CA survivors.
Mion et al. (2020) [120]	Implement the UK's first multidisciplinary follow-up program for OHCA survivors to support psychological and cognitive health.	Retrospective observational service evaluation study	21 survivors	Proof-of-concept, the UK's first multidisciplinary follow-up program for OHCA survivors.
Mion et al. (2021) [121]	Survey on experience of post-discharge care for survivors/family members and their recommended improvements.	Observational: Mixed-method survey-based	123 survivors; 39 family members	The majority of OHCA survivors and families advocated for an early follow-up following hospital discharge and a holistic, multidimensional assessment of arrest sequelae.
Presciutti et al. (2021) [122]	Assess associations between posttraumatic stress and quality of life in CA survivors and caregivers	Retrospective cohort study	169 survivors, 52 caregivers	Posttraumatic stress symptoms were common in survivors and caregivers and were linked to poorer quality of life outcomes.

Study	Objective	Design	Participants	Key Findings
Joshi et al. (2021) [113]	Assess feasibility and effects of residential rehabilitation for fatigue and secondary consequences in CA survivors	Prospective feasibility study	40 survivors	Feasible intervention with high satisfaction. Small to moderate effect size changes for self-reported fatigue, quality of life, anxiety, depression, function, and disability, and for two of the physical capacity tests. The recruitment process needs improvement.
Presciutti et al. (2023) [123]	Explore associations between protective positive psychology factors and emotional distress after CA.	Retrospective cohort study	110 survivors	Higher levels of mindfulness, existential well-being, resilient coping, and perceived social support were each associated with less emotional distress.
Wagner et al. (2024) [124]	Implement the first Danish multidisciplinary guideline-based follow-up program for OHCA survivors and their close family members	Retrospective observational service evaluation study	-	Proof-of-concept, the first guideline-driven, multidisciplinary follow-up program for OHCA survivors and close family members in Denmark.
Wagner et al. (2023) [125]	Explore associations between an early screening procedure and clinical symptoms of anxiety, depression, and PTSD in survivors and co-survivors	Prospective cohort study	297 survivors, 284 co-survivors	Early symptoms of anxiety, depression, and PTSD were associated with unfavorable mental health outcomes at follow-up in survivors. Cognitive impairment in survivors was associated with PTSD in co-survivors.
Bergman et al. (2023) [110]	Determine feasibility, safety, and efficacy of mindfulness-based exposure therapy for PTSD after CA	Open feasibility trial	11 survivors	Acceptance and Mindfulness-Based Exposure Therapy (AMBET) was found feasible and safe for PTSD management in CA survivors, with initial positive indications for efficacy.

Table 51.1 (cont.)

Authors	Purpose of Study	Study Design	Number of Subjects	Summary of Findings
Cornelius et al. (2023) [111]	Test feasibility of an ICU diary intervention targeted toward family member distress	Pilot randomized controlled trial	16 family members, randomized 2:1 to intervention or care as usual	ICU diary intervention was appropriate, feasible, and acceptable. Fear was non-significantly lower in intervention participants (versus control) at the end of hospital care and 30 days later.
Presciutti et al. (2023) [126]	Develop a mindfulness-based resiliency program for caregivers of patients with severe acute brain injury	Open feasibility trial	Mindfulness-Based Resiliency Program (COMA-F)	Intervention not specifically focused on relatives of CA survivors; however, the authors will be trialing it also on family members of patients following hypoxic-ischemic brain injury, therefore could be suitable for some family members of CA survivors.
Agarwal et al. (2024) [127]	Assess intervention preferences to reduce caregiver burden in racially diverse family members of CA survivors	Online survey-based study	550 respondents (close family members of survivors)	Caregiver burden was prevalent among family members, with a preference for interventions that provided more information and support.
Birk et al. (2024) [128]	Test the feasibility of a remote heart rate variability biofeedback (HRVB) intervention for reducing anxiety in CA survivors	Single-arm feasibility trial	10 (out of 12 eligible survivors)	The intervention was acceptable, feasible, and useable for CA with CA-related psychological distress.

Rojas et al. (2024) [90]	Investigate relationships between PICS-relevant domains in CA survivors and psychological distress in their family members	Prospective cohort study	74 dyads (74 survivors and 74 family members)	Both CA survivors and their family members showed substantial evidence of likely PICS. Survivor PTSS (post-traumatic stress disorder) is notably associated with family member distress.
Tincher et al. (2024) [89]	Assess associations of disrupted sleep with psychological distress in close family members of CA survivors	Prospective cohort study	102 close relatives of CA survivors	Significant decline in sleep health among close family members of CA survivors in the acute phase following the event. Psychological distress was associated with this sleep disruption.
Yuan et al. (2024) [90]	Assess associations between social support and psychological distress in family members of CA survivors	Prospective cohort study	102 close family members of CA survivors	Lower perceived social support in family members was linked to greater psychological distress one month after CA.

Table 51.2 Ongoing studies to understand and enhance recovery in cardiac arrest survivors and their families

Authors	Purpose of Study	Study Design	Number of Subjects	Summary of Findings
Agarwal et al. (ongoing)	Characterize psychological and behavioral dimensions of CA survivorship and their association with mortality, cardiovascular disease risk, and quality of life	Prospective cohort study	Target N= 246	To test the associations between negative affect, particularly cardiac anxiety and PTSD, on one-year cardiovascular prognosis and quality of life. To test the mediating role of health behaviors like physical activity and sleep in long-term cardiovascular prognosis.
Birk et al. (ongoing)	Test the association between psychological predictors and long-term recovery outcomes in OHCA survivors	Prospective cohort study	Target N= 228	To test whether positive psychological factors are associated with the measures of disability and quality of life. Test whether positive psychological factors have a potential protective effect on the adverse impact of negative affect on disability and quality of life.
Agarwal et al. (ongoing)	Patterns of Survivors' Recovery Trajectories in the ICECAP Trial (POST-ICECAP)	Prospective cohort study	Aiming to enrol n=1,000 subjects	Ongoing study aiming to describe recovery (functional outcome [primary], cognition, and HRQoL outcomes [secondary]) in a large, well-characterized, racially/ethnically diverse, representative cohort of US OHCA patients (at 6, 9, and 12 months after OHCA).
Mion et al. (2024 – ongoing)	Assess the efficacy of a virtual psychoeducational intervention for OHCA survivors and their families	Randomized controlled trial (sub-study of STEPCARE)	Aiming to recruit at least 25 patients in each arm	Intervention includes psychoeducation, information provision, peer support (in one arm), and a self-management recovery plan.

Study	Aim	Design	Sample	Intervention
Gamberini et al. (2024 – ongoing)	Assess the effect of an internet-based intervention on anxiety, depression, and cognitive impairment in OHCA survivors	Randomized controlled trial	Aiming to recruit 137 patients	Intervention includes information-based emotional support and education on cognitive problems, exercise, and diet. Interactive online physical/cognitive exercises.
Christensen et al. (2024–ongoing)	Evaluate the effectiveness of a multidisciplinary rehabilitation intervention on return to work in OHCA survivors	Randomized controlled trial	Aiming to recruit 137 patients	It is a rehabilitation-based intervention focusing on return to work.
The CARESS-f Study (2024–ongoing)	Develop and test the feasibility of a self-management support intervention for CA survivors and their key supporters	Feasibility study	Up to 25 survivors, 25 supporters	It is a community-based rehabilitation and self-management support intervention.
Agarwal et al. (2024– ongoing)	Evaluate a randomized pilot intervention to reduce uncertainty in surrogates after cardiac events (RESURFACE)	A pilot randomized controlled trial	38 survivors recruited	Feasibility, acceptability, and usability metrics for the web-based informational intervention.

downstream recovery, including the risk for further cardiovascular events. Protective factors, such as resilience, strong social support, and a sense of purpose in life also appear to enhance long-term outcomes. Interventions that target these distinct features of life after CA hold promising early evidence in enhancing physical, mental, and social health for the patient and family unit. It remains ever-important to identify specific clinical interventions that can be leveraged to optimize long-term recovery, quantify the change in patients' recovery trajectories, and identify key social factors that inhibit equitable access to optimal recovery after CA.

Key Points

1. Survival after OHCA and IHCA is increasing due to advances in critical care and effective public health campaigns.
2. Little is known regarding the long-term physical, cognitive, psychiatric, and social outcomes in survivors of CA.
3. The risk factors and mediators of recovery following CA, including societal reintegration, appear to be heavily weighted by psychological well-being.
4. Targeted interventions along the continuum of CA-related critical illness and recovery are much needed.

References

1. E.J. Benjamin, M.J. Blaha, S.E. Chiuve, et al. Heart disease and stroke statistics-2017 update: a report from the American Heart Association. *Circulation* 2017; **135**(10): e146–e603.
2. K. Vellano, Crouch MPH, Rajdev MBA, et al. Cardiac Arrest Registry to Enhance Survival (CARES) Report on the Public Health Burden of Out-of-Hospital Cardiac Arrest. https://mycares.net/sitepages/uploads/2024/2023_flipbook/index.html?page=1. (Accessed on December 5, 2024).
3. R. Deo, C.M. Albert. Epidemiology and genetics of sudden cardiac death. *Circulation* 2012; **125**(4): 620–37.
4. S.M. Al-Khatib, W.G. Stevenson, M.J. Ackerman, et al. 2017 AHA/ACC/HRS guideline for management of patients with ventricular arrhythmias and the prevention of sudden cardiac death: executive summary: a report of the American College of Cardiology/American Heart Association Task Force on Clinical Practice Guidelines and the Heart Rhythm Society. *Heart Rhythm* 2018; **15**(10): e190–e252.
5. K.N. Sawyer, T.R. Camp-Rogers, P. Kotini-Shah, et al. Sudden cardiac arrest survivorship: a scientific statement from the American Heart Association. *Circulation* 2020; **141**(12): e654–e685.
6. G.D. Perkins, C.W. Callaway, K. Haywood, et al. Brain injury after cardiac arrest. *Lancet* 2021; **398**: 1269–78.
7. S. Agarwal S, J.L. Birk, S.L. Abukhadra, et al. Psychological distress after sudden cardiac arrest and its impact on recovery. *Curr Cardiol Rep* 2022; **24**(10): 1351–60.
8. S. van Diepen, S. Girotra, B.S. Abella, et al. Multistate 5-year initiative to improve care for out-of-hospital cardiac arrest: primary results from the heartrescue project. *J Am Heart Assoc*. 2017; **6**(9): e005716.
9. T.J. Bunch, R.D. White, B.J. Gersh, et al. Long-term outcomes of out-of-hospital cardiac arrest after successful early defibrillation. *N Engl J Med* 2003; **348**(26): 2626–33.

10. J.E. Fugate, W. Brinjikji, J.N. Mandrekar, et al. Post-cardiac arrest mortality is declining: a study of the US National Inpatient Sample 2001 to 2009. *Circulation* 2012; **126**(5): 546–50.

11. R.J. Myerburg, J. Fenster, M. Velez, et al. Impact of community-wide police car deployment of automated external defibrillators on survival from out-of-hospital cardiac arrest. *Circulation* 2002; **106**(9): 1058–64.

12. S.A. Bernard, T.W. Gray, M.D. Buist, et al. Treatment of comatose survivors of out-of-hospital cardiac arrest with induced hypothermia. *N Engl J Med* 2002; **346**(8): 557–63.

13. C.W. Callaway, P.J. Coppler, J. Faro, et al. Association of initial illness severity and outcomes after cardiac arrest with targeted temperature management at 36 degrees C or 33 degrees C. *JAMA Netw Open* 2020; 3(7): e208215.

14. T. Cronberg, G. Lilja, M. Rundgren, et al. Long-term neurological outcome after cardiac arrest and therapeutic hypothermia. *Resuscitation* 2009; **80**(10): 1119–23.

15. Hypothermia after Cardiac Arrest Study Group. Mild therapeutic hypothermia to improve the neurologic outcome after cardiac arrest. *N Engl J Med* 2002; **346**(8): 549–56.

16. J. Elmer, J.C. Rittenberger, P.J. Coppler, et al. Long-term survival benefit from treatment at a specialty center after cardiac arrest. *Resuscitation* 2016; **108**: 48–53.

17. K. Sunde, M. Pytte, D. Jacobsen, et al. Implementation of a standardised treatment protocol for post resuscitation care after out-of-hospital cardiac arrest. *Resuscitation* 2007; 73(1): 29–39.

18. R.M. Merchant, A.A. Topjian, A.R. Panchal, et al. Part 1: executive summary: 2020 American Heart Association Guidelines for cardiopulmonary resuscitation and emergency cardiovascular care. *Circulation* 2020; 142(16 suppl 2): S337–S357.

19. J.P. Nolan, I. Maconochie, J. Soar, et al. Executive summary: 2020 international consensus on cardiopulmonary resuscitation and emergency cardiovascular care science with treatment recommendations. *Circulation*. 2020; 142 (16 suppl 1): S2–S27.

20. S. Agarwal, A. Presciutti, T. Cornelius, et al. Cardiac arrest and the subsequent hospitalization-induced posttraumatic stress is associated with 1-year risk of major adverse cardiovascular events and all-cause mortality. *Crit Care Med* 2019; 47(6): e502–505.

21. G.E. Sayde, P.A. Shapiro, I. Kronish, et al. A shift towards targeted post-ICU treatment: multidisciplinary care for cardiac arrest survivors. *J Crit Care* 2024; 82: 154798.

22. D.A. Rojas, C.E. DeForge, S.L. Abukhadra, et al. Family experiences and health outcomes following a loved ones' hospital discharge or death after cardiac arrest: a scoping review. *Resusc Plus* 2023; 14: 100370.

23. T. Ann-Britt, D. Ella, H. Johan, et al. Spouses' experiences of a cardiac arrest at home: an interview study. *Eur J Cardiovasc Nurs* 2010; 9(3): 161–7.

24. B. Grunau, K. Dainty, R. MacRedmond, et al. A qualitative exploratory case series of patient and family experiences with ECPR for out-of-hospital cardiac arrest. *Resusc Plus* 2021; 6: 100129.

25. A. Bremer, K. Dahlberg, L. Sandman. Experiencing out-of-hospital cardiac arrest: significant others' lifeworld perspective. *Qual Health Res* 2009; 19(10): 1407–20.

26. R. Case, D. Stub, E. Mazzagatti, et al. The second year of a second chance: long-term psychosocial outcomes of cardiac arrest survivors and their family. *Resuscitation* 2021; 167: 274–81.

27. L. Whitehead, S. Tierney, D. Biggerstaff, et al. Trapped in a disrupted normality: survivors' and partners' experiences of life after a sudden cardiac arrest. *Resuscitation* 2020; 147: 81–7.

28. A. Ketilsdottir, H.R. Albertsdottir, S.H. Akadottir, et al. The experience of sudden cardiac arrest: becoming

reawakened to life. *Eur J Cardiovasc Nurs* 2014; 13(5): 429–35.

29. A.S. Forslund, K. Zingmark, J.H. Jansson, et al. Meanings of people's lived experiences of surviving an out-of-hospital cardiac arrest, 1 month after the event. *J Cardiovasc Nurs* 2014; 29(5): 464–71.

30. K.N. Sawyer, T.R. Camp-Rogers, P. Kotini-Shah, et al. Sudden cardiac arrest survivorship: a scientific statement from the American Heart Association. *Circulation* 2020; 141(12): e654–e685.

31. POST-ICECAP. https://siren.network/clinical-trials/post-icecap.2023 (Accessed on September 27, 2024). Patterns of Survivors' Recovery Trajectories in the ICECAP Trial.

32. S. Agarwal, A. Presciutti, D. Roh, et al. Abstract 17: Cognitive, psychological, and functional limitations after sudden cardiac arrest among a racially and ethnically diverse United States population. *Circulation* 2019; 140 (Suppl 2).

33. K.D. Raina, J.C. Rittenberger, M.B. Holm, et al. Functional outcomes: one year after a cardiac arrest. *Biomed Res Int* 2015; 2015: 283608.

34. S. Agarwal, A. Presciutti, W. Roth, et al. Determinants of long-term neurological recovery patterns relative to hospital discharge among cardiac arrest survivors. *Crit Care Med* 2018; 46(2): e141–e150.

35. T. Cronberg, G. Lilja, J. Horn, et al. Neurologic function and health-related quality of life in patients following targeted temperature management at 33 degrees C vs 36 degrees C after out-of-hospital cardiac arrest: a randomized clinical trial. *JAMA Neurol* 2015; 72(6): 634–41.

36. Y.J. Kim, S. Ahn, C.H. Sohn, et al. Long-term neurological outcomes in patients after out-of-hospital cardiac arrest. *Resuscitation* 2016; 101: 1–5.

37. G. Lilja, N. Nielsen, J. Bro-Jeppesen, et al. Return to work and participation in society after out-of-hospital cardiac arrest. *Circ Cardiovasc Qual Outcomes* 2018; 11(1): e003566.

38. J. Kearney, K. Dyson, E. Andrew, et al. Factors associated with return to work among survivors of out-of-hospital cardiac arrest. *Resuscitation* 2020; 146: 203–12.

39. K. Smith, E. Andrew, M. Lijovic, et al. Quality of life and functional outcomes 12 months after out-of-hospital cardiac arrest. *Circulation* 2015; 131(2): 174–81.

40. J. Elmer, J. C. Rittenberger, P.J. Coppler, et al. Long-term survival benefit from treatment at a specialty center after cardiac arrest. *Resuscitation* 2016; 108: 48–53.

41. A. Aguila, M. Funderburk, A. Guler, et al. Clinical predictors of survival in patients treated with therapeutic hypothermia following cardiac arrest. *Resuscitation* 2010; 81(12): 1621–6.

42. D.J. Kutsogiannis, S.M. Bagshaw, B. Laing, et al. Predictors of survival after cardiac or respiratory arrest in critical care units. *Cmaj* 2011; 183(14): 1589–95.

43. M.B. Iqbal, A. Al-Hussaini, G. Rosser, et al. Predictors of survival and favorable functional outcomes after an out-of-hospital cardiac arrest in patients systematically brought to a dedicated heart attack center (from the Harefield Cardiac Arrest Study). *Am J Cardiol* 2015; 115(6): 730–7.

44. H.S. Kim, K.N. Park, S.H. Kim, et al. Prognostic value of OHCA, C-GRApH and CAHP scores with initial neurologic examinations to predict neurologic outcomes in cardiac arrest patients treated with targeted temperature management. *PLoS ONE* 2020; 15(4): e0232227.

45. E.J. Benjamin, M.J. Blaha, S.E. Chiuve, et al. Heart disease and stroke statistics-2017 update: a report from the American Heart Association. *Circulation* 2017; 135(10): e146–e603.

46. E. Andrew, Z. Nehme, R. Wolfe, et al. Long-term survival following out-of-hospital cardiac arrest. *Heart* 2017; 103(14): 1104–10.

47. N.A. Morris, M. Mazzeffi, P. McArdle, et al. Hispanic/Latino-serving hospitals provide less targeted temperature management following out-of-hospital cardiac arrest. *J Am Heart Assoc* 2021; 10(24): e017773.

48. R.A. Garcia, S. Girotra, B.F. McNally, et al and CARES Surveillance Group. Racial and ethnic differences in bystander cardiopulmonary resuscitation for witnessed out-of-hospital cardiac arrest. *Circulation: Cardiovascular Quality and Outcomes* 2022; 15: A22.

49. K. Reinier, A. Sargsyan, H.S. Chugh, et al. Evaluation of sudden cardiac arrest by race/ethnicity among residents of Ventura County, California, 2015–2020. *JAMA Netw Open* 2021; 4(7): e2118537.

50. N. Bosson, A. Fang, A. H. Kaji, et al. Racial and ethnic differences in outcomes after out-of-hospital cardiac arrest: Hispanics and Blacks may fare worse than non-Hispanic Whites. *Resuscitation* 2019; 137: 29–34.

51. C.S. Jacobs, L. Beers, S. Park, et al. Racial and ethnic disparities in postcardiac arrest targeted temperature management outcomes. *Crit Care Med* 2020; 48(1): 56–63.

52. S. Moon, B.J. Bobrow, T.F. Vadeboncoeur, et al. Disparities in bystander CPR provision and survival from out-of-hospital cardiac arrest according to neighborhood ethnicity. *Am J Emerg Med* 2014; 32(9): 1041–5.

53. M.Z. Khan, M.U. Khan, K. Patel, et al. Trends, predictors and outcomes after utilization of targeted temperature management in cardiac arrest patients with anoxic brain injury. *Am J Med Sci* 2020; 360(4): 363–71.

54. M.A. Starks, R.H. Schmicker, E. D. Peterson, et al. Association of neighborhood demographics with out-of-hospital cardiac arrest treatment and outcomes: where you live may matter. *JAMA Cardiol* 2017; 2(10): 1110–18.

55. S.D. Casey, B.E. Mumma. Sex, race, and insurance status differences in hospital treatment and outcomes following out-of-hospital cardiac arrest. *Resuscitation* 2018; 126: 125–9.

56. J.R. Lupton, R.H. Schmicker, T. P. Aufderheide, et al. Racial disparities in out-of-hospital cardiac arrest interventions and survival in the Pragmatic Airway Resuscitation Trial. *Resuscitation* 2020; 155: 152–8.

57. S. Agarwal, A. Presciutti, J. Verma, et al. Women have worse cognitive, functional, and psychiatric outcomes at hospital discharge after cardiac arrest. *Resuscitation* 2018; 125: 12–15.

58. V. Jeanselme, M. De-Arteaga, J. Elmer, et al. Sex differences in post cardiac arrest discharge locations. *Resusc Plus* 2021; 8: 100185.

59. A. George, V.F. Mensah. Race, Ethnicity, and cardiovascular disease. *J Am Coll Cardiol* 2022; 78(24): 2457-9.

60. D.M. Needham, J. Davidson, H. Cohen, et al. Improving long-term outcomes after discharge from intensive care unit: report from a stakeholders' conference. *Crit Care Med* 2012; 40(2): 502–9.

61. G.J. Soto, G.S. Martin, M.N. Gong. Healthcare disparities in critical illness. *Crit Care Med* 2013; 41(12): 2784–93.

62. E.P. Havranek, M.S. Mujahid, D.A. Barr, et al. Social determinants of risk and outcomes for cardiovascular disease: a scientific statement from the American Heart Association. *Circulation* 2015; 132(9): 873–98.

63. K.W. Gary, J.C. Arango-Lasprilla, L. F. Stevens. Do racial/ethnic differences exist in post-injury outcomes after TBI? A comprehensive review of the literature. *Brain Inj* 2009; 23(10): 775–89.

64. Z. Javed, H.M. Maqsood, T. Yahya, et al. Race, racism, and cardiovascular health: applying a social determinants of health framework to racial/ethnic disparities in cardiovascular disease. *Circ Cardiovasc Qual Outcomes* 2022; 15(1): e007917.

65. A. Presciutti, J. Shaffer, J.A. Sumner, et al. Hyperarousal symptoms in survivors of cardiac arrest are associated with 13 month risk of major adverse cardiovascular events and all-cause mortality. *Ann Behav Med* 2020; 54(6): 413–22.

66. V.R.M. Moulaert, C.M. van Heugten, T. P.M. Gorgels, et al. Long-term outcome after survival of a cardiac arrest: a prospective longitudinal cohort study.

Neurorehabil Neural Repair 2017; 31(6): 530–9.

67. M.L. Gander, R. von Kanel. Myocardial infarction and post-traumatic stress disorder: frequency, outcome, and atherosclerotic mechanisms. *Eur J Cardiovasc Prev Rehabil* 2006; 13(2): 165–72.

68. C. Copland, K. Joekes, S. Ayers. Anxiety and post-traumatic stress disorder in cardiac patients. *British Journal of Wellbeing* 2011; 2: 21–5.

69. D. Edmondson, L. Falzon, K.J. Sundquist, et al. A systematic review of the inclusion of mechanisms of action in NIH-funded intervention trials to improve medication adherence. *Behav Res Ther* 2018; 101: 12–19.

70. IM Kronish, T Cornelius, JE Schwartz, et al. Posttraumatic stress disorder and electronically measured medication adherence after suspected acute coronary syndromes. *Circulation* 2020; 142(8): 817–19.

71. I.M. Kronish, D. Edmondson, J. Z. Goldfinger. Posttraumatic stress disorder and adherence to medications in survivors of strokes and transient ischemic attacks. *Stroke* 2012; 43(8): 2192–7.

72. C. Southern, E. Tutton, K.N. Dainty, et al. The experiences of cardiac arrest survivors and their key supporters following cardiac arrest: a systematic review and meta-ethnography. *Resuscitation* 2024; 198: 110188.

73. A. Presciutti, E. Sobczak, J.A. Sumner, et al. The impact of psychological distress on long-term recovery perceptions in survivors of cardiac arrest. *J Crit Care* 2019; 50: 227–33.

74. A. Presciutti, J. Verma, M. Pavol, et al. Posttraumatic stress and depressive symptoms characterize cardiac arrest survivors' perceived recovery at hospital discharge. *Gen Hosp Psychiatry* 2018; 53: 108–13.

75. G. Lilja, G. Nilsson, N. Nielsen, et al. Anxiety and depression among out-of-hospital cardiac arrest survivors. *Resuscitation* 2015; 97: 68–75.

76. L. Rosman, A. Whited, R. Lampert, et al. Cardiac anxiety after sudden cardiac arrest: severity, predictors and clinical implications. *Int J Cardiol* 2015; 181: 73–6.

77. A. Hamang, G.E. Eide, B. Rokne, et al. General anxiety, depression, and physical health in relation to symptoms of heart-focused anxiety: a cross-sectional study among patients living with the risk of serious arrhythmias and sudden cardiac death. *Health Qual Life Outcomes* 2011; 9: 100.

78. A. Presciutti, A. Frers, J.A. Sumner, et al. Dimensional structure of posttraumatic stress disorder symptoms after cardiac arrest. *J Affect Disord* 2019; 251: 213–17.

79. S. Agarwal, A. Presciutti, T. Cornelius, et al. Cardiac arrest and subsequent hospitalization-induced posttraumatic stress is associated with 1-year risk of major adverse cardiovascular events and all-cause mortality. *Crit Care Med* 2019; 47(6): e502–e505.

80. A.M. Parker, T. Sricharoenchai, S. Raparla. Posttraumatic stress disorder in critical illness survivors: a metaanalysis. *Crit Care Med* 2015; 43(5): 1121–9.

81. A. Presciutti, J. Verma, M. Pavol, et al. Posttraumatic stress and depressive symptoms characterize cardiac arrest survivors' perceived recovery at hospital discharge. *Gen Hosp Psychiatry* 2018; 53: 108–13.

82. A. Presciutti, E. Sobczak, J.A. Sumner, et al. The impact of psychological distress on long-term recovery perceptions in survivors of cardiac arrest. *J Crit Care* 2019; 50: 227–33.

83. A. Hamang, G.E. Eide, B. Rokne, et al. General anxiety, depression, and physical health in relation to symptoms of heart-focused anxiety: a cross-sectional study among patients living with the risk of serious arrhythmias and sudden cardiac death. *Health Qual Life Outcomes* 2011; 9: 100.

84. L. Rosman, A. Whited, R. Lampert, et al. Cardiac anxiety after sudden cardiac arrest: severity, predictors and clinical implications. *Int J Cardiol* 2015; 181: 73–6.

85. E.M. Wachelder, V.R. Moulaert, C. van Heugten, et al. Life after survival: long-term daily functioning and quality of life after an out-of-hospital cardiac arrest. *Resuscitation* 2009; 80(5): 517–22.

86. H.G. van Wijnen, S.M. Rasquin, C.M. van Heugten, et al. The impact of cardiac arrest on the long-term wellbeing and caregiver burden of family caregivers: a prospective cohort study. *Clin Rehabil* 2017; 31(9): 1267–75.

87. M.J. Douma, T.A.D. Graham, S. Ali, et al. What are the care needs of families experiencing cardiac arrest? A survivor and family led scoping review. *Resuscitation* 2021; 168: 119–41.

88. M. Yuan, I.M. Tincher, D.A. Rojas, et al. Lower perceived social support during hospitalization by close family members may have significant associations with psychological distress 1 month after cardiac arrest. *Neurocrit Care* 2025; 42(2): 440-9.

89. I.M. Tincher, S. Abukhadra, C.E. DeForge, et al. Disruptions in sleep health and independent associations with psychological distress in close family members of cardiac arrest survivors: a prospective study. *J Cardiac Fail* 2024; online ahead of print.

90. D.A. Rojas, G.E. Sayde, J.S. Vega, et al. Associations between post-intensive care syndrome domains in cardiac arrest survivors and their families one month post-event. *J Clin Med* 2024; 13(17): 5266.

91. A. Byron-Alhassan, B. Collins, M. Bedard, et al. Cognitive dysfunction after out-of-hospital cardiac arrest: rate of impairment and clinical predictors. *Resuscitation* 2021; 165: 154–60.

92. S.G. Beesems, K.M. Wittebrood, R.J. de Haan, et al. Cognitive function and quality of life after successful resuscitation from cardiac arrest. *Resuscitation* 2014; 85(9): 1269–74.

93. G. Lilja, N. Nielsen, H. Friberg, et al. Cognitive function in survivors of out-of-hospital cardiac arrest after target temperature management at 33 degrees C versus 36 degrees C. *Circulation* 2015; 131(15): 1340–9.

94. C. Lim, M. Verfaellie, D. Schnyer, et al. Recovery, long-term cognitive outcome and quality of life following out-of-hospital cardiac arrest. *J Rehabil Med* 2014; 46(7): 691–7.

95. A.R. Sabedra, J. Kristan, K. Raina, et al. Neurocognitive outcomes following successful resuscitation from cardiac arrest. *Resuscitation* 2015; 90: 67–72.

96. M. Orbo, P.M. Aslaksen, K. Larsby, et al. Alterations in cognitive outcome between 3 and 12 months in survivors of out-of-hospital cardiac arrest. *Resuscitation* 2016; 105: 92–9.

97. C.V.M. Steinbusch, C.M. van Heugten, S.M.C. Rasquin, et al. Cognitive impairments and subjective cognitive complaints after survival of cardiac arrest: a prospective longitudinal cohort study. *Resuscitation* 2017; 120: 132–7.

98. T. Cronberg, D.M. Greer, G. Lilja, et al. Brain injury after cardiac arrest: from prognostication of comatose patients to rehabilitation. *Lancet Neurol* 2020; 19(7): 611–22.

99. E.B. Nordstrom, J.L. Birk, D.A. Rojas, et al. Prospective evaluation of the relationship between cognition and recovery outcomes after cardiac arrest. *Resuscitation* 2024; 202: 110343.

100. E.B. Nordstrom, G. Lilja. Assessment of neurocognitive function after cardiac arrest. *Curr Opin Crit Care* 2019; 25(3): 234–9.

101. G. Lilja, S. Ullen, J. Dankiewicz, et al. Effects of hypothermia vs normothermia on societal participation and cognitive function at 6 months in survivors after out-of-hospital cardiac arrest: a predefined analysis of the ttm2 randomized clinical trial. *JAMA Neurol* 2023; 80(10): 1070–9.

102. M. Bohm, G. Lilja, H. Finnbogadottir, et al. Detailed analysis of health-related quality of life after out-of-hospital cardiac arrest. *Resuscitation* 2019; 135: 197–204.

103. N. Secher, K. Adelborg, P. Szentkuti, et al. Evaluation of neurologic and psychiatric outcomes after hospital discharge among

adult survivors of cardiac arrest. *JAMA Netw Open* 2022; 5(5): e2213546.

104. R.G. Geocadin, C.W. Callaway, E.L. Fink, et al. Standards for studies of neurological prognostication in comatose survivors of cardiac arrest: a scientific statement from the American Heart Association. *Circulation* 2019; 140(9): e517–e542.

105. E.A. Matthews, J. Magid-Bernstein, A. Presciutti, et al. Categorization of survival and death after cardiac arrest. *Resuscitation* 2017; 114: 79–82.

106. J. Elmer, C. Torres, T.P. Aufderheide, et al. Association of early withdrawal of life-sustaining therapy for perceived neurological prognosis with mortality after cardiac arrest. *Resuscitation* 2016; 102: 127–35.

107. A. Xiao, C.W. Callaway, P.J. Coppler, et al. Long-term outcomes of post-cardiac arrest patients with severe neurological and functional impairments at hospital discharge. *Resuscitation* 2022; 174: 93–101.

108. K. Howell, E. Grill, A.M. Klein, et al. Rehabilitation outcome of anoxic-ischaemic encephalopathy survivors with prolonged disorders of consciousness. *Resuscitation* 2013; 84(10): 1409–15.

109. J.A. Smits, A.C. Berry, C.D. Tart, et al. The efficacy of cognitive-behavioral interventions for reducing anxiety sensitivity: a meta-analytic review. *Behav Res Ther* 2008; 46(9): 1047–54.

110. M. Bergman, J.C. Markowitz, I.M. Kronish, et al. Acceptance and mindfulness-based exposure therapy for PTSD after cardiac arrest: an open feasibility trial. *J Clin Psychiatry* 2023; 85(1): 23m14883.

111. T. Cornelius, M. Mendieta, R.M. Cumella, et al. Family-authored ICU diaries to reduce fear in patients experiencing a cardiac arrest (FAID fear): a pilot randomized controlled trial. *PLoS ONE* 2023; 18(7): e0288436.

112. H. Magne, N. Jaafari, M. Voyer. Post-traumatic growth: some conceptual considerations. *Encephale* 2021; 47(2): 143–50.

113. V.L. Joshi, J. Christensen, E. Lejsgaard, et al. Effectiveness of rehabilitation interventions on the secondary consequences of surviving a cardiac arrest: a systematic review and meta-analysis. *BMJ Open* 2021; 11(9): e047251.

114. A.S. Leon, B.A. Franklin, F. Costa, et al. Cardiac rehabilitation and secondary prevention of coronary heart disease: an American Heart Association scientific statement from the Council on Clinical Cardiology. *Circulation* 2005; 111(3): 369–76.

115. J. Austin, R. Williams, L. Ross, et al. Randomised controlled trial of cardiac rehabilitation in elderly patients with heart failure. *Eur J Heart Fail* 2005; 7(3): 411–17.

116. V.R. Moulaert, J.C. van Haastregt, D.T. Wade, et al. "Stand still ..., and move on", an early neurologically-focused follow-up for cardiac arrest survivors and their caregivers: a process evaluation. *BMC Health Serv Res* 2014; 14: 34.

117. M.J. Cowan, K.C. Pike, H.K. Budzynski. Psychosocial nursing therapy following sudden cardiac arrest: impact on two-year survival. *Nurs Res* 2001; 50(2): 68–76.

118. V.R. Moulaert, C.M. van Heugten, B. Winkens, et al. Early neurologically-focused follow-up after cardiac arrest improves quality of life at one year: a randomised controlled trial. *Int J Cardiol* 2015; 193: 8–16.

119. V.R. Moulaert, M. Goossens, I.L. Heijnders, et al. Early neurologically focused follow-up after cardiac arrest is cost-effective: a trial-based economic evaluation. *Resuscitation* 2016; 106: 30–6.

120. M. Mion, F. Al-Janabi, S. Islam, et al. Care after resuscitation: implementation of the united kingdom's first dedicated multidisciplinary follow-up program for survivors of out-of-hospital cardiac arrest. *Ther Hypothermia Temp Manag* 2020; 10(1): 53–9.

121. M. Mion, R. Case, K. Smith, et al. Follow-up care after out-of-hospital cardiac arrest: a pilot study of survivors and families' experiences and recommendations. *Resusc Plus* 2021; 7: 100154.

122. A. Presciutti, E.E. Meyers, M. Reichman, et al. Associations between baseline total ptsd symptom severity, specific ptsd symptoms, and 3-month quality of life in neurologically intact neurocritical care patients and informal caregivers. *Neurocrit Care* 2021; 34(1): 54–63.

123. A.M. Presciutti, K.L. Flickinger, P.J. Coppler, et al. Protective positive psychology factors and emotional distress after cardiac arrest. *Resuscitation* 2023; 188: 109846.

124. M.K. Wagner, J. Christensen, K.A. Christensen, et al. A multidisciplinary guideline-based approach to improving the sudden cardiac arrest care pathway: the Copenhagen framework. *Resusc Plus* 2024; 17: 100546.

125. M.K. Wagner, S.K. Berg, C. Hassager, et al. Cognitive impairment and psychopathology in sudden out-of-hospital cardiac arrest survivors: results from the REVIVAL cohort study. *Resuscitation* 2023; 192: 109984.

126. A.M. Presciutti, E. Woodworth, E. Rochon, et al. A mindfulness-based resiliency program for caregivers of patients with severe acute brain injury transitioning out of critical care: protocol for an open pilot trial. *JMIR Res Protoc* 2023; 12: e50860.

127. S. Agarwal, I.M. Tincher, S.L. Abukhadra, et al. Prioritizing intervention preferences to potentially reduce caregiver burden in racially and ethnically diverse close family members of cardiac arrest survivors. *Resuscitation* 2024; 194: 110093.

128. J.L. Birk, R. Cumella, D. Lopez-Veneros, et al. Feasibility of a remote heart rate variability biofeedback intervention for reducing anxiety in cardiac arrest survivors: a pilot trial. *Contemp Clin Trials Commun* 2024; 37: 101251.

Chapter 52: PICS in Survivors of Neurological Insult

Julia M. Carlson and Matthew N. Jaffa

Introduction

Post-intensive care syndrome (PICS) describes the physical, cognitive, and psychological impairments develop or persist following critical illness, which often have profound effects on the long-term well-being of patients and their families. To date, PICS is understudied in survivors of acute neurologic injury (ANI) who require intensive care unit (ICU) admission [1]. Distinguishing between the consequences of ANI and the typical symptoms of PICS is difficult and, accordingly, these patients have often been excluded from studies [1]. While limitations for conducting research in the ANI population exist, including higher rates of aphasia and disorders of consciousness (DOC), these survivors likely experience many of the complex symptoms associated with PICS [2,3]. Caregivers of survivors of ANI also experience symptoms consistent with PICS-family (PICS-F), such as depression, anxiety, and post-traumatic stress disorder (PTSD), at rates similar to caregivers of other survivors of critical illness [4,5,6]. Although it is challenging to completely differentiate the influence that critical care treatment has on PICS and PICS-F with the expected recovery trajectory following ANI, survivors and caregivers experience similar symptoms that deserve study and treatment.

There is a growing movement to develop post-neuroICU clinics (also known as NeuroRecovery clinics) to address the issues facing survivors of ANI and to screen for PICS and PICS-F, similar to care provided in other ICU follow-up clinics [3,7]. Post-neuroICU clinics fill a gap in the post-acute care paradigm for these patients by maintaining continuity of care from the acute injury through the resolution of the acute-subacute period and by identifying aspects of care often overlooked by others, including complex medication reconciliation and tapering, addressing ongoing therapy needs, and continued recovery prognostication. A major goal of these clinics is to screen patients for ICU-related complications that primary care physicians and other subspecialists may overlook, including, but not limited to, cognitive changes, mood disorders, weakness, and spasticity. These clinics ensure proper follow-up for medical devices that may need ongoing care or removal, such as tracheostomy tubes, gastrostomy tubes, and inferior vena cava filters, and prescribe additional durable medical equipment to accommodate patients' impairments. Post-neuroICU clinics may also manage medications that require tapering by a specialist other than the primary provider managing follow-up (e.g., vascular neurologist, neurosurgeon, or trauma surgeon), including anti-seizure medications (ASMs), paroxysmal sympathetic hyperactivity (PSH) treatments, anti-psychotics, and neuroendocrine agents. Finally, they can ensure that a patient has appropriate follow-up with primary care, neurology, neurosurgery, physiatry, and therapy services. While there is no standardized way to assess ANI survivors for PICS in a post-neuroICU clinic, clinicians should be aware of disease-specific, long-term symptoms to screen for and treat appropriately.

Disease-Specific Considerations

Patients cared for in the neuro-ICU comprise a multitude of clinical presentations of varying levels of criticality but typically fall into seven main diagnoses: ischemic stroke, subarachnoid hemorrhage (SAH), intracerebral hemorrhage (ICH), traumatic brain injury (TBI), traumatic spinal cord injury (SCI), status epilepticus (SE), and neuromuscular weakness. Each of the above pathologies requires specific acute and post-acute care, and each has its own recovery trajectory. Among these diagnoses, several present unique challenges for clinicians providing care in the subacute and chronic phases of the illness/injury (see Table 52.1).

Table 52.1 Examples of specific recommendations for management of common neuro-ICU conditions and the chronic symptoms that survivors frequently experience

	Disease-Specific Considerations	
Disease	**Challenge**	**Recommendations**
Subarachnoid Hemorrhage	Headache	Opioid avoidance, headache specialist referral, botulinum toxin injections, physical therapy
	Cognitive Dysfunction	Neuropsychiatric evaluation, speech therapy (cognitive), depression screening
	Seizures	Medication tapering/titration
Status Epilepticus	Cognitive Dysfunction	Neuropsychiatric evaluation, speech therapy (cognitive), depression screening, medication reconciliation
Traumatic Brain Injury	Cognitive Dysfunction	Neuropsychiatric evaluation, speech therapy (cognitive), depression screening
	Complex Medication Regimens	Careful medication reconciliation, consultation with clinical pharmacist
	Disorder of Consciousness	Trial of/adjustment of neurostimulants, additional imaging/neurocognitive testing
Traumatic Spinal Cord Injury	Ventilator Management	Interdisciplinary tracheostomy team management, noninvasive mechanical ventilation
	Autonomic Dysreflexia	Reduce bladder/bowel distention
	Neurogenic Bladder	Education, catheterization, anti-cholinergic medications
	Neurogenic Bowel	Increase fiber and water intake, bowel routine, consistent use of stool softeners
	Sexual Dysfunction	Identify noninjury related issues

Subarachnoid Hemorrhage

Survivors of SAH may experience multiple symptoms that affect their long-term quality of life, even among those who achieve good functional outcomes [8]. Ongoing headaches requiring long-term management are among the most common complications experienced following aneurysmal SAH (aSAH) [9]. While there is significant heterogeneity in the management of these headaches, newer studies propose an effective treatment paradigm that minimizes opioids [10]. The variable headache phenotypes present following SAH may benefit from the skillful assessment and treatment of a specialist that can offer both pharmacologic and non-pharmacologic therapies.

Cognitive changes following SAH are prevalent and include mental fatigue, memory deficits, and executive dysfunction, all of which affect quality of life and the ability to return to work [9,11,12,13,14]. Many of these findings may be subtle and are recognized only with an in-depth evaluation of how the patient manages tasks that were a routine part of their pre-injury life; such detailed evaluations may require the assistance of cognitive and occupational therapists and neuropsychologists. Examples include a business executive taking several hours to answer an email that would have previously been completed in minutes or a baker who forgets to turn the oven off at the end of their day. Screening and treatment for depression is also recommended, as cognitive changes can present with mood disorder-type symptoms; however, antidepressants have not been found to improve functional status in aSAH patients without depression [15]. Psychiatrists, sports neurologists, or speech therapists specializing in cognition may help identify deficits and recommend therapies to improve focus and optimize performance.

Twenty-five percent of patients surviving aSAH develop epilepsy requiring long-term ASM treatment [16,17]; however, up to half of patients with stroke complicated by acute seizures may be continued on long-term ASMs unnecessarily [18]. Such patients would benefit from evaluation in a post-neuroICU clinic, where the risks and benefits of continuing or discontinuing ASMs can be thoughtfully weighed.

Finally, further evaluation, management, and counseling for important modifiable risk factors for recurrent aSAH should also be addressed, including hypertension management and smoking cessation [19,20]. Screening first-degree family members for a history of aSAH with potential referral for genetic screening and imaging may also be appropriate [20].

Status Epilepticus

Many patients in the neuro-ICU may experience episodes of SE, either as a complication of their ANI or as the primary admitting diagnosis. Long-term consequences of SE are most commonly cognitive rather than physical impairments [21], and both generalized convulsive and nonconvulsive SE are risk factors for cognitive impairment [22,23]. The pathophysiology of long-term cognitive changes is unknown and an area of active research; potential etiologies include the SE itself, underlying triggers and injuries, and medications used to manage epilepsy [22,24].

Patients treated for SE are often discharged from the hospital with prescriptions for more ASMs than they required prior to hospitalization, even among those with a history of epilepsy [25]. Frequently, depending on the cause of the SE, these additional medications are not required for long-term management and should be evaluated for weaning and discontinuation. It may be possible during hospitalization to safely taper or discontinue one or more of the additional ASMs with careful observation or repeated electroencephalogram

(EEG) monitoring. In the outpatient setting, a slow taper with careful observation by family or caregivers for signs of mental status changes or focal seizures is feasible. It may be of benefit to assess seizure propensity with a routine EEG before or after the decision to make changes to any ASMs.

Traumatic Brain Injury

Similar to survivors of SAH, survivors of TBI frequently experience symptoms in several domains that require ongoing management following hospital discharge. TBI survivors often experience behavioral/emotional dysregulation and personality changes, some of which may be permanent [26]. Management includes screening for problematic behaviors and agitation, referral to appropriate behavioral health clinicians, and appropriate medication initiation and titration. Survivors of TBI may also experience long-term cognitive changes that limit their functioning and affect their ability to return to work or school [27]. The inability to return to prior life roles and development of mood disorders can negatively impact quality of life in survivors of TBI [28].

Survivors of TBI may experience acute symptomatic seizures, central endocrine dysfunction (e.g., adrenal insufficiency, diabetes insipidus, hypothyroidism, and hypogonadism), and/or PSH during the acute phase of their injury. Many of the medications used to treat these disorders, particularly PSH, can have significant side effects and may become unnecessary during recovery as symptoms change and syndromes resolve. Each medication must be reevaluated to determine its benefits and potential risks before being tapered in a rehabilitation or outpatient setting. Many of the medications initially prescribed for management of seizures and PSH may also treat additional presenting symptoms or comorbidities, and special attention must be paid to ensure that the concomitant diagnoses are still being appropriately treated as medication for the primary syndrome is tapered. As an example, clonidine is regularly used to treat PSH, but it also may be used to manage hypertension or liberate patients from dexmedetomidine infusions; if clonidine is tapered because of improvement in PSH symptomatology, the patient may require additional treatments for hypertension and agitation.

Survivors of TBI may also experience DOC in the acute-subacute period and require treatment with neurostimulants such as amantadine [29,30]. With time, the DOC may improve, and the use of stimulants should be reevaluated and potentially discontinued; however, if the DOC does not improve, additional imaging or diagnostic work-up might be considered to assist in prognostication for caregivers [31]. Clinically significant gains in consciousness and level of function have been observed in traumatic DOC generally within two years, although the patients who have the best functional outcomes generally have an earlier recovery trajectory [32,33,34]. Prognostication and time-limited trials of restorative care are addressed later in the chapter.

Spinal Cord Injury

Following the initial life-threatening neurogenic shock associated with a traumatic SCI and the recognition of a life-altering injury, many patients' and families' first thoughts focus on functional capacity. These patients experience ongoing sensorimotor dysfunction, with recovery largely based on the initial injury severity and mechanism of injury (blunt versus penetrating) [35]. The vast majority of recovery occurs in the first three months following traumatic SCI, identifying this time window as an excellent opportunity to provide valuable prognostic information in an ICU follow-up clinic [36]. While quality of life tends to be more favorable in paraplegic versus quadriplegic SCI patients, even among those who attain higher levels of functional independence, many will be affected by a host of long-lasting sequelae that impact daily life [37].

Higher cervical spine injuries and more complete injuries place survivors of SCI at increased risk for long-term tracheostomy and ventilator dependence [38], which significantly impacts where they may receive rehabilitation and long-term care. For example, some states in the United States have stipulations that prevent disposition to skilled nursing facilities if the patient requires both ventilatory support and renal replacement therapy, or there may be a limited number of ventilator-capable beds available within the state's long-term care system. Tracheostomy and long-term ventilator dependence make returning home particularly challenging. There is considerable variation in long-term ventilator management strategies and decannulation protocols, but interdisciplinary tracheostomy team management is the most studied [39]. Ongoing investigation of long-term ventilator management and other strategies, including the use of noninvasive ventilation, may ultimately improve function in patients with SCI.

Autonomic dysreflexia can occur after SCI above the T6 level and consists of episodic rises in systolic blood pressure of at least 20 mmHg and reflexive bradycardia [40,41]. Episodes are typically precipitated by reversible triggers, most commonly bowel or bladder distension [40,41]. Prevention and management are important, as not only can the events occur hourly or more, but they can also be life threatening, with increased rates of both stroke and mortality [40]. Neurogenic bladder management strategies depend on the degree of injury, and they range from intermittent catheterization, botulinum toxin injections, and stenting to permanent indwelling Foley catheter or suprapubic tube placement or surgical options, such as urinary diversion [42]. Neurogenic bowel management relies on consistent laxative use as well as digital stimulation; surgery may be considered as a last resort to limit these events [42].

Neurogenic bowel and bladder symptom management is also important for quality of life after SCI [43]. Constipation is seen in nearly half of SCI survivors, with initial treatment focused on conservative and nonsurgical options [44]. A variety of programs have been developed to improve gastrointestinal transit times and difficulty with evacuation while reducing the need for pharmacologic therapies. These programs include dietary modifications (high fiber, plant-based foods, supplementation), appropriate fluid intake, and timing of the performance of the bowel routine. The early and continued use of stool softeners and stimulants should be instituted to help prevent and regulate chronic constipation.

Neurogenic bladder affects nearly 80% of SCI survivors and increases the risk for significant potential complications, including urinary tract infections, acute kidney injury, and wounds [45]. Management begins with patient education, clean intermittent catheterization, and anti-cholinergic medications, and it may require chronic indwelling catheters and addition of antimuscarinic medications prior to surgical considerations. Active efforts to determine appropriate candidates for aggressive inpatient bladder training programs are ongoing [46].

Sexual dysfunction is a significant recovery priority to improve quality of life among survivors of SCI [47,48]. Despite this, there is significant variability in therapy for sexual dysfunction, which may be driven by a lack of recognition of the noninjury components affecting sexuality, including hormonal changes (e.g., low testosterone or hypothyroidism), depression, altered self-image, pressure sores, and adverse medication effects. Recognizing that sexual dysfunction results from a combination of these factors is important for its comprehensive management in this patient population [47].

Roles of ICU Follow-Up Clinics

Addressing Uncertainty

ANIs often present with a high degree of prognostic uncertainty during the acute phase [49]. Given this uncertainty, early discussions with families and surrogate decision makers to identify therapies and interventions that are most congruent with a patient's known values, goals, and preferences are difficult and have major implications on patient outcomes. How to communicate uncertainty with tact and in a manner that maintains the therapeutic relationship between the medical team and family is an active area of research [50]. For many families and surrogate decision makers, the uncertainty surrounding long-term prognosis is particularly challenging, and they may be differentiated into two distinct perspectives on decision making: those engaged in active decision making and those for whom there is no perceived decision to be made [51]. The concept of time-limited trials (TLT) of critical care is one option that may be presented, but their utility is limited among patients surviving ANIs given their prolonged recovery trajectory, which typically exceeds the conventional time course for placement of tracheostomy and gastrostomy tubes [52]. Visits in post-neuroICU clinics offer additional opportunities for the medical team, patient, and family to assess their current clinical and functional status, recovery trajectory, and goals of care [7].

Emotional Debriefing

Post-neuroICU clinic visits offer an opportunity to debrief with the patient and their loved ones on their survivorship experience. Some survivors of neurological critical illness may not have meaningful memories of their hospitalization or understanding of their illness [53,54]. The clinic visit can provide a time to review their illness and hospital course, view their imaging (often for their first time), and process any memories they have of hospitalization. In some cases, memories must be disentangled from what the person believes they experienced and what occurred in reality. For example, ICU diaries kept by both family and the medical team may be a helpful adjunct in this process, providing a prospective daily summary of events for the patient and family to review (see Chapter 18 for additional information) [55].

Post-neuroICU clinics can also provide an opportunity to check-in on recovery, evaluate new and emerging symptoms that have arisen since hospital discharge, and review challenges at rehabilitation facilities or home [3]. Clinic visits also provide opportunities to mourn the loss of the sense of self, both functional and psychological, and to discuss how life has changed since the illness. Other outpatient visits may offer insufficient time or expertise to reflect on both the injury and the recovery, while an intensivist who has cared for the patient previously is in a unique position to provide valuable support. An intensivist can also use this time to manage goals and expectations for the future and provide reassurance with changes in medications or the benign prognosis of a perimesencephalic SAH, for example.

Readdressing Prognostication and Goals of Care

In the subacute phase, a reevaluation of current level of consciousness and symptoms may provide valuable information for patients and their families regarding the recovery trajectory and inform goals of care moving forward. In some cases, it may be appropriate to obtain additional testing, including neurological evaluation, EEG, somatosensory evoked potentials, and/or neuroimaging, such as magnetic resonance imaging (MRI) or functional imaging (functional MRI, resting state MRI, or positron emission tomography), to assist in this effort [34]. With data generated from a multimodal evaluation, providers, patients, and caregivers can engage in informed discussion regarding the patient's current clinical state, the trajectory of their recovery to date, and their potential for additional recovery, as well as assess possible changes to their current treatment plans and goals of care.

As patients and families reconcile with their "new normal," post-neuroICU clinics can provide opportunities to readdress goals of care. For those survivors and their families engaged in a TLT of restorative care, reevaluation in a post-neuroICU clinic at three or six months is an opportune time, depending on the patient's values, goals, and preferences, to either transition goals from continued restorative care to comfort-focused care or to extend the TLT to see if additional recovery is possible.

Readdressing code status is often the first step taken by patients and their loved ones. Others may prefer an approach that continues current therapies while setting limits on future interventions should complications of their primary injury or comorbid conditions arise. This may mean avoiding future intubations, admission to the ICU, or even admission to the hospital entirely. Importantly, for some survivors, a transition to comfort-focused care will not be as straightforward as it might be during the acute illness, when compassionate extubation and discontinuation of other life-sustaining therapies are commonly performed. Developing relationships with local palliative care clinicians and hospice facilities is paramount to ensuring safe and comfortable transitions of care.

Conclusion

Survivors of critical illness and ANI are steadily increasing, and these survivors, many of whom have complex care needs, would benefit from receiving care in a post-neuroICU clinic to optimize outcomes and reduce distress. Post-neuroICU clinics are beginning to gain traction around the United States and offer patients and their families additional interactions with the healthcare team to ensure that the care they receive is both thorough and nuanced and provides a bridge between the acute and chronic phases of their injury. While the consequences of ANI and non-neurological critical illness have significant overlap and are often indistinguishable, recovery from ANI has unique features that neuro-intensivists can manage and support. Prognostic uncertainty in the acute, and even subacute, phases of ANI requires a different approach to decision making than that which occurs in the ICU, emphasizing the need for potential TLTs of restorative care with benchmarks for reevaluating care decisions only occurring after hospital discharge. The continued evolution of and participation in post-neuroICU clinics is paramount to the continued improvement in long-term care of survivors of ANI.

Key Points

1. PICS has not been well-studied in acute neurologic injury patients because of the overlap between PICS symptoms and expected sequalae of brain injury.
2. There is a growing movement for long-term follow-up of survivors of acute neurologic injury to better address PICS and PICS-F in post-ICU neurorecovery clinics.
3. Patients with acute neurologic injuries such as subarachnoid hemorrhage, status epilepticus, traumatic brain injury, and spinal cord injury all have unique recovery trajectories and considerations for post-acute care.
4. ICU follow-up clinics offer opportunities for re-prognostication and reevaluation of goals of care after acute neurologic injuries.

References

1. J.N. LaBuzetta, J. Rosand, A.M. Vranceanu. Review: post-intensive care syndrome: unique challenges in the neurointensive care unit. *Neurocrit Care* 2019; **31**(3): 534–45.
2. D.Y. Hwang. Is post-neurointensive care syndrome actually a thing? *Neurocrit Care* 2019; **31**(3): 453–4.
3. V. Salasky, M.N. Jaffa, M. Motta, G. Y. Parikh. Neurocritical care recovery clinics: an idea whose time has come. *Curr Neurol Neurosci Rep* 2023; **23**(4): 159–66.
4. D.Y. Hwang, D. Yagoda, H.M. Perrey, et al. Anxiety and depression symptoms among families of adult intensive care unit survivors immediately following brief length of stay. *J Crit Care* 2014; **29**(2): 278–82.
5. S.A. Trevick, A.S. Lord. Post-traumatic stress disorder and complicated grief are common in caregivers of neuro-icu patients. *Neurocrit Care* 2017; **26**(3): 436–43.
6. E.E. Meyers, A. Presciutti, K.M. Shaffer, et al. The impact of resilience factors and anxiety during hospital admission on longitudinal anxiety among dyads of neurocritical care patients without major cognitive impairment and their family caregivers. *Neurocrit Care* 2020; **33**(2): 468–78.
7. M.N. Jaffa, J.E. Podell, M. Motta. A change of course: the case for a neurorecovery clinic. *Neurocrit Care* 2020; **33**(2): 610–12.
8. P.E. Passier, J.M. Visser-Meily, G.J. Rinkel, et al. Life satisfaction and return to work after aneurysmal subarachnoid hemorrhage. *J Stroke Cerebrovasc Dis Off J Natl Stroke Assoc* 2011; **20**(4): 324–9.
9. S.B. Wenneberg, L. Block, A. Sörbo, et al. Long-term outcomes after aneurysmal subarachnoid hemorrhage: a prospective observational cohort study. *Acta Neurol Scand* 2022; **146**(5): 525–36.
10. Z.A. Sorrentino, D. Laurent, J. Hernandez, et al. Headache persisting after aneurysmal subarachnoid hemorrhage: a narrative review of pathophysiology and therapeutic strategies. *Headache J Head Face Pain* 2022; **62**(9): 1120–32.
11. S.A. Mayer, K.T. Kreiter, D. Copeland, et al. Global and domain-specific cognitive impairment and outcome after subarachnoid hemorrhage. *Neurology* 2002; **59**(11): 1750–8.
12. T. Al-Khindi, R.L. Macdonald, T. A. Schweizer. Cognitive and functional outcome after aneurysmal subarachnoid hemorrhage. *Stroke* 2010; **41**(8): e519–536.
13. H.C. Persson, M. Törnbom, O. Winsö, K. S. Sunnerhagen. Symptoms and consequences of subarachnoid haemorrhage after 7 years. *Acta Neurol Scand* 2019; **140**(6): 429–34.
14. E. Western, T.H. Nordenmark, W. Sorteberg, et al. Fatigue after aneurysmal subarachnoid hemorrhage:

clinical characteristics and associated factors in patients with good outcome. *Front Behav Neurosci* 2021; **15**: 633616.

15. H.Y. Chun, A. Ford, M.A. Kutlubaev, et al. Depression, anxiety, and suicide after stroke: a narrative review of the best available evidence. *Stroke* 2022; **53**(4): 1402–10.

16. E. Olafsson, G. Gudmundsson, W. A. Hauser. Risk of epilepsy in long-term survivors of surgery for aneurysmal subarachnoid hemorrhage: a population-based study in Iceland. *Epilepsia* 2000; **41**(9): 1201–5.

17. J. Huttunen, M.I. Kurki, M. von und zu Fraunberg, et al. Epilepsy after aneurysmal subarachnoid hemorrhage. *Neurology* 2015; **84**(22): 2229–37.

18. V. Punia, R. Honomichl, P. Chandan, et al. Long-term continuation of anti-seizure medications after acute stroke. *Ann Clin Transl Neurol* 2021; **8**(9): 1857–66.

19. N. Etminan, H.S. Chang, K. Hackenberg, et al. Worldwide incidence of aneurysmal subarachnoid hemorrhage according to region, time period, blood pressure, and smoking prevalence in the population: a systematic review and meta-analysis. *JAMA Neurol* 2019; **76**(5): 588–97.

20. B.L. Hoh, N.U. Ko, S. Amin-Hanjani, et al. 2023 Guideline for the management of patients with aneurysmal subarachnoid hemorrhage: a guideline from the American Heart Association/American Stroke Association. *Stroke* 2023; **54**(7): e314–70.

21. G. Jacq, B. Crepon, M. Resche-Rigon, et al. Clinician-reported physical and cognitive impairments after convulsive status epilepticus: post hoc study of a randomized controlled trial. *Neurocrit Care* 2024; **40**(2): 495–505.

22. K.N. Power, A. Gramstad, N.E. Gilhus, B. A. Engelsen. Adult nonconvulsive status epilepticus in a clinical setting: semiology, aetiology, treatment and outcome. *Seizure* 2015; **24**: 102–6.

23. K.N. Power, A. Gramstad, N.E. Gilhus, et al. Cognitive function after status epilepticus versus after multiple generalized tonic-clonic seizures. *Epilepsy Res* 2018; **140**: 39–45.

24. A. Gramstad, K.N. Power, B.A. Engelsen. Neuropsychological performance 1 year after status epilepticus in adults. *Arch Clin Neuropsychol Off J Natl Acad Neuropsychol* 2021; **36**(3): 329–38.

25. K. Bauer, F. Rosenow, S. Knake, et al. Clinical characteristics and outcomes of patients with recurrent status epilepticus episodes. *Neurol Res Pract* 2023; **5**: 34.

26. S. Izzy, P.M. Chen, Z. Tahir, et al. Association of traumatic brain injury with the risk of developing chronic cardiovascular, endocrine, neurological, and psychiatric disorders. *JAMA Netw Open* 2022; **5**(4): e229478.

27. D.I. Katz, M. Polyak, D. Coughlan, et al. Natural history of recovery from brain injury after prolonged disorders of consciousness: outcome of patients admitted to inpatient rehabilitation with 1–4 year follow-up. *Prog Brain Res* 2009; **177**: 73–88.

28. S.B. Juengst, L.M. Adams, J.A. Bogner, et al. Trajectories of life satisfaction after TBI: influence of life roles, age, cognitive disability, and depressive symptoms. *Rehabil Psychol* 2015; **60**(4): 353–64.

29. J.T. Giacino, K. Kalmar, B. Eifert, et al. Placebo-controlled trial of amantadine for severe traumatic brain injury. *N Engl J Med* 2012; **366**(9): 819–26.

30. M.E. Barra, S. Izzy, A. Sarro-Schwartz, et al. Stimulant therapy in acute traumatic brain injury: prescribing patterns and adverse event rates at two level 1 trauma centers. *J Intensive Care Med* 2020; **35**(11): 1196–202.

31. J.T. Giacino, D.I. Katz, N.D. Schiff, et al. Practice guideline update recommendations summary: disorders of consciousness: report of the Guideline Development, Dissemination, and Implementation Subcommittee of the American Academy of Neurology; the American Congress of Rehabilitation Medicine; and the National Institute on Disability, Independent Living, and Rehabilitation Research. *Neurology* 2018; **91**(10): 450–60.

32. A. Estraneo, P. Moretta, V. Loreto, et al. Late recovery after traumatic, anoxic, or hemorrhagic long-lasting vegetative state. *Neurology* 2010; **75**(3): 239–45.

33. A. Estraneo, P. Moretta, V. Loreto, et al. Clinical and neuropsychological long-term outcomes after late recovery of responsiveness: a case series. *Arch Phys Med Rehabil* 2014; **95**(4): 711–16.
34. J.M. Carlson, D.J. Lin. Prognostication in prolonged and chronic disorders of consciousness. *Semin Neurol* 2023; **43**(5): 744–57.
35. S. Kirshblum, B. Snider, F. Eren, J. Guest. Characterizing natural recovery after traumatic spinal cord injury. *J Neurotrauma* 2021; **38**(9): 1267–84.
36. J.W. Fawcett, A. Curt, J.D. Steeves, et al. Guidelines for the conduct of clinical trials for spinal cord injury as developed by the ICCP panel: spontaneous recovery after spinal cord injury and statistical power needed for therapeutic clinical trials. *Spinal Cord* 2007; **45**(3): 190–205.
37. D. Cardile, A. Calderone, R. De Luca, et al. The quality of life in patients with spinal cord injury: assessment and rehabilitation. *J Clin Med* 2024; **13**(6): 1820.
38. P.P. Long, D.W. Sun, Z.F. Zhang. Risk factors for tracheostomy after traumatic cervical spinal cord injury: a 10-year study of 456 patients. *Orthop Surg* 2022; **14**(1): 10–17.
39. G.H. Sun, S.W. Chen, M.P. MacEachern, J. Wang. Successful decannulation of patients with traumatic spinal cord injury: a scoping review. *J Spinal Cord Med* 2022; **45**(4): 498–509.
40. H. Cowan, C. Lakra, M. Desai. Autonomic dysreflexia in spinal cord injury. *BMJ* 2020; **371**: m3596.
41. C. Lakra, O. Swayne, G. Christofi, M. Desai. Autonomic dysreflexia in spinal cord injury. *Pract Neurol* 2021;**21**(6): 532–8.
42. T.L. Wheeler, W. de Groat, K. Eisner, et al. Translating promising strategies for bowel and bladder management in spinal cord injury. *Exp Neurol* 2018; **306**: 169–76.
43. C.W. Liu, C.C. Huang, Y.H. Yang, et al. Relationship between neurogenic bowel dysfunction and health-related quality of life in persons with spinal cord injury. *J Rehabil Med* 2009; **41**(1): 35–40.
44. M. Coggrave, C. Norton, J. Wilson-Barnett. Management of neurogenic bowel dysfunction in the community after spinal cord injury: a postal survey in the United Kingdom. *Spinal Cord* 2009; **47**(4): 323–30.
45. W.A. Taweel, R. Seyam. Neurogenic bladder in spinal cord injury patients. *Res Rep Urol* 2015; **7**: 85–99.
46. V. Lim, J.M. Mac-Thiong, A. Dionne, et al. Clinical protocol for identifying and managing bladder dysfunction during acute care after traumatic spinal cord injury. *J Neurotrauma* 2021; **38**(6): 718–24.
47. K.D. Anderson. Targeting recovery: priorities of the spinal cord-injured population. *J Neurotrauma* 2004; **21**(10): 1371–83.
48. L.A. Simpson, J.J. Eng, J.T. Hsieh, D.L. Wolfe. The health and life priorities of individuals with spinal cord injury: a systematic review. *J Neurotrauma* 2012; **29**(8): 1548–55.
49. C.J. Creutzfeldt, W.T. Longstreth, R. G. Holloway. Predicting decline and survival in severe acute brain injury: the fourth trajectory. *BMJ* 2015; **351**: h3904.
50. A. Goss, C. Ge, S. Crawford, et al. Prognostic language in critical neurologic illness: a multicenter mixed-methods study. *Neurology* 2023; **101**(5): e558–69.
51. A.L. Goss, R.R. Voumard, R. A. Engelberg, et al. Do they have a choice? Surrogate decision-making after severe acute brain injury. *Crit Care Med* 2023; **51**(7): 924–35.
52. D.W. Chang, T.H. Neville, J. Parrish, et al. Evaluation of time-limited trials among critically ill patients with advanced medical illnesses and reduction of nonbeneficial icu treatments. *JAMA Intern Med* 2021; **181**(6): 786–94.
53. J.S. Turner, S.J. Briggs, H.E. Springhorn, P. D. Potgieter. Patients' recollection of intensive care unit experience. *Crit Care Med* 1990; **18**(9): 966–8.
54. C. Granja, A. Lopes, S. Moreira, et al. Patients' recollections of experiences in the intensive care unit may affect their quality of life. *Crit Care Lond Engl* 2005; **9**(2): R96–109.
55. A.J. Ullman, L.M. Aitken, J. Rattray, et al. Diaries for recovery from critical illness. *Cochrane Database Syst Rev* 2014; **2014** (12): CD010468.

Chapter 53

The Long-COVID Syndrome

Samuel K. McGowan, Ann M. Parker, and Lekshmi Santhosh

Introduction

The COVID-19 (hereafter simply referred to as COVID) pandemic has been a watershed for the care of critically ill patients with far-reaching impacts on patients, providers, and healthcare systems. As of March 2024, over 700 million people globally have been infected with SARS-CoV-2 [1], with a global mortality of at least 7 million [2]. With the advent of effective treatment regimens, vaccines, less virulent variants, and reduced health systems strain, the survival rate of SARS-CoV-2 infection is fortunately much higher than it had been in the earliest months of the pandemic [3]. Even early in the pandemic, there was recognition that many patients who survived acute COVID developed persistent, debilitating symptoms. Termed "Long COVID (LC)," "Post-COVID Condition (PCC)," or, alternatively, "Post-Acute Sequelae of COVID (PASC)," this syndrome must be understood by clinicians caring for survivors of COVID [4]. Symptoms of post-intensive care syndrome (PICS) and PCC overlap significantly [5], and an integrated, holistic treatment approach is beneficial to facilitate recovery from both PICS and PCC. In this chapter, we define PCC and its disease burden, review principles of diagnosis and management, and explore the relationship between PCC and PICS.

Defining PCC

"Long COVID" is a term that was generated by a specific patient advocacy movement, whereby patients self-identified and found community support in the shared experience of lingering symptoms after COVID. Conceived originally on social media platforms, the term "Long COVID" emerged as a hashtag, leading to millions of likes and shares within months of the onset of the pandemic [6]. In the early phases of the pandemic, the exact definition and timeline of PCC were unclear, but the World Health Organization now defines PCC as occurring in:

> Individuals with a history of probable or confirmed SARS-CoV-2 infection, usually 3 months from the onset of COVID, with symptoms that last for at least 2 months and cannot be explained by an alternate diagnosis. Common symptoms include fatigue, shortness of breath, and cognitive dysfunction, but also others, which generally have an impact on everyday functioning. Symptoms may be new onset, following initial recovery from an acute COVID episode, or persist from the initial illness. Symptoms may also fluctuate or relapse over time. [7]

Clinical trials, such as the NIH-sponsored RECOVER cohort study and the Lifelines cohort study, have aimed to more granularly define PCC and understand its phenotypes [8,9].

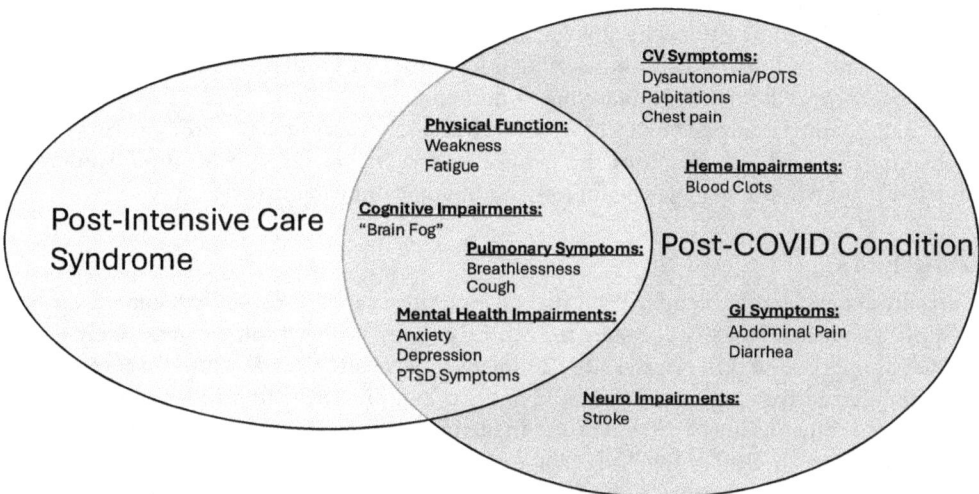

Figure 53.1 PICS-PCC overlap.

Clinical Presentation

Common PCC symptoms identified in the aforementioned studies include post-exertional malaise, fatigue, breathlessness, cough, dizziness, "brain fog," and gastrointestinal symptoms, occurring in approximately 10% of study participants infected with SARS-CoV-2 [8,9]. Patients may also present with diverse symptoms both acutely and chronically, such as venous thromboembolic disease (e.g., deep venous thrombosis and pulmonary embolism) and bleeding events [10], new heart failure or stroke [11], cognitive impairment [12], dysautonomia [13], postural orthostatic tachycardia syndrome (POTS) [14], and abdominal pain and diarrhea [15]. While no specific set of symptoms defines PCC, most patients present with dysfunction across multiple organ systems. One proposed symptom score assesses loss of smell/taste, post-exertional malaise, and chronic cough as common PCC symptoms, but many others are reported [8]. Several of these symptoms also overlap significantly with PICS, as shown in Figure 53.1.

In survivors of SARS-CoV-2 infection requiring intensive care unit (ICU) admission, PICS is prevalent, with approximately two-thirds of patients describing persistent impairments one year after hospital discharge. PCC survivors with PICS are more likely to present with fatigue, dyspnea, and physical impairments, and less likely to experience cognitive impairments or psychiatric symptoms when compared to historical cohorts of critical illness and acute respiratory distress syndrome (ARDS) survivors [16].

Pathophysiology

The pathophysiology of PCC remains under investigation, and the evidence continues to evolve, with several proposed biological mechanisms to explain the wide variety of clinical presentations observed. Patients with PCC have shown evidence of significant immune system dysregulation, including T-cell exhaustion, even after mild infection [17], as well as low antibody production in response to infection [18]. Viral proteins and RNA have been found to persist in tissues throughout the body, including the lung [19], heart, gastrointestinal tract, and endothelium; the spike antigen specifically has been found in up to 60% of survivors with PCC over 12 months after infection [20]. Evidence suggests that COVID causes organ-specific damage, including endothelial dysfunction [21,22], cardiac dysfunction [23], cognitive impairment [12,24], respiratory impairment [25,26], gastrointestinal dysbiosis [27], and alterations of the genitourinary system [28,29]. Multiple studies are underway to further elucidate the underlying biological mechanisms.

Diagnosis

Currently, there are no standardized diagnostic criteria for PCC, leading some experts to propose a data-driven scoring system to identify patients with symptoms most likely related to PCC as opposed to other causes [8]. Clinicians must evaluate each symptom carefully and consider alternative diagnoses [7]. While patients can present with a wide range of unique symptoms, clinicians may find that PCC can fall into specific "phenotypes," in which certain symptoms tend to cluster together. For example, one phenotype overlaps with myalgic encephalomyelitis or chronic fatigue syndrome (ME/CFS), with patients primarily reporting fatigue, weakness, and post-exertional malaise [30]. A respiratory phenotype might include dyspnea, breathlessness, and exercise intolerance, while a cardiac phenotype might include chest pain, palpitations, or POTS [8,31].

Ultimately, PCC is a diagnosis of exclusion, no matter the presenting complaint. While there is currently no specific diagnostic test to evaluate for PCC, many organ-specific tests have been employed to evaluate for certain manifestations of PCC. Advanced imaging modalities have been examined in research studies, including cardiac MRI to identify cardiovascular impairment [23], fluorescence microscopy to image amyloid microclots [32], and 129Xe hyperpolarized MRI to detect pulmonary gas exchange [33]; these tests are not widely used nor routinely available in clinical practice. The tilt table test is an established diagnostic test for POTS that has been used in diagnosing PCC manifesting as dysautonomia [14]. Several biomarkers have been proposed for the diagnosis of PCC, including plasma neuron-derived extracellular vesicles (NDEVs) and astrocyte-derived extracellular vesicles (ADEVs) [18], as well as other immune markers of cytotoxicity and specific autoantibody profiles [34,35], but none have yet been validated for clinical use. Further, given that some patients have a high degree of overlap between symptoms of ME/CFS and PCC, some have suggested adapting the existing diagnostic criteria used for ME/CFS and applying them to patients surviving COVID [30].

Management

Pulmonary Symptoms

Several management considerations should be considered in PCC patients presenting with dyspnea. Clinicians should consider COVID-related causes and non-COVID-related causes of dyspnea when patients present to a PCC-specific or ICU follow-up clinic. Obstructive lung disease, including asthma and chronic obstructive pulmonary disease (COPD), are often exacerbated by COVID; chronic asthma control has been shown to be worse after initial infection [36]. Deconditioning after prolonged acute illness can also contribute to dyspnea. Many PCC patients with critical illness are survivors of ARDS and are at risk for developing post-ARDS fibrosis [37]. Although fibrosis due to COVID is observed, it is unlikely to progress over time, and patients often see improvement in lung function and symptomology [38,39,40]. There is no evidence that prolonged steroid courses are beneficial in COVID-related fibrosis unless there is clear radiographic evidence of organizing pneumonia or other steroid-responsive etiologies. Discontinuing or tapering steroids in ICU follow-up encounters is recommended for patients surviving COVID. Similarly, antifibrotic therapies approved for idiopathic pulmonary fibrosis (IPF) are not routinely recommended for patients with post-COVID interstitial lung disease. Clinicians should compare imaging both before and after COVID to ensure that there were no pre-existing abnormalities, such as evidence of mild interstitial lung disease.

Additional etiologies for dyspnea that should be considered include gastroesophageal reflux disease (GERD), pleuritis, neuromuscular weakness affecting the diaphragm (see Chapter 35 for additional information), cardiogenic causes, vocal cord dysfunction, tracheal stenosis, and tracheomalacia (see Chapter 39 for additional information). Routine testing can include serial pulmonary function tests (PFTs), a six-minute walk test to assess for both exertional hypoxemia and tachycardia, and chest imaging when indicated. The need for supplemental oxygen should be assessed at each visit and weaned as tolerated.

Neurocognitive Symptoms

Many key management principles in the PICS population can be adapted to the care of the PCC patient. As neurological symptoms are common, patients should be screened for cognitive impairment when there is clinical suspicion, and a full neurologic examination should be completed to identify neurologic deficits [41]. A full review of the patient's clinical course should be performed, with attention paid to the identification of reversible causes of cognitive dysfunction. A detailed medication reconciliation should be completed, as polypharmacy is common in the post-ICU setting [42] and may contribute to falls, delirium, progression of cognitive impairment, and rehospitalization, particularly in older patients (see Chapter 32 for additional information) [43]. Polypharmacy and over-prescription are also common in PCC patients that had mild COVID, and neurologic symptoms may improve with de-escalation of psychotropic and overly sedating medications [43], as is already common practice in many ICU follow-up clinics. Patients should be screened for other reversible or treatable causes of cognitive dysfunction, including metabolic disorders and nutritional deficiencies. Many PCC patients present with fatigue and insomnia, and screening for comorbid sleep disorders, such as obstructive sleep apnea, may be beneficial. PCC patients may be susceptible to psychiatric comorbidities, and combination referral to psychiatry and psychology may be superior to medication or therapy alone [44,45,46]. Further, cognitive rehabilitation programs, which involve individualized programs for skill building and metacognitive strategies around cognitive deficits [47], as well as cognitive pacing [48], have shown benefit in the PICS population and can be considered for PCC management [47].

Physical Function Symptoms

Impairments in physical function can be common in PCC. Deprescribing unnecessary medications may positively impact physical deconditioning. For example, many patients are prescribed steroids in the acute setting of COVID in an attempt to prevent or reduce post-ARDS fibrosis. In the absence of clear evidence of an organizing pneumonia, steroids should be tapered or discontinued in the outpatient setting to avoid the development of myopathy. ARDS survivors are particularly prone to developing long-term symptoms, with more than two-thirds describing persistent fatigue up to 12 months after hospitalization [49]. Other mainstays of prevention include early mobility for patients who are mechanically ventilated, which has been shown to improve functional status and reduce disability and ICU-acquired weakness in survivors (see Chapters 11 and 12 for additional information) [50,51].

The evidence for post-discharge physical therapy (PT) and occupational therapy (OT) in PICS is evolving and is described in more detail in Chapters 41 and 42, respectively. While multiple clinical trials evaluating PT and OT in the post-ICU setting have yielded mixed results [52,53,54,55], the emerging evidence base in PCC has shown promise. In a recent, large, randomized trial of COVID patients following hospital discharge, an eight-week online physical and mental health intervention improved health related quality of life when compared to usual care [56]. Recognizing that overextending oneself physically might worsen post-exertional malaise symptoms in some patients, particularly those that fit the ME/CFS phenotype [57], physical rehabilitation, when performed under the guidance of a therapist familiar with PCC, can be beneficial in preventing post-exertional malaise exacerbations. Deconditioning is often invoked as the underlying mechanism for physical dysfunction, and while certainly a component for many with PCC, it is unlikely to fully explain all symptoms, particularly for patients with mild COVID infections [58]. As such, patients would benefit from PT programs with experienced providers that can measure and validate the patient's experience and engage in appropriate resting and pacing. Exercise programs should be carefully designed based on the individual presentation of each patient, and self-management strategies should be considered [59].

Management of Other PCC Symptoms

In addition to the therapies listed above, many treatment modalities across a wide spectrum of disease have been considered for PCC, often targeting specific symptoms. For COVID survivors that develop POTS, non-pharmacological strategies such as volume optimization and recumbent exercise training should be trialed first. If refractory, beta-blockers have well-established efficacy in conjunction with non-pharmacological therapies [60]. In one study, the use of histamine-receptor antagonists (HRAs) reduced the average burden of all PCC symptoms by 72% after several months of treatment [61]. Patients who receive nirmatrelvir during their acute illness are at decreased risk of post-acute adverse health outcomes, regardless of vaccination status or history of prior infection [62].

Anticoagulation

Anticoagulation is not currently recommended in PCC in the absence of confirmed venous thromboembolism or another existing indication, such as atrial fibrillation. Early evidence suggested that prophylactic anticoagulation could reduce both vascular endothelial damage [63] and inflammatory markers [64], particularly in older patients with multiple underlying comorbidities. In one study, prophylactic anticoagulation during hospitalization decreased 30-day mortality risk by 27%, though notably the strongest effects were seen in the non-ICU sub-cohort [65]. Further study, however, has shown that anticoagulation does not improve mortality, reduce blood clots, or decrease cardiovascular events but does confer an increased risk of bleeding events [66]. Current guidelines do not recommend the routine use of either prophylactic or therapeutic anticoagulation after hospital discharge for COVID [67]. Endothelial dysfunction remains an active area of ongoing research in patients with PCC.

Vaccination

Regardless of prior infection history, most patients should be encouraged to receive COVID vaccines as recommended by the Centers for Disease Control and Prevention (CDC). Vaccinated patients, in general, are less likely to have persistent symptoms after acute infection [68], with an approximately 36% risk reduction after one dose and 68% risk reduction after two doses of vaccine [69,70]. While vaccination likely reduces risk for developing PCC, there is currently no evidence that vaccination post-exposure prophylaxis can alter the incidence of PCC [70]. Nevertheless, patients should be counseled that while there is always a small risk of side effects [71], the benefits of vaccination vastly outweigh any risks in the majority of the population [72].

Overlap Between Long COVID Clinics and ICU Follow-Up Clinics

In the spirit of follow-up clinics that care for survivors of critical illness, the growing appreciation of PCC has led to many dedicated clinics to evaluate and manage chronic symptoms related to COVID. These two clinic types are often distinct entities, although in some cases, ICU follow-up and PCC clinics exist under a single program, where providers receive referrals for both survivors of COVID requiring critical care and for survivors of mild to moderate COVID infections. Dedicated PCC clinics or combined ICU follow-up/PCC clinics should include specific expertise in the diagnosis and management of symptoms relating to COVID, including fatigue, dyspnea, exertional intolerance, gastrointestinal discomfort, psychological sequelae, and cognitive dysfunction, and they should be composed of an interdisciplinary team of clinicians with PCC expertise [73].

Many PCC clinics are modeled on ICU follow-up clinics, and as such, are typically multidisciplinary programs composed of a diverse set of healthcare professionals working as a team [74]. Because of their interprofessional nature, these programs offer a diverse array of rehabilitation programs, including physiatry, cognitive therapy, physical therapy, occupational therapy, and rehabilitation psychology. Core team members often include pulmonary-critical care physicians or advanced practice providers, psychiatrists and psychologists, primary care providers, pharmacists, dietitians, social workers, other mental and behavioral health specialists, and subspecialists, including practitioners in palliative care, integrative medicine, neurology, cardiology, and geriatrics [74].

Physical and occupational therapists with PCC experience are an essential component to PCC care. In many clinics, providers may meet as a team prior to seeing patients to coordinate and prioritize care. Physical and occupational therapists with specific PCC experience can be particularly attuned to phenotypes in PCC and can create individualized treatment plans. The American Academy of Physical Medicine and Rehabilitation (AAPMR) provides comprehensive guidance on the care of PCC patients, including consensus statements on the treatment of fatigue [75], breathing discomfort [75], autonomic dysfunction [76], and many other symptoms.

Pharmacists are also an indispensable part of the team, particularly those with ICU training. Pharmacists are useful in addressing polypharmacy, identifying drug-drug interactions, and counseling patients on the risks and benefits of over-the-counter medications, home remedies, supplements, and other treatments patients may try that currently lack a strong evidence base.

Finally, social workers and community health workers are key team members who can assist patients with managing appointments, applying for benefits, engaging in health education, and understanding insurance claims. As PCC patients are often stigmatized by other providers and are disproportionately minoritized, social workers and behavioral health/mental health specialists are particularly helpful in overcoming structural barriers to care.

Disparities in COVID

The COVID pandemic brought into stark focus racial and ethnic inequalities in the United States healthcare system. Black and Latinx Americans are disproportionately more likely to contract COVID and have higher rates of hospitalization and higher mortality [77]. These trends are likely to continue after discharge and impact long-term care of survivors of COVID, as minoritized COVID survivors are more likely to experience cost barriers, receive poor communication from providers, or have other structural or social barriers to obtaining quality healthcare. PCC clinics should consider explicit strategies to reduce such disparities, including adding social workers to their interprofessional teams, engaging in low literacy education strategies, providing flexible office hours, and offering telephone visits [77]. Providing language-concordant care is a particularly important service that will improve access to patients with limited English proficiency, who are at particularly high risk for complications due to COVID [78]. Maintaining and expanding equitable access to both in-person and telehealth services is critical to equitably reach patients with whatever modality is more patient-centered.

Ongoing Research

As new clinics are put into practice and new trial data become available, best practices in the management of PCC will continue to evolve. The NIH RECOVER initiative is an ongoing, patient-centered research collaborative comprising longitudinal observational cohort studies, electronic health record data, and clinical trials to understand the impact and management of PCC [79]. Ongoing clinical trials will explore treatments for autonomic dysfunction, cognitive dysfunction, exercise intolerance, sleep disturbances, and viral persistence. Funding for PCC research continues to grow, including via the US Department of Health and Human Services (HHS), which has announced up to $9 million in grant award funding through the Agency for Healthcare Research and Quality (AHRQ).

Conclusion

As the COVID pandemic wanes, the viral variants change, and the population becomes more vaccinated, the incidence of PCC will hopefully decrease, although its trajectory is still unknown. PCC and ICU follow-up clinics can collaborate to deliver holistic, patient-centered, and multidisciplinary care to a diverse patient population. Finally, the care of PCC survivors is important not only for our patients, but also for clinicians, many of whom continue to recover from the dramatic clinical demands asked of them during the pandemic. Fostering reconnection between clinicians and ICU survivors can not only enhance our understanding of the long term effects of COVID critical illness but also contribute to provider well-being and reduce burnout in a low-cost, high-value clinical intervention [80].

Key Points

1. Post-COVID condition (PCC) describes new or worsening symptoms that develop after initial SARS-CoV-2 infection and are persistent for months without alternative explanations.
2. PCC is common in patients infected with SARS-CoV-2, occurring in as many as 10% of patients enrolled in prospective trials.
3. PCC and PICS symptoms commonly overlap, including impairments in physical, cognitive, and mental health, as well as breathlessness and cough.
4. PCC is a diagnosis of exclusion, as there is no specific diagnostic test to confirm its presence.
5. Many key management principles in the PICS population can be adapted to the care of the PCC patient, including the use of holistic, interdisciplinary clinics that can individualize care to patients based on symptom burden.

References

1. COVID-19 cases | WHO COVID-19 dashboard. *datadot*, https://data.who.int/dashboards/covid19/cases (Accessed March 8, 2024).
2. COVID-19 deaths | WHO COVID-19 dashboard. *datadot*, https://data.who.int/dashboards/covid19/deaths (Accessed March 8, 2024).
3. K. Schwab, E. Schwitzer, N. Qadir. Postacute sequelae of COVID-19 critical illness. *Crit Care Clin* 2022; **38**: 455–72.
4. P.A. Volberding, B.X. Chu, C.M. Spicer (eds). *Long-term health effects of COVID-19: disability and function following SARS-CoV-2 infection*. Washington, DC: National Academies Press. 2024.
5. C.L. Hodgson, A.M. Higgins, M.J. Bailey, et al. Comparison of 6-month outcomes of survivors of COVID-19 versus non-COVID-19 critical illness. *Am J Respir Crit Care Med* 2022; **205**: 1159–68.
6. F. Callard, E. Perego. How and why patients made Long Covid. *Soc Sci Med* 2021; **268**: 113426.
7. J.-W. Seo, S.E. Kim, Y. Kim, et al. Updated clinical practice guidelines for the diagnosis and management of long COVID. *Infect Chemother* 2024; **56**(1): 122-57.
8. T. Thaweethai, S.E. Jolley, E.W. Karlson, et al. Development of a definition of postacute sequelae of SARS-CoV-2 infection. *JAMA* 2023; **329**: 1934–46.
9. A.V. Ballering, S.K.R. van Zon, T.C. Olde Hartman, et al. Persistence of somatic symptoms after COVID-19 in the Netherlands: an observational cohort study. *Lancet* 2022; **400**: 452–61.
10. I. Katsoularis, O. Fonseca-Rodríguez, P. Farrington, et al. Risks of deep vein thrombosis, pulmonary embolism, and bleeding after covid-19: nationwide self-controlled cases series and matched cohort study. *BMJ* 2022; **377**: e069590.
11. E. Xu, Y. Xie, Z. Al-Aly. Long-term neurologic outcomes of COVID-19. *Nat Med* 2022; **28**: 2406–15.
12. D.A. Holdsworth, R. Chamley, R. Barker-Davies, et al. Comprehensive clinical assessment identifies specific neurocognitive deficits in working-age patients with long-COVID. *PLoS One* 2022; **17**: e0267392.
13. N.W. Larsen, L.E. Stiles, R. Shaik, et al. Characterization of autonomic symptom burden in long COVID: a global survey of 2,314 adults. *Front Neurol* 2022; **13**: 1012668.
14. S.M. Jamal, D.B. Landers, S.M. Hollenberg, et al. Prospective evaluation of autonomic

dysfunction in post-acute sequela of COVID-19. *J Am Coll Cardiol* 2022; **79**: 2325–30.

15. H. Meringer, S. Mehandru. Gastrointestinal post-acute COVID-19 syndrome. *Nat Rev Gastroenterol Hepatol* 2022; **19**: 345–6.

16. A.N. Makam, J. Burnfield, E. Prettyman, et al. One-year recovery among survivors of prolonged severe COVID-19: a national multicenter cohort. *Crit Care Med* 2024; **52** (7): e376–389.

17. J. Klein, J. Wood, J.R. Jaycox, et al. Distinguishing features of long COVID identified through immune profiling. *Nature* 2023; **623**: 139–48.

18. M.J. Peluso, S.G. Deeks. Early clues regarding the pathogenesis of long-COVID. *Trends Immunol* 2022; **43**: 268–70.

19. L.J. Ceulemans, M. Khan, S.-J. Yoo, et al. Persistence of SARS-CoV-2 RNA in lung tissue after mild COVID-19. *Lancet Respir Med* 2021; **9**: e78–e79.

20. F. Tejerina, P. Catalan, C. Rodriguez-Grande, et al. Post-COVID-19 syndrome: SARS-CoV-2 RNA detection in plasma, stool, and urine in patients with persistent symptoms after COVID-19. *BMC Infect Dis* 2022; **22**: 211.

21. M. Haffke, H. Freitag, G. Rudolf, et al. Endothelial dysfunction and altered endothelial biomarkers in patients with post-COVID-19 syndrome and chronic fatigue syndrome (ME/CFS). *J Transl Med* 2022; **20**: 138.

22. S. Charfeddine, H. Ibn Hadj Amor, J. Jdidi, et al. Long COVID 19 syndrome: is it related to microcirculation and endothelial dysfunction? insights from TUN-EndCOV Study. *Front Cardiovasc Med* 2021; **8**: 745758.

23. A. Roca-Fernandez, M. Wamil, A. Telford, et al. Cardiac abnormalities in long COVID 1-year post-SARS-CoV-2 infection. *Open Heart* 2023; **10**: e002241.

24. F. Ceban, S. Ling, L.M.W. Lui, et al. Fatigue and cognitive impairment in post-COVID-19 Syndrome: a systematic review and meta-analysis. *Brain Behav Immun* 2022; **101**: 93–135.

25. J.Z. Yu, T. Granberg, R. Shams, et al. Lung perfusion disturbances in nonhospitalized post-COVID with dyspnea: a magnetic resonance imaging feasibility study. *J Intern Med* 2022; **292**: 941–56.

26. J.L. Cho, R. Villacreses, P. Nagpal, et al. Quantitative chest CT assessment of small airways disease in post-acute SARS-CoV-2 infection. *Radiology* 2022; **304**: 185–92.

27. Q. Liu, J.W.Y. Mak, Q. Su, et al. Gut microbiota dynamics in a prospective cohort of patients with post-acute COVID-19 syndrome. *Gut* 2022; **71**: 544–52.

28. E. Kresch, J. Achua, R. Saltzman, et al. COVID-19 endothelial dysfunction can cause erectile dysfunction: histopathological, immunohistochemical, and ultrastructural study of the human penis. *World J Mens Health* 2021; **39**: 466–9.

29. L. Medina-Perucha, T. López-Jiménez, A.S. Holst, et al. Self-reported menstrual alterations during the COVID-19 syndemic in Spain: a cross-sectional study. *Int J Womens Health* 2022; **14**: 529–44.

30. T.L. Wong, D.J. Weitzer. Long COVID and Myalgic Encephalomyelitis/Chronic Fatigue Syndrome (ME/CFS): a systemic review and comparison of clinical presentation and symptomatology. *Medicina (Kaunas)* 2021; **57**: 418.

31. A. Dagliati, Z.H. Strasser, Z.S. Hossein Abad, et al. Characterization of long COVID temporal sub-phenotypes by distributed representation learning from electronic health record data: a cohort study. *EClinicalMedicine* 2023; **64**: 102210.

32. E. Pretorius, C. Venter, G.J. Laubscher, et al. Prevalence of symptoms, comorbidities, fibrin amyloid microclots and platelet pathology in individuals with Long COVID/Post-Acute Sequelae of COVID-19 (PASC). *Cardiovasc Diabetol* 2022; **21**: 148.

33. J.T. Grist, G.J. Collier, H. Walters, et al. Lung abnormalities detected with hyperpolarized 129Xe MRI in patients with

Long COVID. *Radiology* 2022; **305**: 709–17.

34. A. Bodansky, C.-Y. Wang, A. Saxena, et al. Autoantigen profiling reveals a shared post-COVID signature in fully recovered and Long COVID patients. *medRxiv* 2023; 2023.02.06.23285532.

35. M. Galán, L. Vigón, D. Fuertes, et al. Persistent overactive cytotoxic immune response in a Spanish cohort of individuals with Long-COVID: identification of diagnostic biomarkers. *Front Immunol* 2022; **13**: 848886.

36. K.E.J. Philip, S. Buttery, P. Williams, et al. Impact of COVID-19 on people with asthma: a mixed methods analysis from a UK wide survey. *BMJ Open Respir Res* 2022; **9**: e001056.

37. P.M. George, S.L. Barratt, R. Condliffe, et al. Respiratory follow-up of patients with COVID-19 pneumonia. *Thorax* 2020; **75**: 1009–16.

38. M.S. Herridge, A.M. Cheung, C.M. Tansey, et al. One-year outcomes in survivors of the acute respiratory distress syndrome. *N Engl J Med* 2003; **348**: 683–93.

39. X. Han, Y. Fan, O. Alwalid, et al. Six-month follow-up chest CT findings after severe COVID-19 pneumonia. *Radiology* 2021; **299**: E177–E186.

40. B. van den Borst, J.B. Peters, M. Brink, et al. Comprehensive health assessment 3 months after recovery from acute coronavirus disease 2019 (COVID-19). *Clin Infect Dis* 2021; **73**: e1089–e1098.

41. J.S. Fine, A.F. Ambrose, N. Didehbani, et al. Multi-disciplinary collaborative consensus guidance statement on the assessment and treatment of cognitive symptoms in patients with post-acute sequelae of SARS-CoV-2 infection (PASC). *PM&R* 2022; **14**: 96–111.

42. L. Giambattista, R. Howard, R. Ruhe Porto, et al. NICHE recommended care of the critically ill older adult. *Crit Care Nurs Q* 2015; **38**: 223–30.

43. E. Melamed, L. Rydberg, A.F. Ambrose, et al. Multidisciplinary collaborative consensus guidance statement on the assessment and treatment of neurologic sequelae in patients with post-acute sequelae of SARS-CoV-2 infection (PASC). *PM R* 2023; **15**: 640–62.

44. D.J. Kupfer, E. Frank, M.L. Phillips. Major depressive disorder: new clinical, neurobiological, and treatment perspectives. *Lancet* 2012; **379**: 1045–55.

45. P. Cuijpers, J. Dekker, S.D. Hollon, et al. Adding psychotherapy to pharmacotherapy in the treatment of depressive disorders in adults: a meta-analysis. *J Clin Psychiatry* 2009; **70**: 1219–1229.

46. P. Cuijpers, A. van Straten, L. Warmerdam, et al. Psychotherapy versus the combination of psychotherapy and pharmacotherapy in the treatment of depression: a meta-analysis. *Depress Anxiety* 2009; **26**: 279–88.

47. K.D. Cicerone, Y. Goldin, K. Ganci, et al. Evidence-based cognitive rehabilitation: systematic review of the literature from 2009 through 2014. *Arch Phys Med Rehabil* 2019; **100**: 1515–33.

48. H.E. Davis, L. McCorkell, J.M. Vogel, et al. Long COVID: major findings, mechanisms and recommendations. *Nat Rev Microbiol* 2023; **21**: 133–46.

49. K.J. Neufeld, J.-M.S. Leoutsakos, H. Yan, et al. Fatigue symptoms during the first year following ARDS. *Chest* 2020; **158**: 999–1007.

50. D.S. Schujmann, T. Teixeira Gomes, A.C. Lunardi, et al. Impact of a progressive mobility program on the functional status, respiratory, and muscular systems of ICU patients: a randomized and controlled trial. *Crit Care Med* 2020; **48**: 491–7.

51. C. Zhang, X. Wang, J. Mi, et al. Effects of the high-intensity early mobilization on long-term functional status of patients with mechanical ventilation in the intensive care unit. *Crit Care Res Pract* 2024; **2024**: 4118896.

52. J. Mehrholz, M. Pohl, J. Kugler, et al. Physical rehabilitation for critical illness myopathy and neuropathy: an abridged version of Cochrane Systematic Review. *Eur J Phys Rehabil Med* 2015; **51**: 655–61.

53. B.H. Cuthbertson, J. Rattray, M. K. Campbell, et al. The PRaCTICaL study of nurse led, intensive care follow-up programmes for improving long term outcomes from critical illness: a pragmatic randomised controlled trial. *BMJ* 2009; **339**: b3723.
54. T.S. Walsh, L.G. Salisbury, J.L. Merriweather, et al. Increased hospital-based physical rehabilitation and information provision after intensive care unit discharge: the RECOVER randomized clinical trial. *JAMA Intern Med* 2015; **175**: 901–10.
55. K. McDowell, B. O'Neill, B. Blackwood, et al. Effectiveness of an exercise programme on physical function in patients discharged from hospital following critical illness: a randomised controlled trial (the REVIVE trial). *Thorax* 2017; **72**: 594–5.
56. G. McGregor, H. Sandhu, J. Bruce, et al. Clinical effectiveness of an online supervised group physical and mental health rehabilitation programme for adults with post-covid-19 condition (REGAIN study): multicentre randomised controlled trial. *BMJ* 2024; **384**: e076506.
57. J. Wright, S.L. Astill, M. Sivan. The relationship between physical activity and long COVID: a cross-sectional study. *Int J Environ Res Public Health* 2022; **19**: 5093.
58. P.M. Heerdt, B. Shelley, I. Singh. Impaired systemic oxygen extraction long after mild COVID-19: potential perioperative implications. *Br J Anaesth* 2022; **128**: e246–e249.
59. R. Twomey, J. DeMars, K. Franklin, et al. Chronic fatigue and postexertional malaise in people living with long COVID: an observational study. *Phys Ther* 2022; **102**: pzac005.
60. B. Narasimhan, A. Calambur, E. Moras, et al. Postural orthostatic tachycardia syndrome in COVID-19: a contemporary review of mechanisms, clinical course and management. *Vasc Health Risk Manag* 2023; **19**: 303–16.
61. P. Glynne, N. Tahmasebi, V. Gant, et al. Long COVID following mild SARS-CoV-2 infection: characteristic T cell alterations and response to antihistamines. *J Investig Med* 2022; **70**: 61–7.
62. Y. Xie, T. Choi, Z. Al-Aly. Association of treatment with nirmatrelvir and the risk of post-COVID-19 condition. *JAMA Intern Med* 2023; **183**: 554–64.
63. C. Wang, C. Yu, H. Jing, et al. Long COVID: the nature of thrombotic sequelae determines the necessity of early anticoagulation. *Front Cell Infect Microbiol* 2022; **12**: 861703.
64. Y. Arslan, G. Yilmaz, D. Dogan, et al. The effectiveness of early anticoagulant treatment in Covid-19 patients. *Phlebology* 2021; **36**: 384–91.
65. C.T. Rentsch, J.A. Beckman, L. Tomlinson, et al. Early initiation of prophylactic anticoagulation for prevention of coronavirus disease 2019 mortality in patients admitted to hospital in the United States: cohort study. *BMJ* 2021; **372**: n311.
66. J.M. Connors, M.M. Brooks, F.C. Sciurba, et al. Effect of antithrombotic therapy on clinical outcomes in outpatients with clinically stable symptomatic COVID-19: the ACTIV-4B randomized clinical trial. *JAMA* 2021; **326**: 1703–12.
67. A. Cuker, E.K. Tseng, R. Nieuwlaat, et al. American Society of Hematology living guidelines on the use of anticoagulation for thromboprophylaxis in patients with COVID-19: July 2021 update on postdischarge thromboprophylaxis. *Blood Adv* 2022; **6**: 664–71.
68. A. Watanabe, M. Iwagami, J. Yasuhara, et al. Protective effect of COVID-19 vaccination against long COVID syndrome: a systematic review and meta-analysis. *Vaccine* 2023; **41**: 1783–90.
69. P. Gao, J. Liu, M. Liu. Effect of COVID-19 vaccines on reducing the risk of long COVID in the real world: a systematic review and meta-analysis. *Int J Environ Res Public Health* 2022; **19**: 12422.
70. A.R. Marra, T. Kobayashi, G.Y. Callado, et al. The effectiveness of COVID-19 vaccine in the prevention of post-COVID conditions: a systematic literature review and meta-analysis of the latest research.

Antimicrob Steward Healthc Epidemiol 2023; **3**: e168.

71. T. Tsuchida, M. Hirose, Y. Inoue, et al. Relationship between changes in symptoms and antibody titers after a single vaccination in patients with Long COVID. *J Med Virol* 2022; **94**: 3416–20.

72. M. Antonelli, R.S. Penfold, J. Merino, et al. Risk factors and disease profile of post-vaccination SARS-CoV-2 infection in UK users of the COVID Symptom Study app: a prospective, community-based, nested, case-control study. *The Lancet Infectious Diseases* 2022; **22**: 43–55.

73. A.M. Parker, E. Brigham, B. Connolly, et al. Addressing the post-acute sequelae of SARS-CoV-2 infection: a multidisciplinary model of care. *Lancet Respir Med* 2021; **9**: 1328–41.

74. L. Santhosh, B. Block, S.Y. Kim, et al. Rapid design and implementation of post-COVID-19 clinics. *Chest* 2021; **160**: 671–7.

75. J.E. Herrera, W.N. Niehaus, J. Whiteson, et al. Multidisciplinary collaborative consensus guidance statement on the assessment and treatment of fatigue in postacute sequelae of SARS-CoV-2 infection (PASC) patients. *PM&R* 2021; **13**: 1027–43.

76. S. Blitshteyn, J.H. Whiteson, B. Abramoff, et al. Multi-disciplinary collaborative consensus guidance statement on the assessment and treatment of autonomic dysfunction in patients with post-acute sequelae of SARS-CoV-2 infection (PASC). *PM&R* 2022; **14**: 1270–91.

77. N. Thakur, S. Lovinsky-Desir, C. Bime, et al. The structural and social determinants of the racial/ethnic disparities in the U.S. COVID-19 pandemic: what's our role? *Am J Respir Crit Care Med* 2020; **202**: 943–9.

78. K.R. Page, A. Wilson, K.H. Phillips, et al. Responding to the disproportionate impact of COVID-19 among Latinx patients in Baltimore: the JHM Latinx Anchor Strategy. *Health Secur* 2022; **20**: 230–7.

79. L.I. Horwitz, T. Thaweethai, S. B. Brosnahan, et al. Researching COVID to enhance recovery (RECOVER) adult study protocol: rationale, objectives, and design. *PLoS One* 2023; **18**: e0286297.

80. T.L. Eaton, A. Lewis, H.S. Donovan, et al. Examining the needs of survivors of critical illness through the lens of palliative care: a qualitative study of survivor experiences. *Intensive Crit Care Nurs* 2023; **75**: 103362.

Chapter 54

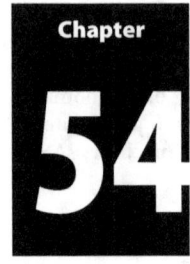

PICS in Pediatric Survivors of Critical Illness

Ericka L. Fink, Aline B. Maddux, Debbie A. Long, Brenda M. Morrow, Julia A. Heneghan, Trevor A. Hall, Karen Choong, Rubén Eduardo Lasso Palomino, Pei Fen Poh, and Joseph C. Manning

Overview of PICS-p

Over the past four decades, significant improvements in medical interventions, therapeutics, and technologies have led to improved survival rates among critically ill and injured infants, children, and adolescents [1]; however, contemporary pathways of pediatric intensive care are often characterized by invasive procedures, prolonged sedation, and exposure to potent medications. While many of these interventions are vital for immediate stabilization and recovery, they can precipitate a cascade of physiological and psychological sequelae that manifest beyond the pediatric intensive care unit (PICU) [2,3,4,5,6]. The experience of critical illness in children is also understood to impact the child's family unit.

While there has been growing recognition of increasing pediatric intensive care-associated morbidity since the mid-1980s, it was not until 2018 that post-intensive care syndrome in pediatrics (PICS-p; see Figure 54.1) was conceptualized. PICS-p provides a framework and nomenclature for the associated new or worsening impairments in PICU survivors [6].

Similar to the adult PICS and PICS-F frameworks, PICS-p categorizes outcomes across several health domains following childhood critical illness, and various trajectories of recovery are possible and dependent on many factors.

From a life-course perspective, childhood is typically a time of significant maturation and growth with respect to capacity and intrinsic ability [7]. PICS-p recognizes that the child's developmental stage when they experience a critical illness may impact their outcome and rehabilitation potential. As such, PICS can last from days to decades for both pediatric patients and their families. The PICS-p framework incorporates the child's developmental age and ability, preexisting health status, and antecedent state, all of which may be protective or exacerbating factors on outcomes [8].

Central to the ethos of care within PICUs, PICS-p is family-centered [9]. The framework recognizes the care continuum and the relationship between the critically ill/injured child and their family unit, which can include parents/caregivers, siblings, and others significant in the child's life (such as grandparents). It recognizes that exposure to the PICU and critical illness/injury is a shared experience, which can result in PICS affecting the family as well as the patient. In turn, PICS-p incorporates the relational and intergenerational impact that family well-being and functioning can have on the child's health outcomes [8].

Understanding and managing PICS-p necessitates a multidisciplinary approach that addresses the diverse needs of pediatric survivors and their families. Addressing the complexities of PICS-p is necessary to optimize long-term outcomes and provide holistic care. This chapter serves as a comprehensive guide to navigate the intricate terrain

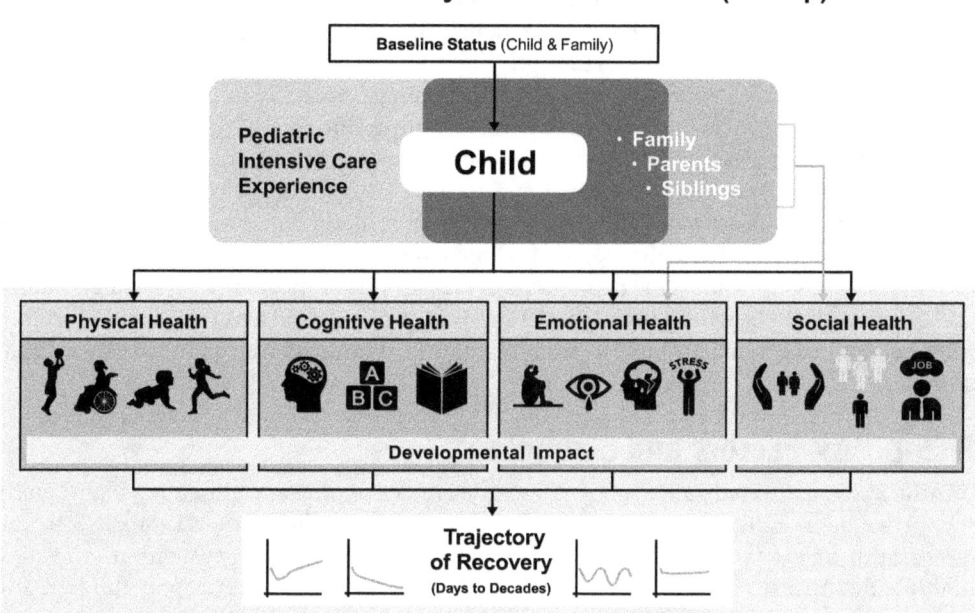

Figure 54.1 Post-Intensive Care Syndrome – Pediatrics conceptual figure. From: J. C. Manning, N.P. Pinto, J.E. Rennick, et al. Conceptualizing Post Intensive Care Syndrome in Children-The PICS-p Framework. *Pediatr Crit Care Med* 2018; **19**: 298–300. Reproduced with permission from Wolters Kluwer Health, Inc.

of PICS-p for the child and their family unit. Through an exploration of risk factors and screening, prevention and treatment in the PICU, outcomes across the four health domains (physical, emotional, cognitive, and social health), impact on the family, developmental aspects, models of care, and future directions, we aim to equip clinicians and other health professionals with the knowledge and tools necessary to identify, prevent, and manage this syndrome effectively.

Clinical Vignette

A previously healthy five-year-old presented to the hospital with four days of abdominal pain. After assessment, he was immediately taken to the operating room for relief of bowel obstruction. He required invasive mechanical ventilation and high-dose vasoactive infusions in the PICU and was ultimately cannulated onto veno-arterial extracorporeal membrane oxygenation (ECMO) due to progressive circulatory failure. On day four, he was decannulated, and upon examination had left-sided upper and lower extremity weakness. A computed tomography scan of the head demonstrated a large right-sided infarct. An intracranial pressure monitor was placed. Rehabilitative interventions were delayed until two weeks into his hospitalization due to the severity of critical illness. His 33-day PICU course was notable for cardiovascular, respiratory, renal, gastrointestinal, and neurologic dysfunction, which required 21 days of continuous renal replacement therapy, 25 days of mechanical ventilation, and 5 abdominal procedures. During this time, his family was divided between the hospital and their home, which was over two hours away. His parents would swap roles of caring for the patient's two siblings, who remained in school and visited on weekends, and experienced financial challenges associated with the loss of wages.

Post-PICU, he was admitted to the rehabilitation medicine inpatient service for one month. At discharge, he was increasingly mobile although wheelchair-dependent, was feeding by mouth without restrictions, and had average neurocognitive functioning with mild attention and processing speed impairments. A modified learning plan was developed at his school prior to returning to in-person instruction. His family arranged for outpatient rehabilitative therapies and six distinct subspecialty outpatient appointments. His goals were to continue to gain motor function skills, participate in community sports activities, and become a physical therapist like his favorite clinician.

This patient's clinical course demonstrates the significant morbidities that can accumulate after a critical illness and highlights the resilience of children and their families as they work to optimize recovery and social reintegration within the structure of their "new normal."

PICS-p Risk Factors and Screening

Identification of affected patients is a cornerstone of developing and evaluating high-quality supportive interventions. Currently, there are no clear diagnostic criteria for PICS-p, and the breadth of domains that can be affected necessitates different evaluation strategies. Multiple putative clinical risk factors exist for the development of PICS-p in children and their families, and specific risk factors vary depending on the PICS-p domain being evaluated. These include severity of illness, ICU length of stay, the need for specific interventions (e.g., medical and surgical procedures, including extracorporeal membrane oxygenation), and the development of delirium. Little is known about the specific interplay between clinical risk factors and an individual patient or family, considering the many preexisting comorbidities that are often present in children prior to critical illness. Although clinicians may have a sense for which patients and families are at greatest risk of long-term sequelae, even patients with acute conditions considered to be low-risk (e.g., bronchiolitis) develop PICS-p [10,11,12].

Given the lack of clear evidence regarding which patients and families may be at the highest risk, screening for the presence and resolution of PICS-p is necessary. This is recognized in several guidelines focused on individual patient populations, including survivors of acute lung injury [12], extracorporeal membrane oxygenation [13,14,15], cardiac arrest [16], and the general PICU population [17,18]. Despite recommendations that screening should occur, there is currently no validated screening tool for PICS-p. Recommendations include a core outcome measurement set designed by multidisciplinary stakeholders [17,18]; however, these screening tools may not apply to all survivors, with many instruments unable to capture the full range of developmental trajectories seen in pediatrics. Children with preexisting physical or intellectual disabilities may also be more difficult to screen due to their limited functional capabilities [19]. Additionally, little is known about the validity and reliability of proxy-report tools in this patient population.

There is currently no standard regarding the optimal location or timing of screening. Screening may be performed by a primary care provider, an ICU follow-up clinic, or a subspecialist, depending on knowledge, resources, and contact with the patient and family [20]. Similarly, the cadence of screening may be impacted by ongoing hospitalization (whether to the general ward or a rehabilitation unit), the familiarity of outpatient providers with PICS-p, and whether adequate time and resources necessary for screening are available. Assessment of PICS-p is also limited by the need for longitudinal data, including pre-illness data, which provide a more comprehensive understanding of a patient's recovery trajectory than measurement at a single time point.

Prevention and Treatment in the ICU

Key strategies to prevent critical illness sequelae and optimize long-term outcomes are targeted as modifiable risk factors for PICS-p, specifically sedation practices, prolonged immobility, and the PICU environment [21]. The "ABCDEF" or "A–F" bundle is recommended as a standard of care based on accumulating evidence of efficacy in reducing critical illness morbidities and the potential for optimizing functional recovery [22,23,24,25]. The ABCDEF bundle components are interdependent, with a potential dose-response with incremental bundle utilization [26]. (A similar ABCDEF bundle is also utilized in the care of adult ICU patients and is described in detail in Chapter 11.)

A Assess, Prevent, and Manage Pain

There is a clear association between pain symptoms experienced by children in the PICU and poor post-discharge health-related quality of life (HRQL), persistent pain, and subsequent psychosocial dysfunction [27,28]. An analgesia-first or analgo-sedation approach advocates for routine pain monitoring and optimizing comfort. Recommended first-line interventions are non-pharmacological (e.g., family participation, non-nutritive sucking, and optimizing the environment) followed by the choice of analgesia and sedation (see "C") [29]. Opioid analgesics are the mainstay of acute pharmacological management of moderate to severe medical and surgical pain, while non-opioid analgesics (e.g., intravenous or enteral nonsteroidal anti-inflammatory drugs and acetaminophen) should be considered as adjuncts to optimize pain control and decrease opioid requirements [24].

B Both Spontaneous Awakening Trials (SATs) and Spontaneous Breathing Trials (SBTs)

The "B" component of the adult ABCDEF bundle involves both SATs and SBTs; however, it has been proposed that the "B" component for pediatric practice should instead focus on "breathing and optimal mechanical ventilation," given that SATs are associated with increased mortality in children [30].

Using a sedation and ventilator liberation protocol has been shown to reduce the time to extubation significantly [31]. Lung protective strategies mitigate against ventilator-induced lung injury by limiting stress and strain during mechanical ventilation, while diaphragmatic protection aims to balance ventilator-induced diaphragmatic strain with dysfunction and atrophy. To achieve the "B" component of the bundle, ventilation and analgo-sedation strategies ("A" and "C") need to be aligned and individualized to promote patient-ventilator synchrony and maintain or restore diaphragmatic activity while avoiding excessive respiratory effort. The role of inspiratory muscle training in pediatric practice is not clear but has been associated with improved exercise tolerance, increased respiratory muscle strength, and reduced dyspnea in different pediatric populations [32]. Inspiratory muscle training could therefore be considered as part of a comprehensive pulmonary rehabilitation program to optimize cardiorespiratory function after critical illness.

C Choice of Analgesia and Sedation

Pain, sedation management, polypharmacy, and disrupted sleep in critically ill children are clear risk factors for the development of adverse neurocognitive sequelae associated with PICS-p [33,34]. Sedation stewardship is therefore an essential strategy for optimizing long-term outcomes. "C" promotes an analgesia-first, benzodiazepine-sparing approach that avoids excessive sedation, allows daytime awakening, and promotes nighttime sleep. This has been shown to reduce sedative exposure and delirium risk, facilitate early mobilization, and enhance patient communication and family satisfaction [22,29]. "C" requires regular assessment of pain and sedation levels and complementary non-pharmacological approaches to comfort management and circadian rhythm regulation [24]. Opioid analgesics and/or alpha agonists may be considered first-line sedative agents; given the association with delirium, benzodiazepine use is minimized [35]. Depth of sedation should be individualized and targets set and reassessed regularly according to the patient's clinical status. The use of sedation protocols and weaning guidelines is suggested to facilitate this goal [24].

D Delirium: Assess, Prevent, and Manage

Delirium in critically ill children is associated with adverse short-term outcomes, including mortality and increased length of PICU stay [36], and is increasingly recognized to have a long-lasting adverse impact on patients and decreased quality-of-life after discharge [37,38]. Noise pollution and considerable nighttime and insufficient daytime light exposures are common in the PICU and are significant risk factors for developing delirium [39,40]. Restricting family presence is a key risk factor for parental stress, delirium, and PICS-p [41,42].

E Early Mobility and Exercise

There is growing evidence that introducing movement and holistic rehabilitation in the PICU may improve patient outcomes and prevent critical illness-acquired morbidities. The goal of early mobilization is to minimize critical illness-acquired deconditioning and delirium and improve long-term physical and neurocognitive outcomes [43]. Mobility-based rehabilitation has been consistently demonstrated to be safe [43,44,45]. Daily risk-based assessment for readiness for mobilization is recommended as soon as possible following PICU admission such that goal-targeted mobilization can occur early [24]. Ambulation may not be feasible or appropriate in children, given the wide range of age and developmental levels in this population. Mobilization activities for critically ill or injured children include a range of graded, age-, and condition-appropriate activities requiring variable levels of assistance [46]. Activities start with passive activities for medically unstable patients requiring maximal assistance, such as positioning, passive exercises, and transfers, followed by progression to more active mobility-associated interventions requiring increasing patient effort.

F Family Engagement and Empowerment

Parent-child interdependence plays a key role in PICS-p outcomes [8]. Parental stress, family satisfaction with care, and family functioning significantly influence a child's longer-term functional recovery from critical illness [41,47,48]. Encouraging family presence and engagement in the care of their critically ill child facilitates analgesia and comfort, improves patient safety and communication, reduces the risk of delirium, and facilitates early mobilization [49,50]. Family engagement impacts a child's recovery from critical illness as well as family functioning after PICU discharge and should be the standard of care in all PICUs [51].

PICU Diaries

In some studies, ICU diaries decrease anxiety, depression, and post-traumatic stress symptoms and improve HRQL among adult ICU survivors (see Chapter 18 for additional information) [52,53]. Diaries are perceived as beneficial by parents and healthcare providers and help to reduce family stress and anxiety [54]. Research is ongoing to understand the effect of PICU diaries on PICS-p.

In summary, the focus of critical care is to actively initiate preventative strategies alongside acute management of organ dysfunction to prevent critical illness-acquired morbidities and provide our patients and families with the best opportunity to optimize functional recovery and HRQL.

Introduction to Functional Outcomes

Functional outcomes include physical, emotional, behavioral, neurocognitive, and social health, including how one participates in activities and interacts with society [8].

Physical Health

Reported physical health outcomes following PICU discharge range from muscle weakness, general fatigue, and sleep disturbances to feeding difficulties, gross and fine motor delays, and impairments in daily activities and mobility [55,56]. Physical health outcomes in critically ill children are important; they impact length of hospital stay and family outcomes, which in turn significantly influence functional recovery and HRQL [57]. Identified risk factors for prolonged physical impairment include higher severity of illness, duration of organ failure, neurologic injury, invasive mechanical ventilation, immobility, and excessive sedation [33,41,58]. The trajectory of physical health recovery in critically ill children is heterogenous and dependent on demographic factors, socioeconomic factors, and family functioning.

Twenty to eighty percent of critically ill children experience functional impairments that can persist for months to years after PICU discharge [41,59–61]. The frequency and nature of physical health impairments vary based on the method and timing of assessment [62]. Furthermore, clinician-applied tools are anchored on disability, do not capture all domains of functioning, and are not as sensitive to change as patient-reported outcome measures [41,63].

Although preexisting conditions are a risk factor for worse functional outcomes, patients with better pre-illness HRQL have been shown to experience longer durations of HRQL impairment [41,61]. Further studies to improve physical health recovery are needed because prolonged impairment may limit a child's ability to participate in activities that foster physical, social, and cognitive development, decreasing the likelihood of maintaining a healthy lifestyle in adulthood.

Emotional Health

A full understanding of post-PICU emotional health in children along with the impact of the interdependent relationship between the child and caregiver is only beginning to emerge. Emotional well-being is particularly important when thinking about the trajectory of recovery in children after a PICU admission.

There is a growing body of evidence demonstrating negative psychological sequelae in pediatric critical care survivors, including increased levels of anxiety, depression, post-traumatic stress symptoms (PTSS) or disorder (PTSD), and pediatric medical traumatic stress (PMTS) [51,64,65,66,67,68,69,70]. In children, these negative outcomes are often colored by fear of future medical care or invasive procedures, the severity of illness, and developmental stage. Results from a systematic review show 16–28% of children experience a deterioration in emotional functioning following PICU hospitalization, regardless of their presenting injury or illness [71]. Another systematic review and meta-analysis of 7,786 children indicates that 5% to 88% of PICU survivors experience long-term psychological issues after discharge, with increased emotional and behavioral problems that impact important cognitive functions (e.g., intelligence and memory) [72], congruent with the PICS-p multimorbidity framework.

Similarly, parents of PICU survivors frequently endorse moderate or severe symptoms of anxiety (45%) and depression (32%) for their child in comparison to their pre-PICU baseline [73]. Further, in a large cohort of parents, 10% received a new mental health diagnosis in the 6 months after their child's PICU hospitalization, representing a 110% increase from pre-PICU rates, and parental diagnosis of PTSS or PTSD increased by 87% from the pre-PICU to the post-PICU period [74]. In addition to negatively impacting parents of children who survive the PICU, parental PTSS interferes with the child's rehabilitative progress; parental mental health struggles impact access to care for children and worsen a variety of child outcomes in physical, cognitive, and emotional domains [74,75,76,77,78,79,80].

While premorbid emotional health status and/or developmental problems have been shown to predict post-admission emotional and behavioral functioning [66,81,82], these are not always predictive of worse mood and anxiety symptoms in children [83]. Further, there is an increasing body of evidence to suggest that experiences that are specifically related to the PICU (see the subsequent section on Cognitive Health) are associated with negative long-term psychological outcomes [68,69,84,85]. As such, it can be argued that children requiring critical care are highly vulnerable to emotional distress given their limited life experience and underdeveloped coping skills for such situations [86]. This highlights the need to assess and address the impact of emotional morbidities both within and after the PICU to provide proactive (instead of reactive) support via a trauma-informed care approach [87].

Although research is limited, emerging data suggest interventions can improve education about PICS and reduce child and family morbidity [64]. Direct intervention studies often focus on educating parents as opposed to children. Educational and anticipatory guidance interventions include handouts, face-to-face communication, videos, computer modules, and directed activities. Simple interventions, like providing informational brochures to parents, are feasible and reduce parental anxiety, which in turn can have a positive impact on the child's emotional health [88,89]. Building on well-established care models for child mental health in the outpatient context (e.g., school resources, home health, psychologic counseling, and out-of-home therapies) is of paramount importance for children who survive the PICU. The primary role of the patient's and family's experience of illness has been integrated into a comprehensive model of PMTS, the Integrative Trajectory Model.

Cognitive Health

Cognitive outcomes are well-studied in children with acquired brain injuries, in whom ongoing cognitive performance deficits are common [90,91,92,93,94]. While cognitive impact is related to severity of the neurological insult, even patients with *mild* brain injury are at risk for chronic cognitive deficits, with age and developmental stage likely affecting response to intervention [90]. PICU survivors admitted for non-neurological disease, such as respiratory failure and sepsis, should also be considered at risk for cognitive sequelae related to secondary neurologic injury. Cognitive impairment may result from inflammation, hypoxia-ischemia, certain medications, and critical care interventions, including mechanical ventilation, central venous access, neurosurgery, intracranial pressure monitoring, and cardiopulmonary resuscitation, all of which have been associated with worsened brain pathology and cognitive outcomes [95,96].

A recent systematic review of cognitive morbidities in PICU survivors found worse outcomes compared with healthy controls or normative population data across the cognitive domains of general intelligence, attention, processing speed, executive functioning, memory, visual motor integration, and motor development [97]. Worse neurocognitive outcomes were associated with those who had direct brain involvement; nonetheless, because children with a history of cardiac arrest, traumatic brain injury, or genetic anomalies associated with neurocognitive impairment were excluded, the systematic review findings show that cognitive morbidities are specifically associated with PICU-related factors and critical illness. Impairments in any of the cognitive domains have the potential to negatively impact school performance and lifelong neurodevelopment [34,91,97,98,99,100,101]. Other research has demonstrated that cognitive impairment is more common among children surviving a PICU admission requiring mechanical ventilation, sedation, and analgesia, and post-discharge cognitive impairment may also be more common among children from lower socioeconomic backgrounds [85,102,103].

Accordingly, the post-PICU population would benefit from follow-up cognitive evaluation and treatment by a qualified specialist (both in the acute recovery phase and in the long-term) to mitigate the risk of long-term cognitive dysfunction [84,104,105]. Interventions for cognitive concerns include cognitive rehabilitation strategies designed to reestablish previously learned behaviors or to develop new compensatory mechanisms in impaired cognitive domains [106,107]. Intervention strategies such as daily attention training, self-instruction, structured workstations, diary training, behavioral coaching, family delivered support, and cognitive behavioral therapy/psychoeducation have been shown to improve attention, memory, adaptive functioning, mood, and stress response in children with a history of critical illness [106,107,108,109]. Moreover, data in PICU survivors also suggest an additional benefit to cognition when physical and cognitive therapies are combined in a multifaceted rehabilitation approach [110,111].

Social Health

Critical illness can have profound and lasting effects on social health, including social activity at home, school, and within the community [112]. These effects may limit social recovery for children and their families. For example, in a cohort of children with acute respiratory failure, two out of three children missed school in the 6 months after discharge, and, of those who missed school, one of four children missed nearly a month or more [113]. Additionally, families report a lack of support for school reintegration with a resultant impact on their child's academic achievement [114]. For caregivers, affected social health domains include employment, housing, economic resources, and family functioning. In the same cohort as above, more than half of caregivers missed work during the 6 months after PICU discharge, and, of those who missed work, one in four missed more than 10 days [113]. This interruption in work can have impacts on social interactions and inflict financial stressors [115,116]. Sibling wellness is not well-studied, but it is recognized that siblings are also at high risk of social health impacts [115]. The rate of childhood traumatic experiences is known to be elevated in critically ill children; prior life experiences and the role of inpatient injury-related factors, such as recurrent invasive procedures or the nature of the illness (e.g., chronic illness of physical trauma), are predictors of trauma symptom trajectories and ongoing PMTS following PICU admission. To date, inadequate attention has been paid to premorbid trauma, how it may interface with the PICU environment, and how it ultimately contributes to PICS-p. Trauma-informed care should be provided to patients and families while in the PICU to enhance care, minimize retraumatization, and facilitate positive coping during the recovery process [87,117].

Evaluation of social health in pediatric survivors of critical illness is challenging, as no comprehensive, validated measures are available to assess this important outcome in critically ill children [63,112]. To date, qualitative studies have identified several barriers and facilitators for children and families to restore social health and to adjust to a "new normal" after critical illness [118]. Families reported using a variety of compensatory or supportive strategies to promote social health for their child and family during and after critical illness [119]. For example, during the hospitalization, caregivers recommended finding time to connect with their significant other or other support persons to ensure maintenance of a strong family unit [120]. After discharge, strategies included changes to the home structure (e.g., adding a ramp) to facilitate the child's functional limitations, a sibling assuming more caregiving responsibilities, and parental employment modification or termination to provide the support needed for their child [118]. Larger studies measuring recovery of social relationships, roles, and activities and evaluating interventions to improve social health are needed [112].

New Technology and Complex Needs

Most pediatric patients ill enough to necessitate PICU admission will survive, yet many emerge with enduring health complications, and some will depend on long-term, life-sustaining advanced medical technologies. Indeed, an increasing number of survivors of pediatric critical illness develop lifelong reliance on medical technologies [121]; for example, in Canada, the incidence of long-term pediatric mechanical ventilation has increased by 37% over a 14-year period. In addition to mechanical ventilation, other long-term support devices include tracheostomy and gastrostomy tubes, central venous and dialysis catheters, and ventricular assist devices (VADs) [122]. Oftentimes, multiple support devices are needed simultaneously, and the duration of support is dependent on a child's trajectory. Tracheostomies, for instance, may facilitate early rehabilitation and discharge to home. This, in turn, may enable a sense of normalcy by allowing home care that includes monitoring, intervention, and consultation regarding the ability to remain at home during periods of future acute illness. Unsurprisingly, this transition introduces challenges for families, including a stressful transition from hospital to home and the heightened risk of medical emergencies at home.

The approach to pediatric patient support requires adjustments for growth and development, including device upsizing. Moreover, the impact of medical technology on children varies by geographic and socioeconomic factors, with higher mortality associated with residence in lower-income areas. Higher income may afford better nutrition and safer housing, mitigating negative environmental impacts such as exposure to cigarettes and low-quality heating [123]. Additionally, disparities in PICU utilization following tracheostomy and gastrostomy tube placements were observed among Black children and those with public insurance [124], underscoring the influence of social determinants of health on outcomes.

VADs, now a standard care element for advanced heart failure, serve as a bridge-to-transplant for 30–50% of candidates [125]. Innovations like the Berlin EXCOR and HeartMate III have revolutionized patient management, permitting discharge from the PICU to less intensive hospital settings or even home care using portable units. A study highlighting the lived experiences of six Canadian school-aged children on VAD support at home reveals their consciousness of an atypical existence, challenges in explaining their condition to peers, and a constant awareness of potential life-threatening events [126]. This mirrors the reported experience of children with tracheostomies and their families, with parents eager for their children to live at home, acknowledging that respiratory technology plays a key role in minimizing hospital admissions [127]. Although technology enables a degree of normalcy, these children and families remain distinct from their peers. Reliance on medical technology and other forms of medical complexity often necessitates repeated interactions with healthcare services. As such, pediatric clinicians of the future must broaden their scope of care for these children, extending their support beyond the confines of the PICU. The role of complex care pediatricians is vital in bridging the gap within traditional health systems accustomed to episodic care, ensuring integrated care for children with complex needs.

The potential impact of recurrent critical illness on children reliant on multiple medical technologies or with neurologic differences are unknown. Methodological challenges to assessing these outcomes include inapplicability of screening instruments and the individual developmental trajectories of all children [122]. Many children with technology dependence may be excluded from ICU research studies due to difficulty in untangling the acute on chronic nature of episodic worsening.

Developmental Aspects

The pediatric brain continues to develop from birth into early adulthood. Interpreting morbidities through the lens of the patient's developmental stage is essential and necessary so that age- and developmental status-appropriate interventions focused on improving long-term outcomes for pediatric survivors of critical illness can be developed and implemented.

Early identification of PICS-p is especially important for infants and young children because they are still in the process of creating foundational brain circuits upon which later development is built, resulting in a unique vulnerability for this population [128]. Relative to other age groups, brain injury is common in infants and young children, who are more likely to suffer severe injuries requiring hospitalization, with a concomitant higher burden of long-term morbidity across physical, emotional, cognitive, and social domains [129,130,131,132,133,134,135,136]. Other critical care conditions and interventions have the potential for negative long-term implications in early childhood. For example, in 2016, a Safety Communication from the United States Food and Drug Administration warned against the prolonged or repeated use of general anesthesia in children under the age of three years and pregnant women [137]. Overall, historical practice trends show that many infants and young children, regardless of their presentation and PICU course, do not receive assessment or interventions until they are older, when impairments are more apparent, a phenomenon called "growing into deficits." The identification of modifiable risk factors and the development of interventions to improve outcomes remain elusive [104,138,139,140].

The impact of PICS-p most certainly extends into functioning at school. Because school is the occupation of childhood for most children, participation often includes primary opportunities for physical, cognitive, and social engagement. Not only are children absent from school due to hospitalization, rehabilitative care, and doctor's appointments, but ongoing symptomatology can impede learning and participation. Even so, it is important to successfully reintegrate a PICU survivor back into their academic environment as soon as it is safe to do so.

Recent work has highlighted the difficulties caregivers face when navigating their child's return to school and the clear advantage when a recovering patient's school attendance is systematically addressed [141]. To that end, outpatient healthcare providers are often tasked with evaluating for PICS-p-related morbidities to inform plans for ongoing care, which often includes suggestions focused on a successful reentry to school [114]. This task is complicated due to the training needed to assess all PICS-p domains with fidelity across the developmental spectrum. In addition to developing patient-specific plans (in cooperation with professionals in the education system as well as parents/caregivers) to facilitate reentry into school with individualized supports, the PICS-p multidisciplinary team can also inform the development of plans to address challenges and create compensatory strategies to optimize function [84].

This chapter's cognitive outcomes section explores the difficulties that PICU survivors face to engage academically and acquire and retain new knowledge and skill sets. Relatedly, emotional and behavioral challenges can exacerbate cognitive weaknesses, hamper peer and teacher interactions, and reduce academic engagement. Consistently, children with a history of brain-related illness or injury show poorer academic functioning, including lower levels of academic achievement and an increased need for educational support. As such, it is important to remember that in the United States, only those students whose disability harms their education are eligible to receive special education services through an Individualized Education Plan (IEP) [142]. Moreover, to be eligible for special education services, the PICU survivor must demonstrate the need for special education and related services to keep their performance from declining and to ensure that they make measurable progress [142]. If a student does not qualify for an IEP, Section 504 offers coverage to address issues that, while not adversely impacting learning, still substantially limit a major life activity. Section 504 plans may also provide an effective means of monitoring potential PICS-p morbidities that take time to emerge [143]. The availability of special educational and related services is limited in many poorly resourced countries.

Barriers to establishing school support are multifactorial and include communication difficulties between medical, educational, and family systems; challenges obtaining medical documentation of the hospital course; inappropriate classification categories for nontraumatic acquired brain injuries; minimal involvement of youth within the identification, evaluation, and implementation process; difficulties accessing resources; and educators' lack of knowledge of brain injury and its sequelae [143]. Solutions for ensuring children and adolescents are properly identified and effectively supported in schools include strategies such as improving hospital-to-school transition services/models, empowering caregivers and clinical providers to enhance communication with schools about the child's educational needs, enhancing professional development and in-service education programs, and engaging in advocacy efforts around policies designed to assist schools in identifying and serving students more efficiently [84,114,141,142,143].

PICS-p-Family

The concept of family includes the patient's parents, siblings, and extended family, such as grandparents [51]. This extended support network plays a crucial role, particularly given the bidirectional interactions that occur among members: between the PICU survivor and their parents, the parents and the unaffected siblings, and the PICU survivor and their siblings [10]. The pediatric context views the family as indispensable participants in the child's recovery, deeply involved in decision-making and the execution of care plans. Pediatric critical illness significantly affects family functioning, impacting the cognitive and physical health of family members.

The caregiving role transition from PICU admission to home discharge marks a significant phase in recovery, signaling not only the resumption of traditional parental roles but also the onset of potential challenges affecting parents' well-being. Reports indicate physical exhaustion and insomnia during PICU stays [161], with continued care demands potentially hindering parental physical recovery. Psychologically, up to 50% of parents experience depression three months after discharge, and 30% exhibit symptoms of post-traumatic stress [161], with maternal stress levels directly influencing the child's stress symptoms up to a year post-discharge [84]. Socially, the impact is profound; traditional caregivers, often mothers, may assume unpaid caregiving roles, with many reporting employment adjustments to meet their child's care needs, alongside a hesitancy to engage socially until a sense of normalcy is regained [162]. The degree and nature of these impacts vary across cultural and economic contexts, underscoring the need for tailored support strategies that address the unique needs of each family to facilitate recovery.

For siblings, having a critically ill or injured brother or sister in the PICU can result in multiple negative reactions, including stress, sadness, and disruptions from parental/child separation [163]. Although evidence is limited, studies highlight the significant impact of a child's critical illness on healthy siblings, with changes in parental attention and shifts in parenting styles leading to behavioral changes in up to 21% of siblings, and alterations in living and schooling arrangements in 40% to accommodate the needs of the PICU survivor [164]. Family dynamics pre-illness and the age of the healthy siblings play pivotal roles in post-illness interactions, with younger siblings often experiencing jealousy and older siblings possibly taking on supportive roles [162].

The adage "It takes a village to raise a child" rings especially true in the context of a PICU survivor's care. Grandparents and the wider family network, regardless of their proximity, often become invaluable in providing support. Extended family can alleviate daily pressures by assisting with household duties, caring for other children, and offering emotional support during challenging times [165]. This involvement, from emotional to instrumental support, such as transportation for medical appointments, helps lessen the financial and emotional burden on parents [162]. In conclusion, healthcare professionals are urged to adopt a holistic approach in the post-intensive care management of families. Despite the scarcity of evidence, the existing research underscores the profound impact of a child's critical illness on parents, healthy siblings, and the extended family, highlighting the necessity of offering support to all family members. An inclusive strategy not only aids in the emotional and social well-being of parents and siblings but may also contribute significantly to the overall resilience of the family unit during challenging times.

After-ICU Models of Care

While there are emerging efforts to provide an integrated, collaborative, and interdisciplinary approach to address the complex multidimensional nature of post-PICU morbidities, to date, very few programs that are designed to specifically detect and address PICS-related challenges in pediatric survivors of critical illness exist [84,104,105,144].

The landscape of post-PICU care is complex, with limited evidence to support the efficacy of any one care model [145]. Despite this, the National Institute for Health and Clinical Excellence (NICE) guidelines on rehabilitation after critical illness recommend that follow-up services should be provided for patients and their families [146]. Unlike for other specific populations, such as neonates and cardiac patients, there are no clear guidelines for the follow-up of children after their admission to the PICU. Various models of care have been proposed, ranging from structured and multidisciplinary follow-up clinics to remote monitoring. Effective models of care are essential to address the multiple areas of need in children and their families; however, the debate on the optimal provision of post-PICU care is multifaceted, with each potential model having its own set of strengths and challenges.

The tertiary care model of PICU follow-up is often coordinated as an outpatient appointment typically run by PICU clinicians with intimate knowledge of PICU interventions and potential complications. This model enables specialized, hospital-based care that includes a review of the PICU admission, ongoing medications, and assessment of PICS-p domains. This model requires the availability of at least one clinician and a physical room for the appointment, but multidisciplinary teams are often utilized to address all domains. Several hospital-based clinics utilize an interdisciplinary approach, including neuropsychology, to review and refer children and their families to relevant treatment providers within the hospital to reduce PICS-p co-morbidities [55,104,141]. The often-centralized nature of this care raises concerns about access and equity, especially for families who live in rural or remote areas. In addition, some patients and families can find revisiting the hospital quite distressing, which makes acceptance of the intervention suboptimal [147]. Difficulty traveling to the hospital and arranging time off from work have been cited as other reasons for nonattendance [148].

The primary care model, on the other hand, emphasizes the role of primary care providers (PCPs), the gateways to child health and well-being, in routine child health screening. A significant benefit for this model is the decreased time to PICS-p evaluation by a healthcare provider who is familiar to the child and family. Models of post-ICU care without in-person attendance at the index hospital potentially have higher rates of recruitment, intervention delivery success, and increased participant retention when compared to hospital-based interventions [149]. PCP models can also offer support for common post-PICU issues like growth, development, and vaccination catch-up; however, the lack of widespread knowledge about PICS-p among PCPs, decreased comfort providing care to complex PICU patients, and inadequate discharge documentation present barriers to effective care [20,150]. Further collaborative work is required to co-design adequate discharge documentation, e-learning content, and identification of PICS-p symptomatology if a primary care model of PICU follow-up is prioritized.

A hybrid care model suggests a shared or integrated care approach, where acute and primary care healthcare professionals collaborate to provide ongoing care. Various versions of hybrid care models have been explored for pediatric chronic illness and typically include a tertiary or primary healthcare provider collaboratively managing child and family care with other healthcare providers and organizations [151,152,153,155]. This model has shown some early benefit in bridging the gap between primary and tertiary care for PICU children [156,157], and it is particularly beneficial in rural, regional, or remote areas, where centralized services pose distance and time barriers. The hybrid model's strength lies in its flexibility and the ability to combine the expertise of specialized clinicians with the accessibility of primary care providers. Considerations for this model of care should include attention to contextual variations in the implementation setting and building cross-sector engagement and buy-in [158].

Regardless of the follow-up care model, several factors are key to optimizing outcomes for both the child and their family. Incorporating socio-ecological theory into the care framework can enhance understanding of the child's recovery within the context of their family, culture, and environment, leading to more effective interventions [159,160]. Assessment should be undertaken across all PICS-p domains, as impairments can span several domains, suggesting that care should be provided by multidisciplinary healthcare professionals [161]. Use of telehealth and other emerging technologies should be integrated to ensure the best engagement and accessibility for all patients, regardless of geography or socio-demographics [162,163]. Finally, there is a global lack of awareness of PICS-p that requires education and training for PICU clinicians, primary healthcare providers, and parents [164,165,166]. A good understanding of the challenges to implementing follow-up care highlights the need for comprehensive planning, adequate funding, and continuous evaluation to ensure that care models are effectively implemented and can meet the needs of children with PICS-p and their families. Ideally, the optimal model for post-PICU care should be tailored to the local healthcare system, the resources available, and the specific needs of the child and family. Integrating models of care, supported by risk stratification and technological advancements, can provide a robust framework for delivering comprehensive care to PICU survivors.

Future Directions and Conclusions

In summary, hundreds of thousands of children and their families around the world are at risk of PICS-p. Stakeholders are calling for more attention to the impact and for more resources to support new, effective preventative and therapeutic interventions to improve PICS-p in children and their families. Table 54.1 highlights some key knowledge gaps and associated recommendations for future research. Optimizing collaborative efforts, innovative strategies, and increased resources are needed to address this next great challenge facing the field of pediatric critical care for surviving children and families.

Table 54.1 Key knowledge gaps and recommendations for future research to improve outcomes for children at risk of PICS-p

Key Knowledge Gaps	Recommendations for Future Research
Risk factors for PICS-p	Identify patient and clinical course characteristics associated with risk for PICS-p (including which domain(s) are impaired) to create screening tools and improve targeted interventions aimed at mitigating or improving these outcomes.
Preventative strategies	Determine factors independently associated with PICS-p to inform preventative interventions and quality improvement.
Approach to assessment	**Timing**: Optimal timing for assessments may differ based on domain affected. It is likely that multiple timepoints after critical illness must be assessed to comprehensively measure PICS-p domains given the undulating recovery course in some patients and families. **Developmental Capacity**: Evaluation of patients at various developmental stages and on varying developmental trajectories complicates the ability to characterize the impact of critical illness on patients. Further studies are needed to understand the trajectory of recovery after critical illness and impact on development. **Location**: The most appropriate setting for evaluation of PICS-p will be different based on patient characteristics and resource availability. Appropriate locations could include the patient's medical home, subspecialty clinics, or post-ICU follow-up clinics.
Impactful interventions	Interventions are needed acutely and during the post-PICU phase aimed at treatment of PICS-p. To optimize study design to test these interventions, it is imperative to target the highest risk populations, which can be identified through patient, clinical course, and biomarker profiles that can be derived from analysis of blood, urine, tracheal aspirate, imaging, or EEG testing.
Personal and neighborhood social determinants of health	Impact of these social determinants of health on recovery and testing of interventions that improve outcomes.
Inequitable access to care	Identify patient populations who lack access to care and identify methods to improve care delivery to these vulnerable populations.

Inclusion of child and family perspectives in prioritizing research strategies	Researchers and funders should systematically seek input from family stakeholders to prioritize programs of research and execution of studies.
Information relating to proxy-report metrics in screening and longitudinal assessment of PICS-p	Evaluation of the most effective method to capture patient-reported outcomes when limitations exist due to patient condition or mental capacity.
Effect of recurrent episodes of critical illness on PICS-p trajectory	PICS-p trajectory, and how it might be affected by hospital and PICU readmission.

Key Points

1. Post-intensive care syndrome in pediatrics (PICS-p) comprises aspects of physical, social, emotional, and cognitive health in children experiencing critical illness and their family units.
2. The child's age, developmental stage, and preexisting conditions at the time of critical illness may affect PICS-p risk, functional domains, and recovery trajectory.
3. Little is currently known about the optimal tools, timing, or location to screen for PICS-p.
4. PICS-p prevention may be assisted with implementation of the principles of ICU liberation. Models of care proposed for the evaluation and treatment of PICS-p range from structured and multidisciplinary follow-up clinics to remote monitoring, but efficacy data are lacking.

References

1. A.G. Woodruff, K. Choong. Long-term outcomes and the post-intensive care syndrome in critically ill children: a North American perspective. *Children (Basel)* 2021; **8**(4): 254.
2. J.D. Wilkinson, M.M. Pollack, U. E. Ruttimann, et al. Outcome of pediatric patients with multiple organ system failure. *Crit Care Med* 1986; **14**: 271–4.
3. M.M. Pollack, U.E. Ruttimann, P. R. Getson. Accurate prediction of the outcome of pediatric intensive care: a new quantitative method. *N Engl J Med* 1987; **316**: 134–9.
4. B.J. Stoll, R.C. Holman, A. Schuchat. Decline in sepsis-associated neonatal and infant deaths in the United States, 1979 through 1994. *Pediatrics* 1998; **102**: e18.
5. P. Namachivayam, F. Shann, L. Shekerdemian, et al. Three decades of pediatric intensive care: who was admitted, what happened in intensive care, and what happened afterward. *Pediatric Critical Care Medicine* 2010; **11**: 549–55.
6. B. Tan, J.J. Wong, R. Sultana, et al. Global case-fatality rates in pediatric severe sepsis and septic shock: a systematic review and meta-analysis. *JAMA Pediatr* 2019; **173**: 352–62.
7. B. Mikkelsen, J. Williams, I. Rakovac, et al. Life course approach to prevention and control of non-communicable diseases. *BMJ* 2019; **364**: 257.
8. J.C. Manning, N.P. Pinto, J.E. Rennick, et al. Conceptualizing post intensive care syndrome in children: the PICS-p framework. *Pediatr Crit Care Med* 2018; **19**: 298–300.
9. J.E. Davidson, R.A. Aslakson, A.C. Long, et al. Guidelines for family-centered care in the neonatal, pediatric, and adult ICU. *Crit Care Med* 2017; **45**: 103–28.
10. E.S.V. de Sonnaville, M. Königs, C.S. H. Aarnoudse-Moens, et al. Long-term follow-up of daily life functioning after pediatric intensive care unit admission. *J Pediatr* 2023; **260**: 113477.
11. S.L. Shein, K.N. Slain, J.A. Clayton, et al. Neurologic and functional morbidity in critically ill children with bronchiolitis. *Pediatr Crit Care Med* 2017; **18**: 1106–13.
12. E.Y. Killien, A.B. Maddux, S.M. Tse, R. S. Watson. Outcomes of children surviving pediatric acute respiratory distress syndrome: from the second pediatric acute lung injury consensus conference. *Pediatr Crit Care Med* 2023; **24**: S28–s44.
13. R.P. Barbaro, D. Brodie, G. MacLaren. Bridging the gap between intensivists and primary care clinicians in extracorporeal membrane oxygenation for respiratory failure in children: a review. *JAMA Pediatr* 2021; **175**: 510–17.

14. H. Ijsselstijn, R.M. Schiller, C. Holder, et al. Extracorporeal Life Support Organization (ELSO) guidelines for follow-up after neonatal and pediatric extracorporeal membrane oxygenation. *Asaio j* 2021; **67**: 955-63.
15. A.R. Lewis, J. Wray, M. O'Callaghan, A. L. Wroe. Parental symptoms of posttraumatic stress after pediatric extracorporeal membrane oxygenation. *Pediatr Crit Care Med* 2014; **15**: e80-8.
16. A.A. Topjian, A. de Caen, M. S. Wainwright, et al. Pediatric post-cardiac arrest care: a scientific statement from the American Heart Association. *Circulation* 2019; **140**: e194-e233.
17. E.L. Fink, A.B. Maddux, N. Pinto, et al. A core outcome set for pediatric critical care. *Crit Care Med* 2020; **48**: 1819-28.
18. N.P. Pinto, A.B. Maddux, L.A. Dervan, et al. A core outcome measurement set for pediatric critical care. *Pediatr Crit Care Med* 2022; **23**: 893-907.
19. J.A. Heneghan, S.A. Sobotka, M. Hallman, et al. Outcome measures following critical illness in children with disabilities: a scoping review. *Front Pediatr* 2021; **9**: 689485.
20. L. Anthony, A. Hilder, D. Newcomb, et al. General practitioner perspectives on a shared-care model for paediatric patients post-intensive care: a cross-sectional survey. *Aust Crit Care* 2023; **36**: 492-8.
21. K. Choong. PICU-acquired complications: the new marker of the quality of care. *ICU Management and Practice* 2019:**19**(2): 85-89.
22. S. Simone, S. Edwards, A. Lardieri, et al. Implementation of an ICU bundle: an interprofessional quality improvement project to enhance delirium management and monitor delirium prevalence in a single PICU. *Pediatr Crit Care Med* 2017; **18**: 531-40.
23. B.T. Pun, M.C. Balas, M.A. Barnes-Daly, et al. Caring for critically ill patients with the ABCDEF bundle: Results of the ICU Liberation collaborative in over 15,000 adults. *Crit Care Med* 2019; **47**: 3-14.
24. H.A.B. Smith, J.B. Besunder, K.A. Betters, et al. 2022 Society of Critical Care Medicine clinical practice guidelines on prevention and management of pain, agitation, neuromuscular blockade, and delirium in critically ill pediatric patients with consideration of the ICU environment and early mobility. *Pediatr Crit Care Med* 2022; **23**: e74-e110.
25. J. Harris, A S. Ramelet, M. van Dijk, et al. Clinical recommendations for pain, sedation, withdrawal and delirium assessment in critically ill infants and children: an ESPNIC position statement for healthcare professionals. *Intensive Care Med* 2016; **42**: 972-86.
26. J.C. Lin, A. Srivastava, S. Malone, et al. Caring for critically ill children with the ICU liberation bundle (ABCDEF): results of the pediatric collaborative. *Pediatr Crit Care Med* 2023; **24**: 636-51.
27. M.B. Smith, E.Y. Killien, L.A. Dervan, et al. The association of severe pain experienced in the pediatric intensive care unit and postdischarge health-related quality of life: a retrospective cohort study. *Paediatr Anaesth* 2022; **32**: 899-906.
28. A.L. Holley, E.A.J. Battison, J. Heierle, et al. Long-term pain symptomatology in PICU survivors aged 8-18 Years. *Hosp Pediatr* 2023; **13**: 641-55.
29. K. Choong, D.D. Fraser, A. Al-Farsi, et al. Early rehabilitation in critically ill children: a two center implementation study. *Pediatr Crit Care Med* 2024; **25**: 92-105.
30. J. Engel, F. von Borell, I. Baumgartner, et al. Modified ABCDEF-bundles for critically ill pediatric patients: what could they look like? *Front Pediatr* 2022; **10**: 886334.
31. B. Blackwood, L.N. Tume, K.P. Morris, et al. Effect of a sedation and ventilator liberation protocol vs usual care on duration of invasive mechanical ventilation in pediatric intensive care units: a randomized clinical trial. *JAMA* 2021; **326**: 401-10.
32. D.M. Bhammar, H.N. Jones, J. E. Lang. Inspiratory muscle rehabilitation training in pediatrics: what is the evidence? *Can Respir J* 2022; **2022**: 5680311.

33. R.S. Watson, L.A. Asaro, L. Hutchins, et al. Risk factors for functional decline and impaired quality of life after pediatric respiratory failure. *Am J Respir Crit Care Med* 2019; **200**: 900–9.
34. R.S. Watson, S.R. Beers, L.A. Asaro, et al. Association of acute respiratory failure in early childhood with long-term neurocognitive outcomes. *JAMA* 2022; **327**: 836–45.
35. A. Amigoni, A. Pettenazzo, P. Biban, et al. Neurologic outcome in children after extracorporeal membrane oxygenation: prognostic value of diagnostic tests. *Pediatr Neurol* 2005; **32**: 173–9.
36. C. Traube, G. Silver, L.M. Gerber, et al. Delirium and mortality in critically ill children: epidemiology and outcomes of pediatric delirium. *Crit Care Med* 2017; **45**: 891–8.
37. G. Silver, H. Doyle, E. Hegel, et al. Association between pediatric delirium and quality of life after discharge. *Crit Care Med* 2020; **48**: 1829–34.
38. J. Moradi, M. Mikhail, L.A. Lee, et al. Lived experiences of delirium in critically ill children: a qualitative study. *J Pediatr Intensive Care* 2022.
39. J.R. Weatherhead, M. Niedner, M.K. Dahmer, et al. Patterns of delirium in a pediatric intensive care unit and associations with noise pollution. *J Intensive Care Med* 2022; **37**: 946–53.
40. K.D. Greenfield, O. Karam, A.M. Iqbal O'Meara. Brighter days may be ahead: continuous measurement of pediatric intensive care unit light and sound. *Front Pediatr* 2020; **8**: 590715.
41. K. Choong, D. Fraser, S. Al-Harbi, et al. Functional recovery in critically ill children, the "WeeCover" multicenter study. *Pediatr Crit Care Med* 2018; **19**: 145–54.
42. B.T. Pun, R. Badenes, G. Heras La Calle, et al. Prevalence and risk factors for delirium in critically ill patients with COVID-19 (COVID-D): a multicentre cohort study. *Lancet Respir Med* 2021; **9**: 239–50.
43. K. Choong, F. Canci, H. Clark, et al. Practice recommendations for early mobilization in critically ill children. *J Pediatr Intensive Care* 2018; **7**: 14–26.
44. B. Wieczorek, J. Ascenzi, Y. Kim, et al. PICU Up!: impact of a quality improvement intervention to promote early mobilization in critically ill children. *Pediatr Crit Care Med* 2016; **17**: e559–e66.
45. E.L. Fink, S.R. Beers, A.J. Houtrow, et al. Early protocolized versus usual care rehabilitation for pediatric neurocritical care patients: a randomized controlled trial. *Pediatr Crit Care Med* 2019; **20**: 540–50.
46. S.G. Ames, L.J. Alessi, M. Chrisman, et al. Development and implementation of pediatric icu-based mobility guidelines: a quality improvement initiative. *Pediatr Qual Saf* 2021; **6**: e414.
47. R.O. Hopkins, K. Choong, C.A. Zebuhr, S.R. Kudchadkar. Transforming PICU culture to facilitate early rehabilitation. *J Pediatr Intensive Care* 2015; **4**: 204–11.
48. K. Zheng, A. Sarti, S. Boles, et al. Impressions of early mobilization of critically ill children-clinician, patient, and family perspectives. *Pediatr Crit Care Med* 2018; **19**: e350–e7.
49. S.R. Kudchadkar, A. Nelliot, R. Awojoodu, et al. Physical rehabilitation in critically ill children: a multicenter point prevalence study in the United States. *Crit Care Med* 2020; **48**: 634–44.
50. K.L. Meert, J. Clark, S. Eggly. Family-centered care in the pediatric intensive care unit. *Pediatr Clin North Am* 2013; **60**: 761–72.
51. J.E. Davidson, C. Jones, O.J. Bienvenu. Family response to critical illness: postintensive care syndrome-family. *Crit Care Med* 2012; **40**: 618–24.
52. P.A. McIlroy, R.S. King, M. Garrouste-Orgeas, et al. The effect of ICU diaries on psychological outcomes and quality of life of survivors of critical illness and their relatives: a systematic review and meta-analysis. *Crit Care Med* 2019; **47**: 273–9.

53. X. Sun, D. Huang, F. Zeng, et al. Effect of intensive care unit diary on incidence of posttraumatic stress disorder, anxiety, and depression of adult intensive care unit survivors: A systematic review and meta-analysis. *J Adv Nurs* 2021; **77**: 2929–41.

54. V. Sansone, F. Cancani, C. Gagliardi, et al. Narrative diaries in the paediatric intensive care unit: a thematic analysis. *Nurs Crit Care* 2022; **27**: 45–54.

55. L. Ducharme-Crevier, K.A. La, T. Francois, et al. PICU follow-up clinic: patient and family outcomes 2 months after discharge. *Pediatr Crit Care Med* 2021; **22**: 935–43.

56. International Classification of Functioning, Disability and Health: Children and Youth version. Geneva, Switzerland; 2007.

57. D. Bossen, R.M. de Boer, H. Knoester, et al. Physical functioning after admission to the PICU: a scoping review. *Crit Care Explor* 2021; **3**: e0462.

58. J.J. Zimmerman, R. Banks, R. A. Berg, et al. Critical illness factors associated with long-term mortality and health-related quality of life morbidity following community-acquired pediatric septic shock. *Crit Care Med* 2020; **48**: 319–28.

59. N.P. Pinto, E.W. Rhinesmith, T.Y. Kim, et al. Long-term function after pediatric critical illness: results from the survivor outcomes study. *Pediatr Crit Care Med* 2017; **18**: e122–e30.

60. R.S. Watson, L.A. Asaro, J.H. Hertzog, et al. Long-term outcomes after protocolized sedation versus usual care in ventilated pediatric patients. *Am J Respir Crit Care Med* 2018; **197**: 1457–67.

61. A.B. Maddux, K.R. Miller, Y.L. Sierra, et al. Recovery trajectories in children requiring 3 or more days of invasive ventilation. *Crit Care Med* 2024; **52**: 798–810.

62. C. Ong, J.H. Lee, L. Yang, et al. A cross-sectional study of the clinical metrics of functional status tools in pediatric critical illness. *Pediatr Crit Care Med* 2021; **22**: 879–88.

63. A.B. Maddux, N. Pinto, E.L. Fink, et al. Postdischarge outcome domains in pediatric critical care and the instruments used to evaluate them: a scoping review. *Crit Care Med* 2020; **48**: e1313–e21.

64. S.C. Baker, J.A. Gledhill. Systematic review of interventions to reduce psychiatric morbidity in parents and children after PICU admissions. *Pediatr Crit Care Med* 2017; **18**: 343–8.

65. L.P. Nelson, J.I. Gold. Posttraumatic stress disorder in children and their parents following admission to the pediatric intensive care unit: a review. *Pediatr Crit Care Med* 2012; **13**: 338–47.

66. D.S. Davydow, L.P. Richardson, D.F. Zatzick, W.J. Katon. Psychiatric morbidity in pediatric critical illness survivors: a comprehensive review of the literature. *Arch Pediatr Adolesc Med* 2010; **164**: 377–85.

67. J.E. Rennick, I. Morin, D. Kim, et al. Identifying children at high risk for psychological sequelae after pediatric intensive care unit hospitalization. *Pediatr Crit Care Med* 2004; **5**: 358–63.

68. G. Rees, J. Gledhill, M.E. Garralda, S. Nadel. Psychiatric outcome following paediatric intensive care unit (PICU) admission: a cohort study. *Intensive Care Med* 2004; **30**: 1607–14.

69. R.J. Gemke, G.J. Bonsel, A.J. van Vught. Long-term survival and state of health after paediatric intensive care. *Arch Dis Child* 1995; **73**: 196–201.

70. National Child Traumatic Stress Network. Medical Trauma. www.nctsn.org/what-is-child-trauma/trauma-types/medical-trauma. Accessed June 2025.

71. J.E. Rennick, J. Rashotte. Psychological outcomes in children following pediatric intensive care unit hospitalization: a systematic review of the research. *J Child Health Care* 2009; **13**: 128–49.

72. M.S.M. Ko, P.F. Poh, K.Y.C. Heng, et al. Assessment of long-term psychological outcomes after pediatric intensive care unit admission: a systematic review and meta-analysis. *JAMA Pediatr* 2022; **176**: e215767.

73. K.R. Bradbury, C. Williams, S. Leonard, et al. Emotional aspects of pediatric

post-intensive care syndrome following traumatic brain injury. *J Child Adolesc Trauma* 2021; 14: 177–87.

74. L.M. Yagiela, E.F. Carlton, K.L. Meert, et al. Parent medical traumatic stress and associated family outcomes after pediatric critical illness: a systematic review. *Pediatr Crit Care Med* 2019; 20: 759–68.

75. M.K. Cousino, K.E. Rea, K.R. Schumacher, et al. A systematic review of parent and family functioning in pediatric solid organ transplant populations. *Pediatr Transplant* 2017; 21(3).

76. J.E. Lambert, J. Holzer, A. Hasbun. Association between parents' PTSD severity and children's psychological distress: a meta-analysis. *J Trauma Stress* 2014; 27: 9–17.

77. V.L. Banyard, L.M. Williams, J.A. Siegel. The impact of complex trauma and depression on parenting: an exploration of mediating risk and protective factors. *Child Maltreat* 2003; 8: 334–49.

78. A.R. Riley, C.N. Williams, D. Moyer, et al. Parental posttraumatic stress symptoms in the context of pediatric post intensive care syndrome: impact on the family and opportunities for intervention. *Clin Pract Pediatr Psychol* 2021; 9: 156–66.

79. A.C. De Young, J.A. Kenardy, V. E. Cobham, R. Kimble. Prevalence, comorbidity and course of trauma reactions in young burn-injured children. *J Child Psychol Psychiatry* 2012; 53: 56–63.

80. D.A. Long, P. Gilholm, R. Le Brocque, et al. Post-traumatic stress and health-related quality of life after admission to paediatric intensive care: longitudinal associations in mother-child dyads. *Aust Crit Care* 2024; 37: 98–105.

81. V.A. Anderson, C. Catroppa, F. Haritou, et al. Identifying factors contributing to child and family outcome 30 months after traumatic brain injury in children. *J Neurol Neurosurg Psychiatry* 2005; 76: 401–8.

82. C. Catroppa, L. Crossley, S.J. Hearps, et al. Social and behavioral outcomes: pre-injury to six months following childhood traumatic brain injury. *J Neurotrauma* 2015; 32: 109–15.

83. C.A. Luis, W. Mittenberg. Mood and anxiety disorders following pediatric traumatic brain injury: a prospective study. *J Clin Exp Neuropsychol* 2002; 24: 270–9.

84. T.A. Hall, R.K. Greene, J.B. Lee, et al. Post-intensive care syndrome in a cohort of school-aged children and adolescent ICU survivors: the importance of follow-up in the acute recovery phase. *J Pediatr Intensive Care* 2022; Article published online: 27 May 2022.

85. J. E. Rennick, C.C. Johnston, G. Dougherty, et al. Children's psychological responses after critical illness and exposure to invasive technology. *J Dev Behav Pediatr* 2002; 23: 133–44.

86. A.E. Kazak, N. Kassam-Adams, S. Schneider, et al. An integrative model of pediatric medical traumatic stress. *J Pediatr Psychol* 2006; 31: 343–55.

87. L.A. Demers, N.M. Wright, A.J. Kopstick, et al. Is pediatric intensive care trauma-informed? a review of principles and evidence. *Children (Basel)* 2022; **9**(10): 1575.

88. S. Linton, C. Grant, J. Pellegrini. Supporting families through discharge from PICU to the ward: the development and evaluation of a discharge information brochure for families. *Intensive Crit Care Nurs* 2008; 24: 329–37.

89. L.R. Bouvé, C.L. Rozmus, P. Giordano. Preparing parents for their child's transfer from the PICU to the pediatric floor. *Appl Nurs Res* 1999; 12: 114–20.

90. T. Babikian, R. Asarnow. Neurocognitive outcomes and recovery after pediatric TBI: meta-analytic review of the literature. *Neuropsychology* 2009; 23: 283–96.

91. T. Babikian, T. Merkley, R.C. Savage, et al. Chronic aspects of pediatric traumatic brain injury: review of the literature. *J Neurotrauma* 2015; 32: 1849–60.

92. L.M. Moran, T. Babikian, L. Del Piero, et al. The UCLA study of predictors of cognitive functioning following moderate/severe pediatric traumatic brain injury. *J Int Neuropsychol Soc* 2016; 22: 512–19.

93. M. Studer, E. Boltshauser, A. Capone Mori, et al. Factors affecting cognitive outcome in

early pediatric stroke. *Neurology* 2014; 82: 784–92.

94. B.S. Slomine, F.S. Silverstein, J. R. Christensen, et al. Neurobehavioral outcomes in children after out-of-hospital cardiac arrest. *Pediatrics* 2016; 137(4): e20153412.

95. M.F. Bone, J.M. Feinglass, D. M. Goodman. Risk factors for acquiring functional and cognitive disabilities during admission to a PICU. *Pediatr Crit Care Med* 2014; 15: 640–8.

96. C.N. Williams, C.O. Eriksson, A. Kirby, et al. Hospital mortality and functional outcomes in pediatric neurocritical care. *Hosp Pediatr* 2019; 9: 958–66.

97. P. Gilholm, K. Gibbons, S. Brüningk, et al. Machine learning to predict poor school performance in paediatric survivors of intensive care: a population-based cohort study. *Intensive Care Med* 2023; 49: 785–95.

98. W. Tomaszewski, C. Ablaza, L. Straney, et al. Educational outcomes of childhood survivors of critical illness: a population-based linkage study. *Crit Care Med* 2022; 50: 901–12.

99. A. Treble-Barna, H. Schultz, N. Minich, et al. Long-term classroom functioning and its association with neuropsychological and academic performance following traumatic brain injury during early childhood. *Neuropsychology* 2017; 31: 486–98.

100. S.A.M. Lambregts, J.E.M. Smetsers, I. Verhoeven, et al. Cognitive function and participation in children and youth with mild traumatic brain injury two years after injury. *Brain Inj* 2018; 32: 230–41.

101. A.B. Arnett, R.L. Peterson, M. W. Kirkwood, et al. Behavioral and cognitive predictors of educational outcomes in pediatric traumatic brain injury. *J Int Neuropsychol Soc* 2013; 19: 881–9.

102. A.G. Kachmar, S.Y. Irving, C.A. Connolly, M.A.Q. Curley. A systematic review of risk factors associated with cognitive impairment after pediatric critical illness. *Pediatr Crit Care Med* 2018; 19: e164–e71.

103. E.A. Herrup, B. Wieczorek, S. R. Kudchadkar. Characteristics of postintensive care syndrome in survivors of pediatric critical illness: a systematic review. *World J Crit Care Med* 2017; 6: 124–34.

104. T.A. Hall, S. Leonard, K. Bradbury, et al. Post-intensive care syndrome in a cohort of infants & young children receiving integrated care via a pediatric critical care & neurotrauma recovery program: a pilot investigation. *Clin Neuropsychol* 2022; 36: 639–63.

105. J.N. Dodd, T.A. Hall, K. Guilliams, et al. Optimizing neurocritical care follow-up through the integration of neuropsychology. *Pediatr Neurol* 2018; 89: 58–62.

106. D.T. Stuss, G. Winocus, I.H. Robertson. *Cognitive neurorehabilitation: evidence and application.* 2nd ed. New York, NY: Cambridge University Press; 2008.

107. B. Slomine, G. Locascio. Cognitive rehabilitation for children with acquired brain injury. *Dev Disabil Res Rev* 2009; 15: 133–43.

108. L.C. Als, S. Nadel, M. Cooper, et al. A supported psychoeducational intervention to improve family mental health following discharge from paediatric intensive care: feasibility and pilot randomised controlled trial. *BMJ open* 2015; 5: e009581.

109. L.W. Braga, A.C. Da Paz, M. Ylvisaker. Direct clinician-delivered versus indirect family-supported rehabilitation of children with traumatic brain injury: a randomized controlled trial. *Brain Inj* 2005; 19: 819–31.

110. J.C. Jackson, E.W. Ely, M.C. Morey, et al. Cognitive and physical rehabilitation of intensive care unit survivors: results of the RETURN randomized controlled pilot investigation. *Crit Care Med* 2012; 40: 1088–97.

111. R.O. Hopkins, M.R. Suchyta, T.J. Farrer, D. Needham. Improving post-intensive care

unit neuropsychiatric outcomes: understanding cognitive effects of physical activity. *Am J Respir Crit Care Med* 2012; 186: 1220–8.

112. H. Daughtrey, K.N. Slain, S. Derrington, et al. Measuring social health following pediatric critical illness: a scoping review and conceptual framework. *J Intensive Care Med* 2023; 38: 32–41.

113. E.F. Carlton, J.P. Donnelly, H.C. Prescott, et al. School and work absences after critical care hospitalization for pediatric acute respiratory failure: a secondary analysis of a cluster randomized trial. *JAMA Netw Open* 2021; 4: e2140732.

114. K. Kastner, N. Pinto, M.E. Msall, S. Sobotka. PICU follow-up: the impact of missed school in a cohort of children following PICU admission. *Crit Care Explor* 2019; 1: e0033.

115. K. Terp, A. Sjöström-Strand. Parents' experiences and the effect on the family two years after their child was admitted to a PICU: an interview study. *Intensive Crit Care Nurs* 2017; 43: 143–8.

116. E.F. Carlton, M.H. Moniz, J.W. Scott, et al. Financial outcomes after pediatric critical illness among commercially insured families. *Crit Care* 2023; 27: 227.

117. E. Defever, M. Jones. Rapid realist review of school-based physical activity interventions in 7- to 11-year-old children. *Children (Basel)* 2021; 8(1): 52.

118. L.M. Olson, G.N. Perry, S. Yang, et al. Parents' experiences caring for a child after a critical illness: a qualitative study. *J Pediatr Intensive Care* 2021; 13(2): 127-33.

119. J.M. Jarvis, K. Choong, M.A. Khetani. Associations of participation-focused strategies and rehabilitation service use with caregiver stress after pediatric critical illness. *Arch Phys Med Rehabil* 2019; 100: 703–10.

120. J.M. Jarvis, T. Huntington, G. Perry, et al. Supporting families during pediatric critical illness: opportunities identified in a multicenter, qualitative study. *J Child Health Care* 2023: 13674935231154829.

121. R.K.H. Shappley, D.L. Noles, T. Spentzas. Pediatric chronic critical illness: validation, prevalence, and impact in a children's hospital. *Pediatr Crit Care Med* 2021; 22: e636–e9.

122. C. Grandjean, M.H. Perez, A.S. Ramelet. Comparison of clinical characteristics and healthcare resource use of pediatric chronic and non-chronic critically ill patients in intensive care units: a retrospective national registry study. *Front Pediatr* 2023; 11: 1194833.

123. A.I. Cristea, V.L. Ackerman, S.D. Davis, et al. Median household income: association with mortality in children on chronic ventilation at home secondary to bronchopulmonary dysplasia. *Pediatr Allergy Immunol Pulmonol* 2015; 28: 41–6.

124. K.N. Slain, A. Barda, P.J. Pronovost, J.D. Thornton. Social factors predictive of intensive care utilization in technology-dependent children, a retrospective multicenter cohort study. *Front Pediatr* 2021; 9: 721353.

125. Y.R. Shin, Y.H. Park, H.K. Park. Pediatric ventricular assist device. *Korean Circ J* 2019; 49: 678–90.

126. M.A. van Manen. The ventricular assist device in the life of the child: a phenomenological pediatric study. *Qual Health Res* 2017; 27: 792–804.

127. T.K. Mitchell, L. Bray, L. Blake, et al. "It doesn't feel like our house anymore": the impact of medical technology upon life at home for families with a medically complex, technology-dependent child. *Health Place* 2022; 74: 102768.

128. L. Ewing-Cobbs, M.A. Barnes, J.M. Fletcher. Early brain injury in children: development and reorganization of cognitive function. *Dev Neuropsychol* 2003; 24: 669–704.

129. J. Haarbauer-Krupa, T. Haileyesus, J. Gilchrist, et al. Fall-related traumatic brain injury in children ages 0–4 years. *J Safety Res* 2019; 70: 127–33.

130. A.V. Ciurea, M.R. Gorgan, A. Tascu, et al. Traumatic brain injury in infants and

toddlers, 0–3 years old. *J Med Life* 2011; 4: 234–43.

131. C.L. Karver, S.L. Wade, A. Cassedy, et al. Age at injury and long-term behavior problems after traumatic brain injury in young children. *Rehabil Psychol* 2012; 57: 256–65.

132. H.G. Taylor, J. Alden. Age-related differences in outcomes following childhood brain insults: an introduction and overview. *J Int Neuropsychol Soc* 1997; 3: 555–67.

133. V. Anderson, C. Catroppa, S. Morse, et al. Functional plasticity or vulnerability after early brain injury? *Pediatrics* 2005; 116: 1374–82.

134. M.C. Dewan, N. Mummareddy, J. C. Wellons, 3rd, C.M. Bonfield. Epidemiology of global pediatric traumatic brain injury: qualitative review. *World Neurosurg* 2016; 91: 497–509.e1.

135. C.N. Williams, J. Piantino, C. McEvoy, et al. The burden of pediatric neurocritical care in the United States. *Pediatr Neurol* 2018; 89: 31–8.

136. E.L. Fink, P.M. Kochanek, R.C. Tasker, et al. International survey of critically ill children with acute neurologic insults: the prevalence of acute critical neurological disease in children: a global epidemiological assessment study. *Pediatr Crit Care Med* 2017; 18: 330–42.

137. FDA Drug Safety Communication: FDA review results in new warnings about using general anesthetics and sedation drugs in young children and pregnant women: FDA; 2019. www.fda.gov/drugs/drug-safety-and-availability/fda-drug-safety-communication-fda-review-results-new-warnings-about-using-general-anesthetics-in-young-women-and-pregnant-women.

138. K.K. Hardy, K. Olson, S.M. Cox, et al. Systematic review: a prevention-based model of neuropsychological assessment for children with medical illness. *J Pediatr Psychol* 2017; 42: 815–22.

139. M.E. Hartman, C.N. Williams, T.A. Hall, et al. Post-intensive-care syndrome for the pediatric neurologist. *Pediatr Neurol* 2020; 108: 47–53.

140. H.T. Keenan, A.P. Presson, A.E. Clark, et al. Longitudinal developmental outcomes after traumatic brain injury in young children: are infants more vulnerable than toddlers? *J Neurotrauma* 2019; 36: 282–92.

141. C.N. Williams, T.A. Hall, V.A. Baker, et al. Follow-up after PICU discharge for patients with acquired brain injury: the role of an abbreviated neuropsychological evaluation and a return-to-school program. *Pediatr Crit Care Med* 2023; 24: 807–17.

142. A.I. Canto, M.A. Crisp, H. Larach, A. P. Blankenship. *General and special education inclusion in an age of change: impact on students with disabilities.* Bradford, UK: Emerald Group Publishing Limited; 2016.

143. W.M. Vanderlind, L.A. Demers, G. Engelson, et al. Back to school: academic functioning and educational needs among youth with acquired brain injury. *Children (Basel)* 2022; 9(9): 1321.

144. C.N. Williams, T.A. Hall, C. Francoeur, et al. Continuing care for critically ill children beyond hospital discharge: current state of follow-up. *Hosp Pediatr* 2022; 12: 359–93.

145. O.J. Schofield-Robinson, S.R. Lewis, A. F. Smith, et al. Follow-up services for improving long-term outcomes in intensive care unit (ICU) survivors. *Cochrane Database Syst Rev* 2018; 11: Cd012701.

146. T. Tan, S.J. Brett, T. Stokes. Rehabilitation after critical illness: summary of NICE guidance. *BMJ* 2009; 338: b822.

147. K.P. Mayer, H. Boustany, E.P. Cassity, et al. ICU recovery clinic attendance, attrition, and patient outcomes: the impact of severity of illness, gender, and rurality. *Crit Care Explor* 2020; 2: e0206.

148. G.A. Colville, P.R. Cream, S.M. Kerry. Do parents benefit from the offer of a follow-up appointment after their child's admission to intensive care? An exploratory randomised controlled trial. *Intensive Crit Care Nurs* 2010; 26: 146–53.

149. S. Dimopoulos, N.E. Leggett, A.M. Deane, et al. Models of intensive care unit follow-up care and feasibility of intervention delivery: a systematic review. *Aust Crit Care* 2024; 37: 508–16.

150. S. Harris-Kober, A. Motzel, S. Grant, et al. Impression of primary care follow-up after a picu admission: a pilot survey of primary care pediatricians. *Crit Care Explor* 2024; 6: e1055.

151. I. Wolfe, R.M. Satherley, E. Scotney, et al. Integrated care models and child health: a meta-analysis. *Pediatrics* 2020; **145**(1): e20183747.

152. R. Blaauwbroek, W. Tuinier, B. Meyboom-de Jong, et al. Shared care by paediatric oncologists and family doctors for long-term follow-up of adult childhood cancer survivors: a pilot study. *Lancet Oncol* 2008; 9: 232–8.

153. J. Simmonds, M. Burch. Shared care in paediatric heart transplantation. *Archives of Disease in Childhood Education and Practice Edition* 2008; 93: 37–43.

154. C. Breen, L. Altman, J. Ging, et al. Significant reductions in tertiary hospital encounters and less travel for families after implementation of paediatric care coordination in Australia. *BMC Health Serv Res* 2018; 18: 751.

155. D.A. Sarik, M.P. Winterhalter, C.J. Calamaro. Improving the transition from hospital to home for clinically complex children. *Pediatric Nursing* 2018; 44: 281.

156. D. Long, K. Gibbons, B. Dow, et al. Effectiveness-implementation hybrid-2 randomised trial of a collaborative Shared Care Model for Detecting Neurodevelopmental Impairments after Critical Illness in Young Children (DAISY): pilot study protocol. *BMJ Open* 2022; 12: e060714.

157. N. Miller Ferguson, L. Lively, T. Sullivan, et al. 805: Inpatient nurse navigator improves communication and follow-up after pediatric TBI admission. *Crit Care Med* 2021; 49: 399.

158. J.L.L. Lin, S. Quartarone, N. Aidarus, et al. Process evaluation of a hub-and-spoke model to deliver coordinated care for children with medical complexity across Ontario: facilitators, barriers and lessons learned. *Healthc Policy* 2021; 17: 104–22.

159. Z. Rahmaty, J.C. Manning, I. Macdonald, et al. Post-intensive care syndrome in pediatrics: enhancing understanding through a novel bioecological theory of human development lens. *Intensive Care Medicine – Paediatric and Neonatal* 2023; 1: 9.

160. D.A. Long, M. Waak, N.N. Doherty, B.L. Dow. Brain-directed care: why neuroscience principles direct picu management beyond the ABCs. *Children (Basel)* 2022; **9**(12): 1938.

161. D.A. Long, E.L. Fink. Transitions from short to long-term outcomes in pediatric critical care: considerations for clinical practice. *Transl Pediatr* 2021; 10: 2858–74.

162. L. Jalilian, M. Cannesson, N. Kamdar. Post-ICU recovery clinics in the era of digital health and telehealth. *Crit Care Med* 2019; 47: e796–e7.

163. A.L. Curfman, J.M. Hackell, N.E. Herendeen, et al. Telehealth: improving access to and quality of pediatric health care. *Pediatrics* 2021; **148**(3): e2021053129.

164. S.A. Esses, S. Small, A. Rodemann, M.E. Hartman. Post-intensive care syndrome: educational interventions for parents of hospitalized children. *Am J Crit Care* 2019; 28: 19–27.

165. J.D. Edwards. Anticipatory guidance on the risks for unfavorable outcomes among children with medical complexity. *J Pediatr* 2017; 180: 247–50.

166. A.L. Alger, T. Owens, E.A. Duffy. Implementing standardized post-intensive care syndrome education by an advanced practice registered nurse in the pediatric intensive care unit. *AACN Adv Crit Care* 2022; 33: 368–71.

Section 7 **Conclusions**

Chapter 55

PICS Advocacy

Sarah Holler and Michael G. Allison

Introduction

Post-intensive care syndrome (PICS) is garnering increased public and professional attention with respect to its prevalence, its impact on survivors of critical illness, and the resources available to help patients and their care partners cope with its burden. Such increased awareness and commitment to further understanding PICS is directly attributable to advocacy efforts by patients, families, healthcare workers, and specialty societies. PICS advocacy has taken many forms, from grassroots movements born on social media, to podcast episodes and books, to formalized task forces in medical societies devoted to enhancing recovery from critical illness.

Toward a Shared Understanding and Definition of PICS Advocacy

The 2002 Brussels Roundtable "Surviving Intensive Care" concluded that survivors of critical illness should be serially followed with standardized assessments to generate data on long-term outcomes following critical illness [1,2], and eight years later, the first formalized definition of PICS was developed in 2010 by the Society of Critical Care Medicine (SCCM) [3]. The subsequent SCCM-sponsored THRIVE initiative, composed of collaboratives of peer support groups and ICU follow-up clinics for survivors of critical illness, provided global collaborators with a source of education, community, and quality improvement and largely set the research agenda for survivorship following critical illness.

Advocacy holds different meanings to the various stakeholders involved in the diagnosis and treatment of PICS. Local advocacy groups, such as those offered at individual hospitals, often focus on improving provider awareness of PICS, identifying patients at risk for PICS, and providing patients and their families resources to cope with the physical, cognitive, and psychological challenges they may face. National and global advocacy has been promoted by specialty societies, such as the SCCM [4], the American Occupational Therapy Association (AOTA) [5], the European Society of Intensive Care Medicine (ESICM) [6], and others. Global advocacy has been further promoted by independent organizations like the Critical and Acute Illness Recovery Organization (CAIRO), an international collaborative of ICU follow-up clinics and peer support groups forged in the tradition of the SCCM's THRIVE initiative, which provides advocacy via development of best practices and interdisciplinary partnerships to improve the care of patients with PICS [7].

A shared understanding of PICS advocacy is not well characterized in the medical literature. For the purposes of this chapter, we define PICS advocacy as an ethical commitment to patient- and caregiver-centered care through: (1) support for those living with PICS, (2) promotion of PICS awareness and prevention in the medical and lay communities, and (3) advancement of the science of PICS.

The Current Landscape of PICS Advocacy

Most advocacy efforts that are focused on supporting patients with PICS are implemented at the local level. Many hospitals and healthcare systems have established ICU follow-up clinics (see Chapter 28 for additional information) and peer support groups (see Chapter 49 for additional information) that provide education and resources to patients and their families, but the current number of such resources available are inadequate to meet the needs of the millions of patients who would derive benefit annually. These diverse groups link patients and their care providers with the information needed to understand and contextualize their constellation of PICS symptoms and provide them with access to helpful medical and community resources. Other support for patients with PICS comes from community resources, care managers, and social workers, who assist patients in navigating post-hospitalization appointments, complex financial decisions, and finding adaptations to help them return to optimal functioning.

Importantly, the vast majority of patients with PICS will receive follow-up care from primary care physicians, most of whom are insufficiently prepared to care for patients with PICS given the lack of education regarding PICS in medical school and primary care training programs and structural barriers in the nature of primary care appointments, which are too limited in time and scope to address the needs of most survivors of critical illness. Accordingly, advocacy efforts must not be limited to the critical care community alone but should include PICS-related education and training to the practitioners who are the most likely to care for survivors of critical illness following hospital discharge. Ultimately, intensivists and the critical care community at large must explore partnerships with primary care physicians to assist them in providing the most sophisticated care possible for patients who do not have access to ICU follow-up clinic services; such engagement likely requires both efforts at the local level as well as collaboration among medical societies at the national and international levels.

The promotion and awareness of PICS has been advanced by leading critical care societies and healthcare institutions, whose efforts have targeted both medical professional and public advocacy. As an example of the former, the SCCM garnered support for the development of a formal International Classification of Diseases, 10th edition (ICD-10) code for PICS and for legislation to fund research and treatment of PICS. These resolutions were presented at the 2022 American Medical Association (AMA) Annual Meeting of the House of Delegates and were recommended for adoption [8], meaning that clinicians are now closer to having a dedicated diagnostic code and support for ongoing PICS research. Other initiatives have raised public awareness, helping PICS become more commonly understood among the general population. Vanderbilt University Medical Center's ICU Recovery Center formed the "Walk4PICS" with the goal of raising awareness of PICS for both the lay public and healthcare professionals [9]. The walk occurs in September of each year, and participants and their supporters are encouraged to walk any distance they are capable of to raise awareness of the challenges of recovering from critical illness. Books and podcasts have also made the concept of PICS more accessible to the general population. A sample of such content, in addition to content created by medical professionals and

Table 55.1 A compendium of existing PICS resources

Resource	Further details
Websites	
Critical and Acute Illness Recovery Organization (CAIRO)	www.cairorecovery.com
Johns Hopkins Outcomes After Critical Illness and Surgery (OACIS)	www.hopkinsmedicine.org/pulmonary/research/outcomes-after-critical-illness
PostICU – a patient-built advocacy and information nonprofit	www.posticu.org
Society of Critical Care Medicine (SCCM)	www.sccm.org
Vanderbilt University Critical Illness, Brain Dysfunction, and Survivorship Center (CIBS)	www.icudelirium.org/the-icu-recovery-center-at-vanderbilt
Walk4PICS	www.walk4pics.com
Podcasts	
Walking Home from the ICU Walking You Through the ICU	Multiple podcasts hosted by Kali Dayton, DNP, AGACNP
Echoes of Trauma: Post Intensive Care Syndrome	Hosted by Health Affairs Podcasts: Narrative matters (Aug 31, 2022), featuring Joanna Bayes
Post-Intensive Care Syndrome in Children (PICS-P)	PedsCrit Podcast (January 22, 2024), featuring Elizabeth Killien, MD, MPH
Post-Intensive Care Syndrome (PICS)	Respiratory Exchange Podcast (January 14, 2024) for the Cleveland Clinic, featuring Michelle Biehl, MD
Post-ICU Clinics and Peer Support Groups to Reduce Post-Intensive Care Syndrome (PICS)	Podcast 396, hosted by SCCM, featuring Kyle B. Enfield, MD and Kimberley J. Haines, PhD, BHSc
Critical Perspective: Management of Post-Intensive Care Syndrome in the Era of COVID–19	Episode 231 of Breathe Easy, sponsored by the American Thoracic Society, featuring Dr. Dale Needham
Books	
You Can Stop Humming Now: A Doctor's Stories of Life, Death and in Between by Daniela Lamas	
Every Deep-Drawn Breath by Wes Ely	
Intensive Care: A Doctor's Journey by Danielle Ofri	

medical societies, is presented in Table 55.1. A shared understanding of the definition of PICS among medical professionals and the lay population will foster collaboration, improve patient outcomes, and drive continued advocacy efforts to address the challenges faced by those affected by critical illness.

Research into PICS takes many forms and has been financed through government, institutional, and specialty society funding. Though there are many areas of active inquiry into PICS, there are certain aspects of the syndrome, such as multimodal treatment and support for patients with lasting symptoms, that would benefit from targeted research. Advocacy to encourage more governmental and institutional research support is needed to increase professional awareness of PICS; the aforementioned efforts of the AMA are one example of advocacy for increased investigator funding.

Promoting Advocacy for PICS

Existing advocacy efforts currently focus on patient support, disease awareness, and research. As awareness of the syndrome grows, healthcare workers, hospitals and healthcare systems, local governments, and large organizations must consider how a comprehensive and coordinated thematic approach to PICS can guide advocacy efforts to areas of greatest need. Developing a well-defined advocacy strategy benefits any individual or organization aiming to address the needs of patients and family members coping with PICS. It is essential to plan and articulate the steps for an advocacy effort in advance to effectively promote the desired change. Answering a few key questions can help transform an advocacy idea into a structured advocacy campaign. Table 55.2 presents sample questions used to structure an advocacy campaign along with sample answers, using the development of a local PICS peer support group as an example.

Table 55.2 A structured approach to developing a PICS peer support group within a regional health system

	Question	Answer
Q1	Can the specific advocacy goal be named?	Creation of a PICS peer support group for a regional health system
Q2	Is the strategy intended to raise awareness, change opinion, or enact action?	Enact action by creation of a peer support group
Q3	Who or what are the targets of the advocacy (policymakers, executive leaders, agencies, organizations)?	Executive leaders within the medical system, inclusive of population health leaders; physician champions; experts in the provision of psychological care; finance executives; and patient experience leaders
Q4	What are the specific objectives that will contribute to achieving the goal?	Establish a program leader Ensure funding for the endeavor Align expectations regarding timing of initiatives Utilize project management tools for structure
Q5	What are the actions that need to be taken?	Create a budget proposal Develop an EMR tool to identify at risk patients Secure a virtual meeting platform and/or physical meeting space Develop meeting agendas for the first year

The questions in Table 55.2, which are based upon an advocacy tool designed to help enact public policy changes [10], may need to be adjusted depending upon the breadth and depth of the advocacy project. Local implementation of a peer support group to enhance community awareness has limited scope, while pursuing a broader change in public policy would require a much larger stakeholder analysis (Question 3) and objectives (Question 4) and actions (Question 5) that would be contingent upon receiving stakeholder support. Key to formulating an advocacy strategy is choosing the correct audience and targeting precise changes in either awareness, opinion, or action. The strategy should be forward-looking enough to envision how current efforts may lead to future endeavors and should utilize outcomes data to track progress and incite change, if needed. For example, the Walk4PICS can track the number of sites hosting a walk and the number of participants that sign up to walk each year as surrogate measures of public awareness.

The Future of PICS Advocacy

Organizations and individuals hoping to advocate for PICS can glean insights from prior successful advocacy campaigns used to enhance awareness, prevention, and treatment of other medical conditions. Efforts in cancer and cardiovascular disease advocacy, for example, have notably increased public awareness and improved patient outcomes. Public media campaigns, such as those by the American Cancer Society (ACS) and the American Heart Association (AHA), have provided education to the public on early detection and prevention of diseases, leading to widespread screening programs and enhanced patient engagement. The ACS's most well-known public awareness and fundraising program is the Relay for Life to support cancer recognition and raise funds for research. Other awareness programs, such as "Coaches vs. Cancer," leverage relationships with other popular entities, in this case the National Association of Basketball Coaches, to promote disease awareness and healthy lifestyle choices. The AHA has their flagship Heart Walk to promote attention to heart disease and to solicit donations for cardiac research. Beyond this, the AHA has a grassroots network entitled "You're the Cure" that has advocated for cardiopulmonary resuscitation training within high school health education curricula [11]. Both the ACS and AHA leverage their networks to influence public policy; the ACS has formalized their policy advocacy efforts through the Cancer Action Network, a nonprofit, nonpartisan affiliate of the ACS [12]. The efforts by organizations such as the ACS and the AHA have enhanced access to care and preventive services for patients, have supported clinical trials and innovative treatment research, and have influenced public health policies. The future of PICS advocacy should be informed by the successes of the advocacy efforts of these organizations. Efforts for PICS advocacy may include pursuing novel partnerships and programs to increase and maintain public awareness and formulating a public policy strategy to enact PICS-specific legislation to support survivors of critical illness.

The targets for PICS advocacy extend from the hyper-local context of a critical care division to the breadth of multinational efforts on a global scale, such as that which is being done by the CAIRO organization. For advocacy to be successful, a variety of targets should be selected for PICS-related awareness and to garner support for PICS. Figure 55.1 depicts potential advocacy targets that range from local (central rings) to global (outer rings), and Table 55.3 provides suggestions for advocacy actions or programs that can be performed at each level. To advance PICS advocacy, examples of past or ongoing

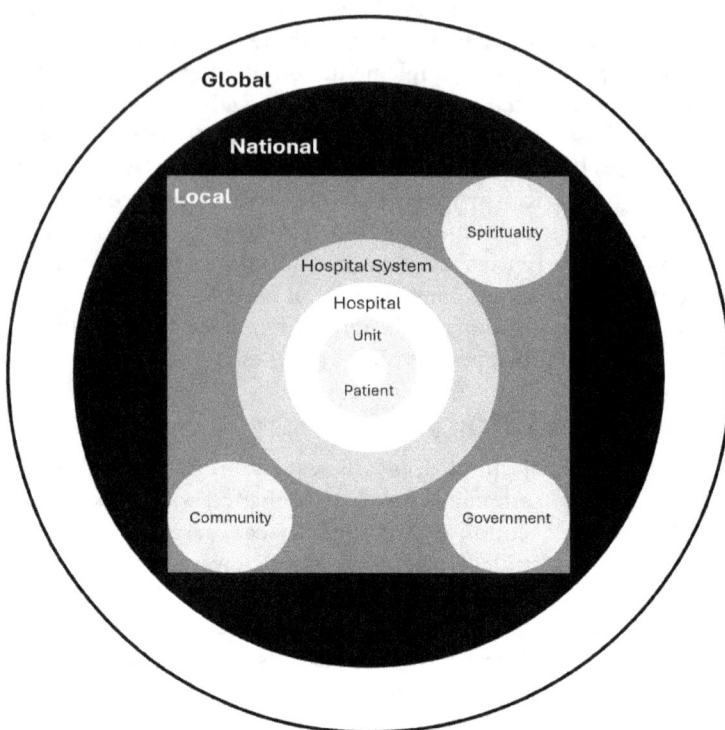

Figure 55.1 Targets for potential advocacy efforts from local to global levels of influence.

initiatives to raise awareness or drive action can serve as valuable guidance for those seeking to advocate for the PICS community. Advocacy can occur at various levels, allowing individuals, groups, or larger organizations to develop strategies to address unmet needs. Furthermore, healthcare professionals and patients interested in supporting this cause may consider joining existing efforts dedicated to promoting PICS awareness and support (see Table 55.3).

Conclusion

There is much to celebrate about the success of PICS advocacy since its recognition and description as a clinical syndrome in 2010. There are multiple examples of individuals and groups working toward a common goal of supporting patients living with PICS, promoting awareness of PICS within professional and nonprofessional communities, and supporting academic work to refine and expand our knowledge of PICS. The emergence of ICU follow-up clinics and peer support groups demonstrates commitment to longitudinal care for patients struggling with PICS. Private and public funding of clinical research has provided new insights into PICS and has laid the academic foundation for continued investigation into assessment and treatment strategies. Continuing to focus advocacy efforts toward enhancing collaboration and removing barriers will undoubtedly lead to improvements in the lives of those living with PICS.

Table 55.3 Advocacy efforts that target awareness or action at various levels of influence

Strategy Impact	Examples of Advocacy
Patient and Caregiver	
Awareness	• Educate other patients and care partners about PICS • Share their experiences via storytelling • Contribute to websites that other patients and care partners can search to find support outside of defined clinics and peer support groups
Action	• Ask for referrals to ICU follow-up clinics and support groups • Participate in patient-lead peer support groups • Engage in grassroots awareness efforts through podcasts, blogs, and social media
Unit Setting	
Awareness	• Educate the multidisciplinary staff caring for patients in the ICU
Action	• Implement preventative strategies, such as the ABCDEF bundle • Create and provide ICU journals for patient families and staff • Create a standard prompt to discuss patient risk for PICS during interdisciplinary rounds • Educate patients and families about PICS prior to ICU discharge • Connect patients with risk factors for PICS to local resources prior to hospital discharge
Hospital Setting	
Awareness	• Educate non-ICU staff about PICS through grand rounds or other large format presentations • Support a local PICS walk • Engage hospital marketing to provide resources for patient, family, and staff awareness
Action	• Collaborate with health information technology teams to create a PICS consult list • Use EMR tools to identify patients with risk factors for PICS • Add discharge instructions that explain PICS • Develop a peer support group • Establish an ICU-follow up clinic

Table 55.3 (cont.)

Strategy Impact	Examples of Advocacy
Hospital System	
Awareness	• Share hospital-based awareness tools though hospital system post-acute care groups, patient experience committees, or cross-functional departments/divisions
Action	• Coordinate patient referrals from hospitals without clinics or support groups to hospitals that have established resources
Local Community	
Awareness	• Coordinate with faith-based resources to provide awareness and community support • Promote awareness at educational institutions such as high schools, colleges, and universities • Perform letter writing campaigns to bring awareness to local elected officials and community organizations
Action	• Add PICS to health curriculums in schools • Provide libraries and community centers with resources to help community members • Encourage hospitals to present on PICS topics at local health fairs • Reach out to community primary care practitioners to provide them with best practices for caring for patients after ICU discharge • Establish relationships with known rehabilitation centers that focus on ICU-acquired weakness and cognitive rehabilitation for survivors of critical illness
National	
Awareness	• Petition media organizations to provide coverage of PICS-related events and PICS stories • Include PICS content in medical texts and communications from specialty societies • Partner with the sports, music, and entertainment industries to bring awareness to PICS • Attend lobbying days on Capitol Hill for healthcare providers, speaking to elected representatives about the impact of PICS on recovery after critical illness • Educate the insurance industry about recovery after critical illness so they may better understand the need for high-intensity care and follow-up to prevent readmissions
Action	• Enact PICS-specific content requirements for continuing medical education for state license recertification

- Join national medical associations to advocate for the inclusion of more content on Post-Intensive Care Syndrome (PICS)
  - National Association of Mental Illness (NAMI) www.nami.org
  - Sepsis Alliance www.sepsis.org
  - American Delirium Society https://americandeliriumsociety.org
  - American Nurses Association www.nursingworld.org
  - Gerontological Society of America www.geron.org
  - American Academy of Critical Care Nursing (AACN) www.aacn.org/
  - American Occupational Therapy Association (AOTA) www.aota.org
  - American College of Chest Physicians (CHEST) www.chestnet.org
  - American Medical Association (AMA) www.ama-assn.org
  - American Thoracic Society (ATS) https://site.thoracic.org
  - American Psychological Association (APA) www.apa.org/
  - National Hospice and Palliative Care Organization (NHPCO) www.nhpco.org
  - National Academy of Medicine (previously Institute of Medicine or IOM) https://nam.edu
  - Patient Centered Outcomes Research Institute (PCORI) www.pcori.org

Global

Awareness
- Utilize collaborations between specialty societies to bring awareness to PICS at international conferences (e.g., ESICM-sponsored conferences in Turkey, Japan, Brazil, and Germany)

Action
- Move for inclusion of PICS in the international classification of diseases (ICD–11) through the WHO
  - To submit questions and suggestions related to ICD–11 contact icd@who.int.
- Join or petition global medical organizations to advocate for the inclusion of more content on Post-Intensive Care Syndrome (PICS)
  - World Health Organization (WHO) www.who.int/
  - ARDS Advisory Board https://ARDSglobal.org
  - United Kingdom Intensive Care Society https://ics.ac.uk

Table 55.3 (cont.)

Strategy Impact	Examples of Advocacy
	○ National Institute for Health and Care Excellence www.nice.org.uk
	○ European Delirium Association www.europeandeliriumassociation.org
	○ American Delirium Society https://americandeliriumsociety.org
	○ Institute for Healthcare Improvement/Age Friendly Health Systems www.ihi.org
	○ ICU Steps: Intensive Care Patient Support Charity https://icusteps.org/
	○ Society of Critical Care Medicine (SCCM) www.sccm.org
	○ Canadian Critical Care Society (CCCS) www.canadiancriticalcare.org
	○ European Society of Intensive Care Medicine (ESICM) www.esicm.org/
	○ Asia Pacific Association of Critical Care Medicine (APACCM) www.apaccm.org
	○ Australian and New Zealand Intensive Care Society (ANZICS) www.anzics.com.au/
	○ National Institutes of Health (NIH) www.nih.gov

Key Points

1. PICS advocacy is an ethical commitment to patient and caregiver-centered care through: (1) support for those living with PICS, (2) promotion of PICS awareness and prevention in the medical and lay communities, and (3) advancement of the science of PICS.
2. Current advocacy efforts have promoted awareness through development of the Walk4PICS and have lobbied for governing body acceptance of PICS as a distinct medical condition with its own diagnostic code.
3. In the future, PICS advocacy can build on successful strategies from established health organizations by leveraging public awareness campaigns, advocating for representative policies, and forming partnerships to improve awareness and outcomes.

References

1. D.C. Angus, J. Carlet. 2002 Brussels Roundtable Participants. Surviving intensive care: a report from the 2002 Brussels Roundtable. *Intensive Care Med* 2003; 29: 368–77.
2. N. Nakanishi, K. Liu, J. Hatakeyama, et al. Post-intensive care syndrome follow-up system after hospital discharge: a narrative review. *J Intensive Care* 2024; **12**: 1–16.
3. D.M. Needham, J. Davidson, H. Cohen, et al. Improving long-term outcomes after discharge from intensive care unit: report from a stakeholders' conference. *Crit Care Med* 2012; **40**: 502–9.
4. SCCM. Society of Critical Care Medicine. www.sccm.org/home. Accessed July 20, 2024.
5. AOTA. American Occupational Therapy Organization. www.aota.org. Accessed July 20, 2024.
6. ESICM. European Society of Intensive Care Medicine. www.esicm.org/. Accessed October 26, 2024.
7. CAIRO. Critical and Acute Illness Recovery Organization. https://criticalacuterecorg.wixsite.com/cairo. Accessed July 20, 2024.
8. American Medical Association. 2022 Annual Meeting. Appendix: Reports of reference committees. 2022. www.ama-assn.org/system/files/a22-reference-committee-reports.pdf. Accessed November 7, 2024.
9. Walk4PICS. www.walk4pics.com. Accessed November 15, 2024.
10. J. Coffman, T. Beer. The Advocacy Strategy Framework: A tool for articulating an advocacy theory of change. [White paper]. https://evaluationinnovation.org/wp-content/uploads/2-15/03/Adocacy-Strategy-Framework.pdf. Accessed June 15, 2024.
11. American Heart Association. At the AHA, advocacy leads to health impact. www.heart.org/en/around-the-aha/at-the-aha-advocacy-leads-to-health-impact. Accessed December 8, 2024.
12. American Cancer Society Cancer Action Network℠ (ACS CAN) www.fightcancer.org. Accessed July 5, 2024.

Chapter 56

A Case Study of PICS

Brad W. Butcher

To integrate the material presented throughout this textbook, we present a case study of post-intensive care syndrome (PICS) that highlights some of the syndrome's defining features: the breadth of disability across physical, functional, cognitive, and psychological domains; the duration of disability despite rehabilitative interventions; the varying degrees of disability over time with the potential for recrudescence, particularly with additional episodes of acute illness; and the social ramifications of the syndrome. This case report also demonstrates the holistic approach taken in intensive care unit (ICU) follow-up clinics and many of the interventions that such a clinic can provide. We follow this patient across more than three years of participation in an ICU follow-up clinic.

The Patient

Auggie is a 57-year-old male with a medical history significant for severe chronic obstructive pulmonary disease (COPD) who was admitted to the hospital from May 18, 2018 until June 15, 2018 for management of the acute respiratory distress syndrome (ARDS) and septic shock secondary to community acquired pneumonia with *Strep pneumoniae*. This 29-day hospitalization included a total of 22 days in the medical ICU. He required intubation and mechanical ventilation for a total of 11 days, and his ARDS was severe enough to require ventilation in the prone position and a continuous infusion of paralytics for 2 days. He required a continuous infusion of norepinephrine for 4 days for the management of hypotension related to septic shock. His course was complicated by acute kidney injury that was not severe enough to require renal replacement therapy, stress-induced cardiomyopathy with an ejection fraction of 35%, new-onset atrial fibrillation, bilateral pulmonary emboli, and anemia that did not require transfusion. He experienced 9 days of delirium that included both hypoactive and hyperactive phenotypes, and he was placed in wrist restraints for 8 days. Elements of the ABCDEF bundle were completed routinely, although not all bundle elements were performed every day during his ICU stay. Following extubation, he was able to walk more than 250 feet prior to transfer out of the ICU.

Prior to hospitalization, Auggie was independent with mobility, did not require assistive devices, and was independent in all activities of daily living (ADLs) and instrumental activities of daily living (IADLs). He endorsed no cognitive concerns prior to his hospitalization, and although he had seen a psychiatrist in the past for periods of depression, he was not taking any psychiatric medications. He was retired, having worked a physical job for the telephone company for decades, and he was capable of driving without difficulty.

Auggie was discharged from the hospital to a skilled nursing facility. Four days after discharge, he returned to the emergency department with abdominal pain, and was sent back to the nursing facility without requiring admission. Six days after hospital discharge, he presented to the ICU follow-up clinic for a comprehensive assessment.

First ICU Follow-Up Clinic Visit

During his first ICU follow-up clinic visit, a thorough assessment of Auggie's physical, cognitive, psychiatric, and social needs was performed. When asked to reflect on his experiences in the ICU, Auggie remembered the need for intubation but suffered a gap in his memory until he was extubated. He was able to remember certain staff members by name, including respiratory therapists, physical therapists, and nurses, particularly one who advocated for him during a moment of crisis when the need for re-intubation was being considered. He recalled numerous vivid dreams and a memory of a "big party in the ICU," but denied scary or troubling dreams, hallucinations, and delusions. He commented on feeling inadequately equipped to make decisions in the ICU, but he felt "safe and watched over" by the ICU staff.

Symptomatically, Auggie complained of shortness of breath, weakness, difficulty sleeping, and feeling that he was unprepared for what was ahead of him. Despite these challenges, he spoke about his faith in God and the solace and comfort that religion brought him. In consultation with the pharmacist, Auggie was started on tiotropium and salmeterol/fluticasone for management of COPD (with instructions on proper use provided by the respiratory therapist), pantoprazole was discontinued as there were no symptoms of gastroesophageal reflux disease, metoprolol tartrate was consolidated to metoprolol succinate for ease of administration, and furosemide was decreased to once daily administration to avoid interruptions in sleep because of nighttime urination. Spirometric evaluation was consistent with severe obstructive lung disease, with a forced expiratory volume in one second to forced vital capacity (FEV_1/FVC) ratio of 40%; although smoking prior to hospitalization, Auggie had not smoked since discharge with no plans to resume. Although Auggie complained of food occasionally feeling stuck in his esophagus, a swallowing evaluation revealed no concern for dysphagia. Physical and functional assessments revealed impairments in strength as assessed by dynamometry and the 5-times sit to stand test, endurance as assessed by the 6-minute walk test, and the ability to perform IADLs as assessed by the Lawton screen. Cognitive and psychiatric assessments, including the Montreal Cognitive Assessment (MoCA) tool, the Hospital Anxiety and Depression Scale (HADS), and the Impact of Events Scale-revised (IES-r), respectively, were within normal limits. Data from ICU follow-up clinic visits can be seen in Table 56.1 and Table 56.2. Upon reviewing his goals of care, Auggie expressed a desire to remain full code, elected his son as his surrogate decision maker, and filled out a Physician Order for Life Sustaining Treatment (POLST) document reflecting those decisions.

At the end of the appointment, Auggie was provided with prescriptions for pulmonary rehabilitation, outpatient physical therapy, and outpatient occupational therapy.

Three-Month Follow-Up Appointment

Since his initial appointment, Auggie had been discharged from the skilled nursing facility and returned home, where he lived with a daughter who assisted with his care. He was engaged with pulmonary rehabilitation, attending two to three sessions per week, had completed 14 sessions of occupational therapy and 13 sessions of physical therapy, and had started driving again. At the visit, Auggie raised concerns about the cost of his medications, and symptomatically, he complained of increasing dyspnea; weakness; difficulty sleeping; feelings of depression, anxiety, and restlessness; and a new tremor in the bilateral upper extremities. He also noted new cognitive challenges, particularly with

Table 56.1 Auggie's concerns and longitudinal pulmonary, physical, and functional data at ICU follow-up clinic visits

Appointment	Major symptoms/concerns	FEV₁/FVC (%)	MRC dyspnea score	Katz ADLs	Lawton IADLs	Grip strength (L/R; KgF)	6-minute walk distance (meters)	Gait speed (m/s)	5 times sit to stand (seconds)
Pre-hospitalization	N/A	No prior PFTs	1	6	8	N/A	N/A	N/A	N/A
Initial (after hospital discharge)	Shortness of breath, weakness, difficulty sleeping, feeling unprepared	40.1	3	6	1	Not tested	354	0.92	16.6
3 months	Medication cost; dyspnea; weakness; difficulty sleeping; depression, anxiety, and restlessness; tremor in the bilateral upper extremities; cognitive challenges	32.2	2	6	7	27/33	361	1.29	14.2
6 months	Poor appetite, worsening dyspnea, lesser ability to carry out daily functions, worsening anxiety and depression	38.2	3	6	7	25/29	384	1.50	15.6
12 months	Poor appetite, a sensation of food getting stuck in the esophagus, breathlessness, lethargy, worsened feelings of depression and restlessness, feeling the need for more support than family and friends could provide	38.4	3	6	8	27/33	436	1.26	8.61

22 months	Mild pain, constipation, significant breathlessness, a lesser ability to carry out daily functions, feeling unprepared for what was ahead of him	Telemedicine	5	6	4			
25 months	Pain, constipation, breathlessness, feeling weak and tired, feeling anxious and depressed, feeling the need for more support than friends and family can provide	40.2	3	6	5	28/31	288	0.95	11.40
28 months	Hair loss, ongoing dyspnea, fatigue, sleep impairments, feelings of anxiety and depression, restlessness, memory deficits, stuttering	26.4	3	6	6	32/41	299	1.25	10.41
31 months	Persistent dyspnea, fatigue, sleeping difficulties, anxiety, depression, and restlessness	28.9	2	6	8	31/37	396	1.15	8.90
39 months	Cognitive concerns, dyspnea, fatigue, confusion, feeling in need of more support than friends and family could provide, challenges with fine motor coordination	25.7	2	6	8	35/39	286	1.20	8.84

L/R = left/right; N/A = not applicable; FEV₁/FVC = ratio of forced expiratory volume in one second to the forced vital capacity; MRC (Medical Research Council) dyspnea score = ranges from 1 to 5, with 1 representing not troubled by breathlessness except on strenuous exercise and 5 representing too breathless to leave the house, or breathless when dressing or undressing; Katz ADLs = screen of activities of daily living, with 6 being the highest score and representing independence in all ADLs; Lawton IADLs = screen of instrumental activities of daily living, with 8 being the highest score and representing independence in all instrumental activities of daily living

Table 56.2 Auggie's longitudinal cognitive, psychiatric, and quality of life data and interventions provided at ICU follow-up clinic visits

Appointment	MoCA	HADS-A	HADS-D	PTSD screen	Clinical frailty score	EQ-5D	Nutrition assessment	Palliative performance score	Interventions
Pre-hospitalization	N/A	N/A	N/A	N/A	2	N/A	N/A	N/A	N/A
Initial (after hospital discharge)	28/30	1	4	8 (IES-R)	Not recorded	45	Not done	80	Several medication changes; inhaler teaching; goals of care conversation; PT, OT, cognitive therapy, pulmonary rehab referrals
3 months	Not tested	6	7	12 (IES-R)	Not recorded	50	Not done	90	Medication fee reduction; furosemide discontinued; pneumococcal vaccine administered; pulmonary rehab, PT, OT, and cognitive therapy referrals; neurology referral
6 months	27/30	8	13	27 (IES-R)	3	56	Not done	80	Pill box provided; influenza vaccination; smoking cessation counseling; PT and cognitive therapy referrals; mental health referral in concert with PCP; referral to support group for survivors of critical illness
12 months	29/30	7	10	28 (IES-R)	3	29	14	80	Bupropion provided; additional smoking cessation counseling; modified barium swallow test ordered; pulmonary rehabilitation referral; pulmonology referral; encouraged to volunteer with ICU journal project

22 months	15/15 (telephone MoCA)	7	8	0 (IES-6)	4	60	11	80	Pantoprazole discontinued, bowel regimen encouraged, goals of care readdressed; PT referral
25 months	29/30	6	10	0.83 (IES-6)	3	40	13	80	Physical therapy referral
28 months	30/30	2	9	0.83 (IES-6)	4	60	11	90	Cognitive therapy referral; dietitian referral; work-up for hair loss initiated with PCP
31 months	30/30	4	11	1.5 (IES-6)	3	60	13	90	Cognitive therapy referral, pulmonary rehab referral
39 months	28/30	6	7	0.83 (IES-6)	3	50	11	90	Goals of care conversation; advance directive packet provided; PT, OT, cognitive therapy referral; pulmonary rehab referral

MoCA = Montreal Cognitive Assessment Tool, with 30 being the highest score (or 15 on the telephone version): scores less than 26 are consistent with cognitive impairment; HADS-A = Hospital Anxiety and Depression Scale – Anxiety subscale: scores 0–7 normal, 8–10 borderline symptoms, 11–21 significant symptoms; HADS-D = Hospital Anxiety and Depression Scale – Depression subscale: scores 0–7 normal, 8–10 borderline symptoms, 11–21 significant symptoms; IES-R = Impact of Events Scale – revised: scores 33–88 are consistent with post-traumatic stress disorder; IES-6 = Impact of Events Scale – 6: mean scores of more than 1.75 concerning for post-traumatic stress disorder; Clinical frailty score: scores range from 1 to 9, with 1 being very fit and 9 being terminally ill; EQ-5D refers to the question "On a score from 0 to 100, with 0 meaning the worst health you can imagine and 100 meaning the best health you can imagine, how would you rate your health today?"; Nutritional assessment = Mini Nutritional Assessments from the Nestle Nutrition Institute: scores range from 0 to 14, with 12–14 representing normal nutritional status, 8–11 representing at risk for malnutrition, and 0–7 representing malnutrition; Palliative performance score = a composite score of ambulation, activity and evidence of disease, self-care, intake, and consciousness level ranging from 0 to 100, with higher scores representing better health; PT = physical therapy; OT = occupational therapy; PCP = primary care physician.

memory, planning, and word finding difficulties. In consultation with the pharmacist, arrangements were made for medication fee reduction, furosemide was discontinued, and a pneumococcal vaccine was administered given his COPD. Despite having started on medications for his COPD and abstinence from smoking, his FEV_1/FVC ratio fell to 32%. Tests of strength and endurance had generally improved compared with his previous visit, and he was far more independent with IADLs. Cognitive testing was deferred at this visit, but scores on the HADS and IES-r increased, consistent with his symptomatology.

At the end of the appointment, Auggie was provided with prescriptions to continue pulmonary rehabilitation, outpatient physical therapy, and outpatient occupational therapy. He was also given a prescription for outpatient cognitive therapy to address his concerns, and a referral was made to neurology for evaluation of the new-onset tremor.

Six-Month Follow-Up Appointment

Since his previous appointment, Auggie resumed smoking, using it as a coping mechanism to manage the worsening depression and anxiety that he was experiencing. He continued to participate in pulmonary rehabilitation, had completed 12 cognitive therapy sessions, and was discharged from both outpatient occupational and physical therapy after 26 and 21 sessions, respectively. He was discharged from occupational therapy because his anticipated goals and expected outcomes had been achieved, and he was discharged from physical therapy because of oxygen desaturation events during therapy sessions. Auggie made plans with the physical therapist to continue workouts in a public gym, but he did not join because he was embarrassed to bring an oxygen tank to the gym. Symptomatically, he endorsed appetite loss, worsening dyspnea, a lesser ability to carry out daily functions, and worsening anxiety and depression.

Auggie asked to discontinue metoprolol, as he felt that it was contributing significantly to his lack of energy. In consultation with his primary care physician, he stopped taking apixaban for his provoked pulmonary embolism, choosing to complete only a three-month course of anticoagulation, and he also stopped melatonin supplementation, as he did not believe that he was deriving benefit from it. Given his cognitive challenges, a pill box was provided to help manage his medications, and given that it was the winter season, the influenza vaccine was administered.

Spirometric evaluation showed a mild improvement in his FEV_1/FVC ratio to 38%. Smoking cessation counseling was provided, but Auggie declined nicotine replacement therapy and other pharmacotherapy to manage his nicotine addiction. Auggie remained independent in ADLs and IADLs except for shopping independently. Despite having resumed smoking, the distance covered on the 6-minute walk test improved compared with the previous appointment, and other physical assessments were relatively unchanged. Scores on the MoCA remained within the normal range despite him not feeling at his premorbid cognitive baseline, and scores on the HADS and IES-r continued to worsen. He was frequently tearful during the clinic visit.

At the end of the appointment, Auggie set personal goals to quit smoking, to create daily chore lists, and to have adequate energy to complete the list. At his request, referrals for additional outpatient physical therapy (despite oxygen desaturations) and cognitive therapy were provided. In collaboration with his primary care physician, Auggie was also referred to a mental health professional; he was offered an anti-depressant medication but declined. He was also referred to our support group for survivors of critical illness and their loved ones.

12-Month Follow-Up Appointment

Since his previous appointment, Auggie continued to participate in outpatient physical therapy and cognitive therapy; he completed 21 physical therapy sessions and 13 cognitive therapy sessions, having been discharged from both after achieving anticipated goals and expected outcomes. He had also been engaged in psychotherapy sessions with a licensed clinical social worker but was dismayed that the provider had never heard of PICS, stating "How can she help me if she doesn't even know what I have?"

Auggie continued to smoke despite having received nicotine replacement therapy by his primary care provider and smoking cessation counseling at his previous appointment. Symptomatically, he complained of persistent poor appetite, a sensation of food getting stuck in the esophagus, worsened breathlessness, worsened lethargy, worsened feelings of depression and restlessness, and feeling a need for more support than family and friends could provide.

In consultation with pharmacy, given his worsening depression and nicotine dependence, a prescription for bupropion was given, and additional smoking cessation counseling was provided. His FEV_1/FVC ratio remained 38%. Although he had been weaned off supplemental oxygen during the day, he continued to require it at nighttime. He remained independent in ADLs and became independent in all IADLs, now capable of shopping independently. His tests of strength and gait speed were consistent with those of age- and sex-matched controls, and his 6-minute walk test improved considerably since his last visit, on par with normative data from other patients with severe COPD. Given the concern for dysphagia, a swallowing evaluation was performed; although normal in the clinic, a modified barium swallow test was ordered for more objective evaluation. A nutrition screen suggested that he was not at risk for malnutrition. His scores on the MoCA remained within normal limits, and his scores on the HADS improved slightly compared with the prior visit, although he endorsed a worsened mood and recurrent thoughts of death but no intent to harm himself.

At the end of the appointment, Auggie set goals to stop smoking, resume an exercise routine, and begin tending his garden with regularity. Per his request, a prescription for pulmonary rehabilitation was provided, a referral to pulmonology was made, and he was strongly encouraged to continue counseling appointments with the social worker. He asked to volunteer with the ICU journal project that was being initiated at the hospital and sought to become a PICS advocate on social media. Given that this was his one-year appointment, Auggie graduated the clinic, but he was encouraged to return if he felt that he needed our assistance.

22-Month Follow-Up Appointment

Since his previous appointment, Auggie was readmitted to the hospital with recurrent bilateral pulmonary emboli, and he requested that he be re-evaluated in the ICU follow-up clinic. His eight-day hospitalization included a total of six days in the ICU, but he did not require mechanical ventilation; a COVID test was negative. This appointment was performed via telehealth, as the COVID pandemic prevented in-person clinic evaluations.

Symptomatically, Auggie complained of mild pain, constipation, significant breathlessness, a lesser ability to carry out his daily functions, and feeling unprepared for what was ahead of him. He had stopped smoking since his last visit, but he required 2L per minute of oxygen around-the-clock, with significant oxygen desaturations when breathing ambient air. Despite his recent hospitalization, he reported a significant improvement in his mood, which he attributed to weekly participation in our support group for survivors of critical illness.

Given that the visit was performed via telehealth, some aspects of the holistic evaluation, including assessments of respiratory and physical function, were limited. Pantoprazole, which had once again been started in the ICU, was discontinued, and over-the-counter polyethylene glycol was recommended for management of constipation. Although he remained independent with ADLs, he had once again developed dependencies in several IADLs, including shopping, food preparation, laundry, and managing transportation. Scores on the MoCA-telephone were normal, scores on the HADS were stable to improved, and scores on the IES-6 suggested no significant post-traumatic stress disorder.

Given his readmission to the hospital, goals of care were reassessed. While Auggie wanted to remain full code, he qualified this by saying that he would only accept a time-limited trial of intubation and critical care. He would not want long-term life support and would not consider long-term dependency on others as an acceptable quality of life. He valued independence, teaching Sunday school, spending time with his children and grandchildren, working in his garden, and taking care of his dog.

25-Month Follow-Up Appointment

Since his previous appointment, Auggie had remained abstinent from cigarettes but continued to require 2–4L per minute of oxygen throughout the day. Symptomatically, Auggie complained of worsened pain, persistent constipation, breathlessness, feeling weak and tired, feeling anxious and depressed, and feeling a need for more support than friends and family could provide. Spirometric evaluation continued to show an FEV_1/FVC ratio of 40%. He remained independent in ADLs and continued to have dependencies in IADLs, including shopping, food preparation, and laundry. There was a significant worsening in gait speed, strength, and endurance compared with the previous in-person visit, with a particularly marked decrease in distance covered during the 6-minute walk test. Scores on the MoCA remained within normal limits, and scores on the HADS were consistent with his previous evaluation; there was no evidence of PTSD on the IES-6.

At the end of the appointment, given the decline in his physical function measures, a prescription for outpatient physical therapy was provided. He was encouraged to continue participating in the support group for survivors of critical illness.

28-Month Follow-Up Appointment

Since his previous visit, Auggie required a four-day hospitalization for acute appendicitis requiring a laparoscopic appendectomy complicated by an exacerbation of COPD. He had participated in physical therapy, having completed 15 sessions since his last visit. Symptomatically, Auggie complained of new-onset hair loss, ongoing dyspnea, fatigue, sleep impairments, and feelings of anxiety, depression, and restlessness. He resumed smoking two cigarettes every day. Spirometric evaluation showed a decrease in his FEV_1/FVC ratio to 26%, and he continued to require 2–4L per minute of supplemental oxygen, depending on his activity level. He remained independent in ADLs and IADLs except for meal preparation and laundry. Physical assessment showed normal handgrip strength, improved gait speed, and persistent endurance impairments based on the 6-minute walk test. He scored a perfect score on the MoCA but complained of memory and concentration impairments and new stuttering. His anxiety had improved on the HADS, but he continued to have scores concerning for depression; there was no evidence of PTSD on the IES-6.

At the end of the appointment, Auggie was encouraged to continue participating in outpatient physical therapy, and a prescription for cognitive therapy was provided given his concerns despite a normal MoCA score. An evaluation was set up with a dietitian to discuss nutritional intake, as a nutritional screen was concerning for malnutrition. The concern for hair loss and a recommended work-up was communicated to his primary care provider.

31-Month Follow-Up Appointment

Since his previous appointment, Auggie had been discharged from outpatient physical therapy, having completed 31 sessions. Although he had been given a prescription for outpatient cognitive therapy at the previous appointment, he decided not to schedule any visits. Symptomatically, his concerns were similar to the previous appointment, including persistent dyspnea, fatigue, sleeping difficulties, anxiety, depression, and restlessness. He continued to smoke, and his FEV_1/FVC ratio remained stable at 29%. He remained independent in ADLs and IADLs, having started preparing meals and doing laundry since his last visit. The physical assessment remained stable compared with the prior visit aside from a marked increase in the distance covered during the 6-minute walk test, despite an oxygen desaturation to 84% while using 4L per minute of supplemental oxygen. Scores on the MoCA, HADS, and IES-6 remained stable compared with his previous appointment. Scores on a nutrition screening tool suggested that he was adequately nourished, an improvement compared with the previous visit.

At the end of the appointment, Auggie was given a new prescription for cognitive therapy and a prescription for pulmonary rehabilitation.

39-Month Follow-Up Appointment

Since his previous appointment, Auggie required an eight-day admission to the hospital for management of community acquired pneumonia and an exacerbation of COPD. He participated in two additional sessions of outpatient physical therapy but then declined to return. Symptomatically, he continued to have concerns about his cognitive function, including an inability to plan, poor concentration, and impaired memory; he also reported dyspnea, fatigue, confusion, and feeling the need for more support than friends and family could provide. He continued to smoke and require supplemental oxygen, and his FEV_1/FVC ratio remained at 26%. Despite his hospitalization, he remained independent in ADLs and IADLs, but he complained of difficulties with fine motor coordination and tremor, making things like getting dressed more challenging. Physical assessment scores remained stable compared with the prior visit except for the distance covered during the 6-minute walk test, which fell to 286 m. Scores on the MoCA, HADS, and IES-6 were generally similar, although scores on the depression subscale of the HADS had improved.

Given another hospitalization, goals of care were revisited. He confirmed that his code status was full, stating that he felt obligated to want future aggressive measures given that he had "beaten the odds" in the past, but he did not want to undergo tracheostomy, have long-term dependence on machines, or reside in a nursing facility. An advance directives packet was provided to him, and he was encouraged to have conversations with his children about his wishes so that the decision-making burden would not be placed on them in the future.

At the end of the visit, he was encouraged to get an influenza vaccination as soon as they became available; he was up-to-date on COVID and pneumococcal vaccinations. He was given prescriptions for physical therapy, occupational therapy, cognitive therapy, and pulmonary rehabilitation. He set the following goals for himself: quit smoking in two months; devise a daily routine for eating, hygiene, exercise, and prayer; and complete the advanced directive documentation.

Auggie never returned to the clinic for another follow-up appointment but continues to remain active in the weekly peer support group, remains an advocate for PICS on social media, and volunteers his time at the hospital when he can.

Major Themes of the Case Study

Auggie's case of PICS highlights a number of important concepts characteristic of the syndrome. Although Auggie had impairments in the three classic domains (physical, cognitive, and psychiatric), there was a progression in their development, and not all of them occurred contemporaneously initially. At the first appointment, Auggie was primarily concerned with physical and occupational deficits. By the second appointment, cognitive impairments had become a significant challenge, and at the third appointment, the psychiatric manifestations of PICS were readily apparent. The combination of these deficits led to significant social disabilities, highlighted by an initial inability to drive and subsequent difficulties resuming previous activities and roles that brought him joy, like gardening, playing with his grandchildren, and teaching Sunday school. It is also important to appreciate that the current screening tools commonly used to assess deficits in these domains are imperfect. For example, Auggie never had a MoCA score that was consistent with cognitive impairment, but symptomatically, he raised concerns about his memory, executive function, and attention frequently, and only he could tell that his presentation was different than his pre-morbid cognitive function.

Auggie's case also demonstrates the frequent interdependency between the physical, cognitive, and psychiatric disabilities of PICS. The psychiatric sequelae of PICS appeared later in Auggie's course, driven largely by his inability to effectively cope with the physical and cognitive challenges he was facing. Worsening depression led to a resumption in cigarette smoking, which negatively impacted his pulmonary function, which in turn prevented him from fully engaging in physical and cognitive therapy. His depression and anxiety contributed to his inability to reintegrate into social roles, which further intensified his sadness and sense of isolation, highlighted in his oft-stated concerns about feeling unprepared for the future and feeling the need for more support than his family and friends could provide.

Patients with PICS are at increased risk for readmission to the hospital, worsening of pre-existing chronic disease, development of new chronic disease, and increased healthcare-related expenditures, all of which were true with Auggie. Furthermore, as a chronic condition, PICS can wax and wane in its intensity and can be exacerbated by acute, intercurrent illnesses, as demonstrated by the declines noticed following Auggie's hospital readmissions.

Auggie's case of PICS is quite typical and demonstrates how difficult managing patients with PICS can be. Patients with PICS benefit from frequent and longitudinal assessment in a multidisciplinary, interprofessional clinic that affords the time and resources that these patients need and deserve. As our knowledge of PICS advances and evidence refines the way we care for patients with it, ICU follow-up clinics can minimize the impact this syndrome has on survivors' lives and help rehabilitate them to the healthiest version of themselves possible.

Chapter 57

In Their Own Words: Perspectives from Survivors and Their Loved Ones

Franziska Herpich, Scott H. Hommel, Sr., Karen A. Korzick, Constance M. Bovier, and Cori Davis

While much of this book has been focused on describing the hazards of hospitalization and post-intensive care syndrome (PICS) in quantitative terms, is if often the personal stories of survivors of critical illness and their loved ones that are so much more revealing than the distance walked during six minutes or a score on a cognitive test. It was not until I began seeing patients in my ICU follow-up clinic that I truly appreciated how life-changing surviving a critical illness could be. Understanding the real-life impact of the physical, functional, cognitive, psychiatric, and social impairments that those suffering from PICS face is a profoundly moving and motivating experience. For that reason, I wanted to close this book with stories of survivors and their loved ones, allowing the reader to integrate and contextualize the objective data that has heretofore been presented in neatly parsed, individual chapters and to more deeply appreciate how that data reflects a much more impactful lived experience.

Franziska Herpich, Neuro-Intensivist and Survivor of Critical Illness Secondary to Stroke

Lying in the back of an ambulance, trying to unsuccessfully unlock my phone, was the last place I would have imagined myself to be on this very busy, fully booked day, just one week before starting my first job as a neurocritical care attending physician.

The morning had started out just as I had planned: I got up at 6am, had a sip of water, put on my running shoes, and headed out into the already hot and humid summer air to go for a short run. I did not know at the time, but this was going to be my last morning run for a long while. At some point in the middle of this fateful morning exercise routine, a blood clot traveled up into one of my major brain arteries, suddenly blocking blood and oxygen supply to the left side of my brain. Due to the resulting immediate right-sided weakness, I tumbled and fell. Some passing runners tried to help me get up and talk to me, but their words were of no use to me. I had absolutely no idea what they were saying. They may as well have spoken a different language; meaningless sounds were escaping their mouths. Peculiarly, I neither noticed nor cared that they were speaking in tongues. I was totally oblivious to the deficit. I had a complete lack of language.

Language is a two-way street: one needs to be capable of speaking in order to communicate, and one also needs to be able to interpret words and sentences into meaning. At that moment, I was incapable of either. I vividly remember feeling mostly embarrassment and annoyance by the entire situation, which only worsened when I realized that my helpers were calling an ambulance. Typically, I am not known for being shy with words, and thankfully, cursing is an emotional response, originating from the right hemisphere and therefore not affected by aphasia. Hence, I was still able to vocalize my frustration via a flurry of swear words.

My biggest stroke of luck was to have a major stroke very close to a comprehensive stroke center, where I was able to quickly receive both intravenous lytic treatment to break up the clot and a mechanical thrombectomy. Despite those prompt measures, I was left with significant expressive aphasia. I had severe difficulties thinking of and saying words, let alone full sentences. Realizing that this would remain a lasting deficit, I was devastated. Life, as I had known it, was over. Everything I had worked hard for over the past decade vanished before my eyes.

From the moment I finished my neurology rotation in medical school, I knew that this would be the specialty I wanted to pursue. One small brain lesion, depending on where it is located, can result in the inability to produce or interpret language, to move half of one's body, to identify faces, or to do math. No other organ fascinated me as much as the brain did. I developed a sharp efficiency during residency and understood that the fast pace and the acuity of the neuro ICU was a wonderful fit for me. The efficiency with which I prided myself, however, was also paired with a fair amount of impatience. Pre-rounding in the morning was mainly a necessary annoyance for me. It was merely something that needed to be done in order for me to fully participate in and lead rounds. Seeing it as an important opportunity to become acquainted with my patients and to update them on their progress hardly crossed my mind. I continued to work hard, and at the age of 33, after one year of internship, three years of neurology residency, and two years of neuro-intensive care fellowship, I was finally ready to take the training wheels off and start my first job as an attending physician.

The sudden transition from a healthy and independent individual to one needing a nurse for nearly everything and finding myself completely reliant on my friends and family as my spokespersons was dizzying. I was in a state of total vulnerability and dependence. My life had been completely turned on its head. Once the shock wore off and I fully internalized that my previously healthy brain was injured, I was determined that I would do anything in my power to facilitate its recovery.

As a neurologist, I am aware that neurons don't replenish, but I know that the brain is both delicate and powerful, with an incredible ability to transform and adjust. I have observed the wonders of neuroplasticity over and over again during my training. Neuroplasticity is an almost magical capacity that our brain has to create new connections and pathways to eventually repossess the lost function of the damaged brain tissue. However, this is not a rapid process! It takes time. It demands both endurance and patience. I knew that my brain needed rest and sleep in order to start this process of transformation and recovery.

Patients in a neuro-intensive care unit are typically bombarded with frequent neuro checks and very little uninterrupted sleep. I recall being woken up every hour to state my name, my birthday, where I was, and the current date. This was frustrating beyond imagination! Not only did I not get the rest that I knew I needed in order to heal, but I was also constantly reminded how inhibited my language production was. Additionally, painful IV sites rendered me nearly sleepless. They pinched and made the IV pump alarm go off every time I bent my elbows during those few hours when I wasn't woken up to remind the nurse of my name.

I was also suffering from the impact of a brain injury on the rest of my body. Upon beginning the recovery process, the entire rest of my body was left completely drained of energy. Something as simple as brushing my teeth seemed like an insurmountable peak to climb. The loud noises from IV pumps or mindless TV shows playing constantly in the hospital were unbearable. Even music, which I loved to listen to, was intolerable. All sounds were essentially causing me physical pain. All I longed for was a calm and silent room in which to rest and let my brain heal.

Thankfully, up to this point in my life, I had never been a person troubled by frequent headaches. However, the overwhelming stress of my life being turned upside down and a mild brain bleed caused by the procedure to get the blood clot out led to an excruciating headache during my hospital stay. The pain was amplified by total lack of sleep and rest. None of the medications that I received seemed to alleviate it. All the pain medications could do was put me in an empty yet still painful daze. These few days were truly a personal hell for me: no rest, no sleep, severe all-consuming headaches, and no words to express the way I felt (swear words aside). This felt like the concoction of the "anti-recipe" for healing a brain.

In neurology, the motto "time is brain" means that we need to act fast on acute brain damage, like strokes or brain bleeds, as every additional elapsed minute leads to further brain damage. Therefore, frequent exams are a necessary evil to detect new brain injury that might require emergent intervention and must not be missed. That being said, now more than ever, I understand how fragile our brain is, and that it requires an inordinate amount of rest in order to equilibrate and to prepare for the upcoming challenges of rehabilitation. Lack of sleep and rest is very counterproductive. We need to find a balance for our brain-injured patients. On the one hand, we need to detect worrisome changes in their exam while also maintaining a higher level of awareness that the constant disturbances interfere with the patient's ability to rehabilitate.

After a couple of days, doctors determined that I was stable enough to have less frequent neuro checks, and thus I was downgraded from the ICU to the regular patient floor. This was great news for my progress, but it also meant that I would be sharing a room with another patient. My roommate was lovely. She was in her 70s and had just undergone spinal surgery. She had a hard time adjusting after surgery, was in severe pain, had frequent nausea and vomiting lasting throughout the night, and she liked her room temperature rather warm. Needless to say, the rest I was longing for was once again hard to come by.

Every stroke patient gets evaluated by an occupational, a physical, and, if indicated, a speech therapist in order to determine what level of therapy is appropriate for them after they leave the hospital. My therapists recommended acute inpatient rehabilitation to help me improve my deficits. I was finally ready for discharge on a Friday. Having worked in a hospital for several years, I knew what that meant. Nothing would be put into motion until Monday, and the earliest I would be able to leave for rehab would be the middle of the following week. This thought was unbearable for me. I was not willing under any circumstances to stay any longer in an environment where I could not get the rest I so desperately needed. Therefore, I decided that, instead of going to an inpatient rehab, I would go home and start an outpatient therapy program.

In the past, I frowned upon my patients who disregarded the recommendations made by our therapists and would just go home and take matters into their own hands. Now having a different perspective, I understand more clearly that no one truly knows their bodies better than patients themselves, and therefore, they should have greater agency over them. We shouldn't be so quick to judge patients who think they know what is best for them. I was very fortunate to have been able to work with incredibly talented, compassionate, and motivated therapists during my outpatient rehabilitation program. My therapists helped me to get back on my feet, literally and figuratively. Miraculously, after a few months, I was even able to, with some delay, start my new job as a neuro-intensive care physician.

This journey of transitioning from a neurologist to a stroke patient and back to a practicing physician has significantly changed both my perspective and my practice. I am now personally and painfully aware that my patients and their families are experiencing the worst moments of their lives when I first meet them. Unfortunately, the day-to-day life in an ICU is busy and hectic, and so we aren't left with an unlimited amount of time to spend with patients and their families. Nevertheless, when I see my patients, I make every attempt to make the interaction personal, even if it is just sharing a word of kindness or giving them the hope and motivation that they so desperately need to begin their recovery journey.

Small needs, like painful IV sites or disturbing noises from the IV pumps, are no longer just petty concerns, but low-hanging fruit that can be fixed easily and improve my patients' hospital experiences and therefore their recoveries. On my checklist for each patient during my daily rounds is the frequency of neuro examinations. This way, I am actively assessing if we can reduce the number of examinations, or if it is still necessary to keep a very close eye on them.

We all know that "time is brain," and this must not be forgotten, yet I had to learn in a very painful way that our brain also requires its own time and rest in order to overcome injury and start the healing process. It is critically important to recognize these two antagonizing forces, find a balance, and treat our patients with understanding and compassion.

Scott Hommel, Survivor of Critical Illness Secondary to Intra-Abdominal Sepsis, and His Wife, Karen Korzick, Intensivist and Expert on Post-Intensive Care Syndrome

On May 7, 2019, our personal journey as future ICU survivors began when I, Scott, woke up with severe abdominal pain. Karen, my wife, kept two journals, one for my hospital stays and experiences and a second for her thoughts and experiences. She played a large role in my care both as my advocate in the hospital and as my primary caregiver at home. We live in a rural area; my care was at the tertiary care hospital and rehabilitation facility operated by the health system at which she works.

From May 8, when I had my first abdominal surgery, to the end of May, I suffered from tremendous delirium driven by recurrent abdominal sepsis and a total of four trips to the operating room. In 30 days, I lost 60 pounds and spent a week in the ICU between surgeries three and four, with three days on the ventilator. I was thought to have an iatrogenic bowel injury from the first surgery that was never localized, which resulted in stool leakage into the abdominal cavity. I lost about 50% of my anterior abdominal wall soft tissues due to recurrent surgeries and was left with a very large ventral hernia defect, a colostomy bag, and an open central wound with a mesh and a vacuum (vacc) dressing. At the inpatient rehabilitation facility in early June, a night shift nurse cross taped my leaking ostomy appliance to my vacc dressing and left me overnight with stool sucking into my open abdominal wound. I could not look at my abdominal wall yet, but knew something was not right, so I asked Karen to look at the situation when she came to visit me the next morning.

In both mid-June and mid-July of 2019, I required repeat hospitalizations for recurrent sepsis from continued intra-abdominal infections. In July, I was discharged home on IV antibiotic and IV antifungal drugs to be given four times a day for six weeks. Karen stayed home with me for most of the summer, and from July to August, she managed the PICC line, not allowing anybody else to touch it. We had developed trust issues by this time, and neither of us felt safe unless we were together and Karen had total control of health devices. With my fifth surgery in January 2020, I had the colostomy reversed, the right half of my colon was removed, and I had a major repair of the large ventral hernia defect. Since then, I have dealt with repeated functional bowel obstruction events two or three times per year, about half of which have required hospitalization. I had no kidney disease prior to all this; now I have stage II chronic kidney disease.

Delirium

I experienced a completely different reality, with its own sights, sounds, smells, and tactile experiences throughout the hospital stay. I talked to people that were not there and watched the walls of my ICU room become something else, placing me in different surroundings. An alien with long tentacles would visit me, floating over my ICU bed and brushing my body with its tentacles. I heard two types of music: happy music and ominous music, matching my mood in the moment. Samples of my delirium experiences are below.

Surgery 2

Scott: I asked my wife to bring in my laptop so I could transmit files to my colleagues at work before the surgery. When she brought it in and asked me for the password to open it, I refused to give it to her "because Agent X would give the secret code to the bad guys and the universe would end." Tuesday night I thought my roommate and his sister were smoking pot in our room. I activated the nurse call button and started pulling off all the medical devices attached to me. I asked the nurses to call security because I did not feel safe.

Karen: I found out the next morning that his roommate had to be transferred to the ICU overnight, but security was never called. We thought the narcotic pain medication was causing his delirium, so I asked for non-narcotic pain medication and arranged for my colleague, an ICU psychologist, to see him.

Surgery 3

Scott: When the IV therapy team came to start a second IV, I thought I was in an alley and the medical team was a bunch of muggers trying to kill me. I cannot overstate how real this was to me. I still remember "standing" in the alley, seeing cars go by at the end, feeling the breeze and watching it stir the debris on the ground. Given the feeling of "they are out to get me" that I had been feeling, being taken into the alley was very threating to me. I therefore cocked my fist and arm back to strike out to defend myself. Karen was able to talk me down and keep me from hitting the staff.

When a patient acts angry, "weird," or even violent, it is possible that they are reacting to things that none of us on the outside can see. I am grateful that Karen and my healthcare team were able to eventually recognize what I was experiencing and that an ICU psychologist was available to help me understand that not everything I was experiencing was real, which allowed me to take the time to evaluate the inputs to my senses before responding to situations that only existed in my mind. The expertise the psychologist brought to both of us was invaluable in my recovery and Karen's sanity. We both wonder what happens to delirious patients when there is no expert behavioral health specialist who is a member of the inpatient care team.

Hopelessness

Scott: By the third surgery, I was feeling weak and hopeless. I thought I was going to die. As I was heading to the operating room, I told Karen to tell everybody that I loved them. Postoperatively, during the week in the ICU, I am told I had a lot of visitors; I remember little of them, but I am grateful they cared enough to visit.

Karen: At this point, I knew that he was thinking he would die without him saying it and that he might be giving up. I ripped him a new one verbally to motivate him to not give up. I told him he had to fight to stay alive because I was not ready to be a widow. His roommate's wife looked at me with eyes wide open in shock from how I spoke. While he was in the operating room, I went to a stairwell to cry for the first time through all these events. Despite all the stress, there were moments of levity: one friend showed up to mow our property numerous times, stuffing himself through the garage dog door when I forgot to leave the main garage door open for him. When he told me this, the visual image of him stuffing himself through that door made me laugh, one of the few times I laughed that summer.

Scott: Hopelessness re-emerged when I developed sepsis again in mid-July. I literally refused to go to the hospital; I told Karen I would rather die than go back to the hospital, and I meant it.

Karen: I gave him a few minutes to think about it. He counter-offered with "let's go in the morning." I knew he was delirious again and tried explaining to him that every hour without treatment increased his risk of death. That did not convince him. So, I had to motivate him with the threat of a phone call to the police and an emergency petition to get him to the hospital. He begrudgingly got in the car.

When things are going wrong repeatedly, hopelessness becomes a real issue for both the patient and their family. Yet we did not recognize this in the moment. We only became aware that this was a theme that we were dealing with in the years of conversation that we have had since 2019. Visits from family, friends, and colleagues were invaluable to both of us. Families need to understand that recovery is not a smooth linear process, especially with respect to the psychological and cognitive effects of prolonged acute severe illness. Reasoning and judgment may be impaired for a long time in the recovering patient, even though physical health is improving, and families need to be educated about this reality and supported through it.

Body Image, Anxiety, Sleep Deprivation, and Discharge Education/Planning

Scott: I would not look at my abdomen until mid-June. Karen cared for my wounds and the ostomy appliance until she started to go into the office for administrative work. It was only because she was no longer home all day that I was forced to look at my abdomen and care for my ostomy appliance. Ostomy education occurred once, for about an hour, the day before my discharge in early June. In retrospect, I was still delirious at that time.

We wonder how well patients and families with no healthcare professionals in the family can learn, while delirious, sleep deprived, and stressed out, about how to care for complex wounds or be compliant with complex discharge instructions. We strongly suspect that some part of morbidity and mortality post discharge from events like mine is driven by the disconnect between what health system process designers, who are not impaired by delirium, acute stress, and sleep deprivation, think patients and family members can learn to do in short periods of time versus what their respectively impaired brains are actually capable of learning on the day of discharge. We both feel this needs to be addressed in transitions of care process design.

Past Experience, Recovery, Emotional Intelligence, and Relationship Health

Scott: Once I was out of the ICU, I agreed to let Karen take me in a wheelchair to the hospital's outdoor serenity garden. The IV pump started beeping, and she could not stop it from beeping, but she did tell me that I was OK. It was beeping because the medication had finished, and the nurse would clear the pump when we got back to my room.

Karen: This really upset Scott, but he was not able to tell me why. He panicked and demanded to return to his room immediately, which we did, and the nurse cleared the pump. It took him weeks to be able to verbalize to me that, as a nuclear submarine veteran, if an alarm goes off on the submarine, you figure out why immediately or you and the whole crew may die. To him, that IV pump continuing to alarm meant that he was going to die in that moment. Weeks later at home, when I was trying to explain to him why it was so important to do his physical therapy exercises every day, Scott responded with "how do you know what you are talking about?" In that particular interaction, I really wanted to throttle him, but instead responded, "you do remember what I do for a living, don't you?" then walked away before a fight ensued. In these two events, it felt to me that he didn't trust my expertise and judgment as a physician, which hurt me. I felt disrespected. What my ICU survivor care provider-trained mind realized is that he really didn't remember what I did for a living, and that the serenity garden experience, while motivated by good intentions on my part, was a terrifying experience on his part.

Again, these are insights that we have gained only through years of ongoing conversations with one another about 2019. We wonder how well families are prepared for what an ICU recovery trajectory really looks like if they are not being cared for by healthcare providers with expertise in ICU recovery. And, we wonder how well life partners are educated about and supported through complex recovery trajectories and how that education and support, or the lack thereof, may result in avoidable damage to some life partner relationships.

Financial and Career Impacts

Scott: My cognitive abilities took until early November 2019 to normalize. I did not start driving until mid-autumn and, even then, only around our neighborhood. I returned to work part-time in early November but could only concentrate for three to four hours at a time and had to take a daily afternoon nap. My job entails travel, but I could not travel from May 2019 until the summer of 2020. Clients agreed to postpone projects that were my primary responsibility until I recovered. In July 2019, I was the minor partner/owner of my company; the senior partner/owner was due to retire, and I was going to buy out the majority ownership interest, with two new colleagues buying into ownership. This was postponed by two years until July 2021, affecting the careers of three of my colleagues.

Karen: My professional life was impacted in several ways. I postponed an expansion of the ICU survivor clinic I ran, postponed planned research projects, and missed months of scheduled ICU shifts to care for Scott, with the associated impact on my colleagues who had to cover my shifts. Due to the iatrogenic bowel injury and nursing care error with the ostomy appliance and my knowledge of health system quality, safety, and risk management processes, we were enrolled in the health system's Candor Program. Our out-of-pocket costs were absorbed by the health system for care received from May 2019 through January 2020, and I had no loss of income while caring for Scott at home. We also missed several once-in-a-lifetime special events for family members during the summer of 2019.

We both wonder what happens to patients injured by gaps in healthcare quality who have no advocate with knowledge of risk management practices or service recovery programs like Candor, which offset the financial impact of my prolonged illness and recovery. Our cash flow was stable throughout while Karen was home taking care of me, but this is not the norm. We worry about the ability of those with no employer support to keep a job and maintain their finances while care is being delivered by family members until the survivor is well enough for them and their family caregiver(s) to return to full-time work. We wonder how families with young children and/or seniors to care for negotiate an ICU stay and recovery at home if they have no help from family or friends. We wonder how many recovering ICU survivors fail to get the care they need and do not recover well due to the financial strain on their household.

The Journey Continues

In addition to the recurrent bowel obstruction events and the need for a nephrologist, I can no longer take non-steroidal anti-inflammatory drugs (NSAIDS) for minor aches and pains, but the acetaminophen that I can take often does not relieve my discomfort. My work continues to be affected by my health. I have missed scheduled work travel due to recurrent bowel dysmotility events. Our family travel plans now always include consideration of the locally available health services and ease of transport back home to my surgeons; we have decided not to travel to certain former "bucket list" destinations due to these concerns. I struggle sometimes to remember clients' names and details of past projects, struggles that I never had prior to 2019.

On the positive side, I have learned to be an advocate for myself with healthcare providers. I watch nurses and insist that IV caps are wiped for a solid 15 seconds before IV medications are administered. I now ask a lot of questions, and if the answers do not make sense, I refuse to proceed until satisfactory explanations are given. I still intensely dislike hospitals, but with time and talking with Karen, her ICU psychologist colleague, and the ICU survivor clinic nurse manager, I no longer have overt panic attacks walking into a hospital or clinic for my care.

Affecting Change
Part of what validated the suffering that I endured is that Karen advocated for change in the healthcare system regarding ostomy care after hours. Now, every adult medical surgical nurse in the main hospital and the rehabilitation hospital has an annual in-service on how to properly care for a leaking ostomy appliance in case the ostomy nurse is not available. Karen was also invited to sit on the health system's patient quality and safety committee as a patient/family representative, a position she holds to this day, and to which she has brought several issues from the patient/family perspective that have been or are being addressed with process changes across the system.

A Note of Thanks to My Nurses
The care of the nurses is so important to patients – I remember the great nurses for their kindness and compassion and willingness to explain things to me as an adult and not as if I were a child. I remember the not-so-great healthcare team members who made my roommate and I feel like we were an annoyance. I do not remember all of their names or faces, but I remember the small acts of kindness provided to me in a way that still brings tears to my eyes. For example, a nurse offered to wash my hair. Afterwards, I felt so normal, so human. These types of small gestures were not small to me. They made all the difference. Good nurses need to be celebrated more than they are at present.

Final Thoughts
We realize how fortunate we were to have the family, friends, colleagues, and financial stability that we had from May 2019 until I recovered from the final surgery in 2020. We are also aware that I may not have survived if Karen was not advocating for me and bringing to bear her expertise in critical care medicine and ICU survivor care to my benefit. We worry about what happens to those ICU patients and their families that have no family members or friends with medical knowledge or no ICU survivor care experts caring for them in recovery.

Our final concern is this: we understand that financial "return-on-investment" is part of the conversation between healthcare system leadership and ICU survivor care provider teams. But as our case illustrates, there is a tremendous return on investment for the patient and their family when expert ICU survivor care is provided, even if the patient needs prolonged, expensive care or is repeatedly readmitted. We are deeply concerned that cost of care, reimbursement rates, and readmission rate reduction in the first 30, 60, or 90 days after discharge are often the only metrics used by health systems to value ICU follow-up clinics. The voices of the patient, their family members, and their employers need to be included in these conversations about finance, value, and return on investment. The 30-to-90-day time frame metric needs to be viewed with a very high degree of suspicion for ICU survivors, particularly those with severe sepsis, prolonged respiratory failure, or prolonged delirium, given the extended time frame needed to fully recover from these pathophysiological conditions. Finally, the value to employers, and to society in general, from returning persons to prior job duties and avoiding prolonged or permanent disability, needs to be part of the return-on-investment calculations of the ICU survivor care process.

Connie Bovier, Survivor of Critical Illness Secondary to Community-Acquired Pneumonia and Acute Respiratory Distress Syndrome

I laughed.

She told me that it would take about a year of rehabilitation for me to recover. And I laughed out loud. Then I realized that she was serious. She, the physical therapist, had just witnessed me walking my first independent lap around the ICU. She heard the encouraging applause from the medical staff that saved my life, and she joined them. She told me this because she knew all about recovering from the ICU, about rehabilitating from death's doorway. OK ... so she knew all about recovering from the ICU, but she didn't know me. I should have told her that I didn't have a year to get back to functioning as I normally do. I had my life waiting for me. Did she know that? I'm already breathing, walking, and eating on my own. Sure, I'm very shaky and weak and tired like I have never been before, but that can't last. Can it?

I've been away from home long enough, and I've got so much to do. I have kids to teach and Bible studies to join and a family who needs me. Why is she talking about rehabilitation facilities or nursing homes before I'll see or do any of that? I'll do whatever it takes to get well and get back to normal. I've risen up above many obstacles in my life, and they only made me stronger. Some people have actually called me the strongest person they know. This wasn't the first time that I nearly died. She didn't know that, I'll bet. I knew, though. How could this be any worse than what I've already overcome? It could only be worse if there were things about my current condition that I didn't know ...

As it turned out, there was so much about getting back to being myself that I didn't know, but I know some things now. My old self wasn't waiting for me at the end of one year of rehabilitation. Or at the end of six years of rehabilitation. She's gone! She's long gone! As my daughter simply stated, "My mom is not my mom anymore."

I came to accept that fact around 18 months after I left the nursing home, which I was miraculously (and happily) able to drive myself home from. Since then, I have come to accept so much of what has happened to me and what is now my life. Learning how to accept this is probably the best thing that came out of my getting sick. Much of that acceptance came with tears, lots of tears. Fearful tears, angry tears. Frustration tears, lonely tears. Tears from fears, tears from memories of a former self, tears from grief. Then there were the tears when I lost a fight with a Ziploc® bag because of my tremors and weakness. I was rescued from that first Ziploc® bag. Today, I laugh at them and don't expect that I will close them easily.

You would think that there would be tears of gratitude for being alive. Naturally, that's what everyone thinks and says, but would they think that and say that if they knew that my brain doesn't work? Would they think that if they knew that I am not OK, even though I tell them that I am? I tell them that I am OK because I am afraid that they wouldn't understand what's going on with me and would reject me if they did. But how could they understand? Even I don't understand why I can't do simple things like put the dishes away when I washed them three days ago or make a to-do list. It's not good to be alive when you can't communicate because you can't process what others are saying to you or remember what they've said. Or you interrupt them because you are afraid that you won't remember what you wanted to say to them. And after the conversation is over, you are afraid that you are going to forget everything that you talked about. I have been afraid of those things so many times and for so long that it makes me not even want to try. I have found myself saying "I can't" to so many things.

The neurologist did an MRI and told me that I have a beautiful brain, but she can't tell me why I have tremors in my arms or why I can't read even the simplest thing. Forget about email. There are over 11,000 waiting for me. I try to read a recipe and focus on completing each step before I forget what I just read. Then I need to read it over again. It's just a cruel joke that I play on myself. Making a meal takes me three times longer than it would have normally taken me to complete. So many hours of the day are lost that I will never get back. Do people with beautiful brains go to their mother's funeral and realize that they forgot to brush their hair? Yes, they do. And it makes them want to cry. Thank God I have learned to laugh at PICS. And I have learned to play the PICS card, which is the excuse that I use when I realize that I have done something wrong or that I can't do what most normal people could. It's my form of self-acceptance.

The neurologist also sent me to have an EMG. The report came back that I was very, very strong. I went there to find out why I was having tremors, not to hear that I was very, very strong. And that's not even the truth. I've been weak since being in the ICU. So weak that I can't even lift a frying pan without using two hands. So weak that I can't hold my granddaughter while I am standing for more than a few minutes. There is so much that I can't do. Would I have laughed if I had known that? Would I have laughed if I had known that it would be such a great struggle to just take care of myself and how impossible it would be to have a daily routine? When your brain doesn't work the way it once did and all that you need to do is not getting done, just living life becomes overwhelming and makes it even harder to think. You want to ask for help, but you can't think to make a list. You can't think to explain why simple things are hard or even impossible.

It's a struggle to not want to end it all, to learn to love this new self. Is there a pill that I can take with the other 11 that could help me love this broken me? The old self only took one pill a day. I could accept that. I also didn't know that a slight sore throat would put me on high alert and send me spiraling with the fear of it happening all over again. I am acutely aware of any twinge that I feel. That's definitely not my old self. I now know that hypervigilance is a symptom of post-traumatic stress disorder (PTSD). I didn't know that I would find various parts of my body clenched tight for seemingly no reason. Maybe my shoulders, or fist, or jaw, or toes. And I can't figure out if it's because my oxygen level is low or because I'm anxious. Both are a struggle for me in this new life. Sometimes I would be clenched so hard that my body would ache and only then would I realize that I was doing it. I didn't know that I would develop a stutter or be unable to convey a cohesive thought regardless of its importance. It's really easy to lose an audience when this happens. Each day is tricky. These days I say that my life is tricky. I can no longer keep promises. Too much comes into play to make things happen, keeping me from what I want or need to do. Forgetfulness. Fatigue. Pain. Depression. Anxiety.

First, you need to remember the date and time. That seems simple enough, right? Wrong! Simply texting a date into your calendar will work only if you can focus long enough to complete it and your tremors don't act up. Setting reminders is a must along with looking at my calendar early and each day. I've learned to choose afternoon appointments and to utilize Alexa (from Amazon) for everything that she's worth.

Also, there is no "simply" in my life. The very first thing that I was taught in occupational therapy, which was the first of many assorted therapies for me, was "You will need to budget your energy." I didn't understand what that meant at first, but I very quickly learned the importance of this and had to accept that I would need to give up so much of my regular routine because nothing was simple anymore, and even the simplest actions were exhausting. I'm talking about self-care, meal preparation, household chores, social activities, and shopping. Just the making of a list and prioritizing and planning the execution could send me back under the sheets. This happened a lot. Unfortunately, this only made matters worse. While under the covers, I stayed isolated, and social events were missed. All of my undone tasks were still waiting for me, along with the ones that piled up while I was in bed, creating an overwhelming mountain for me to face.

Some would say that I should seek help and see a therapist. OK . . . I can't finish what I have for the day already, so I should add something more for me to get done? I did, though. And after a long search and wait, my appointment day came. I had an appointment with a therapist who had never heard of PICS before, and he couldn't understand why I was struggling so much. So sad. I tried to explain what was happening with my brain and the work it took to try to get simple things done, but he couldn't understand. Then the appointment was over, and I was absolutely spent, exhausted, and done for the day. The appointment was the only thing I accomplished that day, and it ended in stress and despair. Despite this, I continue with therapy because living with depression is not the life I want to live.

People don't understand, even those that know me. My adult children don't remember me ever needing help from anyone. These are only a few of the challenges that I encountered after my first ICU stay. There have been three additional illnesses that sent me back there. I have not shared the strife caused by COVID and unvaccinated family members, which kept me isolated in my bedroom until I eventually purchased a new place to live. Being able to successfully accomplish purchasing a home with PICS is a miracle in my eyes. It took me longer than most to pack and move, but I did it with the broken brain method.

PICS affects me physically, mentally, and cognitively every day. I use all that I've learned these past six years from doctors and therapists along with my own trial and error techniques, which I call my "cheats," to overcome obstacles and to accept and love this new me. I've lost so many things about myself and my life that I loved. I now try to reimagine those things and have them back in my life in some form. I may not remember what I read or watch or hear, but I choose to enjoy it still. I refuse to succumb to depression or anxiety and utilize speaking truth to myself when I realize that I'm going in that direction. With all that I've lost, I have not lost hope. These days my heart really aches for all ICU survivors who are being treated by people that don't recognize PICS, the survivors who have the struggles yet are given no explanations or a path forward.

Cori Davis, Survivor of Critical Illness Secondary to SARS-CoV-2 Infection and Acute Respiratory Distress Syndrome

April 8, 2021 was a day that changed my life. It started off as an ordinary day during the pandemic. I woke up, performed my morning ritual, and made a quick breakfast before starting my shift with my former employer. Despite drinking coffee, I still felt exhausted. Initially, I thought that what I was experiencing was a mild case of allergies. I had been taking allergy medicine for a few days, but the medication didn't alleviate my symptoms. Then, I thought that maybe it was a mild cold, so I began taking cold medicine. I didn't see any improvement with the cold medicine either, so I called my primary care doctor, and he told me to take a COVID test. I did, and it came back positive. On the night of April 9, 2021, my oxygen saturation sunk to 30%. I wouldn't have survived the night had it not been for my nephew calling me and then having my oldest daughter check on me because I didn't sound right. She found me passed out on my bed. She called for an ambulance, and I was taken to the hospital, where I was admitted to the ICU due to acute respiratory distress syndrome (ARDS). I was in the hospital for five weeks and two days; over three and a half weeks were spent in the ICU, and for two of those weeks, I was on a ventilator.

After the ICU, I had to learn to eat, talk, walk, and control my bladder and bowels again. It was a second infancy for me. Imagine experiencing a second infancy with the intellect of an adult. It's hard to fathom unless you've experienced it. Having to have my diaper changed because I soiled it was demoralizing, humiliating, and depressing. I had no idea why all of this was happening to me. I needed occupational therapy, physical therapy, cognitive therapy, and speech therapy. I've had many cycles of these therapies since leaving the hospital, and I will go through them again, with the addition of vestibular therapy due to vertigo and with pulmonary rehabilitation added to my physical therapy.

PICS can last for weeks or even years after leaving the ICU. For me, it has been 3 years, 5 months, and 19 days. Some of the symptoms that I am experiencing are: chronic fatigue, generalized weakness, dyspnea on exertion, exercise intolerance, dysphagia, cognitive impairment, impaired balance, vertigo, stuttering, neuropathy, anxiety, depression, changes in taste, and sensitivity to light. PICS is relentless and unforgiving. Each day looks different. My body feels different. I don't know which array of symptoms that I will have deal with from day-to-day. Will I drive to a doctor's appointment and end up in another town without any idea how I got there? Will I forget to turn off the stove or leave the faucet running? Will I even be able to get out of bed tomorrow? I never know what to expect.

Last weekend, I had to go to the emergency room for vertigo. I was fine Friday morning. That afternoon, I dozed off while watching TV. When I awoke, I didn't feel right. I didn't think much of it because I have grown accustomed to not feeling well. I went downstairs to answer the door. As I turned to make my way back upstairs, my legs turned to Jell-o, I felt unsteady, and the room was spinning. This is what life is for me: expecting the unexpected.

Even the simplest things become arduous tasks. It's a chore to schedule a doctor's appointment. Talking on the phone can be exhausting. Doctor's appointments become overwhelming, which is why I have someone accompany me. The next day, I am exhausted from my appointment. I now see a number of specialists for various health conditions as a result of PICS. I'm not as sharp as I once was. I have trouble remembering, paying attention, solving problems, organizing, and working on complex tasks. I used to enjoy Sudoku and word searches. I now find them frustrating. My memory, which I used to take such pride in, is now unreliable. I was once an avid book reader, but now I struggle to read even the shortest articles. I can watch a movie and not remember watching it the next day.

PICS doesn't just affect the patient; it also affects their family. My oldest daughter had to take a leave of absence from work to care for me. She was tasked with making medical decisions on my behalf during my stay in the hospital. It was traumatizing for her to see me in that condition, so close to death. While I was in the hospital, she filed for my short-term disability and managed my bills. When I came home, she combed my hair, assisted me in the shower, continued to manage my bills, cleaned my house, and prepared my food. I could not care for myself. We had switched roles. She became the caretaker, and I became reliant on her. This is something that neither of us expected, nor were we prepared for. She essentially had to run two households. Each of my children accompanied me to doctor's appointments.

My son-in-law would often leave work to take me to my doctor appointments. My oldest son would frequently pop in and out to do chores around the house and to keep my morale up. My youngest son was wracked with guilt because he was across the hall unaware that my life was slipping away. Anytime that I am in the hospital or need a procedure, he gets anxious. Last weekend was no exception. He became my caretaker after he graduated high school and he does so unbegrudgingly.

My personhood has been derailed. I used to love to dress up and wear heels. I have since traded my five-inch heels for sneakers and a cane because I have balance issues. I feel a sense of loss – loss of identity, relationships, employment, and most of all, independence. All of that contributes to the anxiety, depression, and grief that I feel. I feel trapped inside my own body. The woman that I was believed that her capabilities were seemingly endless. The woman that I am today is faced with limitations and uncertainty. My confidence has turned into apprehension and fear. All that remains are the traces of my former self, trapped inside my memories and imagination. I had to adapt to a new normal. I had to grieve the loss of my independence. Three years and five months later, I can no longer participate in many of the things that brought me pleasure. I have not returned to my previous level of functionality. I avoid going to places because I don't like running into people and having to explain why I am now using a cane.

Once the crisis is over, the people around you expect you to return to normal. Sadly, many of us don't, and that can put a strain on both personal and professional relationships due to the lack of awareness surrounding PICS. Some people have disappeared from my life altogether. I am still grieving the woman that I once was, but I have learned to show the woman I am today compassion, patience, and most importantly, grace because, quite honestly, she needs it.

Afterword

Derek C. Angus

Intensive care has been one of the marvels of modern medicine. For centuries, many conditions like septic shock, major trauma, or acute decompensations of chronic pulmonary, cardiac, or liver disease, carried a terrible prognosis. But, with the development and dissemination of modern intensive care systems, the ability to rapidly evaluate and resuscitate patients and to provide vital organ support, such as mechanical ventilation, has led to dramatic reductions in hospital mortality rates. A side-effect of this success, however, is the ever-growing population of individuals who survive life-threatening illness only to face a long and protracted road to recovery.

It is recognition of the lingering burden incurred by survivors of acute illness that has led to the burgeoning field of post-ICU recovery support. This book does an incredible job of summarizing our current understanding of the many challenges patients face and distilling that understanding into the practical steps that clinicians, patients, and their loved ones can take to ensure that patients can best navigate their road to recovery.

But these are still early days, and important challenges lie ahead.

The first challenge is the lack of understanding of the underlying pathophysiology that drives persistent impairment and delayed recovery. Many symptoms incurred by survivors of critical illness are nonspecific, such as fatigue and weakness, and could arise from one of many different disease processes. It is possible that there are specific treatments that would work for one patient but not for another, even when both present with similar symptoms. However, there are still limited studies of patients with post-intensive care syndrome (PICS), and essentially no pre-clinical models of post-ICU recovery exist. A better understanding of the underlying disease processes could aid development of potential therapies.

The second challenge is determining the best way to deploy the resources needed to support patients during their recovery. All healthcare systems are under considerable resource constraint. As is evident in this book, multidisciplinary expertise is required; however, it is unlikely that healthcare systems could routinely provide such expertise to all patients discharged from the ICU. Thus, some form of screening and triage is required. But, how to build (and fund) a referral system that is efficient and accessible is not clear. Here, too, more research evaluating different systems, ideally using study designs that measure the effect of different implementation strategies, would be helpful.

Finally, it is probably a mistake to frame post-ICU recovery in traditional healthcare terms. Survivors of critical illness want their lives back: that means they do not want to remain as "patients," nor do they want to be reliant on healthcare systems any more than necessary. Furthermore, many challenges they face on the road to recovery are not necessarily best addressed by healthcare systems. For example, strategies to get back to work or usual activities may require support from employers or social services. Thus, post-ICU recovery might be best supported by partnerships between healthcare systems and communities. The right way to form and fund such partnerships is, however, unclear and will require pilot projects evaluating novel solutions.

So, this is a big journey – not just for those surviving the ICU, but for the entire field. This book gets us started with a clear-eyed summary of what we know now and what we can do right now. That's a terrific first step, and this book will hopefully become required reading for every healthcare delivery system. I also look forward to future iterations, hopefully incorporating important new updates as we advance knowledge, both on the many aspects of PICS and on the best way to provide care for individuals suffering with PICS. Onward!

Index

Please note: page numbers in **bold type** indicate figures, those in *italics* indicate tables or boxes.

ABC life support checklist, 143
ABCDEF bundle of interventions, 19
  overview, 135
  adherence increased by tele-ICU services, 374
  in delirium management/reduction, 110, 246
  effective ICU rounds, 142
  elements, 19, 135
    assess, prevent, and manage pain, 135–6
    both SATs and SBTs, 137
    choice of analgesia and sedation, 137–9
    delirium assessment, prevention, and management, 139
    early mobility and exercise, 139–40, 150
    family engagement and empowerment, 140–1
  goals, 135
  impact, 19
  implementation challenges, 141–2
  pediatric version, 685–7
    see also under PICS-pediatrics (PICS-p).
  potential for reducing the incidence of PICS, 141
  preservation of habits and routines of daily life, 627
  as preventative strategy against delirium, 630
  recommended by SCCM, 19
  requirements for consistent implementation, 141–2
  and thoughtful use of medication to address pain and agitation, 405
acceptance and commitment therapy (ACT), 575
acid suppressive therapy, complications associated with, 407
acquired brain injury, comparison with PICS-related cognitive impairment, 538
activities of daily living (ADLs)
  definition, 520
  assessment tools, 376, 522, 529
  benefits of adaptive equipment prescription and training for patient independence, 527
  benefits of early active engagement in, 177
  cognitive impairment and independence, 527
  cognitive rehabilitation, 176, 178
  common, *521*
  evaluation of impairment, 522–7
  examples of, *560*
  functional cognition during, **178**
  functional reconciliation and, 559
  impact of fatigue on, 446
  impact of frailty following critical illness on, 63
  impact of functional impairment on, 7–13, 177
  impact of increased dependence in, 521
  impairment in as risk factor for anxiety following critical illness, 569
  interventions for ADL impairment, 527
  Katz ADL screening tool, 376, 522
  potential impact of cognitive impairment on, 527
  requirements of, 520
  role of functional task training, 513
Activity Measure of Post-Acute Care (AM-PAC) (Boston University), 166, 376
acute kidney injury (AKI), risk of for survivors of critical illness, 423
acute neurological injury (ANI)
  difficulties of distinguishing PICS symptoms from consequences of, 660
  lack of study of PICS in survivors of, 660
  see also ANI survivors; post-neuro ICU clinics.
acute rehabilitation services, 289
acute respiratory distress syndrome (ARDS)
  ALTOS study, 16
  case studies, 470, 718
  clinical vignette, 495
  cognitive outcomes study, 1
  corticosteroids and, 406
  COVID-related, pulmonary complications following, 437
  duration of physical impairments, 16
  dysphagia case example, 85
  increased healthcare costs and resource utilization associated with, 424
  persistence of physical impairments following, 16–17
  prevalence of cognitive impairment following, 33
  and prolonged immobility, 449

745

ARDS (cont.)
  and return to work following hospital discharge, 547
  as risk factor for cognitive impairment, 536
  risk factors for development of dysphagia in patients requiring mechanical ventilation, 78
  "What Happens to Survivors of ARDS" (American Thoracic Society), 2
  see also ARDS survivors.
acute respiratory failure
  common causes of, 77
  delirium in mechanically ventilated patients, 102
  EQ-5D-5 L recommended for assessment of physical disability, 504
  physical function study in survivors of, 23–4
adaptive equipment prescription, benefits for patient independence, 527
adolescents, post-intensive care syndrome in, see PICS-pediatrics (PICS-p).
advance care planning
  benefits of Age-Friendly strategies, 636
  ICU follow-up clinics and, 589
  palliative care and, 589
adverse drug events (ADEs), transitions of care as source of, 407
advocacy, role of in increasing awareness of PICS, see also PICS advocacy, 707
Affordable Care Act, 626
Age-Friendly model of care
  components of Age-Friendly Health Systems, 625
  5 Ms of Age-Friendly Healthcare, 625
  preventative, system-based approach, 626 see also

under older adult survivors of critical illness.
agitation in ICU patients
  non-pharmacologic interventions, 174, 184
  pharmacologic interventions, 111, 129, 137, 139, 184, 457
  physical restraint devices, 129
alarmins, 32
alopecia, sepsis as risk factor for, 449
Alzheimer's disease and related dementias (ADRD), delirium as risk factor for development of, 248
ambulation impairment, management of, 565–6
American Occupational Therapy Association (AOTA), PICS advocacy, 707
American Thoracic Society, 2
analgesia and sedation, choice of, 137–9
  for pediatric patients, 686
analgesia-first sedation, recommended for mechanical ventilation, 136, 405
analgesics
  medication management, 405–6
  non-opioid, 136, 685
Angus, D.C., 429
ANI survivors, 660–7
  degree of prognostic uncertainty, 665
  development of post-neuro ICU clinics for, 660
  disease-specific considerations, 661
  examples of specific recommendations, 661
  spinal cord injury, 663–5
  status epilepticus, 662–3
  subarachnoid hemorrhage, 662
  traumatic brain injury, 663

PICS-F symptoms experienced by caregivers, 660
  roles of ICU follow-up clinics, 665–6
  addressing uncertainty, 665
  emotional debriefing, 665
  re-evaluation of prognosis and goals of care, 666
animal assisted intervention (AAI), 255–67
  animals used as therapy animals, 264
  care of animal and handler, 263–4
  case studies
    hospital therapy dog, 264–6
    motivational visit from patient's pet dog, 266
  clinical guidance and risk assessment, 261–3
  diamond model, 263
  evidence of in ICUs, 256–61
  and humanization of intensive care, 264
  mechanisms hypothesized to explain benefits of animal interaction, 255
  physiological changes associated with, 256
  types of, 255
animal naming, as screening tool for cognitive impairment, 23
antibiotics, medication management, 406–7
antipsychotics
  contraindicated for prevention of delirium, 139
  medication management, 406–7
anxiety
  assessment tools, 22, 365, 604
  beneficial effects of music on, 247
  prevalence in survivors of critical illness, 569
  protective factors, 569–70
  as psychological outcome of critical illness, 569–70

Index 747

risk factors following critical illness, 569
screening tools, 377
symptoms, 569
Apple iPhone's Health Kit, 376
Applied Cognitive Inpatient Short Form (ACISF), 166
ARDS survivors
 appropriate timing of physical assessments, 502
 benefits of avoiding steroids during hospitalization, 406
 cognitive impairment in, 536
 common psychiatric symptoms, 17
 dysphagia common in, 463
 first cognitive outcomes study, 1
 impact of critical illness on sense of self, 341
 impairment in QoL, 429
 longitudinal study of psychiatric symptoms, 17
 long-term respiratory disease experienced by, 422
 measurement of long-term outcomes for, 440
 muscle weakness and fatigue experienced by, 423
 outcome measures in studies of, 440
 personal stories, 738–42
 physical impairments experienced by, 1
 prevalence of dysphagia in, 463
 prevalence of hospital readmission within one year, 424
 proneness to developing long-term symptoms, 674
 resumption of employment, 547
 subtypes of disability, 501
 see also acute respiratory distress syndrome (ARDS),
aspiration
 compensatory strategies, 465, 469
 exercises to reduce risk of, 468–9
 implications of inconsistent cough response to, 85
 increased risk of in patients receiving CNS depressants, 80
 intubation-associated risk, 78
 and oral health, 83
 risk of increased by cognitive impairment, 467
 signs and symptoms, 81, 465
 and specialist referral, 467
 surgery and, 479
Assessment of Driving-Related Skills (ADReS), 527
Assessment of Language-Related Functional Activities (ALFA), 173
Assessment of Quality of Life (AQoL-8D), 429
assessment/screening tools
 ADLs and IADLs, 376, 522, 529
 anxiety, 22, 365, 377, 604
 caregiver burden, 607
 cognitive fitness for driving, 554
 cognitive function, 22, 166, 363, 365, 376, 390, 539, 540, 585 *see also* Montreal Cognitive Assessment (MoCA) tool.
 delirium, 103–4, 166, 539
 depression, 22, 365, 605
 driving ability, 551–4
 dysphagia, 376, 466
 executive function, 173, 529, 540, 585
 fatigue, 605
 mental health, 22, 585
 muscle tone, 563
 nutrition, 376, 488, 493
 physical domain, 22, 365, 585
 PICS-F, 22
 psychological symptoms, 573
 PTSD, 365, 377
 quality of life, 22, 23, 429–32, 607
 sedation, 138
 sleep, 22, 457
 social support, 607
 spiritual care, *202–3*
 suitable for clinic settings, 365, 539–40
 two-step PICS screening process, 22–3
assistive technology
 role of in cognitive rehabilitation, 179–80
 role of in physical rehabilitation, 156
Australia
 fresh air therapy study, 271
 history of ICU follow-up clinics, 356
Australia and New Zealand Intensive Care Society (ANZICS), 356
autophagy
 importance of, 39
 myopathies and muscle wasting conditions associated with impairment in, 39
awareness of PICS, strategies to increase, 283
Azoulay, E., 26

Balboni, M.J., 201
"Balcony of Hope," Virgen Macarena University Hospital in Seville, 269
Baseline Dyspnea Index (BDI), 440
Beck Anxiety Inventory (BAI), 605
Beck Depression Inventory-II (BDI-II), 605
bed rest
 association with persistent muscle weakness, 140
 historical perspective, 45
 impact on body systems, 45–6 *see also* immobility and ICU-acquired weakness.
BEERS criteria of potentially inappropriate medications (AGS), 407, 631
behavioral activation, 189, 194, *528*, 631
Behavioral Pain Scale (BPS), 136, *137*

benzodiazepines
  impact on swallow
    function, 80
  and increased risk of
    delirium, 80, 111, 119
Berlin EXCOR, 691
Bermejo, J.C., 208
Berney, S., 157
Bertschi, D., 65
Bienvenu, O. J., 17, 294
"Big Hit" trajectory of
    recovery, 23
biophilia theory, see also fresh
    air therapy 255, 269
blood–brain barrier (BBB),
    33–4, 104
Bloom, S. L., 360
body systems, impact of bed
    rest and immobility
    on, 45–6
Boehm, L. M., 141
Bolton, C. F., 45
Borg Rating of Perceived
    Exertion (RPE), 441
Bovier, Connie, 738–40
brain functional networks,
    effects of music
    on, 249
Branson, S., 256
Bringing Recovery Supports to
    Scale Technical
    Assistance Center
    Strategy (BRSS
    TACS)
    (SAMHSA), 619
Burian, B. K., 143
burnout syndrome
  definition, 213
  caregivers, 346
  COVID-19 pandemic
    and, 221
  mitigation/reduction
    strategies, 224
  connecting with
    survivors, 619
  greenspace exposure,
    271–2
  case study, 272
  humanization of the ICU,
    224
  see also humanization of
    the ICU.
  multidisciplinary
    teamwork and
    planning, 296
  positive feedback, 368

rates of in critical care
    providers, 212,
    224, 235
risk factors, 213, 225
role of
    depersonalization,
    209

Calhoun, L.G., 573
Canadian Occupational
    Performance
    Assessment
    (COPM), 530
Canadian Problem Checklist
    (CPC), 584
Canadian Study of Health and
    Aging, 67
carbon monoxide poisoning,
    research focused on
    neuropsychological
    outcomes following
    hypoxia, 1
cardiac arrest (CA)
  definition, 641
  PICS in survivors of, 641–52
  see also cardiac arrest
    survivors.
  prevalence in the US, 641
  survival rates of OHCA and
    IHCA patients, 641
cardiac arrest survivors,
    641–52
  cardiac rehabilitation
    programs
    recommended
    for, 645
  cognitive impairment
    and, 644
  disorders of consciousness
    and, 644
  the experience of cardiac
    arrest survivorship
    and recovery, 641–2
  impact of prognostic
    uncertainty, 641–2
  increased rates of common
    neurological
    conditions, 644
  psychological distress and,
    643–4
  research requirements for
    long-term recovery
    trajectories, 642–3
  role of the family, 643–4
  sex and racial/ethnic
    disparities, 642–3

studies
  completed studies, 646–9
  ongoing studies, 650–1
targeted interventions, 645
cardiopulmonary exercise
    testing (CPET), 440
cardiovascular disease
  advocacy and public
    awareness, 711
  association with SDOH, 326
  cardiac rehabilitation
    programs, 645
  reducing risk of, 645
  remote patient
    monitoring, 379
  risk of for critical illness
    survivors, 422
Cardiovascular Health
    Study, 64–5
care bundles
  definition and function, 135
  criticisms and caveats, 145
  see also ABCDEF
    bundle of
    interventions.
care plans, for older adults, 635
care providers, impact of
    frequent
    interruptions on
    memory, 141
caregiver burden
  definition, 603
  assessment tools, 607
  family caregivers, 602–3
  measuring, 603
  negative psychological
    outcomes, 603
Caregiver Health Behavior
    Instrument, 605
Caregiver Strain Index
    (CSI), 607
caregivers
  cardiac arrest as traumatic
    and life-altering
    experience for, 641
  importance of emotional and
    social support
    for, 346
  and navigation of the new
    role, 345
  peer support, 617
  support for as principle of
    palliative care, 590
  see also caregiver
    burden; family
    caregivers.

case studies
  animal assisted intervention, 264–6
  ARDS, 85, 470–1, 718, 738–42
  cognitive impairment, 728
  COPD, 718
  dysphagia, 85, 470–1
  fresh air therapy, 272, 274
  medication management in follow-up clinic, *413*
case study of PICS, 718–28
  the patient, 718
  first ICU follow-up clinic visit, 719
  3-month follow-up appointment, 719–24
  6-month follow-up appointment, 724
  12-month follow-up appointment, 725
  22-month follow-up appointment, 725–6
  25-month follow-up appointment, 726
  28-month follow-up appointment, 726–7
  31-month follow-up appointment, 727
  39-month follow-up appointment, 727
  major themes, 728
  patient data at follow-up clinic visits, *720–3*
Center for Epidemiologic Studies Depression Scale (CES-D), 605
central sleep apnea (CSA), comparison with obstructive sleep apnea, 460
CERTAIN (Checklist for Early Recognition and Treatment of Acute Illness) checklist, 144
checklists
  ABC life support checklist, 143
  aviation industry's example, 142–3
  boldface vs non-boldface, 143
  CERTAIN checklist, 144
  'checklist fatigue', 145
  criticisms and caveats, 145
  the E-checklist, 144–5

ICU Family-Centered Care Checklist, **225**
life-cycle, 143–*4*
success stories, 144
types of ICU checklists, 143
WHO Safe Surgery Checklist, 142
Chelsea Critical Care Physical Assessment Tool (CPAx), 54
chemokines, 31, 104
children
  mitigating risk of post-PICU cognitive impairment, 689
  optimization of mechanical ventilation, 685
  pain management, 685
  post-intensive care syndrome in, *see* PICS-pediatrics (PICS-p).
  prevalence of post-PICU cognitive impairment, 689
  prevalence of post-PICU functional impairment, 687
  psychologists' role in preparation for the ICU environment, 191
chronic chest pain, risk of for survivors of critical illness, 438
chronic critical illness (CCI), 32–3, 34, 289
  pathophysiological model, 31
chronic disease, bi-directional relationship with critical illness, 422–3
chronic kidney disease (CKD)
  recognizing early signs of, 423
  risk of for sepsis survivors, 423
chronic obstructive pulmonary disease (COPD)
  case study, 718
  risk of for critical illness survivors, 422
chronic pain
  interventions, 448
  management of, 564–5
  measurement tools, 448

prevalence in survivors of critical illness, 448
as result of mechanical ventilation, 448
circuit training, 513
clinical evaluation of PICS, guidelines on, 20–1
Cognitive Assessment of Minnesota (CAM), 173
cognitive behavioral therapy (CBT), 575
  behavioral strategies, 189
  cognitive restructuring, 189
  grounding and relaxation skills, 189–90
  psychoeducation, 188
  stress reduction findings, 188
cognitive domains, assessment instruments, 22
Cognitive Failures Questionnaire (CFQ), 539
cognitive function
  benefits of early physical rehabilitation for, 158
  benefits of Mediterranean diet for, 492
  positive impact of early physical rehabilitation, 158
  potential impact of bed rest and immobility on, 46
  see also cognitive impairments following critical illness.
  screening tools, 585
cognitive impairment
  definition, 535
  assessment tools, 22, 365, 376, 390
  association with inflammation and cortisol levels, 298
  bi-directional relationship with hospitalization, 166
  case study, 728
  COVID-19 and, 672
  delirium and, 18, 33–4, 101, 103, 106, 139, 166, 246, 536, 539
  and disruption in ADL and IADL independence, 527

cognitive impairment (cont.)
  engendered by limited
    activity and
    mobility, 176
  "gut-brain axis" and, 40
  hepatic encephalopathy
    and, 80
  impairments consistent with
    PICS, 7, 16
  medication and, 405, *634*
  potential consequences
    of, 103
  potential impact on mental
    health, 631
  prevalence in cardiac arrest
    survivors, 644
  prevalence in PICU
    survivors, 689
  remote assessment, 376–7
  and returning to driving, 550
  risk factors, 536, 662, 689
  screening for in long COVID
    patients, 673
  screening tools, 365
  under-diagnosis, 166 *see also*
    cognitive
    impairments
    following critical
    illness; cognitive
    rehabilitation.
cognitive impairments
  following critical
  illness, 535–43
  comparison with acquired
    brain injury, 538
  consequences of delayed
    detection, 539
  definition of cognitive
    impairment, 535
  distinguishing from
    dementia, 538
  domains impacted by, 535
  duration of impairment,
    537
  executive dysfunction, 537
  functional cognitive
    impairment, 527–30
  impacts example, 538
  mitigating risk for
    children, 689
  potential duration,
    535–6, 547
  prevalence, 297, 535–6
    in ARDS survivors, 33
    in children, 689
  protective factors, 536

rehabilitation approaches,
    541–2
  awareness training, 542
  compensatory
    strategies, 541
  pharmacology, 542
  pros and cons of cognitive
    rehabilitation, *542*
  restorative strategies, 542
  research
    recommendations, 537
  risk factors, 18, 364, 536
  screening for, 539–40
    delirium screening
      tools, 539
    outpatient screening tools,
      539–40
    pre-existing cognitive
      impairment
      assessment, 540
    self-report tools, 540
    systematic review, 17, 536
    understanding cognitive
      disability, 537–8
Cognitive Linguistic Quick
    Test Plus
    (CLQT+), 173
cognitive performance, effects
    of music on, 249–50
cognitive rehabilitation,
    166–80
  communication
    improvement
    strategies, 179–80
  consistent screening and
    evaluation of
    cognition, 166–72
  cueing strategy, 178–**9**
  disorders of consciousness,
    173–4
  domains of cognition,
    176
  elements of training, 176
  family members and loved
    ones' role, 175
  feasibility of in ICU and
    hospital settings, 176
  functional cognition, 176–9
  modulating stimulation,
    174–5
  multimodal approach, 175
  orientation assessment, 173
  performing ADLs and
    IADLs, 176, 178
  role of assistive technology,
    179–80

standardized cognitive
    evaluation tools,
    167–72
  standardized functional
    cognition
    assessments, 173
  techniques and
    strategies, 176
Cole, K. M., 256
Coma Recovery Scale –Revised
    (CRS-R), 173
common somatic concerns
    following critical
    illness, *see* somatic
    concerns following
    critical illness.
communication
  about post-ICU
    problems, 7–13
  and humanization of the
    ICU, 211–12
  improvement role of
    psychologists, 192
  improvement strategies,
    179–80, 608
  potential impact of poor
    communication with
    ICU staff, 608
  psychological impact of
    challenges with, 130
  role of family members
    during mechanical
    ventilation, 222
  role of family members in
    acute phase, 608
  VALUE strategy, 222
communication techniques
  "Ask-Tell-Ask," 588
  NURSE Statements, 589
  in palliative care, 588–9
compensatory anti-
    inflammatory
    response syndrome
    (CARS), 31
complementary therapies, 299
Confusion Assessment Method
    (CAM), 103
Confusion Assessment Method
    for the ICU (CAM-
    ICU), 104, **105**, 139,
    166, 539
continuous renal replacement
    therapy (CRRT), 91,
    140, 486, 683
corticosteroids, medication
    management, 406

cortisol levels, association with cognitive impairment, 298
COVID-19 infection
  and cognitive impairment, 672
  dysphagia following, 470–1
  and remote patient monitoring, 379 *see also* SARS-CoV-2 infection.
COVID-19 pandemic
  and disparities in healthcare systems, 676
  impact on patient- and family-centered care, 221
  and implementation of the ABCDEF bundle, 141
  similarity of long-COVID to PICS, **357**, 356, 361
  and virtual peer support groups, 618, 621
  and visiting restrictions, 211
Cox, C. E., 341, 575
Cox, M. C., 32
Critical and Acute Illness Recovery Organization (CAIRO), 360
  peer support, 355, 616
  PICS advocacy, 707
Critical Care Pain Observation Tool (CPOT), 136
Critical Care Recovery Center (CCRC), Indiana University, 354
critical illness
  phases of and key metabolic consequences, **89**
  potential impact on survivors, 6
  as trauma, 306–7
critical illness myopathy (CIM)
  presentation, 560
  sleep and, 460
critical illness polyneuropathy (CIP),
  presentation, 560
critical illness recovery
  five phases, **343**
  phase 1, 341
  phase 2, 342
  phase 3, 342
  phase 4, 342
  phase 5, 342

critical illness survivors
  challenges faced by, 339
  characteristic heightened vulnerability, 6
  chronic disease, mortality, and healthcare utilization, 420–5
  clinical manifestations, 7–**12**
  excess mortality risk, 421–2
  hospital readmission and healthcare resource utilization, 423–5
  percentage of unplanned readmissions, 502
  percentage who develop disabilities requiring caregiver assistance, 217
  percentage who develop PICS, 485
  personal stories, 729–42 *see also* personal stories.
  prevalence of impairment, 36, 547
  prevalence of PICS symptoms, 582
  processing and normalizing of the ICU experience, 296
  prolonged vulnerability exhibited by, 420
  recovery trajectories, variation in, 420
  and research into post-ICU disability, 303
  risk of developing chronic disease, 422–3
  risk of physical disability for, 502
  survival rates one year after hospital discharge, 420
  and the social model of disability, 306–7
  transition challenges, 281
  see also under specific issues e.g. somatic concerns; laryngeal disorders; quality of life.
Cuthbertson, D., 89
cytokines, 31–4, 35, 39, 40, 46, 104–7, 248, 489

Danesh, V., 356, 361, 551, 575
Danon disease, 39

Darden, D. B., 31
Davidson, T. A., 295, 429
Davis, Cori, 740–2
De Bie, A. J. R, 144
decannulation
  considerations for, 481–2
  sequelae of, 482–3
deconditioning
  definition, 560
  causes, 45, 560
  as component of PCC, 674
  and dyspnea, 672
  and exacerbation of neuropathic pain, 565
  potential positive impact of deprescribing unnecessary medications, 673
Decreasing Delirium through Music (DDM), 250
delirium, 101
  definition, 101
  added to DSM-III, 101
  antimicrobials as risk factor for, 407
  antipsychotics
    contraindicated for prevention of, 139
    in ARDS patients requiring mechanical ventilation, 102
  assess, prevent, and manage, 139
  pediatric patients, 686
  assessment tools, 103–4
  beneficial effects of listening to music, 246, 248
  benefits of a diary for hospitalized patients with, 231
  best approach to management of, 139
  changes in terminology, 101
  characteristics of, 126
  and cognitive impairment, 18, 33–4, 101, 103, 106, 139, 166, 246, 536, 539
  consequences and outcomes, 102–3
  decreased by early physical rehabilitation, 158
  dementia associated with, 103
  detection of, 103–4

delirium (cont.)
  diagnostic criteria changes, *102*
  distress mitigating role of psychoeducation, 188
  duration and incidence reduced by early engagement in functional mobility/activity, 178
  family presence restrictions correlated with higher risk of, 221
  geriatric syndromes and, 635
  heterogeneity of, 109–10
  hypotension associated with, 104
  incidence of increased by deep sedation, 138
  intestinal microbiome changes implicated in, 39
  ketamine contraindicated for prevention of delirium, 139
  as key risk factor for PICS, 101
  long-term impact on older adults, 630
  management
    nonpharmacologic, 110–11
    pharmacologic, 111
    limitations of, 246
  opioids and, 405
  PADIS guidelines, 139, 406
  pathophysiology, 104–6, 248
    major mechanisms, **107**
  percentage of mechanically ventilated older adults experiencing delirium, 246
  percentage of mechanically ventilated patients experiencing delirium, 102, 139
  potential long-term complications, 246
  prevalence in sepsis patients, 33
  prevalence of during ICU admission, 125, 126
  prevalence of in critical illness, 101
  protective/preventive factors, 110, 139, 246, 250, 630
  psychological impact, 128
  rates of in older adult ICU patients, 630
  relationship with mortality, 103
  as risk factor for ADRD, 248
  as risk factor for anxiety, 569
  risk factors for, 39, 80, 104, 106–9, 111, 119–20, 138, 221, 405–7
  screening tools, 166, 539
  statins contraindicated for prevention of, 139
  subtypes, 109
  swallow impairments in patients with, 80
Delirium Rating Scale (DRS), 103
Delphi consensus, physical domain assessment tools identified by, 504
dementia
  association with delirium, 103
  beneficial effects of music, 249
  distinguishing PICS-related cognitive impairment from, 538
Denehy, L., 512
Denmark, establishment of first intensive care units, 45
dental health, concerns about following critical illness, 450
deprescribing
  definition, 408
  five step protocol, 408
  for older adults, 631
  for PCC patients, 673
depression
  assessment tools, 22, 365, 605
  bi-directional relationship with physical sequelae of PICS, 570
  prevalence following critical illness compared with general population, 570
  protective factors, 570
  as psychological outcome of critical illness, 570
  risk factors following critical illness, 570
  symptoms, 570
dexmedetomidine, 121
  contraindicated for prevention of delirium, 139
  for management of delirium in mechanically ventilated patients, 139
  for treatment of delirium, 111
  trials investigating treatment of sleep to prevent delirium, 120
diabetes, association with SDOH, 326
diagnosis of PICS, screening and, 20–3
digital health and wearables, 378–80
disability, 303–22
  the biomedical model, 14–**15**
  biomedical vs social models, 304–6
  definition, 303
  definition of physical disability, 500
  difference in prevalence in the US and globally, 303
  equity/equality context, 304
  functional status, 13, 14
  German hiring policies, 307
  human rights and, 303–4
  incidence and prevalence of physical disability, 500–1
  practical strategies for just and inclusive care for people with PICS, 308–13
  social model of in PICS, 306–8
  trajectory of following critical illness, 501–2
  work disability, 550 *see also* post-ICU disability.
disability inclusion
  digital health technologies, 320
  health financing, 316

health policy and systems
  research, 321
models of care, 317–18
monitoring and evaluation,
  320–1
physical infrastructure, 319
political perspectives,
  313–15
practical strategies for
  clinicians, 309–10
quality of care, 320
stakeholder and private
  sector engagement,
  316–17
workforce training and
  education, 318–19
discharge planning, elements
  of a successful
  plan, 630
discrimination, patterns of
  experienced by
  people with PICS, 307
disorders of
  consciousness (DoC)
  cardiac arrest survivors, 644
  and cognitive rehabilitation,
  173–4
  TBI survivors, 663
disrespect, experienced by
  critically ill patients
  and their families, 218
driving, 550–5
  cognitive fitness assessment
  tools, 554
  cognitive impairment
  and, 550
  driving ability assessment
  tools, 551–4
  family support
  initiatives, 555
  literature on driving ability
  after critical illness,
  550–1
  as priority for
  rehabilitation, 550
  rehabilitation programs, 554
  role of occupational
  therapy, 522
dysphagia, 77
  admitting diagnosis and
  hospital course, 77–9
  assessment tools, 376
  background and prevalence
  in PICS, 463
  bedside swallow evaluation
  alertness level, 81

cranial nerve
  examination, 82
current vital signs on
  respiratory status, 81
oral health, 83
patient's social history and
  history of
  dysphagia, 81
benefits of VFSS and FEES
  for patients in the
  ICU, 83
cardiovascular surgery
  patients, 79–80
case example, 85
characteristics of, 463
chest imaging, 79
chronic, 7
considerations prior to SLP
  evaluation
  discussion with medical
  team, 81
  medications, 80
  swallow screen, 80–1
cranial nerves and their
  functions related to
  swallowing, 82
decision-making/synthesis
  for
  recommendations, 84
example treatment plan, 86
geriatric syndromes and, 635
high-flow nasal cannula,
  impact on swallow
  function, 78
instrumental swallow
  evaluation
  best practice in ICU, 84
  flexible endoscopic
  evaluation of
  swallowing, 84
  goals of, 83
  videofluoroscopic swallow
  study, 83
intubation-associated
  risk, 78
lung and liver transplant
  recipients, 80
neurology and neurosurgery
  patients, 79
potential impact on
  nutrition, 88
respiratory disease, 78
risk of spinal surgery for
  development of, 79
tracheostomy tube-related
  risk, 78–9

treatment, 84–5
compensatory
  strategies, 469
dysphagia exercises, 467–9
Expiratory Muscle
  Strength Trainer-150
  (EMST-150), 469
Iowa Oral Performance
  Instrument
  (IOPI), 469
swallowing exercises and
  their intended
  effect, 468
technology's role in
  dysphagia
  rehabilitation, 469 see
  also persistent
  dysphagia following
  critical illness.
Dysphagia Outcome and
  Severity Scale
  (DOSS), 466
dysphonia, laryngeal injury
  and, 477
dyspnea, 437
  interarytenoid adhesion
  and, 478
  measurement tools, 440, 441
  PCC patients, management
  considerations, 672–3
  persistent, 7
  and sleep disruption, 119
  as symptom of tracheal
  stenosis, 438

early mobilization
  definition, 150
  activities, 150
  feasibility for critically ill
  patients, 140
  pediatric patients, 686
  recommendations on
  initiating active
  mobilization in the
  ICU, 157
Eating Assessment Tool
  (EAT-10), 466
Edmonton Symptom
  Assessment System-
  Revised (ESAS-r),
  585, **586**
education and disease
  management
  benefits of early education
  on PICS, 286
fall prevention, 511

education and disease (cont.)
  fatigue, 510–11
  medication, 511
  nutrition, 511
  physical activity, 510
Ehlenbach, W.J., 520
the elderly
  growth in interest in the impact of critical illness on, 2 see also older adult survivors of critical illness.
electronic health records (EHR), integration of checklists and care bundles into, 144–5
Elliott, D., 341
emotional debriefing, ANI survivors, 665
employment, 547–50
  outcomes after critical illness, 548
  return to work
    employers' role in supporting, 548
    functional capacity evaluation, 549
    medical clearance for, 549
    prevalence of failure to, 538, 566
    prevalence of impairments and challenges of, 547
    risk factors associated with failure to, 547–8
    role of physiatrists in, 566
    over time, 548
  vocational rehabilitation, 549
  work disability, 550
end-of-life care
  in fresh air spaces, 272, 274. see also fresh air therapy.
  grief support for family members and loved ones, 191
  humanization of the ICU and, 214
endotracheal intubation, 77
  conversion to tracheotomy, 477
  cuff pressure considerations, 474
  inappropriate tube size, correlation with laryngeal injury, 473
  passage of the tube, 473
  nomograms for, **475**
  positioning of the tube, 476
  risks associated with, 78
  tube size and cuff pressure, 473–4
epilepsy, 33, 422, 550
  percentage of aSAH patients who develop, 662
  risk of for survivors of critical illness, 423 see also status epilepticus.
equality, difference between equity and, 304
Esianor, B. I., 473
ethical decision-making, Jonsen's model, 469
European Society of Intensive Care Medicine (ESICM), PICS advocacy, 707
EuroQol-5 Dimensions (EQ-5D)
  comparison with SF-36, 432
  dimensions explored, 428, 429, 607
  domains of, **431**
EuroQol-5Dimension-5Level (EQ-5D-5 L), 23, 377
  for assessment of physical impairment, 365
  inclusion in core outcome measures, 22
  knowledge gaps, 347
  recommended for assessment of physical disability in acute respiratory failure survivors, 504
  use of via telemedicine, 377
executive function
  definition, 529
  assessment tools, 173, 529, 540, 585
  driving and, 550
  impact of delirium on, 33, 535
  impact of immobility on, 46
  impairment following critical illness, 537
  music therapy and, 249
  older adults, impact of ICU admission on, 536
Executive Function Performance Test (EFPT), 173
exercise
  early mobility and, 139–40, 150
  impaired tolerance of, 7 see also therapeutic exercise.
expectations, management of, 587–8, 591
Expiratory Muscle Strength Trainer-150 (EMST-150), 469
extracorporeal membrane oxygenation (ECMO), 48, 79, 140, 683–4
extubation
  benefits of the ABCDEF bundle for, 405
  delirium as barrier to, 111
  and delirium management, 139
  failure associated with VIDD, 439
  FEES following, 84
  protocol for reduction of time to, 685
  readiness for and mechanical ventilation settings, 121
  relationship with laryngeal injury, 77
  role of anxiety in delaying, 128
  swallow screening and, 80
eyes, concerns about following critical illness, 450

facilitated sensemaking, 295, 609
falling
  evaluation of fall risk with 6MWT, 565
  importance of screening for fear of, 627
  polypharmacy as risk factor in older adults, 511, 631
  risk of heightened by fatigue, 511

role of education and disease management in fall prevention, 511
Family Adaptability and Cohesion Evaluation Scale (FACES), 608
family caregivers
  affected social health domains, 690
  benefits of follow-up care for, 609
  caregiver burden/strain, 602–3
  development of resilience and PTG in as potential area of research in PICS-F, 604
  employment and financial strain, 333, 603
  fatigue assessment tool, 605
  health-risk behaviors, 602
  palliative care and support for, 590
  physical and functional consequences for, 602, 605
  potential for positive experiences, 604
  prevalence of common psychological symptoms, *602*
  prevalence of PTSD after cardiac arrest, 643
  psychological outcomes for, 601–2
  quality of life assessment tools, 607
  recommendations for promotion of social health, 690
  resilience studies, 604
  risk of developing PICS-F, 213
  sleep impairment, 602
  social support assessment tools, 607
  telemedicine assessments and PICS-F, 377
  see also family members and loved ones; PICS-Family (PICS-F).
family members and loved ones
  benefits of unrestricted presence in the ICU, 211
  early engagement and expectation management, 286–7
  engagement and empowerment of, 140–1
  pediatric patients, 686
  fundamental role in the prevention of PICS, 213
  ICU diaries
    benefits of, 235
    purposes, 231
    for coping and grief support, 233
    for memory building, 232–3
  importance of family presence in the ICU, 600, 609
  peer support, 609, 617
  post-intensive care syndrome – family, 600–11, *see also* PICS-Family (PICS-F).
  potential benefits of fresh air therapy, 271
  potential impact of PICS on, 6–7
  potential involvement in pain assessment, 136
  prevalence of anxiety during ICU admission, 602
  prevalence of PICS-F when making end-of-life decisions with inadequate support, 204
  psychological care, 190–1
    dealing with the critical illness, 190
    decision-making and coping with conflicts, 190–1
    end-of-life and grief support, 191
    supporting the patient, 190
  psychological impacts of hospitalization, 126, 132
  risk factors for PICS-F, 132
  role in cognitive rehabilitation, 175
  role in enhancing communication with non-verbal patients, 222
  support provision, 221
  terminology, 600 *see also* family caregivers; PICS-Family (PICS-F).
family-centered care
  components of, 20 *see also* patient- and family-centered care (PFCC).
Fan, E., 140
fatigue, 446–7, 510–11
  definition, 510
  comorbid conditions that overlap with, 447
  falling risk heightened by, 511
  impact on driving, 550–1
  interventions aimed to address, 447
  as manifestation of ICU-AW, 446–7
  measuring tools, 446
  OSA and, 460
  physical and mental impact of, 501
  prevalence following critical illness, 501
  and resumption of employment, 566
  risk of for survivors of critical illness, 423
Ferrante, L. E., 63
Fiatarone, M. A., 69
Fine, Aubrey, 255
Flaatten, H., 352
Fleischmann-Struzek, C., 548
flexible endoscopic evaluation of swallowing (FEES), 84
"four pillars of health" model of care, 296–8
frailty, 61–73
  assessing frailty
    deficit accumulation approach, 65–7
    measurement tools, 65
    phenotypic approach, 65
    predictive validity of questionnaire-based approaches, 65
    symptoms, 65
  bi-directional relationship with critical illness, 62

frailty (cont.)
  Cardiovascular Health
      Study, 64–5
  change in function according
      to frailty status in
      response to minor
      insult, **62**
  Clinical Frailty Scale, 67
  conceptual models of, 63–4
  critical illness-associated
      frailty, 63
  defining, 61
  epidemiology, 62
  evaluation of wearables to
      monitor, 380
  frailty index, 67
  geriatric syndromes and, 635
  and impact of critical illness
      on ADLs and
      IADLs, 63
  influence on ICU treatments
      administered, 72
  management and
      interventions, 67–73
    nutrition, 69–72
    palliative care, 72–3
    physical activity, 69
    pulmonary
        rehabilitation, 69
  mortality risk, 62
  outcomes associated with
      frailty present at ICU
      admission, 62–3
  Precipitating Events Project
      study, 63
  prevalence of, 62
fresh air therapy, 269–77
  benefits of therapy provision
      in fresh air space, 274
  case studies
    end-of-life care, 274
    healthcare workers, 272
  clinical impact and value of
      in intensive care,
      272–4
  common barriers to staff use
      of fresh air
      spaces, 272
  design considerations for
      fresh air spaces,
      275–6
  end-of-life care in fresh air
      spaces, 274
  evidence for benefits of for
      ICU patients and
      families, 269–71

examples of ICU access to
    outdoor spaces,
    269–70
health benefits of greenspace
    exposure, 271
and humanization of
    intensive care, 273
impact of green spaces on
    healthcare workers,
    271–2
Intensive Care Guidance on
    Transfer of Critically
    Ill Patients to the
    Outdoors (UK), 269
optimization of care for
    MDRO patients, 274
potential benefit for family
    members, 271
and recommendations for
    access to outdoor
    spaces, 269
safe transport to fresh air
    spaces, **275**
safety considerations, 274–5
Fried, L. P., 65
Fuermaier, A. B., 554
Functional Activities
    Questionnaire
    (FAQ), 522, 540
functional capacity evaluation
    (FCE), 549
functional cognition, cognitive
    rehabilitation, 176–9
functional impairments
    consistent with
    PICS, 7
functional impairments
    following critical
    illness, 520–32
  common ADLs and
      IADLs, *521*
  energy conservation
      strategies, **529**
  evaluation of ADL/IADL
      impairment, 522–7
  evaluation of physical
      impairment, 522–3
  evaluation role of
      occupational therapy,
      522–3
  functional cognitive
      impairment, 527–30
  interventions for ADL
      impairment, 527
  interventions for physical
      impairment, 527–8

mental health
    impairments, 530
  prevalence in children, 687
  recovery of a patient with
      PICS, **531**
  role of occupational
      therapists, 521–2
Functional Oral Intake Scale
    (FOIS), 466
Functional Outcomes of Sleep
    Questionnaire, 457
functional reconciliation
  the concept of, 374, 559
  as guiding principle for ICU
      follow-up clinics, 365
Functional Status Score for the
    Intensive Care Unit
    (FSS-ICU), 54
functional task training, 513
functional trajectories of
    recovery, 23–4
  acute respiratory failure
      survivors, 23–4
  "Big Hit" trajectory, 23
  disability outcome
      trajectories study, 24
  and prior degree of
      disability, 24
  "Relapsing Recurring"
      trajectory, 23
  "Slow Burn" trajectory, 23
fundamentals of PICS, 6–27
  overview of PICS, *8–11*
  clinical manifestations, 7–**12**
  communication about post-
      ICU problems, 7–13
  degrees of severity, 17–18
  disability
    the biomedical model,
        14–**15**
    functional status, 13, 14
  expanded definition, 7
  functional trajectories of
      recovery, 23–4
  guidelines on clinical
      evaluation, 20–1
  ICU follow-up clinics, 21
  impairments
    co-occurrence of, 16
    duration of, 16–17
    prediction tools, 18–19
    incidence and prevalence,
        14–16
  potential impact of critical
      illness on survivors, 6
  prevention, 19–20

screening and
    diagnosis, 20–3
screening tools/outcome
    measurement
    instruments, 21–3
treatment, 24–6

Gandotra, S., 23
Geense, W. W., 14, 500
Geisinger ICU Survivor Care vs
    usual care, 389
General Sleep Disturbance
    Scale (GSDS), 605
Generalized Anxiety Disorder
    Scale-7 (GAD-7), 23,
    377, 605
genomic storm, role in
    pathophysiology of
    PICS, 34–5
geriatric syndromes, definition
    of, 635
Germany, disability hiring
    policies, 307
Glasgow Coma Scale (GCS),
    evaluation of remote
    assessment, 377
Global Action on Disability
    Network, 307
granulation tissue, formation
    of during prolonged
    intubation, 477
green spaces, see fresh air
    therapy.
guanfacine, 542
Gugging Swallow Screen-
    Intensive Care Unit
    (GUSS-ICU), 81
guidelines on clinical
    evaluation, 20–1
gut microbiome
    beneficial organisms as
        protective factor, 491
    detrimental impact of critical
        illness on, 492
    disruption of in PICS, 39–40
    mental health impact of
        disruption, 40
    potential influence on
        development of ICU-
        AW, 39
    role in cognitive
        impairment, 40
    role in sepsis and
        maintenance of body
        temperature, 39
"gut-brain axis," 39

Haines, K. J., 617, 620
hair
    concerns about following
        critical illness, 449
    sepsis as risk factor for
        alopecia, 449
hallucinations, role of
    psychoeducation in
    mitigating distress
    associated with, 189
haloperidol, 111
    contraindicated for
        prevention of
        delirium, 139
handgrip strength, 23
    impairments in following
        critical illness, 17
    measurement of as
        diagnostic tool for
        ICU-AW, 49
    as objective evaluation of
        muscle strength, 561
healthcare professionals
    benefits of ICU diaries
        for, 235
    caring for, 212–13 see also
        burnout syndrome.
healthcare resource utilization
    by critical illness
    survivors, 423–5
health-related quality of life
    (HRQoL)
    benefits of screening
        tools, 428
    chronic chest pain and, 438
    EQ-5D, 428, 429
    growth in interest in
        measuring across
        populations, 428
    pediatric pain and, 685
    RAND Medical Outcomes
        Study, 428
    SF-36, 428, 429, **431**
Healthy Aging Brain Care
    (HABC) monitor
    tool, 354
hearing loss, 450
HeartMate III, 691
hepatic encephalopathy
    and cognitive
        impairment, 80
    delirium and, 101
Herpich, Franziska, 729–32
Herridge, M. S., 1, 16, 26, 429,
    501, 547, 548
heterotopic calcification, 7

heterotopic ossification (HO),
    448–9
Heyland, D. K., 63
high-flow nasal cannula,
    impact on swallow
    function, 78
high-reliability organizations
    (HRO), 399
Hippocrates, 45
history of PICS, 1–4
holistic approach to care,
    293–300
    benefits of multidisciplinary
        clinics in chronic
        disease, 295–6
    "four pillars of health"
        model, 296–8
    ICU follow-up clinics, 296
    integrative and
        complementary
        therapies, 298–9
    and interrelatedness of
        impairments, 293–5
    outdoor spaces and, 272
        see also fresh air
        therapy.
    patient- and family-centered
        care, 340–1
    requirements for
        a comprehensive
        recovery plan for
        patients with
        PICS, 293
    theoretical model for
        recovery, 295
home healthcare services, 289
Hommel, Scott, 732–7
Hope, A.A., 65, 72, 620
Hopkins Medication
    Schedule, 173
Hospital Anxiety and
    Depression Scale
    (HADS), 365, 573,
    585, 604
    degrees of severity, 17
    inclusion in core outcome
        measures, 22
    incorporation into
        EMRs, 363
    and QoL assessment, 431
    not validated for use in
        telemedicine, 377
Hospital Elder Life Program
    (HELP), 626
    as preventative strategy
        against delirium, 630

hospital readmission
  increased risk for patients with PICS, 7
  percentage of by critical illness survivors, 502
  and resource utilization by critical illness survivors, 423–5
Hospital San Juan de Dios, Spain, ICU access to an outdoor space, 269
hospitalization, bi-directional relationship with cognitive impairment, 166
House, J., 342
human rights, and disability, 303–4
humanization in healthcare, 208–9
  depersonalization of care and its drivers, 208–9
  essential points, 209
  relationship with dignity, 208
  technification and, 208
humanization of the ICU, 209–14, 224
  animal assisted intervention and, 264
  caring for healthcare professionals, 212–13
  communication, 211–12
  and end-of-life care, 214
  enhanced operational and environmental factors, 222
  fresh air therapy and, 273
  HU-CI Project, 209
    strategic components, **210**
  main objective, 210
  open-door policy and family inclusion, 211
  patient well-being, 212
  physical environment, 213–14
  and prevention, detection, and management of PICS, 213
hypotension, association with delirium, 104
hypoxia
  research focused on neuropsychological outcomes following, 1
  as risk factor for cognitive impairment following critical illness, 536

ICD-10 code
  developed for PICS, 708
  disability inclusion restricted by link to a disability diagnosis, 315
  lack of as barrier to services specific to PICS, 307
ICU design, recommended improvements, 223
ICU diaries, 19, 230
  definition, 230
  critical care context, 230
  development, 230–1
  digital diaries, 232
  evidence base
    benefits for family members, 235
    benefits for health care workers, 235
    benefits for patients, 234–5
  examples, 240–3
    diary entry, 230, **234**
    get-to-know-me page, 233
    table of contents, **232**
  and family engagement, 221, format, 231–2
  images as a supplement to, 264
  implementation, 237
    barriers and facilitators, 237–40
  practical aspects
    data protection considerations, 236
    handing over and reading diaries, 236
    indications, 235–6
    writing style, 236
  as protective factor against PICS-F, 609
  as protective factor against PTSS following critical illness, 572
  purposes, 231
    for coping and grief support, 233
    for memory building, 232–3
  research on the effect of PICU diaries on PICS-p, 687
  stress reduction findings, 188
ICU follow-up clinics
  overview, 359
  and advance care planning, 589
  assessing care providers for PICS-Family risk, 290
  attendance and recruitment barriers, 282–3, 286
    solutions, 283
  benefits of for survivors of critical illness, 360–1
  benefits of integrating palliative care techniques into, 582
    see also palliative care.
  benefits of measuring QoL in, 429–32
  benefits of multidisciplinary clinics in chronic disease, 295–6
  brief history, 352–8
  current models and outcomes, 356
  development of peer support and follow-up clinic collaboratives, 354–5
  establishment of clinics in Australasia, 355
  establishment of clinics in the UK and Europe, 352–4
  establishment of clinics in the US, 354–4
  impact of the COVID-19 pandemic, **357**, 356, 361
  review of ICU literature, 352
  roles and responsibilities of MDT at Vanderbilt University ICU Recovery Center, 355
  "Surviving Intensive Care" conference (2002), 352
  timeline, **353**
  case study, 719
  central tenets, 356
  components of successful programs, 286

Index 759

financial considerations, 385–96
 CPT codes for billing, 393
 evaluation challenges, 389–90
 population health management and transitions of care, 386–9
 recommendations to increase presence and accessibility of clinics, 390–3
 research and advocacy recommendations, 395
 stakeholder costs, 391–2
 value-based healthcare, 385–6
"four pillars of health" model, 296–8
fundamentals, 359–70
 collaboration with PCPs, 369
 components, 361–4
 composition of multidisciplinary teams, 362
 the concept of functional reconciliation, 365
 enablers and barriers, 368
 equipment, supplies, and other costs, 362–4
 evidence base, 359–61
 feedback to ICU care, 368
 financial support, 363–4
 finding an appropriate space, 361–2
 in-clinic evaluation, 365
 interventions, 365, 367
 operational characteristics, 361
 patient attendance, 368
 patient perspective, 369
 screening for clinic candidates, 364
 screening tools, 365
Geisinger ICU Survivor Care vs usual care, 389
holistic model of care, 293
 see also holistic approach to care
patient eligibility screening process, 284–6

patient inclusion and exclusion criteria, 285
pharmacists in
 case vignette, 413
 medication management, 409–14
 medication-related problems detected by, 409–14
 summary of interventions, 410–11
 vaccine assessment recommendations, 412
 workflow example, 414
pulmonary aims in, 440–2
role in fostering PTG, 299
role of for ANI survivors, 665–6
role of the registered dietician, 493
telemedicine-based model, assessments, 374–7
 care partner and PICS-F, 377
 cognitive domain, 376–7
 evaluating consciousness and wakefulness, 377
 mental health domain, 377
 physical domain, 374–6
 PICS domains and recommended outcomes, 375
 quality-of-life domain, 377
definition of telehealth, 373
digital health and wearables, 378–80
four principal roles, 374
influence of the COVID-19 pandemic, 373, 374
interdisciplinary collaboration on digital health solutions, 378
percentage of clinics offering, 356
regulatory considerations, 380–1
remote patient monitoring (RPM), 379–80

and tele-ICU services, 373–4
wearables and sensors, 380
workspace requirements, 361
ICU Liberation Campaign (SCCM), 135
ICU Recovery Center, Vanderbilt University, 354
ICU-acquired weakness (ICU-AW), 21
 clinical examination and diagnosis of, 49
 clinical standard for diagnosing, 503
 corticosteroids as risk factor for, 406
 defining, 560
 development of as driver of physical impairment, 7
 diagnosis of, 49–55
 diagnostic and surrogate tools, 50–3
 electrophysiological assessment of, 49
 fatigue as manifestation of, 446–7
 handgrip strength as diagnostic tool, 49
 history of the term, 45
 importance of early mobility for prevention of, 140
 measurement instruments for detecting, 54–5
 mechanisms implicated in development of, 37
 microvascular disruption and, 36
 mortality in patients with, 48
 muscle mass and morphological investigation of, 54
 physical functioning assessment of, 54–5
 potential influence of gut microbiome, 39
 prevalence, 48
 protective role of physical rehabilitation, 151
 respiratory muscle weakness assessment, 54
 risk factors, 55, 405

ICU-acquired weakness (cont.)
  subclassifications, 48
  transcriptomic perturbation and, 35 *see also* immobility and ICU-AW.
ICU steps, 616
immobility, cognitive impairment engendered by, 176
immobility and ICU-AW, 18, 45–57
  defining ICU-AW and its prevalence, 48
  diagnosis of ICU-AW, 49–55
  impact of bed rest and immobility on body systems, 45–6
  impact of critical illness on the musculoskeletal system, 47–8
  potential complications of immobility, **46**
  risk factors for ICU-AW, 55, 405 *see also* ICU-acquired weakness (ICU-AW).
immune system, beneficial effects of music on, 248
immunosuppression, role in pathophysiology of PICS, 34
Impact of Event Scale (IES), 605
Impact of Events Scale – 6 (IES-6), 377, 573, 605
Impact of Events Scale-Revised (IES-R), 22, 365, 605
impairment fundamentals of PICS
  co-occurrence of impairments, 16
  duration of impairment, 16–17
  impairments consistent with PICS, 7
  interrelatedness of impairments, 293–5
  prediction tools, 18–19
  risk factors, 18–19
in-bed cycling, 156
incidence and prevalence of PICS, 14, 16

infants, post-intensive care syndrome in, *see* PICS-pediatrics (PICS-p).
inflammation
  association with cognitive impairment, 33–4, 298
  role in pathophysiology of PICS, 31–2, 33–4
Informant Questionnaire of Cognitive Decline in the Elderly (IQCODE), 540
insomnia
  dedicated worry time technique, 458
  following critical illness, 457–9
  long-term use of sedative-hypnotic agents not recommended, 458
  predisposing factors, 457
  sleep hygiene recommendations, 458
Insomnia Severity Index (ISI), 605
  validated for telemedicine, 377
instrumental activities of daily living (IADLs)
  definition, 175, 520
  assessing performance in, 173
  assessment tools, 376, 529
  cognitive impairment and disruption in independence, 527
  cognitive rehabilitation, 176, 178
  common activities, *521*
  evaluation of impairment, 522–7
  examples of, 176, *521*, *560*
  impact of fatigue on, 446
  impact of frailty on, 63
  impact of functional impairment on, 7–13
  impact of increased dependence in, 521
  Lawton IADL screening tool, 376, 522
  performance of for cognitive rehabilitation, 176, 178

potential impact of cognitive impairment on, 527
requirements of, 520
insulin, medication management, 406
insulin resistance, bed rest and, 46
intensive care, US annual requirements, 6
Intensive Care Delirium Screening Checklist (ICDSC), 104, *106*, 166, 539
Intensive Care Guidance on Transfer of Critically Ill Patients to the Outdoors (UK), 269
Intensive Care Psychological Assessment Tool (IPAT), 186
Intensive Care Unit Delirium Screening Checklist (ICDSC), 139
Intensive Care Unit Mobility Scale (IMS), 54
intensive care units (ICUs)
  common psychological experiences of patients in, 569
  historical perspective, 1, 45
  number of patients admitted annually in the US, 420
interarytenoid adhesion, laryngeal injury and, 478
International Classification of Diseases, 10th edition (ICD-10)398 *see* ICD-10 code.
International Classification of Functioning, Disability, and Health (ICF), 150, 303, 306, 500, 550
International Research Project for the humanization of Intensive Care Units (HU-CI Project), 209
  strategic components, **210**
International Sepsis Forum, 2
interprofessional teams/teamwork, 399–403

aims of interprofessional
education
initiatives, 399
current teaching, 399–400
fostering optimal team
function, 402
HRO principles applicable
to, 399
research
current areas of, 400–1
use of in ICU and post-
ICU settings, 401–2
Sunnybrook Framework,
399–400
TeamSTEPPS system, 400
training frameworks,
399–400 *see also*
multidisciplinary
teams.
Iowa Oral Performance
Instrument
(IOPI), 469
iron depletion, risk of for ICU
patients, 460
Iwashyna, T. J., **421**

Japan, history of ICU follow-up
clinics, 356
Jennings, M. L., 256
Jette, A. M., 14
joint contractures, 7, 448, 562
Jonsen, A. R., 469
Jovell, Albert, 208

Kamdar, B. B., 120, 548
Katz Index of Independence in
Activities of Daily
Living, 376, 522
ketamine, contraindicated for
prevention of
delirium, 139
Kettle Test, 173, 529
Kidd, T., 69
Kim, B., 380
King, J., 342
King's College Hospital,
London, ICU access
to an outdoor
space, 269
Kress, J. P., 137
Kroll, R. R., 380
Kvale, R., 352

laryngeal disorders, 7
laryngeal disorders following
critical illness, 473–83

anatomy of the larynx,
473, **474**
consequences of granulation
tissue formation
during prolonged
intubation, **477**
consequences of ulceration
following prolonged
intubation, **478**
correlation between
endotracheal tube
size and laryngeal
injury, 473–4
definition of acute laryngeal
injury, 473
endotracheal intubation,
passage of the
tube, 473
endotracheal tube cuff
pressure
considerations, 474
minimizing risk of laryngeal
injury, 474, 480
tracheotomy-related issues,
management of,
480–3
vocal cord dysfunction,
475–6 *see also*
endotracheal
intubation;
extubation; laryngeal
injury; paradoxical
vocal fold motion
disorder (PVFMD);
tracheotomy.
laryngeal injury
anatomic sequelae of
dysphonia, 477
interarytenoid
adhesion, 478
posterior glottic
diastasis, 480
posterior glottic
stenosis, 479
subglottic/tracheal
stenosis and
tracheomalacia, 480
vocal process
granulomas, 478
intubation-associated
risk, 78
prevalence of acute injury in
mechanically
ventilated
patients, 473
Lavezza, A., 177

Lawton Instrumental Activities
of Daily Living Scale,
376, 522
Lee's Fatigue Scale (LFS), 605
limitations of the term
PICS, 3–4
Liu, K., 141
Lone, N. I., 424
long-COVID syndrome,
see also post-COVID
condition (PCC);
post-acute sequelae of
COVID (PASC);
SARS-CoV-2
infection 670–7
long-term acute care hospitals
(LTACHs), 289
long-term outcomes
Brussels Roundtable meeting
on, 2, 6, 352, 707
elderly survivors of critical
illness, 2
history of research, 1, 4
increasing international
attention, 2
innovative research
approaches, 2
misaligned expectations of
physicians and
surrogate decision-
makers, 12–13
patient-reported outcome
measures vs
performance-
based, 22
López-Fernández, E., 261
Lovell, T., 256
lower socioeconomic status, as
risk factor for anxiety
following critical
illness, 569

Maiden, M., 270
malnutrition following critical
illness, 485–97
definition of
malnutrition, 487
appetite and weight loss,
489
barriers to optimal nutrition
in patients with
PICS, 485
clinical vignette, 495–6
cognitive disorders, 492
contributing
medications, 486

malnutrition (cont.)
  discharge to post-acute facilities, 488–9
  dysphagia, 490–1
  ICU follow-up clinic experience, 493
  mental health disorders, 491
  nutrition care plan, 493
  nutrition challenges after discharge, 485–8
  nutrition optimization strategies, 494–5
  nutrition screening tools, 376, 488, 493
  physical and functional impairments, 490
  prevalence of malnutrition in patients requiring intensive care, 485
  role of the registered dietitian, 485, 493
  socio-economic barriers and, 492–3
  taste and smell changes, 489–90
manual muscle testing (MMT), 561
Marra, A., 16
Mattioni, M. F., 547
McHugh, L. G., 1
McPeake, J., 341
Mead, Margaret, 208
mechanical ventilation
  adjusting settings to combat sleep impairment, 121
  analgesia-first sedation recommended, 136, 405
  beneficial effects of music, 247–8
  benefits of daily paired SATs and SBTs, 137
  benefits of early physical rehabilitation on cognitive functioning, 158
  chronic pain as result of, 448
  and communication role of family members, 222
  delirium risk in ARDS patients, 102
  diaphragmatic complications of, 54, 438–9
  duration of increased by deep sedation, 138
  dysphagia risk in ARDS patients, 78
  early mobilization trial, 140
  optimizing for pediatric patients, 685
  percentage of older adults experiencing delirium, 246
  percentage of patients developing intubation/extubation-related issues, 77
  percentage of patients experiencing delirium, 102, 139
  percentage of patients with ICU-AW, 140
  polio epidemic and, 45
  potential impact on the eyes, 450
  potential risks for long-term outcomes, 34
  and prevalence of acute laryngeal injury, 473
  psychological impact, 128
  recommended medications for sedation, 406
  relationship of duration with ability to resume work, 548
  relationship with ICU-AW, 48
  as risk factor for anxiety following critical illness, 569
  as risk factor for cognitive impairment following critical illness, 536
  risk factors for development of dysphagia, 78
  and transitions in care location during follow-up, 424
medical errors, number of preventable deaths due to, 142
Medical Research Council Sum-Score (MRC-SS), 49, 50, 55, 503–4
Medicare data, reliance on in the US, 626
medication, and cognitive impairment, 405, 634
medication management, 405–15
  analgesics, sedating medications, and neuromuscular blockade, 405–6
  antipsychotics and antibiotics, 406–7
  case vignette, 413
  corticosteroids and insulin, 406
  discharge counseling, 409
  medication reconciliation at transitions of care, 407–9
  failure to discontinue medications at discharge, 407–8
  failure to initiate home medications during admission, 408
  polypharmacy and deprescribing, 409
  pharmacists in ICU follow-up clinics, 409–14
  sleep impairment, role of prescribed medications in, 457
  vaccine assessment recommendations for adults, 412
medications associated with vitamin deficiencies, 486
Mediterranean diet, benefits for cognitive function, 492
melatonin, 111, 120, 121
melatonin receptor agonists, 111
memory disorders, delivery of music to treat, 249
mental health
  assessment tools, 22, 585
  impairment following critical illness, 530
  potential impact of cognitive impairment on, 631
  remote assessment of, 377
  role of occupational therapy in assessment and interventions, 530
mental illness
  malnutrition and, 491
  role of the microbiome in, 40
Menu Task, 173

Meyer, J., 551
microbiome disruption, mental health impact, 40
microvascular disruption, role in pathophysiology of PICS, 35–6
midazolam, 80, 451
Mikkelsen, M., 354
Millward, K., 347
mind-body interventions, stress reduction findings, 187
Mini Cog, 23, 585
Mini Mental State Examination (MMSE), 166, 539–40
  effectiveness for capturing patients with cognitive impairment, 536
  in physiatry consultation, 560
  telemedicine vs in-person assessment, 376
Mini Nutrition Assessment (MNA), 376
Mini Nutrition Assessment-Short Form (MNA-SF), 493
mitochondrial dysfunction, 37, 47
mobility, management of ambulation impairment, 565–6
Model of Human Occupation (MOHO), 530
Modified Ashworth Scale, 563
modified barium swallow study (MBSS), 83, 465–6, 471
Modified Medical Research Council (mMRC) Dyspnea Scale, 440
monocyte human leukocyte antigen-DR (mHLA-DR), 34
Montreal Cognitive Assessment (MoCA) tool, 166, 363, 365, 376
  alternative versions, 540
  degrees of severity, 17
  incorporation into EMRs, 363
  in physiatry consultation, 560

recommended for screening for cognitive impairment, 540
morphine, 80
Morris, P.E., 155
mortality, relative decrease from 1988 to 2012, 6
movement, role of in recovery of patients experiencing PICS, 297
multi-component or circuit training, 513
multidisciplinary teams
  benefits of for chronic disease, 295–6
  benefits of integrating spiritual care into, 298
  composition of, 362
  importance of for follow-up, 21
  role of effective coordination and communication, 296
  Vanderbilt University model, 354 see also interprofessional teams/teamwork.
multi-drug resistant organisms (MDROs), optimization of care for patients with, 274
Multiple Errands Test, 529
Munn, J., 550
muscle atrophy, 36, 47, 48
muscle dysfunction, contributors to, 38
muscle loss, rates of during a stay in ICU, 88
muscle protein synthesis (MPS), 47, 88
  role of exercise and nutrition, 47
muscle tone, assessment tool, 563
muscle weakness and fatigue, risk of for survivors of critical illness, 423
musculoskeletal system impact of critical illness on, 47–8
  potential impact of bed rest and immobility on, 45
music therapy, 246–51

effects on brain functional networks, 249
effects on cognitive performance, 249–50
effects on pain, anxiety, stress, and sedatives exposure, 247
effects on sleep, 247
implementation considerations, 250
music and cognition, 248
and neurocognitive processing of music, 249
neuromodulatory role, 248
scalability as non-pharmacological intervention for PICS, 250
stress reduction findings, 187
in the context of delirium, 246
"My Life After ICU" (ANZICS, 2022), 356
myeloid-derived suppressor cells (MDSCs), 36

Nagi, S. Z., 14
Nagoya City University West Medical Center, Japan, fresh air therapy study, 270
nails, concerns about following critical illness, 449
Naqvi, I. A., 379
Narváez-Martinez, M. A., 17
National Institute on Aging, 2
Nestle Nutrition Institute
  Mini Nutrition Assessment (MNA), 376
  Mini Nutrition Assessment-Short Form (MNA-SF), 493
Netherlands, examples of ICU access to an outdoor space, 269
Neuro Quality of Life (Neuro-QoL) questionnaire, 376
neurological conditions, increased rates of in cardiac arrest survivors, 644
neuromuscular blockade, medication management, 405–6

neuropathy, 423, 513, 560
"Neuropsychological sequelae in ARDS survivors" (Hopkins et al), 2
New Zealand
 fresh air therapy study, 271
 history of ICU follow-up clinics, 356
NICE (National Institute for Health and Care Excellence)
 guidelines on clinical evaluation, 20
 guidelines on rehabilitation after critical illness, 694
 post-ICU psychological follow-up recommended by, 575
 psychological assessment of all critically ill patients recommended by, 19
nightmares, following critical illness, 459
nocturnal hypoventilation, 460
non-opioid analgesics, 136, 685
Norbeck Social Support Questionnaire (NSSQ), 607
normal activities, resumption of, *see also* driving; employment 547–55
Norway, history of ICU follow-up clinics, 352
Nottingham Health profile, 429
nutrition, 88–97
 clinical consequences of over- or under-provision, 91
 contributing factors to poor nutrition delivery in ICU and post-ICU periods, 88
 energy
  delivery, 90–1
  expenditure, 90
 frailty and, 69–72
 importance of for recovery from critical illness, 88
 metabolic response to critical illness and, 89
 micronutrients, 92

patients at high risk for impaired provision, 93
 obesity, 94
 oral consumption, 93
 potential impact of prolonged under-provision, 88
 process for optimizing nutrition care for critically ill patients, **95**
 protein
  delivery, 92
  requirements, 91
 research recommendations, 96
 role of clinicians in optimizing nutrition therapy, 94
 role of in recovery of patients experiencing PICS, 297
nutrition impairments, *see* malnutrition following critical illness.
nutrition rehabilitation, 297, 485, 489, 493, 496–7
nutritional psychiatry, 491
nutritional status, assessment tools, 376

obesity, and risk of malnutrition, 94
obstructive sleep apnea (OSA)
 comparison with central sleep apnea, 460
 as risk factor for the development of PASC, 459
 screening questionnaires, 459
Occupational Self-Assessment (OSA), 530
occupational therapy
 and driving rehabilitation, 522
 and evaluation of functional impairment, 522–3
 and mental health assessment/ interventions, 530
 recommended for prevention of PICS, 19

 and remediation of functional impairment following critical illness, 521–2
Ohtake, P. J., 520
older adult survivors of critical illness, 625–37
 ageism and ableism, 625–6
 5 Ms of Age-Friendly Healthcare, 625
  medications, 631
   discontinue or use with caution, *632*, *634*
  mind, 630–1
  mobility, 626–30
  multicomplexity, 631–5
   rehabilitation and, 627–30
   and the ABCDEF bundle, 627, *628*, *629*
  what matters most, 635–6
 mortality following ICU and non-ICU hospitalizations, 625
 sepsis survivors' response to rehabilitation, 627
 successful discharge planning, 630
 and the Age-Friendly Movement, 625 *see also entries under* Age-Friendly.
ophthalmologic sequelae of critical illness, 450
opioid analgesics
 adverse effects, 136
 minimizing exposure to, 136
opioids
 adverse effects, 405
 strategies to minimize exposure to, 405–6
orientation assessment, cognitive rehabilitation, 173
outdoor spaces
 recommendations for access to, 269 *see also* fresh air therapy.
Oxygen Cost Diagram (OCD), 441

PADIS guidelines (Clinical Practice Guidelines for the Prevention and Management of Pain, Agitation/

Sedation, Delirium, Immobility, and Sleep Disruption in Adult Patients in the ICU), 405
pain
  assessment, prevention, and management, 135–6
  assessment instruments, 22
  combined approach, 565
  management of in children, 685
  music therapy, 247
  nociceptive vs neuropathic components, 564
  non-pharmacological interventions, 136
  opioids not recommended as primary strategy for chronic pain management, 565
  pharmacotherapy for, 565
palliative care, 582–93
  barriers, 592
  the concept of, 583–4
  frailty and, 72–3
  indicators for referral to specialty palliative care clinic, 591–2
  integration into evaluation and management of patients with PICS, 582
  PICS challenges vs symptoms, 582–3
  principles, 584–91
    advance care planning, 589
    caregiver support, 590
    communication techniques, 588–9
    expectation management and anticipatory guidance, 591
    goal-concordant care and, 587–8
    identifying symptoms, 584–5
    spiritual support, 590
Palliative Performance Scale (PPS), 585
Pandharipande, P.P., 139, 535
paradoxical vocal fold motion disorder (PVFMD)
  management of, 476
  symptoms of, 475
  triggers for attacks, 476
Patel, J., 120
pathophysiology of PICS, 31–40
  definitions of key syndromes related to PICS, 32
  genomic storm and transcriptomic alterations, 34–5
  gut microbiome disruption, 39–40
  immunosuppression, 34
  inflammation, 31–2
    and cognition, 33–4
  microvascular disruption, 35–6
  myopathy, catabolism, sarcopenia, and cachexia, 36–9
  simultaneous inflammation and immunosuppression, 31–4
patient- and family-centered care (PFCC), 217–26, 339–48
  overview, 217–18
  definitions, 218
  addressing patients and their families' experience of disrespect through, 218
  addressing health disparities through, 223
  benefits of PFCC in the research process, 224
  categories of need, 342–7
    appraisal needs, 344
    emotional needs, 344
    family-specific needs, 346–7
    informational needs, 344
    instrumental needs, 344
    patient-specific needs, 345–6
    shared needs, 342
    social/relational needs, 345
    spiritual needs, 345
  five stages of recovery, 343
  fostering meaningful engagement, 224
  guiding principles, 339–42
    holistic approach, 340–1
    proactive, structured, and coordinated care, 339–40
    recovery and resolution centered care, 341
    "timing it right" model, 341–2
  humanization of the ICU, 224
  ICU Family-Centered Care Checklist, **225**
  impact of COVID-19 pandemic on, 221
  increasing interest in, 208
  interventions
    adult ICU family-centered care recommendations, 219, 220
    benefits for both patients and healthcare workers, 220
    communication with family members, 221
    enhanced operational and environmental factors, 222
    ICU diaries, 221–1
    promotion of family presence, 218–21
    support provision for family members, 221–1
    targeted consultations and ICU team members, 222,
    VALUE communication strategy, 222
  Patient and Family Advisory Councils (PFACs), 224
  research recommendations, 347–8
Patient Health Questionnaire-4 (PHQ-4), 22
Patient Health Questionnaire-8 (PHQ-8), 23
Patient Health Questionnaire-9 (PHQ-9), 377, 585
patient-centered goals, management of expectations, 587–8
Patient-Reported Outcome Measurement Information System

(PROMIS)
  questionnaire, 376
PEACE Tool (Physical,
  Emotive, Autonomy,
  Communication,
  Economic, and
  Transcendent
  domains), 585
pediatric medical traumatic
  stress (PMTS), 688
peer support, 616
  benefits, 616-17
  CAIRO network, 355, 616
  for caregivers, 617
  clinic-based groups, 618
  developing a PICS peer
    support group, 710
  development history, 354-5
  for family members and
    loved ones, 609, 617
  holistic approach, 341
  models of, 617
    community-based
      groups, 618
    ICU-based groups, 617
    online groups, 618
    peer mentor model,
      618-19
    social gatherings, 619, 620
    virtual groups, 618, 621
  program development guide,
    620-2
    facilitator selection, 621
    "in-between" time
      planning, 622
    logistical plan, 622
    preparation, 621
    recruitment of
      participants, 620-1
    trauma-informed
      approach, 621
  THRIVE collaborative, 281,
    355, 616
  UK ICUsteps program, 616
  US initiatives, 616
  value of for SDOH, 333-4
  volunteer mentors ship and
    PTG, 619
persistent dysphagia following
  critical illness, 463-71
  background and prevalence
    of dysphagia in
    PICS, 463
  case studies, 470-1
  characteristics of
    dysphagia, 463

discharge considerations,
  469-70
influences on patient
  outcomes, 463
International Dysphagia
  Diet Standardization
  Initiative
  (IDDSI), **466**
outcome measures, 466
outpatient evaluation
  process, 465-7
outpatient SLP therapy
  recommended, 463
referrals, 467
role of patient and family
  training, 463, 470
swallowing phases
  anatomical representation
    of, **464**
  description of, **464**
  treatment, 467-9
persistent inflammation,
  immunosuppression,
  and catabolism
  syndrome (PIICS),
  31, 32, 35
personal stories, 729-42
  Connie Bovier (pneumonia
    and ARDS), 738-40
  Cori Davis (SARS-CoV-2
    infection and ARDS),
    740-2
  Franziska Herpich (stroke),
    729-32
  Scott Hommel (sepsis),
    732-7
physiatry consultation, 559-67
  definition of
    a physiatrist, 559
  examples of ADLs and
    IADLs, *560*
  management of specific
    conditions
    chronic pain, 564-5
    impaired ambulation,
      565-6
    joint contractures, 562
    return to work and
      vocational
      rehabilitation, 566
    spasticity, 563-4
  physiatric history, 559
  physical examination, 560-2
    electrodiagnosis, 562
    muscle weakness
      evaluation, 560

strength evaluation, 560-1
role of the physiatrist in
  PICS, 559
therapy referrals, 562
physical activity, frailty and, 69
physical domain, assessment
  instruments, 22,
  365, 585
Physical Function in Intensive
  Care Test-Scored
  (PFIT-S), 54
physical functioning,
  assessment of in the
  clinical setting, 49-55
physical impairment
  assessment instruments, 22,
    365, 585
  remote assessment, 374-6
physical impairments
  following critical
  illness, 500-15
  definition of physical
    disability, 500
  education and disease
    management, 510-11
    fall prevention, 511
    fatigue, 510-11
    medication, 511
    nutrition, 511
    physical activity, 510
  evaluation of, 522-3
  incidence and prevalence of
    physical disability,
    500-1
  interventions for, 527-8
  management and treatment,
    504-14
    home-based
      treatment, 509
    models of delivery, 509-10
    outpatient (ambulatory)
      physical therapy, 509
    telerehabilitation care,
      509-10
  physical therapy
    interventions, 511-14
    functional task
      training, 513
    multi-component or
      circuit training, 513
    patient safety, 512
    prescription and
      dosing, 514
    therapeutic exercise,
      512-13
  risk factors, 687

Index | 767

screening and evaluation,
502–**8**
assessment tools, 503–4,
505–7
flow diagram of physical
therapist
approach, **508**
timing considerations,
502–3
trajectory of disability, 501–2
physical rehabilitation, 150–60
assessment of physical
functioning, 158–**9**
benefits of early physical
rehabilitation on
cognitive
function, 158
benefits of sedation
interruption paired
with, 151
best practice in the ICU, 151
early mobilization
activities, 150
effects of beyond physical
functioning, 158–60
evidence base, 158
early physical
rehabilitation in the
ICU, 151–5
gaps in, 160
progressive stepwise
rehabilitation and
physical activity in
the ICU, 155
RECOVER trial, 158
rehabilitation across the
hospital, 157–8
safety considerations,
156–7
TEAM study, 152–5
use of assistive
technology, 156
focus of, 150
functional exercises vs non-
functional, 160
goal-directed, 155
implementation of in the
ICU, **161**
implications for clinical
practice, 160
protective role against ICU-
AW, 151
recommendations on
initiating active
mobilization in the
ICU, 157

research
recommendations,
160
risk of adverse events
during, 156
steps for rehabilitation
strategies, **152**
terminology
considerations, 150
physical restraint devices, use
of with agitated
patients, 129
physical therapy,
recommended for
prevention of
PICS, 19
PICS advocacy, 707–17
definition and shared
understanding of,
707–8
compendium of existing
PICS resources, *709*
current landscape, 708–10
developing a PICS peer
support group, *710*
examples of, *713–16*,
725, 728
future of, 711–12
insights from other advocacy
campaigns, 711
promotion of, 707, 710–11
recommendations, 395
and research funding, 709
targets for potential
advocacy efforts,
711, **712**
"Walk4PICS," 708, 711
PICS research, importance of
inclusion of patients
and family
members, 308
PICS-Family (PICS-F), 600–11
definition, 600
after cardiac arrest, 643
assessment instruments, 22
caregiver burden/strain,
602–3
the concept of, 7, **601**
employment and financial
strain of
caregiving, 603
experienced by caregivers of
ANI survivors, 660
focus of research, 601
interventions, 608–10
acute phase

communication
facilitators, 608
facilitated sensemaking
model, 609
family-centered care/
presence, 609
ICU diaries, 609
post-ICU
dyadic intervention,
610
mental health
interventions, 610
peer support
programs, 609
measuring, 604–8
outcomes and measurement
tools, *606, 607*
physical and functional
consequences of
caregiving, 602, 605
positive aspects of
caregiving, 604
potential causes, 601
prevalence, 204
prevalence of common
psychological
symptoms in family
caregivers, *602*
prevalence when making
end-of-life decisions
with inadequate
support, 204
psychological outcomes for
family caregivers,
601–2
risk factors, 132, 213, 608
see also family
caregivers; family
members and loved
ones.
PICS-pediatrics (PICS-p)
overview, 682–3
ABCDEF bundle
components. 682
Assess, prevent, and
manage pain, 685
Breathing and optimal
mechanical
ventilation, 685
Choice of analgesia and
sedation, 686
Delirium assessment,
prevention, and
management, 686
Early mobility and
exercise, 686

PICS-pediatrics (cont.)
    Family engagement and
        empowerment, 686
    benefits of education
        about, 688
    clinical vignette, 683–4
    conceptual figure, **683**
    developmental aspects,
        691, 693
    education and training
        requirements, 695
    functional outcomes
        cognitive health, 689
        emotional health, 687–8
        influence of social
            determinants of
            health on, 691
        physical health, 687
        social health, 689–90
    impact on education, 692–3
    impact on parents, 688, 693
    importance of early
        identification for
        infants and young
        children, 691
    knowledge gaps, *696, 697*
    medical technologies and
        complex needs, 690–1
    PICS-p-family, 693–4
    PICU diaries, 687
    post-PICU models of care,
        694–5
    prevention and treatment
        strategies, 685–7
    research recommendations,
        695–7
    risk factors, 684, 686
    screening for, 684–5
Pillbox Test, 529
Pittsburgh Sleep Quality Index
    (PSQI), 457, 605
polio epidemic, 1
Pollack, L.R., 73
polypharmacy
    in post-ICU settings, 673
    prevalence in long
        COVID, 673
    rates of in older adults, 631
    as risk factor for
        delirium, 109
    as risk factor for PICS-p,
        686
    and risk of adverse health
        outcomes, 408
    risks of for older adults,
        511, 631

Pompe disease, 39
POPPI (Psychological
    Outcomes Following
    a Nurse-Led
    Preventive
    Psychological
    Intervention for
    Critical Ill Patients),
    187–8
Porter, M.E., 386
Post Traumatic Stress Disorder
    Checklist-5 (PCL-
    5), 377
Post-Acute Sequelae of SARS-
    CoV-2 infection
    (PASC), OSA as risk
    factor for the
    development of, 459
post-COVID condition (PCC),
    670–7
    definition, 670
    anticoagulation, 674
    clinical presentation, 671
    common symptoms, 670–1
    diagnosis, 672
    disparities in the COVID-19
        pandemic, 676
    ICU follow-up/long COVID
        clinic overlap, 675–6
    management, 672–4
        neurocognitive
            symptoms, 673
        physical function
            symptoms, 673–4
        pulmonary symptoms,
            672–3
        other PCC symptoms, 674
    ongoing research, 676
    pathophysiology, 671
    polypharmacy and over-
        prescription common
        in, 673
    psychiatric
        comorbidities, 673
    screening for cognitive
        impairment, 673
    symptom overlap with PICS,
        670, **671**
    vaccination, 675
posterior glottic diastasis, 480
    laryngeal injury and, 480
posterior glottic stenosis
    (PGS), 479
    negative QoL impact, 479
    treatment
        early detection, 479

    late detection, 479
    tracheotomy, 479
    transverse cordotomy, 479
post-extubation dysphagia
    (PED) swallow
    screen, 81
post-ICU disability
    age and, 625
    prevalence, 217
    research into, 303
    risk of, 502
    and the social model of
        disability, 306–7
post-intensive care syndrome
    (PICS)
    definition, 14, 660
    characteristics, 293
    development of the term, 3
    expanded conceptualization,
        12
    first formalized definition
        developed, 707
    historical perspective, 1–4
    ICD-10 code developed
        for, 708
    impact on nutritional status,
        485
    see also malnutrition
        following critical
        illness
    increase in awareness of and
        attention to, 707
    limitations of the term
        PICS, 3–4
    number of studies published
        using the term, 3
    potential impact on family
        members and loved
        ones, 6
    prevalence of symptoms in
        survivors of critical
        illness, 582
    related syndromes, *32*
    risk factors, *285*, 303,
        326, 364
    role of advocacy in
        increasing awareness
        of, 707
    see also PICS advocacy
    and societal patterns of
        disparities, 303
    strategies to increase
        awareness of,
        283
    symptoms and
        impairments, 7

and the social model of
disability, 306–8
post-intensive care syndrome
in pediatrics
(PICS-p), *see also*
PICS-pediatrics
(PICS-p) 682–98
post-neuro ICU clinics
development of, 660
function of, 660
post-traumatic growth
(PTG), 299
definition, 299
benefits of peer support
for, 617
cardiac arrest survivors, 645
the concept of, 573, 575
domains of, 299
following critical illness, 573
fostering role of the ICU
follow-up clinic, 299
ICU diaries and, 235
and peer volunteer
mentorship, 619
as potential area of research
in PICS-F, 604
Posttraumatic Stress
Diagnostic Scale
(PDS), 605
post-traumatic stress disorder
(PTSD)
assessment instruments, 22
assessment tools, 605
family involvement as
protective factor
against development
of, 141
ICU-specific examples, *571*
manifestation of in cardiac
arrest survivors, 643
odds ratio for development
reduced by ICU diary
use, 234
prevalence following critical
illness compared with
general
population, 570
prevalence in cardiac arrest
survivors, 643
prevalence in family
members of critically
ill patients, 601
as psychological outcome of
critical illness, 570–2
risk of reduced by facilitated
sensemaking, 295

screening tools, 365, 377
symptoms, 570
Post-traumatic Symptom Scale
(PTSS-10), 605
postural orthostatic
tachycardia
syndrome (POTS),
671–2, 674
potentially inappropriate
medications (PIMs),
407, 409, 414, 631
Potter, K.M., 550
pressure injuries, 7, 449
reducing risk of, 449
prevalence and incidence of
PICS, 14, 16
prevention of PICS, 19–20
primary care physicians
importance of education
about PICS for,
395
importance of targeting
PICS advocacy
towards, 708
lack of understanding of
PICS, 281
limitations on preparedness
to care for patients
with PICS, 708
role in improving clinical
care pathways for
survivors, 576
role of in PICU follow-up,
694–5
privacy, psychological impact
of lack of, 129
progressive universalism, and
disability
inclusion, 316
propofol, 111, 120
as potential driver of
delirium, 119
psychological care, 184–94
cognitive behavioral therapy,
188–90
family members and loved
ones, 190–1
general approaches to care,
186–7
goal of, 184
indirect work by practitioner
psychologists, 191–3
Intensive Care Psychological
Assessment Tool,
186
POPPI trial, 187–8

psychological care of
patients in the ICU,
184–5
psychological first aid, 186
psychological interventions
in intensive care,
187–8
screening for psychological
distress, 185–6
trauma-informed care, 187
psychological first aid
(PFA), 186
psychological impacts of
hospitalization,
125–33
impact on family members
and loved ones,
126, 132
percentage of patients
experiencing long-
term psychological
difficulties after
discharge, 125
positive reactions and
coping, 125, 131–2
psychological experiences in
the ICU, 126–7
risk factors for long-term
psychological
distress, 125, 127
sedation and, 125
stressors experienced in the
ICU, 127–31
environment-related, 129
illness-related, 128–9
interpersonal
stressors, 130
other stressors, 130–1
psychological interventions,
recommendations
for, 19
psychological outcomes
following critical
illness, 569–78
anxiety, 569–70
assessment, 573
depression, 570
early screening of
psychological
symptoms
recommended, 573
evidence on risk and
protective factors of
psychological
distress, **572**
example questions, *574*

psychological outcomes (cont.)
  interventions, 574–8
    stepped care framework, 574–5
  physical manifestations of psychological distress, 572–3
  post-traumatic growth and resilience, 573
  proposed psychological process, **577**
  PTSD, 570–2
  resources, *576*
  screening tools, 573
  self-report measures, *574*
psychological stress, family involvement as protective factor against, 141
psychologists
  incorporation of into multidisciplinary ICU teams, 184
  indirect work in the ICU, 191–3
    communication improvement, 192
    consultation provision, 192–3
    therapeutic environment creation, 193
  role of in intensive care, **185**
Psychologists in Intensive Care-UK (PINC-UK), 184
Psychosocial Screen for Cancer (PSSCAN), 584
psychosocial screening tools, 584–5
PTSD Checklist-5 (PCL-5), 605
pulmonary and diaphragmatic complications following critical illness, 437–43
  clinical vignette, 442–3
  diaphragmatic complications, 438–9
  evaluating pulmonary function, 439–40
  measurement tools for dyspnea, 440, *441*
  measuring pulmonary function, 437
  pulmonary aims in ICU follow-up clinics, 440–2
  pulmonary complications, 437–8
  respiratory status assessment tools, 440
pulmonary function, measuring, 437
pulmonary rehabilitation, frailty and, 69

quality of life
  assessment instruments, 22
  family caregivers, 607
  remote assessment, 377
quality of life following critical illness, 428–34
  assessment tools, 23
  benefits of measuring in ICU follow-up clinics, 429–32
  comparison of measurements with general population controls, **430**
  comparison of SF-36 and EQ-5D, **432**
  domains of EQ-5D and SF-36 QoL measures, **431**
  historical perspective, 428–9
  patient-specific nature of assessment, 432–4
  screening tools, 429–32
  limitations, 432
  WHO classification of functioning after critical illness, **433**
quetiapine, 111

Rahman, A., 71
ramelteon, 120, 121
Rapid Pace Walk Test (RPW), 522
RECOVER trial, evaluating post-ICU rehabilitation on general wards, 158
Recovering Together, 610
recovery
  five stages of, **343**
  trajectory variation, 420
registered dietician (RD), role in ICU follow-up clinic, 493
rehabilitation
  definition, 150
  cognitive, 166–80
  gym environments, challenges for infection prevention and control measures, 274
  nutrition, 297, 485, 489, 493, 496–7
  physical, 150–60
  vocational, 549
"Relapsing Recurring" trajectory of recovery, 23
Remington, P.L., 326
remote patient monitoring (RPM), 379–80
renal disease, risk of for survivors of critical illness, 423
renal replacement therapy, 48
Repeatable Battery for the Assessment of Neuropsychological Status (RBANS), 23, 173, 376
research recommendations, ICU follow-up clinics, 395
resilience
  definition, 604
  as potential area of research in PICS-F, 604
  prevalence in survivors of critical illness, 573
resistance training, 155
respiratory disease, risk of for critical illness survivors, 422
respiratory muscle weakness, 54
respiratory status, assessment tools, 440
restless leg syndrome (RLS), 460
  exacerbated by SSRIs, 457
resumption of normal activities, *see also* driving; employment 547–55
returning to work, *see under* employment.
Richards-Campbell Sleep Questionnaire (RCSQ), 380
Richmond Agitation Sedation Scale (RASS), 138
Riddersholm, S., 548

Rijnstate Hospital,
    Netherlands, ICU
    access to an outdoor
    space, 269
Riker Sedation Agitation Scale
    (SAS), 138
risk factors for the
    development of
    PICS, 18
rivastigmine, 111
robotic devices, physical
    rehabilitation
    and, 156
Roy's Adaptation Model, 295

sarcopenia, nutritional
    prevention
    measures, 72
SARS-CoV-2 infection,
    case study, 470–1
    global infection and
        mortality rates, 670
    prevalence of dysphagia at
        hospital
        discharge, 463
    prevalence of PICS in
        survivors, 671
    as risk factor for
        delirium, 109
Schulte, P. J., 536
Schweickert, W. D., 151
Scotland, integrated health and
    social care
    intervention trial, 307
screening and diagnosis of
    PICS, 20–3
Screening for Distress Toolkit
    Working Group, 585
Screening Tool of Older
    People's
    Prescriptions
    (STOPP), 631
Screening Tool to Alert to
    Right Treatment
    (START), 631
screening tools, see assessment/
    screening tools.
sedation
    assessment tools, 138
    benefits of interruption
        paired with physical
        rehabilitation, 151
    choice of analgesia and,
        137–9
    exposure to reduced by
        music, 247

impact comparison of light
    vs deep, 138
medication
    management, 405–6
    as risk factor for cognitive
        impairment, 536
    optimizing for children, 686
    role of in sleep
        impairment, 120
    role of music in reducing
        exposure to, 247
sepsis
    as a risk factor for
        alopecia, 449
    definition, 32
    and co-occurrence of PICS
        impairments, 294
    disruption to
        microvasculature, 35
    effects on membrane
        properties of skeletal
        muscle, 36
    and immunosuppression, 34
    impact of sepsis-induced
        systemic
        inflammation, 33
    increased healthcare costs
        and resource
        utilization associated
        with, 424
    inflammatory biomarkers
        studies, 31–2
    MDSCs associated with
        adverse clinical
        outcomes, 36
    prevalence of delirium in
        patients with, 33
    and prevalence of
        ICU-AW, 48
    as risk factor for cognitive
        impairment, 536
    as risk factor for delirium,
        104, 109
    role of the gut microbiome
        in, 39
    severity associated with
        inability to return to
        work, 548
sepsis survivors
    excess mortality risk, 421
    functional impairment
        studies, 520
    hospital readmission
        rates, 424
    older adults' response to
        rehabilitation, 627

personal story, 732–7
prevalence of PICS, 15–16
risk of cardiovascular
    disease, 422
risk of chronic kidney
    disease, 423
risk of hospital readmission
    and mortality, 502
risk of stroke, 423
septic encephalopathy,
    delirium and, 101
severity, degrees of in PICS,
    17–18
sexual dysfunction, 450, 451
Short Form 36 item health
    survey (SF-36), 14,
    428, 429, **431**
    comparison with EQ-
        5D, 432
    domains, **431**
    evaluation of caregivers'
        quality of life, 607
    inclusion in core outcome
        measures, 22
    knowledge gaps, 347
Short Memory Questionnaire
    (SMQ), 14
Short Physical Performance
    Battery (SPPB),
    23, 504
Sickness Impact Profile, 429
Sickness Insight in Coping
    Questionnaire
    (SICQ), 131
six-minute walk test
    (6MWT), 376
    as assessment of physical
        functioning, 16–17,
        22, 365, 439, 503–4
    as assessment of pulmonary
        function, 439–41,
        673
    and evaluation of fall
        risk, 565
Skei, N. V., 548
skilled nursing facilities
    (SNFs), 289
skin, concerns about following
    critical illness, 449
sleep
    assessment instruments, 22
    enhancement of nighttime
        sleep, 193
    Functional Outcomes of
        Sleep
        Questionnaire, 457

sleep (cont.)
  Pittsburgh Sleep Quality
      Index, 457
  potential impact of bed rest
      and immobility on, 46
  role of in recovery of patients
      experiencing
      PICS, 297
sleep disturbances, remote
    assessment, 377
sleep impairment, 117–22
  delirium and, 109, 119–20
  examples of sleep
      fragmentation in ICU
      patients, **118**
  family caregivers, 602
  interventions
    mechanical ventilation
        settings, 121
    medication, 120–1
    non-pharmacological, 121
    monitoring with
        wearables, 380
    music therapy, 247
  prevalence of following
      critical illness, 572
  psychological impact, 129
  reasons for poor sleep in the
      ICU, 119
  role in the development of
      PICS, 117
  role of sedation, 120
  sleep in the ICU, 117
    comparison with normal
        sleep, 117–18
sleep impairments following
    critical illness, 456–61
  overview of sleep
      problems, 456
  approach to sleep in the PICS
      clinic, **457**
  assessing sleep problems,
      456–7
  common sleep disturbances,
      457–60
  insomnia, 457–9
    dedicated worry time
        technique, 458
    sleep hygiene
        recommendations,
        458
  nightmares, 459
  nocturnal
      hypoventilation, 460
  obstructive sleep apnea,
      459–60

prevalence of post-ICU sleep
    disturbances, 456
restless leg syndrome, 460
role of prescribed
    medications, 457
"Slow Burn" trajectory of
    recovery, 23
Snell, K.P., 360
social determinants of health
    (SDOH),
  the concept of, 325–8
  County Health Rankings
      Model, **327**
  helpful interventions, 332–3
  impact on critical illness,
      328–9
    financial stress, 329
    neighborhood residence,
        328–9
    race and ethnicity,
        328, 329
  importance of screening for
      SDOH, 325–34
  influence of in outcomes of
      critical illness
      survivors, 299
  policy implications, 332
  relationship with
      development and
      recovery from critical
      illness, 325
  research implications, 331–2
  risk factors for myriad
      adverse SDOH, 326
  role of social workers in
      addressing SDOH for
      survivors of critical
      illness, 330–1
  screening tool, *330*
  social work practice
      implications, 332–4
  three-tiered model, 325,
      326, 328
  value of peer support,
      333–4
social model of disability
    contrasted with the Age-
        Friendly model, 626
  older adult survivors of
      critical illness
      and, 626
  in PICS, 306–8
social stressors of the ICU,
    examples of, 193
Society of Critical Care
    Medicine (SCCM)

A-F bundle,
  see also ABCDEF bundle
      of interventions **136**
  conclusions of the 2012
      stakeholders
      meeting, 359
  definition of PICS developed
      by, 707
  goals of the 2010 meeting,
      3, 6
  guidelines on clinical
      evaluation, 20–1
  launches ICU Liberation
      Campaign, 135
  PADIS guidelines, 405
  PICS advocacy, 707
  THRIVE post-ICU clinic
      and peer support
      collaboratives, 281,
      355, 616
sodium channel
    inactivation, 47
somatic concerns following
    critical illness, 446–51
  chronic pain, 448
  dental health, 450
  fatigue, 446–7
  hair, 449
  hearing loss, 450
  heterotopic ossification,
      448–9
  joint contractures, 448
  nails, 449
  ophthalmologic
      sequelae, 450
  pressure injuries, 449
  sexual dysfunction, 450–1
  skin, 449
  urinary complications,
      451
Spain, examples of ICU access
    to an outdoor
    space, 269
spasticity
  management of, 563–4
  with botulinum toxin,
      564
  Modified Ashworth Scale for
      assessment of muscle
      tone, *563*
speech-language pathologists
    (SLP), evaluation role
    in the ICU, 77
spinal cord injury (SCI),
    663–5
spiritual care, 197

Index

ACCM
  recommendations, 197
  assessing spiritual needs of patients and families, 201
  barriers to delivery of, 197
  beyond the ICU, 204
  chaplaincy training and education, 200-1
  evaluation of remote delivery, 377
  palliative care and, 590
  practices and interventions, *199*
  resources for patients and families, 205
  role of spirituality and religiosity in critical care, 197
  SCCM recommendations, 198
  spiritual assessment tools, *202-3*
  spiritual competency and training for clinicians, 201-3
  spiritual crisis and spiritual distress in the ICU, 204
  spiritual history-taking, 201
  spirituality in critical care, 198-9
  spirituality vs religiosity, 197
spontaneous awakening trials (SATs), 19, 137
spontaneous breathing trials (SBTs), 137
Stamatelos, P., 554
statins, 111
  contraindicated for prevention of delirium, 139
status epilepticus, 138, 662-3
  sedation requirements, 138
stimulation, modulating, 174-5
STOP-BANG questionnaire, 459
stress management
  beneficial effects of music for, 187, 247, 248
  role of in recovery of patients experiencing PICS, 298

stressors experienced in the ICU, 127-31
  environment-related, 129
  illness-related, 128-9
  interpersonal stressors, 130
  other stressors, 130-1
stroke
  likelihood of dysphagia following, 79
  personal story, 729-32
  remote patient monitoring, 379
  risk of for survivors of critical illness, 423
sub-acute rehabilitation, 289
subarachnoid hemorrhage (SAH), 662
subglottic/tracheal stenosis, laryngeal injury and, 480
Substance Abuse and Mental Health Services Administration (SAMHSA), 619
Substance Abuse and Mental Health Services Administration (SAMHSA), BRSS TACS initiative, 619
suicide, risk of in critical illness survivors compared with general population, 570
Sunnybrook Framework, 399-400, 402
"Surviving Intensive Care" (2002 Brussels Roundtable), 2, 6, 352, 707
swallow function, evaluation of, *see* dysphagia, instrumental swallow evaluation.
symptom identification in PICS, 584-5
  cognitive screening tools, 585
  mental health assessment tools, 585
  physical screening tools, 585
  psychosocial screening tools, 584-5
symptoms of PICS, 7
synchronous neuromuscular electrical stimulation (NMES), 156

syndromes related to PICS, definitions of, *32*
systemic inflammatory response syndrome (SIRS), 31, 55

tachycardia, detection of with wearables, 380
TEAM study, comparison of high-dose and low-dose physical rehabilitation, 152-5
Tedeschi, R. G., 299, 573
Teisburg, E. O., 386
telehealth, definition of, 373
Telehealth After Stroke Care (TASC), 379
telemedicine, *see also* ICU follow-up clinics, telemedicine-based model 284, 373-81
Telephonic Montreal Cognitive Assessment tool (T-MoCA), 376
temperature regulation, role of the gut microbiome in, 39
ten-meter walk test (10MWT), 376
"The Sepsis Aftermath: Repair, Recurrence, Recovery, and Rehabilitation," 2
therapeutic environment, psychologists' role in creation of, 193
therapeutic exercise, 512-13
  definition, 512
  aerobic/endurance training, 513
  muscle strength/resistance training, 512-13
  neuromotor exercise, 513
THRIVE Peer Support Collaborative (SCCM), 281, 355, 360, 616, 707
Timed Up and Go test (TUG), 23, 504, 565
Tosto-Mancuso, J. M., 379
tracheal stenosis
  presenting symptoms, 438
  risk of for survivors of critical illness, 438
  treatment, 438

tracheomalacia, laryngeal
    injury and, 480
tracheostomy tubes
    placement-attributable
        risks, 78
    role of post-neuroICU
        clinics, 660
tracheotomy
    definition, 480
    conversion of endotracheal
        intubation, 477
    laryngeal injury reduced by
        early
        tracheotomy, 480
    "open" vs "percutaneous"
        approaches, 480–1
    placement, 480, 481
    speaking valve trial, 481–2
    as treatment for PGS, 479
    tube capping trial, 481–2
    tube size selection, 482
tracheotomy-related issues,
    decannulation
    management
    considerations for, 481–2
    sequalae of decannulation,
        482–3
Trail Making Test (TMT), 23
transcriptomic perturbation
    and development of ICU-
    AW, 35
    role in pathophysiology
        PICS, 34–5
Transition Dyspnea Index
    (TDI), 440
transition from ICU, 281–90
    benefits of early education
        on PICS, 286
    challenges faced by survivors
        of critical illness and
        their caregivers,
        281–2
    critical illness survivors and
        caregivers studies,
        281–2
    discharge locations, 287–90
    family engagement and
        expectation
        management, 286–7
    follow-up clinics, see ICU
        follow-up clinics.
    patient recovery
        pathways, **283**
    research limitations, 282
    transition-related phone
        calls, 287–9

transitions of care, as source of
    adverse drug
    events, 407
transverse cordotomy, as
    treatment for
    PGS, 479
trauma
    critical illness as, 306–7
    procedure-related, 7
trauma-informed care
    (TIC), 187
traumatic brain injury
    (TBI), 663
treatment of PICS,
    contradictory
    literature on efficacy
    of, 24–6
Trzepacz, P. T., 103
two-minute walk test (2MWT),
    23, 504

ubiquitin proteasome system
    (UPS), 36, 47–8
ulceration, following
    prolonged
    intubation, **478**
Ulrich, R., 271
United Kingdom (UK)
    examples of ICU access to an
        outdoor space, 269
    history of ICU follow-up
        clinics, 352–4
    peer support program, 616
    review of ICU literature, 352
    see also NICE
        (National Institute
        for Health and Care
        Excellence).
United Nations Convention on
    the Rights of Persons
    with Disabilities
    (CRPD), 304
United States
    adults requiring intensive
        care annually, 6
    COVID and racial/ethnic
        inequalities in
        healthcare, 676
    data sources on survivors of
        critical illness, 626
    peer support initiatives, 616
University Hospitals Plymouth
    ICU access to an outdoor
        space, 269
    ICU Secret Garden, **273**
urinary complications, 451

value-based healthcare
    comparison with fee-for-
        service models, 385–6
    comparison with zero-sum
        competition
        model, 386
    stakeholders, metrics, and
        targets, *387, 388*
van Beusekom, I., 422
venous thromboembolism
    (VTE), risk of for
    survivors of critical
    illness, 438
ventricular assist devices
    (VADs), 691
Verbrugge, L.M., 14
videofluoroscopic swallow
    study (VFSS), 83
Virgen Macarena University
    Hospital in Seville,
    Spain, ICU access to
    an outdoor space, 269
visual impairment, concerns
    about following
    critical illness, 450
vitamin and mineral
    deficiencies,
    medications
    associated with, *486*
vocal process granulomas,
    laryngeal injury
    and, 478
vocational rehabilitation, 549
    return to work and, 566
Vukoja, M., 144

Walden, M., 256
"Walk4PICS," awareness
    raising initiative,
    708, 711
wearables, digital health and,
    378–80
Weekly Calendar Planning
    Activity (WCPA), 173
Weick's Organizational
    Sensemaking
    Model, 295
Weiss, C. H., 145
well-being of patients
    benefits of ICU diaries for,
        234–5
    humanization of the ICU
        and, 212
"What Happens to Survivors of
    ARDS" (American
    Thoracic Society), 2

work, returning to, *see under* employment.
work disability, 550
World Health Organization (WHO) Disability Assessment Schedule (WHODAS 2.0), 23

International Classification of Functioning, **433**
Quality-of-Life Scale (WHOQOL-BREF), 347
Safe Surgery Checklist, 142

Xue, Q. L., 64

Yale Swallow Protocol (YSP), 81, 465

Zarit Burden Interview (ZBI), 607
Zarit Burden Inventory, 603
ziprasidone, 111

For EU product safety concerns, contact us at Calle de José Abascal, 56–1°,
28003 Madrid, Spain or eugpsr@cambridge.org.

www.ingramcontent.com/pod-product-compliance
Lightning Source LLC
LaVergne TN
LVHW021941060526
838200LV00042B/1887